INFORM

Toxics Watch 1995

Contributors

Barbara F. Bass, Ph.D.
Diane Benjamin
Mark H. Dorfman
John Howay
Lois Lobo
Sharon Martin
Catherine G. Miller, Ph.D.
Warren R. Muir, Ph.D.
Thomas E. Natan, Jr., Ph.D.
Carolyn Nunley
Costas Pappas
Bonnie A. Scarborough
Hilary V. Sheevers, Ph.D.
Daniel L. Tuttle II
John S. Young, Ph.D., Project Manager

Carroll L. Bastian, Editor

INFORM, Inc.
120 Wall Street
New York, NY 10005
Tel 212 361-2400
Fax 212 361-2412
E-mail Inform@igc.apc.org

Printed in the United States of America

Toxics Watch 1995 is the first in a new series of reports from INFORM covering the full range of data on toxics in the environment, toxics in commerce, and toxics in waste. The series will provide a comprehensive analysis of annually available data on toxics conditions and trends; discuss current and future influences on such trends; and include a current and visionary examination of progress in source reduction.

Series: *Toxics Watch*
ISSN 1079-6118

This volume: *Toxics Watch 1995*
ISBN 0-918780-64-0

INFORM, Inc., is a nonprofit environmental research organization that examines business and municipal practices that threaten our environment and public health; assesses changes business and government are making to improve their performance; and identifies new business strategies and technologies moving the United States toward an environmentally sustainable economy. INFORM's research currently focuses on strategies to reduce industrial and municipal wastes and to preserve air and water quality.

Hampshire Research Institute (HRI) is a not-for-profit scientific, engineering, and computer-programming firm located in Alexandria, Virginia. HRI uses its technical expertise to promote environmental goals by conducting analyses in support of sound public policies and better public understanding.

Printed on recycled paper

Preface

Three decades ago, the first photographs from outer space gave us a new view of earth, a small orb spinning in infinite space. In the years since we first saw those photographs, we have become increasingly aware of the fragility of life on this small planet. And we have come to realize that it is our responsibility to protect the magnificent diversity of Earth's life forms — and to preserve the health of the air, water, and lands on which they depend.

Our challenge is a formidable one: to create a way of life that is economically and environmentally sustainable. And millions of people around the globe are rising to the challenge, debating environmental solutions in forums that range from tiny village meetings to the U.S. President's Council on Sustainable Development to international assemblies in cyberspace. The information superhighway pulses with data on environmental conditions, enabling millions of humans seeking answers to participate in a dialogue that is personal yet global. Not only government and scientific leaders, but citizens from around the world are taking part in the vital debate over the Earth's future.

The fundamental relevance of our global environmental dialogue depends greatly on both the quality of the information that is available to us and the sophistication with which this data is analyzed. And it is here that this new *Toxics Watch 1995* report seeks to break new ground. It delves into a sea of data on a crucial environmental challenge: the rising tide of toxic chemicals that threatens our environment and the health of our species.

In *Toxics Watch 1995*, the first in a series of reports, INFORM has explored a broad range of U.S. data on the use and presence of toxic substances in our environment, looking for answers to important questions. Just how prevalent are toxic substances in the environment? What are the major sources of toxic contaminants? What industries contribute the greatest share of toxic substances and waste? What has been the impact of government and industry programs designed to reduce toxic exposure? Are we managing toxic materials in the most environmentally sound way possible? Perhaps of greatest importance, is the United States meeting its national goal of reducing toxic waste at the source by preventing its creation in the first place?

Toxics Watch offers new perspectives on the problems we face and the progress we are making in solving these problems. In addition, it offers insights about gaps in our current data, drawn from analyses of the U.S. Toxics Release Inventory, of reports compiled under the Resource Conservation and Recovery Act and the Toxic Substances Control Act, of other national environmental databases, and of scientific analyses from around the country. We hope that this *Toxics Watch* analysis will help inform not only the myriad decisions about policies and programs made by government, business, and environmental leaders and communities across the United States, but that it will also aid all industrialized and developing nations that are shaping systems for tracking and regulating toxic substances.

There is no more essential task than that of moving the United States and our world toward an environmentally sustainable economy. We hope that *Toxics Watch* will contribute to this process, helping us target our efforts to preserve our ecosystems and to create a viable way of life for future generations.

Joanna D. Underwood
President
INFORM

Acknowledgements

INFORM and our colleague in preparing *Toxics Watch 1995,* Hampshire Research Institute, want to thank the many individuals and institutions, without whose generous help this report would not have been possible. Many contributed long hours of effort to provide the data that we requested in the form we needed. Many agreed to review one or more chapters of the book in draft. To each, we are indebted and offer special thanks.

Among those who provided data or other information, or who arranged access to data, for Toxics Watch 1995 are:

at the U.S. Environmental Protection Agency

Darryl Ballard
Kent Benjamin
Doris Bloch
Michael Burns
Frank V. Caesar
Richard Clements
Maria Doa
David Eng
Kathleen Franklin
John Harman
Louis H. Hoelman II
Steve Hoffman
David Levy
Joanne M. Martin
Donna Perla
Larry Rosengrant
John Sager
David J. Sarokin
Douglas Sellers
Scott M. Sherlock
Chris C. Tirpak
David Updike
Dina J. Villari
Lance Wallace
Linda Wunderlich

Individuals at Other Organizations

Jackie Alderman, Dow Chemical Company
Bruce Alexius, Dow Chemical Company
Jose Alvarez, The Upjohn Company
Jeff Appel, U.S. General Accounting Office
Keith Bergseid, Star Enterprises
Frank Bevacqua, International Joint Commission
Douglas Bice, Doe Run Company
Nick Bock, Kerr McGee
Janetta Bowden, Fina Oil & Chemical Co.
Margit Brazda, Monroe County Department of Health
Dona Brock, Computer Sciences Corp.
Kirk Brown, Texas A&M University
Marise Burger, American Journal of Industrial Medicine
Alan Dalpias, Hill Air Force Base
Gary Davis, Energy, Environment, and Resources Center, University of Tennessee
R. W. Dement, Elkem Metals Company
Ronald Edwards, Revere Copper Products
Susan Ellis, Gates Rubber Co.
Danny Flack, Lyondell Petrochemical Co.
Michael Garvey, Novacor
Patrick Godfrey, MathTech
Connie Harrison, Atochem NA Inc.
Jeff Hartman, Champion International Corp.
Anthony A. Hermann, Johnson & Johnson
D. F. Hunter, Phillips 66 Co.
Gregory Keoleian, National Pollution Prevention Center, University of Michigan

Individuals in Other Organizations (cont'd.)

Jay Kress, Reilly Industries
Bruce Kurchner, Regional Office of the International Joint Commission
Philip J. Landrigan, Mount Sinai Medical Center
Haines Lockhart, Eastman Kodak
Mary Logue, Cosmar Co.
Deborah Mark, ITT Rayonier
Dan Marks, First Chemical Corporation
Carl Martin, RJR Nabisco
Pat McLaine, National Center for Lead-Safe Housing
Gretchen Meng, Computer Sciences Corp.
Joseph Mon, AT&T Network Cable Systems
Robert Murphy, National Center for Health Statistics
Cynthia Osmola, Forbo Industries
Al Pagano, DuPont Chambers Works
Brian Pistali, Wyman Gordon Co.
Fred Powers, Computer Sciences Corp.
Ron Rosendorn, Coastal Eagle Point Oil Co.
Nelson Sabogal, Ozone Secretariat United Nations Environment Programme
Tim Saylor, International Paper
Diane Schwartz, Environmental and Energy Study Institute
Michael Sparago, BASF Corporation
Dale Stehley, Corning Asahi Video Products
Mark Sullivan, Hercules (Radnor Air Force Base)
Sandy Sustin, Agency for Toxic Substances and Disease Registry
Thomas Swulius, Chevron Corporation
Duane Tolle, Batelle Columbus Laboratories
Donna Tomlinson, Carolina Eastman Company
John Wagner, American Petroleum Institute
Jan Whitfield, Dow Chemical Company
Daisy Wong, ARCO
Rosemary Younts, GenCorp

The following people graciously provided reviews of one or more draft chapters. Every reviewer provided important insights that have improved this book, although INFORM assumes full responsibility for the final content.

at the U.S. Environmental Protection Agency

Paul Bickart
Howard Cantor
Carol Christensen
John Fogerty
Loren Hall
Susan Hazen
Richard Healy
Nora Lopez
Barbara Mandula
Melinda Pearce
James Pendergast
John Schaeffer
Anning Smith
Alexandra Tarnay
Pauline Wagner
Andrew Wheeler
James Willis

Individuals in Other Organizations

Michael Aucott, New Jersey Department of Environmental Protection
Douglas Bannerman, National Electrical Manufacturers Association
Vicki Been, New York University School of Law
Cynthia Chavez, Toxics Use Reduction Institute, University of Massachusetts
Janet Clark, Toxics Use Reduction Institute, University of Massachusetts
Theo Colborn, World Wildlife Fund
J. Ronald Condray, Monsanto Company
Christopher J. Daggett, William E. Simon and Sons
Betsy Elzufon, Larry Walker Associates
Benjamin Goldman, Jobs and Environment Campaign
Hillel Gray, National Environmental Law Center
Linda E. Greer, Natural Resources Defense Council
Charles Griffith, Ecology Center of Ann Arbor
Shelley Hearne, The Pew Charitable Trusts
Jeanne Herb, New Jersey Department of Environmental Protection
Edward Hopkins, Citizen Action
Frances H. Irwin, World Wildlife Fund
Edwin Mongan, E. I. du Pont de Nemours and Co.
Andrew J. Opperman, New Jersey Department of Environmental Protection
Paul Orum, Working Group on Community Right-to-Know
Suzi Peck, Massachusetts Department of Environmental Protection
Ann Pistell, Office of Pollution Prevention, Maine Department of Environmental Protection
James Reisa, National Research Council, National Academy of Sciences
Nikki Roy, Environmental Defense Fund
Philip Shabecoff, Greenwire
Jodi Siegel, Toxics Use Reduction Institute, University of Massachusetts
Paul Templet, Institute for Environmental Studies, Louisiana State University

We also want to acknowledge and thank the organizations and foundations that provided the funding to enable research to go forward and this first *Toxics Watch* report to be prepared. Those sources include:

W. Lyons Brown Foundation
The Nathan Cummings Foundation
W. Alton Jones Foundation
The Joyce Foundation
Charles Stewart Mott Foundation
The Pew Charitable Trusts
The Schumann Fund for New Jersey

Partial financial support was also provided by the U.S. Environmental Protection Agency under cooperative agreement 822086-01-0. This publication has not been reviewed by EPA and does not necessarily represent the views of the Agency.

Contents

Chapter 3 - Toxics in Commerce

Chapter 4 - Toxics in Waste: Overview and Key Facilities

Chapter 5 - Chemicals in Waste

Chapter 6 - Toxics in Waste by Industry

Chapter 7 - Geography and Waste

Chapter 8 - Toxics in the Environment

Chapter 9 - Environmental Justice

Chapter 10 - State Databases: Use, Materials Accounting, and Pollution Prevention in New Jersey and Massachusetts

Chapter 11 - Tackling Industrial Toxic Waste Through Voluntary Action: EPA's 33/50 Program and Preliminary Findings of INFORM's Research

Appendix A

Appendix B

Appendix C

Appendix D

Appendix E

Appendix F

Appendix G

Appendix H

Appendix I

Appendix J

Appendix K

Appendix L

Appendix M

Appendix N

Appendix O

Appendix P

Appendix Q

Boxes

Maps

Figures

Tables

Tables in Appendices

Chapter 1

Introduction

Environmental Toxics: A Major Issue

Toxic chemical environmental contamination is anything but an obscure issue for Americans. For more than 100 years, one toxics crisis after another has blind-sided the public. For example:

- In the 1800s, hatmakers and furriers developed "Mad Hatter's" disease that results from nerve damage caused by mercury used in treating furs and pelts.[1] Methylmercury has been found in recent years in remote lakes in Michigan, Wisconsin, and Minnesota, resulting from long-range deposition of air pollution from the combustion of mercury-laden fossil fuels and from various industrial sources.[2]
- In the 1930s, a large incidence of bladder tumors was reported among dye workers, which was much later linked to exposure to benzidine.[3]
- In 1962 Rachel Carson published her award-winning book *Silent Spring*, describing major ecological damage from the use of persistent bioaccumulative pesticides.[4] Of the hundreds of pesticides now in use that were registered before November 1984, few (about 17 percent) have been re-registered to conform to more modern standards of testing.[5]
- In the early 1970s, PCBs (polychlorinated biphenyls), which are toxic and extremely persistent in the environment, were discovered to be a contaminant of everything from fish to cereal boxes to human breast milk. Manufacture of PCBs was banned in 1979, but large pre-existing inventories of certain enclosed uses of PCBs, primarily in electrical equipment, are still legally in use and have not been safely disposed of. In addition, environmental contamination remains widespread.[6]
- In the mid-1970s, chlorofluorocarbons (CFCs), found in aerosol sprays, air conditioners, and refrigerators in nearly every home, were reported to be depleting the stratospheric ozone layer, which would allow greater levels of ultraviolet radiation to reach the earth with attendant increases in skin cancer and certain adverse ecological effects.[7] The United States banned aerosol propellant uses of CFCs in 1978, and international treaties are phasing out all uses of those and other ozone-depleting chemicals, but significant uses still exist.[8]

- The National Priorities List of Superfund sites identifies more than 1,200 sites contaminated with hazardous waste.[a]

Life expectancy in the United States is going up, and toxic environmental chemicals have been a very small constraint on that expectancy. This does not mean that public concerns over toxic chemicals are misplaced; rather, it means that this country has done a better job of isolating its citizens from contaminated environments and of treating toxic chemical waste entering the environment. For example, people are advised not to eat fish from the Hudson River because of PCB contamination[9] or, until recently, from the James River because of Kepone pesticide pollution.[10] Identified hazardous waste sites are routinely fenced off from public access. Reservoirs or underground aquifers found to be contaminated are either condemned or must undergo extensive treatment before they can be used as public water supplies.

In some cases, protective measures are incomplete or fail — leaving communities exposed to toxics from local waste sites or factories, workers exposed to health-threatening chemicals in their workplaces, or families consuming pesticide-laden foods or breathing contaminated indoor air. Often such communities consist disproportionately of minority or lower-income individuals.

Different toxic chemicals exhibit a wide range of adverse health and environmental effects. Many of the human health effects suffered at the current levels of exposure are nonlethal though very serious. For example, the federal Centers for Disease Control and Prevention estimate that 1.7 million children aged one to five in the United States (9 percent of all children in that age group) have blood lead levels associated with developmental delays and deficits in intellectual performance.[b] These exposures are believed to result most often from contact at home with deteriorating lead-based paint or with water that has flowed through lead or lead-soldered pipe. (See Chapter 2.) In other cases, individuals seem to be suffering severe reactions, including allergies, asthma, headaches, and dizziness, to low levels of chemicals to which they have become sensitized, such as those often found in synthetic carpets, adhesives, and building materials. These apparent chemical reactions have come to be known as multiple chemical sensitivity (MCS).[11]

Toxics in the environment and in products are an increasing public issue in the United States, as they are elsewhere in the world, and they will continue to be until they are adequately addressed.

[a] According to the EPA Superfund/RCRA/CERCLA Hotline, the total number of National Priorities List (NPL) sites as of September 26, 1994 was 1,231 (information obtained via telephone on October 27, 1994). The comprehensive NPL list was last published on May 31, 1994 (59FR27989), and there have been some amendments since.

[b] Calculated from figures provided in Debra J. Brody *et al.*, "Blood Lead Levels in the US Population: Phase 1 of the Third National Health and Nutrition Examination Survey (NHANES III, 1988 to 1991)," *Journal of the American Medical Association*, 272, no. 4 (July 27, 1994): 277-283.

This *Toxics Watch 1995* Report

Purpose

This *Toxics Watch 1995* report inaugurates what is expected to be a series of biennial reports on environmental toxic chemical issues. *Toxics Watch* reports are intended to be a resource to anyone concerned about or involved in addressing these issues.

The emphasis of this and future *Toxics Watch* reports is to provide the fullest possible overview of what can and cannot be ascertained about the conditions and trends of:

- toxics in the environment,
- toxics in industrial waste, and
- toxics in commercial products.

Toxics Watch reports will cover many types of topics, including:

- in-depth analysis of particular aspects of key toxic chemical problems;
- analysis of baseline data on the status of these problems and of the country's efforts to reduce or eliminate them;
- information on new databases that may expand insights into toxics sources and on initiatives that may influence data in the future;
- analysis of key public and private sector policies and programs addressing environmental toxic chemical challenges in the United States and, in some cases, abroad.

The goal of these reports is to help U.S. leaders and citizens address environmental toxic chemical problems by being better informed about the state of knowledge regarding both problems and solutions.

Each report will be grounded in data analyses, seeking to identify the major insights possible from available data. Note that the date in the title of the *Toxics Watch* report, in this case 1995, is the date of publication. The data used in the report are the latest available on a particular topic. This report includes 1992 Toxics Release Inventory data, for example, which were submitted by facilities in 1993 and made publicly available in the spring of 1994. Key data used in the *Toxics Watch* reports will be provided in appendices to facilitate further analyses by readers.

Although the principal focus of the data analysis is intended to be what the data show about environmental toxics, consideration of the adequacy of existing data systems to answer important questions is also included. Although these reports are intended for a general rather than a technical audience, some discussion of the intricacies of data systems is necessary for an understanding of just what the data do and do not reveal. In some cases, analyzing the gap between what seems reasonable and important to know on the one hand, versus what can be ascertained from available quantitative and qualitative information, requires more space and time than describing environmental conditions and trends.

Scope

This *Toxics Watch* report addresses the problems related to the use of major industrial toxic chemicals. These primarily synthetic chemicals have experienced explosive growth beginning in the mid-1940s and now involving 200,000 facilities in the United States alone — from small operations with a handful of employees to giant multinational corporations with tens of thousands of workers, such as DuPont, Procter and Gamble, and 3M. Now over 72,000 chemical compounds are in commerce, produced in nearly 6-trillion-pound quantities each year, serving as a foundation of this country's advanced lifestyle. They include plastics, adhesives, semiconductors, pharmaceuticals, dyes, and resins. In this country, 24,000 manufacturing plants produce or use some 340 toxic chemicals that make them subject to federal reporting requirements, and they had waste generation of almost 38 billion pounds of those chemicals in 1992.

This report does not discuss issues associated with more conventional pollutants such as carbon monoxide, sulfur oxides, and smog in air, or biological oxygen demand, suspended solids, and pH in water (even though those pollutants are made up of chemicals, like all other matter). The toxic chemical issues addressed in this report rest on the definition of toxic substances as found in many governmental toxic chemical lists. The lists include chemicals that have been deemed hazardous to humans or ecosystems. They include chemicals with a potential to reduce stratospheric ozone, but do not include gases that are suspected of contributing to global warming. The report does not cover radioactive substances and their effects.

Within the chemical lists identifying toxic substances, this 1995 *Toxics Watch* report focuses on general industrial chemicals, the problems related to their use in manufacturing and in commercial and consumer products, and their impacts on human beings and ecosystems. Many other substances and issues will be addressed in future *Toxics Watch* issues, such as food, drugs, cosmetics, and pesticides, and exposures in the workplace and indoor environments.

The report gives special attention, where appropriate, to chemicals that are halogenated (i.e., that contain fluorine, chlorine, bromine, or iodine). This focus is to provide illustrative examples of the more general points and conclusions of the report, using a group that includes chemicals broadly represented in commerce and that contains several chemicals of environmental concern. For example, Greenpeace, the environmental watchdog group, has called for a phase-out of most uses of chlorine and chlorinated compounds, and the International Joint Commission, the joint U.S.-Canadian body addressing cooperation over the Great Lakes, has called for a phase-out of toxic, persistent, bioaccumulative compounds, many of which are halogenated organics.[12] Future *Toxics Watch* reports are likely to focus on additional groups of chemicals of interest to readers.

Although all matter consists of chemicals, and many naturally occurring substances, such as metals, are toxic, this report concentrates on manufactured or processed chemicals for several reasons: These chemicals, unlike those that are part of the natural background, are more directly under our control. We can choose to make or not make them. We can choose how to make them and how to use them, so as to limit the risks they pose. Many of these chemicals pose unknown risks to humans, other animal species, or ecosystems because they are relatively new and being poured into our society in great quantities. Also, they are unlike toxic chemicals that have existed in nature for millions of years, against which ecosystems and life forms have had a chance to evolve defenses.

The questions that this *Toxics Watch* report specifically addresses are these:

- What are the main causes of environmental toxic contamination by industrial chemicals? Chapter 2 explores a variety of contaminated settings to assess the extent to which the contamination comes from industrial manufacturing or formulating operations or from commercial and consumer products.
- How do toxic chemicals move through commerce and at what stages may what kinds of environmental impacts result? Chapter 3 examines the full flow of toxic chemicals through commerce, from extraction of the raw materials to processing and manufacturing of products and then to use and disposal, to identify the types of chemical uses that may generate the greatest risks.
- What information do the major databases provide about waste generation, pollution prevention, and waste management of industrial toxics, both overall and for specific facilities (Chapter 4)? What conclusions can be drawn about the trends in waste generation for specific chemicals and chemical groups (Chapter 5), the industries and companies that are the main sources (Chapter 6), and the geographic nature of the distribution of waste (Chapter 7)?
- What do available national data reveal about the conditions and trends of toxic chemicals in air, water, and land? Even more important than what Chapter 8 is able to present on conditions and trends of toxics, is what it shows about what cannot be concluded for lack of data.

The final three special-feature chapters in this year's report describe certain public and private initiatives that seek to address toxics problems. Chapter 9 provides an overview of the rise of the environmental justice movement, a topic attracting increasing attention. Chapter 10 looks at data from innovative state programs in Massachusetts and New Jersey, whose data collection systems provide more extensive perspectives on industrial waste and pollution prevention than the federal data systems in existence today. Chapter 11 reports on the 33/50 Program, the first major initiative taken by the U.S. Environmental Protection Agency to launch a program seeking voluntary and cooperative efforts by manufacturers to significantly reduce the releases and transfers of 17 key toxic chemicals.

Appendices provide more extensive tables and information than can be included in the text of the report.

Setting the Stage for Pollution Prevention

A common framework of understanding is helpful for people to work together on assessing problems related to toxic chemicals and evaluating solutions. Although scientific knowledge is incomplete, much is being learned about why many chemicals are toxic, how toxic materials reach and affect ecosystems and living organisms, and what approaches can be taken that will enable this country to enjoy the many benefits that manufactured chemicals provide without incurring unnecessary risks caused by exposures of environments and populations to them. The following section and material elsewhere in the report present some of the many facets of this framework.

Pathways to Environmental Chemical Risks

Assessing Toxic Chemical Risks

Assessing environmental risks is a complex process. Environmental risks occur at specific times and places, based upon 1) the ability of the environmental chemicals present to cause one or more adverse effects, 2) the susceptibility of the target species or environmental setting to such effects, and 3) the degree to which humans or the ecosystem are exposed to levels of the chemicals that will cause such effects.

It is not as simple as it sounds. First, while it is clear that death, cancer, severe nerve damage, and species extinction are devastating adverse effects, other effects are less clearly so devastating. For example, the nature and extent of adverse biological effects in humans or other living species have not been determined for many chemicals (e.g., changes in enzyme levels, modest changes in sperm motility, or toxicity to the weaker members only of an abundant animal or plant species). There is currently no consensus on the effects of concern for neuro-behavioral effects (e.g., visible cell damage, versus alterations in mood or behavior, versus nerve conduction changes). The answers are value-laden and will continue to evolve over the foreseeable future. This issue of *Toxics Watch* focuses on well-accepted effects of concern that are either explicitly included in the language of federal statutes (e.g., "cancer, gene mutation, or birth defects" in the Toxic Substances Control Act) or that are inherent in the toxic chemical lists established under their implementing regulations (e.g., priority pollutants under the Clean Water Act or the chemicals subject to reporting to the Toxics Release Inventory).

Chemicals are evaluated, often in laboratory toxicological experiments, for their ability to cause different adverse effects over a range of exposures. This information is then compared to the exposures encountered in the particular environmental setting being assessed. The experiments must generally be performed using chemical exposures far in excess of those encountered in the environment, in order to see a significant effect with the number of animals feasible in a laboratory experiment. Moreover, for several reasons, not the least of which are moral and legal prohibitions against human experimentation, the experiments are typically performed on small rodents or other animals seemingly only distantly related to humans.[c] Estimating the magnitude of the uncertainties involved in comparing laboratory data with real human exposures requires considerable scientific judgment. Deciding how cautious to be in the face of the uncertainties relies on value judgments.

Assessing the environmental effects of chemicals is, in some ways, even more difficult. There is less agreement on defining what effects are "adverse." Much human activity seeks to alter ecosystems (e.g., agriculture, mosquito control, fishing, and forestry). Species extinction, although often the matter of vast debate, is clearly an adverse effect; so is significant depletion or destruction of economically or ecologically valuable resources (e.g., a forest stand or a fishery). The adverse effect of other impacts on species is less clear. Is a great reduction of mosquitoes in a suburban area an adverse effect or is it acceptable? What about a great reduction in a local plant population or an algae? Where are the lines to be drawn?

Compounding the difficulty is that most adverse ecological effects of concern relate to populations of species, whereas human health effects even to individuals are of concern. Most environmental standards are designed to prevent *any* human death or injury. People were horrified in December 1984 when more than 2,000 citizens of Bhopal, India, were killed and many more severely injured by the effects from an explosion releasing methyl isocyanate from the local Union Carbide plant.[13] People cared deeply about these deaths, even though they represented essentially no measurable impact on the human population, which is in the billions and growing by a greater number each day than died in the Bhopal incident.

In contrast, only when an animal population has been reduced to a few, such as is the case for the dozen or so remaining whooping cranes in the United States, does the public seem to care about the fate of individual members of a species. Large mammals attract sympathy more readily (whales, for example, and pandas), although smaller animals might have direct and specific benefits for humans (for example, the need for a sufficient population of honey bees to pollinate fruit trees). As more is learned about the ecological interconnections between human life and the environment, the debate over toxic chemicals is expected to continue and broaden to combine scientific and technological issues with ethical and spiritual ones.

Being concerned about populations, instead of individuals, makes laboratory data on a limited number of animals even more difficult to employ for environmental risks than for health risks. There are, again, few alternatives, because it is generally difficult and unwise to experiment on an ecosystem.

[c] Although some raise ethical concerns over such animal experimentation.

Identifying Exposure Pathways

Evaluating human and environmental exposures to chemicals in particular settings is often as complex as trying to compare information on the toxicity of a chemical in various animal species to an exposed human population. As people do not live in a controlled laboratory environment, each person has a distinct life style, living in any of widely varying locations, eating many different types of foods, and working in occupations that may engender extremely different chemical exposures, both qualitatively and quantitatively. All of these settings can, and usually do, change over the course of a lifetime.

Each day individuals are exposed to an often ill-defined stew of chemicals in each of these settings. Exposures to any chemical are almost always extremely varied from person to person, from one time to another, and are never isolated from exposures to other chemicals.

To estimate risks, one must estimate exposures chemical by chemical. To do so requires adding up the predicted or measured exposures to the chemical from all the applicable pathways. Just a few of the many possible significant exposure pathways include:

- drinking water,
- showering (exposure through skin contact and/or inhalation of vapors),
- eating meat or dairy products,
- eating fruits or vegetables,
- eating fish or shellfish,
- breathing vapors or particulates (dust) indoors,
- breathing vapors or particulates outdoors,
- ingesting soil (e.g., from grimy hands), and
- swimming (swallowing water or skin contact).

Exposures result from a combination of specific scenarios over time where individuals come in contact via different exposure pathways with toxic chemicals in the environment. Clearly, estimating such exposures is seldom easy.

Determining Sources and Environmental Fate

The chemicals in the environment that pose risk in cases of human and ecosystem exposures come from three different sources: some exist in nature, others are generated as industrial waste, and still others are in products. Countless numbers of chemicals are present naturally in the Earth's crust, oceans, and atmosphere. Probably even more are associated with the millions of different living species on Earth. These many millions of chemicals and the products of their decay constitute what is normally referred to as natural background.[d]

Added to the natural background are the many tens of thousands of chemicals that are manufactured and used by humans. Some toxic chemicals enter the environment as waste from industrial activities,

[d] As indicated later in this report, "natural background" is often used to include amounts of some chemicals, originating from human activities, that are so pervasive in space and time that they have become inseparable from the truly natural amounts of the same chemicals.

others through use or disposal of chemical-containing products. Once in the environment, these chemicals may last a long time or may be transformed into other chemicals. Some chemicals that degrade quickly to common simple molecules (by sunlight, by reaction with air or water, or by other means) only create immediate and direct exposures to humans and the ecosystem. But if chemicals or their degradation products are persistent, they may be transported through the air or down streams and rivers, sometimes to distant locations, where they may be a source of exposure for a very long time. If they are very soluble in fat or otherwise bind to living cells, they may bioaccumulate in animals and plants at concentrations far in excess of levels found in the soil, water, or air. Such bioaccumulation may lead to long-term and elevated exposures, increasing the risk from such chemicals.

Three Approaches to Reducing Risks of Environmental Toxics

There are three fundamental approaches to reducing the risks of environmental chemicals. Two tackle risks of toxic chemicals *in the environment*. The other tackles them *at their source*. They involve:

1. cleaning up the environment by trapping and treating or disposing of chemical contaminants,
2. isolating people from contact with the environment, and
3. preventing contamination of the environment by avoiding the creation of toxic chemicals at their source, preventing exposures in the first place.

Clean-up

Cleaning up the environment after toxic chemical contamination occurs is, at best, difficult and costly or, at worst, an impossible task. To remove asbestos — a human carcinogen — from public buildings, for example, could cost many billions of dollars, as would removing lead — a neurotoxin — from homes. To clean up or even stabilize contaminated hazardous waste sites in the United States may cost as much as 1 trillion dollars.[14] Cleaning up the Great Lakes completely of its many toxic contaminants or cleansing the stratosphere of ozone-depleting substances seems inconceivable at any expense. "End-of-the-pipe" strategies, even if they could be 100 percent effective, also remain an inefficient use of resources and dollars.

There are not enough dollars in the U.S. economy to resolve all the contamination problems posed directly by industries and products, and, over the last 15 years, efforts have intensified to use risk assessments to decide how the limited available financial resources and expertise can most effectively be spent. Such assessments seek to identify the situations in which clean-up actions are most important.

Isolation

An alternative strategy to environmental clean-up is to prevent exposures to toxic chemical contaminants by isolating humans from the contamination. Uses of this strategy include treating contaminated drinking water, fencing off hazardous waste sites, providing impervious suits for workers in

Figure 1-1.

Environmental Management Hierarchy

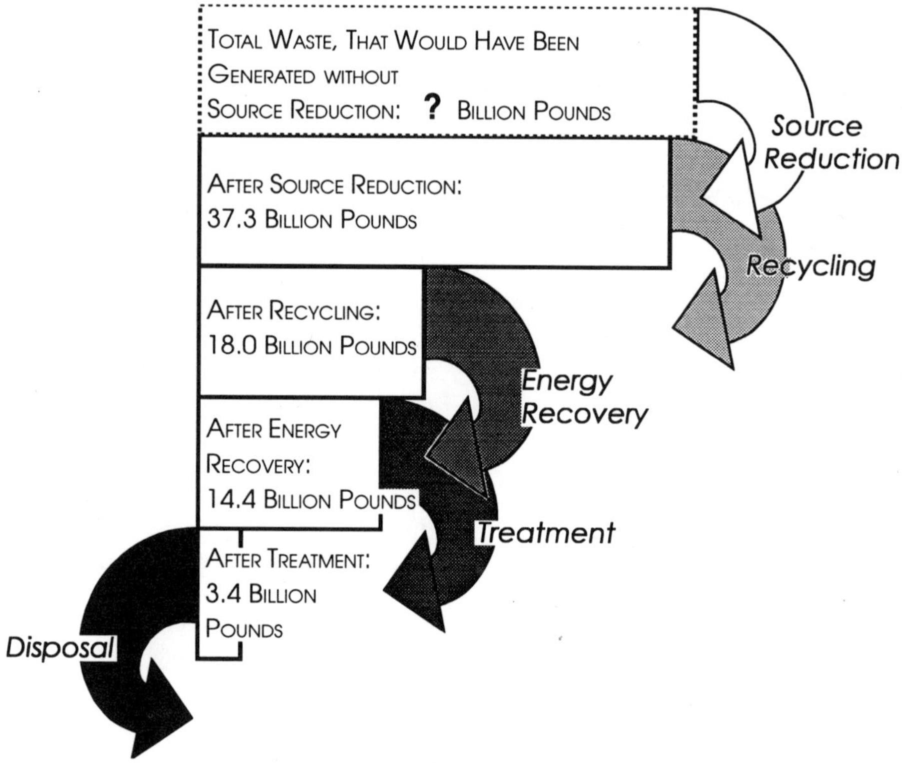

1992 Toxics Release Inventory (TRI) data

hazardous workplaces, and prohibiting fishing or swimming in polluted waters. This approach often can be implemented quickly, at much less expense and with greater certainty of success, than cleaning up the environment.

Isolation strategies, however, deny access to and enjoyment of the Earth's natural environment. Most provide no ecological protection, and they do not result in environmental restoration, so environmental insults from today are passed on to future generations. They also may be the source of environmental injustice to predominately minority or lower-income communities.

Prevention

The third strategy for addressing toxic contamination, and the one that business, governmental, and environmental leaders now solidly agree is the best choice, is to prevent contamination in the first place. Since this country's first national environmental laws were enacted, mostly in the early 1970s, effort has been devoted to establishing a broad pollution control framework to limit present and future environmental contamination. Up until the mid-1980s, the emphasis was on waste and pollution clean-up. But as the cost of pollution control skyrocketed and it became clear that toxic wastes were often just moved from one environmental medium to

Box 1-A. Source Reduction and Pollution Prevention

In this report, the terms "source reduction" and "pollution prevention" are used interchangeably, as defined in the Pollution Prevention Act of 1990:[a] "any practice which 1) reduces the amount of any hazardous substance, pollutant, or contaminant entering any waste stream or otherwise released into the environment (including fugitive emissions) prior to recycling, treatment, and disposal; and 2) reduces the hazards to public health and the environment associated with the release of such substances, pollutants, or contaminants. The term [source reduction] includes:

- equipment or technology modifications,
- process or procedure modifications,
- reformulation or redesign of products,
- substitution of raw materials, and
- improvements in housekeeping, maintenance, training, or inventory control [bullets added]."

Source reduction does not entail any form of waste management (e.g., recycling or treatment). A hazardous substance, pollutant, or contaminant must be integral and necessary to the production or a product or providing of a service for any change in its physical, chemical, or biological characteristics or volume to be considered source reduction.

[a] Omnibus Budget Reconciliation Act of 1990, Public Law 101-508, 104 Stat. 1388-321 *et seq.*

another, rather than safely disposed of, the focus shifted to pollution prevention.

The unanimously passed federal Pollution Prevention Act of 1990 states that "source reduction is fundamentally different and more desirable than waste management and pollution control." This Act establishes a national policy of hierarchical environmental protection, singling out prevention at the source as the top priority for addressing industrial waste problems. Pollution that could not be prevented should be recycled in an environmentally sound manner. The Act further states that, in the absence of feasible prevention and recycling opportunities, pollution should be treated and that disposal of waste or its release into the environment should be used only as a last resort. (See Figure 1-1 and Box 1-A.)

Source reduction represents improved industrial process efficiency and often greater process and product consistency. Therefore, in contrast to the impossibly large costs of attempting to clean up toxic contaminants from the environment, source reduction often promises to save companies money, while reducing risks with greater certainty. In contrast to isolating humans from their environment, this approach aims at avoiding ecological impacts and at preserving the environment intact for future generations.

For these reasons, the analyses in *Toxics Watch* emphasize the status and trends of source reduction in industry today. Greater attention is paid to the amount of waste produced, for example, than to releases to the environment, relative to earlier reports on these topics.

Please Comment

We hope that you find this report of value. We welcome ideas for future *Toxics Watch* topics, comments on the report, and other suggestions. Please send them either to:

Toxics Watch INFORM 120 Wall Street, 16th Floor New York, NY 10005-4001 Fax: 212/361-2412 E-Mail: Inform@igc.apc.org	or:	*Toxics Watch* Hampshire Research Institute 9426 Forest Haven Drive Alexandria, VA 22309-3151 Fax: 703/684-7704

---

1 Ethel Browning, *Toxicity of Industrial Metals*, London: Butterworth & Co., Ltd., 1961, 204.

2 Robert Collins and Henry S. Cole, *Mercury Rising: Government Ignores the Threat of Mercury from Municipal Waste Incinerators*, Clean Water Action/Clean Water Fund Research and Technical Center, September 1990, 16-17.

3 L.J. Goldwater, *et al.*, "Bladder Tumors in a Coal Tar Dye Plant," *Archives of Environmental Health*, 11 (1965): 814-817; National Institute of Environmental Health, U.S. Department of Health and Human Services, *Seventh Annual Report on Carcinogens 1994: Summary*, Washington, DC, 1994, 37-39.

4 Rachel Carson, *Silent Spring*, New York: Houghton Mifflin Company, 1962.

5 Office of Prevention, Pesticides and Toxic Substances, U.S. Environmental Protection Agency, *Pesticide Reregistration Progress Report*, Washington, DC, EPA 783-R-94-014, July 1994.

6 Telephone conversation with Tom Simmons, Environmental Protection Specialist, Operations Branch, Office of Pollution Prevention and Toxics, U.S. Environmental Protection Agency, November 2, 1994.

7 F.S. Rowland and M.J. Molina, "Stratospheric Sink for Chlorofluoromethanes: Chlorine Atom-catalyzed Destruction of Ozone," *Nature* (London), 249 (1974): 810.

8 For information on the history of CFC and halon use, see Sheila A. Ferguson, Warren R. Muir, and John S. Young, "Technology Trends in CFC and Halons Replacement, *Technology Trends Series: No. 11*, United National Industrial Development Organization," May 3, 1990. For the most recent international agreements, see Ozone Secretariat, United Nations Environment Programme, *Handbook for the Montreal Protocol on Substances that Deplete the Ozone Layer*, Third Edition, Nairobi, Kenya, August 1993.

9 Telephone conversation with Don Brown, Public Health Specialist, Bureau of Toxic Substance Assessment, New York State Department of Health, October 27, 1994; Center for Environmental Health, New York State Department of Health, "Health Advisory: Chemicals in Sportfish and Game, 1994-1995," Albany, NY, August 1994.

10 Office of the Governor, Commonwealth of Virginia, press release, March 18, 1988.

11 Nicholas Ashford and Claudia Miller, *Chemical Exposure: Low Levels and High Stakes*, New York: Van Nostrand Reinhold, 1991. For a skeptical account of MCS, see Gregory E. Simon, *et al.*, "Immunologic, Psychological, and Neuropsychological Factors in Multiple Chemical Sensitivity," *Annals of Internal Medicine*, 19, no. 2 (July 15, 1993): 97-103.

12 Bette Hileman, Janice Long, and Elizabeth Kirschner, "Chlorine Industry Running Flat Out Despite Persistent Health Fears," *Chemical and Engineering News*, November 21, 1994, 12-26.

13 Mary O. Amdur, "Air Pollutants," *Casarett and Doull's Toxicology: The Basic Science of Poisons*, Fourth Edition, Mary O. Amdur *et al.*, eds., New York: Pergamon Press, 1991, 855.

14 Milton Russell, *et al.*, *Hazardous Waste Remediation: The Task Ahead*, Report by Waste Management Research and Education Institute, Knoxville, TN: University of Tennessee, 1991 as cited in National Research Council, National Academy of Sciences, *Ranking Hazardous Waste Sites for Remedial Action*, Washington, DC, 1994, 51.

Chapter 2

Tracking the Sources of Environmental Toxics

Introduction

The history of determining the causes and cures of toxic chemical pollution in the environment during the past few decades reads like a detective story, but one in which the "crime" as well as the "culprit" changes in every chapter. At first, the main purpose of investigation was to improve basic scientific understanding of the nature of the crime. Why were bird eggshells thinning? Why were fish dying in the Great Lakes? Why was the incidence of a serious and rare lung disease much higher than normal among former asbestos workers? One by one such questions about chemical sources of human health and environmental problems entered the public consciousness and the front page, as well as the agendas of policymakers.

By the 1970s, it became clear that the legal and administrative mechanisms for dealing with all these issues were inadequate, and so began a decade of developing legislative and governmental programs to confront them. Some focused on environmental media (e.g., the Clean Air Act in 1970; Clean Water Act, 1977 amendments to 1972 and earlier legislation; and Safe Drinking Water Act in 1974) or on types of contaminants (e.g., the Federal Insecticide, Fungicide, and Rodenticide Act, amendments in 1972 and 1978 to the 1947 legislation). Other legislation covered broader categories of hazardous and toxic substances and activities (the Resource Conservation and Recovery Act and the Toxic Substances Control Act, both in 1976).

Pollution control programs took the most obvious and easiest route to begin to address environmental contaminants — by limiting releases of certain chemicals to the environment from identifiable industrial sources and from other controllable sources, such as automobiles. Requirements could be set on what a factory emits into the air from its smokestack or discharges into a river through an effluent pipe or on what anti-pollution devices manufacturers install on new cars. Monitoring of the chemical constituents of the air around the plant and in the river around the discharge pipe was technically possible; emissions inspection could be required for vehicles. Fines and other penalties could be levied for non-compliance.

Such "end-of-the-pipe" programs were effective in reducing certain kinds of pollution to a certain degree, and they continue to be needed, but environmental chemical pollution is still a serious problem. Aside from the technological and economic problems involved in extending the degree of pollution control achieved by such programs (e.g., requiring higher levels of treatment at sewage treatment plants or raising the standards for land disposal sites and what could be sent there), whole other source areas have hardly been addressed. These include "nonpoint" sources, such as urban and agricultural storm runoff, and chemicals dispersed to the environment through the use of commercial products by consumers, businesses, and industry. People began to recognize that such problems, as well as many aspects of chemical pollution from industrial processes, could be addressed only through pollution prevention. The Pollution Prevention Act of 1990 made official this growing recognition that the best solution is to prevent the generation and release of toxic substances in the first place, to the fullest extent possible, rather than destroy or recapture them after they have entered the environment.

As crime prevention may be aided by improved understanding of the sources of criminal behavior, pollution prevention may be aided by improved characterization of the sources of toxic pollution and their roles. Characterizing the source of environmental toxics involves finding answers to such questions as:

- What are the types and levels of contaminants in various environmental settings?
- Who or what is responsible for particular types of contamination — industries, individuals, nature?
- What are the pathways by which the pollutants reach human and environmental targets?
- What is the relative contribution of the various sources?
- How are the contaminants generated and released?

Case Study Approach of This Chapter

This chapter examines a number of important environmental settings to find out what is known about the kinds of contamination in them and to assess the relative contributions from different sources. The settings chosen for study were those where sufficient data are available to begin answering the who, what, where, when, and how of chemical contamination. Although these settings are presented as illustrative examples, rather than as representative of the whole range of toxics settings, they are situations that in and of themselves are worthy of serious attention because of the potentially significant health or environmental consequences of exposures to the contaminants in them.

The settings covered by the case studies includes different environmental media (air, water, land) as well as quite different areas of physical scope. They range from the human body, with data on blood lead levels in children, to a large regional area of the Great Lakes, with data identifying a significant variety of environmental problems and sources. (See Table 2-1.)

Summary of Findings

The discussion of each environmental setting that follows draws upon some of the studies whose data are helpful in characterizing the sources of toxic chemical pollution. The particular supporting studies are by no means comprehensive or definitive. Each has both inherent and methodological limitations; each leaves unanswered questions and unsolved riddles. The qualitative conclusions that can be drawn are often more persuasive than the data, which are insufficient in amount and coverage for comprehensive characterization. Nevertheless, these studies point strongly to the following findings:

- Without in any way diminishing the seriousness of the problem of toxics in industrial waste, the role of product use as a source of chemical contamination was found to be significant and in some cases predominant in the settings covered by the studies examined in this chapter. In some cases (such as lead, indoor air toxics, and ozone depletion), products are the primary source of the problem; in other environmental settings (such as the Black River Watershed in Ohio), their role is secondary to industrial process waste, but still significant.
- Examining some of the particular environmental settings turns up some counter-intuitive results concerning the role of product use, such as: 1) indoor air pollution is a more dangerous contributor of toxic contaminants to many people than outdoor air pollution, and 2) the materials in municipal landfills in many cases are at least as hazardous as those in industrial landfills. In both cases — indoor air and municipal landfills — the presence of toxics stems primarily from the intentional use of toxic chemicals in widely distributed commercial products.
- Even when the environmental setting itself is generally perceived as industrial — for example, many Superfund sites — much of the contamination there does not originate directly from waste generated by chemical manufacturing and processing, but from the use and disposal of the commercial products made by these processes.
- The impact of pollution arising from product use is particularly significant when assessing the total body burden in a human being of a particular toxic chemical or group of chemicals. Without denying the importance of occupational exposure or exposure to certain types of

Table 2-1. Contaminated Settings and Contributing Sources

Environmental Setting	Source Designations
1. Blood Lead Poisoning	●▲
2. Outdoor Air Carcinogens	●▲✻
3. Indoor Air Contaminants	
Volatile Organics	●▲
Asbestos	●
Lead/Mercury	●
Radon	✻●
Formaldehyde	●
4. Stratospheric Ozone Depletion	
Refrigerants	●
Foams	●▲
Solvents	●▲
Aerosol Propellants	●▲
Fire Protection	●
Sterilants	●
5. Superfund Sites	▲●✻
6. Landfill Leachate	▲●
7. Great Lakes	
Black River AOC	▲●✻
Rochester Embayment AOC	▲●✻

Key: ● - Commercial/Consumer Product Use
▲- Industrial/Manufacturing Process Waste
✻ - Natural Sources
AOC - Area of Concern

Symbols indicate types of contributing sources. Multiple symbols indicate either multiple types of contributing sources or sources that fall between listed designations.

industrial waste, it can nevertheless be said that the cumulative effects of exposure through product use create hidden hazards that are difficult for the individual to avoid.

- One of the clearest examples of unavoidable exposure is the case of lead, which is ubiquitous in the environment, partly from natural and industrial sources but mostly from centuries of human use of products containing lead. Emissions of lead to the environment primarily reflect commercial use rather than industrial waste. For example, while EPA estimates that industrial processes such as lead smelting and battery manufacturing released a combined total of 5,200 metric tons of lead to the environment in 1979, more than 94,600 metric tons were released via transportation sources alone in that same year.

  Despite a dramatic decrease in exposure during the past two decades (median blood levels in children aged one to five fell 75 percent between 1976 and 1991 as the result of curtailment of lead in gasoline, paint, and plumbing materials), dangerous levels of exposure to lead continue, especially in children. As many as 16 million children under the age of seven may be exposed to elevated levels of environmental lead., and more than 1.7 million children between the ages of one and five have blood lead levels in excess of the target set by the Centers for Disease Control and Prevention (10 ug/dl).

- EPA's estimates of cancer risks from various sources of air pollution provide approximate information on the relative importance of product use and industrial process wastes for this category of contamination. While the induction of cancer is only one of many risks to human health and the environment, the data indicate that product use may contribute substantially more to this risk (between 54 and 90 percent of the total risk from all sources considered by EPA) than do production wastes (between 3 and 25 percent).

- An individual's exposure to toxics results from that person's general geographic location, the chemicals present in the indoor air of that person's home, and particular personal habits and activities. Activities that contribute significantly to personal exposure to certain organic toxics, for example, include smoking and passive smoking, visiting commercial establishments of high toxic-chemical use such as dry-cleaning establishments and gas stations, and working in settings or occupations of high chemical exposure.

- Over six years of EPA studies of individual exposures to airborne contaminants found that not only were half of the 20 chemicals studied prevalent in indoor air, but that levels were consistently higher indoors than outdoors. Further, indoor air concentrations of these chemicals were better predictors of exposure (as measured by chemical concentration in exhaled breath) than were outdoor concentrations. While increased understanding of all aspects of indoor air pollution is important, the predominant causes are product-related, including exposures from products such as room deodorizers, paints and adhesives, and non-occupational uses of pesticides.

- Releases of ozone-depleting chemicals to the atmosphere occur during their manufacture, during the manufacture and processing of products containing ozone depleters, and throughout the period of product use and disposal, in some cases for several decades. The phase-out of ozone-depleting substances mandated by the Clean Air Act domestically and the Montreal Protocol internationally (see Box 2-A) requires the development of substitutes for ozone depleters in important uses, including aerosol propellants, solvents, coolants in refrigeration and air conditioning, and fire retardants. Reducing the amount of these chemicals that reach the stratosphere will even require recovering ozone depleters already in products. While the amount of ozone-depleting chlorofluorocarbons (CFCs) released from use in an individual product may be small, cumulative effects may be substantial. For example, an automobile air conditioner releases only about 400 grams of CFCs each year, but there are 140 million such vehicles on the road in the U.S. alone. Total releases (56,800 metric tons) from these vehicles are more than five times as large as the estimated quantity of all ozone depleting chemicals released from chemical production and processing operations.

- INFORM's analysis of Superfund sites in three states found that contamination of 18 of 36 sites was attributable primarily or in part to commercial product use and disposal, rather than industrial process waste. A study of 58 landfills by Texas A & M scientists found that of 143 toxic chemicals found, 60 were found in municipal waste samples, 31 in industrial waste landfills, and 39 in both. Half the chemicals found in landfill leachate had higher concentrations in municipal landfill leachate than in industrial waste landfill leachate. For example, the suspected carcinogen isophorone was found in municipal solid waste leachate at levels 30 times higher than those in samples from industrial waste landfills.

- Studies of large geographic settings including the Great Lakes region reveal contamination resulting from all three categories of toxic chemical sources (industrial process waste, commercial product use, and natural causes), but knowledge of these sources is very incomplete. Although many facilities contribute waste that is characteristic of their industries, industrial process waste is not easy to trace. Moreover, once all known industrial waste sources are identified, much pollution remains unaccounted for. For example, less than 1 percent of the lead that enters Lake Ontario from the Genesee River can be traced to permitted discharges to that river; the remaining 99 percent comes from sources that are difficult to measure, including airborne emissions from motor vehicles and incinerators and urban stormwater runoff.

- Considering the amount of study resources and attention being given the Great Lakes Basin (one of two environmental settings addressed in this chapter) by two

Box 2-A. Montreal Protocol Sets Accelerated Timetable

Depletion of the earth's stratospheric ozone, which has already created a "hole" in that protective layer, is a global problem. Recognition of this worldwide condition and of the need to act unilaterally led 23 nations to sign the precedent-setting Montreal Protocol on Substances that Deplete the Ozone Layer on September 16, 1987. The initiative originally placed limits on the worldwide production and use of certain ozone-depleting chemicals, including the fully halogenated chlorofluorocarbons (CFCs), and halons, later adding 1,1,1,-trichloroethane (methyl chloroform), carbon tetrachloride, and bromomethane (methyl bromide). Ultimately these and other chemicals with lower ozone-depletion potentials are to be completely phased out of production. By December 1994, more than 140 countries and the European Community had ratified the Protocol.

Comprehensive in nature, the Protocol includes measures of control, reporting of data, non-compliance, research, public awareness, exchange of information, technical assistance, financial provisions, withdrawal from the Protocol, and transfer of technology for all member countries.

The Montreal Protocol is an evolving document. The original called for a freeze in CFC use at 1986 levels and a 50-percent reduction by 1998. With this scenario, ozone levels would have continued to decline indefinitely, so in 1990 at the London meeting, the Protocol was amended to accelerate the reduction with a complete phase-out at the end of the century. By the 1992 meeting in Denmark, the phase-out in use had been moved to January 1, 1996, and other chemicals with lower ozone-depleting potentials were added to the controlled list. These include the hydrobromofluorocarbons, hydrochlorofluorocarbons (HCFCs), and bromomethane. The first two will be phased out by 1996 and 2030, respectively. In January 1995, a cap will be placed on bromomethane that will limit production and consumption to 1991 levels.[1] In June 1994, the European Union environment ministers agreed to phase out HCFCs and bromomethane more rapidly than the Protocol requires, with their phase-out coming by the end of 2014.[2]

Since the implementation of the Protocol, production and use of these ozone-depleting substances has steadily decreased. However, these chemicals have very long lifetimes in the stratosphere, ranging anywhere from 50 to over 200 years. As a result, the ozone hole is not expected to start diminishing until the turn of the century, even with these latest Protocol amendments, and will probably continue to expand over the next few years. Ozone levels are expected to return to normal sometime in the second half of the next century.

The Protocol has always granted developing countries more time to phase out these chemicals because of their special needs for access to appropriate technology and financial assistance.

The Industry Cooperative for Ozone Layer Protection (ICOLP) is a nonprofit consortium of leading electronic and aerospace companies devoted to sharing technology to reduce the use of ozone-depleting substances that they have successfully implemented. Working in voluntary partnership with government, ICOLP is assisting developing countries to eliminate the use of ozone-depleting solvents by holding technology cooperation workshops and providing information on substitute chemicals and alternative process and technologies. The seven countries that ICOLP currently works with are Brazil, China, India, Malaysia, Mexico, Thailand, and Turkey.

[1] Ozone Secretariat, UNEP, *Handbook for the Montreal Protocol on Substances that Deplete the Ozone Layer*, Third Edition, August 1993, 12.

[2] *International Environment Reporter*, 17:16:659.

nations and several provinces and states, the deficiencies in quantifiable information and the resulting absence of precise knowledge about the sources of toxic chemical contamination are sobering. Even less must be known about geographic areas that are experiencing some of the same types of chemical-related environmental problems, but which have no special focus on these matters.

Potential Sources of Chemicals in the Environment

The case studies presented in this chapter examine what is known about the three principal sources of the chemicals found in several specific, but important, environmental settings: 1) waste and releases from industrial processes, 2) commercial product use, and 3) "natural" sources (some enhanced by human activity). The distinctions among these sources are not always clear-cut, and their relative importance can often be described but not quantified. Awareness of the importance and complexity of the second category, product use, is growing and is perhaps not as well understood as industrial process waste. The attention given to product use in this chapter is not intended to diminish the significance of industrial process waste, but rather to suggest that product use is also a major environmental concern requiring pollution prevention.

Industrial Process Waste

Industrial process waste, in the context of this report, is a waste containing one or more toxic chemicals that is generated either deliberately or inadvertently as the direct result of the manufacture or processing of a product. Some process waste is a planned part of the process whose nature and amount is well known in advance. A metals fabricator that stamps a rounded shape out of a rectangular piece of sheet metal may know, for example, that 5 percent of each sheet is left over as scrap metal. Other industrial process waste is inadvertently produced as the result of accidents or inefficiencies. These include spilled, leaked, unreacted, or otherwise wasted raw materials; spilled, residual, defective, or otherwise wasted finished product; contaminants, intermediates, or other byproducts generated as a result of the process; and catalysts and processing aids that are an *essential* part of the process.

Industrial process waste excludes chemical waste resulting from incidental use of a chemical product at an industrial facility, such as chemicals used to clean up after other chemicals or paint used to paint facility structures. For the purposes of this report, such waste is considered waste from product use.

The variety of chemicals included in industrial waste is vast, in its range of toxicity and potential health and environmental effects, its composition, and its physical and chemical characteristics. In some cases, the waste consists of a pure chemical or chemical compound; in other cases, the waste is a complex mixture of substances of varying composition at different times. Certain industries tend to produce certain kinds of waste, nevertheless, and improved characterization of "typical" waste streams aids in reducing pollution as well as in tracking the release of chemicals from industrial facilities.

Equally varied are the ways that the chemicals enter the environment. Some will be released deliberately, such as by venting to the air through stacks or by permitted wastewater discharges directly to surface water, by incinerator, by being landfilled or put in a storage lagoon, or by many other methods of release, treatment, or disposal. Other industrial process waste is sent away from the facility for recycling, energy recovery, treatment, or disposal, and part or all of its chemical constituents may be released to air, water, or land during those activities. Some industrial waste enters the environment indirectly, such as through discharge to the public sewage treatment system or by runoff from storage areas or from hazardous waste sites.

In some instances, the characteristic of the chemical or chemical waste will dictate the avenue of its release: volatile liquid or gaseous chemicals such as 1,1,1,-trichloroethane (methyl chloroform) or chlorine will generally end up in the air, whereas scrap metal that is not recycled will probably end up in some type of land disposal. The original part of the environment into which the chemical is introduced is not necessarily its final destination. For example, atmospheric deposition occurs when pollutants emitted into the air by smokestacks and other sources are deposited from the atmosphere, alone or in rainfall, into surface water or onto land; from land they could be washed into streams in stormwater runoff.

Investigation of industrial process waste is sometimes easy and sometimes extremely difficult. The waste disposal or treatment method might be quite legal, appropriate, and well known, and the constituents of the waste monitored on a regular basis. In many cases, what is done with the waste may be entirely legal, but unknown and undocumented outside the company responsible. There may be no applicable federal or state reporting requirement because of the size of the facility, the amount of waste, or other circumstances. In still other cases, the disposal may have been illegal or surreptitious or done before restrictions covered the situation, but a clue is found (for example, a leaking drum with the company's name still on it found at a Superfund site).

When a chemical problem is found in the environment, the source may be close at hand geographically and in time, or quite the opposite. Many air pollutants may travel hundreds of miles from their original source. Certain chemicals, such as polychlorinated biphenyls (PCBs), are so persistent in the environment that they may be discovered and still produce adverse effects long after the original industrial source has gone out of business or the chemical has been banned. Metal tailings from mines abandoned in the nineteenth century still contaminate land and water in many western states.

All these complexities in characterizing and tracing industrial process waste have stymied both pollution prevention and clean-up efforts in many areas, despite progress in others. Similarly, successes in correcting some contamination problems stemming from commercial product use, discussed below, represent a small portion of the myriad of environmental concerns relating to this type of environmental chemical source.

Commercial Product Use

Once raw chemicals are incorporated into products for industrial or consumer use, the potential for environmental contamination is by no means over. Some products, such as pesticides or cleaning sprays, are specifically designed to be released to the environment during use. Whether that release causes a harmful effect depends on the nature of the chemical and the conditions of use and exposure. Much of the product can be expected to be released within a reasonably short time after marketing, although some may remain in containers a long time before it is needed, and residues in containers can contaminate the environment when they are eventually discarded. Some chemicals designed for release are relatively harmless (except under conditions of acute overexposure); others are extremely toxic and may persist in the environment and may also bioaccumulate in certain organisms.

Other chemical-containing products are not designed for release but nevertheless may slowly emit contaminants during their long product lives. These include many paints, adhesives, and building products commonly found in homes, schools, and offices. For example, formaldehyde, a probable human carcinogen as defined by EPA, is found in particleboard, insulation, and carpeting, from which it slowly escapes into the air.

Still other products are reasonably safe under normal conditions of use, but eventually will cause a problem when discarded at the end of their useful lives, such as some types of batteries and mercury-filled thermometers. Asbestos contained within insulation in older structures does not cause a problem so long as the materials are intact, but once this insulation begins to deteriorate or is removed, as during building renovation, the asbestos fibers are released to the air and pose a serious health threat. The same is true of lead in paint in older structures that were painted before lead was banned for such use. Some of the lead is released as dust to the air during deterioration of painted surfaces and may be ingested, especially by small children putting hands contaminated by lead-laden dust into their mouths; children also may eat chips of peeling paint.

Manufacturing and service industries and business establishments use products that generate potential toxic chemical hazards, either directly and immediately or eventually after waste disposal. Tetrachloroethylene (perchloroethylene) is a toxic chemical commonly used at dry-cleaning establishments. Pentachlorophenol was formerly widely used by the lumber industry as a wood preservative. The pentachlorophenol then contaminated the industrial waste from that industry and frequently caused soil contamination in the area. Facilities categorized as electroplaters and metal finishers are heavy users of organic solvents such as trichloroethylene and 1,1,1-trichloroethane, but such solvents are also used by many other manufacturing industries and business consumers.

Industrial releases from product use may occur through volatilization during use or disposal, by incineration, by leaching from land into groundwater, and by other routes, depending on the particular chemical and chemical process used. Industrial waste from industries that do not normally manufacture and process chemicals (e.g., textile mills, food canneries, plumbing fixture manufacturers, transportation industries, clock makers) can be assumed to be predominantly in the "product use" category, whereas industrial waste from facilities in such industries as Chemicals, Petroleum Refining, Plastics, and Primary Metals will produce industrial process waste plus some waste from product use. Uses of given chemicals sometimes overlap at an industrial facility, so the distinction between industrial process waste and product use is often not at all clear-cut either industry-wide or for an individual facility.

Natural Sources

To further complicate the mystery, pollutants may also be generated and/or released to the environment by natural processes that may occur on their own or be exacerbated by human activities. Cadmium, a probable human carcinogen, naturally occurs in low levels in soil and in high levels in igneous rocks and western phosphate ores, in addition to its industrial uses and product sources such as metal alloys, paints, and batteries. Radon, a dangerous indoor air pollutant, originates in natural rock, with varying concentrations and degrees of hazard depending on very localized geological conditions.

These naturally occurring chemicals include both some that are nonessential or harmful to the human body (like lead and cadmium) and some that are essential and beneficial in appropriate quantities but toxic in higher amounts (like chromium). Natural pollutants may be mobilized by natural occurrences to accumulate in a certain place in an excessive amount, such as by leaching from the soil or by natural erosion and sedimentation. Human activity may also increase pollution from natural sources, such as when construction or mining waste concentrates the loading of metals and other inorganic toxic chemicals in inappropriate locations, or when the use of building materials containing natural toxics such as radon increases human exposure to such chemicals.

Some chemicals whose sources are primarily or entirely of human rather than natural origin are today so persistent and ubiquitous in the environment that they have come to be classified as part of a "natural background level" of exposure that some studies use as the starting point against which any additional loadings are compared. Trace levels of the man-made pesticide DDT are found all over the world, for example. This contamination is more correctly characterized as a commercial product use source than a "natural" source, however, and is so considered in this report.

Exposure to Lead and Blood Lead Poisoning

Lead has come to be known as one of the most damaging and pervasive of toxic chemicals. The toxic effects of human exposure to lead range from kidney failure and death at high doses to digestive problems and neurological damage at lower doses. Clinical lead poisoning (i.e., with symptoms that are readily noticed in routine clinical exams) is a small part of the problem of lead, because it is comparatively rare and readily treated. More serious are the subtle effects of subclinical poisoning from lower-level exposures to lead. The effects of these lower-level exposures in young children cause the greatest concern and are just beginning to be understood. Even small amounts of lead may have serious effects on a child's developing nervous system, causing irreparable harm to cognitive and behavioral functioning, including ability to learn.

An estimated 9 percent of U.S. children aged one to five years, 1.7 million children, have elevated levels of lead in blood that exceed 10 micrograms per deciliter (ug/dl), and as many as 16 million children under the age of seven may be exposed to elevated environmental concentrations of lead.[1] The question of what constitutes elevated and dangerous levels is a tricky one, because over the past several decades evidence of effects at very low levels has caused re-evaluation of issues of safety. The Centers for Disease Control and Prevention (CDC) now indicate that children's blood lead levels should not exceed 10 ug/dl.[a] EPA has taken the position that there is no safe blood level. Thus lead, a ubiquitous chemical that occurs throughout the environment from numerous human and natural sources, is a toxicant with no safe threshold level of exposure.

Lead contamination and resulting health effects are not a recent phenomenon resulting from modern industrialization. Populations throughout history have suffered from lead's effects. While lead occurs naturally in soil, signs of man-made lead contamination have been traced back some 5,000 years to when early civilizations first discovered how to separate silver from lead ore. Anthropologic artifacts such as beads and statues indicate that lead use dates back even further, to 6500 BCE. Lead was used in products ranging from medicinal and food additives to wine stabilizers and pottery glazes. Anthropologists even speculate that exposure to lead through food and wine was a primary factor that led to the decline of the Roman Empire.

A historical record of environmental lead levels is sealed in the layers of Arctic ice cores and sediment cores from streams and lakes, which shows that the problem has worsened as people have repeatedly made the poor choice of lead as a primary constituent of many widely used products. Analysis of these cores reveals a 230-fold increase in annual lead

[a] Because of the difficulty of accurate testing, the uncertainty of intervention, and the large numbers of children who would be involved, CDC does not recommend intervention at blood lead levels between 10 and 14 ug/dl.

deposition rates over the last 3,000 years, from 0.03 nanograms per cubic centimeter in 800 BCE to about 7 nanograms per cubic centimeter in the last 20 years. Levels in the body have also increased dramatically since that time. Bone samples from North American Indians who lived during the pre-Columbian period show that current average body burdens are 100 to 1,000 times greater now than then.[2]

Once absorbed by the body, lead circulates in the bloodstream. Most is eventually stored in bone, where it may remain for years until it is mobilized back into the bloodstream by metabolic processes such as pregnancy or aging. During pregnancy, bone is often desorbed, and accumulated lead can be transferred with it to the bloodstream, where the lead can affect the fetus.[3]

Despite the fact that encountering some lead is inescapable, the challenge is to limit exposures resulting from its widespread use and release to the environment. These exposures today result primarily from the past extensive use of lead worldwide in such products as gasoline, paint, plumbing materials, and food packaging, and from the disposal of these products; from the continuing widespread uses of lead in many countries; and from the much more limited remaining uses in this country. Exposure to lead also results from its release from industrial processes such as smelting operations and lead-acid battery manufacturing.

What is the relative importance of the many sources of environmental lead? How have recent efforts to reduce the amount of the lead in the environment, such as through drastically reducing the use of lead additives in gasoline and paint, affected the prevalence and severity of blood lead levels in children? This section summarizes the findings of several research efforts to answer these and other important questions.

Study Characterization

Research on the human effects of lead in the environment includes two major areas of exploration:

- Studies characterizing the environmental concentrations of lead and the exposure pathways from different sources, and
- Studies of actual human uptake from these pathways, to assess the impact of varying levels of exposure.

A number of researchers have analyzed relevant data, particularly those gathered in a series of studies included in the National Health and Nutrition Examination Surveys (NHANES). The National Center for Health Statistics/Centers for Disease Control and Prevention (NCHS/CDC) conducted NHANES to ascertain the general state of health and nutrition in the U.S. population. The work included standardized cross-sectional[b] surveys of blood contaminants such as lead. National estimates of blood lead levels were first made in the second NHANES (conducted 1976-

[b] A cross-sectional study examines representative members of all groups (e.g., age classes) at a given point in time, as opposed to a longitudinal study in which members of a certain group are monitored as they move through different ages.

1980) and again in NHANES III (1988-1991) and in the Hispanic Health and Nutrition Examination Survey (HHANES, 1982-1984).

These studies are important because they make it possible to demonstrate relationships among sources of lead in the environment, potential exposure pathways associated with multiple major and low-level sources, and actual measurements of lead in the bloodstream.

Study Methodology

The NHANES studies target civilian, non-institutionalized residents of the United States for the purpose of monitoring health and nutritional status. The HHANES sample included only Mexican Americans residing in southwestern states, whereas the NHANES II and III were based on national samples representative of the entire U.S. population.[c] These studies analyzed lead in blood samples collected from persons in the following age groups: 6 months to 74 years (NHANES II), 4 to 74 years (HHANES), and 1 year and older (NHANES III). National trends were then developed across these studies for the age group 1 to 74 years.[d]

Each study involved administering a questionnaire to participants and a detailed medical examination at a mobile center. The questionnaire sought information on participants' demographic and socio-economic status sufficient to stratify results of blood lead sampling according to age, sex, race/ethnicity, urban status, and income level. This information is particularly useful in determining how people are exposed to lead and what behavioral or lifestyle factors affect the degree of exposure that different groups experience.

In 1989 researchers Mushak and Crocetti summarized the findings of a report to the U.S. Congress on childhood lead poisoning with a focus on the relative importance of various sources to overall exposure. Using NHANES data and other sources (including EPA, the U.S. Census Bureau, and the U.S. Department of Housing and Urban Development), they developed a quantitative assessment of the estimated contributions from different sources. They also reviewed the methods available for measuring these contributions and for predicting their impact on blood lead levels. The exposure estimates compiled for a number of different sources include the number of children in contact with potentially dangerous environmental lead levels, those at risk of having elevated[e] blood lead levels as a result of this contact, and the number of children who are likely to have measurably elevated levels of lead in their blood as a result of exposure to a particular source.[4]

Authors Pirkle and Brody, *et al.*, recently published findings from the latest NHANES studies. Their

[c] The samples consisted of 9,832 participants for NHANES II and 12,119 participants for NHANES III, representative of the U.S. population. The HHANES included 5,682 participants representative of Mexican Americans in the southwestern United States.

[d] The trends analysis included five variables: age, sex, race/ethnicity, urban status, and income level. Age groups were 1-5 (4-5 for Mexican Americans), 6-19-, and 20-74.

[e] There was no single number for "elevated" used in these studies, but the level varied for different types of exposures, although in all cases exceeded 10 ug/dl. In any case, the terminology may be somewhat misleading, in view of the absence of a safe blood level.

works examine trends during the time period 1976 to 1991 for the U.S. population as a whole and for specific minority and socio-economic subgroups. They also evaluate what these trends indicate about the relative importance of various sources and the success of various control initiatives that have been implemented over the course of these studies.[5]

Study Findings

These studies show that while lead exposure from industrial process waste has been significant in certain geographic locations, those exposures are dwarfed in magnitude by exposure caused by the use of commercial products that were made with lead despite its inherent toxicity. Although blood lead levels have decreased dramatically as the result of curtailment of lead in gasoline, paint, and plumbing materials, clearly dangerous levels of exposure to lead continue, especially in children. This exposure stems primarily from soil and dust contaminated by past vehicular emissions and from deteriorating paint in older buildings. Minority populations experience greater levels of lead exposure because of the nature and location of present-day sources.

Industrial Process Waste

Primary and secondary lead smelters and lead-acid battery manufacturing operations have been the principal contributors of lead contamination from industrial process waste. Other less significant industrial sources include manufacture of ceramic-coated capacitors and resistors by the electronics industry, rubber products manufacturing, and munitions manufacturing and use.[6] EPA estimates that industrial sources emitted to the atmosphere a combined total of 5,200 metric tons of lead per year in 1979.[7]

People living in the immediate geographic vicinity of these facilities are particularly susceptible to exposure to lead from industrial process waste (although others may be as well). An EPA study done in 1985 estimated that 233,000 children in the United States were potentially affected by emissions from smelters and lead-acid battery plants by virtue of their residence.[8] Applying the prevalence rates of blood lead poisoning observed in children living near smelters in Montana and Idaho, Mushak and Crocetti determined that between 210 and 5,500 children in the United States could experience blood lead levels of 25 ug/dl or greater, caused by emissions from primary smelters, and up to 7,500 could have levels greater than 20 ug/dl from secondary smelter emissions. (See Table 2-2.)

Commercial Product Use

Much larger numbers of people have been and continue to be exposed to lead from the past use of such products as leaded gasoline, paint, lead solder, and plumbing materials than have been exposed from industrial uses. In 1979, the year in which EPA estimated that 5,200 metric tons of lead was generated by industrial facilities, at least 18 times this amount, 94,600 metric tons, was generated just by transportation sources.[9] The estimates by EPA of children exposed to lead from smelters and lead-acid battery plants are dwarfed by the number of potential childhood

Table 2-2. Estimated Number of Children (under Age Seven) Potentially Exposed to Lead From Various Sources and Estimated Number with Elevated Blood Lead Levels

Source	**Potentially Exposed** Thousands	**With Source-Specific Elevated Blood Lead Levels** Thousands
Dust and Soil	11,700	NA
Paint	12,043 - 6,000	1,200
Gasoline	5,600	1,200
Stationary Sources	230	NA
Primary Smelters	21	0.21 - 5.5
Secondary Smelters	187	7.5
Lead-acid Battery Plants	25	NA
Plumbing Fixtures and Solder	21,000 - 3,800	241.1
Food	973	973

Source: Developed from information reported in Mushak and Crocetti, "Determination of Numbers of Lead-Exposed American Children." See Appendix G-1 for an explanation of how these estimates were determined.

exposures and poisonings that may be caused by the use of lead in commercial products. (See Table 2-2.)

Substantial reductions in blood lead levels have followed the near elimination of the sale and new uses of lead-containing products. Federal initiatives aimed at preventing exposure to lead in products began in 1970 with the Lead-Based Paint Poisoning Prevention Act,[10] which made available funds to remove lead paint from homes and to screen children for blood lead poisoning. Under the amended act, the Consumer Product Safety Commission limited the level of lead in paints to 0.06 percent.[11] More recently, the Residential Lead-Based Paint Hazard Reduction Act of 1992 (Title X)[12] established new standards for lead risk abatement in federally financed housing that came into effect on January 1, 1995; defective painted surfaces containing lead are to be abated, with controls to minimize exposure to dusts generated by abatement procedures. Lead levels remain high in specialty paints used on roads and bridges, thus posing a continuing occupational and environmental risk for exposure and poisoning.

EPA promulgated regulations in 1973 that initiated the reduction of lead in gasoline.[13] Hydrocarbon emissions, a target of the Clean Air Act, not childhood lead poisoning, provided the impetus for these regulations that were intended to encourage the use of catalytic converters, whose parts are damaged by leaded gasoline. Lead levels were further reduced by later regulations to a final limit of 0.1 grams per gallon in leaded gasoline and 0.05 grams per gallon in unleaded gasoline.[14] Total elimination took effect January 1, 1995, in areas required to use reformulated gasoline, and will become effective for the rest of the country by January 1, 1996.[15] Other regulatory and legislative initiatives include a 1986 prohibition on the use of lead connectors and service pipes in new

Figure 2-1.

Blood Lead Levels for Children Aged One to Five Years

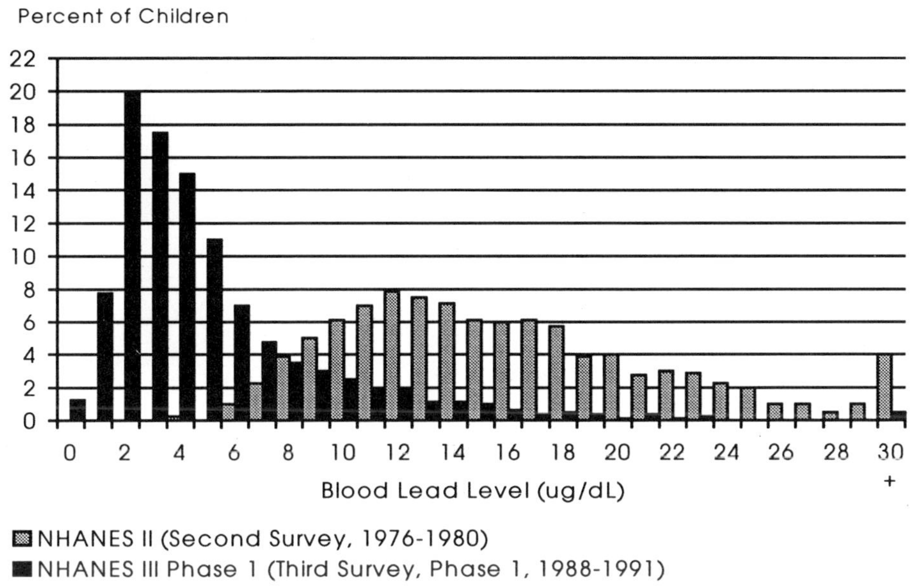

Source: National Health and Nutrition Examination Surveys (NHANES)

construction,[16] and the virtual elimination of lead solder in food and beverage cans, beginning in 1972 with limits on lead in evaporated milk cans.[17]

Between 1976 and 1991, median blood lead levels of United States children between the ages of one and five dropped 75 percent. (See Figure 2-1.) These reductions in blood lead levels parallel reductions in the use of leaded gasoline during the same period.[18] As a result of gasoline reformulation, emissions of lead from automobiles decreased from 94,600 to 2,200 tons per year (a 98 percent reduction) from 1979 to 1989, according to EPA estimates.[19]

Lead levels in food also declined during this time, both as a result of reduction in the United States of lead in gasoline, which enters the food supply through soil and other pathways, and virtual elimination in this country of the use of lead solder in cans for food and beverages. Based on their Total Diet Food Studies, the Food and Drug Administration estimates that these measures reduced young children's daily intake of lead in food from approximately 45 micrograms in 1980 to 4.3 micrograms in 1990 (a 90 percent reduction).[20]

What is also compelling about the findings from these studies is that greatly reducing the use of leaded products has reduced but not eliminated all pathways of exposure resulting from their use. The phase-out of lead in gasoline drastically reduced direct exposure from automobile exhaust and helped to reduce blood lead levels for everyone. This action did nothing, however, to reduce secondary exposure to lead that had already accumulated in soil and dust in urban and suburban areas where vehicular emissions were particularly high. As many as

5.6 million children are potentially exposed to dust and soil contaminated with lead as a result of leaded gasoline use.[21]

Despite regulatory actions against the use and sale of leaded paint, significant exposure from this source continues today, as leaded paint deteriorates in homes where it was used. The developmental stage that young children go through of putting everything in their mouths makes them particularly vulnerable to ingesting peeling leaded paint. Leaded dust generated by general deterioration of painted surfaces or home renovation activities may pose an even greater hazard, particularly when ingested, as when children put dusty hands in their mouths. In the HANES surveys, blood lead levels were consistently higher for younger children than for older children.[f] At least 6 million young children remain vulnerable to lead exposure from the past use of paint and plumbing materials that are no longer on the market. (See Table 2-2.)

These materials are designed to be long-lasting. Leaded paint and plumbing materials often remain longer in deteriorated condition in low-income housing, where regular maintenance and renovation is less affordable for owners and often not provided by landlords. Low-income children are already more susceptible to the effects of lead as a result of poor nutrition, a condition that increases the amount of ingested lead that the body absorbs and retains. Minority populations also experience greater levels of exposure to lead: for example, according to the NHANES data, 21 percent of non-Hispanic black children have blood lead levels greater than 10 ug/dl, compared to 6 percent for non-Hispanic white children.[22] Because of these and other factors, disproportionate exposure to lead has become a target for action by environmental justice organizations.

Unanswered Questions

Ranking the importance of the various sources of lead exposure is complicated by the fact that lead comes from so many sources, is persistent in the environment, and accumulates in the body. All sources are therefore important because of the contribution each source adds to the total body burden, the number of exposure pathways involved, and the size of the exposed population.

Governmental and academic research is continuing to quantify more specifically the relative contributions of the various sources of lead that remain in industrial process waste and in commercial products and to determine the effectiveness of different measures to prevent further exposure. The problems resulting from past use of lead-containing products are the most difficult. As the NHANES studies show, taking lead out of

[f] As mentioned earlier, the lead in blood eventually migrates to the bone, as well as the hairs, nails, and teeth. The older children may once have had high blood lead levels as the result of exposure when they were younger. The difference in blood lead levels between older and younger children at a particular point in time means that the younger children have a greater present exposure to lead. This does not indicate whether the older children may have already experienced harmful effects from prior exposure or may experience effects in the future resulting from those past exposures. More needs to be understood about the effects of lead in bone; it may cause problems during pregnancy or in old age.

these products is just the first step. A complete solution requires finding ways to take these products out of the environment, to prevent exposure to the lead that remains, and to ensure that lead or equally toxic chemicals are not used for such purposes in the future.

The NHANES studies also identified the need for more work on characterizing the effects of low-level exposure to lead and a greater focus on vulnerable risk groups such as urban minorities and the poor.[23]

Toxic Chemicals in Air

Concern about toxic chemicals in the air has been particularly high compared with some other types of environmental pollution because air is impossible for people or ecosystems to avoid. Toxic chemicals in the air can cause a variety of health and environmental effects, including respiratory diseases such as asthma and bronchitis, various forms of cancer, stratospheric ozone depletion, and ecosystem damage. These and other effects can result from releases that occur from indoor and outdoor sources.

Since chemicals may become airborne through volatilization, combustion, or activities that generate gases or dust, a large variety of activities contributes to air contamination. Outdoor sources include stationary "point" sources such as smokestacks; fugitive emissions such as from leaks in pipes; agricultural and home garden use of pesticides; mining operations; and mobile or intermittent "nonpoint" sources such as the use of automobiles. Indoor sources include building materials, the use of commercial products such as paints and cleaning solvents, and appliances such as stoves or kerosene heaters. These sources exist both in residential environments and occupational settings, where they may be combined with sources that are more closely related to industrial process waste. (See Table 2-3.)

This section explores what is known about the relative significance of the various sources of airborne pollutants to human health by examining measurements of carcinogenic risk from various outdoor sources and data characterizing exposures to airborne chemicals from indoor and outdoor sources.

Carcinogens in Outdoor Air

Study Characterization

In 1990 EPA's Office of Air Quality Planning conducted a national source-specific analysis of the risks associated with releases of more than 90 chemicals generated by 60 source categories.[24] Its analysis built on an initial scoping study, published in 1985, to characterize the impact of toxic chemicals in air in terms of potential excess cancer incidence, to assess the relative contributions of specific sources and pollutants, both regionally and nationally, and to identify any data gaps that require more research.[25] The findings are being used to focus federal and state air quality programs on those sources and pollutants that cause the greatest risks to human health and

Table 2-3. Typical Sources of Some Indoor Air Pollutants Grouped by Origin

Pollutants	Sources
Group I—Sources Predominantly Outdoor	
Sulfur oxides (gases, particles)	Fuel combustion, smelters
Ozone	Photochemical reactions
Pollens	Trees, grass, weeds, plants
Lead, manganese	Automobiles
Calcium, chlorine, silicon, cadmium	Suspension of soils of industrial emission
Organic substances	Petrochemical solvents, natural sources, vaporization of unburned fuels
Group II—Sources Both Indoor and Outdoor	
Nitric oxide, nitrogen dioxide	Fuel-burning
Carbon monoxide	Fuel-burning
Carbon dioxide	Metabolic activity, combustion
Particles	Resuspension, condensation of vapors and combustion products
Water vapor	Biologic activity, combustion, evaporation
Organic substances	Volatilization, combustion, paint, metabolic action, pesticides, insecticides, fungicides
Spores	Fungi, molds
Groups III—Sources Predominantly Indoor	
Radon	Building construction materials (concrete, stone), water
Formaldehyde	Particleboard, insulation, furnishings, tobacco smoke
Asbestos, mineral, and synthetic fibers	Fire-retardant, acoustic, thermal, or electric insulation
Organic substances	Adhesives, solvent cooking, cosmetics, solvents
Ammonia	Metabolic activity, cleaning products
Polycyclic hydrocarbons, arsenic, nicotine, acrolein, etc.	Tobacco smoke
Mercury	Fungicides, in paints, spills in dental-care facilities or laboratories, thermometer breakage
Aerosols	Consumer products
Viable organisms	Infections
Allergens	House dust, animal dander

Source: Committee on Indoor Air Pollutants, National Academy of Sciences, *Indoor Air Pollutants*, Washington, DC, 1981.

the environment and to support more effective control programs. National estimates of excess annual cancer cases are based on data from a variety of sources that include 10 area-specific or national air quality reports and 14 source- and pollutant-specific studies.

The American Cancer Society reported that in 1993 approximately 1.2 million new cancer cases were diagnosed in the United States.[26] EPA estimates that exposure to airborne pollutants could cause as many as 1,700 to 2,700 excess cancer cases per year in the United States.[g] [27] Cancer is just one of many adverse effects that these chemicals can have on human health and quality of life; therefore, it provides a very incomplete indicator of the costs, in either health or economic terms, imposed by toxic air pollutants. It is, however, the only effect for which source-specific releases have been characterized in a standardized way. Until such releases can be evaluated for other adverse effects such as asthma and other respiratory diseases, cancer risk serves as a surrogate measure for toxic effects.

Because cancer is a complex set of diseases caused by many different factors, the effort to define the actual or potential number of excess cancer cases caused by just one factor like airborne pollution is by no means a straightforward or precise activity. Estimated excess cancer rates derived for air pollutants are theoretical and relative. They are based on statistical probabilities that reflect many assumptions about how much chemical exposure the general population experiences as a result of airborne releases and about the toxicity of the chemicals themselves. For example, EPA's analyses for airborne carcinogens assume that average outdoor concentrations of these chemicals remain relatively constant throughout the United States and that the entire U.S. population experiences the same level of exposure to them. In reality, average outdoor concentration and level of exposure are known to vary considerably from region to region, depending on the density of the population and the commercial character of the area.[28] Thus, estimates of excess national cancer cases simply provide a measure of risk by which to compare chemicals and sources. The estimates are relative in nature and will change, perhaps significantly, as more information becomes available on additional chemicals and sources.

Reliable data characterizing source-specific releases and resulting outdoor air concentrations and other parameters to define the impact of air toxics on cancer rates are generally unavailable. Rather, predictions are based on theoretical models of releases and resulting exposures from the more-than-60 source categories that generate substantial quantities of airborne pollutants. The resulting risk estimates are therefore more useful for comparing the relative importance of different chemicals and sources than for predicting the actual impact of these emissions on cancer rates.

[g] While the EPA study may be reliable for estimating the relative contribution of various sources, it should not be used for assessing the absolute number of cases attributable to airborne pollutants as compared with other causes of cancer.

Study Methodology

EPA researchers based their risk estimates on release and air quality data from a number of regional and national studies that together identified more than 60 source categories contributing to regional and national air toxics problems. Most pollutant-source combinations evaluated in the EPA analysis had been included in at least one nationwide study. Many were analyzed by more than one study, and in some cases, estimates of resulting excess cancer cases differed significantly among these studies. To resolve these discrepancies and derive national estimates, EPA researchers evaluated factors such as carcinogenic potency estimates, emission factors, and mathematical models, which can vary substantially, altering the estimates of chemical concentrations in outdoor air and resulting excess cancer cases. EPA eliminated some studies from further consideration because of data inadequacies or inconsistencies, and combined some source categories to develop a list of 43 source categories for which national cancer estimates could be developed.[29] The EPA authors emphasize that this list is in no way comprehensive. It simply reflects those categories for which sufficient data were available to estimate ambient air concentrations and cancer risk. As more categories are identified, the relative risk estimates will change accordingly.[30] (See Table 2-4.)

Many of the sources characterized in the study involve the widespread use of commercial products such as motor vehicles, asbestos releases from building renovation and demolition activities, gasoline marketing, drycleaning operations, pesticide use, chlorinated drinking water, and paint stripping. The study also evaluated airborne releases of industrial process waste from chemical production and processing facilities such as smelters, polybutadiene and ethylene oxide production facilities, pharmaceutical manufacturing operations, and petroleum refineries.

Study Findings

EPA's data indicate that between 54 and 90 percent of the cancer cases from airborne pollutants covered by this set of studies are caused by emissions from use of commercial products. In contrast, cases that reflect releases of industrial process waste account for between 3 and 25 percent of the total. (See Table 2-4 and Appendix G-2.)

If one excludes those sources that may represent either product use or process waste, between 54 and 77 percent of the cancer cases reflect product use. Most of these additional cancer cases are attributed to motor vehicle emissions, which account for between 42 and 69 percent of the total attributed to all airborne pollutants. Other significant product use-related sources include asbestos released from building demolition activities (3.2 to 5.7 percent), gasoline marketing (1.0 to 5.1 percent), chromium emissions from cooling towers (0.0 to 7.2 percent), and solvent use/degreasing operations (0.9 to 2.5 percent). (See Table 2-4 and Appendix G-2.)

Source categories that generate pollutants that may be associated with either industrial process waste or product use contribute between 8 and 20 percent of the overall risk

Table 2-4. Summary of Estimated Cancer Cases Based on Modeled Ambient Concentrations by Source Category

Source Category	Source Type	Annual Cancer Cases	Percent of Total*	Principal Pollutants
Motor Vehicles	U	769 - 1,461	41.58 - 68.81	PIC,** 1,3 - butadiene
Secondary Formaldehyde***		106 - 154	4.25 - 10.41	Formaldehyde
Electroplating	U/P	120	4.72 - 8.38	Hexavalent chromium
TSDFs****	U/P	49 - 140	2.00 - 9.20	Dioxin
Woodsmoke	U/N	89	3.50 - 6.22	PIC
Asbestos, Demolition	U	81	3.19 - 5.66	Asbestos
Unspecified (point)		27 - 92	1.09 - 6.15	Arsenic, formaldehyde
Cooling Towers	U	0.01 - 111	0.00 - 7.20	Hexavalent chromium
Gasoline Marketing	U	24 - 75	0.96 - 5.06	Gasoline vapors, Benzene
Solvent Use/Degreasing	U	22 - 36	0.87 - 2.49	Tetrachloroethylene, Dichloromethane
Unspecified (area)		21	0.83 - 1.47	Carbon tetrachloride
PVC/EDC/ Vinyl Chloride	P	19	0.75 - 1.33	Vinyl chloride
Iron and Steel	P	17 - 18	0.67 - 1.26	Coke oven emissions, Benzene, PIC
Sewage Sludge Incinerators	U/P	13	0.51 - 0.91	Cadmium, Vinyl chloride
Municipal Waste Combustors	U/P	2 - 22	0.08 - 1.52	Dioxin
Petroleum Refineries	P	8 - 14	0.32 - 0.97	Gasoline vapors, Formaldehyde
1,3-Butadiene Production	P	10	0.39 - 0.70	1,3 - Butadiene
Styrene - Butadiene Rubber Production	P	10	0.39 - 0.70	1,3 - Butadiene
Coal and Oil Combustion	U/N	8 - 10	0.32 - 0.70	Arsenic
POTWs****	U/P	6	0.24 - 0.42	Vinyl chloride
Smelters	P	3 - 4	0.12 - 0.28	Formalehyde
Commercial Sterilization/Hospitals	U	3 - 4	0.12 - 0.28	Ethylene oxide
Pesticide Production/Usage	U/P	3.4	0.13 - 0.24	Benzene
Dry-cleaning	U	3	0.12 - 0.21	Perchloroethylene
Pulp and Paper Manufacturing	P	2.1	0.08 - 0.15	Chloroform
Chlorinated Drinking Water	U	1.7	0.07 - 0.12	Chloroform
Ethylene Dibromide Production	P	1.5	0.06 - 0.10	Ethylene dibromide
Polybutadiene Production	P	1.2	0.05 - 0.08	1,3 - butadiene
Ethylene Oxide Production	P	1.2	0.05 - 0.08	Ethylene oxide
Ethylene Dichloride Production	P	0.8	0.03 - 0.06	Ethylene dichloride
Waste Oil Burning	U/P	0.6	0.02 - 0.04	Arsenic
Asbestos Manufacturing	P	0.5	0.02 - 0.03	Asbestos
Asbestos Renovation	U	0.4	0.02 - 0.03	Asbestos
Glass Manufacturing	P	0.4	0.02 - 0.03	Arsenic
Hazardous Waste Combustors	U/P	0.3	0.01 - 0.02	Hexavalent chromium
Paint Stripping	U	0.22	0.01 - 0.02	Dichloromethane
Pharmaceutical Manufacturing	P	0.2 - 0.4	0.01 - 0.03	Chloroform
Benzene Fugitives	U/P	0.2	0.01 - 0.01	Benzene
Nitrile Elastomer Production	P	0.16	0.01 - 0.01	Acrylonitrile
ABS/SAN Production	P	0.13	0.01 - 0.01	Acrylonitrile
Asbestos Fabrication	P	0.13	0.01 - 0.01	Asbestos
Benzene Storage	U/P	0.1	0.00 - 0.01	Benzene
Other		6 - 13	0.24 - 0.90	Hexavalent chromium, Radon

Note: Values in this table are not absolute predictions of cancer occurrence and are intended to be used in a relative sense only. The dose-response relationships and exposure assumptions have a conservative bias, but omissions due to uncharacterized pollutants (either directly emitted or secondarily formed) and emission sources, the long-range transport of pollutants, and the lack of knowledge of total risk from multi-pollutant exposures counteract this bias to an unknown extent.

* See Appendix G-2.

** PIC - Products of incomplete combustion

*** Secondary formaldehyde - Formaldehyde that forms in the atmosphere by the reaction of other chemicals emitted from a variety of undefined sources.

**** TSDFs: Treatment, Storage, and Disposal Facilities (hazardous waste); POTWs Publicly Owned Treatment Works

Source: Adapted from EPA, *Cancer Risk from Outdoor Exposure to Air Toxics*, Vol. I, Final Report. Office of Air Quality Planning and Standards, Research Triangle Park, NC, EPA-450/1-90-004a, 3 - 25.

from the sources covered by EPA's studies. These categories include electroplating (4.7 to 8.4 percent), waste treatment, storage and disposal facilities (2.0 to 9.2 percent), sewage sludge incinerators (0.5 to 0.9 percent), municipal waste combusters (0.1 to 1.5 percent).

Releases from industrial process source categories, excluding those that may also be attributable to product use, appear to contribute between 3 and 6 percent of the total cancer cases attributed to exposure to airborne pollutants. The most important process categories in the EPA study include polyvinyl chloride (PVC)/ethylene dichloride (EDC)/vinyl chloride production processes (0.8 to 1.3 percent), iron and steel manufacturing (0.7 to 1.3 percent), and petroleum refining (0.3 to 1.0 percent).

Two other categories included in the EPA study emit pollutants generated by the use of natural products for fuel and contribute between 4 and 7 percent of the overall risk from air pollutants from sources covered by the study. These are emissions from wood combustion and from coal and oil combustion.

The majority of cancer cases associated with each of the 60 source categories in the EPA study could be attributed to relatively few types of chemical releases. For example, the analysis of hazardous waste combusters found that while more than 70 pollutants are emitted from these sources, cadmium and hexavalent chromium together account for almost 90 percent of the risk from this source category.[31]

Unanswered Questions

1. What percentage of the carcinogens contributing significantly to overall risk from airborne pollutants has been characterized?

The 90 chemicals for which source contributions and relative cancer risk have been characterized represent just a small fraction — less than 4 percent — of the more-than-2,800 pollutants that have been detected in the atmosphere. EPA estimates that for thousands of these chemicals, toxicity and exposure profiles have not yet been adequately evaluated and sources have not been identified. As more information on currently uncharacterized chemicals and sources becomes available, the relative risks for all chemicals and sources will likely change substantially.[32]

2. What other major sources of airborne carcinogens have not yet been characterized?

There is great difficulty in determining the extent to which all the significant contributing sources have been identified and accurately characterized. Because there is no national chemical use inventory to track actual or potential emissions for all sources or all chemicals in commerce, it is not possible to determine whether all major contributing sources have been assessed. This is especially true for sources that involve the use of a variety of commercial products.

3. How accurate are the estimates of national excess cancer cases caused by carcinogenic air pollutants?

As mentioned earlier, cancer is a complex set of many different diseases, and until all the various causes are better understood, quantifying the impact of environmental pollutants will remain an uncertain process. Exposure to environmental pollutants is just one causal factor that contributes to cancer incidence. Others include diet, lifestyle, and heredity. This complexity makes it extremely difficult to separate and measure the impact of any one factor such as exposure to airborne pollutants. The many simplifying assumptions used to estimate exposure to these pollutants could overstate the actual impact of these releases on cancer rates. However, the fact that many sources and chemicals have not been included in the analysis may mean that the impact of airborne carcinogens has been grossly underestimated. For these reasons, currently available data and methods for estimating the impact of releases of carcinogenic air pollutants on national cancer rates at best can provide only a rough picture of their potential impact.

Total Exposure Assessment Methodology: Comparing Exposures from Indoor and Outdoor Sources

As people have come to spend more time indoors and buildings have been designed to be more airtight for the purpose of energy conservation, and as greater numbers and quantities of toxic chemicals have been put in commercial products, the quality of indoor air has become a more serious public health concern. Traditionally, outdoor sources, particularly industrial processes, received primary blame for human exposure to air pollutants. Not until researchers began to investigate the sources of actual human exposure to airborne pollutants was the importance of indoor air contamination identified. The discussion below relies primarily on the findings of a series of EPA-directed studies called Total Exposure Assessment Methodology (TEAM).

Study Characterization

The National Academy of Sciences (NAS) reviewed and summarized early work on sources of indoor air contamination in 1981, at the request of EPA. This and later work by NAS addressed indoor air issues that were explored in the EPA-sponsored TEAM studies that are the subjects of this case study. In its report, NAS concluded that "indoor pollution in residences, public buildings, and offices is created for the most part by the occupants' activities and their use of appliances, power equipment, and chemicals, by wear and tear and outgassing of some structural or decorative materials, by thermal factors, and by the intrusion of outdoor air."[33] While the NAS report is not a comprehensive review of all hazardous pollutants found in indoor air, it provides a wide range of examples from a diverse set of sources. The report examines chemicals and conditions for which there is direct circumstantial evidence that the chemical or condition causes or is reasonably likely to cause human stress, illness, or material damage indoors.

Factors known to influence the relative concentrations of airborne contaminants include the generation rate for pollutants generated indoors, the ambient concentration for pollutants originally generated outdoors, the volume of the indoor environment, the air-exchange rate, and the circulation of the indoor air. The report discusses how these various factors differ significantly among different building structures. Because of these differences, the NAS report concludes that the most dependable approach to controlling indoor air quality is to concentrate on reducing the generation of these contaminants at the source, rather than controlling contaminant levels through engineering controls such as increasing ventilation or air filtration or altering building structures. Indoor air quality can be improved universally by eliminating materials intended for use indoors or by reformulating or substituting others for them in ways that prevent contaminants from entering the airspace, such as by using less volatile chemicals.

Because the database on indoor air contamination was at that time limited primarily to pilot and anecdotal studies, NAS recommended that a national coordinated research effort be established. Its mission would be to determine various sources of selected pollutants and their relative contributions, to understand the fate of indoor air pollutants inside a building, to develop effective control strategies, and to characterize the effects of energy-conservation measures on indoor air quality.

Meanwhile, EPA had begun a series of studies known as the Total Exposure Assessment Methodology (TEAM) studies, described below, that were intended to begin to unravel the mystery of where the greatest exposures to airborne contaminants originate. The first TEAM study was designed to compare exposures among people who live close to chemical plants and petroleum refineries with exposures experienced by people who live farther away from these point sources. The TEAM studies that followed began to look more closely at sources of exposure in indoor environments.

Study Methodology

The first three phases of TEAM studies examined personal exposure of 600 residents in seven communities in New Jersey, North Carolina, North Dakota, and California. The participant-selection process was designed to be statistically representative of the 717,000 people in those communities.[h] Communities were selected to represent a range of ambient environments, including those which were considered to contain relatively "large" point sources (Elizabeth and Bayonne, New Jersey) and others considered to have far less significant point sources (Greensboro, North Carolina, and Devils Lake, North Dakota). The studies measured

[h] The seven cities include Elizabeth and Bayonne, New Jersey; Greensboro, North Carolina; Devils Lake, North Dakota; Antioch and Pittsburg, California, and selected communities in and around Los Angeles, California, including El Segundo, Manhattan Beach, Redondo Beach, Torrance, Hermosa Beach, Carson, Lomita, and Dominquez.

exposure to chemicals in air and water in and around participants' homes. The study objectives were to identify major sources and exposure pathways of toxics and to assess their relative importance in overall exposure to toxics.

These first three studies measured exposure to toxic volatile organic chemicals (VOCs) by measuring their presence in outdoor air, "personal air" (air breathed by an individual in a normal living and working environment, primarily indoors), water, and expired air. Contaminants in outdoor air were measured by analyzing samples taken from fixed points outside the participants' homes over two 12-hour sampling periods: during the daytime from 6 A.M. to 6 P.M., and overnight from 6 P.M. to 6 A.M. Contaminants in personal air were measured during the same periods with monitoring devices that the participants carried with them as they went about their normal activities. While the personal air samples reflect some exposure to outdoor air as well as to indoor air in the household and workplace, contamination from occasional outside air exposure was not significant, based on additional study of results from participants who stayed indoors throughout the 12-hour sampling period. Overnight measurements from all participants primarily reflect contaminants in household air. The studies were limited to volatile organic chemicals because this was the only category for which adequate analytical techniques were available for all media tested.

Several phases of the TEAM studies explored the hypothesis of the NAS report that most indoor sources of air pollutants (in the non-industrial environments that NAS studied) result from the use of commercial products. The TEAM studies also attempted to further characterize indoor sources of airborne pollutants. To determine what types of materials and activities contributed to daytime personal air exposure, participants in the first two phases of the TEAM studies completed questionnaires indicating the types of activities and exposures they experienced.

Study Findings

The first three TEAM studies, conducted over a six-year period, found that people are actually exposed to greater levels of a wider range of chemicals from indoor sources than outdoor sources, regardless of their proximity to outdoor sources. These findings support the conclusion of the NAS report regarding sources: sources of indoor air pollutants contribute more to personal contaminant exposure than sources of outdoor air pollutants. The findings further suggest that the elevated indoor levels are due to a variety of sources including consumer products, building materials, and personal activities. Half of the 20 chemicals that were included in the analyses of indoor air were found to be consistently prevalent in the indoor air of all seven communities.

The first TEAM study surprisingly found no relationship between proximity to chemical plants and petroleum refineries and degree of exposure to VOCs, suggesting that most exposures to airborne contaminants originate from sources other than outdoor point sources.[34] This finding was based on a stratified analysis of data from

New Jersey according to participants' proximity to point sources. Participants living within at least 1.5 kilometers of at least one point source were included in the "high proximity" group. "Moderate proximity" was defined as living on the border of a high proximity area, intersected by major highways, and "low proximity" was defined as living more than 1.5 kilometers from a point source. A serious limitation of this phase of the TEAM studies was the failure to account for wind patterns. True exposure differences are not well represented by distance alone, since some of the people who live close to a facility will be upwind most of the time, while some of the people living farther away will be downwind most of the time and may have higher exposures.

The TEAM studies further reported that in the study communities for which outdoor air data were reported (in New Jersey and California), air concentrations of the prevalent chemicals were consistently higher inside participants' homes than in the outdoors. (See Appendix G, Tables G-3 and G-4.) With few exceptions, the ratios of concentrations in daytime personal air and daytime outdoor air were greater than one, indicating that levels were greater in personal than outdoor air. (See Figure 2-2.)

Levels of many chemicals were also higher in exhaled breath than in outdoor air, indicating that the bulk of exposure resulted from indoor sources. Statistically, for 10 of the 11 prevalent chemicals in New Jersey, levels in exhaled breath correlated significantly with personal air levels, but did not correlate with outdoor air levels. The 11th chemical, chloroform, was significantly correlated with drinking water concentrations, indicating that most personal exposure to this chemical results from drinking chloroform in tap water and inhaling chloroform as it evaporates from household water (cold water in toilets, warm tap water used for showering, cooking, and washing clothes, etc.).[35] Chloroform is frequently formed in drinking water when chlorine, which is added to kill microbial organisms in drinking water, reacts with natural organic material in the water. (See Appendix G, Table G-3.)

Analyses showed that certain activities involving contact with products and processes that contain or use toxic chemicals contributed significantly to personal exposure as measured in personal air and expired breath. These include visiting a dry-cleaning establishment, visiting a gas station, and working in occupations of high chemical exposure such as a chemical laboratory or print shop. People who indicated on the questionnaire that they participated in one of these type of activities (those in the "exposed" group) had higher levels of organic compounds in exhaled breath than people who did not (those in the "unexposed" group). Most of these activities involve the often unavoidable use of or contact with commercial products, such as gasoline, metal-working solvents, and furniture-refinishing agents (See Figure 2-3.) However, some of the activities that caused higher exposure levels involved occupational contact with industrial process waste such as from chemical plant and plastics manufacturing processes.

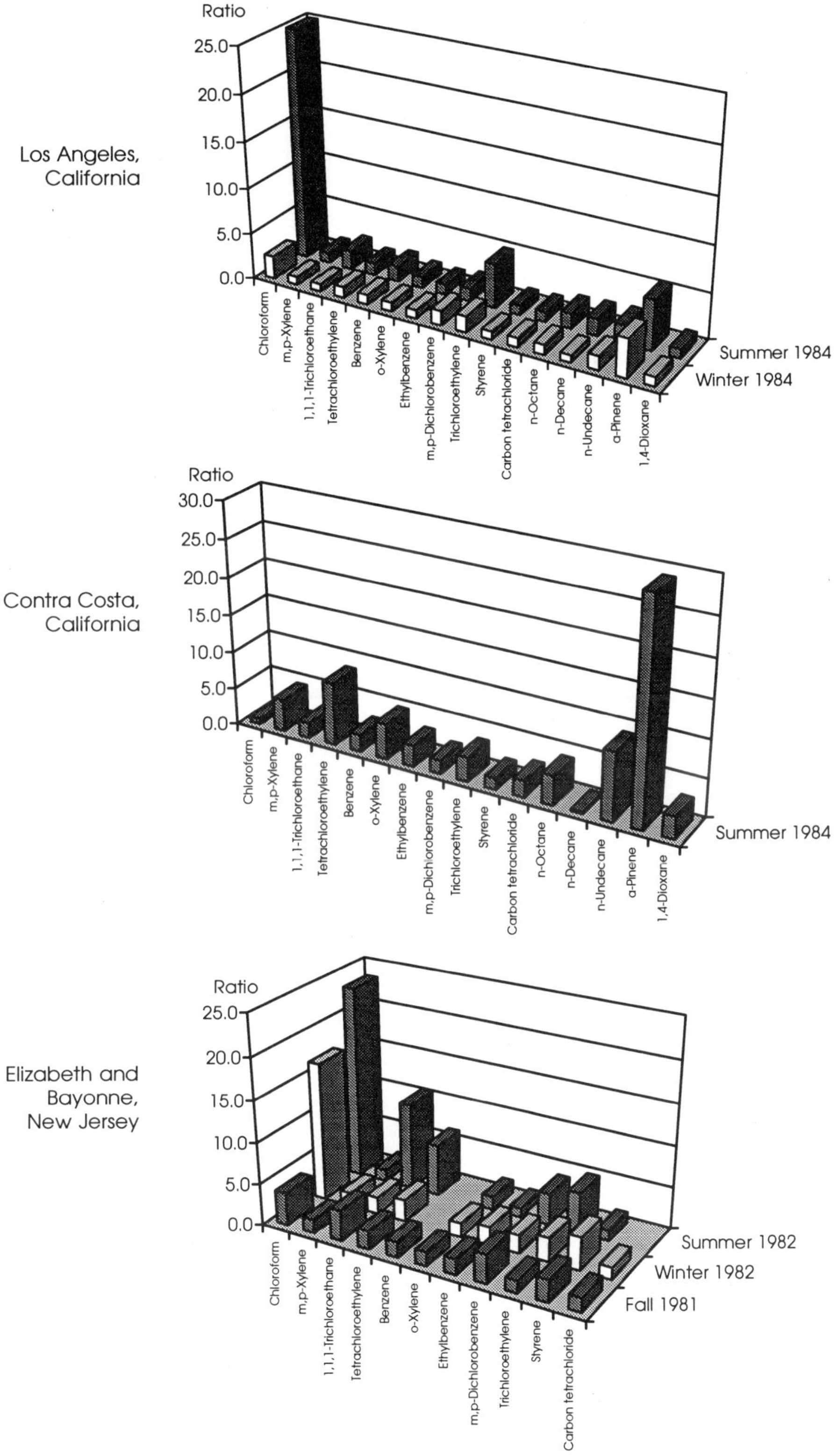

Figure 2-2.

Summary of Indoor and Outdoor Air Concentrations (Ratio of Median Overnight Personal Exposures to Overnight Outdoor Concentrations)

Figure 2-3.

Selected Volatile Organic Chemicals (VOCs) with Significantly Higher Concentrations in Air and Breath of Persons Recently Exposed to Potential Sources Compared to Persons Not Exposed to Any Source

New Jersey, 1981-1982, and California, 1984

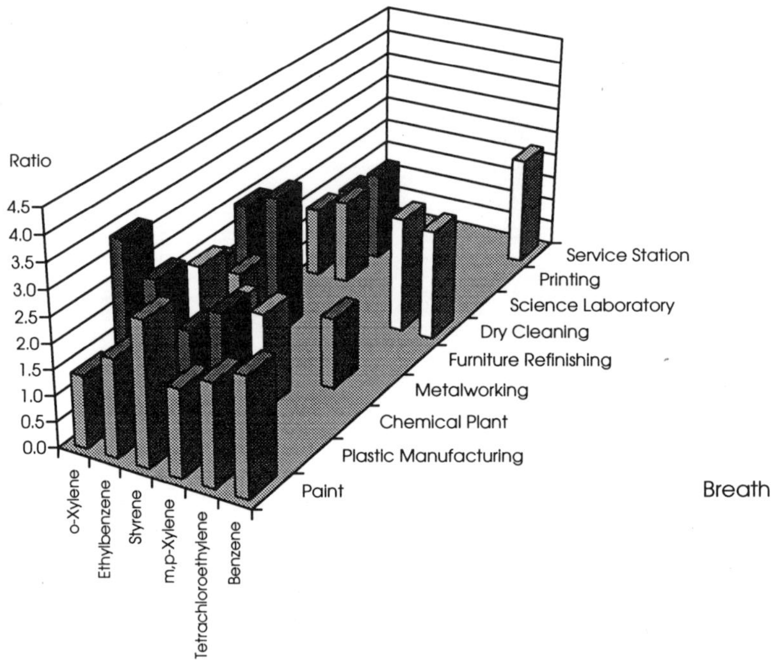

Ratio of Mean Concentrations for Exposed vs. Unexposed Groups

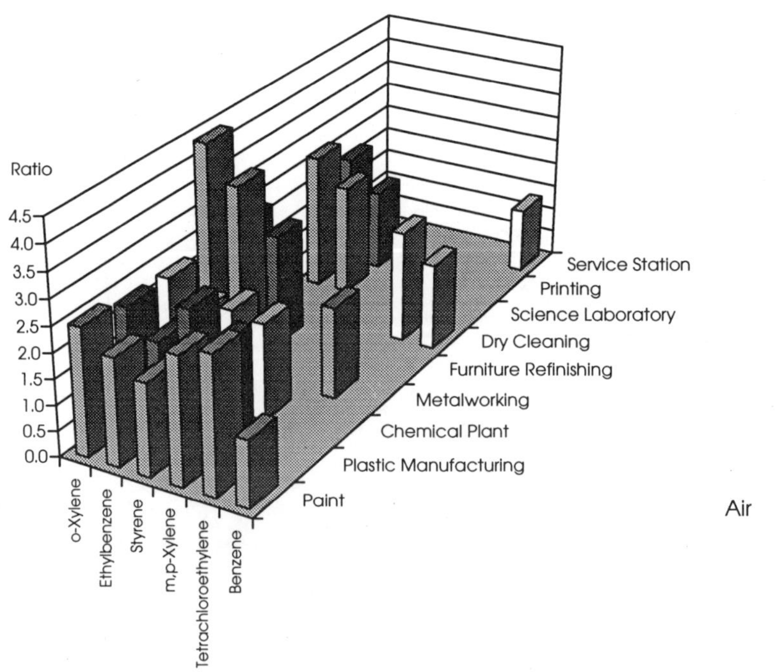

Ratio of Mean Concentrations for Exposed vs. Unexposed Groups

Since the completion of the first three TEAM studies, TEAM authors have conducted several more specialized studies characterizing sources of individual chemicals, classes of chemicals, and contributions from specific sources and personal activities, which included:

- exposure to 1,4-dichlorobenzene from bathroom air deodorizers;
- exposure to dry-cleaning chemicals from bringing home freshly dry-cleaned clothes;
- levels of common chemical constituents in paints and adhesives in indoor air of new buildings compared to older ones;
- specific sources of carbon monoxide in indoor air;
- non-occupational exposure to pesticides; and
- exposure to particulates from indoor and outdoor sources.

Each of these studies confirmed that chemicals in commercial products contribute significantly to personal chemical exposure.

For example, 1-4-dichlorobenzene, the active ingredient in many bathroom deodorizers, could be measured in blood samples of residents collected three days after a fresh deodorizer was placed in the home. Levels of dry-cleaning chemicals such as tetrachloroethylene were found to exceed outdoor levels by about 100 times in homes where freshly dry-cleaned clothes were taken. Concentrations remained elevated in these homes as long as one week after the clothes were delivered. The study of exposure to airborne pesticides in Florida and Massachusetts found that indoor sources accounted for 90 percent or more of the total airborne exposure to most pesticides. A number of the pesticides detected in these homes have been banned or their use restricted, yet they continue to be found in indoor air. The study reports that in cases where homes or the surrounding neighborhoods have been historically treated for termites or other common pests, pesticides that were used in the past and are now no longer used may continue to enter the indoor air either from soil gas that moves into basements or from soil that is tracked into the house from the yard.[36]

Unanswered Questions

1. What are the specific sources and pathways of indoor and personal exposure and how can these be predicted in given situations?

Based on their first three studies, TEAM authors recommended follow up in several areas. Subsequent TEAM studies began to explore limited aspects of these areas, but more work remained to be done at the completion of the TEAM studies. Study areas for future work might include:

- Studies of high-exposure participants to determine specific reasons for elevated exposures;
- Development of emission inventories of major sources of indoor and personal exposure that emphasize consumer products, building materials, and personal activities; and
- Development of models to predict exposures from specific products, activities, and building designs, for large populations.

EPA has developed a prototype database, IACS (for Indoor Air Chemical Sources Tracking System) that addresses the presence of toxic chemicals in household and other commercial products. The system contains information obtained from 11 reports published between 1986 and 1990 and can be searched either by product or by chemical. The system appears to be in a prototype stage; the completeness of its coverage is unclear, and it is not possible to fully identify the reference documents upon which it is based. The status of plans for further development of the database is unknown.

The latest EPA initiative in this area is the National Human Exposure Assessment Study (NHEXAS), which will attempt to develop a comprehensive view of exposures to between 20 and 30 pollutants. The project will begin with three pilot field studies that are intended to identify study designs, analytical techniques, and potential problems for a nationwide study. One field study will examine exposures in EPA's Region V (Illinois, Indiana, Michigan, Minnesota, Ohio, and Wisconsin), one will involve a statewide assessment in Arizona, and one will examine exposure variability in a small group (approximately 50 people) studied repeatedly. NHEXAS is an effort to examine all pathways of exposure, including food and water, air, soil, and dust, coupled with estimates of body burdens.

2. What are the effects of indoor air contaminants, singly and in combination?

The TEAM studies address the presence and sources of indoor air contaminants, but not their effects on human health. The effects of chronic elevated exposure to a few chemicals, such as benzene and lead, have been clearly documented, and there is a relatively strong level of consensus in the scientific community about these effects. For some other chemicals, effects of chronic exposure to levels measured in indoor air are not well characterized. Furthermore, there is the question of how the various indoor air contaminants behave and cause effects when a human being is exposed to them in combination in a given environmental situation. Further studies may be helpful to explore some suspected relationships and interactions, but just to look at all aspects of exposure to the 11 VOCs included in the TEAM studies would be virtually impossible, let alone studying all of the products and chemicals that may play a role in indoor air pollution.

Ozone Depleters

Chemicals that deplete the stratospheric ozone layer constitute another group of environmentally damaging chemicals that are found throughout society in industrial processes and commercial products. Damage to the ozone layer allows higher levels of ultraviolet radiation to enter the lower atmosphere, where it can cause human health effects such as skin cancer, eye cataracts and retina damage, and possibly weakened immune response. Possible ecological effects include harm to aquatic organisms living near the surface of water bodies and limited plant growth.

The chemicals of most serious concern for their ozone-depleting effect are chlorofluorocarbons (CFCs). These chemicals have been widely used as coolants in refrigerators and air conditioners, as propellants in aerosol spray cans, and as sterilants for health care equipment. CFCs also have been used to manufacture polystyrene and polyurethane foam for packaging and various other uses. Other chemicals that contribute to ozone depletion include carbon tetrachloride, 1,1,1-trichloroethane, bromomethane, and halons.

When discovered in the early 1930s, CFCs were heralded as miraculous substances, because they had extremely low toxicity and were highly stable, odorless compounds. They seemed to be the perfect substitute for ammonia, a toxic and moderately flammable chemical in widespread use as a refrigerant at the time. Unfortunately, the chemical stability that accounts for their low toxicity is the very factor that allows CFCs to migrate far up into the stratosphere rather than degrade in the lower atmosphere. Once in the stratosphere, they are broken up by the high levels of ultraviolet radiation and participate in a chain reaction that upsets the natural balance between ozone and oxygen, resulting in a decrease in the protective ozone layer. The emergence of the theory of ozone depletion in the early 1970s and its subsequent confirmation by research and monitoring was a great shock to scientists, industry, and government. Concern about ozone depletion continues to have wide repercussions for manufacturers and consumers, as the important uses of ozone depleters are affected by domestic regulations under the Clean Air Act and by international treaty obligations under the Montreal Protocol of 1987.

Study Characterization

International efforts to eliminate the production and use of ozone-depleting chemicals have included intensive study of the range of sources that cause their release. In 1987, a treaty known as the Montreal Protocol called for international cooperation to eliminate the production and use of ozone-depleting substances. Since then more than 130 nations and the European Union have ratified the Protocol and have agreed to a series of reductions and elimination of the various ozone depleters, until all ozone depleters are eliminated by the year 2030. (See Box 2-A.)

To evaluate the feasibility and implications of reaching these goals, especially for developing countries, and to measure progress in meeting them, the United Nations Environment Programme (UNEP) has organized a series of assessment panels whose reports document use applications and quantitative estimates for the different categories of use of ozone-depleting substances. These reports provide a picture of the relative contribution of various commercial products and industrial processes to the overall problem of ozone depletion based on annual global production and use estimates.

Study Methodology

The process of eliminating such a large class of chemicals from such a broad range of product use and industrial applications has not been straightforward. To continue making and using these products, substitutes must be developed for each ozone-depleting chemical and each application. As in the case of lead, eliminating further production of ozone depleters is just the first step toward solving the problem. Existing products that contain these chemicals remain scattered throughout the environment, causing lingering releases. Many of these products, such as cars, refrigerators, and air conditioners, are designed to last 10 to 20 years or longer.

The committees of the Montreal Protocol evaluated a variety of factors for each use category of each identified ozone depleter. These factors include worldwide use estimates, availability of safe substitutes, and the technical feasibility and economic impacts of various alternatives for eliminating production and use and for reclaiming and recycling existing supplies of Protocol substances. After considering these and other factors, the committee members recommended the earliest achievable target dates for phasing out the production and use of each chemical and its various applications and for granting any exemptions for specific uses.

Study Findings

The manufacture, processing, and use of commercial products is the greatest potential source of ozone-depleting chemicals released to the atmosphere. Of the nearly 2,400,000 metric tons manufactured and used in 1991, approximately 57 percent was used for commercial products. Carbon tetrachloride accounts for the remaining 43 percent of worldwide use of ozone depleters. Although it is also used as a solvent and cleaning product, approximately 95 percent of all carbon tetrachloride produced worldwide is used as a feedstock (raw material) to make chlorofluorocarbons. (See Table 2-5.)

There is little information to compare how much of these chemicals is actually released 1) during their manufacture (e.g., releases of carbon tetrachloride during its use in the manufacture of CFCs), 2) during the manufacture of products containing ozone-depleting chemicals, and 3) throughout the use and disposal of such products in industrial, commercial, and household settings. UNEP estimates that inadvertent emissions of ozone-depleting chemicals from chemical production and processing operations total only 0.5 percent of worldwide production (approximately 12,000 metric tons based on 1991 estimates), but this amount does not include releases associated with waste management and disposal.[37]

A wide range of products used in manufacturing, commercial, and household applications contain ozone-depleting substances, of which solvents are the largest category. Although most solvents do not contain ozone depleters, those that do account for approximately 30 percent of the worldwide use of ozone-depleting substances. Their largest use is in manufacturing applications that involve cleaning metal or electronic parts. In the electronics industry, they are used for defluxing — the removal of residues from assemblies after soldering. Solvents containing ozone depleters are also used in commercial dry-cleaning operations and in many other service industries such as automotive and electronic maintenance operations. Since ozone-depleting substances evaporate quickly, their use results

Table 2-5. Ozone-depleting Substances, Types and Quantities of Worldwide Use

Application	Controlled Chemicals*	Total Use Metric Tons	Year of Estimate	Percent of Total Use Percent	Type
Carbon tetrachloride	Carbon tetrachloride	1,000,000	1988	43%	▲●
Solvents	CFC-113* (30%) 1,1,1-Trichloroethane (70%)	773,500	1989	34%	●▲
Electronics Cleaning		201,000			
Metal cleaning		173,000			
Precision Cleaning		260,000			
Dry-cleaning		10,500			
Aerosol Application		60,000			
Coatings and Ink		21,000			
Adhesives		48,000			
Refrigerants (56.4% mobile)	CFCs-11, 12-13, 114, 115*	260,000	1991	11%	●
Foams	CFCs-11, 12, 114*	174,150	1990	8%	●▲
Aerosol Propellants	CFC-11, 12* and 1,1,1-Trichloroethane	115,000	1991	5%	●▲
Fire Protection Halons**	Halon 1211 and 1301*	25,000	1990	1%	●
Sterilants	CFC-12*	20,000	1991	1%	●
Total		2,367,650		103%	

Key:
▲- Industrial/Manufacturing Process Waste
●- Commercial/Consumer Product Use
* - CFC-11: Trichlorofluoromethane
CFC-12: Dichlorodifluoromethane
CFC-13: Chlorotrifluoromethane
CFC-113: Freon 113
CFC-114: Dichlorotetrafluoroethane
CFC-115: Monochloropentafluoroethane
Halon 1211: Bromochlorodifluoromethane
Halon 1301: Bromotrifluoromethane
** - Quantity listed is a production estimate

Source: Derived from United Nations, *Montreal Protocol on Substances that Deplete the Ozone Layer 1991 Assessment*. Report of the Technology and Economic Assessment Panel, December 1991.

in release to the ambient air and eventually to the stratospheric ozone layer, unless vapor recovery systems are in place. Solvent-use operations recover[i] less than 20 percent of the total amount purchased, so more than 80 percent of solvents used is apparently lost to the atmosphere. Control technologies are now available to reduce this atmospheric loss to 30 or even 10 percent.[38] Major electronics companies are working to make these technologies available to companies throughout the world and to promote their use.

[i] "Recover" here means the amount available for reuse or recycling plus the amount in waste that is treated or disposed of.

As components of commercial products, ozone-depleting chemicals are used primarily as coolants in refrigerators and air conditioners, blowing agents in Styrofoam packaging and insulation, propellants in aerosol products (where such uses have not yet been banned), and flame retardants in fire protection equipment. (See Table 2-5.)

In 1978 the United States and several other countries banned the use of CFCs as aerosol propellants (except for some essential medical uses), and soon thereafter companies reformulated their foam packaging products to reduce or eliminate the use of CFCs. A high level of public awareness of the ozone problem and its causes contributed to both of these actions. These uses were not discontinued in every country, however; and foam and aerosol uses of CFCs still account for 8 percent and 5 percent of the total worldwide market for ozone-depleting chemicals, respectively. (See Table 2-5.)

Worldwide production volumes did not continue to decrease after an initial decrease in the mid-1970s. This decrease was the result of both economic factors and actions taken by the United States and other countries against certain CFCs and their uses, in response to ozone-depletion concerns. In fact, world production of all CFCs peaked again in 1986 at levels exceeding 1974 output figures.[39] Only recently, as a result of the 1987 Montreal Protocol, have production levels substantially declined.

Approximately 260,000 metric tons of CFCs and other ozone-depleting substances are used annually as coolants and refrigerants, accounting for 11 percent of worldwide use of ozone-depleting chemicals. (See Table 2-5.) Quantities that do not leak from refrigerators and home or automotive air conditioners during the useful life of these appliances reach the atmosphere when the appliances are disposed of in landfills or dismantled by scrap-metal reclamation processes. Domestic refrigerators contain only a small quantity of cooling fluid — typically less than 200 grams. But with the world market producing an estimated 56,330,000 refrigerators each year (based on a 1990 estimate), the total quantity of CFCs produced and therefore potentially released from this application alone totals more than 9,526 metric tons. Releases from commercial refrigeration units are even greater. Typical losses from supermarket units vary from 45 kilograms per year to more than 300 kg/year depending on the size of the unit and quality of preventive maintenance. Releases occur throughout the life of the unit during manufacturing and installation (11 percent), leakage (8 percent), during service (54 percent), and disposal (27 percent).[40]

Automotive air conditioning systems are particularly prone to leaks. Most vehicles lose more than half the total amount of CFCs in the system before a noticeable loss of performance causes the owner to have the system serviced. Because of such leakage, in-use vehicles require approximately 0.4 kg of new CFC per year to maintain the air conditioning unit.[41] With an estimated 140 million CFC-carrying vehicles on the road in the United States alone, releases from this source pose a substantial risk to the ozone layer.[42] Historically, regular maintenance procedures for automobile air conditioning have been a large source of emissions. Because CFCs were safe and inexpensive, service workers generally did not take any special precautions to conserve the fluid or prevent exposure. Thus, reclamation and conservation measures require a tremendous amount of education to change habits among the people who service appliances that contain CFCs.

With so many different ozone-damaging chemicals in so many products and with such a diversity of applications for each one, commercial product use is also the most difficult source to eliminate. Researchers from nearly every commercial sector are working to find substitutes that are safe, effective, and affordable. In some cases, such as domestic refrigerators and automobile air conditioners, ozone-friendly hydrofluorocarbons can be used after expensive alterations in equipment. For many large-scale applications, transitional substitutes such as hydrochlorofluorocarbons (HCFCs) will need to be used until better alternatives are found. These transitional chemicals also damage the ozone layer, but to a lesser extent than CFCs, and will be permitted under the terms of the Montreal Protocol until 1996, when production will be capped and a 35-year phase-out initiated. Because CFC systems are known to leak over time, early retrofitting is important — even if transitional substances must be used.

No ozone-safe alternatives have yet been identified for halons that match their effectiveness at extinguishing fires with low toxicity. Production of halons is stopped and recycling is currently filling the demand until a satisfactory substitute is available.

Unanswered Questions

Although more needs to be understood about the chemistry and physics of stratospheric processes and about the effects of increased ultraviolet radiation, these matters are outside of the scope of this report. What is relevant is the question of the chemical sources of ozone depletion, and those sources are well characterized. The "solution" is also well understood — to eliminate the production and use of ozone depleters as soon as possible and to recover and prevent the release of as great a quantity as possible of such chemicals already in existence. The timing and practical methods for arriving at that solution, or coping with the tremendous costs involved, are not so clear.

The principal unanswered questions within the scope of this study relate to the chemicals that will be substituted for present ozone depleters in various uses. Will reclamation and recovery programs for existing ozone-damaging chemicals be effective? Which of the available alternatives to these chemicals will prove to be acceptably effective, safe, and affordable? For those substitutes that are more toxic to humans or more damaging to the earth's environment (below the stratosphere) than the chemicals they replace, how can such effects be prevented or mitigated or exposure reduced?

Chemicals in Waste

The final discharge point for chemicals in products and process waste is wherever these materials are ultimately disposed of — in landfills or other waste sites. Two major EPA regulatory programs cover hazardous and other solid waste disposal sites. The Comprehensive Environmental Response, Compensation and Liability Act (CERCLA), otherwise known as Superfund, evaluates and remediates uncontrolled hazardous waste sites at which contaminants are found at levels that present danger to public health or welfare or the environment. The National Priorities List (NPL) now numbers 1,242 sites for remediation, plus another 46 proposed sites.[43] These Superfund sites have resulted both from negligent and illegal practices, many in the past, and from legal practices where environmental consequences were unknown or disregarded.

The Resource Conservation and Recovery Act (RCRA) regulates hazardous waste generation, as well as municipal, commercial, and industrial treatment, storage, and disposal facilities (TSDFs). Landfills are one type of solid waste disposal facility that comes under RCRA jurisdiction. The RCRA program is designed to prevent pollutants from entering the environment both through regulations and permits that limit the disposal of hazardous waste and by requiring groundwater monitoring, leachate collection systems, and proper design and operation of landfills.

The contaminated leachate that is often found at Superfund sites and solid and hazardous waste landfills is usually a complex mixture of many toxic and hazardous substances originating from many sources. The following discussion provides examples of the difficulties in identifying and tracing these contaminants and their sources, but nevertheless indicates the apparently major role of everyday product use.

Superfund Hazardous Waste Sites

Study Characterization

To learn more about the major sources that contributed hazardous chemicals to Superfund sites, INFORM examined summary data on sites in three arbitrarily selected states: Delaware, New York, and Michigan. To limit the analysis to a manageable number of seriously contaminated sites, only sites on the National Priorities List with a Hazard Ranking System Score of 50 or greater (out of a possible score of 100) were included. The Hazard Ranking System Score is a standard measure of the severity of contamination at hazardous waste sites, which EPA uses to prioritize sites. The NPL sites undergo further investigation by EPA to characterize the contamination and the human health and environmental risks posed, identify parties responsible for generating the waste, and set goals for cleaning up the contamination.[j]

Study Methodology

INFORM used the summary site and waste descriptions given in EPA's NPL database to categorize each site according to source category (industrial process waste, commercial product use, both, or other) and type of site (landfill/

[j] See Appendix Q for information on public access to RTK-Net, which includes summary information from EPA Superfund site investigations.

disposal site, manufacturing facility, recycling facility, or other). (See Appendix G, Table G-5.)

The source data are limited in usefulness in several ways. The listed sources are usually those organizations or individuals held responsible for the contamination, which may not in all cases be the ones who generated the waste or caused the contamination. There does seem to be strong agreement between the contaminants listed and the sources, however (i.e., one would expect the contaminant profile from the sources listed). The exact method by which the contaminants were generated and the pathway by which they entered the environment are often obscure, particularly at mixed disposal sites with both municipal and industrial waste. For such sites, the NPL database does not offer a clear picture of waste sources.

Where possible the source and site-type designations were interpreted from the list of chemicals of concern and from those parties listed as potentially responsible for the contamination or liable for site remediation. For other sites, where the summary information did not adequately describe waste constituents and sources, the further investigation with local officials and others that would be required to make more accurate assessments was outside the scope of this study.

Study Findings

Most people probably picture a Superfund site as a dump full of leaking drums of industrial process waste, and, indeed, half of the 36 sites in the sample appear to be predominantly contaminated by industrial process waste, although details are sketchy. Sources at 8 of the 36 sites, however, relate primarily to commercial product use, and product use plays an important role at 10 other sites that have mixed sources of industrial process waste and product use.

Of the 18 sites designated as caused by industrial process waste, chemical manufacturing operations were the type of source associated with 12. Some of these sites are either former or currently operating manufacturing facilities, but most contamination seems to have arisen from process waste disposal operations, such as unlined lagoons, landfills, and surface impoundments. The other six sites in the process waste category are industrial waste landfills or incinerators that accepted wastes generated by industrial processes.

Of the eight sites that were primarily contaminated as a result of commercial product use, one, Thermo-Chem in Muskegan, Michigan, had been operated as a recycling facility. There the treatment of paint wastes, antifreeze, dry-cleaning solvents, and other products to reclaim solvents for reuse caused the contamination of local groundwater, presumably from spills, leaks, and other types of releases.

Another clear-cut case of product-related contamination is the Wide Beach Development Corporation site in Brant, New York, where environmental degradation resulted from pouring PCB-contaminated waste oil on the access road to control dust. (This practice is now prohibited.)

The remaining six sites whose contamination source is designated product-related are mixed municipal and industrial hazardous waste disposal sites, where multiple types and generators of waste make the nature of the sources and their relative contributions more difficult to establish. The strong connection with product use can be established by the nature of the contaminating materials found there, which include paints, oil and grease, and other such product-related waste.

Sources of contamination at the 10 remaining sites in the sample of 36 could not be categorized on the basis of the information available. Of these, three handled mixed municipal/industrial waste; three handled primarily industrial waste that includes waste from commercial product use; and four are presently operating or former manufacturing facilities that probably generated both process and product waste. The last group includes three companies using electroplating processes and one that manufactures universal joints for the automotive industry, all of which are types of facilities that are likely to entail heavy product use.

Unanswered Questions

1. How well do EPA site characterizations of Superfund sites reflect the range and relative contribution of various sources of contamination?

Because many sites were abandoned long before they were put on the National Priorities List, every site investigation is indeed a true detective story to piece together evidence to identify potentially responsible parties and to determine how the waste was generated. For many sites with multiple sources and multiple contaminants, the true nature and quantitative contributions of each of the sources will probably never be known, whether measured by amount of waste, concentrations of contaminants, or risk to human health and the environment. With so much mystery shrouding each individual site, efforts such as this INFORM study to draw national conclusions from a sampling of sites are bound to be inconclusive. Further investigation does appear to be worthwhile, however, particularly if focused on how smaller contributors to the contamination (households and small business and industries) generate product waste. This would not be an easy task, but it does get to the heart of the whole complex set of questions surrounding the role played in contamination and exposure by toxics in commerce.

2. What sources and practices are causing sites to be contaminated today?

Contamination at many sites currently on the National Priorities List occurred prior to the passage of most environmental regulations, by hazardous material handling and disposal practices that have since been prohibited. Are current regulations effective in preventing site contamination or is contamination occurring today by different sources and pathways?

Leachate from Landfills

Old solid and hazardous waste landfills still provide a major source of environmental contamination, which is why many of them are on the National Priorities List. Releases from these sites occur as chemicals leach out of material buried in the landfills, as rainwater flows through the site, and as the material degrades, resulting in pollution of groundwater, surface water, and soil near the landfill. Since the passage of RCRA, landfills have been subject to regulations requiring a variety of engineering controls designed to limit the generation of leachate and the release of chemicals into the environment by these pathways; such measures have reduced but not removed the environmental problems from leachates. Any landfill or other type of land disposal site that existed prior to the passage of RCRA had to meet the new RCRA requirements or cease operation and follow RCRA closure procedures.

Investigation of sources of contaminants in landfill leachates is in its infancy. The study reported below looked at a sample of industrial hazardous waste landfills and municipal solid waste landfills that are currently operating to compare the chemical profiles of their leachates. Although that study's purpose was to compare chemical profiles of leachates from the sites rather than to trace sources of waste, some aspects of the findings are nevertheless relevant to the subject of this chapter.

Study Characterization

Researchers at Texas A & M University examined chemical analyses of leachate and groundwater samples from landfills across the country.[44] Their purpose was to understand more about the chemical composition and toxicity of leachate and, hence, the potential contamination that can result from municipal solid waste and industrial hazardous waste landfills. While these data do not allow one to characterize the specific sources generating the waste at these facilities or the proportion contributed by product vs. process sources, they do help to assess the relative polluting potential of material in municipal solid waste and industrial hazardous waste.

Study Methodology

The Texas A & M researchers reviewed chemical analyses of leachate and groundwater reported in the literature in nine studies published between 1979 and 1988. The dataset is comprised of samples taken at 19 municipal solid waste landfills and 39 industrial and mixed waste landfills. The data are more useful for making general qualitative comparisons than for any precise quantitative results, because of several limitations. Different types of chemical analysis were conducted at different sites, and chemicals may not have been detected at some sites simply because the analyses did not test for them. The composition of waste at municipal solid waste landfills is always particularly difficult to verify because of the very wide range of possible contaminants. Other problems outside the scope of this chapter make the information on the presence of a certain chemical at a certain site somewhat more reliable than the actual concentration.

Study Findings

Of the 143 chemicals that were detected at one or more of these sites from among the various sets of chemicals tested for at each site, 60 were found in municipal solid waste sites, 31 in industrial sites, and 39 in both. (Another 13 chemicals were detected only at or below the limits of reliable detection, 12 of which were found only in municipal landfills.) Of the 39 chemicals detected in both types of sites, 19 were found at higher concentrations in municipal waste leachate, and 20 were higher in leachate from industrial sites. For example, isophorone, classified by EPA as a possible human carcinogen, was found in municipal solid waste leachate at levels over 30 times higher than levels in industrial and mixed waste leachate. Isophorone is a solvent that is widely used in a variety of industrial processes and commercial products, including lacquers, coatings and finishes, inks, pesticides, and photographic supplies. (See Figure 2-4.)

As one would expect, the chemical profile of leachate from municipal solid waste landfills reflects the broad range of chemicals that comprise commercial and consumer products. This municipal leachate is not only as complex, but also contains as many toxic chemicals, as the leachate generated by industrial hazardous waste or mixed industrial and municipal waste landfills. Municipal leachate may be comparable in toxicity as well, although further study is needed to determine this. This suggests that efforts to reduce the environmental hazard posed by landfill leachate must also address the amount and toxicity of chemicals used in commercial products that are found in the municipal solid waste stream.

Unanswered Questions

1. What are all of the sources of environmental toxics generated by the disposal of municipal solid waste?

Much work has been done to characterize the constituents of what has come to be recognized as household hazardous waste — materials that are already recognized as toxic at levels used in household products, such as paints, batteries, and cleaners. What is less understood is the long-term, cumulative impact of the many chemicals that may or may not be recognized as toxic in the myriad of commercial products that are discarded into municipal solid waste. These are not necessarily toxic in the form in which they are used, but they may pose a risk when concentrated in waste and/or when they decompose after disposal. Such materials include building products, adhesives, paper coatings, inks, dyes, plastics, and preservatives. Research is underway at several institutions, including the University of Tennessee and EPA (see the earlier description of the IACS database), to evaluate and characterize the chemical content of commercial products and the relative risk and potential fate of these materials in use and disposal.

Figure 2-4.

Concentration of Selected Compounds Identified in Industrial and Municipal Landfill Leachate or Groundwater Plume

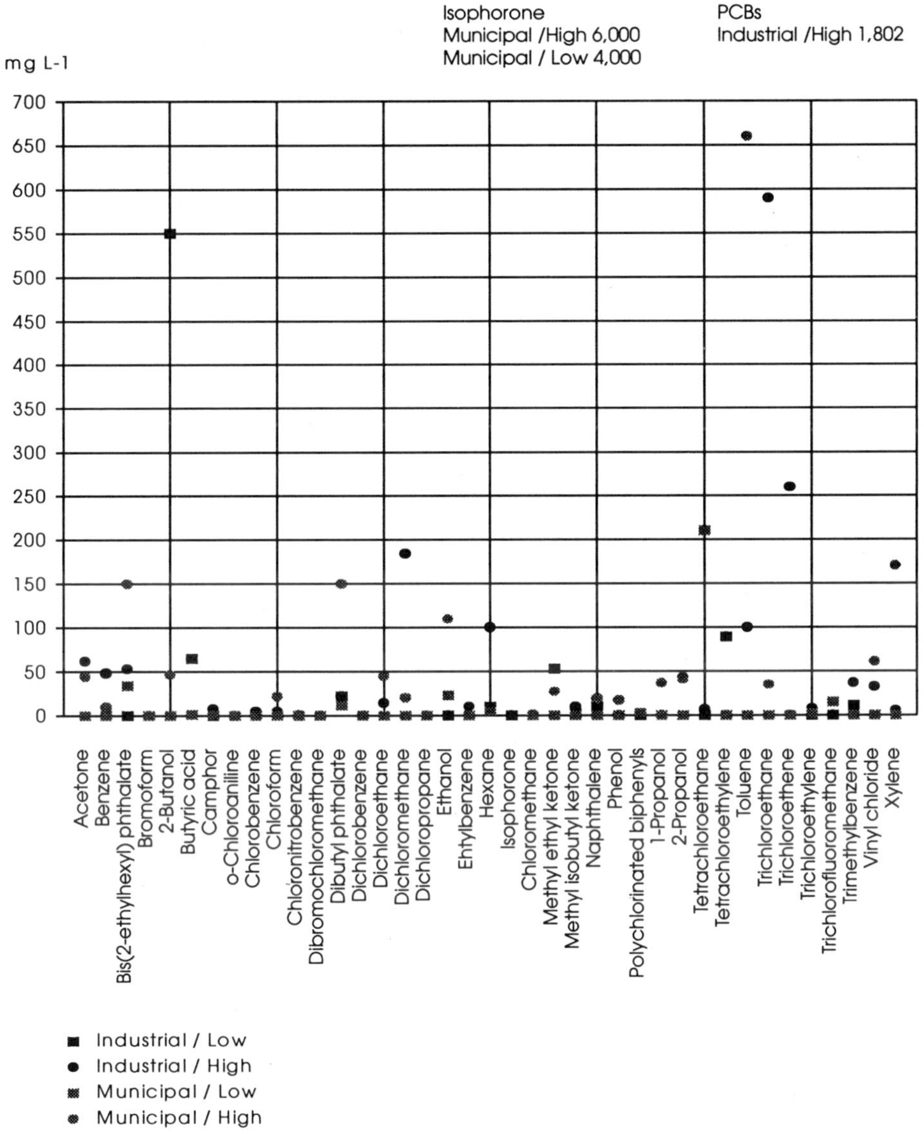

2. What is the ultimate fate of chemicals that leach from hazardous waste and municipal solid waste and what is the relative risk they pose?

Hazardous chemicals in leachate, whether industrial or municipal, represent just one stage in the complex pathway from source to waste disposal site to environmental contamination to resulting effects on human health and the environment. The actual risk occurs when these chemicals reach, or accumulate in, media that contact humans, plants, or animals at levels and under conditions that are toxic to these populations. Is there a difference in contribution to actual risk to health and the environment from industrial/mixed hazardous waste and municipal solid waste? Which products and processes contribute the most seriously toxic chemicals and which are relatively benign? How much is known about the toxicity of chemicals that leach from these wastes? A number of chemicals such as 2,6-dichlorobenzamide and bromoethane that were detected at more than 100 milligrams per liter of leachate have not been fully evaluated for long-term effects on human health and the environment.

Great Lakes Basin Areas of Concern

The Great Lakes Basin has come to be recognized as one of the more severely contaminated regions of the country. Looking broadly at a large geographic area to identify many types of pollution and their many sources is obviously a very large undertaking. The Great Lakes area was chosen for inclusion in this chapter both because of the recognized seriousness of the toxic chemical contamination there and because the area is subject to considerable scrutiny and data collection.

The following discussion summarizes what has been learned about two regions within the Great Lakes Basin, which have been identified as "Areas of Concern" under the Great Lakes Water Quality Agreement of 1972. This agreement commits the United States and Canada to develop and implement programs and other measures to restore and maintain the integrity of the waters of the Great Lakes Basin ecosystem.[45] The Agreement, as amended in 1987, calls upon the eight Great Lakes Basin states[k] in the United States and the Canadian Province of Ontario to prepare Remedial Action Plans (RAPs) in areas of chronic pollution within the Basin, known as Areas of Concern (AOCs). The scope of interest of the RAP process is much broader than that of this chapter, which focuses only on toxic chemical contamination and its sources. Source and contaminant data from two Areas of Concern, the Black River Watershed in Ohio and the Rochester Embayment in New York, are summarized below to demonstrate the pathways and describe the sources of contamination that have been identified to date. (See Map 2-1.)

[k] New York, Pennsylvania, Ohio, Michigan, Indiana, Illinois, Wisconsin, and Minnesota.

Map 2-1.

Great Lakes Basin Showing Black River Watershed Area of Concern (AOC) and Rochester Embayment AOC

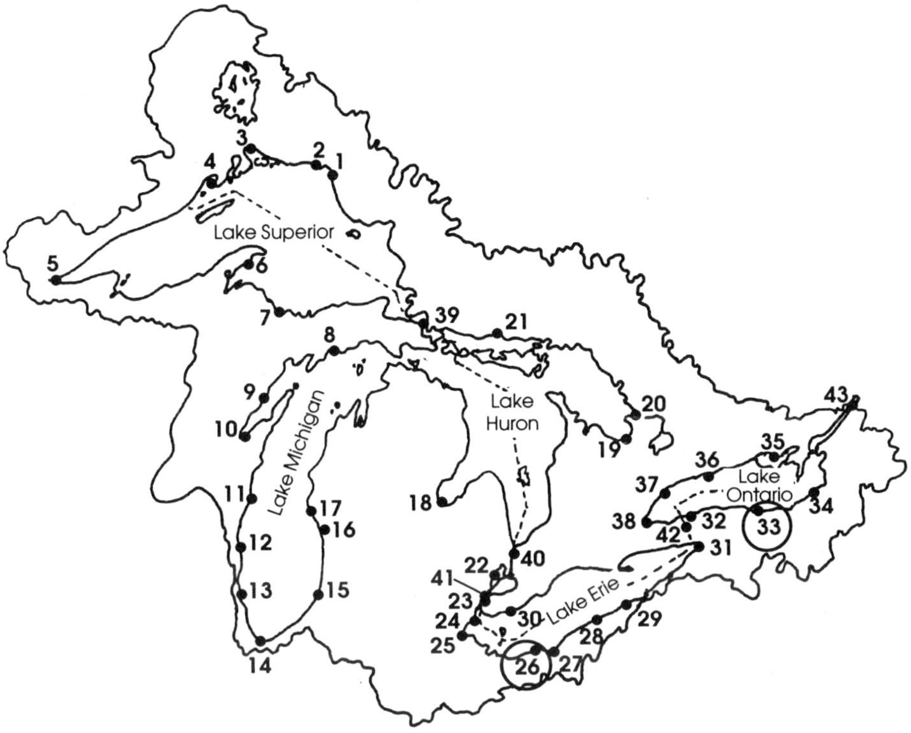

Lake Superior
1 Peninsula Harbour
2 Jackfish Bay
3 Nipigon Bay
4 Thunder Bay
5 St. Louis Bay / River
6 Torch Lake
7 Deer Lake-Carp Creek / River

Lake Michigan
8 Manistique River
9 Menominee River
10 Fox River / Southern Green Bay
11 Sheboygan River
12 Milwaukee Estuary
13 Waukegan Harbor
14 Grand Calumet River / Indiana Harbor Canal
15 Kalamazoo River
16 Muskegon Lake
17 White Lake

Lake Huron
18 Saginaw River / Saginaw Bay
19 Collingwood Harbour
20 Severn Sound
21 Spanish River Mouth

Lake Erie
22 Clinton River
23 Rouge River
24 River Raisin
25 Maumee River
26 Black River
27 Cuyahoga River
28 Ashtabula River
29 Presque Isle Bay
30 Wheatley Harbour

Lake Ontario
31 Buffalo River
32 Eighteen Mile Creek
33 Rochester Embayment
34 Oswego River
35 Bay of Quinte
36 Port Hope
37 Metro Toronto
38 Hamilton Harbour

Connecting Channels
39 St. Marys River
40 St. Clair River
41 Detroit River
42 Niagara River
43 St. Lawrence River (Cornwall / Massena)

Source: Review and Evaluation of the Great Lakes Remedial Action Plan Program 1991, *Great Lakes Water Quality Board, International Joint Commission, 1991*

Study Characterization

Although the concerns in this chapter are narrower than the scope of the Remedial Action Plans, the material here is taken from the "Stage I" documents of the Black River and Rochester Embayment RAPs, completed in 1994 and 1993, respectively.[46] Stage I is the first of a three-stage RAP process:

- Stage I: to characterize the contamination in each area in terms of the use impairments outlined by the International Joint Commission (IJC)[l] and to identify sources causing the contamination;
- Stage II: to develop remedial strategies to restore beneficial uses by cleaning up contaminated areas and preventing further releases; and
- Stage III: to confirm the restoration of beneficial uses.

Use impairments are defined by the Great Lakes Water Quality Agreement as a change in the chemical, physical, or biological integrity of the Great Lakes System sufficient to limit or prevent beneficial uses of the waters in any of 14 specified ways.[m]

The Black River Watershed is located in north-central Ohio. (See Map 2-2.) The AOC includes the lower portion of the Black River and the harbors of the City of Lorain, on Lake Erie. The IJC Water Quality Board first designated the Black River as an Area of Concern in 1985, due to its probable contribution to water-quality degradation in adjacent Lake Erie. Although the primary portion of the AOC includes the lower 6.5 miles of the river, the Stage I document addresses additional upstream areas, due to the significance of contributing sources located in these areas.

The Rochester Embayment is an area along the southern shore of Lake Ontario near Rochester, New York, which includes six miles of the Genesee River. (See Map 2-3.) The IJC identified it as an Area of Concern in 1981, on the basis of moderate violations of water-quality objectives and indications of fish and sediment contamination in Rochester Harbor and Irondequoit Bay.

Study Methodology

While the RAP process in every AOC is unique, each involves the participation of a stakeholder group comprised of representatives from

[l] The IJC is a bi-national (United States and Canada) permanent body that was convened by the Boundary Waters Treaty of 1909 to prevent and mitigate disputes regarding the use of waters between the two countries. It provides a framework for cooperation on issues of air and water pollution and the use and flow of boundary waters.

[m] The 14 use impairments are: restrictions on fish and wildlife consumption; tainting of fish and wildlife flavor; degradation of fish and wildlife populations; loss of fish and wildlife habitat; bird or animal deformities or reproduction problems; degradation of benthos (organisms living on the lake bottom); restrictions on dredging activities; eutrophication or undesirable algae; restrictions on drinking water, or drinking water taste and odor problems; beach closings; degradation of aesthetics; added costs to agriculture or industry; degradation of phytoplankton and zooplankton populations; and loss of fish and wildlife habitat.

Map 2-2.

Black River Watershed Area of Concern

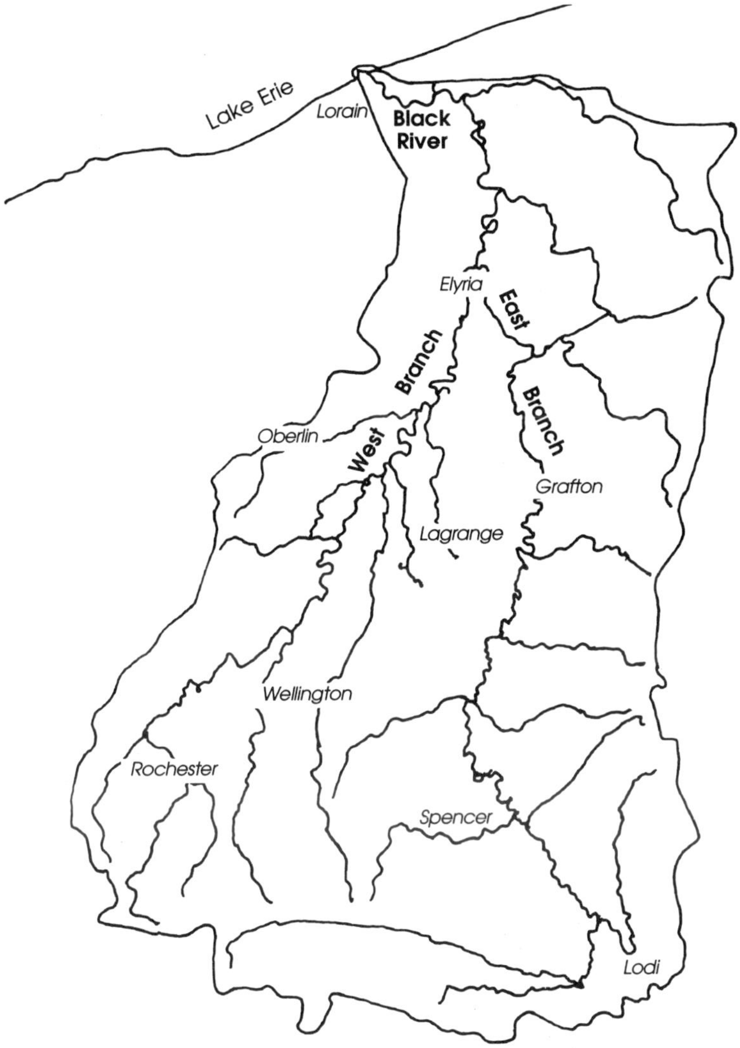

Source: Black River Remedial Action Plan Stage One Report, *Black River Remedial Action Plan Coordinating Committee, 1994*

Map 2-3.

Rochester Embayment Area of Concern

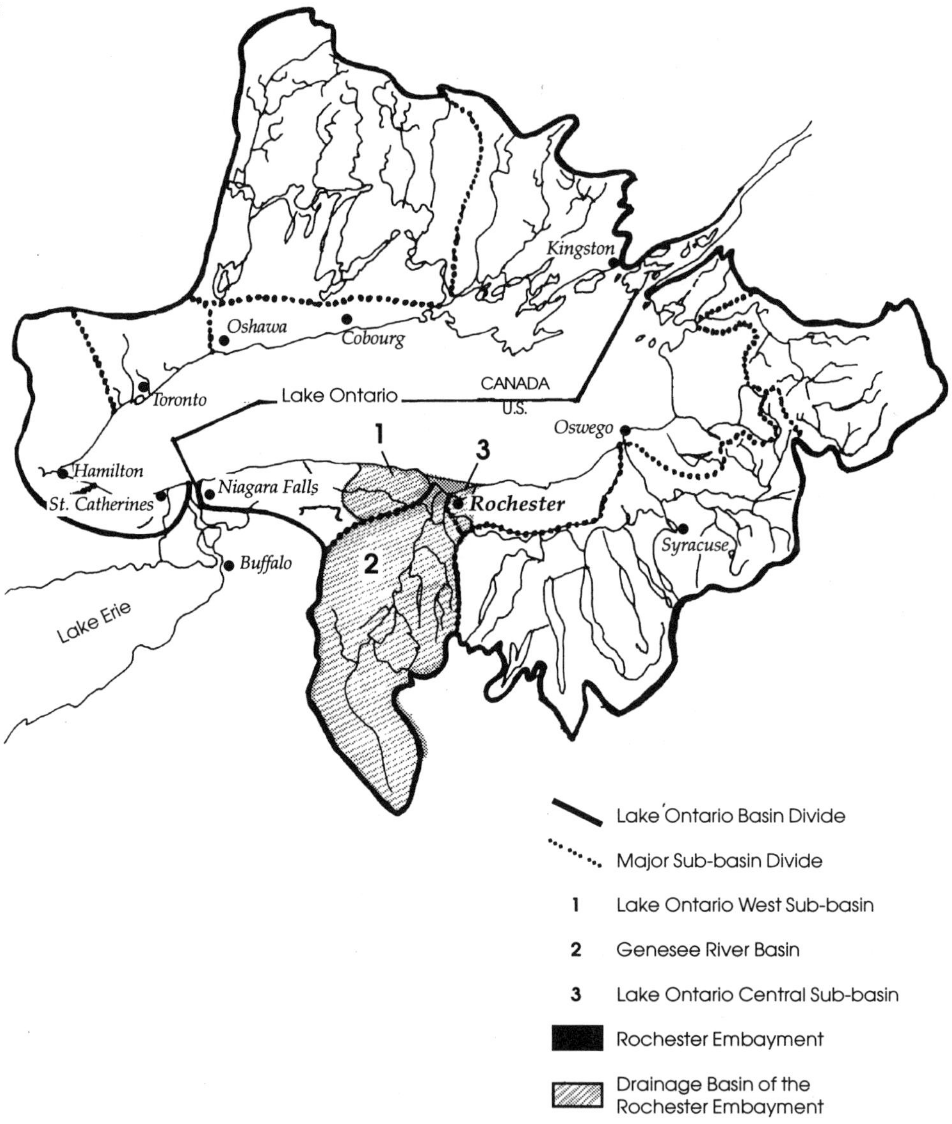

Source: New York State Department of Environmental Conservation and Monroe County Department of Planning and Development, Rochester Embayment Remedial Action Plan Stage I Document, *1993*

local public agencies, state and federal agencies, industries, private commercial groups, and grassroots citizen groups. The groups develop the Stage I document using qualitative and quantitative information from regulatory programs and published research to characterize water quality and use impairments, the pollutants causing the impairments, known and suspected sources of those pollutants, and the relative contributions from each source.

Members of the Black River Coordinating Committee (BRCC) and its study team first identified 10 categories of concern associated with impaired beneficial uses of the watershed. Next they attributed a level of concern to each category based on evaluation of available sediment, fish tissue, and surface water monitoring data for each portion of the river. The BRCC evaluated the major historical and present day sources of contamination by conducting an inventory of point and nonpoint sources discharging to the AOC. In addition to its own evaluation, the BRCC drew heavily on the results of the 1992 Ohio EPA Biological and Water Quality Study of the Black River.

The RAP technical committee for the Rochester Embayment used similar methodology to identify use impairments, "priority pollutants,"[n] and likely sources of those pollutants. Their study focused even more on problems specifically associated with toxic chemicals, because that type of pollution was more of a problem in this AOC than in the Black River AOC. The only sources that the committee could easily quantify were wastewater discharges from point sources, whose data are in the New York State Pollutant Discharge Elimination System. Since these sources do not account for a significant portion of the contamination entering the region, investigators had to use chemical-specific studies in the literature to characterize other contributions, especially those from nonpoint sources.

As noted before, the RAP documents of both AOCs are considerably broader in scope than the chemical contaminants that are the main focus of this chapter. The analysis of findings below does not include some of the major findings of the Stage I documents, such as those associated with conventional pollutants (pathogens, biological oxygen demand, chlorides, oil and grease, sediment volume) or nutrients (phosphorous and nitrogen compounds).

Study Findings: Black River Watershed

The study team qualitatively estimated the relative contributions of pollutants associated with impairments of beneficial watershed use as major, intermediate, possible, or minor amounts. The Black River Remedial Action Plan identified many pollutant contributions outside the scope of this report, since contamination by toxic chemicals is only a part of the area's environmental problems. Pathogens

[n] When used in this Great Lakes section of the chapter, "priority pollutant" refers to the terminology used by the RAP process to define pollutants of concern, but is not the same as the particular designation of "priority pollutants" in the Clean Water Act and associated regulations.

and sediment volume are of high concern throughout the watershed, for example, and phosphorous and chlorides are of moderate concern in Lake Erie. The pollutants of greatest concern within the scope of this report are organic toxics and heavy metals. The BRCC considers organic toxics to be of moderate concern in the main channel of the Black River and nearshore areas, especially polycyclic-aromatic hydrocarbons (PAHs) and polychlorinated biphenyls (PCBs). Heavy metals are a high concern in the sediments in the lower river basin, including cadmium, chromium, lead, mercury, zinc, and copper.[47]

The results for toxic contaminants suggest that present and historical releases generated by industrial process waste, commercial product use, and natural occurrences all contribute significantly to the environmental toxics problems in the watershed. (See Table 2-6.)

Industrial process sources identified in the RAP document to be of particular concern include industrial stockpiles related to the steel industry in the area, which contribute to metal loadings through stormwater runoff. Fly ash, foundry sand, slag piles, and iron ore pellets contribute major loadings of heavy metals to the watershed.[48]

Contributions from direct industrial wastewater discharges have declined significantly in recent years, largely as a result of the National Pollutant Discharge Elimination System (NPDES) as well as plant closings and process changes. Nevertheless, the BRCC attributes major loadings of organic toxics and heavy metals (as well as of certain nutrients and conventional pollutants) to industrial dischargers in the region, based on NPDES permit data and sediment and water quality monitoring data characterizing areas around industrial outfalls. Industrial dischargers within the Black River Watershed include automotive manufacturers, metal finishers, and steel manufacturing and processing companies. Note that the wastewaters of the first two industries especially are likely to contain both process waste and chemicals that originate in the use of products not manufactured or processed by those industries.

Municipal wastewater treatment plants (POTWs) are another potential source of contaminants, both from household waste and from industrial wastewater that is discharged indirectly through the municipal sewer system. The quality of releases from POTWs has improved considerably in the last decade, however, as wastewater treatment plant capacity has been enlarged, POTWs have been upgraded, and industrial wastewater pretreatment programs have been implemented. Despite these improvements, pollutants can still escape treatment by leaks in sewer conduits and by sewer overflows from systems with combined sewers, when a system's capacity is overwhelmed by heavy rainstorms. The Stage I RAP document attributes major levels of contamination from metals to wastewater system failures like these and to discharges made before POTW upgrades and improvements.[48]

Differentiating the relative contributions from households, industrial process waste, industrial product use, and other specific sources of this metals contamination would require extensive study of

Table 2-6. Sources of Toxic Pollutants in the Black River Area of Concern and Their Estimated Relative Contributions

	Toxic Pollutants		
Source Categories	**Pesticides (herbicides, insecticides, fungicides)**	**Organic Toxics (PCBs, PAHs, others)**	**Metals (cadmium, chromium iron, lead, mercury, others)**
Background Contribution	major	no	intermediate
Atmospheric Deposition	minor	major	major
Hazardous Waste Sites	intermediate	major	intermediate
Industrial Stockpiles	no	minor	major
Home Sewage Systems	possible	possible	minor
Chemical Spills	possible	possible	possible
Crop Land*	major	no	no
Rural Non-crop Land*	minor	no	no
Metropolitan/Suburban*	minor	intermediate	major
Streets/Highway runoff	minor	minor	major
Urban-construction	minor	minor	no
Industrial Wastewater Discharges	no	major	major
Municipal Wastewater	no	no	intermediate

No, major, intermediate, minor, and possible categories refer to the estimated relative contribution from each source as reported in the Black River Remedial Action Plan, April, 1994. Designations reflect the qualitative evaluation conducted by the RAP study team.
* Refers to releases related to land use designation

the loadings to each POTW in the AOC. Such a detailed study was not conducted as part of the RAP process, but a survey of industrial dischargers to the two main municipal wastewater treatment plants in the region provides some information on the relative contributions from industrial sources. Information on the quantities of specific chemicals released by each user is not available.[50]

The RAP document also identifies hazardous waste sites as an important source of nonpoint source pollution within the Black River AOC, causing intermediate loadings of pesticides and metals and major loadings of organic toxics. The Stage I document lists 18 sites on the Comprehensive Environmental Response, Compensation, and Liability Information System (CERCLIS), which lists all potential sites for federal cleanup assistance, most of which are under investigation by the Ohio EPA. Of the 18 sites on the State I list, those that can be characterized from their names are six industrial and municipal waste landfills, one chemical recovery facility, two manufacturing plants, and one plating company. While a detailed analysis of their specific contributions to the watershed has not been conducted by the RAP study team, the team's review of the general information available suggests that these sites contribute major quantities of organic toxics and intermediate amounts of pesticides and metals to the watershed.[51]

Atmospheric deposition contributes pollution throughout the Great Lakes Basin, carrying contaminants as far as 500 miles from their points of origin, which include both stationary sources such as industrial smokestacks and mobile sources, especially automobiles. The relative contribution of these sources is not given in the RAP documents, nor is it possible to distinguish between industrial process and product sources. Based on a recent study of the contribution of atmospheric deposition to Lake Erie as a whole, the RAP document indicates that such deposition contributes major quantities of PAHs (especially benzo(a)pyrene) and cadmium to the basin.[52]

Other significant nonpoint sources of toxic contamination in the Black River Watershed from commercial products are stormwater runoff from streets and highways and a variety of urban and suburban activities relating to use and disposal of chemical-containing products. The Stage I document estimates that these sources contribute minor amounts of pesticides; but metropolitan/suburban activities contribute intermediate amounts of organic toxics and major quantities of metals. Runoff from streets and highways also contributes major loadings of metals. The major sources of pesticide loadings to the watershed are agricultural practices from the approximately 1,860 farms that cover 60 percent of the land in the watershed area.

The main contaminant categories attributed to natural sources by the study team are certain heavy metals and other inorganic pollutants. In the Black River watershed, background levels of iron and arsenic in the soil are particularly high. They enter the water through leaching and sedimentation and violate water quality standards in some areas. The study team also included the trace levels of DDT found in the AOC as natural background pollution, even though DDT is a commercial pesticide, because of its worldwide distribution from past use.[53]

Study Findings: Rochester Embayment

The use impairments described in the Rochester Stage I document whose known or potential causes are specifically associated with toxic chemical pollutants include restricted fish and wildlife consumption from high PCB, mirex, chlordane, and dioxin levels in animal tissues; degraded wildlife populations from PCB contamination; and degraded river and lake bottoms also related to PCBs.[54] The RAP technical committee included in its list of priority pollutants those chemicals that it knew or suspected cause use impairments within the Embayment itself, others that violate water quality criteria in Lake Ontario, and others that the IJC had identified as critical pollutants within the entire Great Lakes System. The Stage I document focuses mainly on those chemicals known to be or suspected of causing damage in the Embayment itself.

The data in the Stage I document indicate that the usual broad range of sources all contribute to the overall pollutant load in the Embayment, but the data are not sufficient to determine the relative contributions of those sources. (See Table 2-7.) Although estimated loadings for some of these sources are

Table 2-7. Known or Suspected Sources of Priority Pollutants in the Rochester Embayment Area of Concern

Source Category	Organics	PCBs	Dioxin	Pesticides	Metals	Nutrients	Designation*
Point Sources		X(1)	X	X	X	X	▲●✻
Atmospheric Deposition	X	X	X		X	X	▲●
Local Air Emissions	X						●▲
Hazardous Waste Sites/ Landfills	X	X			X		▲●
Nonpoint Sources	X (PAHs)				X		●▲✻
Spills	X						●▲
Electrical Equipment in Use		X					●
Agricultural Runoff				X			●

Key: ▲ - Industrial/Manufacturing Process Waste
● - Commercial/Consumer Product Use
✻ - Natural Sources
* Designation based on INFORM's interpretation of source descriptions listed in the RAP
(1) sources are outside the Embayment area

More than one symbol together indicates multiple designations contribute or distinctions are unclear.
Source: Adapted from Table 4 of the Rochester Embayment Remedial Action Plan Stage I Document, August 1993.

available, the data are incomplete. It is apparent that currently permitted industrial wastewater discharge contributions are relatively minor and that these and other known point source discharges to the Genesee River and from the river to Lake Ontario do not account for a significant portion of the contamination entering the region. For example, permitted discharges account for less than 1 percent of the total amount of lead that enters Lake Ontario from the Genesee River. The difference is considered mostly to be loadings from nonpoint sources that are difficult to characterize fully.

Determining the industrial sources of chemical contamination in the Embayment area required combining limited specific information with more general information and assumptions to fill in the gaps. The study was able to determine, for example, that mirex, a persistent toxic pesticide, probably originated from process wastes at the Hooker Chemical Company (a subsidiary of Occidental Petroleum) in Niagara Falls, where it was produced from 1959 to 1967. The study team also identified former coal gas production facilities in the Genesee Gorge and nearby landfills containing fly ash and other waste from industrial combustion processes as possible local sources of polycyclic aromatic hydrocarbons (PAHs), which are detected widely throughout the Embayment.[55]

In the case of dioxin, specific source sites could not be identified. The RAP study team speculated that levels found in fish in the Embayment area may have been generated by chemical companies in the Niagara River basin, as a byproduct of trichlorophenol manufacturing. Combustion processes and fly-ash disposal sites adjacent to the Genesee River may have been contributing sources of dioxin in addition to PAHs.[56]

Tracing the industrial process sources of heavy metals contamination (including mercury, alkylated lead, cadmium, and silver) required reviewing data from all environmental media, since such loadings may come from discharges to water, air deposition of stack or fugitive emissions, or land disposal of process wastes. According to data from the State Pollutant Discharge Elimination System, there are few significant permitted wastewater discharges from individual facilities. The Eastman Kodak facility at Rochester is the only facility named in the Stage I document as a large, permitted industrial discharger of heavy metals. Most other heavy metal contamination appears to come from air deposition and nonpoint sources. The Kodak facility reported to EPA's Toxics Release Inventory on chromium, lead, silver, and zinc compounds. For the year 1992, it reported 21,865 pounds of air emissions, 52,887 pounds of surface water discharges, 33 pounds of on-site land releases, and 238,017 pounds of off-site transfers mainly to recycling facilities. This represents a 1991-1992 decrease in air emissions of 46 percent and an increase in surface water discharges of 12 percent, with transfers to recycling being about the same as in 1991.

The RAP study team examined the sources of waste at three hazardous waste sites, selected because of their proximity to the Embayment or its major tributaries: the Genesee River Gorge in the City of Rochester, the Rochester Fire Academy site, and the inactive 28-acre Old Rochester City Landfill. Although the first is primarily an industrial waste site and the other two municipal, all three appear to contain both industrial process waste and commercial product waste.

The Genesee River Gorge extends from the Upper Falls to the Lower Falls, which form the southern boundary of the Embayment. The ravines of the gorge were used to dispose of process wastes from early mill operations and a variety of industries that manufactured coal gas, furniture, lanterns, ink, and fabricated metal products. Other operations contributed wastes associated with the use of commercial products, such as dying operations, lithography, and industrial laundries with toxic-contaminated waste. Historically, chemical seeps released PAHs, benzene, toluene, and xylene from the gorge area, although measures have been taken more recently to prevent further discharge from this site to the river.

The Rochester Fire Academy site, located on the west bank of the Genesee River, is a 21-acre site used as a training area by the Rochester Police and Fire Departments. Between 1955 and 1980, the burning of hazardous waste from local generators in training procedures reportedly caused the groundwater contamination at the site. That contamination consists primarily of chlorinated solvents and volatile aromatic compounds, but low levels of semi-volatile organics, iron, and manganese, and trace levels of PCBs, were also detected. Some of the chemical contaminants such as

PCBs are commonly associated with product use, but the generators probably handled industrial process waste as well, although the RAP documentation provides no details.

Groundwater from this site flows to the Genesee River, contributing an estimated 77 kilograms per year of volatile organics and a total of 278 kilograms per year of iron and manganese, based on computer modeling. These contributions did not, however, cause measurable differences between contaminant concentrations in river water samples taken from points upstream and downstream of this location.

The third site, the Old Rochester City Landfill, operated from 1956 to 1962 as a municipal solid waste disposal facility, suggesting that contamination is largely derived from commercial products. However, buried drums containing PCB- and lead-contaminated wastes found at the site indicate that industrial process waste may also have been buried there. The landfill is located on the east side of the Genesee River, approximately one-half mile south of the Lake Ontario shoreline. Contaminants of concern in soil include nine volatile and semi-volatile organic compounds and three pesticides. Groundwater samples contain low levels of PCBs and concentrations above drinking water standards for several heavy metals and volatile organic chemicals. The site investigation did not include an assessment of the impact of this contamination on the river.

Many of the priority pollutants in the Rochester Embayment appear to have been released at least partly from the wide use of commercial products. Chemicals associated with product use and disposal in the Embayment area include PAHs, PCBs, pesticides, lead, and cadmium, mercury, and other metals.

The study team could not quantify all the contributors to PAH contamination, because these chemicals, discussed above as a component of industrial process waste, are widely used and generated from many different sources. All of the common sources of PAHs (combustion and releases of petroleum and its derivatives, coal tar, bitumen-based paints and coatings, diesel engine exhaust, used crankcase oil, incinerator residues, fly ash, asphalt runoff to the storm sewers, and airborne releases from vehicle exhaust and stationary sources) were assumed to be involved in the Embayment area.

The most likely source of much of the PCB contamination in the Embayment is the now-discontinued widespread use of PCBs in electrical equipment, appliances, medical equipment, transformers, capacitors, electric motors, and other products. The RAP document cites an IJC study that estimates that, of all the PCBs manufactured and used in the United States, 54 percent are still in use and 21 percent are buried in landfills.[57] (The remaining 25 percent presumably consists of PCBs that are somewhere in the environment, or have been recovered and safely treated or disposed of, or have been incinerated or otherwise destroyed.) The IJC Advisory Board determined that releases from these and other sources enter the Great Lakes ecosystem by a number of pathways, including atmospheric deposition throughout the watershed and direct discharges to the lakes themselves and upstream lakes and tributaries. Tributary input and direct discharge to upstream lakes is deemed responsible for 82 percent of the total PCB load; but most tributary input in turn is thought to come from atmospheric deposition, since PCBs cycle constantly between air and water. The IJC estimates that up to 53 percent of the PCBs that reach Lake Ontario volatilize back to the atmosphere, compared to 30 percent which accumulates in sediment and 17 percent which flows out to the St. Lawrence River.[58]

Health advisories limiting the consumption of fish are in effect for most areas of Lake Ontario due to hazardous levels of the pesticides chlordane and mirex in fish tissue samples. Although most of the mirex contamination is thought to have originated from Hooker Chemical process waste outside the Embayment area, as described above, chlordane and other pesticide contamination in the area is believed to stem from nonpoint sources of product waste, including runoff from the agricultural and household uses of pesticides.

Data on sources of metals contamination are spotty. Air appears to be the major pathway of lead contamination in the Embayment area, with loading estimates from atmospheric deposition of lead ranging from 42,000 to 179,000 pounds per year. Origins of the airborne lead include the use of lead paint on bridges, combustion of waste oil and trash, and some lingering uses of lead-based fuels. Hazardous waste sites and landfills in the Embayment area were also considered contributors of undefined quantities of heavy metals, in addition to other toxic chemicals, but again the composition of waste from such sites was not documented sufficiently to determine the relative roles of process and product waste.

Although some mercury is found in wastewater discharges, both from industrial process waste and product origins, more results from atmospheric deposition. Because there are few facilities in the local area that are permitted to discharge mercury to air, mercury loadings may come from point sources outside the watershed, most likely from elsewhere in New York or from Ohio. Coal-fired power plants and municipal waste incinerators are additional point sources of airborne metal emissions, although the Stage I document does not include monitoring data from such facilities in the Embayment. The RAP cites the literature to conclude that a large portion of the mercury in the area may come from biocides in latex paint, fossil fuel combustion, and fluorescent lamp disposal. Note that mercury emissions from coal combustion are a natural source (because the mercury is present in the naturally originating coal), but one that reaches the environment only as the result of human activity.

Unanswered Questions

Although the specific pollutants and degrees of contamination from toxic chemicals vary, the unanswered questions in the Black River and Rochester Embayment areas, and presumably in other AOCs of the Great Lakes Basin, are similar when trying to characterize sources of chemical pollution:

1. What is the actual degree of harm caused by toxic contamination and how is it related to specific chemicals and pathways of contamination?

More research is needed to assess the degree of impairment of certain beneficial uses within each watershed, such as the extent of contamination of waterfowl in the Black River main channel and the relationship of that chemical contamination to chemical sources.

2. What are the specific causes and contributions of nonpoint source pollution?

Some of the many questions about nonpoint sources include how much contamination is coming from automobile emissions, from incinerator and power plant emissions, and from specific products in solid waste. In the Rochester Embayment, the gap between known industrial point sources of pollution, many of which have been controlled, on the one hand, and total contamination in a geographic area on the other hand, is particularly clear. The RAP suggests that nonpoint sources may be largely responsible for the unaccounted contamination, when comparing the measured upstream inputs to the Genesee River from identified sources and total river discharges of contaminants to Lake Ontario as measured at the mouth of the river. Although the Stage I document identifies probable general categories of these nonpoint sources, a great deal more work would need to be done to specifically characterize individual sources or the relative share coming from product uses and industrial process wastes.

3. What improved mechanisms of cooperative study and pollution prevention activities are needed to address long-distance sources of chemical contamination, in which the original generator of the chemical is outside of the area where the contamination is causing a problem?

While the social, political, economic, and legal dimensions of such a question are outside the scope of this report, it is impossible to look at chemicals in the environment and their sources without bumping into this problem at some point. Mercury contamination in the Rochester Embayment, for example, apparently results largely from airborne sources outside that area and would need to be addressed on a regional basis. This is not just a problem for contaminated waterways; ozone depletion is an example of an environmental chemical problem that can only be addressed effectively on a worldwide basis.

---

1 Estimates for children ages one to five: Debra J. Brody, *et al.*, "Blood Lead Levels in the U.S. Population: Phase 1 of the Third National Health and Nutrition Examination Survey (NHANESIII, 1988 to 1991)," *Journal of the American Medical Association*, 272, no. 4 (July 27, 1994): 277-283; estimates for children under age seven: Paul Mushak and Annemarie F. Crocetti, "Determination of Numbers of Lead-Exposed American Children as a Function of Lead Source: Integrated Summary of a Report to the U.S. Congress on Childhood Lead Poisoning," *Environmental Research*, 50, no. 2 (1989): 210-229.

2 Committee on Measuring Lead in Critical Populations, National Research Council, *Measuring Lead Exposure in Infants, Children, and Other Sensitive Populations*, Washington, DC: National Academy Press, 1993.

3 *Toxicological Profile for Lead,* Report prepared by Clement International Corporation for Agency for Toxic Substances and Disease Registry, Public Health Service, U.S. Department of Health and Human Services, TP-92/12, April 1993.

4 Mushak and Crocetti, "Determination of Numbers of Lead-Exposed American Children," 210-229.

5 James L. Pirkle, *et al.*, "The Decline in Blood Lead Levels in the United States: The National Health and Nutrition Examination Surveys (NHANES)," *Journal of the American Medical Association*, 272, no. 4 (July 27, 1994): 284-291.

6 *Toxicological Profile for Lead,* Clement International Corporation, 196.

7 *Toxicological Profile for Lead,* Clement International Corporation, 186.

8 Mushak and Crocetti, "Determination of Numbers of Lead-Exposed American Children," 222.

9 *Toxicological Profile for Lead,* Clement International Corporation, 186.

10 P.L. 91-695, amended in 1973 (P.L. 93-151), and 1976.

11 42FR44193, September 7, 1977.

12 P.L. 102-550.

13 U.S. Environmental Protection Agency, "Regulation of Fuels and Fuel Additives," *Code of Federal Regulations*, 40CFR80, 1973.

14 50FR9386, March 7, 1985

15 Clean Air Act (1990 Amendments P.L. 101-549), Section 211n.

16 Safe Drinking Water Act Amendments of 1986 (P.L. 99-330).

17 Samuel Merrill, Michael M. Simpson, and Wilbur Johnson, *Lead Exposure: Health Effects, Regulatory Actions, and Congressional Options*, Congressional Research Service, Washington, DC, 1984.

18 J.S. Annest, J.L. Pirkle, *et al.*, "Chronological Trend in Blood Lead Levels between 1976 and 1980," *New England Journal of Medicine,* 308 (1983): 1373-1377, cited in Pirkle and Brody, 1994.

19 *Toxicological Profile for Lead,* Clement International Corporation, 186.

20 *Toxicological Profile for Lead,* Clement International Corporation, 199.

21 Mushak and Crocetti, "Determination of Numbers of Lead-Exposed American Children."

5 Pirkle, *et al.*, "The Decline in Blood Lead Levels in the United States," 284.

23 Brody, *et al.*, "Blood Lead Levels in the U.S. Population," 277, 282, 283.

24 Office of Air Quality Planning and Standards, U.S. Environmental Protection Agency, *Cancer Risk from Outdoor Exposure to Air Toxics,* Vol. I Final Report, EPA-450/1-90-004b. Research Triangle Park, NC, September 1990, 1-1.

25 Office of Air Quality Planning and Standards, *Cancer Risk from Outdoor Exposure,* Vol. I, Final Report, 1-1.

26 American Cancer Society, *Cancer Facts and Figures — 1993.*

27 Office of Air Quality Planning and Standards, *Cancer Risk from Outdoor Exposure,* Vol. I, Final Report, ES-7.

28 Office of Air Quality Planning and Standards, *Cancer Risk from Outdoor Exposure,* Vol. I, Final Report, 2-40.

29 Office of Air Quality Planning and Standards, *Cancer Risk from Outdoor Exposure,* Vol. I, Final Report, 2-17

30 Office of Air Quality Planning and Standards, *Cancer Risk from Outdoor Exposure,* Vol. I, Final Report, 3-24

31 Office of Air Quality Planning and Standards, *Cancer Risk from Outdoor Exposure,* Vol. I, Final Report, ES-10.

32 Office of Air Quality Planning and Standards, *Cancer Risk from Outdoor Exposure,* Vol. I, Final Report, 2-37.

33 Committee on Indoor Pollutants, National Academy of Sciences, *Indoor Pollutants*, Washington, DC: National Academy Press, 1981, ES-1.

34 Lance Wallace, "The TEAM Studies: Hot Showers Produce Elevated Levels of Chloroform," *EPA Journal*, 19, no. 4 (October-December 1993): 23.

35 Lance A. Wallace, *The Total Exposure Assessment Methodology (TEAM) Study: Summary and Analysis*, Vol. I, Report by Office of Research and Development, EPA/600/6-87/002a, Washington, DC: U.S. Environmental Protection Agency, June 1987, 59

36 Lance Wallace, "The TEAM Studies: Hot Showers Produce Elevated Levels of Chloroform."

37 United Nations Environment Programme, *Montreal Protocol on Substances That Deplete the Ozone Layer*, 1994 Report of the Technology and Economic Assessment Panel , March 1994, Executive Summary, 12.

38 United Nations Environment Programme, *Montreal Protocol on Substances That Deplete the Ozone Layer*, Chapter 8, 4.

39 *Preserving the Global Environment: The Challenge of Shared Leadership*, Jessica T. Mathews, ed., New York: W.W. Norton & Company, 1991, 117.

40 Technical Options Committee, United Nations Environment Programme, *Technical Progress on Protecting the Ozone Layer: Refrigeration, Air Conditioning and Heat Pumps*, RWR-570-LK-91423-al, December 1991, 79

41 Technical Options Committee, United Nations Environment Programme, *Technical Progress on Protecting the Ozone Layer: Refrigeration, Air Conditioning and Heat Pumps*, 177.

42 Pamela S. Zurer, "Looming Ban on Production of CFCs, Halons Spurs Switch to Substitutes," *Chemical and Engineering News*, 71, no. 46 (November 15, 1993): 12-18

43 59FR65206, December 16, 1994.

44 K. W. Brown and K. C. Donnelly, "An Estimation of the Risk Associated with the Organic Constituents of Hazardous and Municipal Waste Landfill Leachates," *Hazardous Waste and Hazardous Materials*, 2, no. 1 (1988).

45 Great Lakes Water Quality Board, *Great Lakes Water Quality Board Report to the International Joint Commission*, Windsor, Ontario, 1989.

46 *Black River Remedial Action Plan Stage One Report: Impairments of Beneficial Uses and Sources of Pollution in the Black River Area of Concern*, Report by Black River Remedial Action Plan Coordinating Committee to Ohio Environmental Protection Agency, April 1994; New York State Department of Environmental Conservation and Monroe County Department of Planning and Development, *Rochester Embayment Remedial Action Plan Stage I: Executive Summary*, Rochester, NY, August 1993.

47 Black River Remedial Action Plan Coordinating Committee Study Team, "Statement of Degree of Contaminant Concerns within the Black River Watershed," in *Black River Remedial Action Plan*, June 29, 1993.

48 *Black River Remedial Action Plan Stage One Report*, 5-38.

49 *Black River Remedial Action Plan Stage One Report*, 5-2.

50 *Black River Remedial Action Plan Stage One Report*, 5-17 - 5-24.

51 *Black River Remedial Action Plan Stage One Report*, 5-30.

52 *Black River Remedial Action Plan Stage One Report*, 5-35.

53 *Black River Remedial Action Plan Stage One Report*, 5-31.

54 *Rochester Embayment Remedial Action Plan Stage I: Executive Summary*, 17-21.

55 New York State Department of Environmental Conservation and Monroe County Department of Planning and Development, *Rochester Embayment Remedial Action Plan Stage I Document*, Rochester, NY, August 1993, 5-11, 5-14.

55 *Rochester Embayment Remedial Action Plan Stage I*, 5-11, 5-14.

57 Virtual Elimination Task Force, International Joint Commission, *Persistent Toxic Substances: Virtually Eliminating Inputs to the Great Lakes*, Windsor, Ontario, July 1991, cited in *Rochester Embayment Remedial Action Plan Stage I Document*, Rochester, NY, August 1993, 5-13.

58 *Rochester Embayment Remedial Action Plan Stage I Document, Chapter Five*, 5-12.

Chapter 3

Toxics in Commerce

Introduction

All ordinary matter is made of "chemicals." These consist of large numbers of one or more molecules, each in turn made up of combinations of one or more atoms of the 88 naturally occurring elements.[a] The abundance of the elements in the Earth's crust, oceans, and atmosphere is uneven: Just 10 elements account for 99.2 percent of all matter. Oxygen (a major component of air, water, and sand) is by far the most plentiful, followed by silicon (a major component of most sand and stone). (See Table 3-1.)

Each of the elements helps to impart physical properties (e.g., brittleness, color, electrical conductivity, physical state, solvent characteristics, and solubility) and chemical properties (e.g., reactivity, acidity, and flammability) to the molecules that they make up. Molecules that make up a homogeneous compound, therefore, have physical and chemical properties that are caused by, but quite different from, those of their constituent elements.

Some combinations of elements make molecules that are essential for life. As a component of hemoglobin, for example, iron enables the blood to carry oxygen throughout the body. Cobalt is a constituent of Vitamin B12, carbon is a component of most biological molecules in human and other living bodies, and phosphorus is contained in most of the molecules involved as energy carriers in cells. (See Table 3-2.) Other combinations of elements (whether found in nature or synthesized by humans) impart to their compounds physical and chemical properties that make these chemicals or mixtures valuable in commerce (e.g., the color, sheen, and durability required for an automobile paint, or the ability to kill certain pests). On the other hand, some combinations of elements have chemical and physical properties that are very toxic to humans and/or to other forms of life. For example, most compounds of lead are nerve poisons, and most containing cadmium have significant kidney toxicity. Some of these chemicals (e.g., methylmercury, dioxin, and DDT) pose problems when present in the environment even in trace amounts.

[a] To date, 111 elements have been identified; 88 occur naturally, and the rest are unstable elements made in high-energy nuclear reactions.

Table 3-1. The 20 Most Abundant Elements (Earth's Crust, Oceans, and the Atmosphere)

Rank	Element	Percent	Cumulative Percent
1	Oxygen	49.50	49.5
2	Silicon	25.70	75.2
3	Aluminum	7.50	82.7
4	Iron	4.70	87.4
5	Calcium	3.40	90.8
6	Sodium	2.60	93.4
7	Potassium	2.40	95.8
8	Magnesium	1.90	97.7
9	Hydrogen	0.87	98.6
10	Titanium	0.58	99.2
11	Chlorine	0.19	99.3
12	Phosphorus	0.12	99.5
13	Manganese	0.09	99.6
14	Carbon	0.08	99.6
15	Sulfur	0.06	99.7
16	Barium	0.04	99.7
17	Chromium	0.03	99.8
18	Nitrogen	0.03	99.8
19	Fluorine	0.03	99.8
20	Zirconium	0.02	99.8
	All 89 Others*	0.16	100.0

* Of the 89 unlisted elements, only 68 occur naturally.

Source: Raymond E. Davis, Kenneth D. Gailey, and Kenneth W. Whitten, *Principles of Chemistry*, Philadelphia, PA: Saunders College Publishing, 1984, 9.

This chapter seeks to provide an overview of chemicals, natural and synthetic; to describe the stages in commerce through which chemicals flow; and to summarize what is known and not known about commercial chemicals and their uses, as they relate to health and environmental concerns. The compounds of one group of elements — the halogens, including fluorine, chlorine, bromine, and iodine — are used throughout this chapter to present specific chemical examples.

The purpose of this chapter is to set a general framework for looking at chemicals in commerce, in terms that everyone can understand, whether from industry, environmental groups, government, academic institutions, or the general public. This overview has two aims: 1) to show the wide range of information that would be useful for analyzing the complex set of issues relating to chemicals in commerce — very little of which is actually available — and 2) to fill any gaps in the reader's understanding of the role of chemicals, as an aid in understanding the rest of this *Toxics Watch* report.

A common understanding is needed of the variety and complexity of the ways in which

Table 3-2. Elements that Make Up the Human Body

Chemical*	Symbol	Approximate Composition of Human Body by Mass	Importance or Function
Oxygen	O	65%	Required for cellular respiration; present in most organic compounds; component of water.
Carbon	C	18%	Forms backbone of organic molecules; can form four bonds with other atoms.
Hydrogen	H	10%	Present in most organic compounds; component of water.
Nitrogen	N	3%	Component of all proteins and nucleic acids
Calcium	Ca	1.5%	Structural component of bones and teeth; important in muscle contraction, conduction of nerve impulses, and blood clotting.
Phosphorus	P	1%	Component of nucleic acids; structural component of bone; important in energy transfer.
Potassium	K	0.4%	Principal positive ion (cation) within cells; important in nerve function; affects muscle contraction.
Sulfur	S	0.3%	A component of most proteins.
Sodium	Na	0.2%	Principal positive ion in interstitial (tissue) fluid; important in fluid balance; essential for conduction of nerve impulses.
Magnesium	Mg	0.1%	Needed in blood and body tissues; a part of many important enzymes.
Chlorine	Cl	0.1%	Principal negative ion (anion) of interstitial fluid; important in fluid balance.
Iron	Fe	Trace amount	Component of hemoglobin and myoglobin; component of certain enzymes.
Iodine	I	Trace amount	Component of thyroid hormones.

* Other elements, found in very small amounts in the body (the trace elements), include manganese (Mn), copper (Cu), zinc (Zn), cobalt (Co), fluorine (F), molybdenum (Mo), selenium (Se), and a few others.

Source: Claude A. Villee, Eldra Pearl Soloman, and P. William Davis, *Biology*, Philadelphia, PA: Saunders College Publishing, 1985, 27.

chemicals permeate our society, to consider at what stages chemicals might affect the environment and what options are available to industry and to policymakers to reduce adverse impacts. Later editions of *Toxics Watch* will build on this groundwork to identify, for example, obstacles and opportunities for pollution prevention at particular points in the universe of chemicals in commerce.

This first *Toxics Watch* largely frames the environmental issues of toxics in commerce qualitatively, because few data resources provide a quantitative description of the conditions and trends of toxic chemicals in commerce. It focuses on chemicals that are not used as pesticides, foods, drugs, or cosmetics. This report also focuses on organic chemicals that are subject to EPA review when they are introduced and to periodic production reporting provisions thereafter, under the Toxic Substances Control Act (TSCA).

Summary of Findings

- More than 13 million chemicals have been characterized and reported on in the scientific literature. An additional 685,000 chemicals are identified each year. Many chemicals present in nature remain unidentified.
- There are more than 72,000 chemicals in commerce in the United States, excluding foods, drugs, cosmetics, and pesticides. Each year, as reported to EPA, nearly 6 trillion pounds (5,905.0 billion pounds in 1989) of chemicals are manufactured in or imported to the United States.[b]
- Thousands of chemicals in commerce are of undefined or variable composition. Their environmental and health hazards are often undefined as well.
- Almost none of the 72,000 chemicals in commerce in the United States have been fully characterized for their ability to cause environmental and health effects.[c]
- Fuels dominate chemical production in the United States. Their composition is often undefined or variable, and many liquid fuels, such as benzene and polynuclear aromatic hydrocarbons, contain cancer-causing agents. Fuels represent the use of chemicals most often involved in chemical accidents.
- Each year, EPA receives proposals for manufacture or import of another 1,000 to 2,000 new chemicals. New chemicals enter commerce through manufacture or import at the rate of 200 to 1,000 per year.
- Of the 20,100 new chemicals proposed for manufacture or import between 1979 (when EPA

[b] Data from the 1989 update to the Toxic Substances Control Act (TSCA) Chemical Inventory. The reported figure does not include chemicals produced or imported in amounts less than 10,000 pounds per year, and it excludes polymers and inorganics unless they are specifically regulated under other sections of TSCA.

[c] The National Research Council in *Toxicity Testing: Strategies to Determine Needs and Priorities* (Washington, DC: National Academy Press, 1984), which studied a statistical sample of chemicals, found no chemicals adequately characterized and only 20 percent with *any* health or safety data.

began to monitor new chemicals under TSCA) and 1993, the Agency restricted 4 percent and submitters withdrew 5 percent. Although EPA took no action to restrict or ban the remaining 91 percent, only half of these (45 percent of the total) were ever introduced into commerce.

- New chemicals introduced into commerce since 1979 account for less than 0.03 percent (between 0.5 and 1.7 billion pounds[d]) of the amount of chemicals manufactured or imported in 1989, as reported to EPA. Chemicals brought into commerce before 1979 constitute more than 99.9 percent of production, and they are marketed with few restrictions on use. Moreover, they account for most of the growth in chemical production.
- Seven percent of the chemicals introduced into commerce since 1979 is governed by EPA restrictions to protect human health and the environment. Those 7 percent accounted for more than half (55 percent) of the production of new chemicals, as reported to EPA in 1989.
- No clear picture of U.S. chemical production or use can be had. The paucity of data on the manufacture and use of chemicals makes quantification impossible. With no database providing the public or the government with a national overview, it is also not possible to track product stewardship efforts by companies or facilities.
- Only a portion of the chemical production and use information that can be found in government databases are available to the public —how much is uncertain. Industry submits much of its data with claims of confidentiality, and those data are withheld from the public.
- The properties that make a chemical attractive for practical and commercial purposes are often the properties that give rise to environmental concerns. For example, the high reactivity which makes some chemicals useful for disinfection and in industrial processes also makes those chemicals harmful in the tissues of humans and wildlife.
- Preventing toxic substances from entering commerce presents the best prospect for addressing the environmental and health concerns they raise. Risks that may be posed by toxic chemicals are difficult to address once such chemicals enter the market. The more fully integrated a chemical is into the economy, the more complex are both the regulatory task of acting to remove it from use and the industrial task of identifying and applying less harmful substitutes. Chlorine, for example, is integral to the manufacture of hundreds, even thousands, of commercial products, and its market is intertwined with markets for table salt (raw material for chlorine gas manufacture) and sodium hydroxide (a byproduct). Both factors complicate prospects for reducing its use.

[d] Most quantitative data in this chapter are reported in ranges because much of the data has been submitted to EPA with Confidential Business Information claims. In some cases, the mid-point of the range is used to facilitate graphical presentations. The use of a mid-point, however, should not detract from the clear findings available from the data.

Chemicals in Commerce and Their Health and Environmental Effects

Chemicals in Nature and in Manufacture

More than 13 million chemicals have been characterized and reported on in scientific publications, but many of the chemical substances in nature have yet to be isolated and identified. About 680,000 additional chemical substances are reported on each year.[1] The vast majority of chemicals occur naturally. Some are present as gases in air, others as materials dissolved in oceans and lakes, and still others as minerals in the Earth's crust. By far the greatest number and range of chemical substances are associated with the myriad forms of life that inhabit this planet or inhabited it in the past. Most compounds of biological origin have yet to be identified.

The elements most used in chemicals in commerce are those with the greatest ability to bond with one another, such as hydrogen and carbon. (See Table 3-3 and Figure 3-1.) Of all the elements, carbon is undoubtedly the most versatile. Carbon atoms can bond with more types of atoms than any other element, and they can bond with other carbon atoms in several ways. Carbon atoms form the backbone of most chemicals found in living organisms. They provide the energy value of most fuels in use today, and carbon is the key element in most of the chemicals manufactured and used in commerce. Any chemical containing carbon is considered an "organic chemical." The organic chemical industry — by far the largest segment of the Chemical and Allied Products manufacturing industry — could therefore be called the "carbon chemical industry."

Equipped with knowledge about the chemical and physical properties of the elements alone and in combination, chemists seek to design and synthesize or mix chemicals to obtain particular combinations of chemical and physical properties of commercial value at a price that is economically competitive.

Health and Environmental Effects of Chemicals

Industrial chemists and engineers have long focused primarily on the nature and behavior of chemicals in deciding when and how to make new chemical substances and introduce them into commerce. Increasingly, however, health and environmental effects, safety risks, and other unintended side effects have emerged as critical factors — not only for industry, but for the public, government regulators, and future generations. The challenge is to determine which chemicals under what circumstances pose significant risks — from their inherent toxicity and the conditions of their use that expose people or the environment to toxic quantities — and to take steps to avoid or mitigate such risks.

Table 3-3. Production Amount of Chemicals Containing the 20 Most Naturally-Abundant Elements, 1989

Element	**Production Amount of Chemicals Containing Element** Pounds	**Percent of Total Production Amount*** Percent
Oxygen	4,683,843,273,409	79.32056
Silicon	2,406,161,148	0.04075
Aluminum	7,330,210,810	0.12414
Iron	4,574,145,022	0.07746
Calcium	19,656,149,998	0.33288
Sodium	12,757,430,344	0.21605
Potassium	645,561,900	0.01093
Magnesium	3,934,921,666	0.06664
Hydrogen	5,789,184,639,236	98.03943
Titanium	12,289,392	0.00021
Chlorine	77,437,854	0.00131
Phosphorus	6,845,126,342	0.11592
Manganese	29,661,222	0.00050
Carbon	5,742,079,723,841	97.24172
Sulfur	396,551,252,410	6.71557
Barium	89,788,772	0.00152
Chromium	176,814,446	0.00299
Nitrogen	67,302,370,637	1.13976
Fluorine	2,891,123,004	0.04896
Zirconium	5,397,146	0.00009

* Many compounds contain more than one element.
Source: 1989 TSCA Inventory Update.

Some of the very properties that make a chemical attractive for commercial purposes give rise to its environmental concern. For example, reactive chemicals often make good intermediates,[e] but their ability to react readily with other substances may also allow them to react harmfully with molecules in the tissues of humans and wildlife. In another example, the stability of many chlorinated organic chemicals makes them less flammable in commercial applications, but more persistent in the environment.

Concerns about chemicals shift and expand as knowledge grows. Just as stratospheric ozone depletion was not even a suggested concern with chemicals in commerce in the 1960s, only recently have possible health and environmental concerns arisen over the suspected estrogenic effects of chemicals, many of them man-made. (See Chapter 5, Box 5-D.)

To determine whether a chemical has the potential to cause adverse effects, toxicity testing is performed.

[e] An intermediate is a substance formed as a necessary stage in the change from reactants to products during a chemical reaction.

Figure 3-1.

TSCA Inventory Compounds Containing the 20 Most Naturally Abundant Elements, 1993

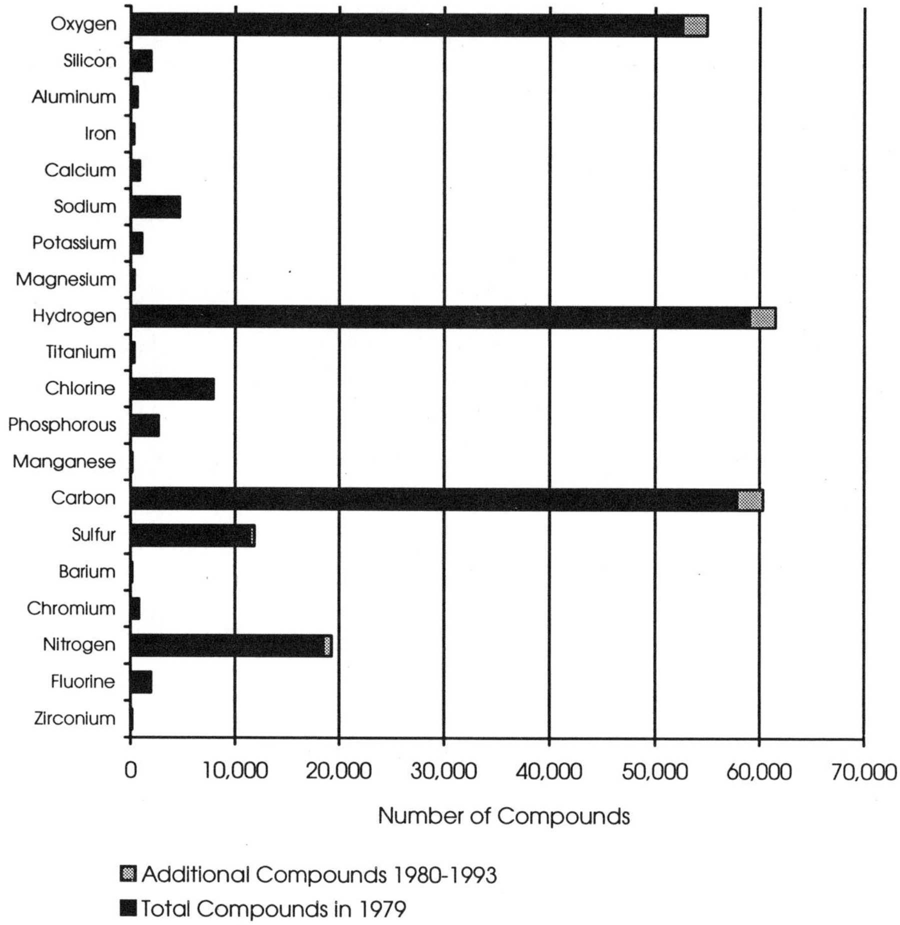

Test subjects are usually laboratory animals (e.g., rats, mice, and rabbits), because most human and ecosystem experimentation is considered unethical; increasingly microbes or other substitutes for higher animals are now tested, because of similar ethical concerns, cost, and time. Only a small percentage of chemicals in commerce, however, have undergone much testing for health effects, and even fewer have had adequate laboratory evaluations for ecological hazards. Such tests can be very expensive, often costing more than a million dollars for a single chemical and requiring several years to complete. In the absence of such tests, both EPA and industry more often are attempting to compare untested chemicals to structurally similar compounds that have more test data available, in the belief that the existing test results may be used to predict the toxicity of untested substances. Time will tell whether this approach will give satisfactory results.

Lack of information on chemical toxicity may be somewhat less troubling for chemicals that are used in ways that do not expose humans or for chemicals that cannot enter the body. These circumstances pose little risk to human health. For example, the many chemicals present in layers below the surface of photographic film result in virtually no human contact and thus pose little risk to humans during consumer use. In fact, film manufacturers are much more concerned about human contact with these chemicals because of damage to the film than because of health effects. Similarly, very large polymers (e.g., nylon, cellulose, and polyethylene) tend to pose little direct health risk because they cannot be easily absorbed into the bodies of humans or wildlife. If eaten, they tend to pass quickly through the digestive system untouched.

Risks from chemical hazards may result from direct exposures, as in the workplace or through the ingestion of food additives, or from indirect exposures via the environment. Indirect exposures result when chemicals are released to the environment, persist long enough to be transported through the air, in surface water, on sediment, or through soil to groundwater, and then reach humans who, for example, consume fish and other foods in which the chemicals have accumulated or in other ways come into contact with the chemicals in the environment. Chemicals in the environment are converted over time into other substances (although elements do not degrade); sometimes the degradation products of these conversions are more persistent, more able to accumulate in biological tissues, and more toxic than the original chemicals.

Other Environmental Effects

In addition to human health and ecological hazards, high on the list of environmental concerns about chemicals in commerce are the two interrelated issues of energy consumption (and generation) and resource implications. Chemicals contain energy to varying degrees. Those containing large amounts of such energy may be used as fuels. To create chemicals containing large amounts of energy requires either using raw materials that themselves contain large amounts of energy or

Box 3-A. Ozone Depleters

Twenty years ago, one of the more surprising adverse effects of certain chemicals was discovered. This was the ability of chlorofluorocarbons (CFCs), and a few other chemicals to affect the amount of ozone in the stratosphere.

Drs. Rowland and Molina at the University of California at Irvine first put together the pieces of a theory of ozone destruction by chlorofluorocarbons. These CFCs were considered a threat to the ozone layer because they would:

- last long enough to reach the stratosphere after circulating several years in the lower atmosphere;
- decompose there in sunlight, releasing chlorine atoms;
- precipitate a chain reaction, because chlorine atoms can react catalytically with ozone, each one converting thousands or more ozone molecules into oxygen;
- be used and ultimately released into the environment in large enough quantities to result in a several percent reduction in stratospheric ozone;
- thereby lead to an even greater percent increase in harmful ultraviolet light from the sun (that is normally screened by stratospheric ozone) reaching the Earth's surface; and
- thereby cause an increase in exposure to ultraviolet light that would be expected to cause increases in skin cancers and important, but difficult to predict, ecological effects.[1]

using large amounts of energy (usually in the form of heat) to bring about their synthesis.

Generally, the lower the concentration of the desired chemical in the starting materials, the higher the energy required to separate and refine elements and chemical substances. This applies to raw materials that are extracted from the earth, air, or water and to materials that are refined, manufactured, and processed. It also applies equally to starting materials that are waste and to products destined for recycling. In general, the lower the concentration of the desired element or chemical substance in a starting material, the greater the other environmental impacts as well. For example, the lower the iron content of an ore, the larger the volume that must be excavated to obtain the same amount of iron — and the greater the waste byproducts that can be expected from refining.

Because the amount of each element on Earth is fixed, no element is used up. What matters is the energy needed to obtain the element in the form and purity desired. Using up the energy content of raw materials in creating products that consist of complex mixtures of many different substances, each in lower and lower concentrations, raises the ante for the energy required to recapture their chemical constituents in high concentration.

Such a chain of consequences, which seems all the more likely to be occurring as further atmospheric monitoring and research are conducted, could not have been foreseen by the chemists, chemical engineers, and product marketers who introduced the chlorofluorocarbon into commerce as a safe and effective fluid for refrigeration and air conditioning and as a non-flammable gas to make bubbles in foams and to propel aerosols.

Interestingly, both chlorine and fluorine atoms play a role in the ability of chlorofluorocarbons to carry out such a scenario. The fluorine-carbon bonds are so strong that they are not degraded by light, water, or air. The chlorine-carbon bonds are strong enough to withstand the degrading forces in the lower atmosphere, but eventually can be broken by the higher-energy ultraviolet sunlight in the stratosphere. Thus, carbon-based compounds that are attached only to chlorine and fluorine atoms are susceptible to such a scenario. (The same is true for carbon-based compounds that also have bromine atoms with fluorine and chlorine, but these have had much less commercial use. If one or more of the bonds to carbon is with an element other than chlorine or bromine, the compound will tend to be destroyed in the lower atmosphere. When the chemical is totally fluorinated, it is expected not to degrade at all, even in the stratosphere.)

Needless to say, industrial chemists now know what to include and not to include in a chemical to avoid stratospheric ozone threats.

[1] F.S. Rowland and M.J. Molina, "Stratospheric Sink for Chlorofluoromethanes: Chlorine Atom-catalyzed Destruction of Ozone," *Nature* (London), 249 (1974): 810.

Other environmental effects associated with chemicals span widely different types of problems — e.g., the ability of certain chemicals to mar the paint on cars or homes, or to spoil the taste of fish, or to present unpleasant odors in the air surrounding industrial facilities, or to contribute to global warming. This open-ended category can be defined only as miscellaneous effects broader or different than health or ecological effects. What portion of all such possible effects has even been contemplated, let alone studied is utterly unclear. From time to time, scientists, industrialists, and policymakers are caught entirely by surprise, as in the case of ozone depleters. (See Box 3-A.)

Safety

Concern about the health effects of toxic chemicals in the environment usually focuses on the consequences of long-term, relatively low-level exposures. However, accidents and other forms of direct short-term exposures can produce severe health damage. Hazards are greatest in industrial operations that:

- use gases under high pressure that may cause containment vessels to explode;
- use chemicals under conditions where they may either burn or explode;

- employ highly acidic, caustic, or corrosive chemicals;
- contain large amounts of heavy gases that could displace air near the ground and suffocate individuals; or
- contain chemicals with high acute toxicity (effects that result from short-term exposures) that may disable or kill those briefly exposed to them.

EPA has identified 701 chemicals that it considers acutely toxic and for which accident reports must be made and emergency plans developed.[f] Because far more chemicals have been tested for acute toxicity than for any other effect, this list is relatively more complete than for other adverse effects.

Chemical safety is no small issue. From 1988 to 1992, the federal Emergency Response Notification System (ERNS) received reports of 34,575 toxic chemical accidents, of which 2,186 involved fatalities.[2] The ERNS database provides the best available overview on toxic chemical accidents, but understates the total number of accidents because not all accidents are in fact reported to this federal system and overstates the total when more than one report is made on the same accident.

Sources of Information on Toxic Chemicals in Commerce

Analyses in this chapter focus on data in three categories:

- the numbers of chemicals in commerce and the amounts of their production;
- uses of chemicals that may lead to human or environmental exposure and the production amounts associated with those uses; and
- the new chemicals being proposed for manufacture in or import into the United States, their types, their anticipated uses, and their expected production amounts.

The type of information sought in this report is on trends in the production of environmentally relevant chemicals and in uses of existing and new chemicals. *Toxics Watch* sought to examine the situation from a national perspective, as well as from a company and facility point of view.

The quantitative analyses that are possible from accessible data fall short of this scope. The amount of information is extremely limited, and there are few sources of it. For narrow questions involving a single

[f] 40 CFR 302.4 Appendix A. Appendix A gives the CAS numbers of Hazardous Substances identified in the Comprehensive Emergency Response, Compensation, and Liability Act of 1980 (CERCLA). Table 302.4 actually lists more than 1,000 Hazardous Substances and their reportable quantities; this includes common industrial solvents and other mixtures that have no CAS number.

chemical, manufacturer, or use, an *ad hoc* study can sometimes collect the needed information. There are also companies that prepare and sell proprietary research reports on chemicals, at considerable cost and with restrictions on their circulation and use.[g] Periodicals such as *Chemical and Engineering News, Chemical Week,* and similar trade publications often include feature articles on segments of the chemicals business that provide valuable insights into conditions and trends of the sector from an overall business perspective. These have been used for many of the examples provided in this chapter.

Government programs have the greatest repositories of information on the production of chemicals in commerce in the United States. Some of the main information sources include:

- The Bureau of Mines in the U.S. Department of Interior collects data on the amount of minerals extracted from the earth each year. Numerous Bureau publications summarize the information.
- The Energy Information Agency in the U.S. Department of Energy collects and publishes information on petroleum, coal, natural gas, and other energy-rich material production and consumption.
- The Census Bureau in the U.S. Department of Commerce collects chemical production data from manufacturers and provides summary results to the public.
- The Office of Pollution Prevention and Toxics of EPA collects information on the production of chemicals already in commerce and on anticipated production and uses of new chemicals being proposed for manufacture or import into the United States. The Toxic Substances Control Act (TSCA) of 1976 gave rise to three sources of such information — the TSCA Chemical Inventory, the 1985 and 1989 TSCA Inventory Updates, and the Premanufacture Notifications submitted under TSCA:
  - — an inventory of chemicals in commerce, created in 1979, from reports by manufacturers of all chemicals (except foods, drugs, cosmetics, pesticides, and materials gathered from nature and used unaltered, such as sand), to which have been added new chemicals manufactured and imported since then;
  - — 1985 and 1989 updates to the chemical inventory, consisting of the production amounts by facility of all organic non-polymers, from manufacturers and importers of more than 10,000 pounds of each such chemical per year; and
  - — notifications by companies of new chemicals that are not pesticides, foods, drugs, or cosmetics and that are not already on the existing chemical inventory. These notifications occur at least 90 days prior to manufacture or

[g] For example, the Stanford Research Institute prepares and sells *The Chemical Economics Handbook* for $37,500 per year (telephone confirmation, Joan Bergquam, November 1994); the *Handbook* covers the production and uses of many of the more important chemicals in commerce.

Box 3-B. What's in Commerce?

Prior to the enactment of the Toxic Substances Control Act of 1976 (TSCA), only wild guesses existed as to how many chemicals were in commerce, much less what they were. Because the law sought a review by EPA of all new chemicals entering commerce, the need arose to know what chemicals were already present in commerce that would not require such a review.

Therefore, EPA required every manufacturer or importer of chemicals covered by the Act[1] to report the identity of the chemical and the number of pounds of manufacture or import by facility. Excluding chemicals gathered and used in an unaltered form (such as clay, stone, sand, air, and water), EPA compiled the submissions into a consolidated list of existing chemicals known as the TSCA Chemical Inventory. To this inventory are added new chemicals, after they go through premanufacture review by EPA and enter commerce. Even when a chemical is no longer manufactured or imported, it remains on the TSCA Chemical Inventory.

In 1986, 1990, and every four years thereafter, EPA requires manufacturers and importers of chemicals on the Inventory to update the amount that they manufacture or import, if they do so in quantities of more than 10,000 pounds (TSCA Chemical Updates). Such updating is not required for the more than 3,800 inorganic chemicals on the Inventory, nor for polymers; EPA exempted these because it views them as of lesser concern. Any or all the data submitted to EPA in the updates, as well as the original Inventory, may be claimed confidential. (See Box 3-C.) Therefore, this *Toxics Watch* report often provides summary data in broad ranges or with omissions of data claimed as confidential.

[1] TSCA excludes foods, drugs, cosmetics, and pesticides — all of which are regulated under other laws.

import (except for substances excused under low-volume, test-market, or polymer exemptions), and they contain information on the chemical identity, anticipated production and use of the chemical, expected exposures, and any existing health or environmental data. (See Box 3-B.)

This report focuses on data derived from these confidential TSCA databases and represents only a beginning exploration of the information they contain.

Other federal agencies with data on chemicals in commerce include the Food and Drug Administration, the U.S. Department of Agriculture, and the Drug Enforcement Agency.

Each of these government sources collects a wealth of data, only some of which is publicly available. Even though these government agencies collect the information from individual companies and facilities, chemical production data from these sources are available to the public only in national summaries. Information on individual chemicals is often not released. Claims of confidentiality covering business submissions to the government keep other data from public view. (See Box 3-C.) These limitations permit at best only a cloudy picture of the status and trends of chemicals in commerce.

Box 3-C. Confidential Business Information Claims

A major issue in data availability and interpretation is Confidential Business Information (CBI) claims, which prevent public disclosure of data reported to the government. The legal policies and procedures vary from one government program to the next.[1] However, all allow companies to claim that any or all of their chemical production data are company secrets that should not be publicly disclosed. In some cases, the government (usually as required by law) has responded to the tension between the public interest in the data and company claims of secrecy by releasing for each chemical only aggregated production data in which the contribution of a single company or facility cannot be discerned, even by the submitter. In other cases, the government aggregates whole groups of chemicals and releases data only for the class.

Perhaps the most deleterious situation occurs when data cannot be disclosed at all in any form, and there is no way of knowing whether or not or to what degree data are being withheld. For example, the U.S. Environmental Protection Agency, a sponsor of this report, was asked to provide the production amounts for the 25 chemicals with the largest production amounts in its 1989 TSCA Inventory Update. The Agency, however, could release only a table of 25 chemical entries; with the production amounts given in broad ranges. This practice prevents anyone from "reverse engineering" the data to estimate quantities in any individual submission claimed as confidential. The identities of 20 to 30 percent of the submitters to the inventory update and 3 to 4 percent of the chemicals are confidential; therefore, the number of facilities submitting (20 percent of which are held confidential) and the production amounts (60 to 65 percent are claimed as confidential) are presented in broad ranges. However, if all submitters claim confidentiality for the identity of a chemical, then EPA will not disclose any information about the chemical. Thus, while 25 chemicals appear on the table with large production amounts, these are probably not the 25 with the largest production, as requested, depending upon the number of confidential chemicals with larger production amounts whose identities cannot be disclosed. (EPA indicates that of the 853 confidential chemicals on the 1989 inventory update, 31 are produced in excess of 10 million pounds.)[2]

Thus, while some government programs have some information about the production of toxics in commerce, the public has very little, largely as the result of policies toward protecting data claimed as confidential by submitters.

[1] An overview of the impacts of confidential business information claims under the Toxic Substances Control Act is provided in Sheila A. Ferguson, *et al.*, *Influence of CBI Requirements on TSCA Implementation*, Report prepared by Hampshire Research Associates, Inc., for the U.S. Environmental Protection Agency, Alexandria, VA, March 1992.

[2] Personal communication, Scott Sherlock, Information Management Division, Office of Pollution Prevention and Toxics.

Chemicals in Commerce — Amounts and Trends

The amount[h] of chemicals in commerce is growing. The amount of minerals, petroleum, coal, natural gas, and other raw materials consumed absolutely, as well as per capita, has grown continuously over the 20th century. The amount of solid household waste per person[i] has risen 50 percent over the past 30 years to 4.3 pounds per person per day.[3] Data from the Bureau of Mines on "materials" added to fuel consumption data from the U.S. Department of Energy roughly depicts the dramatic growth of chemicals in commerce over the last half century. (See Figure 3-2.)

Total production of the top 50 chemicals in commerce in 1993, as tracked by the American Chemical Society (ACS), was 684.8 billion pounds, up 3 percent from 1992. Average growth in this total from 1983 to 1993 was 3 percent per year. ACS, which supplements government, trade association, and industry estimates, reports annually in *Chemical and Engineering News* the amounts and trends for the top 50 chemicals. These chemicals do not include those introduced for use as fuels. Inorganic chemicals constituted 62 percent of the total (428.0 billion pounds), with sulfuric acid, nitrogen, oxygen, lime, and ammonia produced in the largest amounts. Organic chemicals constituted 38 percent (256.8 billion pounds), with the five highest-production chemicals being ethylene, methyl tert-butyl ether, propylene, sodium carbonate, and ethylene dichloride.[4] (See Figure 3-3.)

The TSCA Chemical Inventory listed 61,948 chemicals in 1979, and it grew with the addition of 9,512 new chemicals to 71,460 as of October 1, 1994. Not all of these chemicals are currently in commerce, as chemicals are not removed when they are no longer produced. As a result, the total represents the number of chemicals that at some point have been produced in or imported to the United States since 1979. Halogenated compounds represent a substantial number of chemicals on the TSCA inventory. (See Figure 3-4 and Boxes 3-B and 3-D.)

The total production/import of the chemicals on the 1989 TSCA Inventory Update was 5,905.0 billion (nearly 6 trillion) pounds.[j] Each of these chemicals is produced or imported by the reporting facility in quantities of at least 10,000 pounds a year. This excludes pesticides, foods, drugs, cosmetics, other substances not covered by TSCA (e.g., tobacco and firearms), and minerals gathered and used in

h "Amount" in this chapter generally refers to quantity by weight, usually stated in pounds. The amount most often discussed here is production amount (other sources often refer to this as "production volume").

i A crude measure of per capita materials consumption, although it does not take into account industrial waste associated with product manufacture, the amount dissipated in use, the increasing amount of materials in use, and other factors.

j All TSCA Inventory Update data were compiled and supplied by the U.S. Environmental Protection Agency. Another update covering 1993 has been submitted by companies and will be fully compiled by EPA in 1995.

Figure 3-2.

U.S. Material and Fuels Consumption, 1950-1990

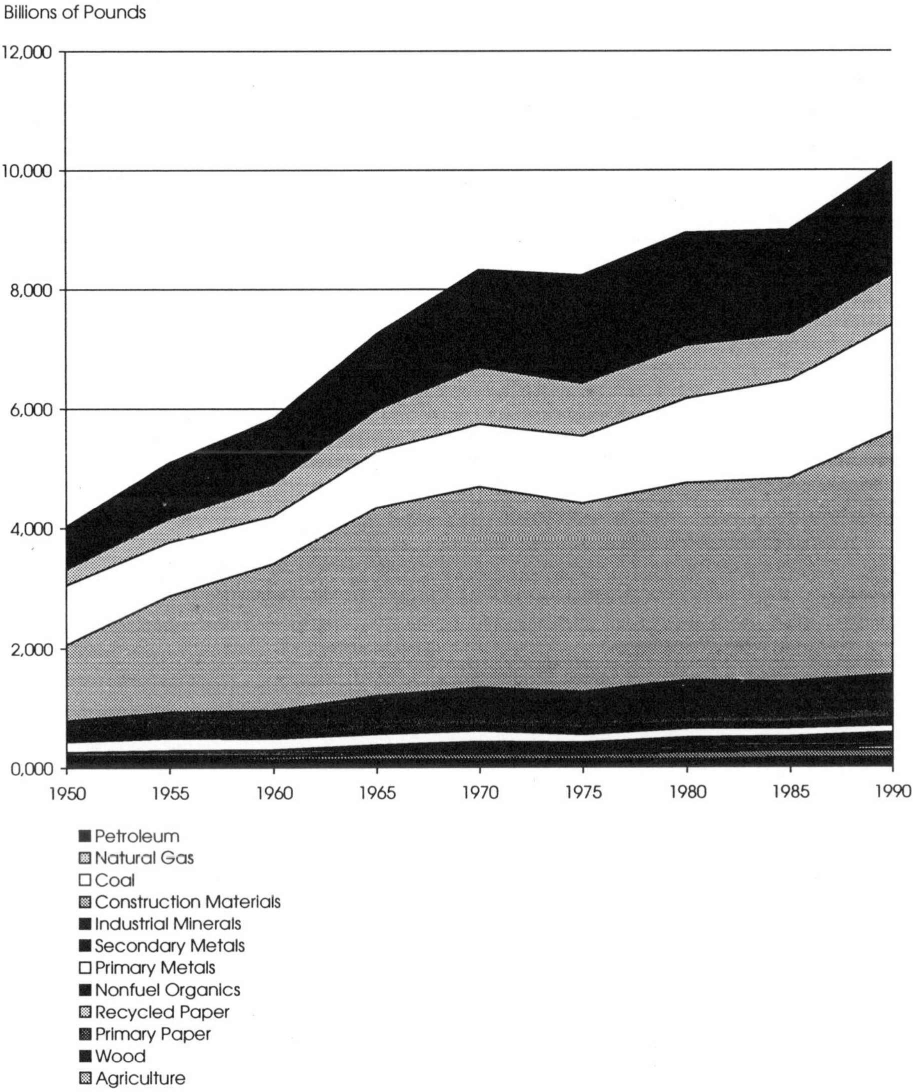

Data for primary and recycled paper from 1960; secondary metals from 1965

Data for non-fuel materials provided by U.S. Bureau of Mines; data for fuels from Energy Information Administration, U.S. Department of Energy, Annual Energy Review, 1993, *July 1994*

Figure 3-3.

Top 50 Non-fuel Chemicals for Production Amount, 1983-1993

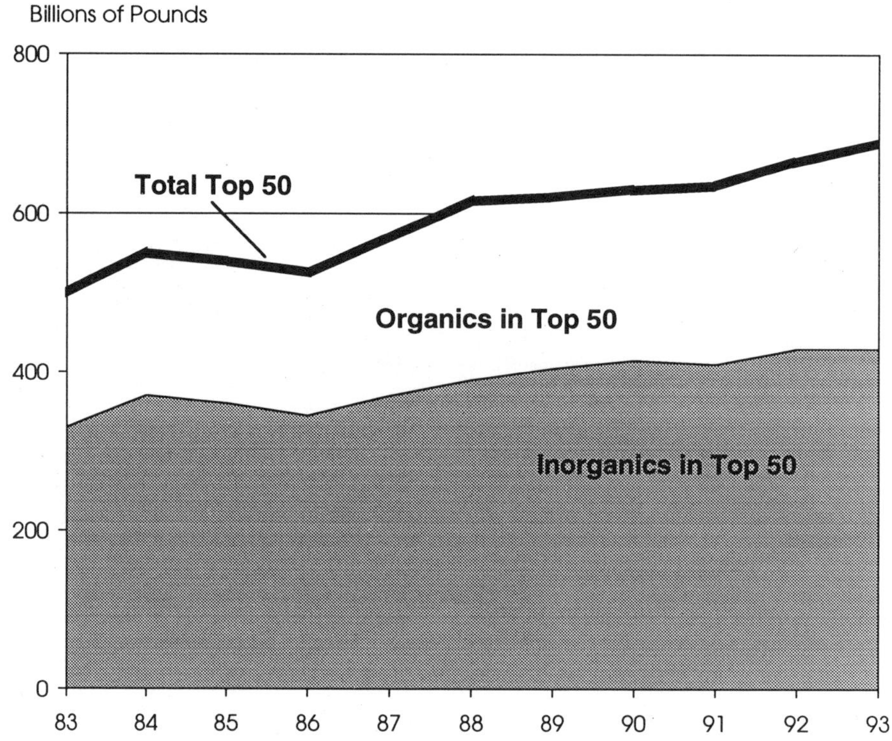

Reprinted with permission from Chemical and Engineering News, *72, no. 15 (April 11, 1994): 14. Copyright 1994 American Chemical Society.*

unaltered form. It also excludes polymers and 3,816 inorganic compounds on the inventory, unless they are subject to testing or control regulations under TSCA.

The pattern of chemical production in the United States is one of large quantities of a limited number of chemicals and quite small quantities of many others. Only 3,022 chemicals were reported as being produced/imported in the United States in amounts greater than 1 million pounds, and 313 chemicals in amounts greater than 1 billion pounds, in 1989. (See Table 3-5.)

The top 100 chemicals on the TSCA Inventory Update that are not confidential[k] had production amounts ranging from 11 billion to 642 billion pounds. The chemical with the largest reported production amount in 1989 was produced/imported at a level between 450 billion and 834 billion pounds. (See Table 3-6.) Appendix H provides similar data for the chlorinated chemicals on the 1989 TSCA Inventory Update with non-confidential identities and the largest production amounts.

[k] An unknown number of chemicals were not disclosed because their identity and/or production amount were claimed as confidential by the companies submitting them to the update. (See Box 3-B.)

Figure 3-4.

Total Number of Chemicals on the TSCA Inventory, by Year, 1979-1993

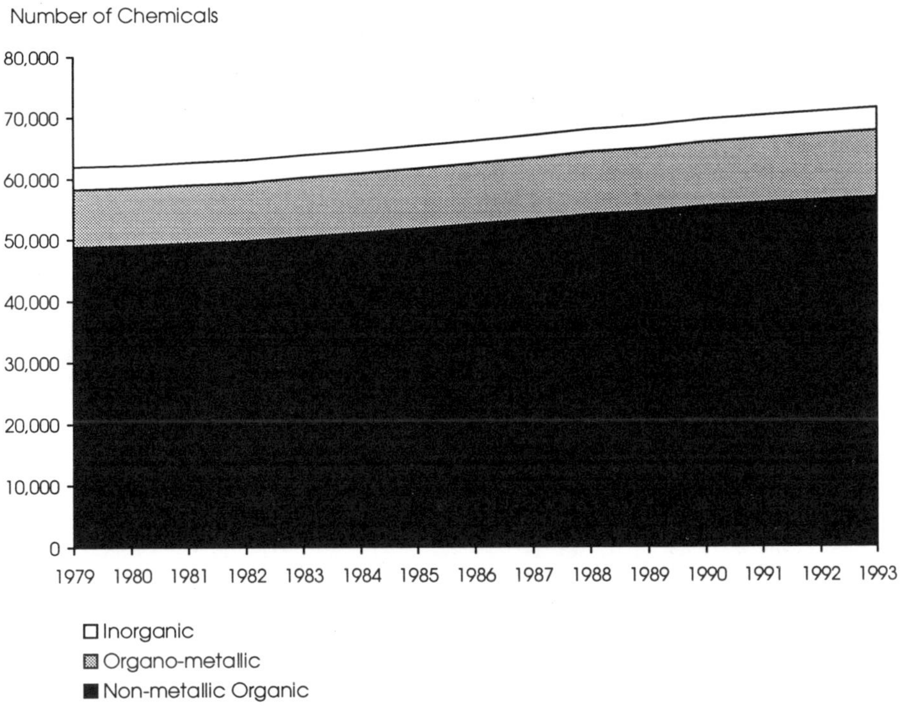

Box 3-D. Halogens in Commerce - I

The four naturally occurring halogens (the elements fluorine, chlorine, bromine, and iodine) represent less than one-quarter of 1 percent of the matter on Earth and an even smaller percentage of the human body. But the four elements are found in hundreds to thousands of chemicals each on the TSCA Chemical Inventory, and they are contained in more than 3,000 of the new chemicals submitted to EPA for premanufacture review. Of these four elements, organic chemicals containing chlorine have by far the largest production amount in 1989 (77.4 billion pounds) followed by fluoro-, bromo-, and iodocarbons (2.9 billion pounds, 738 million pounds, and 67 million pounds respectively). Thus, halogenated compounds are of major commercial significance. (See Table 3-4; see also Box 3-E.)

Table 3-4. Halogens in Nature vs. Commerce

	Abundance in Nature* Percent	Content of the Human Body** Percent
Fluorine	0.03	trace
Chlorine	0.19	0.1
Bromine	<0.023	—
Iodine	<0.023	trace

	Chemicals with the Element on the TSCA Inventory Update		New Chemicals with the Element Proposed for Manufacture	New Chemicals with the Element Entering Commerce		Chemicals with the Element on the TSCA Inventory
	(CUS) 1989 Number	(CUS) 1989 Pounds	(PENTA) 1979-1993 Number	(CICIS) 1979-93 Number	(PENTA) 1979-93 Number	(CICIS) 1993 Number
Fluorine	198	2,891,123,004	805	85	442	1,840
Chlorine	958	77,437,854,980	2,610	316	1,306	7,655
Bromine	118	738,376,032	331	42	156	1,414
Iodine	45	67,452,494	57	4	36	625

CUS Chemical Update System — Inventory Update Rule (confidential and non-confidential data)
CICIS Chemicals in Commerce Information System (non-confidential data only)
PENTA PENTA, The Section 5 System (confidential and non-confidential data)

* Source: Raymond E. Davis, Kenneth D. Gailey, and Kenneth W. Whitten, *Principles of Chemistry*, Philadelphia, PA: Saunders College Publishing, 1984, 9.
** Source: Claude A. Villee, Eldra Pearl Soloman, and P. William Davis, *Biology*, Philadelphia, PA: Saunders College Publishing, 1985, 27.

Toxics in Commerce — Amounts and Trends

There is no definitive list of the chemicals in U.S. commerce that are considered "toxic," since most have not been tested extensively for their potential to cause health and environmental effects. But looking at the production of chemicals listed for Toxics Release Inventory (TRI) reporting[1] offers some insights into the amounts and trends of toxic chemicals in relationship to their waste generation and environmental disposal by manufacturing facilities. The ratio of TSCA inventory production amounts to TRI waste generation quantities can indicate uses, efficiency, and other characteristics of chemical production and handling.

The amount of production on the 1989 TSCA Inventory Update for some chemicals is more than 1,000 times larger than the amount of

[1] Manufacturers report to the Toxics Release Inventory their direct environmental releases and transfers off site for some 340 specified chemicals and chemical categories. Reported data include quantities recycled, used for energy recovery, treated, and released/disposed of; these can be summed as total production-related waste. See Chapter 4.

*Table 3-5. Production Amount Distribution for TSCA Inventory Update Chemicals, 1989**

Production Amount Pounds	Number of Chemicals
10,000 - 100,000	3,608
100,000 - 1,000,000	2,843
1,000,000 - 10,000,000	1,576
10,000,000 - 100,000,000	792
100,000,000 - 1,000,000,000	341
More than 1,000,000,000	313

* For chemicals produced in excess of 10,000 pounds.

production-related waste reported to TRI. Such a large difference may result for chemical reagents or in instances where the use of the chemical falls outside of the manufacturing industries that report to TRI. A ratio close to one is indicative of an industrial use chemical that sooner or later becomes waste, such as an industrial solvent or other process aid. The higher the ratio, the greater the efficiency of the facility in its use of the substance —and the greater the amount of the chemical in commerce per unit of industrial waste. (See Table 3-7.) Production amounts similarly do not correspond to TRI release and transfer quantities. (See Table 3-8.)

Trends in production, waste generation, and environmental release and disposal are noteworthy. While the amounts of TRI chemicals being released and disposed in the environment show a steady decline, waste generation reported to TRI is much larger and is projected to continue increasing. Chemical production on the TSCA Inventory Update of TRI chemicals is much larger still and, if the rate of increase indicated by the 1985 and 1989 updates continues, rising faster. In other words, TRI chemical use is increasing significantly over time in comparison to a smaller increase in waste managed by manufacturing facilities and a steady decline in environmental disposal and releases. (See Figure 3-5.)

New Chemicals in Commerce

Trends reported in this section do not include new chemicals being registered as pesticides, food additives, drugs, and cosmetics, because they are not reported to the TSCA Inventory. Instead this section focuses on new chemicals reported to EPA under TSCA.

New chemicals reported under TSCA far outnumber those introduced as pesticides, food additives, drugs, and cosmetics (these are reported under other legislation). On the other hand, chemicals in the latter categories are either designed to be toxic or intended for direct human or environmental exposure, whereas most industrial chemicals are neither designed to be toxic nor

*Table 3-6. Top 100 Non-confidential Chemicals by Production Amount, 1989**

CAS Number	Chemical	Production Lower Bound Pounds	Production Upper Bound Pounds	Production Mid-point Pounds
64741-57-7	Gas oils (petroleum), heavy vacuum	449,951,200,000	834,329,400,000	642,140,300,000
74-98-6	Propane	157,736,700,000	430,056,400,000	293,896,550,000
64741-45-3	Residues (petroleum), atm. tower	195,855,400,000	344,258,000,000	270,056,700,000
64741-56-6	Residues (petroleum), vacuum	133,504,600,000	328,864,800,000	231,184,700,000
64741-47-5	Natural Gas condensates (petroleum)	136,962,500,000	300,099,900,000	218,531,200,000
106-97-8	Butane	75,425,840,000	346,216,700,000	210,821,270,000
8008-20-6	Kerosene (petroleum)	46,866,850,000	209,684,000,000	128,275,425,000
64741-54-4	Naphtha (petroleum), heavy catalytic cracked	81,500,340,000	170,789,800,000	126,145,070,000
64741-44-2	Distillates (petroleum), straight-run middle	33,112,880,000	200,492,100,000	116,802,490,000
64741-59-9	Distillates (petroleum), light catalytic cracked	66,863,870,000	133,838,600,000	100,351,235,000
64741-55-5	Naphtha (petroleum), light catalytic cracked	41,231,000,000	132,308,800,000	86,769,900,000
64741-41-9	Naphtha (petroleum), heavy straight-run	29,712,170,000	141,879,700,000	85,795,935,000
64741-63-5	Naphtha (petroleum), light catalytic reformed	23,722,320,000	145,550,100,000	84,636,210,000
64741-43-1	Gas oils (petroleum), straight-run	27,077,160,000	114,519,000,000	70,798,080,000
64741-46-4	Naphtha (petroleum), light straight-run	16,799,360,000	120,120,300,000	68,459,830,000
115-07-1	Propene	45,527,030,000	78,732,230,000	62,129,630,000
64742-80-9	Distillates (petroleum), hydro-desulfurized middle	18,036,700,000	98,018,670,000	58,027,685,000
64742-48-9	Naphtha (petroleum), hydrotreated heavy	41,922,190,000	73,687,240,000	57,804,715,000
64742-59-2	Gas oils (petroleum), hydrotreated vacuum	41,316,280,000	72,573,480,000	56,944,880,000
64742-79-6	Gas oils (petroleum), hydrodesulfurized	32,307,620,000	75,772,190,000	54,039,905,000
64741-58-8	Gas oils (petroleum), light vacuum	34,607,110,000	71,208,940,000	52,908,025,000
64742-81-0	Kerosene (petroleum), hydrodesulfurized	33,747,070,000	70,434,150,000	52,090,610,000
68955-27-1	Distillates (petroleum), petroleum residues vacuum	33,366,660,000	67,679,150,000	50,522,905,000
8030-30-6	Naphtha	16,751,880,000	84,020,780,000	50,386,330,000
74-82-8	Methane	14,780,390,000	84,294,830,000	49,537,610,000
64741-42-0	Naphtha (petroleum), full-range straight-run	12,267,560,000	86,293,340,000	49,280,450,000
64741-68-0	Naphtha (petroleum), heavy catalytic reformed	19,749,600,000	77,727,820,000	48,738,710,000
70592-78-8	Distillates (petroleum), vacuum	28,319,850,000	63,680,020,000	45,999,935,000
64741-87-3	Naphtha (petroleum), sweetened	13,446,870,000	72,344,610,000	42,895,740,000
8002-05-9	Petroleum	14,646,900,000	68,512,710,000	41,579,805,000
68955-35-1	Naphtha (petroleum), catalytic reformed	19,155,590,000	63,267,530,000	41,211,560,000
64741-78-2	Naphtha (petroleum), heavy hydrocracked	23,787,710,000	53,489,070,000	38,638,390,000
74-85-1	Ethene	22,988,360,000	48,712,390,000	35,850,375,000
64741-64-6	Naphtha (petroleum), full-range alkylate	11,824,480,000	59,705,470,000	35,764,975,000
64742-86-5	Gas oils (petroleum), hydrodesulfurized heavy vacuum	11,948,010,000	57,363,000,000	34,655,505,000
64742-73-0	Naphtha (petroleum), hydrodesulfurized light	20,999,090,000	47,218,570,000	34,108,830,000
64741-48-6	Natural Gas (petroleum), raw liq. mix	11,429,760,000	56,646,540,000	34,038,150,000
64741-69-1	Naphtha (petroleum), light hydrocracked	23,004,370,000	44,269,330,000	33,636,850,000
64741-79-3	Coke (petroleum)	9,113,427,000	57,914,480,000	33,513,953,500
68410-63-9	Natural gas, dried	11,999,130,000	54,916,700,000	33,457,915,000
64741-60-2	Distillates (petroleum), intermediate catalytic cracked	23,754,020,000	41,191,960,000	32,472,990,000
64741-81-7	Distillates (petroleum), heavy thermal cracked	13,381,430,000	51,546,290,000	32,463,860,000
64741-82-8	Distillates (petroleum), light thermal cracked	10,152,900,000	54,470,420,000	32,311,660,000
64742-46-7	Distillates (petroleum), hydrotreated middle	10,588,330,000	49,528,250,000	30,058,290,000
68478-32-0	Tail gas (petroleum), saturate gas plant mixed stream, C4-rich	20,367,800,000	37,872,110,000	29,119,955,000
68410-00-4	Distillates (petroleum), crude oil	17,219,470,000	38,166,810,000	27,693,140,000
65996-77-2	Coke (coal)	10,996,560,000	42,462,390,000	26,729,475,000
57-13-6	Urea	7,886,487,000	44,568,060,000	26,227,273,500
68333-25-5	Distillates (petroleum), hydrodesulfurized light catalytic cracked	16,940,060,000	28,995,030,000	22,967,545,000

* 1989 TSCA Chemical Update System data.

Table 3-6. Top 100 Non-confidential Chemicals by Production Amount, 1989, (cont'd.)*

CAS Number	Chemical	Production Lower Bound Pounds	 Upper Bound Pounds	 Mid-point Pounds
65996-68-1	Flue gases, ferrous metal, blast furnace	4,805,863,000	41,016,950,000	22,911,406,500
64742-82-1	Naphtha (petroleum), hydrodesulfurized heavy	9,550,678,000	36,166,730,000	22,858,704,000
68477-85-0	Gases (petroleum), C4-rich	5,916,973,000	38,433,710,000	22,175,341,500
66071-92-9	Pulping liquors, spent	12,685,250,000	30,738,310,000	21,711,780,000
68476-46-0	Hydrocarbons, C3-11, catalytic cracker distillates	12,918,430,000	29,508,090,000	21,213,260,000
75-28-5	Propane, 2-methyl-	5,495,578,000	36,730,440,000	21,113,009,000
124-38-9	Carbon dioxide	6,793,145,000	34,760,870,000	20,777,007,500
68410-97-9	Distillates (petroleum), light distillate hydrotreating process, low-boiling	13,201,170,000	27,396,560,000	20,298,865,000
64741-62-4	Clarified oils (petroleum), catalytic cracked	6,565,178,000	33,594,350,000	20,079,764,000
8006-61-9	Gasoline, Natural	11,997,410,000	27,312,100,000	19,654,755,000
68603-08-7	Naphtha (petroleum), arom.-contg.	13,474,790,000	24,725,340,000	19,100,065,000
64742-47-8	Distillates (petroleum), hydrotreated light	12,416,080,000	25,200,720,000	18,808,400,000
64741-86-2	Distillates (petroleum), sweetened middle	8,187,218,000	28,513,770,000	18,350,494,000
8052-42-4	Asphalt	5,897,489,000	30,731,810,000	18,314,649,500
70592-77-7	Distillates (petroleum), light vacuum	4,519,232,000	31,433,840,000	17,976,536,000
68915-96-8	Distillates (petroleum), heavy straight-run	4,735,474,000	30,241,700,000	17,488,587,000
65996-81-8	Fuel gases, coke-oven	6,161,184,000	28,421,770,000	17,291,477,000
68783-08-4	Gas oils (petroleum), heavy atmospheric	9,574,875,000	24,803,860,000	17,189,367,500
68919-37-9	Naphtha (petroleum), full-range reformed	5,166,936,000	28,267,490,000	16,717,213,000
64742-23-0	Naphtha (petroleum), chemically neutralized light	11,066,530,000	21,584,910,000	16,325,720,000
64741-88-4	Distillates (petroleum), solvent-refined heavy paraffinic	11,541,450,000	20,304,080,000	15,922,765,000
68476-33-5	Fuel oil, residual	8,640,534,000	23,167,770,000	15,904,152,000
64742-10-5	Extracts (petroleum), residual oil solvent	11,344,270,000	20,201,880,000	15,773,075,000
64742-22-9	Naphtha (petroleum), chemically neutralized heavy	6,274,577,000	24,228,810,000	15,251,693,500
64742-87-6	Gas oils (petroleum), hydrodesulfurized light vacuum	4,979,017,000	24,622,210,000	14,800,613,500
68606-11-1	Gasoline, straight-run, topping-plant	4,558,625,000	23,246,190,000	13,902,407,500
68333-22-2	Residues (petroleum), atmospheric	7,666,115,000	20,100,330,000	13,883,222,500
74-84-0	Ethane	7,401,068,000	18,951,350,000	13,176,209,000
64741-66-8	Naphtha (petroleum), light alkylate	8,159,497,000	18,085,460,000	13,122,478,500
107-06-2	Ethane, 1,2-Dichloro-	3,360,254,000	22,756,410,000	13,058,332,000
64742-78-5	Residues (petroleum), hydrodesulfurized atmospheric tower	2,841,869,000	22,818,050,000	12,829,959,500
64741-51-1	Distillates (petroleum), heavy paraffinic	4,184,257,000	21,411,060,000	12,797,658,500
64741-49-7	Condensates (petroleum), vacuum tower	6,759,862,000	18,734,310,000	12,747,086,000
64741-77-1	Distillates (petroleum), light hydrocracked	4,705,548,000	20,584,180,000	12,644,864,000
64741-84-0	Naphtha (petroleum), solvent-refined light	8,424,473,000	16,497,640,000	12,461,056,500
64741-61-3	Distillates (petroleum), heavy catalytic cracked	7,448,379,000	17,401,130,000	12,424,754,500
68308-27-0	Fuel gases, refinery	2,825,210,000	21,762,510,000	12,293,860,000
68606-28-0	Hydrocarbons, C5 and C10-aliph. and C6-8-arom.	8,259,274,000	16,238,190,000	12,248,732,000
68476-50-6	Hydrocarbons, C5, C5-6-rich	5,714,266,000	18,356,290,000	12,035,278,000
64741-75-9	Residues (petroleum), hydrocracked	5,904,876,000	17,963,810,000	11,934,343,000
68915-97-9	Gas oils (petroleum), straight-run, high-boiling	5,753,899,000	17,504,510,000	11,629,204,500
68514-79-4	Petroleum products, hydrofiner-powerformer reformates	7,860,001,000	15,125,690,000	11,492,845,500
64742-65-0	Distillates (petroleum), solvent-dewaxed heavy paraffinic	6,883,488,000	15,890,000,000	11,386,744,000
68334-30-5	Fuels, diesel	4,547,184,000	17,788,340,000	11,167,762,000
68131-33-9	Pulping liquors, white	3,098,516,000	19,139,520,000	11,119,018,000
68476-30-2	Fuel oil, no. 2	6,340,301,000	15,865,900,000	11,103,100,500
64741-92-0	Naphtha (petroleum), solvent-refined heavy	7,759,889,000	14,388,900,000	11,074,394,500
	Total	2,559,019,066,000	7,163,010,000,000	4,861,014,533,000

*Table 3-7. Top 10 Chemicals with Largest and Smallest Production/Waste Ratios**

Largest Production/Waste Ratios			Smallest Production/Waste Ratios		
CAS Number	**Chemical**	**Ratio**	**CAS Number**	**Chemical**	**Ratio**
134-32-7	alpha-Naphthylamine	96,662	75-05-8	Acetonitrile	0.007
95-80-7	2,4-Diaminotoluene	25,499	86-30-6	N-Nitrosodiphenylamine	0.011
606-20-2	2,6-Dinitrotoluene	24,200	87-68-3	Hexachloro-1,3-butadiene	0.037
120-58-1	Isosafrole	16,875	91-22-5	Quinoline	0.071
60-34-4	Methyl hydrazine	4,170	540-59-0	1,2-Dichloroethylene	0.071
106-42-3	p-Xylene	1,929	120-80-9	Catechol	0.159
79-21-0	Peracetic acid	1,621	75-25-2	Bromoform	0.177
99-59-2	5-Nitro-o-anisidine	1,346	542-75-6	1,3-Dichloropropylene	0.178
541-41-3	Ethyl chloroformate	1,215	88-89-1	Picric acid	0.345
106-93-4	1,2-Dibromoethane	1,052	67-72-1	Hexachloroethane	0.380

* Production amounts from the 1989 TSCA Inventory Update for 183 organic TRI chemicals included in the Update. TRI production-related waste is that reported in 1991 for the previous year 1990 and does not include seven TRI chemicals in the TSCA Update for which no production-related waste was reported.

meant to directly expose individuals and the environment. Therefore, TSCA new chemicals, discussed below, are not environmentally comparable to the lesser number of chemicals in these inherently higher hazard or exposure uses.

TSCA Premanufacture Notification

TSCA treats existing and new chemicals differently. The main purpose of the TSCA Chemical Inventory in 1979 was to list existing chemicals. For these existing chemicals, EPA has the burden to show that an unreasonable risk exists before it can act to restrict their production, distribution, or use. Moreover, it is up to EPA to determine when it requires information on an existing chemical, to make the case for any additional testing, and to carry out the assessments of unreasonable risk.

For new chemicals, fewer burdens hinder EPA from action, but the Agency still does not control the agenda. Rather, any firm proposing to manufacture or import any chemical not on the TSCA existing chemical inventory must notify EPA at least 90 days in advance of doing so. The manufacturer or importer need not test the proposed new substance nor assess its expected health or environmental consequences. Rather, the premanufacture notification (PMN) must contain —only to the extent "reasonably ascertainable" — the identity of the substance, its expected use and exposure, its expected production amount, and any available health and safety information.

If EPA finds, within the review period, that the proposed chemical may pose an unreasonable risk and that further data are necessary to determine whether it does or not, the Agency can restrict the chemical (by banning it or by imposing use

Table 3-8. Production Amount and Production-related Waste for Top 50 TRI Chemicals for Off-site Transfers and Quantity Released, 1989 and 1990*

CAS Number	Rank	Chemical	1990 Released/ Disposed of * Pounds	1990 Total Production-related Waste * Pounds	1989 TSCA Inventory Update Production ** Pounds
67-56-1	1	Methanol	275,338,517	2,189,119,531	7,565,219,500
108-88-3	2	Toluene	221,541,451	1,258,653,606	7,923,053,500
67-64-1	3	Acetone	188,347,707	726,719,540	3,136,990,000
71-55-6	4	1,1,1-Trichloroethane	144,740,342	382,691,144	627,007,200
1330-20-7	5	Xylene (mixed isomers)	119,050,362	586,560,571	12,370,781,500
78-93-3	6	Methyl ethyl ketone	118,201,287	479,528,275	614,563,750
75-15-0	7	Carbon disulfide	99,661,638	128,784,363	382,587,500
75-09-2	8	Dichloromethane	91,101,891	313,778,510	560,879,000
	9	Glycol ethers	47,762,850	116,228,955	NA
76-13-1	10	Freon 113	38,728,807	290,590,007	NA
74-85-1	11	Ethylene	38,724,801	1,010,672,523	21,447,896,500
79-01-6	12	Trichloroethylene	38,193,885	280,465,751	179,223,350
71-36-3	13	n-Butyl alcohol	33,602,948	147,208,014	779,849,000
100-42-5	14	Styrene	31,144,339	214,399,341	8,354,619,000
108-10-1	15	Methyl isobutyl ketone	26,892,038	325,596,795	124,672,750
107-21-1	16	Ethylene glycol	23,541,528	537,957,202	5,082,495,000
67-66-3	17	Chloroform	23,189,204	65,015,287	801,292,900
71-43-2	18	Benzene	23,180,838	219,455,791	17,736,780,000
115-07-1	19	Propylene	22,880,906	1,660,554,587	58,449,715,000
79-10-7	20	Acrylic acid	22,129,270	68,417,706	914,184,750
75-05-8	21	Acetonitrile	21,155,784	2,987,508,195	20,480,256
50-00-0	22	Formaldehyde	20,736,221	314,879,119	2,575,356,600
110-82-7	23	Cyclohexane	20,167,577	83,683,922	2,373,047,800
463-58-1	24	Carbonyl sulfide	19,201,958	28,879,361	NA
127-18-4	25	Tetrachloroethylene	19,181,095	205,007,701	712,321,200
108-95-2	26	Phenol	13,797,910	106,657,379	4,678,170,000
75-71-8	27	Dichlorodifluoromethane (CFC-12)	11,658,046	12,705,512	317,065,650
100-41-4	28	Ethylbenzene	9,715,197	74,140,530	6,079,117,500
75-07-0	29	Acetaldehyde	9,300,784	19,087,611	706,310,450
75-69-4	30	Trichlorofluoromethane (CFC-11)	8,221,523	62,752,194	121,619,710
74-87-3	31	Chloromethane	8,074,938	20,052,951	932,416,700
107-13-1	32	Acrylonitrile	7,935,512	41,588,074	2,720,610,000
108-05-4	33	Vinyl acetate	6,748,336	34,029,440	3,203,138,000
107-06-2	34	1,2-Dichloroethane	6,286,993	155,250,948	18,334,790,000
8001-58-9	35	Creosote	5,589,361	17,147,886	271,217,850
95-63-6	36	1,2,4-Trimethylbenzene	5,312,729	18,098,955	47,253,325
106-99-0	37	1,3-Butadiene	5,203,457	319,899,886	5,314,046,500
79-06-1	38	Acrylamide	5,114,812	5,467,706	61,623,075
106-42-3	39	p-Xylene	4,762,008	5,312,343	10,248,188,000
91-20-3	40	Naphthalene	4,658,116	63,872,859	NA
98-82-8	41	Cumene	4,444,075	301,714,108	2,912,932,000
108-90-7	42	Chlorobenzene	4,349,878	13,208,286	358,769,700
75-00-3	43	Chloroethane	4,046,196	99,068,309	104,772,925
74-83-9	44	Bromomethane	3,127,590	3,700,633	39,009,660
62-53-3	45	Aniline	2,988,185	22,082,419	619,770,750
1634-04-4	46	Methyl tert-butyl ether	2,904,788	4,742,265	4,459,400,500
109-86-4	47	2-Methoxyethanol	2,795,646	13,214,365	NA
76-14-2	48	Dichlorotetrafluoroethane (CFC-114)	2,790,283	4,640,283	23,983,490
75-65-0	49	tert-Butyl alcohol	2,699,340	77,046,179	2,027,609,950
80-62-6	50	Methyl methacrylate	2,673,621	11,591,012	1,247,407,400
		Total	1,873,596,568	16,129,427,930	217,562,239,191

* Amount for 1990 as reported on the TRI 1991 Form R.

** Production amounts based on mid-point from 1989 TSCA Inventory Update data.

NA Amount not available from the TSCA database due to confidential business claims except for glycol ethers which is a combination of chemicals under TRI.

Figure 3-5.

Quantity Released, Production-related Waste, and Production Amount for Organic Chemicals in TRI, 1985-1989, 1990-1994

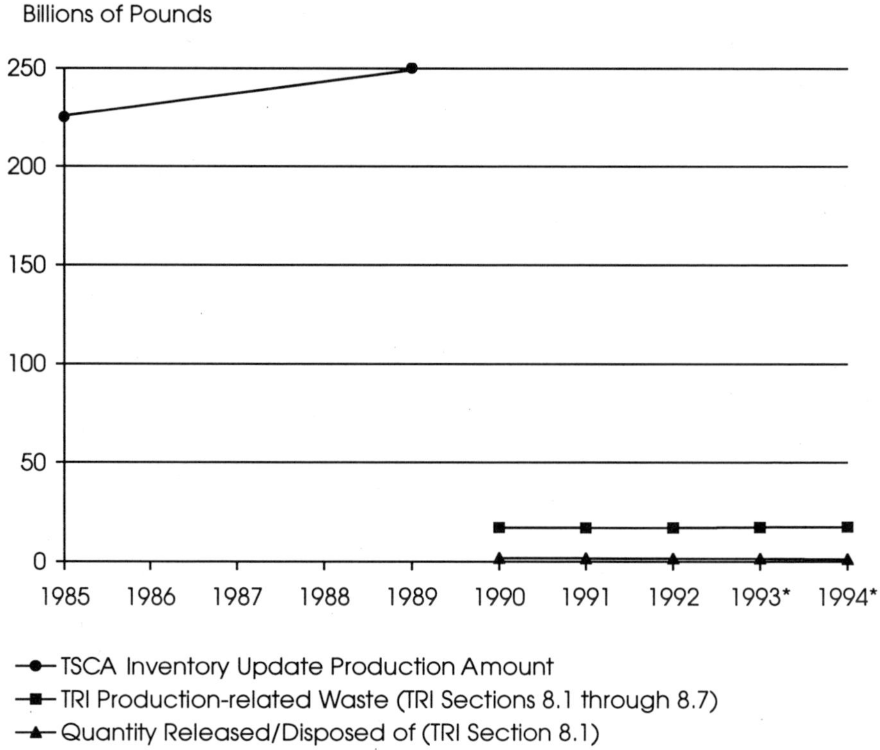

* *Projected*

Sources: Data for "Quantity Released/Disposed of" and "Production-related Waste" for 1990 as reported for previous year on 1991 TRI Form Rs; for 1991-1994 from 1992 TRI Form Rs. Production amounts from 1985 and 1989 TSCA Inventory Updates. Production amounts may contain production from facilities that do not report to TRI (for example, facilities that produce, but do not use, more than 10,000 pounds per year of the chemical being reported would be included in the TSCA Inventory Update but would not be required to report under TRI). While TRI reporting started in 1987, the first waste data were reported under Section 8 in 1991 and included 1990 (previous year) data.

restrictions), pending the development of additional data. Such actions are known as "5(e) actions," named for the relevant section of TSCA. If a manufacturer or importer proposes to introduce a new chemical that is found to pose an unreasonable risk, based upon the information available, Section 5(f) of TSCA requires EPA to restrict or ban the chemical to eliminate such unreasonable risk. These "5(f) actions" occur much less frequently.

Given that EPA must provide submitters with at least 45 days of notice prior to taking either a 5(e) or 5(f) action, the Agency has a very short period in which to act. If EPA does not act to restrict the proposed new chemical during PMN review,[m] the chemical can be manufactured or imported without restriction. Upon entering commerce, it is added to the existing chemical inventory, once EPA receives a notice of commencement of manufacture/import (NOC).

[m] Extendible to 180 days by EPA, with a showing of cause.

What has happened with TSCA PMNs since 1979 could not have been predicted when the law was enacted, because prior to TSCA there were no good estimates of the number and types of existing chemicals in commerce, nor of the new ones entering commerce. Many expected EPA to be able to act only rarely within the short 90-day PMN review period; subsequent history has instead proved this arena one of the most active under TSCA. This section provides an overview of this history and the information gained on the role in commerce of new chemicals introduced over the past 15 years.

Proposed New Chemicals

From 1979, the beginning of the TSCA new chemical review process, until 1985, all new chemicals proposed for manufacture or import required a PMN.[n] Only manufacturing for test marketing purposes was excluded (with notice to EPA). After 1985, large polymers and chemicals proposed for manufacture in very low amounts were exempted from review (also with notice to EPA). Since 1979, therefore, EPA has the primary record of new chemicals entering commerce in the United States.

Number of Premanufacture Notifications

In the first year of the program, 1979,[o] EPA received eight PMNs. For the next three years of the program, the number of PMNs each year totaled less than 1,000. The number of new chemicals in these years appears to be artificially low as manufacturers may have sped up initial production of contemplated new chemicals to get them on the existing chemical inventory or postponed manufacture to observe how EPA would handle new chemical review. (See Figure 3-6.)

Over the next five years, the total number of PMNs per year rose to nearly 2,500 in 1988 and has hovered around 1,500 per year since. In other words, EPA receives an average of seven or eight new chemical notices each work day of the year.

From 1979 through 1993, EPA received 23,071 PMNs. Since 1985, EPA has received 2,507 low-production exemption notices and 1,890 large-polymer exemption notices.

EPA Actions Prior to Manufacture

Despite (some might argue because of) the short 90-day review period for the approximately 1,500 PMNs received annually, EPA has imposed Section 5(e) restrictions pending additional data on over 4 percent (828) of the PMNs reviewed from 1979 to 1993. Four other PMNs were restricted as unreasonable risks under Section 5(f). Meanwhile, usually upon questioning by EPA, submitters withdrew or suspended the review of another 5 percent (1,020) of PMNs during the review period.

[n] For use as other than a food, drug, cosmetic, or pesticide.

[o] Fiscal Year 1979, ending September 30, 1979. All years cited here are federal fiscal years, ending September 30.

Figure 3-6.

Notifications of New Chemicals Received by EPA, 1979-1993

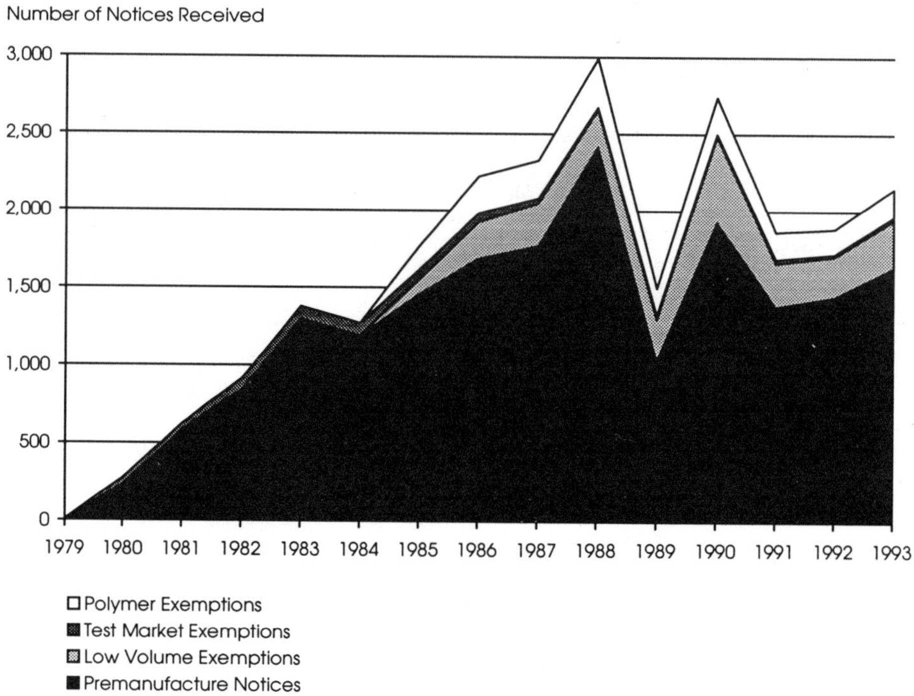

Therefore, nearly 10 percent of new chemicals (1,852 of 20,100) have been either voluntarily withheld from the market by the submitter or restricted by EPA as a result of PMN review. (See Figure 3-7.)

New Chemicals Entering Commerce

Number of New Chemicals Entering Commerce

Over the life of the program, only about half the chemicals submitted to EPA for new chemical review have entered commerce so far. More than 50 percent of the chemicals for which PMNs were received in each year from 1979 to 1985 have entered commerce. Since then, only in 1989 have as many as half the submissions entered commerce, although the number may rise for more recent years because of the lag time between premanufacture notification and actual commencement of manufacture. Most chemicals enter commerce within a few years after PMN review, dropping off rapidly each year. Few chemicals are introduced later than six years after PMN submission. (See Figures 3-8 and 3-9.)

These new chemicals entering commerce brought the TSCA Chemical Inventory total to 71,460 by 1993. Of the nearly 10,000 additions to the inventory, only 86 have been inorganic chemicals, in contrast to 9,426 that have been organic chemicals (1,300 were

Figure 3-7.

Regulatory Actions on Chemicals with Premanufacture Notifications (PMNs), 1979-1993

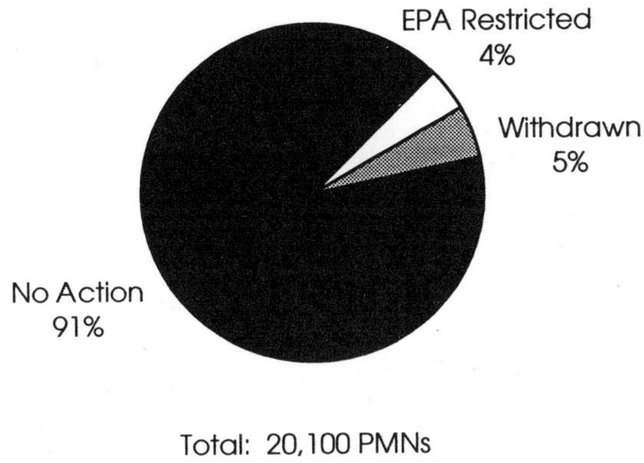

organo-metallic, containing both carbon and metal atoms). While over 5 percent of the initial 1979 inventory were inorganic chemicals, less than 1 percent of the additions have been inorganic. These TSCA data make clear that most new chemical innovation involves organic chemicals. (See Figure 3-4.)

Approximately 2 percent of the chemicals for which EPA has issued 5(e) orders during PMN review are now in commerce. Under certain 5(e) orders,[p] EPA may allow a chemical to enter commerce but restrict either the amount of production or the conditions of use pending the development of the data being sought. (See Figure 3-10.)

New Chemical Production

In the 1985 update to the TSCA Inventory, only those new chemicals with PMNs submitted in 1983 were produced in the aggregate in excess of 150 million pounds. In the 1989 inventory update, new chemicals with PMNs in both 1982 and 1986 were produced in excess of 150 million pounds. For these years, the aggregate production amount was higher than any in the previous update, more than 350 million pounds. No year exceeded 400 million pounds. Thus, only a small fraction of the PMN chemicals on the inventory account for the vast majority of all production of new chemicals. (See Figure 3-11.)

In 1989 more than half of the new chemical production (by amount produced) took place under 5(e) restrictions by EPA, pending the development of additional data. In that year, about 450 million pounds of chemicals that entered commerce after 1979 were used without restriction. (See Figure 3-12.)

In reviewing new chemicals, EPA seeks to employ its TSCA authority to prevent chemicals from entering commerce, when it finds that they are not as environmentally sound as the chemicals being replaced. Based upon this objective and the relative production figures of restricted and

[p] Such restrictions often include either or both use limitations and worker protections.

Figure 3-8.

Percentage and Number of Chemicals with Premanufacture Notifications (PMNs) That Have Entered Commerce, 1979-1993

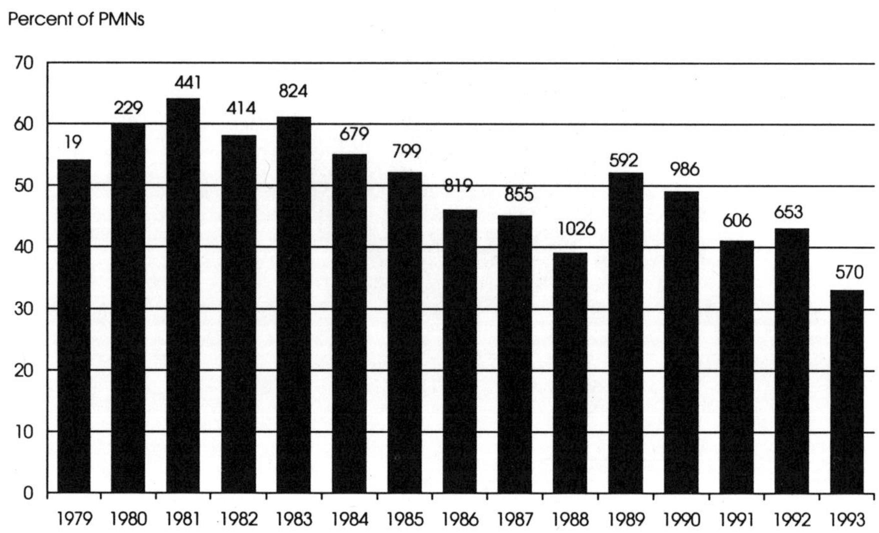

Chemicals with PMNs are considered to have entered commerce when a Notice of Commencement of Manufacture/Import (NOC) is received

Figure 3-9.

Length of Time for New Chemicals from Premanufacture Notification (PMN) to Notice of Manufacture/ Import (NOC), 1979-1993

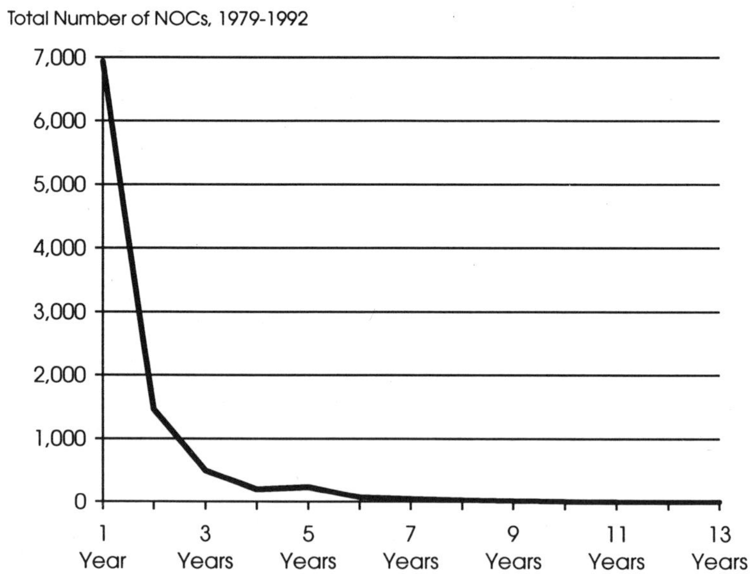

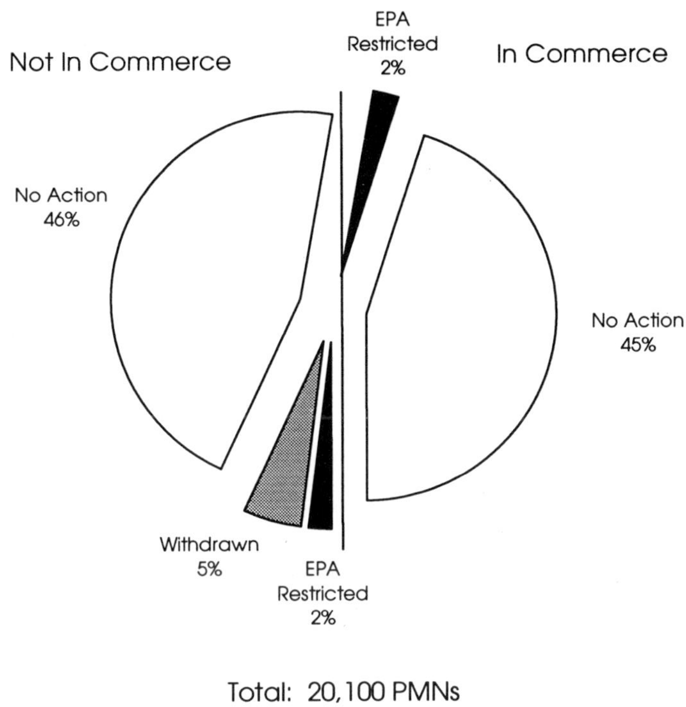

Figure 3-10. Regulatory Actions on Chemicals with Premanufacture Notifications (PMNs) for Those in Commerce and Those Not in Commerce, 1979-1993

non-restricted new chemicals, it is clear that the greatest environmental and health risks from chemicals in commerce come from those chemicals grandfathered as existing chemicals under TSCA in 1979. In fact, there are few examples of important environmental problems with chemicals that were not in use before 1979.

Total production of all new chemicals introduced since 1979 and reported to the 1989 TSCA Inventory Update was a little over 1 billion pounds. This compares to a total for all reported chemicals of 5,905.0 billion pounds (nearly 6 trillion pounds). Chemicals entering commerce since 1979, therefore, constitute less than 0.02 percent of chemical production. Moreover, all the new chemicals together would not rank in the top 100 chemicals on the basis of production. New chemicals, therefore, represent an insignificant fraction of chemicals in commerce, and practically none of the 3.2 percent growth in chemical production arises from the addition of new chemicals; rather it must result from expansion in the use of chemicals in commerce before 1979. These percentages would increase were the huge production amounts of fuels excluded from consideration.

Findings in this section are based upon the use of the mid-point in the range of production provided by EPA. However, use of either of the extremes of the range brings no change at all in the basic findings.

Figure 3-11.

1985 and 1989 TSCA Inventory Update Production Amounts for Chemicals with Premanufacture Notifications (PMNs), by Year of PMN Notification, 1978-1989

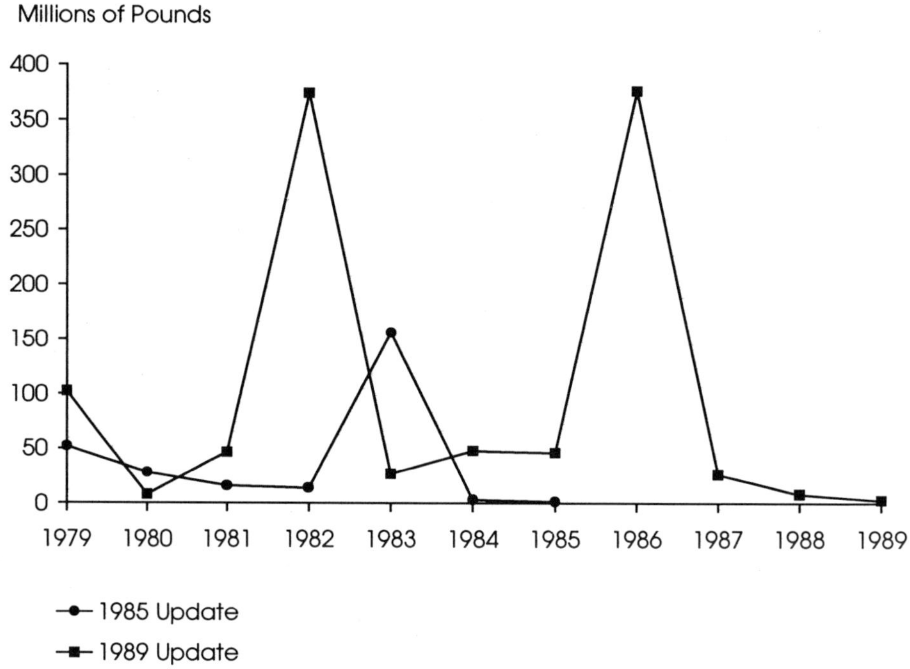

Based on mid-points of production ranges used to mask confidential data

New Chemical Functions

In contrast to the 62,000 chemicals on the original TSCA inventory, for which only fuel uses can be inferred, new chemical PMNs contain information on the proposed functions of the chemical.[q] When a chemical completes PMN review successfully, without EPA acting to restrict or ban it, it may be manufactured or imported by anyone for any purpose. Actual uses may not equate to the proposed functions in all cases, but are likely to in most cases.

New chemical functions are an indication of the directions of innovation in the design of new chemicals. They are also important for EPA's review, so that the expected risks of the proposed new chemical can be compared with those of existing substances for which it may substitute. There are distinct differences between the chemical functions proposed in the greatest numbers and those representing the greatest amounts of projected production.

The function category proposed in the greatest *number* of PMNs is a series of different dye and pigment

[q] The term "function" refers to the particular engineering purpose for the chemical (e.g., emulsifier or lubricating agent). The function often does not provide insight into the condition of use (e.g., whether it is in a dispersive consumer use or is an essential industrial process aid).

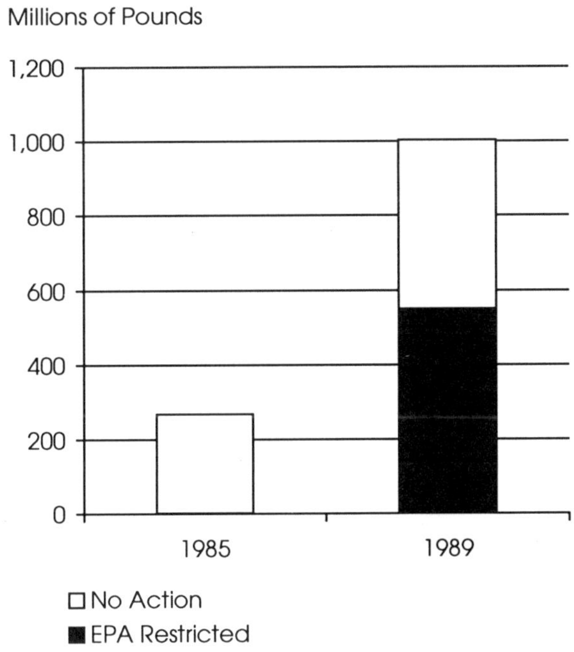

Figure 3-12.

1985 and 1989 TSCA Inventory Update Production Amounts for Chemicals with Premanufacture Notifications, by Regulatory Action

functions (9 of the top 50 proposed functions in non-polymeric submissions, totaling 1,717 PMNs). Only one dye function was in the top 50 in 1990 on the basis of expected *production,* and that (dyes–type unknown) ranked 45th for production with 14 million pounds. A disparity in the opposite direction applies to the function of asphalt additives, for which there are only two new chemical additions to the inventory but for which 385 million pounds were produced in 1990 (ranked fourth). (See Tables 3-9 and 3-10.)

In contrast to the disparity between number of submissions and production for dyes and asphalt additives, intermediates rank relatively high both in number of PMNs submitted (754, ranked first) and pounds of expected production (453 million pounds, ranking third). While fuel and fuel additives appear in the top 50 functions in terms of production, new chemical manufacture and import amounts of chemicals in these functions do not dominate, as they do for the chemicals in commerce prior to 1979.

Halogenated compounds differ from the new chemical group as a whole both in proposed functions and in the restrictions resulting from premanufacture review. (See Box 3-E and Appendix H.)

Table 3-9. Top 50 Primary Functions of Non-polymer Organic Chemicals Entering Commerce, 1979-1993

Rank	Primary Function	**Premanufacture Notices Submitted** Number	**Notices of Commencement of Production** Number
1	Intermediates	754	337
2	Reactive dyes	502	220
3	Dyes (type unknown)	473	308
4	Curing agents	403	175
5	Catalysts	394	205
6	Surfactants	335	108
7	Lubricating agents	324	117
8	Fragrances	317	243
9	Corrosion inhibitors	294	134
10	Photographic chemicals (unspecified)	194	129
11	Surface coating additives	158	79
12	Acid dyes	153	84
13	Not elsewhere classified	152	61
14	Emulsifiers	150	49
15	Stabilizers	144	74
16	Monomers	141	48
17	Herbicides	137	82
18	Dispersants	137	83
19	Antiseize agents	136	54
20	Adhesion promoters / adhesives	124	80
21	Antioxidants	121	58
22	Color former	121	69
23	Coupling agents	118	88
24	Fuels	111	105
25	Additives / processing aids	111	77
26	Direct dyes	108	66
27	Pigments	99	59
28	Lubricant additives	98	41
29	Basic dyes	95	47
30	Disperse dyes	91	31
31	Antistatic agents	88	37
32	Photosensitive agents	87	55
33	Solvents	86	43
34	Viscosity adjustors	83	41
35	Plasticizers	81	31
36	Softeners	78	33
37	Reagents	75	36
38	Sensitizing dyes	75	55
39	Flame retardants	73	33
40	Pesticides	72	48
41	Binders	69	35
42	Prepolymers	68	31
43	Functional fluids	67	33
44	Initiators	66	34
45	Light stabilizers	63	41
46	Reactive diluents	59	28
47	Wetting agents	57	22
48	Scavengers	56	23
49	Modifiers	55	23
50	Agricultural chemicals (type unknown)	53	32
	Subtotal	7,906	4,025
	All Others	1,871	900
	Total	9,777	4,925

Source: Based on data from U.S. EPA, Regulatory Impact Branch.

Table 3-10. Top 50 Primary Functions for Non-polymer Organic Chemicals Produced in Greatest Amount in 1989

Rank	Primary Function	Notices of Commencement of Production Number	Production Amount Pounds
1	Fuel additives	19	713,467,572
2	Surfactants	108	480,184,026
3	Intermediates	337	453,156,848
4	Asphalt additives	2	385,808,955
5	Absorbents / adsorbents	5	331,155,157
6	Agricultural chemicals (type unknown)	32	202,881,713
7	Lubricant additives	41	201,323,980
8	Complexing agents	21	153,178,852
9	Solvents	43	146,201,751
10	Cleaner / detergent additives	10	118,436,581
11	Binders	35	112,554,934
12	Fuels	105	111,112,979
13	Antiseize agents	54	83,912,497
14	Flame retardants	33	83,735,542
15	Lubricating agents	117	81,321,192
16	Curing agents	175	76,126,191
17	Flotation agents	15	73,972,200
18	Corrosion inhibitors	134	73,119,203
19	Dispersants	83	70,275,140
20	Antioxidants	58	69,874,085
21	Antiknock agents	1	66,138,678
22	Herbicides	82	63,850,593
23	Pesticides	48	59,378,494
24	Plasticizers	31	52,199,109
25	Softeners	33	46,842,504
26	Catalysts	205	46,350,282
27	Blowing agents	6	46,282,249
28	Prepolymers	31	41,355,552
29	Functional fluid additives	5	40,884,726
30	Viscosity adjustors	41	37,173,906
31	Bleaching assistants	2	36,817,197
32	Emulsifiers	49	34,309,746
33	Monomers	48	33,087,525
34	Additives / processing aids	77	30,015,435
35	Degreasers	3	29,169,362
36	Fluxing agents	4	28,994,425
37	Bleaching agents	8	26,403,001
38	Fire extinguishing agents	2	21,682,022
39	Wetting agents	22	20,994,775
40	Not elsewhere classified	61	20,862,491
41	Vulcanizing agents	4	16,152,719
42	Surface coating additives	79	15,669,645
43	Brighteners	14	14,676,066
44	Coagulants	2	14,638,694
45	Dyes (type unknown)	308	14,044,096
46	Thickeners	22	13,937,644
47	Photographic chemicals (unspecified)	129	13,574,852
48	Initiators	34	13,280,812
49	Adhesion promoters / adhesives	80	12,828,604
50	Reducers	2	12,812,411
	Subtotal	2,860	4,946,207,013
	All Others	2,065	329,674,338
	Total	4,925	5,275,881,351

Source: Based on data from U.S. EPA, Regulatory Impact Branch.

Table 3-11. Functions of New Halogenated Organic Chemicals Entering Commerce, 1979-1993

Rank	Primary Function	Notices of Commencement	TSCA Inventory Update Production	
			Production Amount	Cumulative Percent
		Number	Pounds	Percent
Fluorinated Organics				
1	Blowing agents	4	46,112,605	22.67
2	Fluxing agents	2	28,867,300	36.86
3	Degreasers	1	28,864,000	51.06
4	Fire extinguishing agents	2	21,636,560	61.69
5	Pesticides	11	19,715,729	71.39
6	Additives / processing aids	3	17,701,200	80.09
7	Refrigerants	3	12,291,565	86.13
8	Herbicides	29	11,441,340	91.76
9	Intermediates	18	4,981,342	94.21
10	Solvents	6	2,264,350	95.32
Chlorinated Organics				
1	Binders	3	64,801,000	13.20
2	Agricultural chemicals (type unknown)	10	60,615,496	25.55
3	Blowing agents	4	46,112,605	34.94
4	Bleaching assistants	2	36,740,000	42.43
5	Pesticides	23	34,136,408	49.38
6	Degreasers	1	28,864,000	55.26
7	Fluxing agents	1	28,864,000	61.14
8	Herbicides	44	21,486,034	65.52
9	Antiseize agents	3	17,046,920	68.99
10	Intermediates	65	15,581,459	72.16

Box 3-E. Halogens in Commerce - II

Halogens are components of thousands of new chemicals proposed and used. For premanufacture review of new chemicals, the manufacturer or importer indicates the intended functions for the chemical. The proposed functions differ from one halogen to another and from those of chemicals with premanufacture notifications as a whole. For example, brominated compounds are used significantly in fire extinguishing (owing to the ability of bromine atoms to react with other chemicals in flames, thereby quenching a fire) and iodinated compounds have special uses in photography (owing to the ability of iodine in certain compounds to react with light). (See Table 3-11 and Appendix H.)

New halogenated compounds proposed for manufacture and import have come under scrutiny by EPA. Chemicals containing halogens have been either withdrawn by the submitter or restricted by EPA to a greater degree than the average new chemical. In the case of proposed new iodinated chemicals, 27 percent have been withdrawn or restricted. (See Figure 3-13.)

Rank	Primary Function	Notices of Commencement Number	TSCA Inventory Update Production: Production Amount Pounds	TSCA Inventory Update Production: Cumulative Percent Percent
Brominated Organics				
1	Flame retardants	13	39,911,482	64.69
2	Fire extinguishing agents	1	11,000,000	82.52
3	Pesticides	2	4,983,000	90.60
4	Antiscaling agents	1	999,999	92.22
5	Insecticides	1	866,800	93.62
6	Corrosion inhibitors	2	826,399	94.96
7	Herbicides	2	748,000	96.18
8	Photographic chemicals (unspecified)	16	490,732	96.97
9	Softeners	1	349,250	97.54
10	Color former	5	319,471	98.06
Iodinated Organics				
1	Corrosion inhibitors	2	469,997	39.10
2	Catalysts	3	396,000	72.05
3	Antiseize agents	1	169,998	86.19
4	Stabilizers	1	88,000	93.51
5	Curing agents	3	41,998	97.01
6	Surfactants	1	22,000	98.84
7	Sensitizing dyes	4	10,703	99.73
8	Ink additives	1	1,760	99.87
9	Initiators	1	986	99.96
10	Photosensitive agents	2	286	99.98

Figure 3-13.

Regulatory Actions on Halogenated Compounds with Premanufacture Notifications (PMNs), 1979-1993

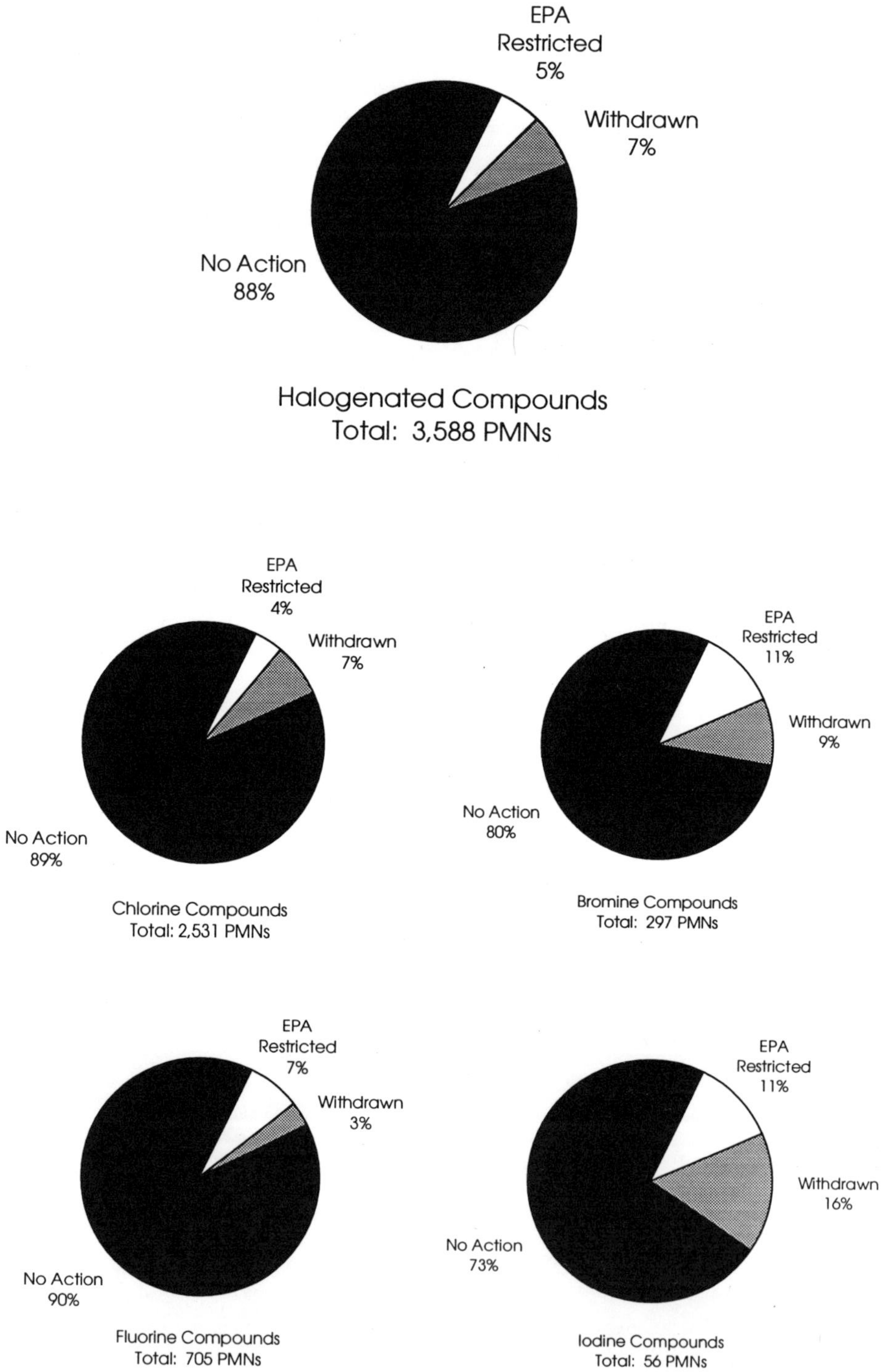

Issues with Chemical Substitutions

Because exposures to less toxic chemicals pose less risk than exposures to more toxic ones, the environmental community advocates a strategy of toxics use reduction. This strategy includes substituting non-toxic and less toxic chemicals for the chemicals of concern. Substitutions for toxic chemicals in commerce raise several important issues, however, some of which are outlined below. It should be pointed out, that when a toxic chemical is banned or regulated, often it is not clear what will replace it.

What is a Substitute?

Usually a chemical is in use because it has a cost, engineering, or marketing advantage over the alternatives. If a chemical occupies its place on the market merely because of a marketing advantage, then other chemicals may easily take its place if it is removed. When this is not the case, substitution is likely to entail a disadvantage either in cost or efficacy. These disadvantages are weighed against the environmental benefit of the substitution. For example, asbestos has long been used in brake linings, but asbestos causes cancer. Substitution for the asbestos by some automobile companies has resulted in linings that cost automobile owners much more and wear out much faster than those containing asbestos.

The issue of what constitutes a substitute has at least one other important, but often overlooked, dimension. Most people think of one-for-one chemical substitution using the same or a similar commercial chain of suppliers and customers. Often, substitution can occur by a completely different approach to the role served by the toxic chemical that is being replaced. For example, many computer and electronics manufacturers in search of a solder substitute for the neurotoxin lead have devised, instead of another solder, simple snap connections requiring no solder at all. Automobile manufacturers in search of substitutes for the highly volatile organic chemical solvents in their paints that pollute the air have developed powders that do not require solvents and liquids that cure under high-intensity light instead of through solvent evaporation. It is often difficult to predict how the market will respond when an opportunity, such as the elimination of a chemical from commerce, presents itself.

Hazardous Substitutes

One of the first issues that arises in substituting one chemicals for another in a particular use is the toxicity of the substitute. Is it worse than that of the chemical it replaces? Does it raise new concerns? How well are its health and environmental effects known?

There are numerous examples of merely switching from one problem substance to another. For example, other fibrous materials are being substituted for cancer-causing asbestos. Concerns are now being raised that some of these substitute fibers, especially those that are small and easily inhaled, may pose problems similar to those of the asbestos that they are replacing.

Clearly, manufacturers and users of toxic chemicals need to consider a wide array of possible ramifications of substitutions to address toxic concerns. Moreover, they must contend with a greater range of possible effects (e.g., trans-generational and immune system effects) as knowledge of chemical toxicity increases.

Linkage Between Chemicals

Chemical linkages also influence the feasibility and efficacy of chemical substitution. For example, one chemical may be inextricably linked to another as part of a mineral resource. Such is the case for cadmium metal, which is most often derived from zinc ore. Toxic cadmium is a common lesser constituent of such ores and can be separated as part of the refining process. The amount of cadmium being mined is therefore almost completely linked to the supply and demand for zinc ore. Were cadmium not isolated for use on its own, it would most likely be carried in commerce in the same quantities, but as a contaminant in zinc-galvanized articles.

Similarly, chlorine gas is a major chemical commodity, made from electrolysis of common table salt. While chlorine is used directly in numerous applications and converted into thousands of manufactured chemicals, its market is linked to sodium hydroxide (lye), because two molecules of sodium hydroxide are formed for every one molecule of chlorine made from salt. Thus, any change (market-driven or regulatory) in the supply of either chlorine or sodium hydroxide affects the other.

A final example of linkage is the substitution of less-toxic bismuth for lead in solder. Although such a substitution would reduce the risks to workers in soldering and to the environment in which the soldered product is disposed, the substitution may not be environmentally desirable. Most bismuth is derived as a minor constituent of lead ore. To get a pound of bismuth, much more lead will generally be mined and refined than would have been the case if the ore was being mined for a pound of lead.

New vs. Existing Chemicals

It is much easier to address a toxic chemical concern prior to the manufacture and sale of the substance than after the chemical has been engineered into different applications on the market. Before marketing, the environmental consequences have not occurred, the manufacturer has not invested in equipment and personnel to produce the substance, and users have neither designed their products and processes based upon the chemical and physical properties of the chemical nor evaluated the substance for its benefits.

For this reason, Congress, in enacting TSCA, decided to address existing chemicals and new chemicals differently. EPA reviews chemicals before manufacture and faces relatively low hurdles to action to restrict or ban them. In contrast, for existing chemicals (those listed on the initial inventory in 1979), EPA must conduct a lengthy risk-benefit analysis and rule-making process to address unreasonable risks. Similarly, existing pesticides can continue to be marketed while pertinent health and environmental data are reviewed by the government, but new pesticides must be approved by EPA before they can legally be sold or used in the United States. The distinction recognizes the opportunity to forestall damage to health and the environment from chemicals not yet entrenched in the marketplace, but leaves chemicals brought to commerce before 1979 in the market with, overall, little government review.

Issues of substitution make clear that toxics in commerce are a major environmental issue that is best addressed by prevention. Once a chemical is fully integrated into the economy it becomes more difficult to address than before it is introduced. At present, new chemicals entering the market have been neither a major environmental scourge nor a major solution to toxic pollution. It is in the production and use of chemicals that have been in use for decades that most concerns lie.

Types of Chemicals in Commerce

Often it is hard to produce or obtain chemical substances with a high degree of purity without great effort and expense. Most chemicals in commerce have measurable, and sometimes large, amounts of unintended impurities, the nature of which depends upon the way in which the compound is manufactured or isolated. Approximately 85 percent of manufactured and imported chemicals on the TSCA inventory have a defined structure, but are marketed in varying degrees of purity.

Most chemicals in commerce do not consist of pure chemical compounds. Most involve either:

- blended mixtures (formulations),
- undefined and/or variable mixtures,
- polymers,
- fabricated combinations, or
- naturally occurring materials used in an unaltered form.

To some extent, the nature of the compounds may represent not only different conditions of use, but quite different environmental challenges.

Blended Formulations

Because the chemical and physical properties of chemical compounds vary with their atomic structure, processors often blend chemicals together to create combinations with a desired mix of properties. For example, laundry detergents are formulated mixtures of chemical substances that often contain compounds that:

- dissolve grease and oil, like soap (surfactants),
- soften hard water (builders),
- whiten (whiteners),
- degrade food stains biologically (enzymes), and
- smell good (fragrances).

Other examples include the chemical compounds of different colors blended together as dyes or as pigments to give a wide variety of hues to nearly all consumer products. Such formulated mixtures are used when there are no inexpensive single-compound alternatives.

A blended mixture, indeed any mixture, presents problems at the end of its product life-cycle, unless all components and their degradation products are relatively nontoxic. Mixtures can present challenges in recycling because of the tendency to yield much lower-grade products than purer substances do when recycled.

There is no national database available on the types and amounts of chemicals in commerce in this form. Various trade associations or consultant studies may have figures for a specific type of product (e.g., for pesticides, for spot-removers, or for liquid detergents).

Undefined and/or Variable Mixtures

Approximately 9,230 manufactured chemicals in commerce have an undefined or variable molecular structure. An undefined or variable structure comes about most often when the material is manufactured from a complex raw natural material that has had little refinement (e.g., coal, petroleum, wood, or shale; or coconut, linseed, and other seed oils). Many of these undefined and variable compounds are fuels derived from petroleum, such as gasoline, kerosene, and Diesel #2. These contain thousands of chemicals in amounts that vary depending upon the composition of the crude oil used to make them. Each is refined to meet certain performance specifications, but the chemical composition varies from refinery to refinery and from one period of time to the next. Chemicals with an undefined or variable structure dominate the top 100 chemicals for production amount on the 1989 Inventory Update. (See Table 3-6.)

Unlike formulated mixtures, which tend to be used to achieve a commercial purpose only when unblended compounds are not economically available to meet the purpose, most undefined and variable composition mixtures are used because they can meet the intended application without going to the time and expense of purifying the component chemicals. Pure compounds are not needed for chemicals used as fuels, for example. Variable and undefined mixtures usually suffice, so long as the energy value is within an acceptable range for the combustion equipment being employed, and so long as the mixtures do not contain chemicals with undesirable properties such as corrosivity, odor, or elemental toxicity. The expense of additional refining to separate and purify the chemical compound components of such mixtures may not be warranted.

Polymers

Polymers are chemical compounds created by linking together one or a few smaller chemicals (monomers) into much larger structures. Polymers, like undefined and variable composition mixtures, are usually mixtures with a distribution of sizes and an average composition of monomers. Unlike

Table 3-12. Top 10 Polymers by Production Amount, 1992

Polymer	Production Amount Pounds
Low density polyethylene	11,917,000,000
High density polyethylene	9,808,000,000
Polyvinyl chlorine	9,989,000,000
Polypropylene	8,421,000,000
Polystyrene	5,096,000,000
Phenolic	2,923,999,000
Styrene copolymers	2,723,000,000
Thermoplastic polyester	2,413,000,000
Urea	1,548,000,000
Unsaturated polyester	1,175,000,000

Derived from Society of Plastics Industry, *1992 Statistical Yearbook.*

undefined and variable composition mixtures, the polymer's composition is defined by the identity of its monomer constituents. (Sometimes, depending upon the monomers involved, the relative monomer composition is fixed, because they can bond together in only one way.)

Polymers may have valuable properties such as flexibility, slipperiness, and high strength relative to weight. When monomers are highly chlorinated or brominated, the resulting polymer is often flame resistant. For example, vinyl chloride monomer, with four chlorine and two carbon atoms, results in PVC (polyvinylchloride) plastic, which is generally flame resistant.

A few polymers represent the overwhelming majority of polymer production. Polyethylene, polyvinylchloride, polypropylene, and polystyrene are each produced in excess of 5 billion pounds per year. (See Table 3-12.) The American Chemical Society reports that polymer production rose an average of 4 percent per year between 1983 and 1993, with plastics accounting for the majority of this growth. The production of polymers in the United States in 1993 was 67.4 billion pounds.[5] (See Figure 3-14.)

While most high-molecular-weight polymers pose little health hazard, because they are not easily absorbed into the body, many polymer-containing products also contain large amounts of additives, some of which may migrate from the product and some of which are highly toxic (e.g., heavy metals such as cadmium or mercury). In other cases, if the reaction creating the polymer is not run to completion, reactive and potentially toxic monomers may remain in the product.

Fabricated Combinations

Fabricated combinations are similar to formulated mixtures, in that they represent the intentional combination of different compounds to achieve a design

Figure 3-14.

U.S. Production of Plastics, Synthetic Rubber, and Synthetic Fibers, 1983-1993

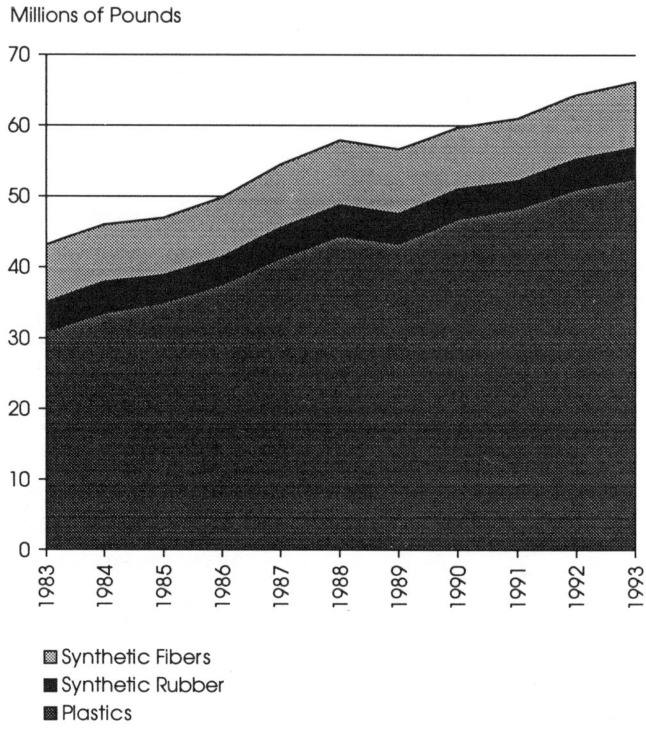

Sources: Society of the Plastics Industry, International Institute of Synthetic Rubber Producers, and Fiber Economics Bureau

purpose, except that the chemical compounds are not blended into a mixture. Rather, the chemicals in fabricated combinations may be layered or otherwise physically, rather than chemically, combined so that different locations in the final article have different concentrations of the constituent compounds. For example, an electronic circuit board is fabricated from many chemicals, in such a way that some locations have chemicals that conduct electricity in specific ways and some locations have chemicals that do not. An automobile is fabricated from thousands of chemical compounds, from chromium-plated steel bumpers to PVC seat covers.

Such fabricated combinations pose similar environmental challenges upon product retirement as blended mixtures. The main exception is the extent to which fabricated products can be disassembled or "defabricated" into relatively pure substances for reuse or recycling.

Naturally Occurring Materials Used in Unaltered Form

Almost certainly the largest quantities of chemicals in commerce are in an unaltered form as collected from nature. Sand, air, slate, water, marble, clay, and granite are all examples of materials used widely throughout the economy without chemical alteration. Although such materials are not without their environmental consequences (e.g., the radioactivity present in some thorium-containing stone used to build homes and the cancer-causing ability of some sands), naturally occurring materials that are used unaltered are not discussed further in this report in order to focus upon materials being chemically designed and introduced into commerce.

Considerations in Choosing Chemicals for Commerce

Many factors influence the choice of chemicals that might be successful in commerce. These include chemical and physical properties and environmental and safety considerations discussed above, chemical and engineering feasibility, property rights, costs, and market demand.

Chemical and Engineering Feasibility

Many factors determine the technical feasibility of introducing a chemical into commerce. The first issue is one of possibility, or whether the chemical can be made at all. For some applications, there may be many chemical options (e.g., general use as an antifreeze); in others, there may be no substitute (e.g., for certain pharmaceuticals and biological molecules).

The next issue is one of practicality, or figuring out a way to synthesize the chemical to obtain a significant yield economically. Making large, complex molecules, such as pharmaceuticals, often requires many sequential chemical reactions. Often there are several conceivable sequences of reactions that might be considered. The chemist needs to find the best synthetic pathway to convert a large fraction of the starting material to the desired product with little yield lost along the way.

Once chemists identify a viable synthetic pathway in the laboratory, the challenge for chemical engineers is to scale up the synthesis to commercial proportions. Seldom is the process of scale-up straightforward. Often it does not work at all. The engineers must devise means of adding ingredients to one another, mixing them during reaction, separating the desired product from undesired ones, and then purifying it to the required specification —all in much larger amounts than in the laboratory. Issues such as storing and transferring chemicals, cleaning during shutdowns in production, and handling waste must be worked out satisfactorily. All of this must be done with commercially available raw materials to give a product with enough uniformity to meet customer specifications at a competitive price.

Property Rights

Chemical and process patents, as well as process knowledge, can be important factors in the commercialization of chemicals. A chemical or process that is unique and new may be eligible for patent protection, in which the government grants a 17-year marketing monopoly. Such patents are granted to create an incentive for companies and individual scientists and engineers to make the effort and to take risks to develop new technologies and products. On the other hand, if another company has already patented the desired chemical or process, it may not be possible to make, use, or modify the product or technology without paying for a license from the patent holder.

Even for unpatented chemicals and processes, the chemical and engineering knowledge gained by a company in deciding to make and use chemicals in particular ways or under particular operating conditions may offer a company a significant competitive advantage over others. Such chemical and process knowledge can be quite proprietary.

Costs

A major consideration in making any chemical or in using any chemical process is cost. If costs become too high, the company cannot rationalize moving forward on the commercial venture for business reasons. Even when a project can be economically justified, competitive pressures always create an incentive to find less costly ways of making substances. Thus, engineers continue to fine-tune processes in an effort to gain efficiency.

When a chemical must meet only a general specification (e.g., to dissolve varnish applied to furniture), several chemical substances might quality. Cost and availability will often dictate the choice of chemicals used in such cases. For example, the refining of petroleum generates numerous petrochemical streams. Depending upon the demands from the various fuel markets (e.g., gasoline, jet fuel, industrial boiler fuel), some of these streams may be more abundant and thus less expensive than others, as the oil companies try to find markets for as many of their refinery streams as possible. As a result, manufacturers of furniture strippers may shift the petroleum-based solvents in their product formulations in response to the changing markets of the oil refiners.

Market Demand

No chemical can be important in commerce without market demand. Sometimes this market demand arises first from the customers of chemical manufacturers and processors. Examples include customer demand for water-based cleaners and degreasers for industrial processes or for paints and coatings with fewer volatile organic compounds. At other times, the product chemist in the chemical industry can invent chemicals or new uses for existing chemicals that stimulate new markets. The early development of plastics exemplifies this case. Finally, effective marketing may increase demand for particular chemicals. In the end, no more of a chemical will be sold than there is market demand.

Chemical Uses — Commercial Stages and Conditions of Use

The economy is made up of goods and services. As all goods are made of chemicals, chemicals pervade the economy. Chemicals flow through many stages of commerce from extraction to manufacture to use, recycling, and retirement. Their conditions of use in part determine the amount of waste generated in each stage; a "condition of use" may indicate the role of the chemical in a process (raw material, chemical reagent) or the context in which it performs its role (use by consumers vs. industrial applications, use indoors or out). Each combination of stage in commerce and condition of use has its own business and environmental significance. Some conditions of use are peculiar to a particular stage in commerce (e.g., use of chemicals as intermediates is inherently a characteristic of manufacturing), but others apply across the economy (e.g., use of chemicals as fuels occur at all stages in commerce).

This section describes the stages of commerce in relationship to environmental impacts and includes descriptions of several different roles and environmentally relevant conditions of use of chemicals in the economy. (See Table 3-13.) This section may seem elementary to readers well acquainted with the many roles of chemicals. Its contribution toward a general framework for looking at chemicals in commerce is quite basic. This descriptive framework will provide a basis for more detailed and more closely focused analyses in later editions of *Toxics Watch*. Except as noted, there is a general lack of quantitative data to support the qualitative description of this framework.

Mining/Extraction

Any material having the requisite elemental composition can in theory be used as a raw material for chemical production. However, relative abundance and the energy and expense required to obtain chemicals that are in low concentration or in difficult-to-separate mixtures limit the choice of raw materials. Raw materials can be either renewable resources (those that are restored over time, such as timber or sea water) or non-renewable, in the sense that the particular raw material form is limited (such as petroleum, which is believed to form only after millions of years of decay of organic material).[r] Natural resources that are currently most widely used to produce chemicals are petroleum, natural gas, coal, metals, industrial minerals,[s] water, and air products.

[r] Many of the Earth's renewable resources such as fish and timber are being depleted more rapidly than non-renewable resources. Renewable resources that are derived from living organisms may be depleted beyond the point of recovery, in the absence of responsible resource management.. In contrast, non-renewable resources could be "renewed" in theory, with the application of enough energy. Care must therefore be exercised in the relatively rapid use of any resource.

[s] Industrial minerals are non-metal minerals used primarily in chemical production as opposed to energy production or construction applications.

Table 3-13. Conditions of Use and the Commercial Stages to Which They Most Often Apply

Condition of Use / Commercial Stage	Mining/Extraction	Refining	Chemical Manufacturing	Processing and Fabricating	Distribution	Product Use	Product Retirement
Raw Material	✓						
Refinery Feedstock		✓					
Heterogeneous Catalyst		✓	✓				
Batch vs. Continuous vs. Semi-batch Process		✓	✓	✓			
Chemical Reagent/Intermediate			✓				
Specific Process Aid	✓	✓	✓	✓			
General Process Aid	✓	✓	✓	✓			
Open vs. Closed System		✓	✓	✓	✓	✓	
Fuel	✓	✓	✓	✓		✓	
Commercial/Industrial vs. Consumer						✓	✓
Dispersive vs. Closed Use						✓	✓
Indoor vs. Outdoor			✓	✓		✓	

Organic Raw Materials

Petroleum, natural gas, and coal are organic materials and are primarily used to generate energy as fuels. They are also the raw material sources for organic chemical production.

By far the largest source of carbon and hydrogen for organic chemicals is petroleum. The environmental consequences associated with petroleum extraction are inherently significant because of the large scale on which petroleum extraction occurs. Mud generated during the drilling of wells may contain many toxic materials; those materials may lead to soil contamination. Chemicals injected into the wells to increase yield may contaminate groundwater sources. Petroleum is also, by far, the chemical most often reported as accidentally released to the environment; these releases range from small pipeline leaks to massive spills, such as the dramatic rupture of the *Exxon Valdez* supertanker in the coastal waters of Alaska. Safety concerns are always present, because petroleum is both flammable and often under great pressure.

Natural gas, a mixture of hydrocarbon gases, is the predominant fuel gas. Commercially important products from natural gas are methane, ethane, propane, butane, and gasoline. Coke, which is used to make steel, is the product produced in the largest quantities from coal. Liquid products from coal are tar and crude light oil, which are used to make organic chemicals, aromatics in particular. Gaseous products from coal include hydrogen, methane, and ethylene.

Inorganic Raw Materials

Inorganic chemicals are derived from industrial minerals, metals, and air products. Those sources also contribute elements contained in organic chemicals other than the prerequisite carbon. For example, nitrogen is an air product and sulfur is an industrial mineral. These are two elements that are seen in many organic chemicals (e.g., amino acids) but they are also the primary constituents of inorganic chemicals (e.g., sulfuric acid, ammonia).

Metals and industrial minerals (as well as coal) are extracted through mining techniques. Mining involves removing the desired material or ore from the ground and separating it from the associated bulk materials. Typically, the first step in mining is removal of the soil and rock called "overburden" that covers the ore. While not necessarily hazardous, large quantities of waste can be generated, particularly in open pit mining. In 1992, 1.1 billion tons of overburden was produced at non-fuel mines.[6]

Finely ground materials generated in the next step, concentration of the ore, make contaminants such as arsenic or cadmium that were bound up in solid rock more accessible to water. Sulfur is also often mined with metals, and acid drainage results as it is released. Tailings, which are solid residues from the concentration step, are also waste that can contaminate the ground in the mining area and surface and groundwater. In addition to residual metals, tailings can contain organic chemicals, such as toluene, that are used in the mining process.

To the extent that these raw materials are not refined, this production is not covered by the reporting requirements of the TSCA Chemical Inventory, nor are the wastes captured by the Toxics Release Inventory (as the extraction industries are currently excluded from TRI reporting).

Conditions of Use: Raw Materials — Status and Trends

When lead or any other element or chemical is required, a raw material from which it can be extracted or made is essential. Yet extraction of resources is not without environmental consequences. Therefore, the role "raw material" is an environmentally relevant and commercially distinct condition of use which is unique to extraction operations.

The United States used approximately 1.9 trillion pounds of petroleum in 1993; 56 percent came from domestic sources and the rest was imported from abroad. Approximately 910 billion pounds of natural gas was extracted from the earth in 1993 for use in this country, 91 percent of it from domestic sources. Approximately 1.9 trillion pounds of coal was consumed in the United States in that year; 99 percent of this came from domestic mines. (See Table 3-14.)

The metallic inorganic raw materials produced in the largest quantities are iron followed by aluminum, copper, lead, magne-

Table 3-14. Petroleum, Coal, and Natural Gas Production and Consumption, 1993

	Domestic Production Pounds	**U.S. Consumption** Pounds	**Percent Imported** Percent
Petroleum*	1,065,000,000,000	1,908,000,000,000	44
Coal	1,892,000,000,000	1,852,000,000,000	0.8**
Natural Gas*	828,000,000,000	909,000,000,000	9

* Pounds of petroleum were calculated by assuming an average density of 0.869g/ml. Pounds of natural gas were calculated by assuming an average density of 0.045 lbs/ft^3. Calculations based on data from Energy Information Administration, Department of Energy.

** Because of an open market system and competitive prices, a small amount of coal is imported from Colombia, Venezuela, Indonesia, and Canada although U.S. production does, in fact, exceed consumption. Approximately 15 billion pounds of coal were imported in 1993.

sium metal, and zinc. In 1990 approximately 124 billion pounds of iron ore were extracted, with the other metals ranging from 8.9 billion pounds of aluminum to 1.2 billion pounds of zinc. Industrial minerals produced in the largest quantities in the United States include phosphate rock used to make phosphoric acid, sulfur used to make sulfuric acid, limestone, and salt. In 1990, 102 billion pounds of phosphate rock were produced, 80 billion pounds of salt, 35 billion pounds of lime, and 26 billion pounds of sulfur.[7] (See Table 3-15.)

Nitrogen and oxygen, the two elements present in air (as a mixture) in much the greatest quantities, are commercially separated through cooling (as they liquefy at different temperatures); they are major chemicals in commerce. In 1993 U.S. production of nitrogen and oxygen was 65.3 billion pounds and 46.5 billion pounds, respectively.[8]

Refining

Petroleum Refining

The largest waste streams from refineries are the aqueous waste streams, since water usage is quite high, especially for cooling. Other aqueous waste streams include storm runoff and streams — contaminated with chemicals such as hydrogen sulfide, ammonia, cyanides, metals, and salts.

Air emissions come largely from combustion and evaporation due to the volatile nature of petroleum products. Refineries can prevent evaporation largely by improved equipment maintenance to prevent leaks. Combustion can be relatively clean, producing only water and carbon dioxide, but certain fuel compositions result in emissions of sulfur and nitrogen oxides as well.

The Petroleum industry reported 2.9 billion pounds of production-related waste to TRI in 1992,

Table 3-15. Top U.S. Non-fuel Minerals by Production Amount, 1990

Mineral	**Production** Million Tons
Crushed stone	1,222.0
Sand and gravel (construction)	910.6
Cement (Portland, masonry, other)	77.1
Iron ore	62.2
Phosphate rock	51.1
Clays	47.4
Salt	40.6
Sand and gravel (industrial)	28.4
Lime	17.5
Gypsum	16.4
Ammonia (fixed Nitrogen)	14.0
Sulfur	12.7
Soda ash	10.1
Aluminum	4.5
Potash	1.9
Copper	1.8
Talc and pyrophyllite	1.4
Dimensional stone	1.2
Diatomite	0.7
Feldspar	0.7
Boron	0.7
Zinc	0.6
Magnesium compounds	0.6
Lead	0.5
Pumice and pumicite	0.5
Barite	0.5
Silicon	0.5

Source: Compiled from *1994 Mineral Commodity Summaries*, Bureau of Mines.

ranking 3rd of the 22 industry groups reporting. Given that almost all of the huge amounts of petroleum extracted are being refined, this represents a tiny percent of process loss. Moreover, the industry has little choice in what raw materials it uses and what products it produces. Refining of natural gas has even fewer residuals, so options for further pollution prevention may be even more limited. So long as petroleum is needed in enormous quantities as a feedstock for fuel and petrochemicals, the Petroleum industry will probably continue to be a major toxic waste generator, despite efficiencies that are high relative to most other industries.

Metal and Mineral Refining

Metal and mineral (and coal) refining often have much greater environmental consequences than does petroleum refining. Such impacts can include the disruption to land caused from surface mining, acid run-off, and toxic chemical air and water pollution. In some cases, alternatives for process technology

Box 3-F. The Environmental Midas Touch

The concentration of gold from low-grade ore using cyanide leaching is one example of a refining process with the potential for significant environmental consequences. This relatively common process involves placing thousands or millions of tons of crushed ore on pads lined with clay or plastic in heaps tens of feet high over many acres. Then a cyanide-containing solution is sprayed over the heap, percolating through and dissolving the gold, carrying it to collecting ponds. The gold-laden cyanide solution then goes through a multi-step process to remove the gold. The process, which can take weeks or months to complete, is continued until little further gold can be leached from the heap.

Environmental concerns arise when the cyanide liquid escapes through cracks or holes in the clay or plastic or when toxic heavy metals (lead, cadmium, and/or mercury) are liberated by the process; either event leads to contamination of the soil and of water supplies. Other processes that use cyanide in vats to contain leaks or that eliminate the use of cyanide altogether may avoid some of the adverse effects this method of gold refining.

result in differing environmental consequences. Metals in ores that have been extracted from the ground are usually concentrated and/or chemically converted before use. Depending upon the process, concentration may be highly polluting. (See Box 3-F.) After concentration the ores are often reduced to crude metal at high temperatures in a smelter. Smelting may also be highly polluting, often producing large quantities of air pollution, particularly sulfur dioxide, which causes acid rain. Arsenic, lead, cadmium, and other heavy metals can also be released to the air as part of the smelting process.

Status of Uses in Refining

Refinery Feedstock

The refining of an element of chemical requires an appropriate feedstock, just as refined metal requires a metal-bearing ore as raw material. If an organic chemical is needed, petroleum or some other hydrocarbon-based feedstock is required. Particular feedstocks and how they are refined may lead to widely differing environmental consequences. Therefore, the role "refinery feedstock" is an environmentally relevant and commercially distinct condition of use that is specific to refining operations.

As noted above, virtually all petroleum extracted is refined. Approximately half the petroleum refined is used to make gasoline, while another 40 percent goes to making other fuels. A relatively small portion of refined petroleum (less than 5 percent) is used as feedstock for the organic chemical industry.[9] Similarly, most natural gas is refined prior to use, although the refining process is much more modest and more than 97 percent goes to fuel use, with the rest being used as a chemical feedstock, particularly in the manufacture of ammonia.[10]

In contrast, very little coal is refined, as most coal is used directly as a fuel. The largest portion of coal that is refined (4 percent of the 900 million tons of coal mined) is used to make coke, a key ingredient in the most common steelmaking process. Only a small portion is refined into other chemical feedstocks.

Most minerals tend to fall into either a processed or unprocessed category. This report does not focus on the use of minerals used for their physical properties in an unprocessed form such as granite and slate. Rather, it focuses on those minerals that are generally processed prior to use (such as iron ore, copper ore, bauxite, and phosphate rock). For these materials, the amount processed is essentially the same as that extracted, except for changes in stockpiles of the unprocessed mineral.

Heterogeneous Catalyst

Another condition of use in the refining industry that should be distinguished from that of feedstock is the "heterogeneous catalyst," which facilitates chemical reactions without in the end being changed itself. The refining of petroleum and natural gas relies heavily upon such chemicals, which typically are insoluble solids across which large volumes of the liquid or gaseous feedstocks are passed (hence the term heterogeneous, referring to the different phases of the materials involved). Most catalysts are highly specialized chemicals or combinations of chemicals.

Heterogeneous catalysts are not intended to be incorporated into products and can often be restored after they have lost their effectiveness over time. A heterogeneous catalyst, if it operates effectively, should process large quantities of product and should not enter the environment, except in very small quantities at the very end of its life cycle. Heterogeneous catalysts are used not only in refining operations but also heavily in chemical manufacturing and to a limited extent in chemical processing. Heterogeneous catalysts are included in the pollution control systems of most automobiles sold in the United States today.

Chemical Manufacturing

"The Chemistry Industry"

Chemical manufacturers use extracted and refined substances as starting materials to create more than 72,000 other substances. Often it takes many steps in sequence to create the desired product. For example, the major cyclic[t] chemicals — benzene, xylene, toluene, and naphthalene — are converted through many steps into a wide variety of dyes, pigments, pesticides, medicinal chemicals, rubber-processing chemicals, and plasticizers.

Similarly, large volume acyclic chemicals (such as acetylene, ethylene, propylene, butylene, and their related alcohols), chlorinated

[t] *Cyclic* compounds are those that exist as rings of three or more carbon atoms. Benzene, a six-carbon hexagonal ring, and those compounds that are similar to benzene, make up an important class of cyclic chemicals known as "aromatics." *Acyclic* organic chemicals have "open-chain" structures, or strings of carbon atoms that do not bond together in closed rings.

hydrocarbons, amines, and amides are converted through several reactions into products such as surface active agents (e.g., detergents, emulsifiers, foaming agents), elastomers (e.g., synthetic rubber), flavors, and fragrances. These products are then sold either to processors, fabricators, and users, or to other chemical manufacturers for conversion into yet another compound. Figure 3-15 shows just some of the many products in commerce derived from chlorine. Some of these are not chlorinated themselves (e.g., polycarbonates), but are the result of reactions by one or more chlorinated intermediates.

Companies involved in chemical manufacturing could be said to represent a "Chemistry Industry," since this is the stage in commerce where chemical design is most involved. It is also a stage constrained, on the one hand, by the availability and cost of appropriate raw materials and by scientific and engineering feasibility and, on the other hand, by market demands.

Usually there is more than one technically feasible method for making any given chemical product. The challenge to companies is to find the most economical way, in order to compete effectively against others who may offer the same or similar product. Sometimes there are significant differences in the environmental, health, and safety considerations among the alternatives. Increasingly, chemical manufacturers are having to consider such factors in their choice of approach. Sometimes the choice lies between two sequences of chemical conversions. In other cases, it involves deciding among process methods. As chemical facilities collectively are by far the largest producers of toxic waste and the sources of the largest amounts of releases to the environment, the environmental stakes in these decisions are high. Recent developments in chemical design consciously address environmental factors. (See Box 3-G.)

Batch vs. Continuous vs. Semi-batch Processes

The most fundamental choice in process method for a chemical manufacturer is between a batch process, a continuous process, and a semi-batch process. Batch process operations are like making a cake. The various ingredients are added to a relatively standard piece of equipment. The ingredients are mixed; the mixture is heated, cooled, or pressurized, as appropriate; the results are removed, and purified as necessary; and the equipment is cleaned prior to being used again, often to make a different product.

Most chemicals are manufactured in batch process operations. Batch processing is almost always used when less than 100,000 pounds per year is needed or when production is episodic because dedicated equipment would be too expensive. But batch processes can generate relatively large amounts of waste per unit of product (leaving the equivalent of a sink full of dirty dishes and utensils after every batch). Batch process operations also often involve manual efforts either to prepare a batch or to collect the product. If conditions are not quite right, an entire batch may produce an off-specification product. Sometimes trial and error is required, especially if the product is made infrequently.

Chemicals with larger production amounts and relatively constant demand are typically made in continuous processes. In continuous processes, specialized equipment is designed so that the ingredients may be fed in continuously at one end with product being removed at the same rate from the other end of the process. Because the equipment is dedicated to production of one product, every effort is made to keep it running continuously. Typically, a continuous process is designed to be shut down only once a year or less for maintenance, avoiding all the waste associated with batch clean-up. The ongoing nature of a continuous-process operation lends itself to monitoring and refinement to increase yield and to improve product quality and uniformity. Continuous-process operations are typically much less wasteful per unit of product than are batch processes. As equipment utilization goes up, continuous processes become more economical. Continuous processes account for the vast majority of chemical production amounts.

Semi-batch processes are those that cannot be classified as either batch or continuous. In a semi-batch process, some reagents are added to a batch-like reaction vessel and other chemicals are added continuously without removal of the products. Such processes are typically used to regulate the speed of a reaction that results in a very homogeneous product. Semi-batch processes tend to share most of the environmental characteristics of batch processes.

General knowledge about a process, such as whether it is batch, continuous, or semi-batch and about the identity of the major chemicals involved can provide important insights into its likely environmental and safety consequences. Information on detailed operating parameters (e.g., temperature, concentration, mixing procedures, and pressure) is generally of lesser interpretative value.

Conditions of Use Unique to Chemical Manufacturing

While several of the environmentally relevant conditions of use discussed before, such as heterogeneous catalyst, apply to chemical manufacturing, others are particularly relevant to this industry.

Chemical Reagent/ Intermediate

Chemical reagents (i.e., those chemicals converted into different chemicals) are significant in several respects. First, because they are being converted to other chemicals, the process may result in little or none of the reagent chemical remaining upon completion. The extent to which this is true depends on the particular reactions involved and the conditions under which they are run. For example, extremely toxic phosgene gas may be used as a reagent to produce much less toxic carbonyl-containing (CO) products; virtually all the phosgene is consumed in the process.

Second, chemical reagents are significant because they are reactive. If they are small and can enter biological systems and react with biological molecules, this reactivity can be a source of toxicity. Most reagents have some form of

Figure 3-15. Overview of Chemicals Derived from Chlorine and End-product Uses

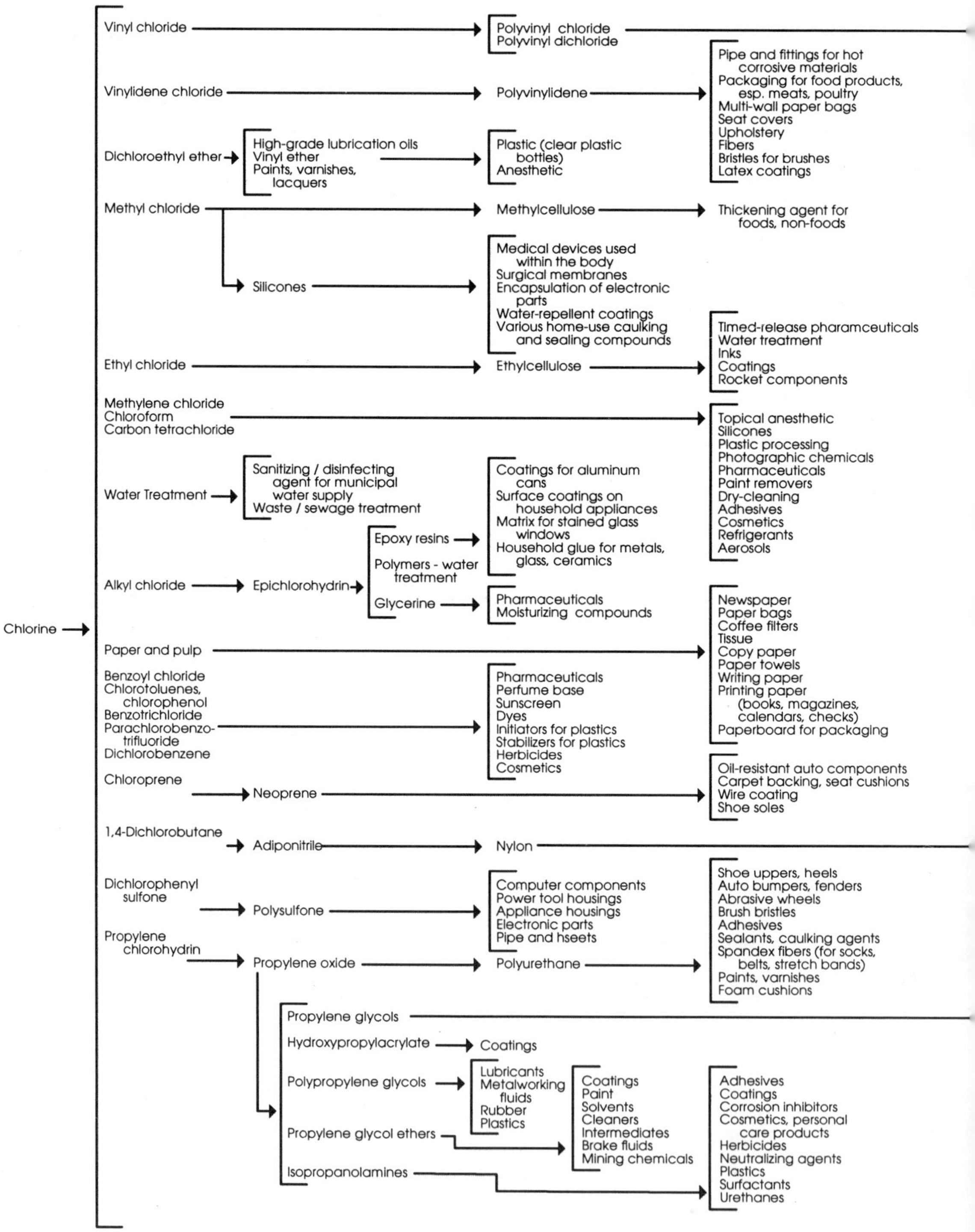

Sources: The Dow Chemical Company; The Chlorine Institute, Inc.

→ Luggage
Handbags
Watchstraps
Billfolds
Shoes, belts
Textile fabric coatings
Raincoats, rainsuits, parks
Magnetic recording tape
Golf bags
Bicycle seats, handlebar grips
Exercise equipment pad coverings
Inflatable boats, water floats
Floor coverings, decorative molding strips
Wallpaper
Siding, gutters, gutter leaf guards
Window, door frames
Plumbing fittings
Film, sheeting
Solar reflective film
Electricdal insulation
Baby strollers
Baby bibs, crib bumper pads, mattress covers
Toys
Card tables, chairs
Wood-grain vinyl coating for stereo cabinets, radio/TV cabinets, TV carts, bookshelves, table tops, counters
Cases for cosmetics, cameras, binoculars, hunting rifles, musical instruments
Containers for food products, cosmetics, toiletries, household chemicals
Coating for paper
Adhesive/bonding agent base for synthetic turf
Swimming pool liner, covers
Garden hoses
School/office supplies, e.g., ring bnider covers pencil cases, book totes
Automobile vinyl tops, upholstery, floor mats
Seat coveringss
Umbrellas
Electrical, decorative vinyl tapes

Tire cord
Wearing apparel (shirts, blouses, lingerie, hosiery, jackets, swimwear
Jogging shoes, sneakers
Flotation vests for boating
Fishing boots, nets, line
Cordage, bowlines, rope
Tents
Window screens
Tarpaulins, canopies, awnings
Sleeping bags, camping equipment
Tennis racket strings
Guitar strings
Bristles for toothbrushes, hairbrushes, paintbrushes, carpets, rugs
→ Artificial turf
Parachutes
Sails
Automotive upholstery
Furniture fabrics
Gears, bearings
Wire insulation
Surgical sutures
Pen tips

→ Plastics
Solvents
Coatings
Paint
Food additivies
Plasticizers
Antifreeze, coolants
Flavoring extracts
Soft-drink syrups
Lotions, creams
Cosmetics
Cleansing creams
Suntan lotions
Brake fluids
Pharmaceuticals
Insecticides
Natural gas treatment

Hydrochloric acid →
- Food processing → Sugar refining, Corn syrup, Gelatin, Monosodium glutonate, Brewing
- Desulfurization agent for petroleum
- Production of aklyl chlorides → Electronic silicone
- Oil well acidizing
- Production of metallic chlorides → Photoflash bulbs, Refractories, Alloys, Pyrotechnics
- Water treatment
- Pickling in steel manufacture
- Production of hydrochlorides → Rubber accelerator, Plastics stabilizer, Rocket propellants, Pharmaceuticals
- Latex coagulating agent

Methyl chloroacetate
Chloroacetic acid → Permanent wave solutions, hair-care products; 2,4,D, other herbicides; Synthetic caffeine; Vinyl stabilizer; Pharmaceuticals

Trichloroacetaldehyde → Liniments, pharmaceuticals

Tetrachlorophthalic anhydride → Flame retardant for plastics

Chlorinated paraffins → Highway stripe paint; High-pressure lubricants; Flame retardants; Cable insulation; Plasticizers for polyvinyl chloride; Detergents

Sulfur dichloride
Sulfur monochloride
Thionyl chloride
Sulfuryl chloride → Photographic chemicals; Dyes; Rubber antioxidants; Purifying sugar juices; Bandaids; Erasers; Oil additives; Pacemaker batteries; Fungicide

Phosphorus trichloride
Phosphorus pentachloride
Phosphorus oxychloride → Gasoline additives; Hydraulic fluids; Semiconductor manufacture; Fire-retarding agents; Herbicides

Ferric chloride → Photography; Etching, engraving; Printed circuitry; Pharmaceuticals

Stannous chloride → Silvering mirrors; Stabilizer for perfume in soaps

Zinc chloride → Soldering fluxes; Deodorant preparations; Dental cements, dentifrices

Chlorinated isocyanurates → Sanitizers for swimming pools; Household, commercial bleaches; Detergents for automatic dishwashers; Scouring powders

Sodium hypochloride → Bleaching pulp, paper, textiles; Water purification; Pharmaceuticals; Household bleach; Disinfectant for swimming pools

Calcium hypochloride → Algaecide; Bactericide; Deodorant; Potable water purification; Disinfectant for swimming pools

1,1,1-Trichloroethane
Perchloroethylene
Ethylene dichloride
Trichloroethylene → Paper de-inker; Transformer fluid; Circuit boards; Drain cleaners; Textile manufacture; Leather finishing; Pigments; Dyes; Refrigerants; Spot remover; Insecticides; Pesticides; Solvents; Adhesives; Degreaser; Dry-cleaning

Titanium dioxide → Electrical components; Semiconductors; Corrosion-resistant paint; Synthetic gemstones; Catalyst; Paint pigment

Box 3-G. Green Chemistry: Benign by Design

Much attention has focused on pollution prevention in the last five years, and, more recently, there has been a move afoot to achieve pollution prevention through "green chemistry" or "benign by design" chemicals. This approach takes into consideration the environmental impact of a chemical that is being made for a particular purpose, as well as the impact of the process used to manufacture the chemical, and then intentionally designs environmentally benign chemicals and chemical processes. Not only is this approach applicable to new chemicals, but also to existing ones.

Often, many different chemical pathways could theoretically be taken in the synthesis of a desired chemical compound. Traditional chemical design approaches have emphasized the pathway obtaining the greatest yield at the lowest cost. The results have often included the use of high-risk substances as feedstocks, solvents, and catalysts and the generation of hazardous byproducts that require the implementation of various waste management options. The development of alternative pathways to create chemical products cost-effectively in a more environmentally preferable manner presents a new challenge to chemists.

Green chemistry has advanced slowly, with government, academia, scientific organizations, and industry participating to varying degrees. EPA has developed a "designing safer chemicals" program to encourage research based on an understanding of the mechanism of toxicity of chemicals. EPA has also been working with the National Science Foundation in establishing grants for research to develop processes that are environmentally preferable to existing ones. Numerous academic research facilities have become involved in the search for green chemistry, and some have joined with industry in specific ventures. The American Chemical Society has sponsored several symposia on green technology, as well as other pollution prevention approaches. Industry,

significant toxicity. Handling toxic chemicals is thus an inherent characteristic of chemical manufacturing — perhaps more so than for any other stage in commerce.

Third, while there may be alternative pathways, usually they are limited, and in any case they must contain the necessary elements to synthesize the desired product. For example, if an application requires polyvinylchloride (PVC) plastic, almost inevitably cancer-causing vinyl chloride will be needed as a reagent.

There is no database that permits an overview of the status and trends of reagent use from the national, company, or facility level. The 1979 TSCA Chemical Inventory provided for reporting of site-limited intermediates[u] (i.e., reagents that are produced and consumed at the same site), but this served as a criterion for excluding them from reporting in subsequent updates.

Process Aids — Specific and General

While reagents containing the necessary elements are required to make the intended product, large amounts of other chemicals are usually involved in the process. A chemical that facilitates the desired reaction but that is neither produced or consumed in the process is a

[u] Production amounts for site-limited intermediates on the TSCA Chemical Inventory are not available.

overall, has approached green chemistry with caution, due to concerns about such issues as efficiency, cost, and patent infringements (e.g., modifying another company's patented chemical). However, some results have been positive not only for the environment, but also for the efficiency and cost of manufacturing, thus making green chemistry potentially more attractive to industry in the future.

Projects that have been developed include:

- A new process to produce quinoic acid incorporates the use of bacteria. The process releases sugar instead of benzene, a known carcinogen and problem pollutant.
- Supercritical carbon dioxide (carbon dioxide between the liquid and gaseous state) has been used as a solvent for various reactions, substituting for environmentally problematic solvents such as benzene and chlorofluorocarbons (CFCs).
- The metabolism of benzo(a)anthracene to a carcinogen can be disrupted by replacing a hydrogen atom on the molecule with a fluorine atom, without reducing the compound's efficacy.

Sources: Joe Breen, "Green Chemistry: Benign by Design," *Chemicals in Progress,* 15, no. 1 (Spring 1994): 18-21; Faye Flam, "EPA Campaigns for Safer Chemicals," *Science,* 265 (September 9, 1994): 1519; U.S. Environmental Protection Agency, "Design for the Environment: Chemical Design Project," April 1993; "DfE Project Updates," *Chemicals in Progress,* 15, no. 2 (Summer 1994): 21-22.

process aid. Process aids may be specific and important or essential to the process, or they may be general and easily substituted in the process.

A heterogeneous catalyst, mentioned earlier, is one special example of a specific process aid. Often homogeneous catalysts (i.e., those dissolved in a reaction solution) fall into the same category. While chemists and chemical engineers continually seek better catalysts, they are not easily substituted. Many times acidic or caustic reaction conditions are essential. If so, the presence of an acid or base as a processing aid is essential.

General process aids usually have significant alternatives possible. For example, many solvents serve a general purpose, such as to clean a reaction vessel or to bring reagents together in solution. What solvent is used may not matter, so long as it cleans the vessel or dissolves the ingredients. If a general processing aid has adverse environmental consequences, substitutes can usually be considered, in contrast to essential processing aids for which few substitutes, if any, can serve. Research efforts for a limited number of process aids aim to identify alternatives. Chlorinated solvents (particularly those that deplete stratospheric ozone) are probably the most well-known topics for such research, where many alternatives are being identified and implemented.

Open vs. Closed Systems

A very important environmental consideration is whether a use is open or closed. In an open system the chemicals can be released to one or more environmental media. For example, the outdoor piles of salts and other reagents at chemical plants represent open systems. On the other hand, a reaction vessel in which the chemical is contained, thus preventing human and environmental exposures and resulting risks, is a closed system. Most gas extractions are done in closed systems if for no other reason than to prevent loss of the product to the air.

The environmental importance of open vs. closed systems applies at every stage in commerce. It is particularly important in chemical manufacturing, however, because choices between open and closed methods are often available, the toxicity of the materials being used is often high, and the materials involved are often liquids or gases that can easily escape.

Processing and Fabricating

After chemicals are manufactured, if they are not used to make other chemicals, they often are processed (formulated) into mixtures or fabricated into articles. Processing is the blending of multiple chemicals into a product. Examples include the formulation of paints, detergents, furniture strippers, pesticides, aerosol sprays, and cake mixes. Fabrication is the assembly of different components, each with its own chemical composition, into a hybrid product. Examples of fabrication include radio and computer assembly, metal plating, plastic coating, and the painting of metal parts.

In either case, processing or fabrication, this is the stage in commerce in which toxic chemicals most often get incorporated into end-use applications. Therefore, being a formulation ingredient and being a fabricating component are two important environmentally relevant conditions of use. It is useful to keep formulation and fabrication distinct, because formulated products usually must be chemically separated for recycling, whereas fabricated articles can often be physically disassembled.

Distribution

The distribution phase of commerce also raises environmental issues where chemicals are concerned. Whenever more than one facility or place of use is involved in the commercial flow of a chemical and its derivatives, transportation and distribution must occur. Chemicals are moved in bulk by a variety of means, including truck, barge, train, and pipeline. An accident or a spill can release chemicals to the environment and potentially expose people. In processed form and in articles, chemicals flow around, as well as in and out of, the country by every possible mode of transportation.

The Chemical Manufacturers Association maintains the *Chemtrek* database on chemical shipments. In the event of an accident, this system is available to identify the contents of a shipment, its possible health and environmental consequences, and the most appropriate clean-up method. Otherwise, the shipment data in the system are considered proprietary. Therefore, *Chemtrek* is not available for national analyses of trends in shipment methods, such as which chemicals are being shipped where and by what means, nor is it available for company- or facility-level analysis and accountability.

The other national database related to distribution is the Emergency Response Notification System (ERNS) discussed earlier, which contains accident reports relayed to the federal government.

Product Use

While many of the environmental consequences of toxic chemicals relate to the industrial processes in which they are used and the manner in which such processes are operated, many chemicals are used as or in products. These uses can have major environmental consequences, again depending upon the nature of the chemicals involved and their conditions of use. Fuel use, commercial/industrial vs. consumer use, dispersive vs. closed system use, indoor vs. outdoor use, and direct human exposure uses are all important environmentally distinct conditions of end use. (See Table 3-13.) Note that many chemicals, even a batch of a single chemical made at a single time by a single facility, are subsequently used in many different types of products and under different conditions. It is the diversity of chemical use that makes this stage of chemicals in commerce particularly difficult to characterize and track for information-gathering and policy analysis purposes.

Fuel

The use of chemicals as fuels in the United States is huge. Fuels dominate the manufactured chemicals reported to the 1989 TSCA Inventory Update. Although the update does not classify chemicals by their use, a great proportion of the top 100 chemicals (by production amount) on the list are clearly fuels. In fact, it is clear that fuel uses are the dominant ones in terms of production amount and use of chemicals in commerce. (See Table 3-6.)

Much of the focus on fuels to date has been on energy use, carbon dioxide emissions and their global-warming potential, and combustion products. Less attention has centered on the health and environmental effects from human exposures to unburned fuels and releases to the environment; yet given the huge quantities of fuels being used, population exposures are likely to be higher than for practically any other uses of chemicals.

Data availability on fuels greatly exceeds that on other chemicals. The Department of Energy has numerous databases on fuel and energy use in the United States and worldwide.

Commercial/Industrial vs. Consumer Use

User knowledge of the risks of chemicals can differ substantially from industrial to commercial to public use of a product. The setting is therefore an important distinction in the condition of use. Consumers range widely in age, literacy, and physical ability. In the workplace, workers are on average healthier than the general population and can be informed of and trained to address the hazards associated with different chemicals and work practices in a way that would be impossible for the general public. Therefore, the presence of some hazardous chemicals in some products may be more problematic in consumer products than industrial ones. This is the underlying philosophy of allowing persons certified as pesticide applicators to use certain chemicals although they are banned for use by the general public.

Dispersive vs. Closed System

Whether a chemical product is used in dispersive conditions or in a closed system has considerable environmental significance, parallel to the potential consequences of open- vs. closed-system manufacture. An agricultural pesticide or aerosol spray designed to deliver chemicals directly into the environment poses issues quite different from those of chemicals on the inner layers of photographic film or inside a home smoke detector, neither of which should come into direct contact with humans or the environment. Production data without end-use data cannot provide the total picture. Knowing that Company X increased its production of Chemical Y, a highly toxic substance and suspected carcinogen (e.g., formaldehyde), would give more cause for alarm if the intended use were a household room deodorizer than if it were a completely enclosed use. Presently available data do not provide this picture.

Indoor vs. Outdoor

As people lead most of their lives indoors, yet the ecosystem is largely outdoors, the distinction between indoor and outdoor uses is important. A chemical that harms fish but not humans may be more dangerous if used in an agricultural pesticide than if used in carpeting, at least in regard to consequences stemming from the use stage. A chemical that may not be particularly hazardous to humans when dispersed in the outdoor air may be extremely hazardous when humans are exposed to it for many hours a day in indoor air.

Direct Human Exposure Uses and Poisons

Clearly, chemicals designed for intentional direct human exposure, such as pharmaceuticals, foods, water additives, and cosmetics, represent an important condition of use, as do chemicals designed to be toxic and used as poisons (e.g., pesticides and warfare agents). Long-standing government programs cover the chemicals used in these capacities, and each program has its own databases and means of tracking progress.

Type of Product Retirement

While humans and the environment are exposed to chemicals from industrial waste and product use, such exposures also occur from products as they are retired from use. Here the environmental management hierarchy applies, as it does for industrial waste — source reduction being the much-preferred option, followed in decreasing preference by recycling, energy recovery, treatment, and disposal to land, air, or water. (See Chapter 1.) As for most other stages and conditions of use, there is no national database available to assess the status and trends in the disposition of products at the end of their life cycle.

Analyses in Future Editions of *Toxics Watch*

Future *Toxics Watch* reports will build on the groundwork laid in this chapter. Many databases remain to be analyzed for their contributions to a national overview of toxics in commerce, although none promises both the scope and the detail needed to establish a clear view of present conditions and future prospects. Future editions of *Toxics Watch* will review:

- other databases in EPA, especially those covering pesticides, food, drugs, and cosmetics;
- data on inorganic chemicals and polymers, excluded from TSCA coverage;
- data on toxic chemical spills and accidents reported to the federal Emergency Response Notification System (ERNS);
- information on minerals (collected by the Bureau of Mines), fuels (Energy Information Administration), and chemical production (Census Bureau), identified earlier in this chapter.

The universe of toxics in commerce is so broad, so little understood, and so important for human health and the environment, that topics for further exploration abound. In particular, future *Toxics Watch* reports will look closely at uses of chemicals that pose likely threats to the environment and offer fruitful opportunities for intervention. They will explore ways to address concerns about the overwhelming predominance in commerce of chemicals unreviewed for their potential to cause harm. And they will examine emerging developments in government, industry, and commerce that respond to concerns about chemicals in the environment and in the marketplace.

---

1 Chemical Abstracts Service, Columbus, OH.

2 Joel A. Tickner and Hillel Gray, *Accidents Do Happen*, National Environmental Law Center and United States Public Interest Research Group, August 1994.

3 *Characterization of Municipal Solid Waste in the United States, 1992 Update*, Report prepared by Franklin Associates, Ltd., for the U.S. Environmental Protection Agency, Prairie Village, Kansas, 1992.

4 Marc S. Reisch, "Top 50 Chemicals Production Rose Modestly Last Year," *Chemical and Engineering News*, 72, no. 15 (April 11, 1994): 12-15.

5 Marc S. Reisch, "Output of Polymers Increased Almost 3%," *Chemical and Engineering News*, 72, no. 15 (April 11, 1994): 15-16.

6 Bureau of Mines, U.S. Department of the Interior, *Mining and Quarrying Trends in the Metals and Industrial Minerals Industries*, Washington, DC, 1992.

7 Bureau of Mines, U.S. Department of the Interior, *Mineral Commodities Summaries 1994*, Washington, DC, January 1994.

8 Reisch, "Top 50 Chemicals Production Rose Modestly Last Year," 13.

9 Energy Information Administration, U.S. Department of Energy, *Manufacturing Consumption of Energy, 1991.*

10 Mike Conner, Energy Information Administration, telephone conversation, January 23, 1995.

Chapter 4

Toxics in Waste: Overview and Key Facilities

Introduction

With the passage of the Pollution Prevention Act of 1990 (PPA),[a] Congress established as statute a national policy of preventing pollution or reducing waste at its source. According to the Act, source reduction "reduces the amount of any hazardous substance, pollutant, or contaminant entering any waste stream or otherwise released into the environment . . . prior to recycling, treatment, or disposal." This focus on source reduction is part of the broader concept of an environmental management hierarchy in which source reduction should be considered first so that waste is not generated. Once the waste exists, management options in priority order include: recycling, energy recovery, and treatment. Release and disposal to the environment is the last and least desirable option. (See Box 4-A.)

The PPA also mandated the collection of data leading to an estimate of toxic waste generation at facilities (see Toxics Release Inventory Reporting Categories, below). Previously, the data collected on toxic chemicals in waste at industrial facilities by U.S. EPA since 1987 were limited primarily to environmental releases and transfers: direct discharges of toxic or hazardous chemicals to air, land, and water, as well as shipments of waste to other locations.

Passage of the PPA was a milestone making pollution prevention a national policy objective. (See Box 4-B.) To underscore this policy shift, EPA was given the tasks of developing standardized methods of measuring source reduction and providing a biennial report to Congress that, among other topics, evaluates the usefulness and validity of the data collected by the Agency under the PPA for estimating source reduction. In a similar vein, *Toxics Watch 1995* examines in Chapter 6 the progress made toward the goal of integrating pollution prevention into business and regulatory practice. This Section of the report examines the

[a] Omnibus Budget Reconciliation Act of 1990, Public Law 101-508, 104 Stat. 1388-321 *et seq.*

Box 4-A. Environmental Management Hierarchy, Source Reduction Activities, and Waste Management Options

Environmental Management Hierarchy

The environmental management hierarchy stresses the importance of pollution prevention by making *source reduction* the first priority. Source reduction makes waste management unnecessary, since waste is not generated. When source reduction is not possible or has been implemented, the remaining waste should first be managed by *recycling*. The quantity not recycled should be used for *energy recovery*, if possible. The next waste management option is *treatment*. Only when all other waste management options have been employed should waste be *released or disposed of*.

The hierarchy places the focus on doing the least harm to the environment. Business decisions may alter the order of consideration of waste management options for a particular company or facility, but a company seeking to practice superior environmental management will examine and maximize use of source reduction.

Source Reduction Activities

Process or procedure modifications allow a manufacturer to operate the manufacturing process more efficiently, either by using less raw material or by making more efficient use of the raw material. For example, process parameters could be varied (e.g., operating temperature), or the order of operations in the manufacturing process could be changed. *Operational modifications* such as improvements in housekeeping, maintenance, training, and inventory control are all measures to use, handle, and track toxic chemicals more effectively. *Equipment or technology modifications* are changes in the equipment or production technology that result in more efficient use of raw materials or elimination of certain raw materials. *Substitution of raw materials* is switching from a toxic chemical as a raw material to a non-toxic alternative without a change in product. *Redesign of products* results in manufacturing a new product that may or may not meet the same specifications as the previous product, but is an acceptable substitute. The product may use non-toxic raw materials in manufacturing or may be produced by a manufacturing process that results in less waste.

Definitions of Waste Management Options

Recycling is the extraction of a chemical from a stream that would otherwise have been waste. By definition, a recycling process yields the same chemical that went into the recycling process, as opposed to another chemical or substance. If "Chemical A" is used to make a product, and the waste stream contains "Chemical A" and other substances, "Chemical A" is recycled if it is extracted from the waste stream as "Chemical A" and not "Chemical B." The recycled chemical can be returned to the original production process, used in other processes, or sold as a separate product.

Energy recovery is the combustion or burning of a chemical to produce heat. To be considered energy recovery, the chemical must produce enough heat to keep burning. The heat not used to sustain combustion can be used for a variety of purposes, such as in a boiler to produce hot water or electricity. The chemical is destroyed by the energy recovery process. Energy recovery differs from incineration because incineration generally does not sustain combustion on its own, and heat may not be extracted.

Treatment can involve a variety of processes that change a chemical into another substance. As with energy recovery, the chemical is essentially destroyed through treatment — even though some substance may remain after treatment, it will not be the original chemical. The treated chemical may be used for other purposes, but will not be used in its original form.

Release/disposal is the direct discharge of waste to air, water, or land, including fugitive air emissions, point source air emissions, surface water discharges, injections of waste underground into deep wells, and disposal in landfills.

Box 4-B. Making Pollution Prevention a Priority: Selected Quotations

Our long term strategy invests more in pollution prevention, energy efficiency, and solar energy.
— President Bill Clinton, April 1993[1]

I have four priorities for the Agency. First, pollution prevention . . . . Pollution prevention is our best hope for the future of environmental protection: not just environmental regulation, but environmental protection.
— Carol Browner, Administrator, U.S. EPA, April 1993[1]

We have learned the inherent limitations of treating and burying wastes. A problem solved in one part of the environment may become a new problem in another part. We must curtail pollution closer to its point of origin so that it is not transferred from place to place.
— William Reilly, Administrator, U.S. EPA, December 1990[1]

EPA should shift the focus of its environmental protection strategy from end-of-the-pipe controls to preventing the generation of pollution.
— U.S. EPA Science Advisory Board, September 1988[1]

New Jersey has already enacted restructuring measures that will be hallmarks of a new era of environmental protection, where agencies will promote pollution prevention, public access, efficiency, and a 'holistic' environmental awareness.
— Scott A. Weiner, Commissioner, New Jersey Department of Environmental Protection[1]

We are working to emphasize pollution prevention, reduce and eliminate waste, and make our products safer to produce and use.
— Frank Popoff, Chairman and CEO, The Dow Chemical Company[2]

Source reduction is fundamentally different and more desirable than waste management and pollution control . . . . there are significant opportunities for industry to reduce or prevent pollution at the source through cost-effective changes in production, operation and raw materials use. Such changes offer industry substantial savings in reduced raw material, polluti9on control, and liability costs as well as help protect the environment and reduce risks to worker health and safety.
— H.R. 5931, Pollution Prevention Act of 1990 [3]

[1] Reprinted from *Industrial Pollution Prevention Handbook*, Harry M. Freeman, ed., New York: McGraw-Hill, Inc., 1995.
[2] Dow Chemical Company, *Dow Environment, Health and Safety Annual Report*, October 1993.
[3] Introduced by Representative Howard Wolpe.

Box 4-C. TRI and BRS Data Reporting Systems

	TRI	BRS Data
Legislative acts and important amendments	Superfund Amendments and Reauthorization Act of 1986 (SARA), Public Law 99-499, Title III, Sec. 313. Also the Pollution Prevention Act of 1990, 42 U.S.C. 13101 *et seq.*	Resource Conservation and Recovery Act of 1976 (RCRA), 42 U.S.C. §6901 *et seq.* Also the Hazardous and Solid Waste Amendments of 1984 (HSWA), Public Law 98-616
Reporting chain	Facilities report to EPA	Facilities report to states, states report to EPA
Summary reports	For 1987 through 1992 data	For 1987, 1989, and 1991 data
First year of publicly available data	1987 1991 Pollution Prevention Act data	1985 state summaries 1987 facility data
How often data are reported	Annually	Biennially
Latest available reporting year	1992	1991
Frame of reference for reporting	Chemical-specific, multimedia, facility-wide	Waste-stream-specific, facility-wide; does not include air emissions
Number of facilities in latest year	23,630	24,378 (not including facilities claiming data as confidential)
Percent of facilities reporting to one system that also report to the other in latest available year[a]	46%	43%
Number of report forms in latest year	81,016	304,796 (forms reporting on waste generation)
Industries that report	Manufacturers in SIC codes 20-39	Treatment, storage, and disposal facilities under RCRA, regardless of industry
Facilities that report[b]	Manufacturers of the chemical: produce 25,000 pounds per chemical per year. Other users: use 10,000 pounds per chemical per year	Depends on waste management methods used or "large quantity generator" status (See BRS Reporting Requirements, in text)
Number of chemicals reported in latest year	316 chemicals and 20 chemical categories	Approximately 700 single and multiple chemical waste codes; also waste codes based on waste characteristics, rather than specific chemicals
Number of chemicals reported to one system also reported to the other in latest year	All	Not all waste codes are comprised of specific chemicals, so number cannot be determined

[a] Percent calculated by finding number of facilities reporting to TRI in 1992 that also reported valid EPA Identification Numbers (used to identify facilities in BRS). The EPA Identification Numbers were checked against the 1991 BRS data to see which facilities had actually reported.

[b] Each system excludes certain facilities or wastes. For further details, consult the legislative acts.

national environmental data currently available to the public with an eye toward estimating waste generation and amounts of source reduction in the United States.

National Data Reporting Systems

EPA currently administers two national reporting systems for collecting multimedia data from facilities on toxics in waste: the Toxics Release Inventory (TRI) and the Resource Conservation and Recovery Act (RCRA) Biennial Reporting System (BRS).[b] Both TRI and BRS provide potentially valuable information for examining toxics in waste at the local, state, and national levels, and both are publicly accessible. (See Box 4-C.)

Since 1987 TRI has collected data from industrial manufacturing facilities operating under Standard Industrial Classification (SIC) codes 20-39. (See Appendix L.) A facility must complete a TRI form for each reportable chemical used in quantities at or above the reporting threshold.[c] (See Box 6-C for further information on SIC codes covered by TRI and BRS reporting.) TRI requires reporting quantities of toxic chemicals on a chemical-specific basis in environmental releases to air, water, underground injection, and land; off-site transfers; and on- and off-site waste management by type of waste management activity. For the purposes of this report, waste generation under TRI is calculated as the sum of releases, off-site transfers to disposal, and amounts managed on-and off-site. This is called "production-related waste" and is the sum of Sections 8.1 through 8.7 on TRI Form R. Facilities must also submit information on types of source reduction activities undertaken and the methods used to identify source reduction opportunities, but not the amount of waste reduced as a result of the source reduction activities.

In contrast, BRS collects data from reporting facilities on the generation and management of individual liquid and solid hazardous waste streams at reporting facilities. BRS does not include air emissions. Facilities must report to BRS if they are "large quantity generators" or if they treat, store, or dispose of RCRA hazardous waste on site by methods that require RCRA permits.

BRS considers waste streams to be hazardous based in part on toxicity but also on other properties. Individual waste streams at facilities are reported to BRS if they exhibit RCRA characteristics for toxicity, ignitability, corrosivity, or reactivity. BRS waste streams may or may not contain TRI chemicals. Although the universe of chemicals reported to BRS is larger than the TRI universe due to the various criteria for definition as "hazardous waste" in RCRA, *quantities* of the individual chemical constituents are

[b] TRI legislation: Superfund Amendments and Reauthorization Act of 1986 (SARA), Public Law 99-499, Title III, Sec. 313. Also the Pollution Prevention Act of 1990, 42 U.S.C. 13101-13109. BRS legislation: Resource Conservation and Recovery Act of 1976 (RCRA), Public Law 94-580, 42 U.S.C. 6901-6992. Also the Hazardous and Solid Waste Amendments of 1984 (HSWA), Public Law 98-616.

[c] Current threshold amounts are 25,000 pounds per year for manufacturers or processors of the chemical and 10,000 pounds per year for facilities that otherwise use the chemical.

not reported to BRS, nor do the quantities of individual chemicals determine whether a given waste stream is "hazardous." Instead, the total volume of each waste stream, including any water, soil, or other material, must be reported. The entire stream is considered hazardous and must be reported on the BRS form if any portion of the stream meets any of the RCRA hazard characteristics described above.

Not all waste streams reported to BRS contain toxic chemicals. This *Toxics Watch* report focuses on specific toxic chemicals, and so it includes only those BRS waste streams containing TRI chemicals or waste streams defined as toxic by RCRA. (See Appendix E.) It excludes waste streams defined solely as ignitable, corrosive, or reactive, but not designated as toxic or as containing toxic chemicals, because those waste streams cannot be grouped or compared with other toxics in waste. BRS data classified as confidential also had to be excluded.[d] Even with these exclusions, the pounds of BRS waste containing toxic chemicals dwarf the pounds of TRI waste because BRS waste volumes include water, soil, and other materials mixed with the toxic constituents of BRS waste, while only the amount of the toxic chemical itself is included in TRI. (See Box 4-D.)

In 1991, the latest year for which BRS data are available, TRI waste generation totaled 36.3 billion pounds, while BRS toxic waste generation was an order of magnitude higher, totaling 948.2 billion pounds.[e] The differences in the raw data for the two reporting systems lead to considerable confusion in characterizing toxics in waste. Also, large amounts of waste or changes in waste at a handful of key facilities dominate both TRI and BRS. These facilities are largely responsible for the trends in geographic, chemical, and industry distribution of waste visible in the data that are reported to the systems. To the extent that any inaccuracies or anomalies exist in the data from these key facilities, misleading conclusions might be drawn from the overall data picture.

This chapter and Chapters 5, 6, and 7 examine the TRI and BRS data to evaluate the types of information available from both systems and to present what those data reveal about past, current, and projected toxic waste management and pollution prevention. Wherever possible, the data have been explained or adjusted to account for the undue effect of individual facilities.

[d] John Sager of EPA's Office of Solid Waste estimates that waste generation that is considered to be Confidential Business Information (CBI) amounted to no more than 40 billion pounds in the 1991 BRS. This figure is for all BRS waste, not just BRS toxic waste as defined in this report.

BRS CBI data are not used in this report; however, CBI data in TRI are included in the totals. The total production-related waste for which the chemical identity is claimed as trade secret is 689,138 pounds for 1991. TRI Section 8 data for 1991 is the data reported as "previous year" on the 1992 Form R, unless otherwise specified.

[e] This report uses TRI data from EPA's public data release in April 1994 and BRS data made available by EPA June 30, 1994.

Summary of Findings

- TRI and RCRA BRS are the two major sources of national, multimedia data on toxics in waste, although the focus of each system is different. Facilities report amounts of specific chemicals in waste to TRI. In contrast, facilities report total amounts of materials in waste streams to BRS, including toxic chemicals and carrier materials such as water or soil.

- Generation of toxic waste, as reported to both TRI and BRS, increased between the last two reporting years of data available for this report.

  — TRI production-related waste increased by 3 percent between 1991 and 1992, from 36.3 billion pounds to 37.3 billion pounds. More facilities showed decreases between the two years than increases, but the size of the average increase exceeded the size of the average decrease. Facilities have projected a further increase in production-related waste of 0.3% by 1994 from 1992 levels.

  — Generation of BRS toxic waste increased 9 percent between 1989 and 1991, from 482.6 billion pounds to 526.3 billion pounds. These figures represent those waste codes reported in both years. Additional waste codes were added for 1991 reports, and these new codes generated an additional 421.9 billion pounds of toxic waste.

- Neither TRI nor BRS allows clear measurement of changes in amounts of generation of specific chemicals in waste due to source reduction.

  — TRI facilities report whether or not source reduction activities were undertaken during a reporting year, but not the pounds of toxic chemicals reduced.

  — The production or activity index reported to TRI cannot be used in conjunction with changes in production-related waste to calculate the amount of source reduction as a substitute for direct reporting of the amount of source reduction by facilities.

  — BRS facilities report amounts of individual waste streams reduced by source reduction, but this quantity does not allow calculation of reductions in specific chemical waste.

- Amounts of waste generated, as reported to TRI and BRS, decreased at facilities reporting source reduction activities, but this decrease was more than offset by increases at facilities not reporting source reduction activities.

  — 36 percent of TRI facilities reported undertaking source reductions in 1992, and these facilities were responsible for 28 percent of 1992 total production-related waste. Production-related waste decreased by less than one-half of 1 percent between 1991 and 1992 at facilities reporting source reduction activities to TRI in 1992. In contrast, production-related waste increased by 4 percent

Box 4-D. Waste Generation, Source Reduction, and Waste Management in TRI and BRS

The data elements reported to TRI and BRS relate directly to the flow of input materials, product, and waste in manufacturing facilities. (See Figure 4-1.) Input material enters the facility and goes through a production process. This production process results in product and waste. The product leaves the facility. Some of the waste may go back into the production process or leave the facility in the form of on-site releases and off-site transfers without any waste management. The remaining waste is managed on site; some of the managed waste is returned to production, and the waste still remaining after management leaves the facility as on-site releases and off-site transfers. *Source reduction* decreases the amount of waste that is generated before waste management takes place and before any on-site releases or off-site transfers. Source reduction activities are associated with input material, production, and product. (See Box 4-A for an explanation of waste management options and source reduction activities).

Amounts of waste generation, source reduction, and waste management at facilities are reported in different ways to TRI and BRS. The table in this box describes the data elements reported to each system and how waste generation is calculated.

Figure 4-1. Waste Generation, Source Reduction, and Waste Management

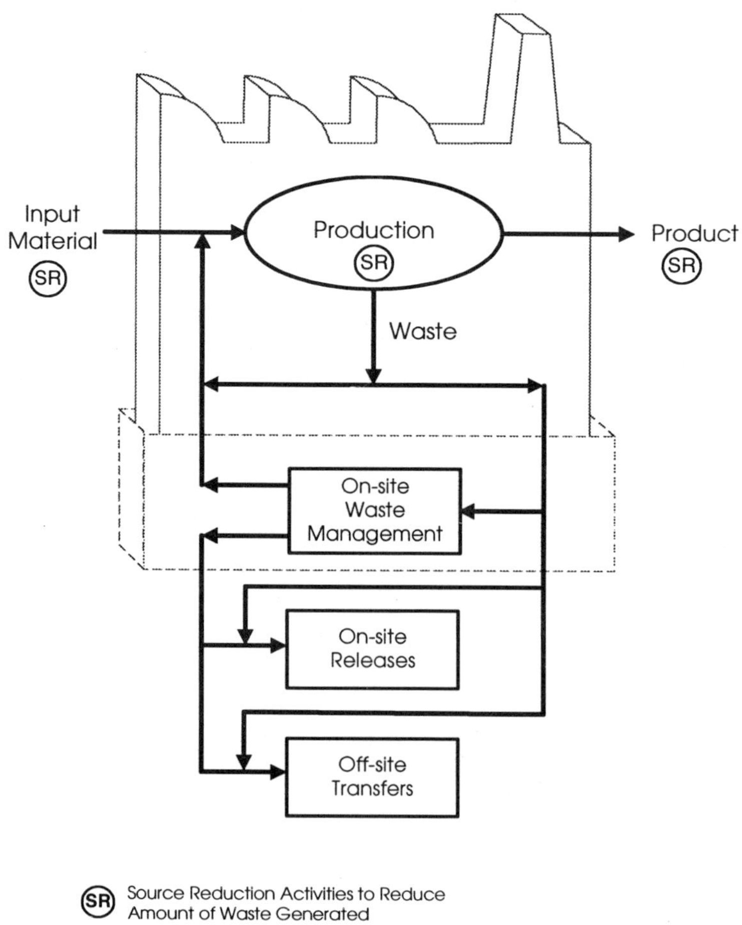

	Data Element Reported to TRI	Data Element Reported to BRS
Source Reduction	Quantity not reported	Amount of waste stream reduced by source reduction
On-site Waste Management	Quantity of chemical in waste stream recycled on site	Amount of waste stream recycled on site
	Quantity of chemical in waste stream used for energy recovery on site	Amount of waste stream used for energy recovery on site
	Quantity of chemical in waste stream treated on site	Amount of waste stream treated on site
On-site Releases	Quantity of chemical in fugitive air emissions	Not reported
	Quantity of chemical in point source air emissions	Not reported
	Quantity of chemical in surface water discharges	Amount of surface water discharges of waste stream*
	Quantity of chemical injected underground in deep wells	Amount of waste stream injected underground in deep wells*
	Quantity of chemical discharged to land	Amount of waste stream discharged to land*
	Quantity of chemical in waste stream sent off site for recycling	Amount of waste stream sent off site for recycling*
Off-site Transfers	Quantity of chemical in waste stream sent off site for energy recovery	Amount of waste stream sent off site for energy recovery*
	Quantity of chemical in waste stream sent off site for treatment	Amount of waste stream sent off site for treatment*
	Quantity of chemical in waste stream discharged to publicly owned treatment works (POTWs)	Amount of waste stream discharged to POTWs*
Waste Generated	Calculated as quantity of on-site waste management of chemical plus quantity of releases of chemical plus quantity of off-site transfers of chemical	Reported directly as amount of waste stream generated on site; does not include air emissions

* Data element reported to BRS but not used in this report.

between 1991 and 1992 at facilities reporting no source reduction activities to TRI in 1992.

— 51 percent of BRS facilities reporting toxic waste also reported undertaking source reduction activities in 1991, and these facilities were responsible for 78 percent of 1991 BRS toxic waste. However, their gains were marginal.

— 12.1 billion pounds of BRS toxic waste were reported as not generated due to source reduction activities in 1991, just 2 percent of the amount of BRS toxic waste that would have been generated without any source reduction activities.

- TRI facilities report a movement toward more desirable waste management options.

— Recycling is the most widely used waste management option reported to TRI and is projected to increase. Fifty-two percent of production-related waste was managed by recycling in 1992, and is expected to rise to 55 percent by 1994.

— Releases to the environment and off-site transfers to disposal is the least widely used waste management option reported to TRI and is projected to decrease. Nine percent of production-related waste was managed by release and disposal in 1992, and is expected to decline to seven percent by 1994.

- Large facilities represent a disproportionately large fraction of TRI production-related waste. Out of 23,630 facilities reporting to TRI in 1992, the 50 facilities reporting the largest amounts of production-related waste to accounted for 43 percent of all such waste. The top 50 represent only 0.2% of TRI facilities. Hence, both the practices of these facilities and the way in which they are reporting waste management activities are of paramount importance in getting a clear picture of TRI production-related waste.

— The five facilities reporting the largest increases and the five reporting the largest decreases in production-related waste to TRI for 1991-1992 had total increases of 292 million pounds and total decreases of 431 million pounds in production-related waste for those years due *solely* to changes they made in calculation of quantities of on-site management of waste, rather than a change in activity (especially recalculating on-site recycling as part of the manufacturing process). These same 10 facilities had increases of 171 million pounds and decreases of 142 million pounds due solely to reporting or database errors.

— Among those facilities contacted to clarify their TRI data, the various reporting issues do not seem to affect nationally aggregated production-related waste reported in this chapter more for increases than for decreases. So, while they may not affect changes from year to year on a national bases, how reporting is done can have a dramatic effect on analyses of local facilities or analyses by chemical, industry, or geography.

Toxics Release Inventory Data

TRI Reporting Categories

The data collected for TRI, in addition to descriptive information about the facility, the chemical, and the activities and uses applying to that chemical, include:

- the quantity of the toxic chemical released on site to air, surface water, underground injection wells, and land (reported in Section 5 of TRI Form R);
- the quantity of the toxic chemical transferred to off-site locations such as publicly owned treatment works (POTWs) or other facilities for the purposes of treatment or disposal, and (since 1991) the quantity transferred to off-site locations for recycling or energy recovery (reported in Section 6 of TRI Form R);
- also since 1991, under the mandates of the 1990 Pollution Prevention Act:
  - — source reduction activities associated with the chemical undertaken in the reporting year (optional until 1991);
  - — quantities of the chemical recycled on site and recycling activities associated with the chemical undertaken in the reporting year;
  - — quantities of the chemical used for energy recovery on site and energy recovery activities associated with the chemical undertaken in the reporting year;
  - — quantities of the chemical treated both on and off site;
  - — quantities of the chemical released/disposed of; and
  - — projections of the quantities expected to be recycled, used for energy recovery, treated on site or off site, and released/disposed of over the next two-year period, as well as those for the previous reporting year (reported in Section 8 of TRI Form R).

(See Appendix A and Box 4-E.)

These data are discussed individually below, beginning with releases and transfers. At the time of this report, announced changes to TRI for the 1994 and 1995 reporting requirements will not expand the kinds of data reported. (See Boxes 4-F and 4-G.)

Box 4-E. Reporting On- and Off-site Waste Management to TRI

The quantities of waste management reported in Section 8 of TRI Form R seem relatively straightforward, but are in fact calculated differently for waste managed on site and waste transferred off site for management.[1] The difference in calculation comes about for two reasons: to avoid reporting the same waste in more than one on-site waste management category, and because a facility knows more about what happens on site than off site.

On-site waste management (recycling, energy recovery, and treatment) is calculated as the amount of a given chemical that is recycled, transformed, or destroyed by the waste management process, as opposed to the total amount of the chemical sent to a waste management unit. In other words, if 1.0 million pounds of "Chemical A" were sent for on-site waste management, and 99 percent was actually recycled, used for energy recovery, or treated, the quantity reported in the on-site waste management options in Section 8 would be 990,000 pounds. If the remaining 10,000 pounds were released to air or disposed of as sludge, it would be accounted for as the "quantity released" — the amount of the chemical released on site or sent off site for disposal. If the full 1.0 million pounds had been reported as managed on site, and the 10,000 pounds also reported as the "quantity released," then there would have been an over-reporting of 10,000 pounds.

Off-site waste management is calculated differently. In this case, it is impossible to know how much of the waste shipped off site is recycled, used for energy recovery, or treated, and how much is released/disposed of after waste management. Therefore, the entire quantity of the chemical shipped off site to be managed by recycling, energy recovery, or treatment is reported in Section 8. The amount sent off site for treatment includes the quantity sent to publicly owned treatment works (POTWs) as well as to other treatment locations.

[1] U.S. Environmental Protection Agency, *1992 Toxics Release Inventory Public Data Release*, EPA 745-R-94-001, April 1994.

Box 4-F. Changes to TRI for 1995

Two rule changes will modify TRI reporting requirements for reporting year 1995, although these changes will affect the number and amounts of chemicals reported rather than existing data elements. The first expands the list of chemicals required to be reported, adding 286 chemicals to the current list of 316 chemicals and 20 chemical categories. The decision to require TRI reporting of these additional chemicals was based on various criteria, including carcinogenicity and other human health effects and effects on the environment.[1] (See Appendix C.)

The second modification is an exemption from TRI reporting requirements reports from a facility on a chemical for which its production-related waste totals 500 pounds or less per year.[2] This modification would result in a 21 percent decrease in the number of forms submitted based on 1992 data. While 36 percent of TRI facilities (8,533 out of 23,630 facilities) reported at least one form with 500 pounds or less of production-related waste in 1992, a total of 13 percent (3,097 out of 23,630 facilities) would be completely exempt from TRI reporting, based on 1992 data. The others use one or more chemicals with a large volume of waste generation and, therefore, would still have to report for the other chemicals.

In 1992 those forms reporting less than 500 pounds of production-related waste accounted for 1.9 million pounds of total production-related waste, or 0.005% of the 37.3 billion pounds of production-related waste reported to TRI that year. These forms also accounted for 1.4 million pounds of releases and transfers to disposal, or 0.04% of the 1992 total.

[1] 59FR61432, November 30, 1994.
[2] 59FR61488, November 30, 1994.

Box 4-G. Federal Compliance with the Right-to-Know Laws and Pollution Prevention Requirements

On August 3, 1993, President Clinton signed Executive Order 12856 into law committing the federal government to report publicly its toxic waste and to reduce its environmental releases of such waste by 50 percent by 1999. The requirements of this Executive Order bring the federal government into step with what has been required of industry under the Emergency Planning and Community Right-to-Know Act (EPCRA) and the Pollution Prevention Act (PPA). The order is intended to provide the public with information on toxic chemicals in their communities, to help communities with emergency planning and notification, to ensure that federal agencies practice pollution prevention in managing their facilities, and to encourage markets for clean technologies and safe alternatives for toxic chemicals.

To achieve the requirements of Executive Order 12856, each federal agency must develop a pollution prevention strategy and is encouraged to do so with the help of the public. The strategy should contain a policy statement that reflects a commitment to pollution prevention through source reduction in the management of its facilities, in its acquisitions, and as the primary means of complying with federal, state, and local environmental requirements.

Executive Order 12856 requires federal facilities to report annually to the Toxics Release Inventory (TRI) such information as is required under Section 313 of EPCRA and PPA. This includes information on TRI waste generated by the facilities, as well as their releases and transfers. Criteria for determining which facilities must report to TRI are the same for *federal* facilities as for *industrial* facilities except in the case of the Standard Industrial Classification (SIC) codes. Only *industrial* facilities that fall within certain SIC codes are subject to TRI reporting. As SIC code delineation does not apply to *federal* facilities, none are excluded on the basis of industrial classification.

Reporting is to be no later than for the 1994 calendar year with reports due by July 1, 1995. Federal facilities must also meet the other emergency planning and notification provisions of EPCRA (Sections 301 through 312), which include submission to the appropriate State Emergency Response Commissions (SERCs) and the Local Emergency Planning Committees (LEPCs) of relevant information on chemicals stored or used at the facility.

Pollution prevention action is another key component of this executive order. Each federal agency must develop voluntary goals to reduce by 50 percent by December 31, 1999, the agency's total releases of toxic chemicals to the environment and off-site transfers of such chemicals for treatment and disposal. This 50-percent reduction should, to the greatest extent practicable, be due to the implementation of source reduction practices. The baseline for measuring the 50-percent reduction is the first year in which a federal agency reports TRI data, but not later than the 1994 reporting year. These pollution prevention goals (except for the baseline year) are similar to those of EPA's voluntary 33/50 Program for industry.

Pollution prevention is further encouraged by requiring each federal agency to establish plans and goals for eliminating or reducing unnecessary acquisition of products that contain extremely hazardous or toxic chemicals as well as an agency's own manufacturing, processing, or use of such chemicals. Steps taken by each agency to achieve these goals shall include review of the agency's standardized documents such as specifications and standards. Federal agencies are encouraged to develop and test innovative pollution prevention technologies, to help expand the markets for these cleaner technologies.

Overview of TRI Releases and Transfers, 1992 and 1988-1992

In 1992, 23,630 facilities reported to TRI, submitting a total of 81,016 individual chemical forms. The average facility thus reported to TRI for three chemicals; the range was one to ninety.

This chapter concentrates on the reasons for changes in the data between years than on the characteristics of the data at any one time. Information on the distribution of the 1992 TRI data by chemical, by industry, and by geographic location can be found in Chapters 5, 6, and 7. Readers are also encouraged to consult EPA's *1992 Toxics Release Inventory Public Data Release* for further detailed analyses of TRI releases and transfers.[1]

The 1988 data are generally superior in quality to the 1987 data, and EPA, most companies, and this report use 1988 TRI figures as the baseline for releases and transfers. In evaluating changes during the 1988-1992 period, *Toxics Watch* includes data on only those chemicals that were reported in each of the years 1988-1992, revealing trends in comparable data. Amounts for chemicals that have been removed from the TRI reporting list (delisted) or added in years after 1988 are not included, nor are transfer categories that were not required for reporting prior to 1991 (see next section). Later sections of this chapter comparing 1991 and 1992 *include* the added chemicals and transfer categories.

A strikingly different picture of the trends in releases and transfers emerges using the two different frames of reference. A restricted look at the type of data reported prior to 1991 shows decreases, not only for 1988-1992 but also for the 1991-1992 portion. By contrast, once broader transfer categories had to be reported and chemicals taken into account that were not reported each of the five years, the data reveal that releases and transfers are increasing.

Prior to addition of the transfer categories added in 1991 and chemicals not reported in each year, TRI releases and transfers decreased by 35 percent from 1988 to 1992 and by 4 percent from 1991 to 1992. The extent of the continuing decrease results from the decline in on-site releases, because releases represent 75 percent of the total. (See Figure 4-2.)

From 1988 to 1992, TRI *releases* of toxic chemicals (for the chemicals reported in every one of the five years dropped from 4.9 billion pounds to 3.2 billion pounds (35 percent). From 1991 to 1992, the corresponding decrease was 216.0 million pounds (6 percent of the 1991 figure). Although there have been fluctuations both up and down in amount of release, the percentage share for each type of release (air, surface water, underground injection, on-site land) has remained steady with over 50 percent of releases being air emissions. (See Figure 4-2 and Table 4-1.)

TRI off-site *transfers* from 1988 to 1992 dropped from 1.6 billion pounds to 1.0 billion pounds, a decrease of 529.7 million pounds (34 percent) from 1988. From 1991 to

Figure 4-2.

TRI Releases and Transfers, 1988-1992

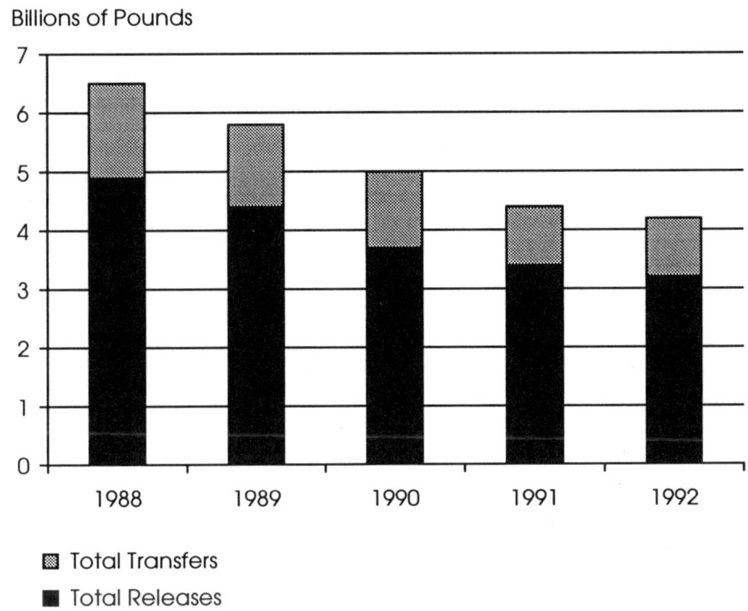

Excludes transfers to recycling and energy recovery

*Table 4-1. Toxics Release Inventory Data, 1988-1992**

	1988 Number	1989 Number	1990 Number	1991 Number	1992 Number	Percent Change 1991-1992 Percent	Percent Change 1988-1992 Percent
Total Facilities	22,395	24,366	24,713	24,181	23,533	- 2.68	5.08
Total Forms	77,873	86,497	86,051	82,658	79,979	- 3.24	2.70
	Pounds	Pounds	Pounds	Pounds	Pounds	Percent	Percent
Form R, Section 5							
Total Air Emissions	2,683,451,601	2,573,987,161	2,304,480,107	2,005,088,636	1,820,965,216	- 9.18	- 32.14
Fugitive Air	829,601,355	796,011,966	713,869,291	616,663,149	536,680,299	- 12.97	- 35.31
Point Source Air	1,853,850,246	1,777,975,195	1,590,610,816	1,388,425,487	1,284,284,917	- 7.50	- 30.72
Surface Water	311,236,419	187,704,802	198,131,625	243,331,324	272,905,180	12.15	- 12.32
Underground Injection	1,343,657,667	1,175,506,563	754,523,494	710,237,637	725,820,874	2.19	- 45.98
On-site Land Releases	514,592,116	440,197,787	436,018,244	414,576,639	337,590,822	- 18.57	- 34.40
Total Releases	4,852,937,803	4,377,396,313	3,693,153,470	3,373,234,236	3,157,282,092	- 6.40	- 34.94
Form R, Section 6							
Transfers to Treatment	492,538,569	467,883,861	374,810,144	351,112,534	389,675,327	10.98	- 20.88
Transfers to POTWs	581,038,548	568,915,677	469,486,355	394,421,377	380,708,363	- 3.48	- 34.48
Transfers to Disposal	484,882,422	400,239,337	433,105,439	262,810,417	256,005,214	- 2.59	- 47.20
Other Off-site Transfers**	14,475,986	8,129,769	12,991,803	10,288,734	16,876,490	—	—
Total Transfers	1,572,935,525	1,445,168,644	1,290,393,741	1,018,633,062	1,043,265,394	2.42	- 33.67
Total Releases and Transfers	6,425,873,328	5,822,564,957	4,983,547,211	4,391,867,298	4,200,547,486	- 4.36	- 34.63

* Excludes delisted and added chemicals and transfers to recycling and energy recovery reported in any year
** No valid code given

1992, the decrease was 191.3 million pounds (4 percent). Unlike the stable distribution of TRI releases, TRI transfers have changed direction. The amount of transfers to disposal and to POTWs decreased, and while the largest amounts were transferred to POTWs in 1988, the largest amounts are going instead to private waste management facilities for treatment in 1992. (See Table 4-1.)

But what appeared to be a trend of decreasing releases and transfers between 1988 and 1992 took on quite a different look when more data were required in 1991.

TRI Releases and Transfers, 1991-1992

Prior to 1991, while off-site transfers to POTWs and disposal facilities were reported to TRI, transfers to recycling or energy recovery facilities were not.[f] Beginning in 1991, companies were required to report this additional information about their management of TRI chemicals in waste, and the expansion of TRI to include these types of transfers shows that the generation of waste was not decreasing, but increasing from 1991 to 1992. (Compare Figures 4-2 and 4-3.)

TRI off-site transfers in 1992, including those wastes destined for recycling and energy recovery, totaled 4.4 billion pounds, an increase of 630.8 million pounds (17 percent) from 1991. (See Table 4-2.)

While transfers to POTWs and to disposal declined by 4 percent and 3 percent, respectively, it became clear that the majority of toxic chemicals in waste transferred off site are being transferred to recycling. In 1992 facilities reported they had transferred off site for recycling 2.8 billion pounds of TRI chemicals, which represents 65 percent of all reported transfers. Transfers to recycling increased from 1991 to 1992 (by 25 percent), as did transfers to treatment (11 percent) and transfers to energy recovery (8 percent). (See Table 4-2.)

Although TRI releases decreased from 1991 to 1992, by 7 percent (from 3.4 to 3.2 billion pounds), these decreases did not offset the increases in transfers to recycling, energy recovery, and treatment. Overall, total TRI releases and transfers increased by 6 percent from 1991 to 1992. (See Figure 4-3 and Table 4-2.)

The net increase in releases and transfers occurred not because relatively large numbers of TRI facilities are reporting increases. Actually, more TRI facilities reported decreases than increases from 1991 to 1992; 39 percent of TRI facilities reporting in both years reported decreases. But the decreases totaled 27 percent while those facilities that did report

[f] Some facilities had reported these off-site transfers prior to 1991 anyway in a manner enabling them to be identified as transfers for recycling or energy recovery. They are excluded from Table 4-1 and the discussion in the previous section, but are included in Table 4-2 and this section along with all chemicals added to the TRI list since 1988. Other facilities in previous years reported these transfers as "other" without identifying them as recycling or energy recovery. Though this number is small overall, an individual facility's totals may not be, making year-to-year comparisons before 1991 difficult for such facilities.

Figure 4-3.

TRI Releases and Transfers, 1991-1992

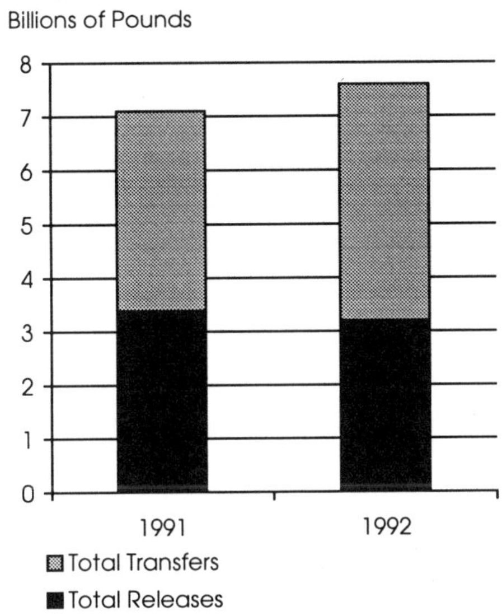

Includes transfers to recycling and energy recovery

Table 4-2. Comparison of TRI Releases and Transfers, 1991-1992

	1991	**1992**	**Change from 1991 to 1992**	
	Number	Number	Number	Percent
Total Facilities	24,294	23,630	-664	-2.7
Total Forms	83,815	81,016	-2,799	-3.3
	Pounds	Pounds	Pounds	Percent
Form R, Section 5				
Total Air Emissions	2,036,678,204	1,844,958,336	-191,719,868	-9.4
Fugitive Air	633,586,799	549,351,729	-84,235,070	-13.3
Point Source Air	1,403,091,405	1,295,606,607	-107,484,798	-7.7
Surface Water Discharges	243,351,148	272,932,953	29,581,805	12.2
Underground Injection	710,366,770	725,946,415	15,579,645	2.2
Releases to Land	414,844,420	337,809,053	-77,035,367	-18.6
Total Releases	3,405,240,542	3,181,646,757	-223,593,785	-6.6
Form R, Section 6				
Transfers to Recycling	2,266,829,164	2,839,825,919	572,996,755	25.3
Transfers to Energy Recovery	443,311,526	477,639,264	34,327,738	7.7
Transfers to Treatment	353,150,798	393,466,540	40,315,742	11.4
Transfers to POTWs	395,560,966	381,096,823	-14,464,143	-3.7
Transfers to Disposal	267,586,409	258,642,577	-8,943,832	-3.3
Other Off-site Transfers*	10,316,150	16,933,490	6,617,340	64.1
Total Transfers	3,736,755,013	4,367,604,613	630,849,600	16.9
Total Releases and Transfers	7,141,995,555	7,549,251,370	407,255,815	5.7

* No valid code given

increases shows a large increase (50 percent). Eleven percent remained the same for both years. (See Figure 4-4 and Table 4-3.)

New TRI Reporting on Production-related Waste, 1991 and Beyond

The additional data reported on the on- and off-site management of TRI chemicals in waste beginning in 1991, as mandated by the Pollution Prevention Act of 1990, is reported in Section 8 of TRI Form R. The slightly different way that releases and transfers are totaled under these requirements than in the past and in other sections of the form, plus varying interpretations of those requirements by facilities, complicates making comparisons among facilities in a given year or between years for the same facility. The next several sections explain the requirements and the confusion, and what this report has done to adjust the data, so that the direction and extent of the changes in production-related waste can be better understood. (See Appendix A.)

How Production-related Waste is Calculated

Production-related waste is the amount of a chemical used at a facility in the manufacture of one or more products that does not end up in those products, either in its original form or as another substance. It may also include the amounts of the chemical that may be generated during manufacture of the products; if these quantities are not used in products or sold as byproducts, they are considered waste. Subsequently, the waste can be released/disposed of or managed on- or off-site by recycling, energy recovery, or treatment. Facilities must report the amounts released/disposed of or managed by each method in Section 8 of TRI Form R. (See Boxes 4-A and 4-E.)

Total production-related waste in *Toxics Watch* is calculated by adding the quantity released/disposed of to the amounts of on- and off-site recycling, energy recovery, and treatment for each chemical. While the quantity of production-related waste reported as released/disposed of in Section 8 should equal the quantity of total releases in Section 5 plus total off-site transfers to disposal in Section 6 minus those releases and off-site transfers for disposal that occurred because of a one-time event not associated with production, the actual data in the TRI database do not balance so neatly. In 1992 the net discrepancy between the Section 8 and Sections 5 and 6 data on releases and off-site transfers to disposal came to 55.8 million pounds. The similar discrepancy for off-site transfers for recycling, energy recovery, and treatment came to 688.3 million pounds. In relationship to the total reported quantities, these numbers are small; EPA attributes the discrepancies to misunderstandings in filling out the form and expects improvement in data quality with time.

Quantities of *non-production-related* waste are aggregated and reported separately in Section 8. Such waste results from remedial actions, spills, catastrophic events, or other one-time events not associated with production processes. (See Chapter 5.)

Figure 4-4.

Change in TRI Releases and Transfers, 1991-1992

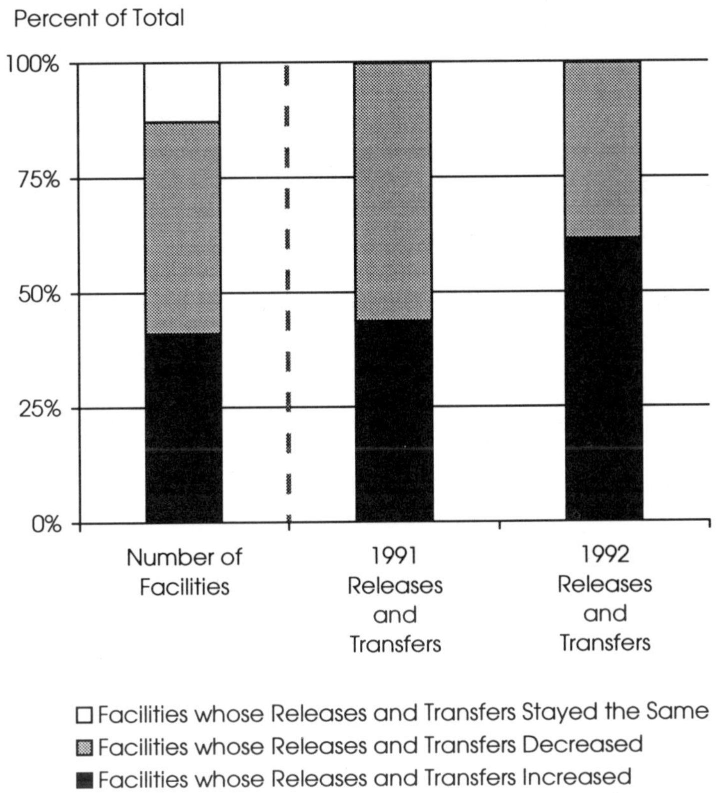

Includes only those facilities reporting in both years

Table 4-3. Comparison of Change in TRI Releases and Transfers between Facilities Reporting Increases and Facilities Reporting Decreases, 1991-1992

			1991 Total Releases and Transfers			1992 Total Releases and Transfers			Percent Change in Average Pounds per Facility
Change from 1991 to 1992	**Facilities** Number	**Percent of Total** Percent	**Pounds** Pounds	**Percent of Total** Percent	**Average Pounds per Facility** Pounds	**Pounds** Pounds	**Percent of Total** Percent	**Average Pounds per Facility** Pounds	Percent
Increased	8,990	34.54	3,051,125,197	42.72	339,391	4,587,283,207	60.76	510,265	50.35
Decreased	10,100	38.80	3,910,714,473	54.76	387,199	2,847,823,279	37.72	281,963	-27.18
Stayed Same	2,803	10.77	18,696,619	0.26	6,670	18,696,619	0.25	6,670	0.00
Did not report in 1991	1,737	6.67	0	0.00	0	95,448,265	1.26	54,950	—
Did not report in 1992	2,401	9.22	161,459,266	2.26	67,247	0	0.00	0	—
Total	26,031	100.00	7,141,995,555	100.00	274,365	7,549,251,370	100.00	290,010	5.70

TRI Production-related Waste and the Environmental Management Hierarchy

Looking at how facilities manage their production-related waste gives an indication of how much emphasis they are placing on the environmental management hierarchy. As stated previously, the "environmental management hierarchy" describes the various options for avoiding or managing waste in an order of preference, starting with the one most beneficial to the environment (source reduction) and proceeding in order through recycling, energy recovery, treatment, and finally disposal, the last resort and the least desirable option. A facility seeking the best environmental management will try to maximize the use of source reduction to avoid generating waste. When waste generation is unavoidable, a facility moves "down" the hierarchy, seeking to manage as much waste as possible by the methods that are the least undesirable. (See Chapter 1 and Box 4-A.)

Although in certain cases facilities may be required to use a certain manufacturing process or manage their waste in a prescribed manner (and therefore cannot switch from one waste management activity to another),[g] this is not usually the case. Calculating the individual amounts of recycling, energy recovery, treatment, or release/disposal as a percentage of production-related waste over the years gives an indication of whether the facilities are making progress in implementing the hierarchy.

TRI Production-related Waste 1991-1992

On- and off-site recycling together represented 52 percent of total waste generated in 1992 by TRI facilities reporting in that year,[h] while energy recovery accounted for 10 percent and treatment of waste for 30 percent. Facilities released and disposed of the final 9 percent of production-related waste. (See Table 4-4.)

A few facilities generate the lion's share of all TRI chemicals in waste. The 50 facilities with the largest total production-related waste accounted for 43 percent of all such waste in 1992. These facilities (0.2 percent of those reporting to TRI in 1992) accounted for 68 percent of all on-site recycling. (See Table 4-5.)

This distribution of types of waste in 1992 is essentially unchanged from 1991 to 1992. (See Table 4-4.) Total production-related waste increased 3 percent from

[g] Facilities manufacturing products for federal use may be required to use specific processes or chemicals (e.g., Defense Department procurement; however, Executive Order 12873 requires the federal government to change procurement specification and standards, so this may not be the case for much longer). The same may also be true for federally regulated products such as pharmaceuticals.

[h] All facilities submitting TRI forms in 1992 are required to report their waste generation amounts for both 1991 and 1992 on the 1992 form, even if they did not submit a form in 1991.

Table 4-4. TRI Production-related Waste by Waste Management Type, 1991-1992

Waste Management Type	1991 Production-related Waste		1992 Production-related Waste	
	Pounds	Percent	Pounds	Percent
Recycled On-site	15,852,682,387	43.7	15,884,194,888	42.5
Recycled Off-site	2,976,812,329	8.2	3,473,894,509	9.3
Energy Recovery On-site	2,842,457,939	7.8	2,941,222,113	7.9
Energy Recovery Off-site	580,710,271	1.6	627,954,600	1.7
Treated On-site	9,868,146,903	27.2	10,326,749,494	27.7
Treated Off-site	680,368,098	1.9	678,373,850	1.8
Released/Disposed Of	3,515,785,150	9.7	3,401,386,170	9.1
Total	36,316,963,077	100.0	37,333,775,624	100.0

36.3 billion pounds in 1991 to 37.3 billion pounds in 1992. This increase was due to more facilities reporting increases than decreases in waste generation from 1991 to 1992. Of all TRI facilities reporting in 1992, 49 percent reported increases in production-related waste from 1991, while 40 percent reported decreases and 11 percent reported no change. The absolute increase was fairly small (1.0 billion pounds), because those facilities whose waste amounts decreased had on average a larger decrease (26 percent) than the average increase for those reporting increases (21 percent). (See Figure 4-5 and Table 4-6.)

Factors in Interpreting TRI Production-related Waste Amounts and Changes

National data on production-related waste and changes in waste management activities may be useful indicators of these trends for the United States as a whole, but certain facilities and industries have a disproportionate effect on the data. The data, as they appear in the publicly available TRI database, appear to show an increase in production-related waste and no change in relative amounts of waste managed by different waste management options for 1991-1992. Before stating categorically that these conclusions reflect how toxic waste is generated and managed throughout the nation, however, it is important to have a clear focus on what is happening at the small number of facilities with the largest amounts of waste or the largest changes in waste.

Influence of Facilities with Largest Increases and Decreases

Four main questions arise when evaluating the effect of individual facilities:

- To what extent do facilities with large amounts (or reporting large changes in amounts) affect the national data?

Table 4-5. The 50 TRI Facilities with Largest Total Production-related Waste, 1992

Rank	Facility	City	State	SIC Code	Recycled On-site Pounds	Recycled Off-site Pounds
1	First Chemical Corp.	Pascagoula	MS	28	4,039,035,000	2,500,000
2	Goodyear Tire & Rubber Co.	Beaumont	TX	28	2,518,250,000	5,400,000
3	Uno-Ven Co.	Lemont	IL	29	5,669,430	65,704
4	Solvay Polymers Inc.	Deer Park	TX	28	397,000,000	0
5	Cyprus Miami Mining Corp.	Claypool	AZ	33	390,075,000	1,715,000
6	Texaco Refining & Marketing	El Dorado	KS	Mult	292,852,030	0
7	Goodyear Tire & Rubber Co.	Houston	TX	28	307,000,000	10,900,000
8	Kemira Inc.	Savannah	GA	28	260,000,000	0
9	National Cooperative Refinery	Mc Pherson	KS	29	0	0
10	Dow Chemical Co.	Freeport	TX	28	91,957,359	9,838
11	SCM Chemicals	Baltimore	MD	28	0	0
12	Coulton Chemical Corp.	Oregon	OH	28	270,000,000	1,009,000
13	Citgo Petroleum Corp.	Lake Charles	LA	Mult	67,000,000	160,036,000
14	Texasgulf Inc.	Aurora	NC	28	0	0
15	Doe Run Co.	Boss	MO	33	110,003,980	121,363,200
16	Allied-Signal Inc.	Chesterfield	VA	28	0	34,000
17	Amoco Oil Co.	Whiting	IN	29	28,900	221,338,573
18	Gates Rubber Co.	Iola	KS	30	218,896,396	376,277
19	Zeneca Inc.	Bucks	AL	28	0	186
20	Bristol-Myers Squibb Co.	Syracuse	NY	28	202,100,000	64,900
21	Celanese Engineering Resins	Bishop	TX	28	184,005,000	16,000
22	Quaker State Corp.	Newell	WV	29	200,000,000	0
23	Courtaulds Fibers Inc.	Axis	AL	28	136,000,000	0
24	Upjohn Co.	Portage	MI	28	161,200,000	0
25	Hoechst-Celanese Corp.	Spartanburg	SC	Mult	180,000,000	710,000
26	Star Ent. Inc.	Union	LA	Mult	0	390
27	PPG Ind. Inc.	Lake Charles	LA	28	98,428,000	92,000
28	Shintech Inc.	Freeport	TX	28	169,780,000	0
29	American Cyanamid Co.	Westwego	LA	28	9,020	217,000
30	Star Ent. Inc.	Port Arthur	TX	29	411,616	141,755,642
31	Dow Chemical Co.	Plaquemine	LA	28	0	0
32	Copper Range Co.	White Pine	MI	None	0	0
33	Westlake Petrochemicals Corp.	Sulphur	LA	28	0	8
34	Du Pont Beaumont Plant	Beaumont	TX	28	38,901,463	0
35	Sterling Chemicals Inc.	Texas City	TX	28	6,000	12,500
36	East Penn Mfg. Co. Inc.	Lyon Station	PA	Mult	123,050,068	2,856,989
37	ARCO Prods. Co.	Carson	CA	29	101,837	0
38	Elkem Metals Co.	Marietta	OH	33	102,000,000	32,000
39	Magnesium Corp. Of America	Rowley	UT	33	4,000	2,926,000
40	PVS Chemicals Inc. of NY	Buffalo	NY	28	104,000,000	0
41	Holnam Inc.	Clarksville	MO	Mult	0	0
42	Eastman Kodak Co.	Kingsport	TN	28	0	21,000
43	Agrico Chemical Co.	Saint James	LA	28	0	30,500
44	Material Service Corp.	Chicago	IL	32	0	0
45	Timken Co.	Canton	OH	33	0	0
46	Rouge Steel Co.	Dearborn	MI	33	289,800	73,360,400
47	Monsanto Co.	Alvin	TX	28	25,080,000	0
48	ARCO Cherry Point Refinery	Ferndale	WA	29	241,840	41,727
49	Pfizer Inc.	Groton	CT	28	76,527,000	45,300
50	Revere Copper Prods. Inc.	Rome	NY	33	87,602,000	1,073,000
	Subtotal				10,857,505,739	748,003,134
	Percent of Total				68.35	21.53
	Total				15,884,194,888	3,473,894,509

Energy Recovery On-site Pounds	Energy Recovery Off-site Pounds	Treated On-site Pounds	Treated Off-site Pounds	Released/ Disposed of Pounds	Total Production-related Waste Pounds
5,024,025	470	0	0	79,216	4,046,638,711
2,505,320	0	569,848	0	130,357	2,526,855,525
127,953,156	24,500,475	329,924,293	4,117	112,117	488,229,292
590,000	0	14,300,000	0	372,000	412,262,000
0	0	0	0	3,165,000	394,955,000
59,223,000	700,000	2,919,996	91,244	1,495,461	357,281,731
0	280,000	888,010	2,800	836,070	319,906,880
0	0	55,518,000	22,250	982,020	316,522,270
312,068,268	0	324,178	0	464,265	312,856,711
47,333,393	0	153,491,817	126,841	8,844,715	301,763,963
0	0	286,910,210	0	897,586	287,807,796
140,000	0	2,278,000	0	42,050	273,469,050
0	4,059	24,334,780	0	6,022,370	257,397,209
0	0	240,568,700	0	14,440,660	255,009,360
0	0	0	0	133,678	231,500,858
0	0	230,000,000	1,400	178,170	230,213,570
0	0	4,144,510	0	1,273,973	226,785,956
0	0	0	143	213,628	219,486,444
0	1,808	208,432,000	495,260	6,386,151	215,315,405
0	552,300	6,560,000	1,714,500	3,438,610	214,430,310
11,007,022	0	14,105,960	8,800	3,047,440	212,190,222
0	0	35,480	1,000	341,275	200,377,755
0	0	14,707,000	0	43,497,458	194,204,458
0	19,183,200	2,596	5,814,770	5,486,728	191,687,294
0	240,000	1,242,390	12,910	895,391	183,100,691
0	0	180,193,300	491	110,770	180,304,951
6,360,843	20	67,695,320	109,674	2,053,157	174,739,014
0	0	0	0	148,062	169,928,062
8,278,210	0	10,010,420	5,369	146,669,560	165,189,579
4,904,984	0	1,516,582	1,531	1,737,288	150,327,643
35,006,000	0	109,861,437	44,001	3,926,076	148,837,514
0	0	140,152,000	0	8,114,000	148,266,000
124,306,722	562,922	16,004,796	0	35,027	140,909,475
17,906,365	0	41,664,360	833,819	40,222,129	139,528,136
78,738,130	19,633	14,688,410	84,483	37,192,950	130,742,106
0	0	962,000	247,530	317,663	127,434,250
908,070	123,020,000	1,740,684	917,590	603,120	127,291,301
0	0	17,000	0	16,575,331	118,624,331
0	0	53,800,000	98	60,762,763	117,492,861
0	0	1,122,118	0	21,672	105,143,790
101,900,000	0	0	0	9,080	101,909,080
21,485,436	3,170,000	43,999,626	127,733	33,072,598	101,876,393
3,555,000	0	6,279,704	0	90,799,975	100,665,179
0	0	99,982,822	0	0	99,982,822
0	0	97,000,000	0	0	97,000,000
0	62,310	15,105,000	0	7,871,221	96,688,731
0	180,000	15,349,150	0	55,852,659	96,461,809
91,000,423	572	3,340,111	0	768,191	95,392,864
1,093,300	439,100	6,631,069	1,841,233	3,521,763	90,098,765
0	0	577,210	36	26,388	89,278,634
1,061,287,667	172,916,869	2,518,950,887	12,509,623	613,187,832	15,984,361,751
36.08	27.54	24.39	1.84	18.03	42.81
2,941,222,113	627,954,600	10,326,749,494	678,373,850	3,401,386,170	37,333,775,624

Figure 4-5.

Change in TRI Total Production-related Waste, 1991-1992

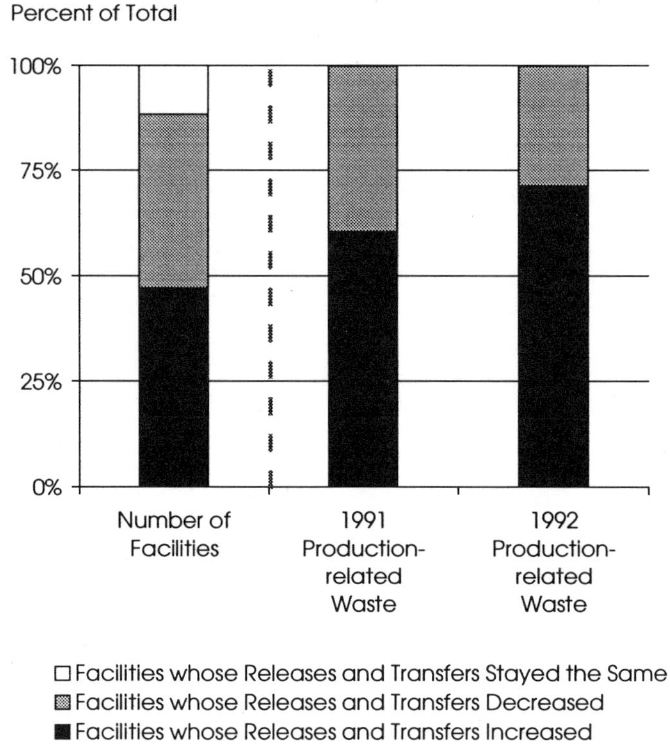

Table 4-6. Change in TRI Production-related Waste, 1991-1992

Change from 1991 to 1992	Facilities: Number	Facilities: Percent of Total	1991 Production-related Waste: Pounds	1991: Percent of Total	1991: Average Pounds per Facility	1992 Production-related Waste: Pounds	1992: Percent of Total	1992: Average Pounds per Facility	Percent Change in Average Pounds per Facility
	Number	Percent	Pounds	Percent	Pounds	Pounds	Percent	Pounds	Percent
Increased	11,557	48.91	21,970,203,405	60.50	1,901,030	26,656,508,746	71.40	2,306,525	21.33
Decreased	9,412	39.83	14,301,448,135	39.38	1,519,491	10,631,955,341	28.48	1,129,617	-25.66
Stayed same	2,661	11.26	45,311,537	0.12	17,028	45,311,537	0.12	17,028	0.00
Total	23,630	100.00	36,316,963,077	100.00	1,536,901	37,333,775,624	100.00	1,579,931	2.80

- To what extent are the trends shown by the key facilities typical of the larger group, or are there identifiable differences between them and the rest?
- Do the characteristics and trends indicated in the data from these facilities accurately portray how they actually manage their waste? If so, their potential effect on the environment is real, whether or not their waste management practices are "typical" of facilities nationwide. If not, their potential effect on the environment might be entirely different than the data seem to show.
- If the large-facility data were disregarded in certain analyses or corrected where they contain significant errors, how would the overall results differ?

The answer to the first question is easy: individual facilities greatly influence the overall data. The average increase between 1991 and 1992 for production-related waste at more than 11,500 TRI facilities reporting increases was 405,000 pounds per facility. (See Table 4-6.) Just 25 facilities reporting the largest increases reported total increases of 1.7 billion pounds, however, which makes their average increase 68.4 million pounds. The total increase in production-related waste from these 25 facilities was 35 percent. Similarly, the 25 facilities with the largest decreases reported decreases of 1.8 billion in production-related waste. This is a decrease of 50 percent from these 25 facilities and represents an average decrease of 70.6 million pounds, where as the average decrease for all facilities reporting decreases was 390,000. (See Tables 4-7 and 4-8.)

The significant influence of these key facilities is evident if one looks at the TRI data excluding them. Setting aside the data of all 50 of the facilities, the result would be a slightly greater increase in waste between the two years (4 percent instead of 3 percent). If the data of the 25 facilities with the largest *increases* were removed, but not those of the 25 largest decreasers, the change would be an overall 2 percent *decrease* in production-related waste (decrease of 696 million pounds); if the data of the 25 facilities with the largest *decreases* were removed, but not those of the 25 largest increasers, the change would be a 8 percent *increase* (2.8 billion pounds).

These two groups of 25 facilities, then, appear to account for the changes observed in the national TRI waste generation data. Their data will also greatly influence any analysis of the data by chemical, by industry sector, or by geographic area. (See Chapters 5 through 7.)

Table 4-7. TRI Production-related Waste for the 25 Facilities with Largest Increase from 1991 to 1992

Rank	Facility	City	State	Total Production-related Waste 1991 Pounds	Total Production-related Waste 1992 Pounds	Increase 1991 to 1992 Pounds	Percent Increase 1991 to 1992 Percent
1	Doe Run Co.	Boss	MO	50,358,284	231,500,858	181,142,574	359.71
2	Star Enterprises Inc.	Union	LA	9,652,137	180,304,951	170,652,814	1,768.03
3	Goodyear Tire & Rubber Co.	Beaumont	TX	2,423,678,742	2,526,855,525	103,176,783	4.26
4	Elkem Metals Co.	Marietta	OH	17,565,510	118,624,331	101,058,821	575.33
5	Revere Copper Prods. Inc.	Rome	NY	1,771,521	89,278,634	87,507,113	4,939.66
6	Dow Chemical Co.	Freeport	TX	215,678,049	301,763,963	86,085,914	39.91
7	ARCO Cherry Point Refinery	Ferndale	WA	14,020,197	95,392,864	81,372,667	580.40
8	Westlake Petrochemicals Corp.	Sulphur	LA	62,669,023	140,909,475	78,240,452	124.85
9	Chevron USA Products Co.	Port Arthur	TX	6,086,761	69,087,239	63,000,478	1,035.04
10	Quantum Chemical Corp.	La Porte	TX	11,825,939	70,556,476	58,730,537	496.62
11	Uno-Ven Co.	Lemont	IL	430,919,553	488,229,292	57,309,739	13.30
12	Du Pont Beaumont Plant	Beaumont	TX	83,788,966	139,528,136	55,739,170	66.52
13	Upjohn Co.	Portage	MI	138,252,387	191,687,294	53,434,907	38.65
14	SCM Chemicals	Baltimore	MD	234,486,858	287,807,796	53,320,938	22.74
15	Union Carbide C & P Co.	Institute	WV	16,951,078	70,121,286	53,170,208	313.67
16	Goodyear Tire & Rubber Co.	Houston	TX	272,059,600	319,906,880	47,847,280	17.59
17	Zeneca Inc.	Bucks	AL	168,773,359	215,315,405	46,542,046	27.58
18	Star Enterprises Inc.	Port Arthur	TX	105,923,573	150,327,643	44,404,070	41.92
19	El Paso Refinery L.P.	El Paso	TX	31,839,021	76,220,876	44,381,855	139.39
20	Johnson Controls Inc.	Garland	TX	9,888,204	52,472,277	42,584,073	430.66
21	Gates Rubber Co.	Iola	KS	177,302,326	219,486,444	42,184,118	23.79
22	Copper Range Co.	White Pine	MI	106,477,000	148,266,000	41,789,000	39.25
23	Material Service Corp.	Chicago	IL	59,067,966	99,982,822	40,914,856	69.27
24	Mississippi Phosphates Corp.	Pascagoula	MS	43,042,844	82,171,447	39,128,603	90.91
25	Allied-Signal Inc.	Chesterfield	VA	193,370,000	230,213,570	36,843,570	19.05
	Subtotal			4,885,448,898	6,596,011,484	1,710,562,586	35.01
	Percent of Total			13.45	17.67		
	Total for All TRI Facilities			36,316,963,077	37,333,775,624	1,016,812,547	2.80

Table 4-8. TRI Production-related Waste for the 25 Facilities with Largest Decrease from 1991 to 1992

Rank	Facility	City	State	Total Production-related Waste 1991 Pounds	Total Production-related Waste 1992 Pounds	Decrease 1991 to 1992 Pounds	Percent Decrease 1991 to 1992 Percent
1	DuPont Chambers Works	Deepwater	NJ	243,531,644	69,782,276	-173,749,368	-71.35
2	Corning Asahi Video Products	State College	PA	163,842,990	21,869,850	-141,973,140	-86.65
3	Phillips 66 Co.	Sweeny	TX	154,483,279	21,901,036	-132,582,243	-85.82
4	Reilly Industries Inc.	Indianapolis	IN	191,028,072	67,283,187	-123,744,885	-64.78
5	Carolina Eastman Co.	Columbia	SC	130,703,470	9,683,370	-121,020,100	-92.59
6	Atochem N.A. Inc.	Calvert City	KY	101,292,955	11,778,204	-89,514,751	-88.37
7	Cosmar Co.	Carville	LA	102,041,342	16,994,607	-85,046,735	-83.35
8	AT&T Network Cable Sys.	Norcross	GA	89,113,151	6,514,275	-82,598,876	-92.69
9	Lyondell Petrochemical Co.	Channelview	TX	128,955,947	49,099,531	-79,856,416	-61.93
10	GNB Inc.	Frisco	TX	72,883,740	4,179,363	-68,704,377	-94.27
11	ITT Rayonier Inc.	Jesup	GA	85,727,750	23,132,105	62,295,645	72.67
12	Champion International Corp.	Courtland	AL	73,753,400	16,195,600	-57,557,800	-78.04
13	Fina Oil & Chemical Co.	Port Arthur	TX	140,704,719	83,207,724	-57,496,995	-40.86
14	Cargill Corn Milling	Eddyville	IA	110,347,077	55,420,940	-54,926,137	-49.78
15	Texaco Refining & Marketing	El Dorado	KS	409,156,000	357,281,731	-51,874,269	-12.68
16	Solvay Polymers Inc.	Deer Park	TX	463,273,000	412,262,000	-51,011,000	-11.01
17	DSM Chemicals N.A. Inc.	Augusta	GA	73,033,964	25,003,522	-48,030,442	-65.76
18	GNB Inc.	Vernon	CA	53,844,964	6,701,475	-47,143,489	-87.55
19	General Battery Corp.	Reading	PA	81,723,701	35,177,717	-46,545,984	-56.96
20	Occidental Chemical Corp.	Gregory	TX	114,313,998	72,469,986	-41,844,012	-36.60
21	Cyprus Miami Mining Corp.	Claypool	AZ	435,264,000	394,955,000	-40,309,000	-9.26
22	Cox Creek Refining Co.	Baltimore	MD	34,539,227	45	-34,539,182	-100.00
23	Midstates Wire	Crawfordsville	IN	29,268,549	3,284,591	-25,983,958	-88.78
24	Eastman Kodak Co.	Batesville	AR	35,801,223	11,675,537	-24,125,686	-67.39
25	Rexene Corp.	Odessa	TX	30,540,993	8,202,047	-22,338,946	-73.14
	Subtotal			3,549,169,155	1,784,355,719	-1,764,813,436	-49.72
	Percent of Total			9.77	4.78		
	Total for All TRI Facilities			36,316,963,077	37,333,775,624	1,016,812,547	2.80

Influence of Methods of Classifying and Calculating On-site Waste Management Activities

To evaluate what underlies an individual facility's waste generation data in a given year requires knowing 1) what components the facility counts in its waste generation amounts and 2) how the facility calculated those amounts. To make sound comparisons of what's happening in different years for a group of facilities requires also knowing whether facilities changed their methods of waste classification or calculation from year to year without revising the previous years' numbers for consistency. This would lead to apparent changes in waste generation that are not attributable to any real changes in activity.[i]

Of on-site recycling, energy recovery, and treatment, on-site recycling is the least well defined. A survey of facilities reporting large quantities of on-site recycling to TRI in 1991 or 1992 revealed three main calculation methods used, and a fourth method is possible. Use of one method as opposed to another can result in reporting widely divergent quantities of on-site recycling, and switching calculation methods from one year to the next can make it appear as though the facility has changed waste generation levels or waste management strategies when no change in activity has occurred. Users of on-site recycling data cannot tell from the TRI database how the data have been calculated or if a facility has changed calculation methods.

The four methods count on-site recycling by calculating either 1) the pounds of the chemical in the waste stream sent to the recycling process; 2) the pounds of recycled chemical used to manufacture the product (as long as the recycling took place on site); 3) the amount of recycled chemical used for any purpose at the facility (reused to manufacture product, sold as coproduct, or used elsewhere, as long as the recycling was done on site); or 4) nothing, because the facility considered what it was doing an integral part of the production process (called "in-process recovery" in this report[j]) or the recycled material is used elsewhere (not in the original product, but still used at the same facility) or sold as product. (See Appendix B.) Some facilities also incorrectly report the total pounds

[i] Section 8 of TRI Form R provides no instructions for classification and calculation of on-site waste management activities, so there is no requirement for facilities to use the same classification or calculation method each year. The report "More Reliable Source Reduction Data Needed" by the General Accounting Office (GAO/RECD-94-93, September 23, 1994) describes the history of revisions to TRI Form R Section 8. Because the quantity of waste managed on site is not duplicated in other sections of the form, there is no self-consistency check. As described earlier in this chapter, facilities are required to report quantities of waste transferred off site for recycling, energy recovery, and treatment in Section 6 of Form R as well as in Section 8. Recycling, energy recovery, and treatment operations at off-site locations can provide some guidance for classification of on-site activities as well.

[j] Many technical terms are commonly used to describe recycling processes that are "integral to and necessary for" a production process under the Pollution Prevention Act of 1990. "Closed-loop recycling," "hard-piped recycling," and "recirculation" are a few of these. "In-process recovery" was chosen for this report to distinguish it from on-site recycling that must be reported in TRI Section 8 and to avoid possible confusion with too many kinds of recycling.

of the waste stream sent to the recycling process, instead of the TRI-chemical component.

Choice of calculation method for on-site recycling can lead to over-reporting or under-reporting the amount of production-related waste to TRI. Appendix B shows how counting the entire waste stream sent to the recycling process, used in 1992 by First Chemical Corporation of Pascagoula, Mississippi, made that facility appear to have the largest amount of production-related waste reported for that year: 4.0 billion pounds or 11 percent of all U.S. production-related waste in 1992.

Eastman Kodak's Kodak Park facility in Rochester, New York, by reclassifying some of its on-site recycling to in-process recovery (the fourth method) and not counting the waste, appeared to have had a major decrease. In 1991 Kodak Park reported 2.7 million pounds of dichloromethane recycled on site and 2.7 million pounds treated on site. The plant's 1992 Form R for dichloromethane listed 4.9 million pounds treated on site and zero on-site recycling. The apparent reduction of 500,000 pounds of dichloromethane was actually just the amount reclassified as in-process recovery, although the facility had not changed the way it used or processed the chemical. Eastman Kodak in fact did nothing wrong by reclassifying its waste management activities — the lack of reporting instructions for the Section 8 data leaves facilities free to choose any chemical-specific method of calculating the data.

TRI Facilities with the Largest Changes in Production-related Waste, 1991-1992

For the facilities that are the leading five in either increasing or decreasing production-related waste for 1991-1992, most of the apparent increases or decreases result either from reporting errors or from changes in waste management definition by the facilities and not from any change in activity. Examining the data from these 10 facilities, however, reveals that the changes in production-related waste attributable to recalculation, reporting errors, and non-standard operating conditions do not appear to favor increases more than decreases or vice versa. This finding indicates that reporting variations at individual facilities may be responsible for trends in analyses of production-related waste by chemical, industry, or geographic area. (See Table 4-9.)

An investigation by Hampshire Research Institute, as part of the research for this edition of *Toxics Watch,* of the 15 facilities reporting the largest decreases in production-related waste between 1991 and 1992 revealed only four plant-wide decreases attributable to changes in a manufacturing process while still maintaining production levels: Lyondell Petrochemical Company of Channelview, Texas; ITT Rayonier of Jesup, Georgia; Champion International Corporation of Courtland, Alabama; and the reduction in on-site treatment of hydrochloric acid made by DuPont Chambers Works of Deepwater, New Jersey (see below).

Table 4-9. Corrections to TRI Production-related Waste

SIC Code	Facility	City	State	Chemical
28	Carolina Eastman Company	Columbia	SC	Methanol
28	DuPont Chambers Works	Deepwater	NJ	Sulfuric acid
28	DuPont Chambers Works	Deepwater	NJ	Chloroethane
28	DuPont Chambers Works	Deepwater	NJ	Acetone
28	DuPont Chambers Works	Deepwater	NJ	n-Butyl alcohol
28	DuPont Chambers Works	Deepwater	NJ	Methanol
33	Elkem Metals Company	Marietta	OH	Manganese compounds
28	Goodyear Tire & Rubber Co.*	Beaumont	TX	Acetonitrile
28	Reilly Industries	Indianapolis	IN	Benzene
33	Revere Copper Products	Rome	NY	Copper compounds
	Total for 1991			
28	Goodyear Tire & Rubber Co.*	Beaumont	TX	Acetonitrile
	Total for 1992			

* Analyses in this report based on EPA database as released to the public in April 1994; Goodyear's revisions will be reflected in subsequent data releases.

Lyondell decreased the amount of on-site treatment of ethylene from 85.0 million pounds in 1991 to 6.7 million pounds in 1992. Ethylene is a product sold by the facility, and therefore any ethylene waste is a monetary loss. Lyondell undertook several housekeeping, inspection, and process efficiency improvement measures to reduce unanticipated shutdowns, since these require purging the system of ethylene before maintenance and thus result in product loss. The other two large reducers are paper manufacturers. ITT Rayonier installed new equipment to increase production of chlorine dioxide on site. The new equipment changed the manufacturing process so that less sulfuric acid was required to produce each pound of chlorine dioxide. This allowed the facility to decrease its on-site recycling of sulfuric acid by 63.0 million pounds between 1991 and 1992. Similarly, Champion International installed new bleaching processes to change over some of its chlorine-based pulp bleaching process to chlorine dioxide, reducing on-site treatment of chlorine by 51.4 million pounds between 1991 and 1992. This process modification is a source reduction activity, even though the substitute chemical, chlorine dioxide, must be reported to TRI.

The following facilities among the top five increasers and decreasers of production-related waste achieved their status by reclassifying waste management activities as reported in 1991 and 1992 (presented in alphabetical order):

- Carolina Eastman Company in Columbia, South Carolina, reported eliminating on-site recycling of methanol in 1992, a

Year	Production-related Waste Before Pounds	After Pounds	Difference Pounds	Type of Waste
1991	122,000,000	0	-122,000,000	Recycled on-site
1991	58,680,200	0	-58,680,200	Recycled on-site
1991	36,806,754	0	-36,806,754	Recycled on-site
1991	23,759,000	0	-23,759,000	Recycled on-site
1991	16,000,000	0	-16,000,000	Recycled on-site
1991	6,272,369	0	-6,272,369	Recycled on-site
1991	0	102,000,000	102,000,000	Recycled on-site
1991	2,423,678,742	0	-2,423,678,742	Recycled on-site
1991	120,000,000	1,300,000	-118,700,000	Recycled on-site
1991	0	87,585,000	87,585,000	Recycled on-site
	2,807,197,065	190,885,000	-2,616,312,065	
1992	2,526,855,525	0	-2,526,855,525	Recycled on-site
	2,526,855,525	0	-2,526,855,525	

decrease of 122.0 million pounds from 1991, by reclassification its activity as in-process recovery.

- DuPont Chambers Works in Deepwater, New Jersey, reported several reductions in on-site waste management activities for specific chemicals between 1991 and 1992, including elimination of on-site recycling of acetone, n-butyl alcohol, chloroethane, methanol, and sulfuric acid. Of these five, four resulted from reclassification to in-process recovery: only chloroethane processing was actually eliminated as part of a phase-out of tetraethyl lead production, a 36.8 million pound reduction in production-related waste. A decrease of 18.3 million pounds in on-site treatment of hydrochloric acid was caused by substituting a reprocessing step for some of the treatment and selling the reprocessed acid or using it on site in other processes.

- Elkem Metals Company in Marietta, Ohio, changed its on-site recycling of manganese compounds from zero pounds in 1991 to 102.0 million pounds in 1992. Before 1992 the company had considered its reuse of scrap and product not meeting quality standards to be part of the manufacturing process rather than on-site recycling.

- Goodyear Tire & Rubber Company in Beaumont, Texas, reported an increase in on-site recycling of acetonitrile from 2.4 billion pounds in 1991 to 2.5 billion pounds in 1992. Subsequently, the facility revised its 1991 and 1992 Form R submissions, eliminating all on-site recycling of acetonitrile in both years, reclassifying the on-site recycling to in-process recovery.[k]

- Reilly Industries in Indianapolis, Indiana, reported a decrease in on-site recycling of benzene from 120.0 million pounds in 1991 to 1.3 million pounds in 1992, due to a change in calculation method. The facility now counts only the benzene recovered via solvent extraction, instead of its previous method of considering the total amount of the extraction feed stream. (See recycling method 3 in Appendix B.)

- Revere Copper Products in Rome, New York, reported no on-site recycling of copper compounds in 1991 and 87.6 million pounds in 1992 with no apparent change in production. The company had always reincorporated scrap and product not meeting specifications into new production and did not consider this activity recycling. The 1992 report, however, reflects a change in classification to on-site recycling. (See Table 4-9.)

Of the other four facilities among the top five increases and decreases in production-related waste for 1991-1992, two have reporting errors confirmed by the facilities. The precipitous drop in on-site recycling of lead compounds by Corning Asahi Video Products of State College, Pennsylvania, from 160.0 million pounds to 17.0 million pounds from 1991 to 1992 resulted from an error in the 1991 figure that should have been 16.0 million pounds. Hence, the facility actually had an increase of 6 percent rather than a decrease of 89 percent. Similarly, a large increase in on-site treatment of ammonia from 9.3 million pounds to 180.0 million pounds from 1991 to 1992 by Star Enterprises of Union, Louisiana resulted from an error in the 1992 figure, which should be 18.0 million pounds.

The remaining two facilities are among the five largest increasers and decreasers for process-related reasons. Doe Run Company of Boss, Missouri, began operations at the site during the last third of 1991. Because 1992 was the first full year of operation, the "increase" in production-related waste between 1991 and 1992 represents the difference between the start-up activity in 1991 and the full year's operations in 1992. Phillips 66 Company of Sweeny, Texas, reported a decrease in on-site recycling of xylene between 1991 and 1992 caused by a temporary (and, according to the facility, inexplicable) increase in process efficiency of xylene extraction in 1992. According to plant representatives, the 1993 figures are back up to 1991 levels.[2]

These 10 facilities represent a 292-million-pound increase and 431-million-pound decrease in production-related waste between 1991 and 1992 due mainly to recalculation of on-site recycling. An additional 171-million-pound increase and 142-million-pound decrease are attributable to reporting errors, and increases of 181 million pounds and decreases of 124 million pounds are attributable

[k] All TRI data in this report were taken from the database released to the public by EPA in April 1994. EPA accepts revisions to the database as submitted by facilities throughout the year; these revisions are then reflected in the next annual public data release.

to non-standard operating conditions. The net sum of the changes in production-related waste for these 10 facilities is a decrease of 53.1 million pounds — an amount smaller than the largest single confirmed reduction in production-related waste. Considering that production-related waste totaled 37.3 billion pounds in 1992 for 23,630 facilities, these 10 facilities clearly had a disproportionate effect on the TRI Section 8 data.

TRI Source Reduction and Changes in Production

Information Collected on Source Reduction

A decrease in production-related waste for a given chemical at a facility without an accompanying decrease in production may be attributable to source reduction activities. However, further information is needed to determine the true nature of changes in production-related waste and to separate the effects of source reduction from those changes. The TRI Form R collects information about *types* of source reduction activities undertaken at a particular facility for a specific chemical, but not the change in the *amount* of waste due to those source reduction activities alone.

The amount of waste reduced due to source reduction activities cannot be quantified using TRI data because of the nature of production processes and the difficulty in characterizing changes by a single index. TRI requires a facility to report an index number for each TRI chemical used at the facility that represents the ratio of the amount of production associated with the chemical in the current year divided by the amount of production in the prior year. A number less than one represents a decrease in production; a number greater than one an increase in production. The assumption is that a decrease in waste greater than that expected given the change in production is due to source reduction.

Several problems arise. Changes in production may not relate to changes in waste generation. For example, if several different products are manufactured, one index number may not reflect changes in the product mix and, hence, changes in the use of the toxic chemical. Variations in the efficiency of the production process unrelated to source reduction may cause changes in waste generated without any change in production levels. The method used to estimate the amount of waste generated may change without any production changes. Facilities may not report source reduction activities when actually applying such methods to increase yields or improve efficiency because the activities were undertaken for reasons other than pollution prevention.

For these reasons, this *Toxics Watch* report uses the TRI production index to group TRI chemical forms into categories of increases and decreases in relation to source reduction activity but does not calculate the amount of waste reduced by these source reduction activities. (See Chapter 10 for additional analysis of the type of data needed for determining the quantity of source reduction.)

Table 4-10. TRI Source Reduction Activity and Production-related Waste, 1991 and 1992

	1992 Forms		**Total 1991 Production-related Waste on 1992 Forms**	
	Number	**Percent of Total**	**Pounds**	**Percent of Total**
	Number	Percent	Pounds	Percent
With Source Reduction Activity	20,508	25.31	10,279,645,214	28.31
No Source Reduction Activity	60,508	74.69	26,037,317,863	71.69
Total	81,016	100.00	36,316,963,077	100.00
Type of Source Reduction Activity				
Good Operating Practices	9,357	11.55	3,890,462,544	10.71
Inventory Control	2,473	3.05	327,726,568	0.90
Spill/Leak Prevention	5,957	7.35	4,371,790,881	12.04
Raw Material Modifications	3,860	4.76	928,516,408	2.56
Process Modifications	7,570	9.34	4,459,533,605	12.28
Cleaning and Degreasing	2,815	3.47	521,580,292	1.44
Surface Preparation and Finishing	2,308	2.85	189,995,034	0.52
Product Modifications	1,853	2.29	277,300,619	0.76

Figure 4-6.

TRI Source Reduction Activity, Number of Forms and Total Production-related Waste, 1992

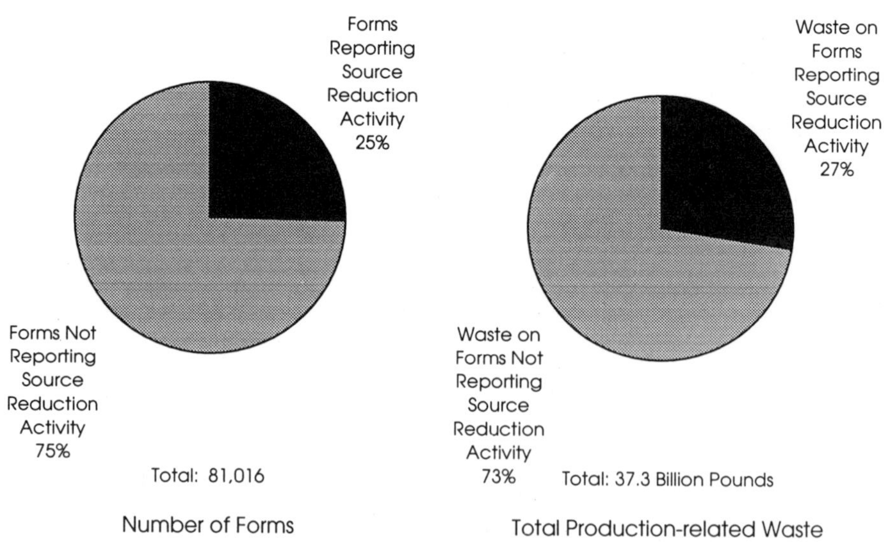

Total 1992 Production-related Waste		Change from 1991 to 1992	
Pounds	Percent of Total	Pounds	Percent
Pounds	Percent	Pounds	Percent
10,247,165,333	27.45	-32,479,881	-0.32
27,086,610,291	72.55	1,049,292,428	4.03
37,333,775,624	100.00	1,016,812,547	2.80
3,948,373,652	10.58	57,911,108	1.49
371,399,047	0.99	43,672,479	13.33
4,558,228,304	12.21	186,437,423	4.26
804,882,984	2.16	-123,633,424	-13.32
4,459,483,165	11.94	-50,440	-0.00
472,239,580	1.26	-49,340,712	-9.46
165,162,512	0.44	-24,832,522	-13.07
270,728,932	0.73	-6,571,687	-2.37

Source reduction activities undertaken by facilities may actually be under-reported in TRI. If a facility has undertaken one or more source reduction activities that reduce use or production of a chemical below the TRI reporting threshold, no form will be filed for that chemical. Thus, a facility that reported a particular chemical in 1991 may have undertaken a source reduction activity in 1992 that eliminated the use of that chemical. The source reduction activity would normally be reported on the 1992 Form R, but in this case, no 1992 form would be filed, and information on the source reduction activity would be lost to TRI. As of 1993, Massachusetts asks for voluntary information on chemicals that were reported in the previous year but not in the current year including information on source reduction activities and declines in business. These data can then be used to account for source reduction activities not reportable to TRI. (See Chapter 10.)

Source Reduction Related to Production-related Waste

In 1992, 25 percent of TRI forms indicated some kind of source reduction activity. The production-related waste reported on these forms was 27 percent of the total from all forms. (See Figure 4-6 and Table 4-10.)

Those TRI forms reporting source reduction activity collectively showed a small (less than one-half of 1 percent) decrease in total production-related waste from 1991 to 1992, while those forms with no source reduction reported had an increase in such waste of 4 percent. The group of source reduction activities classified as "good operating practices" was reported on the greatest number of forms (12 percent), but these practices did not result in an overall reduction in production-related waste. For raw material modifications, while reported on only 5 percent of the forms, those forms achieved the greatest reductions, a total decrease of 123.6 million pounds (13 percent). (See Table 4-10.)

For TRI facilities reporting source reduction activities for the same chemical in both 1991 and 1992, the decrease in total production-related waste was larger but still quite small, a decrease of 96.9 million pounds or 1 percent. For those forms with source reduction activity indicated in 1992 but not in 1991, the decrease was even smaller (5.7 million pounds or 0.2 percent). For those reporting source reduction activity only in 1991, or not reporting it in either year, total production-related waste increased, by 3 percent and 4 percent respectively. (See Figure 4-7 and Table 4-11.)

Source Reduction and the Environmental Management Hierarchy

The waste management data for 1991 and 1992 also indicate that facilities reporting source reduction activities for a given chemical seem to be managing the waste associated with that chemical in such a way that there appears to be a shift toward more environmentally desirable methods of waste management. (See Box 4-A.) Forms reporting source reduction in 1992 showed a combined 1991-1992 decrease of 155.3 million pounds (10 percent) in the quantity released/disposed of. In contrast, facilities showed an increase of 40.9 million pounds (2 percent) in the quantity released/disposed of on forms reporting no source reduction activity. Thus, the use of the least desirable option, release/disposal to the environment, was reduced for the waste associated with source reduction activities, but was increased for waste not associated with such activities.

Furthermore, those forms reporting source reduction practices collectively showed an increase in the quantity of waste recycled or used for energy recovery and a decrease in waste treated or released/disposed of. In contrast, the forms reporting no source reduction activities collectively reported an increase in every type of waste management option, with the largest absolute increase (545.6 million pounds) as well as largest percent increase (8 percent) in the treatment option, which is the second-least desirable waste management option. (See Figure 4-8 and Table 4-12.)

Interestingly, in many cases, facilities do not consider improvements in process efficiency to be source reduction, especially when the reduction in waste was not the intended effect. ITT Rayonier did not identify its large reduction of sulfuric acid as a source reduction activity on the Form R, because the facility considered the reduction a byproduct of its program to increase chlorine dioxide production. ITT Rayonier's unintentional omission is a common one — a study of

Figure 4-7.

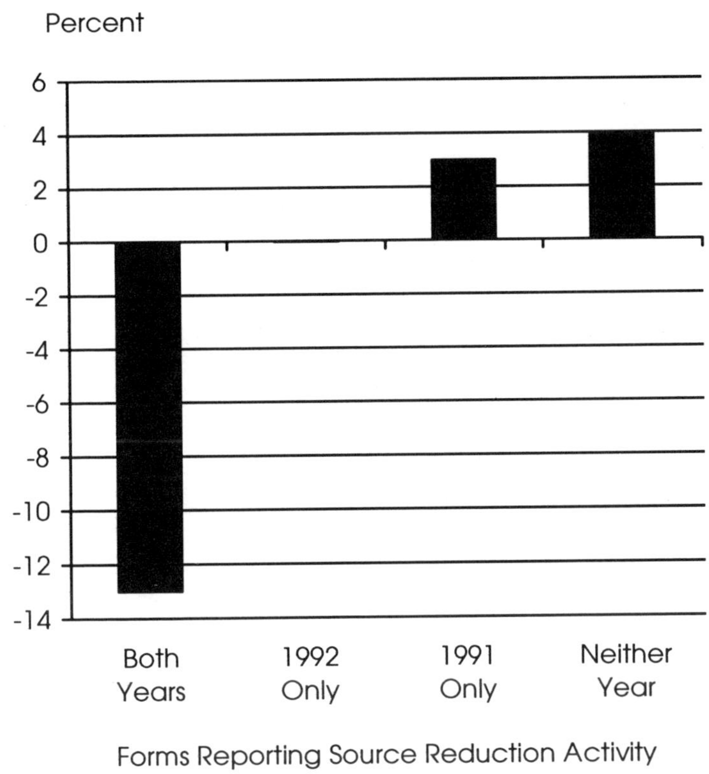

Percent Change in Total TRI Production-related Waste for Forms Reporting and Not Reporting Source Reduction Activity, 1991-1992

*Table 4-11. TRI Source Reduction Activity Reporting in 1991 and 1992**

Reporting Source Reduction Activity	**Forms** Number	**Total Production Related Wastes** **1991** Pounds	**1992** Pounds	**Difference in Waste from 1991 to 1992** Pounds	**Percent Difference in Waste from 1991 to 1992** Percent
Both years	13,282	7,542,209,700	7,445,325,524	-96,884,176	-1.28
1992 only	5,319	2,535,284,851	2,529,544,541	-5,740,310	-0.23
1991 only	4,624	2,533,173,259	2,599,786,183	66,612,924	2.63
Neither year	47,589	23,179,458,128	24,033,327,575	853,869,447	3.68
Total	70,814	35,790,125,938	36,607,983,823	817,857,885	2.29

* Source Reduction Reporting was identified on 1991 forms and on 1992 forms. The "waste" is determined from the 1992 form for both years, that is "1991" figure is reported as previous year and the "1992" figure is reported as current year. There are 10,082 forms in 1992 with no matching form in 1991. These forms are not included in this analysis.

Figure 4-8.

Change in Types of TRI Waste Management, 1991-1992

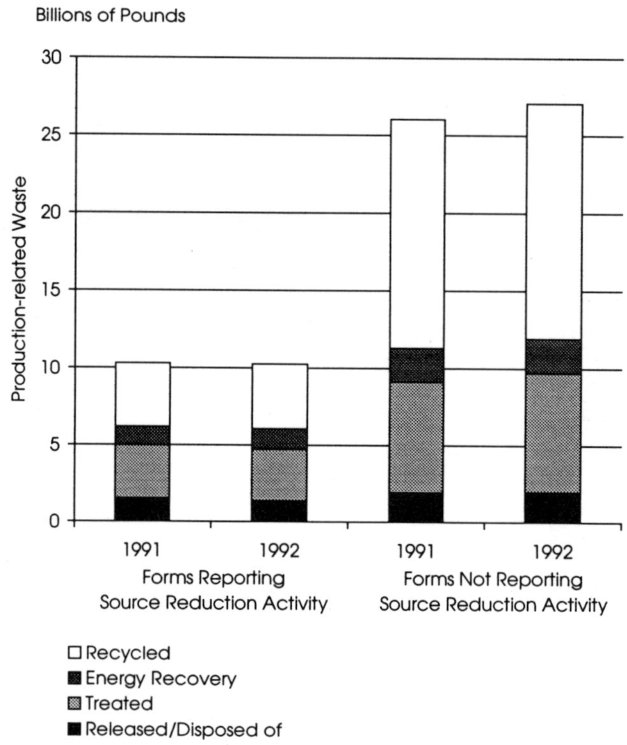

Table 4-12. TRI Waste Management for Forms with and without Source Reduction Activity Reported, 1991-1992

Waste Management Type	**1991** Pounds	**1992** Pounds	**Change 1991 to 1992** Pounds	**Percent Change 1991 to 1992** Percent
With Source Reduction Activity Reported				
Recycled on-site	3,234,519,492	3,212,785,140	-21,734,352	-0.67
Recycled off-site	876,641,058	988,959,621	112,318,563	12.81
Energy Recovery on-site	865,964,164	982,967,058	117,002,894	13.51
Energy Recovery off-site	326,361,441	330,591,427	4,229,986	1.30
Treated on-site	3,195,700,589	3,152,087,775	-43,612,814	-1.36
Treated off-site	233,312,925	187,961,807	-45,351,118	-19.44
Released/disposed of	1,547,145,545	1,391,812,505	-155,333,040	-10.04
Total Production-related Waste	10,279,645,214	10,247,165,333	-32,479,881	-0.32
With No Source Reduction Activity Reported				
Recycled on-site	12,618,162,895	12,671,409,748	53,246,853	0.42
Recycled off-site	2,100,171,271	2,484,934,888	384,763,617	18.32
Energy Recovery on-site	1,976,493,775	1,958,255,055	-18,238,720	-0.92
Energy Recovery off-site	254,348,830	297,363,173	43,014,343	16.91
Treated on-site	6,672,446,314	7,174,661,719	502,215,405	7.53
Treated off-site	447,055,173	490,412,043	43,356,870	9.70
Released/disposed of	1,968,639,605	2,009,573,665	40,934,060	2.08
Total Production-related Waste	26,037,317,863	27,086,610,291	1,049,292,428	4.03

facilities in New Jersey indicates a significant probability that companies implementing source reduction will not report it under TRI.[3]

Source Reduction, Waste Generation, and Changes in Production

The decreases discussed above do not measure the amount of waste reduced due to source reduction because source reduction activities are not the only reason that production-related waste may change from year to year. Production levels will also affect the amount of waste generated, as can be seen in the examples of Doe Run Company and chloroethane at DuPont Chambers Works above. TRI Form R requires reporting of a production activity index indicating how much production changed from one year to the next.[1] Given the possibility for multiple products and uses of a given chemical at a facility, it can be difficult to apply a facility-wide production activity index to a waste generation figure to normalize for production. The New Jersey study mentioned above concluded that for more than 60 percent of facilities, the normalization is not valid.[4]

Accepting that normalization of production-related waste will not allow reliable comparisons from year to year, it is still reasonable to assume that the direction of change in production-related waste at a facility will normally follow the same directional trend as the production activity index. Index values less than or greater than 1.0 should be accompanied by corresponding decreases or increases in production-related waste, although the magnitudes of the changes would probably not be equivalent.

One way to look at the relationship between source reduction and production is to divide the TRI data on production-related waste into categories of production activity change (decrease, no change, increase) and source reduction activity (any reported or not reported). The majority of those forms reporting source reduction, as well as a majority of those forms reporting no source reduction, indicate an increase in production, and both of those groups that are increasing production also report an increase in total production-related waste. However, the increase is one-fourth as large for those reporting source reduction as for those not reporting source reduction (3 percent versus 12 percent). On the other hand, forms showing decreases in production without source reduction outnumbered forms with both decreases in production and with source reduction (18,319 versus 7,024) and achieved a larger percentage reduction in production-related waste (11 percent versus 7 percent). Again, this finding is consistent with the New Jersey study, in which facilities cited production changes at the operating plant rather than source reductions as the primary reason for reductions in production-related waste.[5] (See Table 4-13.)

This look at production-level changes and source reduction activity indicates that source

[1] The activity index is a ratio. If production in a given reporting year is unchanged from the previous year, the index would be 1.0. Decreases in production result in an index less than 1.0, while increases in production result in index values greater than 1.0.

Table 4-13. Comparison of TRI Production-related Waste to Change in Production Level and Source Reduction Activity, 1991-1992

Production Level*	Forms		Total Production-related Waste				Change 1991 to 1992	Percent Change 1991 to 1992
			1991 Pounds	Percent	1992 Pounds	Percent		
	Number	Percent	Pounds	Percent	Pounds	Percent	Pounds	Percent
With Source Reduction Activity Reported								
Decrease	7,024	9.57	3,102,054,532	9.73	2,894,648,078	8.84	-207,406,454	-6.69
No change	1,479	2.02	644,391,874	2.02	582,664,102	1.78	-61,727,772	-9.58
Increase	10,916	14.87	6,428,013,308	20.17	6,631,168,587	20.24	203,155,279	3.16
Subtotal	19,419	26.46	10,174,459,714	31.93	10,108,480,767	30.86	-65,978,947	-0.65
With No Source Reduction Activity Reported								
Decrease	18,319	24.96	6,090,266,801	19.11	5,446,879,475	16.63	-643,387,326	-10.56
No change	5,453	7.43	2,050,545,693	6.43	2,085,599,865	6.37	35,054,172	1.71
Increase	30,201	41.15	13,553,416,672	42.53	15,114,650,496	46.14	1,561,233,824	11.52
Subtotal	53,973	73.54	21,694,229,166	68.07	22,647,129,836	69.14	952,900,670	4.21
Total	73,392	100.00	31,868,688,880	100.00	32,755,610,603	100.00	886,921,723	2.78

* Production level according to reported Production Index. Forms with no Production Index or Index >= 100 not included in analysis.

Figure 4-9.

Comparison of TRI Production-related Waste, for Production Level and Source Reduction Activity, 1991 and 1992

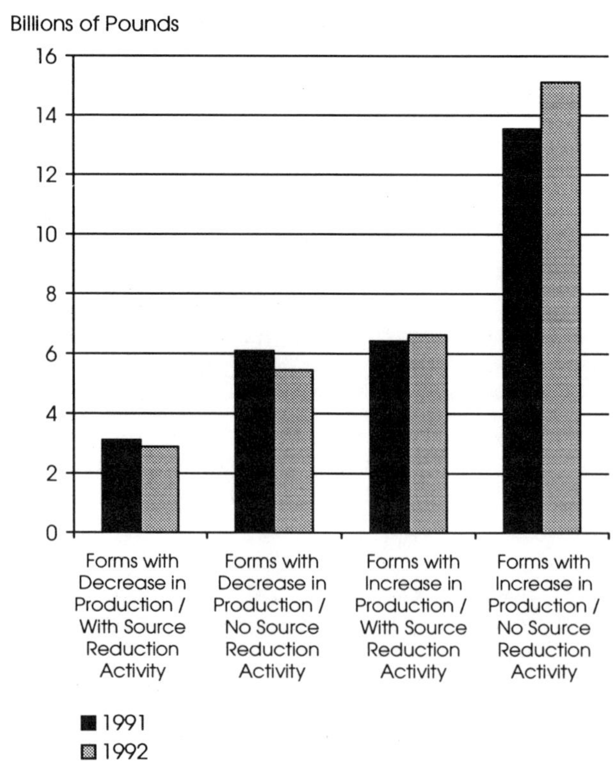

reduction in the face of decreasing production is undertaken less often and with less dramatic results, but that source reduction activity undertaken during increases in production levels can help keep production-related waste from increasing proportionately. (See Figure 4-9.)

Comparison of 1992 to 1994 Projections

Projected Changes in Waste Generation, 1992-1994

Facilities are required to report in Section 8 their projections of waste generation for each of the next two years. The projections made for 1993 and 1994 indicate that the amount of total production-related waste is expected to change little between 1992 and 1994. These projections amount to an increase from 37.3 billion pounds to 37.5 billion (0.3 percent increase). About half of all facilities expect to be able to reduce production-related waste, and these facilities account for about half of the total production-related waste in 1992. Facilities projecting increases, however, expect an average increase of 19 percent. These increases cancel out the decreases, because the decreases are projected to be less, on average 17 percent per facility. (See Figure 4-10 and Table 4-14.)

How Facilities Calculate Projections

Data for the 10 facilities with the largest increases or decreases in production-related waste between 1991 and 1992 suggest that projections for 1993 and 1994 seem to be based on 1992 calculation methods.[m] In other words, projections for on-site recycling are more likely to be made based on the present year's reporting method, whereas past years' reporting may have used a different estimation method.

One way to evaluate TRI projections is to check the accuracy of past projections. Facilities must report production-related waste for the current year, the prior year, and the following two years. On the 1991 form, then, 1992 figures are projections. Comparing the 1992-year quantities (projections made on the 1991 forms to those reported on the 1992 forms) shows that the initial projections were somewhat low. The actual 1992 total was 1.3 percent higher than the projection made the year before. Since the reporting deadline for 1991 data with 1992 projections was June 30, 1992, it is likely that much actual 1992 data were used in making 1992 projections. By the same reasoning, the one-year projections are likely to be more accurate than the two-year projections. The projections for 1993 as made in 1991 are 3.7 percent lower than projections for 1993 made in 1992. (See Figure 4-11.)

[m] All facilities questioned by HRI for this report indicated that they were using their 1992 methodology to estimate 1993 and 1994 data.

Figure 4-10.

Projected Change in TRI Production-related Waste, 1992 -1994

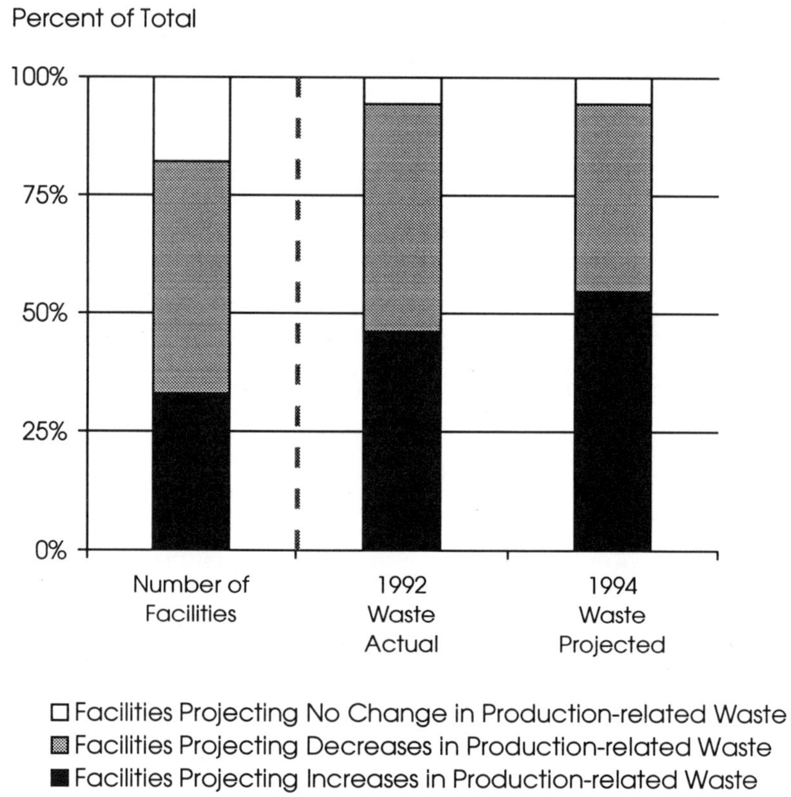

Table 4-14. Change in TRI Production-related Waste, Actual 1992 to Projected 1994

Projected Change from 1992 to 1994	Facilities		1992 Production-related Waste			1994 Production-related Waste			Percent Change in Average Pounds per Facility
	Number	Percent of Total	Pounds	Percent of Total	Average Pounds per Facility	Pounds	Percent of Total	Average Pounds per Facility	
	Number	Percent	Pounds	Percent	Pounds	Pounds	Percent	Pounds	Percent
Increased	7,810	33.05	17,202,080,212	46.08	2,202,571	20,474,314,623	54.66	2,621,551	19.02
Decreased	11,615	49.15	18,035,839,118	48.31	1,552,806	14,890,240,615	39.75	1,281,984	-17.44
Stayed same	4,205	17.80	2,095,856,294	5.61	498,420	2,095,856,294	5.59	498,420	0.00
Total	23,630	100.00	37,333,775,624	100.00	1,579,931	37,460,411,532	100.00	1,585,290	0.34

Figure 4-11.

Comparison of TRI Production-related Waste for 1991, 1992 and 1993

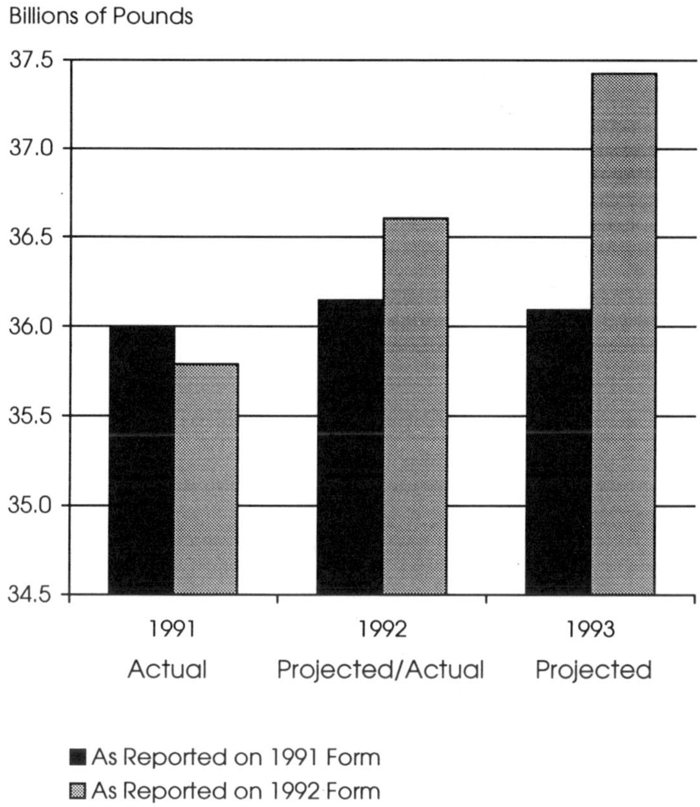

For 74,375 forms that reported in both years

In addition to the data, anecdotal evidence suggests that companies are conservative in making projections on TRI Form Rs — conservative, in this case, meaning production-related waste numbers that do not change much up or down. International Paper Company, for example, does not want its facilities to project decreases they are not absolutely certain will be met. Representatives of the company's environmental division cited reports such as this one that examine company data as one reason for this conservative approach: the company expects to be held accountable with ever-increasing scrutiny of its Section 8 data.[6] Also, companies may find it difficult to project the effects of new products or processes on their TRI data. So although GenCorp reported to EPA's 33/50 Program that the company has undertaken significant new production at its facility in Columbus, Missouri, company representatives indicate that the new activities are not reflected in Section 8 projections.[7]

Projections and the Environmental Management Hierarchy

In spite of forecasting difficulties, it is useful to examine whether facilities expect to manage waste differently, given that little change is

Table 4-15. TRI Production-related Waste, 1992-1994

Waste Management Type	Actual 1992 Pounds	Projected 1994 Pounds	Change 1992 to 1994 Pounds	Percent Change 1992 to 1994 Percent
Recycled On-site	15,884,194,888	16,911,850,011	1,027,655,123	6.47
Recycled Off-site	3,473,894,509	3,454,654,976	-19,239,533	-0.55
Energy Recovery On-site	2,941,222,113	3,091,684,371	150,462,258	5.12
Energy Recovery Off-site	627,954,600	589,834,167	-38,120,433	-6.07
Treated On-site	10,326,749,494	10,097,658,804	-229,090,690	-2.22
Treated Off-site	678,373,850	598,615,840	-79,758,010	-11.76
Released/Disposed of	3,401,386,170	2,716,113,363	-685,272,807	-20.15
Total Production-related Waste	37,333,775,624	37,460,411,532	126,635,908	0.34

expected in the total quantity of waste. In total, a positive movement up the environmental management hierarchy appears to be projected from 1992 to 1994. Facilities estimate that the quantity of waste released/disposed of will decrease by 20 percent (685.3 million pounds) and that waste that is treated will decrease by 3 percent (308.8 million pounds) while the amount used for energy recovery will increase by 3 percent (112.3 million pound) and the amount recycled by 5 percent (1.0 billion pounds). (See Table 4-15.)

Biennial Reporting System Data

BRS Reporting Requirements

Facilities that generate and/or manage hazardous solid or liquid wastes must report to BRS every two years on the quantity, management, and minimization of these wastes. Those sites considered to be treatment, storage, and disposal facilities (TSDFs) must report to the BRS if any of the waste was managed by methods requiring RCRA permitting. If a TSDF meets that requirement, then it must report all of its hazardous waste streams to the BRS. Facilities generating hazardous waste must also report to BRS if they meet one or more of the large quantity generator criteria:

- generate 2,200 pounds or more of RCRA hazardous waste in a single month;
- generate 2.2 pounds of RCRA acute hazardous waste in a single month or accumulate that amount at any time; or
- generate or accumulate more than 220 pounds of spill clean-up material contaminated with RCRA acute hazardous waste.

Waste management activities are classified as "RCRA managed" or "exempt" based on whether the type of waste management requires a RCRA permit. Among other methods, exempt types of waste management include any waste-water treatment in tanks regardless of toxicity or hazard; consequently, nearly half of the waste generated and reported to the BRS is exempt waste. The waste management activity is also considered when determining large quantity generator status, since exempt waste is not counted when calculating amounts on site.

Because they are not tied to individual chemicals, RCRA waste streams are described by means of RCRA waste codes. A RCRA waste code is an identification number assigned to a type of waste stream regulated under RCRA. Some waste codes name chemical constituents (e.g., waste code P021, calcium cyanide), some describe the output of a manufacturing process (e.g., K132, spent absorbent and waste-water separator solids from the production of methyl bromide), and some describe specific properties (e.g., D002, corrosive waste).

Many of the waste codes contain a mix of toxic chemicals, some of which may also appear in other waste codes. For example, the waste code F003 describes the waste stream of spent non-halogenated solvents. Such a waste stream could contain xylene, acetone, and methanol, but the BRS report does not specify how much of any of the chemicals might be in the waste stream. Xylene is also in waste code U239, acetone is in U002, and methanol is in U154, all waste codes covering discarded commercial chemical products. In addition, an individual stream can be described by multiple waste codes and may contain several toxic chemicals and non-toxic substances as well (such as water). For example, a facility might use carbon tetrachloride as a cleaner. The resulting waste stream could be described by the waste codes F001, spent halogenated solvents used in degreasing, and D019, hazardous waste containing carbon tetrachloride. (See Chapter 5 for examples of waste streams reported to BRS designated as hazardous because of the presence of specific chemicals). In this report, a "toxic" waste reported in BRS is a waste stream containing a TRI chemical or waste code defined as toxic by RCRA. (See Appendix E.)

The waste codes are assigned in five groups:

- *Characteristic Hazardous Waste* is classified by ignitability, corrosivity, reactivity, or toxicity (waste codes begin with "D");
- *Hazardous Waste from Nonspecific Sources* consists mostly of waste-water, solvents, and outputs of treatment processes (waste codes begin with "F");
- *Hazardous Waste from Specific Sources* are waste streams resulting from defined production process activities and usually contain identifiable chemicals (waste codes begin with "K");
- *Discarded Commercial Chemical Products, Off-Specification Species, Container Residuals, and Spill Residues Thereof — Acute Hazardous Waste* consists of single chemicals or chemical groups (waste codes begin with "P"); and
- *Discarded Commercial Chemical Products, Off-Specification Species, Container Residues, and Spill Residues Thereof — Toxic Wastes* also consists of single chemicals or chemical groups (waste codes begin with "U").

In addition to these waste code categories, facilities may report certain laboratory waste separately.

Table 4-16. RCRA Biennial Report Data, Summary, 1991

	1991 All Reports	1991 Toxic Reports	Percent Toxic of Total
	Number	Number	Percent
Number of Facilities	24,378	22,344	91.66
Number of Reports	304,796	201,566	66.13
	Pounds	Pounds	Percent
Waste Generated	1,117,734,012,000	948,243,750,120	84.84
Quantity Managed On-site	1,130,537,974,620	963,917,566,300	85.26
Managed in RCRA units	515,827,550,180	478,110,746,580	92.69
Managed in exempt units	610,054,264,840	481,518,364,160	78.93
Storage	4,656,159,600	4,288,455,560	92.10
Quantity Sent Off-site	25,359,700,000	22,109,496,000	87.18

1991 BRS Data

The 1991 BRS contains reports from 24,378 facilities, of which 92 percent (22,344 facilities) reported on toxic waste generated, as defined above. The 948.2 billion pounds of toxic waste they reported represents 85 percent of all BRS waste for 1991.[n] (See Table 4-16.)

Facilities also report how the waste was managed, whether and how it was treated on site, or if it was sent off site. (See Appendix D.) For 1991 RCRA facilities *managed* 963.9 billion pounds and sent off site another 22.1 billion pounds of toxic waste streams. (See Table 4-16.) Note that quantities of *waste generated* and *waste managed* as reported to BRS for a given year may not be equal. A facility may not manage all of its waste on site (and so its waste generated would exceed its waste managed), and the facility may manage or treat waste in one calendar year that was generated and stored in the previous calendar year (and so its waste managed would exceed its waste generated). A facility may also be a treatment, storage, and disposal facility (TSDF), in which case waste management would far exceed waste generation.

Most RCRA waste generation occurs at a few facilities. In 1991, 50 facilities reported 72 percent of all the RCRA toxic waste generated. This is an even higher degree of concentration than for TRI, where the largest 50 facilities reported 43 percent of all TRI production-related waste. (See Tables 4-17 and 4-5.)

[n] No data for which the facility claimed Confidential Business Information are included in this report.

Figure 4-12.

RCRA Toxic Waste Generated for Waste Codes Added in 1991

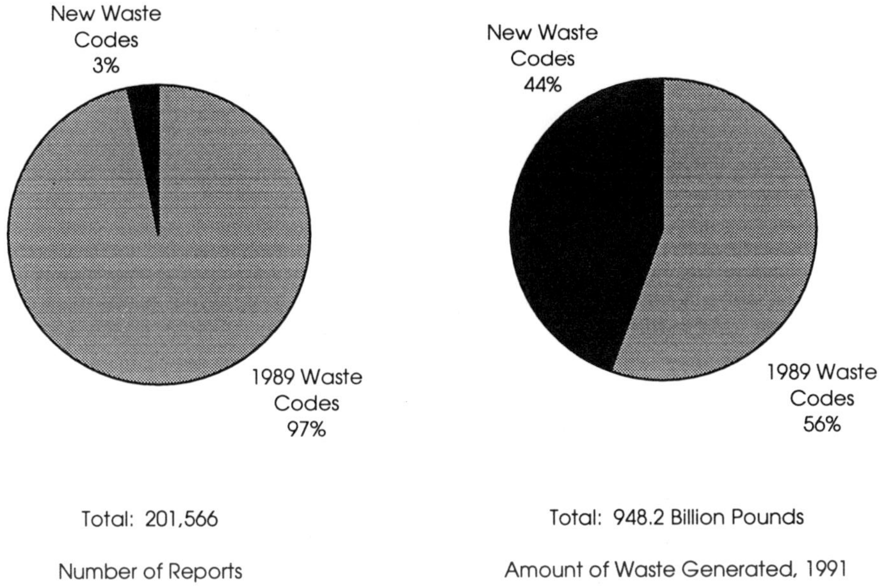

Waste Generation in BRS, 1989 and 1991

Comparing Years of BRS Data

This report compares the 1989 BRS data to the 1991 data for those data elements with reasonably large coverage nationwide.[o] Publicly available BRS data were first collected in 1985, but these were collected by states using their own forms. Uniform data elements on a nationwide basis were not available until the 1989 reporting year. Even for 1989, many common data elements are missing from some states, particularly identifiers such as SIC codes, descriptions of wastes beyond the waste codes, and some waste minimization data.

Expansion of Waste Codes in 1991

In 1991 new hazardous waste codes were required to be reported, which almost doubled the amount of toxic waste reported. The new codes cover characteristic waste of specific chemicals, including such TRI chemicals as benzene, carbon tetrachloride, chloroform, cresol, methyl ethyl ketone, and vinyl chloride, as well as waste from nonspecific sources such as residues from the treatment of waste including wastewater, sludge, and leachate. (See Figure 4-12 and Appendix E.)

[o] Each BRS may actually cover two years, since the 1991 form allows voluntary reporting of 1990 data as well as 1991 data. However, the data for 1990 do not appear to be complete and are not used in this report.

Table 4-17. The 50 RCRA Facilities with Largest Total RCRA Toxic Waste Generated, 1991

Rank	Facility	City	State	1991 Toxic Waste Generated Pounds	1991 Toxic Waste Managed Pounds
1	Kodak Park	Rochester	NY	83,225,844,980	83,209,211,720
2	The Dow Chemical Company	Midland	MI	60,274,801,720	60,259,302,940
3	Amoco Oil Company Refinery	Texas City	TX	52,275,053,600	52,288,196,680
4	E.I. Dupont-Chambers Works	Deepwater	NJ	48,843,789,760	49,830,189,760
5	Shell Oil Company	Deer Park	TX	38,738,555,340	38,858,036,000
6	Citgo Petroleum Corporation	Lake Charles	LA	27,121,056,040	27,118,164,600
7	Chevron USA Products Company	Philadelphia	PA	24,434,042,460	24,419,204,000
8	Shell Oil Co/Martinez Mfg Comp	Martinez	CA	21,547,852,000	21,535,389,400
9	Shell Oil Co	Roxana	IL	18,882,321,460	18,838,008,000
10	Amoco Chemical Company	Alvin	TX	16,503,998,360	16,486,739,660
11	Phillips Petroleum Sweeny Complex	Old Ocean	TX	15,005,072,500	15,280,699,000
12	Chevron	Pascagoula	MS	13,528,679,760	13,527,246,960
13	Rhone-Poulenc Ag Company	Institute	WV	13,313,468,980	13,308,711,880
14	Union Carbide Chemicals & Plas. Co.	Taft	LA	13,021,427,200	13,020,968,540
15	Sun Company, Inc.	Marcus Hook	PA	12,000,230,120	12,000,000,000
16	Eastman Chemical	Longview	TX	11,348,671,660	11,348,501,560
17	Hercules,Incorporated	Radford	VA	11,241,373,400	11,240,348,800
18	BP Oil Company - Alliance Ref.	Belle Chasse	LA	10,681,891,800	10,681,762,000
19	ARCO Products Co	Ferndale	WA	10,220,819,820	10,220,323,200
20	Sun Refining & Mktg. Co.	Tulsa	OK	8,717,414,960	8,706,740,400
21	Coastal Refining & Marketing, Inc.	Corpus Christi	TX	8,441,243,760	8,440,812,000
22	E I Dupont De Nemours & Co.	Victoria	TX	7,890,537,600	7,902,101,020
23	Dow Chemical U.S.A.	Freeport	TX	7,486,554,200	6,974,822,800
24	Robins AFB	Warner Robins	GA	7,379,602,300	7,376,146,240
25	Sun Company, Inc.	Philadelphia	PA	7,009,089,600	7,003,864,000
26	Mobil Chemical Co O/A Plant	Beaumont	TX	6,846,048,420	6,849,091,240
27	Kemira Inc	Savannah	GA	6,716,824,000	6,716,692,000
28	Shell Oil Company	Anacortes	WA	6,680,620,620	6,680,010,400
29	Crown Central Petroleum Corp.	Pasadena	TX	6,625,361,860	6,623,981,500
30	Champlin Refining & Chemicals, Inc.	Corpus Christi	TX	6,323,361,700	6,424,923,440
31	Unocal-San Fran Refinery	Rodeo	CA	6,281,453,440	6,279,305,440
32	Koch Refining Co.	Corpus Christi	TX	6,191,808,000	6,188,356,000
33	Texaco Refining & Marketing	Anacortes	WA	5,745,785,660	5,745,100,720
34	Lyondell Petrochemical Co.	Chennelview	TX	5,647,578,800	5,647,563,160
35	3M Company	Cottage Grove	MN	5,336,152,080	5,323,499,060
36	Ashland Petroleum Company	St. Paul Park	MN	5,237,316,280	5,236,464,460
37	DSM Chemicals North America Inc	Augusta	GA	5,168,570,440	5,168,565,440
38	Puerto Rico Sun Oil Co.	Yabucoa	PR	5,019,950,600	5,019,104,900
39	Lederle Laboratories Division	Pearl River	NY	4,946,542,660	4,944,630,000
40	Armco Advanced Materials Co.	Lyndora	PA	4,931,192,360	4,908,785,280
41	Monsanto Company	Alvin	TX	4,812,338,740	4,806,230,860
42	U.S. DOE Idaho Nat. Engr. Lab	Scoville	ID	4,660,975,840	4,659,744,640
43	J&L Specialty Products Corp.	Midland	PA	4,657,012,480	4,629,643,620
44	E I Du Pont De Nemours & Co. Inc.	Richmond	VA	4,428,655,540	4,426,013,600
45	B.F. Goodrich Chemical Group	Calvert City	KY	4,334,409,420	4,330,764,440
46	Sterling Chemicals, Inc.	Texas City	TX	4,320,216,400	6,770,554,200
47	Eli Lilly & Co.	Shadeland	IN	4,261,128,980	4,794,516,380
48	Merck Manufacturing Division	Albany	GA	4,102,230,600	4,095,237,700
49	Williamette Industries	Johnsonburg	PA	3,855,217,360	3,855,212,680
50	The Dow Chemical Co	La Porte	TX	3,830,770,200	3,853,867,960
	Subtotal			680,094,915,860	683,853,350,280
	Percent of Total			71.72	70.95
	Total			948,243,750,000	963,917,566,000

Quantity Managed			Quantity Recycled due to WM	WM Source Reduction Quantity
in RCRA Units Pounds	**in Exempt Units** Pounds	**by Storage** Pounds	Pounds	Pounds
65,175,000	83,144,036,720	0	0	41,440
60,259,302,940	0	0	0	0
51,745,700,540	127,020,640	415,475,500	0	0
49,830,189,760	0	0	0	0
21,189,466,000	17,518,900,000	149,670,000	0	0
27,081,572,800	36,591,800	0	0	0
3,018,000	24,416,186,000	0	0	19,428,000
14,520,795,600	7,014,593,800	0	111,800	1,326,800
18,838,008,000	0	0	17,834,580	8,418,540
16,486,718,760	0	20,900	0	0
15,280,537,000	0	162,000	0	0
22,776,300	13,504,470,660	0	0	87,670,200
13,308,711,880	0	0	0	0
13,020,968,540	0	0	0	0
0	12,000,000,000	0	0	0
11,347,974,100	0	527,460	0	0
1,531,600	11,238,817,200	0	0	0
10,681,762,000	0	0	0	0
165,200	10,220,158,000	0	0	0
2,740,400	8,704,000,000	0	10,163,800	0
39,992,000	8,400,000,000	820,000	0	0
7,896,306,820	0	5,794,200	0	0
6,970,178,000	967,200	3,677,600	0	0
0	7,376,146,240	0	0	0
1,864,000	7,002,000,000	0	0	0
0	6,843,100,500	5,990,740	0	0
0	6,716,692,000	0	0	0
10,400	6,680,000,000	0	0	0
0	6,623,961,600	19,900	0	0
6,303,930,780	0	120,992,660	0	0
0	6,279,305,440	0	3,464,880	0
3,232,000	6,185,124,000	0	0	0
0	5,745,100,720	0	0	0
5,625,043,480	0	22,519,680	0	0
5,323,499,060	0	0	0	0
5,236,464,460	0	0	0	0
3,335,240	5,165,230,200	0	0	0
5,018,765,100	339,800	0	0	0
0	4,944,630,000	0	0	0
0	4,908,785,280	0	0	415,893,980
41,696,020	4,678,676,900	85,857,940	0	0
4,659,744,640	0	0	0	9,980
0	4,629,643,620	0	0	0
0	4,426,013,600	0	0	0
0	4,330,764,440	0	0	0
4,312,880,000	2,403,738,000	53,936,200	0	0
137,130,160	4,657,386,220	0	321,560	569,140
0	4,095,237,700	0	0	0
0	3,855,212,680	0	0	0
1,599,440	3,819,720,000	32,548,520	0	0
375,262,786,020	307,692,550,960	898,013,300	31,896,620	533,358,080
78.49	63.9	20.94	10.22	4.53
478,110,746,000	481,518,364,000	4,288,456,000	312,188,000	11,780,506,000

Table 4-18. RCRA Biennial Report Data, Summary, 1989 and 1991

	1989 Toxic Reports	1991 Toxic Reports*	Change 1989 to 1991	Percent Change 1989 to 1991
	Number	Number	Number	Percent
Number of Facilities	21,069	21,792	723	3.43
Number of Reports	94,862	195,069	100,207	105.63
	Pounds	Pounds	Pounds	Percent
Waste Generated	482,554,451,140	526,314,995,300	43,760,544,160	9.07
Quantity Managed On-site	481,727,504,000	535,708,103,700	53,980,599,700	11.21
Managed in RCRA units	330,136,692,200	213,765,122,600	-116,371,569,600	-35.25
Managed in exempt units	151,588,343,740	318,343,322,220	166,754,978,480	110.01
Storage	2,468,060	3,599,658,880	3,597,190,820	145749.73
Quantity Sent Off-site	16,204,698,000	17,744,016,000	1,539,318,000	9.50

* Only for waste streams required to be reported in both years.

To compare changes in toxic waste generated from 1989 to 1991, it is necessary to remove waste stream records that cover wastes reported under the newly added waste codes. While only an additional 552 facilities (a 2 percent increase) had to report under the new waste codes, the amount of waste generated that had to be reported was an additional 421.9 billion pounds (an 80 percent increase) because of these added waste codes. (See Tables 4-16 and 4-18.)

Changes in Number of Facilities and Waste Managed, 1989 - 1991

The number of facilities reporting to BRS on toxic waste common to both years increased by 3 percent from 1989 to 1991, and the total amount of such waste generated increased by 9 percent. Waste managed under exempt processes rather than RCRA-regulated management methods primarily accounted for this increase, however. The amount of RCRA-managed waste decreased by 35 percent, while the amount of waste managed under exempt processes more than doubled (increasing 110 percent). (See Table 4-18.)

Which facilities report each year changes quite dramatically. Reports from facilities reporting in both 1989 and in 1991 represent only about half of all reports in either year. Over 10,000 facilities reporting in 1991 did not report in 1989. However, facilities reporting in both 1989 and 1991, while small in numbers, represent 95 percent of the waste

Figure 4-13.

RCRA Toxic Waste Generated, 1989 and 1991

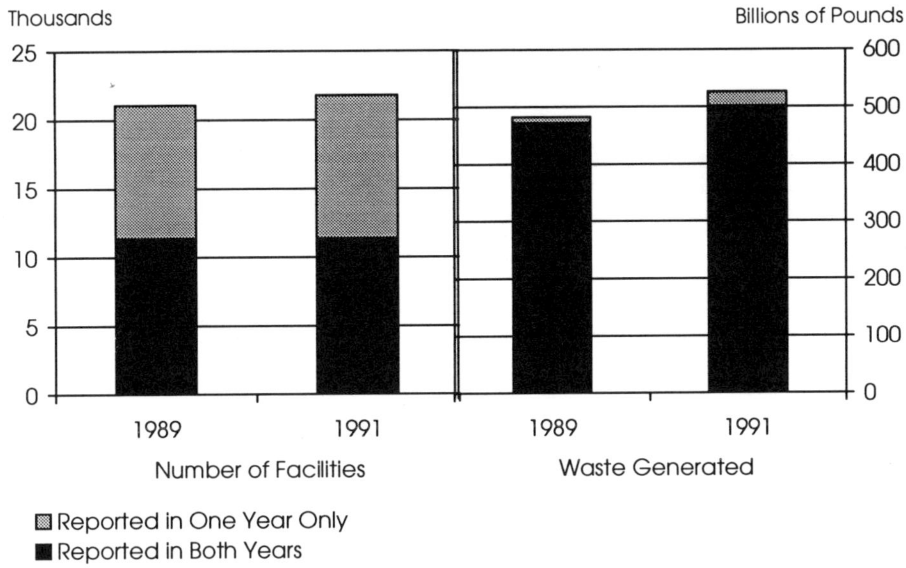

generated. This is because the facilities with the largest waste streams dominate the amount of toxic waste generated, and the larger facilities tend to meet RCRA reporting requirements each year. The 50 facilities that reported the largest amounts of RCRA toxic waste generated in 1991 (excluding the reports with the added waste codes) account for 58 percent of all such waste generated in 1989 and 71 percent of the 1991 total. (See Figure 4-13 and Table 4-19.)

Facilities with Largest Reported Amounts of BRS Waste, 1991

For this *Toxics* Watch report, the five facilities reporting the largest amounts of toxic waste generation to BRS in 1991 were contacted to identify changes in operations that might be responsible for changes in the amount of waste reported to BRS since the 1989 reports.[8] (See Box 4-H.) These five facilities show various changes including significant increases in the number of waste streams and reporting more multiple waste codes in waste streams. Since many of the waste streams reported to BRS are high-volume wastewater streams, small changes in methods of estimating the volume of those streams can result in large changes in reported amounts.

Most facilities contacted for this report agree that their 1991 reporting improved over the 1989 BRS, due in part to increased EPA guidance and, in some cases, guidance from parent companies or trade associations. The facilities also

*Table 4-19. The 50 Facilities with Largest 1991 Toxic Waste Generated with 1989 BRS Data**

Rank	Facility	City	State
1	Kodak Park	Rochester	NY
2	The Dow Chemical Company	Midland	MI
3	E.I. Dupont-Chambers Works	Deepwater	NJ
4	Texas Eastman Division, Eastman Chemical	Longview	TX
5	Hercules,Incorporated	Radford	VA
6	Dupont De Nemours & Co.	Victoria	TX
7	Robins AFB	Warner Robins	GA
8	Kemira Inc	Savannah	GA
9	Shell Oil Company	Anacortes	WA
10	Crown Central Petroleum Corporation	Pasadena	TX
11	Unocal-San Fran Refinery	Rodeo	CA
12	Lyondell Petrochemical Company	Chennelview	TX
13	3M Company	Cottage Grove	MN
14	Lederle Laboratories Division	Pearl River	NY
15	Armco, Inc. Armco Advanced Materials Co.	Lyndora	PA
16	U.S. DOE Idaho National Engineering Lab	Scoville	ID
17	J&L Specialty Products Corporation	Midland	PA
18	Monsanto Company	Alvin	TX
19	E I Du Pont De Nemours & Company Inc.	Richmond	VA
20	Sterling Chemicals, Inc.	Texas City	TX
21	Eli Lilly & Co.-Tippecanoe Laboratories	Shadeland	IN
22	Merck Manufacturing Division	Albany	GA
23	Williamette Industries Pennetch Mill	Johnsonburg	PA
24	The Dow Chemical Co	La Porte	TX
25	Uniroyal Chemical Co Inc	Naugatuck	CT
26	ARCO Chemical Company/Channelview	Channelview	TX
27	GMC Cadillac Motor Car Clark Plant	Detroit	MI
28	American Cyanamid	Waggaman	LA
29	Pratt & Whitney Aircraft Group	East Hartford	CT
30	National Semiconductor Corp	Santa Clara	CA
31	Merck & Co., Inc. Cherokee Plant	Riverside	PA
32	Occidental Chemical Corp	Montague	MI
33	Nalco Chemical Co	Bedford Park	IL
34	Carpenter Technology Corp.	Reading	PA
35	LTV Aerospace & Defense Co.	Dallas	TX
36	Occidental	Niagara Falls	NY
37	Du Pont Sabine River Works	Orange	TX
38	Vulcan Materials Company	Wichita	KS
39	E.I. Du Pont De Nemours & Co., Inc.	Nederland	TX
40	Boeing - Auburn	Auburn	WA
41	Buckbee-Mears Cortland	Cortland	NY
42	Vulcan Chemicals	Geismar	LA
43	U.S. Steel Corporation Fairless Works	Fairless Hills	PA
44	American Telephone & Telegraph	Richmond	VA
45	Rollins Environmental Services	Bridgeport	NJ
46	Quanex Corp Michigan Seamless	South Lyon	MI
47	National Semi Conductor	West Jordan	UT
48	Dupont Washington Works	Washington	WV
49	Zycon Corporation	Santa Clara	CA
50	Mobil Oil Corporation	Chalmette	LA
	Subtotal		
	Percent of Total		
	Total		

* Only reports with waste codes required to be reported in 1989.

1989 Toxic Waste Generated Pounds	1991 Toxic Waste Generated Pounds	Change in Toxic Waste Generated From 1989 to 1991 Pounds
75,613,200	83,225,651,660	83,150,038,460
67,506,060,820	60,269,680,500	-7,236,380,320
93,388,715,940	42,615,144,100	-50,773,571,840
8,905,552,000	11,348,671,660	2,443,119,660
8,099,941,700	8,800,005,200	700,063,500
7,266,890,000	7,890,537,600	623,647,600
1,725,600	7,379,602,300	7,377,876,700
7,442,200,000	6,716,824,000	-725,376,000
5,203,438,000	6,680,610,220	1,477,172,220
326,000	6,624,299,860	6,623,973,860
3,711,440	6,281,257,840	6,277,546,400
32,000	5,647,578,800	5,647,546,800
5,171,972,700	5,336,152,080	164,179,380
1,673,600	4,946,542,660	4,944,869,060
9,094,554,120	4,931,190,960	-4,163,363,160
12,014,900	4,660,945,680	4,648,930,780
4,715,860,080	4,657,012,480	-58,847,600
4,131,660,000	4,497,080,180	365,420,180
5,075,200	4,428,595,440	4,423,520,240
2,397,606,000	4,316,842,400	1,919,236,400
20,163,280	4,261,100,940	4,240,937,660
4,306,148,440	4,102,230,600	-203,917,840
3,450,483,740	3,855,217,360	404,733,620
3,552,148,000	3,830,689,040	278,541,040
4,662,898,900	3,785,845,580	-877,053,320
71,640,000	3,635,358,060	3,563,718,060
2,172,180	3,572,200,600	3,570,028,420
4,086,587,000	3,445,172,120	-641,414,880
2,977,727,540	3,366,810,600	389,083,060
3,020,423,040	3,210,291,980	189,868,940
3,290,470,200	3,183,225,180	-107,245,020
3,106,641,840	3,001,569,440	-105,072,400
147,280	2,852,049,520	2,851,902,240
3,193,764,200	2,570,861,600	-622,902,600
2,230,848,000	2,516,839,500	285,991,500
6,210,200	2,473,887,580	2,467,677,380
3,128,454,000	2,437,071,440	-691,382,560
3,185,546,560	2,429,631,480	-755,915,080
2,763,708,000	2,392,820,180	-370,887,820
1,239,838,920	2,323,739,160	1,083,900,240
2,652,600	2,101,036,060	2,098,383,460
10,119,000	2,075,513,660	2,065,394,660
3,404,031,480	2,057,337,640	-1,346,693,840
2,864,785,860	2,035,042,800	-829,743,060
15,230,400	1,806,177,380	1,790,946,980
2,029,537,400	1,784,240,860	-245,296,540
1,518,004,440	1,739,225,980	221,221,540
64,700	1,674,848,400	1,674,783,700
319,272,420	1,640,436,620	1,321,164,200
21,659,000	1,633,479,000	1,611,820,000
281,906,001,920	373,048,175,980	91,142,174,060
58.42	70.88	
482,554,451,140	526,314,995,300	43,760,544,160

Box 4-H. Five Facilities Reporting the Largest Amounts of Toxic Waste Generated to BRS in 1991

The five facilities reporting the largest amounts of toxic waste generated to BRS in 1991 are Eastman Kodak's Kodak Park facility in Rochester, New York; Dow Chemical Company in Midland, Michigan; DuPont Chambers Works in Deepwater, New Jersey; Texas Eastman Division, Eastman Chemical Company in Longview, Texas (operated by Eastman Kodak until 1993); and Hercules, Inc., in Radford, Virginia. (See Table 4-19.) Three of the five facilities reported increases in the amount of waste generated from 1989, and two reported decreases. Comparisons of data from different reporting years in this report use only waste streams with waste codes required to be reported in both years.)

These five facilities or their corporate parents were contacted to determine how amounts of waste generated were calculated in 1989 and 1991, and to see if the changes in waste between those years were due to actual changes in activity that would have an effect on waste generation.

- Eastman Kodak did not consider most of its on-site wastewater treatment at the Kodak Park facility to be reportable to BRS in 1989, because of existing wastewater exemptions. In preparing the 1991 report, however, the Kodak Park facility reexamined the wastewater exemptions and decided that they no longer applied to the facility. The 1991 report reflects the amount of wastewater treated on site. Eastman Kodak also reports that the much smaller increase reported by the Texas Eastman Division facility was most probably due to changes in amounts of wastewater.

- Dow Chemical Company treats approximately 18 to 20 million gallons of wastewater per day at its Midland facility. Although the company has undertaken several initiatives to reduce the generation of hazardous waste, these reductions are dwarfed by the sheer volume of the plant's wastewater stream. Amounts of wastewater treated from year to year can vary without changes in activity, due to factors such as the amount of rainfall, since runoff becomes part of the wastewater treated on site.

- DuPont Chambers Works undertook several projects to decrease waste generation between 1989 and 1991. Most of these projects concentrated on wastewater, resulting in a decrease in the amount of wastewater generated by the facility. The facility also received less wastewater from other facilities for treatment. In addition, the facility discontinued a business activity involving lead, resulting in shutting down an incinerator that had been used on site. Chambers Works also decreased the generation of waste that is sent to an on-site landfill.

- Hercules, Inc., manages the Radford Air Force Base's operations for the U.S. Department of Defense. Facility representatives state that it has decreased generation of waste steadily since 1988; the increase in toxic waste generation from 1989 to 1991 was due to a change in estimating the flow rate of a D002 waste code waste stream (corrosive waste).

indicated that they are not generally confident about using their own BRS data to compare waste generation for 1989 and 1991.[p] International Paper, which was contacted for background information on BRS and TRI data for the Paper industry, stated that even with improved reporting for 1991 and 1993, the company would not compare even its own 1993 BRS reports to 1991 forms.[9]

Waste Minimization in RCRA

BRS Waste Minimization Reporting Requirements

The BRS collects information on waste minimization that includes recycling and source reduction. The type of reporting on recycling and source reduction is different from TRI in that BRS forms, in contrast to TRI Form R, require a facility to report the amount of waste that was reduced due to source reduction activities. Second, for recycling, the amount of recycling that is new in the year of reporting is included as a separate item. The waste generation amount includes amounts recycled but these amounts are not itemized or reported by chemical constituent, as they are on the TRI form.

Information about source reduction and about new recycling due to waste minimization activities is reported to BRS on two forms. Form IC is a facility-wide report that asks for qualitative information about plans and activities involving source reduction or recycling and about any obstacles that limit such activities. Form GM requires quantitative as well as qualitative information about actual 1991 source reduction and recycling efforts for each waste stream affected. (See Appendix D.) The BRS goes beyond TRI by requiring the facility to report how much waste was reduced due to source reduction. TRI requires the facility to report only whether it undertook any source reduction activities, but not the results of that activity.

The waste-stream-specific Form GM asks whether new activities implemented in 1991 resulted in a minimization of the waste stream. If the answer is positive, the facility reports the quantity recycled and the amount reduced due to source reduction. Facilities also report other effects of the waste minimization activity, such as increased toxicity of the waste or increased releases to air, water, or land, although no quantitative information is requested for these.

[p] Twelve facilities were contacted with questions about their BRS data or about BRS data in general. All of the facilities asked (9) agreed that the 1991 data were more accurate than the 1989 data. Ten indicated that they have their own accounting systems for waste and do not use BRS data to track waste generation at the facilities. In a telephone conversation on August 14, 1994, Al Pagano of DuPont Chambers Works in Deepwater, New Jersey, explained that part of the reason that BRS data cannot be used for this purpose is that the data the facility had reported to the state was not the same data that ended up in EPA's database, and that Chambers Works was not told which data had been changed. Ken Ratzman of New Jersey's Department of Environmental Protection confirmed this on September 19, 1994, although Mr. Ratzman said that the amount of waste was not changed, but rather individual waste stream classifications were altered.

Figure 4-14.

BRS Waste Minimization Data Reported by Facilities, 1991

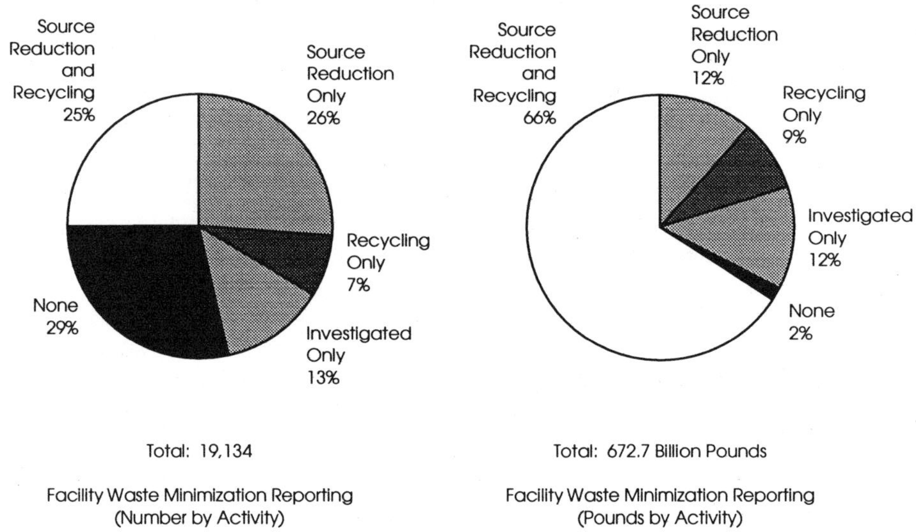

Excludes facilities in Ohio, Texas, and Washington

Data for three states — Ohio, Texas, and Washington State — were not available at the time of this report.[q] Therefore, the waste minimization analysis in this chapter excludes all reports and all facilities in these three states. This analysis covers 86 percent of facilities (19,134 out of 22,344) and 71 percent of the toxic waste generated (672.7 out of 948.2 billion pounds).

Source reduction activities resulting in waste minimization may be under-reported in BRS. If a facility undertakes one or more source reduction activities for a waste stream that result in elimination of the waste stream or change it in such a way that it is no longer reportable, the facility will not file a Form GM for that waste stream. Thus, a waste stream that was reported in 1989 but then was the subject of source reduction activities may not appear in a facility's 1991 report, but there would be no indication of the reason.

Facilities Reporting Waste Minimization

In 1991 a total of 71 percent of facilities (in all states except Ohio, Texas, and Washington) reported either implementing or investigating source reduction or recycling during the reporting period (1990 and 1991). More than half the facilities reported implementing source reduction during 1990 or 1991, either alone or in combination with recycling. Another 13 percent of the facilities reported investigating source reduction or recycling but not implementing these activities. (See Figure 4-14.) These results

[q] Data on waste minimization was not reported on the federal Form GM in these states. Under the BRS, states may use their own forms for collecting data.

Figure 4-15.

BRS Waste Minimization Data Reported for Waste Stream, 1991

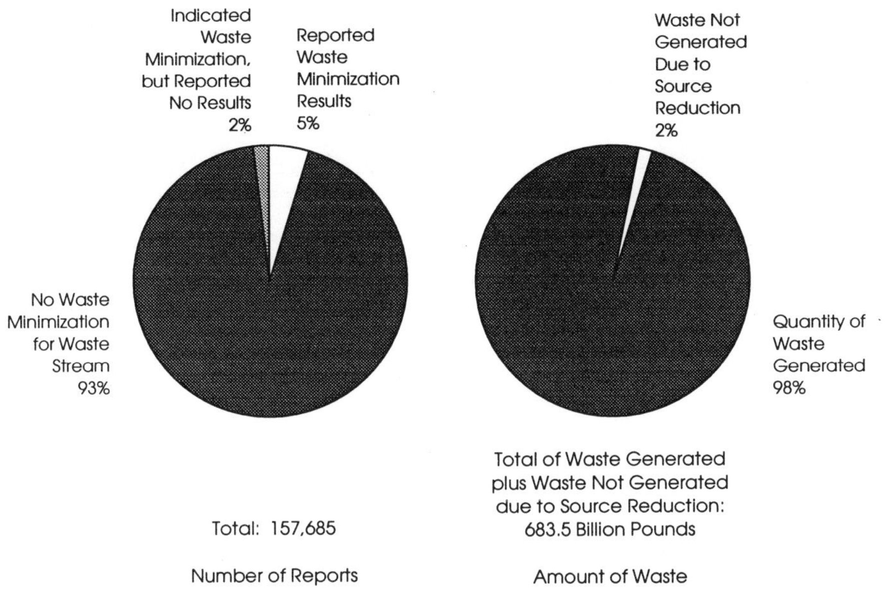

Excludes facilities in Ohio, Texas, and Washington

indicate somewhat more source reduction activity among BRS than among TRI facilities. In TRI 36 percent of facilities reported implementing source reduction activities.

While 51 percent of BRS facilities reported undertaking source reduction alone or in conjunction with recycling, these facilities generated 78 percent of all toxic waste generated. (See Figure 4-14.) Thus, over three-quarters of the total toxic waste generated was generated at facilities that indicate they undertook source reduction. However, the source reduction activities reduced this generated waste by only a small amount.

Results of Waste Minimization Activities

Although most waste generation came from facilities either implementing or investigating source reduction or recycling, the reported results (in reducing waste generation) of these waste minimization activities yield very much smaller numbers. As reported on 5 percent of the toxic waste stream reports, the amount of waste not generated in 1991 because of source reduction activities was just 2 percent (11.8 billion pounds) of all waste generated. (See Figure 4-15.) Indeed, one facility accounted for one-third of the reduction reported: Hill Air Force Base, on the west side of the Great Salt Lake in Utah, reported reducing its "main base industrial wastewater line flow" by 3.5 billion pounds, leaving 406.2 million pounds generated in 1991. Hill Air Force Base implemented several projects to reduce the amount of waste and wastewater generated at the facility. Among these was a new aircraft paint stripping system, replacing the organic solvent/water wash with a high pressure plastic bead stripping process.[10]

*Table 4-20. BRS Waste Minimization Data, 1991**

As Reported on BRS Form GM	**All Reports**		**Wastewater Wastestreams**		**Non-wastewater Wastestreams**	
	Number	Percent	Number	Percent	Number	Percent
Reports on Results of Waste Minimization (WM)						
Facilities						
Total	19,134	100.00	6,405	100.00	18,123	100.00
Indicate WM Results	5,155	26.94	1,053	16.44	4,102	22.63
Reports						
Total	157,685	100.00	17,799	100.00	139,886	100.00
Indicate WM Results	10,578	6.71	1,471	8.26	9,107	6.51
Amount Indicated	7,253	4.60	472	2.65	6,781	4.85
No Amount Indictated	3,325	2.11	0.00	0.00		
	Pounds	Percent	Pounds	Percent	Pounds	Percent
Quantity of Waste Generated						
Total	672,702,542,000	100.00	653,985,578,000	100.00	18,716,964,000	100.00
Reporting Waste Minimization	74,633,032,000	11.09	71,528,036,120	10.94	3,104,995,880	16.59
Quantity Recycled Due to WM	312,188,000	0.05	113,512,000	0.02	198,676,000	1.06
WM Source Reduction Quantity	11,780,506,000	1.75**	10,842,256,000	1.66**	938,250,000	5.01**
Average Pounds per Report						
Quantity of Waste Generated						
Total	4,266,116		36,742,827		133,802	
Reporting Waste Minimization	7,055,496		48,625,449		340,946	

* Totals exclude reports from Ohio, Texas, and Washington because these states did not collect this data on the BRS Form GM.

** These percentages represent percent of waste not generated because of source reduction. For example in the column "All Reports," 672.7 billion pounds plus 11.8 billion pounds (683.5 billion pounds total) of waste *would* have been generated without source reduction. The 11.8 billion pounds is 1.75 percent of this total.

The quantities actually recycled as a result of new activities in 1990 or 1991 were even smaller. The total amount of toxic waste reported generated by the facilities was 672.7 billion pounds, and the amount recycled was only 312.2 million pounds (less than 0.05 percent). (See Table 4-20.)

Since wastewaters represent 97 percent of the reported quantity of toxic waste generated but only 11 percent of the reports, the waste minimization data are broken down into wastewater waste streams and non-wastewater waste streams. A higher portion of the toxic waste generated from non-wastewater waste streams is subject to source reduction and/or recycling: 17 percent compared to 11 percent for toxic wastewater waste streams. The average amount of waste generated for reports of wastewater waste streams was 48.6 million pounds, which is higher than the average for all non-wastewater waste streams. The fact that those forms reporting waste minimization results had higher average pounds of waste generation than those not reporting such results shows that the larger waste streams, in spite of efforts to minimize them, were more likely to remain reportable even after minimization activities in 1991. Waste minimization results might not appear in BRS for smaller, successfully minimized streams if the result was elimination or other changes that eliminated reporting for those streams. (See Table 4-20.)

Obstacles to Waste Minimization Reported

The qualitative information form, BRS Form IC, is a facility-wide report that asks if source reduction and/or recycling was begun or expanded at the site and if the site systematically investigated implementing such activities. The same form also presents a list of possible obstacles to source reduction and recycling and asks the facility to check off any that apply. These questions apply to the facility as a whole, not to individual waste streams.

Almost two-thirds of facilities with toxic waste stream reports indicated that they encountered obstacles to both source reduction and recycling. These obstacles do not appear to have kept facilities from undertaking source reduction. About the same percentage of facilities that reported undertaking source reduction also indicated no obstacles to source reduction and recycling. (See Figure 4-16.)

The obstacles to source reduction mentioned by the most facilities were technical limitations (31 percent) and product quality concerns (28 percent). The fact that source reduction had been undertaken previously was mentioned by 26 percent of all facilities. Regulatory burdens were mentioned by the fewest number of facilities (13 percent). (See Figure 4-17 and Table 4-21.)

Figure 4-16.

BRS Facilities Reporting Obstacles to Source Reduction, 1991

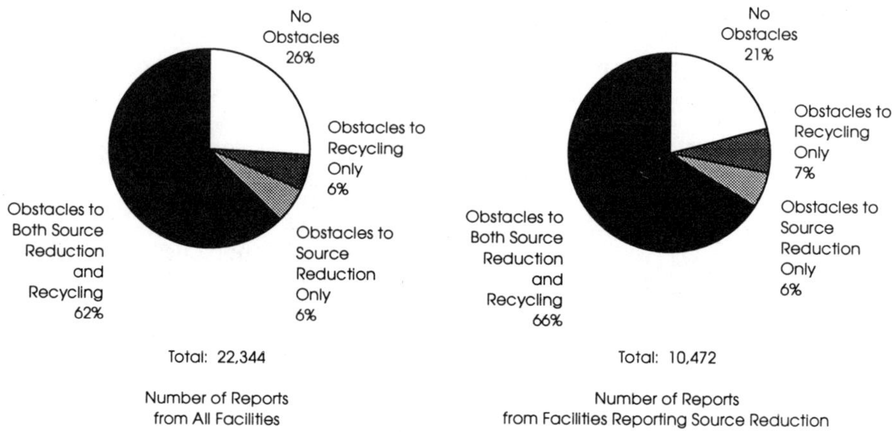

Figure 4-17.

BRS Obstacles to Source Reduction Activity, 1991

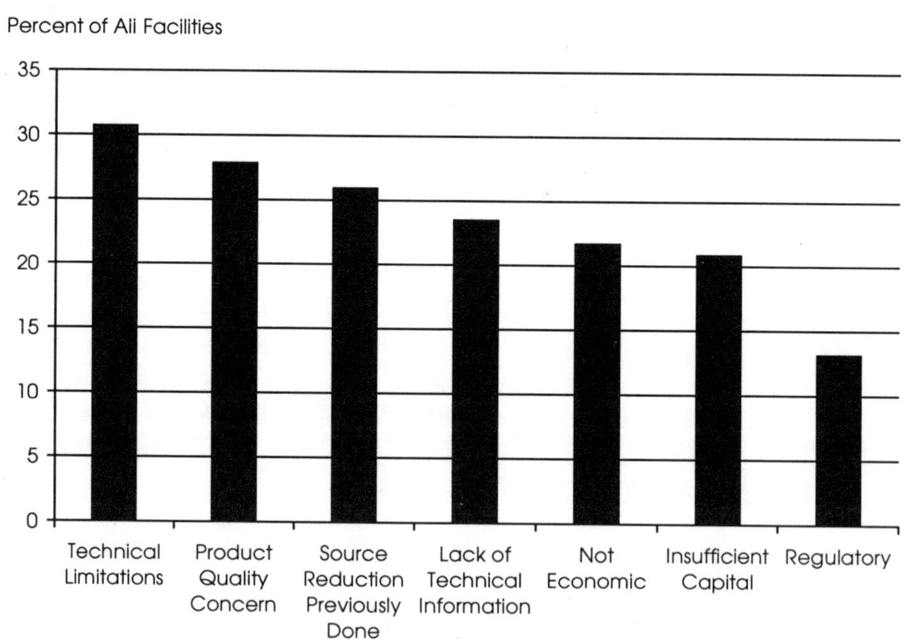

Table 4-21. BRS Waste Minimization Reporting by Facilities with Toxic Reports, 1991

	Number*	Number*	Yes as Percent of Total
Number of Facilities	22,344		
	Yes	**No**	
Waste Minimization Activity during 1990/1991			
Began/expanded source reduction activity	10,472	11,872	46.87
Began/expanded recycling	6,531	15,813	29.23
Investigated source reduction/recycling	12,182	10,162	54.52
Obstacles to Source Reduction			
Insufficient capital	4,664	17,680	20.87
Lack of Technical Information	5,253	17,091	23.51
Not economic	4,855	17,489	21.73
Product quality concern	6,223	16,121	27.85
Technical limitations	6,861	15,482	30.71
Permitting burdens	2,938	19,406	13.15
Previously done	5,794	16,550	25.93
SR previously done-technical limits	3,780	18,564	16.92
SR previously done-economic limits	3,059	19,285	13.69
SR previously done-permitting limits	1,529	20,815	6.84
Other	2,206	20,138	9.87
Obstacles to Recycling			
Insufficient capital	4,218	18,126	18.88
Lack of technical information	4,953	17,391	22.17
Not economic	5,060	17,284	22.65
Product quality concern	4,923	17,421	22.03
Manifests regs limitations	1,499	20,845	6.71
Financial liability limitations	1,824	20,520	8.16
Technical limitations for offsite recycling	2,281	20,063	10.21
Technical limitations for onsite recycling	4,794	17,550	21.46
Permitting burdens	4,156	18,188	18.60
Lack of offsite recycling facilities	3,820	18,524	17.10
No market for recyclable materials	5,454	16,890	24.41
Previously done	6,576	15,768	29.43
Recycling previously done-technical limits	4,446	17,898	19.90
Recycling previously done-economic limits	4,121	18,223	18.44
Recycling previously done-permitting limits	2,673	19,671	11.96
Other	2,903	19,441	12.99

* For all items, a facility reports yes or no. Therefore, items within a section do not add.

Assessment of Nationwide BRS and TRI Waste Generation Data

TRI and BRS data provide different glimpses of waste generation nationwide. Each contributes useful information; each has limitations. Box 4-I lists some of these. Differences in what is reported and how make the data in the two systems difficult to compare directly.

Does either system or a combination of both provide an adequate picture of waste generation and waste management trends to answer important environmental questions? Two studies have pointed out the need for additional data beyond those currently reported to TRI in order to gain greater insight into pollution prevention issues. The first is INFORM's 1991 report, *Toward a More Informed Public*, which provides a list of specific recommendations for improving TRI reporting, including specific data that would quantify source reduction.[11] The other is a 1995 study by Hampshire Research Institute (HRI) and World Wildlife Fund (WWF) that examines the ability of TRI and pollutant release and transfer registries in other countries to answer 11 common environmental questions, ranging from releases to various media to amounts of chemicals used in products and amounts of reductions in waste generation due to source reduction.[12] (See Box 4-J and Appendix F.) Both studies identify the strengths and weaknesses of TRI and indicate additional data elements and policies that would greatly expand the utility of the database (e.g., to track product stewardship and to inform workers of hazards).

One way to explore the ability of national data systems is to postulate environmental questions and see if the answers are available from the data. For example, a recent *Wall Street Journal* article commented on the decline in numbers and profitability of hazardous waste dumps in the past two years.[13] The waste data as they exist presently are not capable of forecasting these types of events. With regard to toxic waste disposal, the TRI data indicate that off-site transfers to disposal decreased by 3 percent between 1991 and 1992. Additionally, the Section 8 quantity released/ disposed of is projected to decrease by 20 percent by 1994 from 1992 levels. While it is not known what portion of the decrease will be attributable to transfers to disposal, on- and off-site recycling are expected to increase from 1992 to 1994, as is on-site energy recovery. All other waste management techniques are expected to decrease, which may indicate a general shift toward on-site activities. The BRS data for 1993 are not yet available, but BRS toxic waste showed an increase from 1989 to 1991, even excluding the newly added waste codes. These data would not necessarily lead to the conclusion that toxic waste disposal facilities will decrease in number, and the time lapse between reporting and public availability of the data makes it difficult to predict environmental trends.

BRS and TRI data have been available since the mid-1980s and have greatly increased the amount of knowledge about toxic chemicals

Box 4-I. Contributions of TRI and BRS to a National View of Waste Generation

TRI	BRS
Provides amounts of specific chemicals leaving facilities as releases or transfers; but does not consider the whole waste stream, so in that sense underestimates the total volume of waste	Non-specific in characterizing waste in regard to chemical constituents; looks at waste stream as a whole to determine hazard; captures information on material that may not appear in TRI data
Only national source of data on air emissions that includes fugitive emissions	Excludes air emissions
Includes no data on waste received by treatment and disposal facilities	Includes reporting of waste received by facilities as well as waste generated and managed at the facilities
Provides data on types of source reduction activities undertaken, but not the amount of waste that was reduced as a result of those activities	Provides the amount of a waste stream reduced by source reduction, but not the amount of specific chemicals reduced
Confusion by facilities on how to classify on-site management activities, particularly recycling, and how to calculate their amounts leads to inconsistencies and largely different amounts of waste reported among facilities and for the same facility from year to year	Not as likely as TRI to pick up low amounts of toxic substances: RCRA toxicity standard may exclude waste streams from BRS reporting because of low concentrations of toxic chemicals, yet the waste streams contain enough of the toxic chemicals to trigger TRI reporting
Although database contains many errors in facility reporting, facilities are generally able to understand and clarify their data, more so than for BRS	Reporting is complex according to facilities contacted for this report, various ways to report waste streams are permissible, and data are difficult to interpret, resulting in difficulty explaining the data or making year-to-year comparisons, even by a facility for its own data
Data have been publicly available since 1989, disseminated and analyzed in many forms	Data available through Freedom of Information Act (FOIA) requests, have become more widely available through RTK-Net in the past year

Box 4-J. National Reporting Systems for Industrial Pollutant Releases and Transfers

One of the key outcomes of the 1992 UN Conference on Environment and Development was Agenda 21, which, among other things, addresses prevention of pollution at the source. The agenda promotes the idea that reducing the amount of energy and materials used in the production of goods and services can both alleviate environmental stress and contribute to productivity. Substances that are less toxic or non-toxic can be substituted as input materials, resulting in reduced pollution and waste disposal.[1] Over 150 countries participating at the conference agreed to Agenda 21 which, in Chapter 19, also advocates that countries develop public "emissions inventories" or pollutant release and transfer registries (PRTRs) to allow for monitoring conditions and trends of pollutants.

Following the 1992 UN Conference, the Organisation for Economic Cooperation and Development (OECD) has been holding a series of workshops on Pollutant Release and Transfer Registers since January 1994. The aim of the workshops is to develop guidance for countries implementing this provision of Agenda 21 and at creating PRTR data that can be shared internationally with little difficulty. Data elements such as common identifiers of chemical names and facility locations, data collection methods, and data collection frequency are being discussed in light of the Agenda 21 goal of reducing toxics at the source.

The Hampshire Research Institute (HRI) and World Wildlife Fund (WWF) developed a study recommending key data elements for facility-level PRTRs that has been presented at the OECD workshops.[2] The benchmark contains four types of data elements: identification, energy and water use, releases and transfers of specific chemicals in waste, and transfers of chemicals in production and products. Identification elements name the facility, give its location, its links to parent companies, and specific information on the chemical being reported, including reporting units. Energy and water use are included because they are important interfaces between facilities and the environment, and because changes amounts of chemicals in waste and in products will affect their use as well. Releases and transfers of specific chemicals in waste include on-site waste management activities and amounts of chemicals in waste reduced by specific source reduction methods.

in waste, particularly in releases and off-site transfers. The shift in national environmental policy toward source reduction and examining waste generation means that uses of the data systems are evolving. At this writing, TRI Section 8 data have been reported for only 1991 and 1992. Two years of data are not enough to discern trends in waste generation or source reduction activity. There are also two effects which may occur as facilities report in future years. First, there is the learning curve as facilities become more familiar with reporting Section 8 data. More important, however, is the effect that having to assemble and report the production-related waste data will have on facilities' future source reduction activities. This effect occurred with the 1987 TRI data on releases and transfers: the task of collecting these data and making them public showed facilities how high their releases and transfers actually were. Johnson & Johnson of New Brunswick, New Jersey, reports that collection and publication of the 1987 TRI data was a major factor in the company's subsequent reductions in releases and transfers.[14] The 1991 data on production-related waste may serve a similar function as an impetus to source reduction.

Finally, transfers of chemicals in products provides information on the flow of chemicals into and out from facilities in non-waste forms, allowing assessment of the effects of transportation activities of chemicals on the environment, as well as providing data on what is by far the largest source of chemicals in the environment — products containing those chemicals (see Chapter 8). These four data element categories contain the information necessary to answer a wide range of environmental questions commonly encountered on pollution prevention.

This study compared seven currently existing state and national reporting systems to their benchmark. The seven inventories include three from the United States (Massachusetts, New Jersey, and the U.S. TRI), as well as inventories from Canada, the Netherlands, Sweden, and the United Kingdom. (See Appendix F.) The study judges TRI to be the most useful of the national inventories for answering questions on the amounts of chemicals in releases and off-site transfers, as well as the amounts of chemicals managed on-site by various methods. TRI does not provide data on chemicals in products, however, while the Netherlands' inventory does. The Netherlands' inventory also provides quantitative source reduction data at the facility level, although its characterization of on- and off-site waste management does not allow calculation of waste generation. Canada and Sweden provide less quantitative data compared to the other national inventories, although Canada does require facilities to explain changes in releases of chemicals from one year to the next. Sweden's inventory is voluntary at this writing, and is being tested in a single county. While it collects the least amount of information among the national inventories in the study, it does gather some information on toxic chemicals in products.

The study showed New Jersey's inventory to be the most complete of all those examined, and Massachusetts' inventory also provides useful data for measuring source reduction progress. (See Chapter 10.)

[1] Agenda 21, Chapters 4 and 19.
[2] Frances H. Irwin, *et al.*, *A Proposed Benchmark for Industrial Pollutant Release and Transfer Reporting,* World Wildlife Fund, January 1995.

---

1 U.S. Environmental Protection Agency, *1992 Toxics Release Inventory Public Data Release*, EPA 745-R-94-001, April 1994.

2 Facility information from telephone conversations with company representatives, July-November 1994:

Carolina Eastman Company: Donna Tomlinson
Champion International Corporation: Jeff Hartman
Corning Asahi Video Products: Dale Stehley
Doe Run Company: Doug Bice
DuPont Chambers Works: Al Pagano
Elkem Metals Company: R. W. Dement
First Chemical Corporation: Dan Marks
ITT Rayonier: Deborah Mark
Lyondell Petrochemical Company: Danny Flack
Phillips 66 Company: D. F. Hunter
Reilly Industries: Jay Kress
Revere Copper Products: Ronald Edwards
Star Enterprises: Keith Bergseid

3 Shelley A. Hearne, "Potential Modifications to the US EPA Toxics Release Inventory to Better Assess Pollution Prevention," unpublished doctoral dissertation submitted to Columbia University, 1994.

4 Hearne, "Potential Modifications."

5 Hearne, "Potential Modifications."

6 Telephone conversations with Tim Saylor, International Paper Corporation, August 4, 1994, and November 3, 1994.

7 Meeting with GenCorp environmental personnel and staff of EPA's 33/50 Program, January 12, 1994.

8 Facility information from telephone conversations with facility representatives, July-November, 1994:

The Dow Chemical Company: Jan Whitfield
DuPont Chambers Works: Al Pagano
Eastman Kodak: Dr. Haines Lockhart
Hercules: Mark Sullivan

9 Telephone conversation with Tim Saylor, International Paper Company, August 4, 1994.

10 Telephone conversation with Alan Dalpias, Hill Air Force Base, November 7, 1994.

11 Jacqueline B. Courteau and Nancy Lilienthal, *Toward a More Informed Public*, New York: INFORM, Inc., 1991.

12 Frances H. Irwin, *et al.*, *A Proposed Benchmark for Industrial Pollutant Release and Transfer Reporting*, World Wildlife Fund, January 1995.

13 Jeff Bailey, "Slump at Hazardous-Waste Dumps Raises Concerns," *Wall Street Journal*, August 5, 1994.

14 Conversation with Anthony A. Herrmann, M.D., Johnson & Johnson, January 18, 1994.

Chapter 5

Chemicals in Waste

Introduction

To examine specific chemicals in waste and how such waste is managed, this chapter looks at the Toxics Release Inventory (TRI) for the 1992 reporting year.[a] While the RCRA Biennial Reporting System (BRS) contains reports on the amounts of entire hazardous waste streams, it does not contain information on quantities of specific chemicals, as does TRI. (See Chapter 4 and the last section of this chapter.) The TRI data are useful for identifying individual chemicals, chemical categories, chemical classes, and groups of chemicals of special concern due to specific health and environmental effects.

This chapter addresses key questions about the chemicals in TRI waste. It looks at these chemicals in three time-frames: first, it looks at TRI waste in 1992; then it focuses on changes that took place between 1991 and 1992; and finally it looks at changes projected by TRI reporting facilities to occur between 1992 and 1994.

Toxics Watch analyzes the waste profiles from several points of view for each time period. The questions addressed first for 1992 include:

- What chemicals were generated in waste in the largest amounts?
- What were the wastes associated with five specific chemical classes: non-halogenated organics, acids/bases/salts, metals, halo-organics, and non-metallic inorganics? *Toxics Watch* chose to divide the TRI chemicals into these five groups both because they are often associated with different conditions of use in industry and because they behave differently in the environment.
- How prevalent were wastes in three special groups of environmental concern: carcinogens, ozone depleters, and chloro-organics?
- How did TRI facilities manage chemically different types of waste?
- What chemicals were managed in the least desirable way — through release and disposal?

[a] Because this chapter focuses on chemicals in waste, the primary data analyzed are the data reported in Section 8 of the TRI Form R in 1992. 1991 TRI Section 8 data is reported on 1992 Form Rs as data for the previous year (see Chapter 4). A limited evaluation of information on releases and transfers to disposal as reported in Sections 5 and 6 is presented, in order to examine the environmental distribution of such releases.

- How much influence did source reduction have on the generation of waste?

Toxics Watch also looked at how reliable the TRI data were with regard to major increases or decreases in specific chemicals reported to TRI by contacting facilities to assess the reasons for reported changes.

Although all chemicals reported to TRI are of environmental concern, not all are subject to the same level of concern and scrutiny by government, communities, and industry. Some chemicals raise different issues and are greater hazards than others. That is why this chapter features three special groups of concern: carcinogens, because of their potential to cause cancer; stratospheric ozone depleters, even though their release through use is much greater than as waste from industrial facilities (see Chapter 2); and finally chloroorganics, not because all chemicals in this group represent a common environmental hazard, but rather because the group is the focus of an active debate involving a wide range of adverse environmental effects. It is especially valuable to know the amounts of such chemicals in waste and to be able to evaluate whether and how much such chemicals have decreased in waste, as well as how much they are projected to increase or decrease in future years.

Overall, TRI data show that relatively few chemicals account for the majority of waste generated. Just 25 chemicals out of the 336 TRI chemicals and chemical categories accounted for 84 percent of the total amount of TRI production-related waste in 1992. It is only necessary to look at those 25 chemicals to gain a broad national overview of toxic chemicals in manufacturing-facility waste. However, a resident near a factory releasing significant amounts of a chemical locally that is unimportant on a nationwide basis, or an official of an industry or facility using such a chemical, will need to plunge further into the data than is done in this chapter. (See Chapter 7 for major geographical patterns in the data.)

Looking at the summary data alone, moreover, does not always reveal why the data are the way they are. Numerous factors may be involved. For example, the physical-chemical properties of a chemical can influence how a chemical is released to the environment; the way a chemical is used can determine the nature of its waste and how that waste is managed; or one or two facilities might dominate the data on a particular chemical so much that how other facilities deal with the chemical is lost in the aggregate information. While investigating each finding in detail is beyond the scope of this report, this chapter provides explanations for many of the observations that are presented.

Many kinds of chemical-specific information and analysis can be derived from the publicly available database. Although the analyses presented here are on an aggregate national level and valuable in informing national policy decisions, similar analyses can be conducted on a regional, state, or local level, where the findings can inform decisions on the waste activities of relevant facilities.

Summary of Findings

- In 1992 TRI facilities reported a total of 37.3 billion pounds of production-related waste containing 272 of the 336 TRI chemicals and chemical categories.
  - — Of the 37.3 billion pounds of production-related waste, 3.0 billion pounds (8 percent) was composed of carcinogens; 738.1 million pounds (2 percent) was ozone depleters, and 2.3 billion pounds (6 percent) was chloro-organics.
  - — Just 25 TRI chemicals accounted for the vast majority (84 percent) of all production-related waste in 1992.
  - — Similarly, the top 25 chemicals based upon the amounts released/disposed of account for more than 84 percent of all TRI release and disposal (2.8 billion pounds out of 3.4 billion pounds).
  - — Of all the 37.3 billion pounds of TRI waste, 9 percent is released or disposed of — the least environmentally desirable option. In general the three chemical groups of special concern had as great or greater percentages of environmental release and disposal: 8 percent for carcinogens, 22 percent for ozone depleters, and 14 percent for chloro-organics.
- Most patterns of waste management and of environmental distribution for chemical classes are consistent with their common chemical and physical properties (e.g., nonflammable metals are seldom sent to energy recovery and volatile ozone depleters are mostly released to the air). The relative cost of the chemicals is also a factor.
  - — 81 percent of production-related waste for metals was managed by recycling in 1992. Metals do not burn and so cannot be used for energy recovery, and regulations restrict their release and disposal. In addition, metals are relatively expensive as raw material when compared to other chemical classes.
  - — Recycling accounted for 53 percent of production-related waste associated with acids/bases/salts in 1992, and treatment for another 41 percent. These chemicals are generally inexpensive and easily recycled or treated, but usually do not burn and have restrictions on their release and disposal.
  - — 98 percent of 1992 releases and disposal of halo-organics emerged as air emissions, consistent with their uses as solvents and their relatively high volatility.
  - — 46 percent of 1992 production-related waste for non-halogenated organics was managed by recycling, and an additional 22 percent was managed by energy recovery — the highest percentage of waste management by energy recovery among the chemical classes in this report. This high percentage occurred because most of these chemicals burn well.

- All of the chemical classes showed an increase in production-related waste between 1991 and 1992 except for halo-organics, which showed a decrease. Among the special groups, carcinogens showed an increase in production-related waste between 1991 and 1992, while ozone-depleters and chloro-organics showed a decrease. These decreases in production-related waste for ozone depleters, halo-organics, and chloro-organics are consistent with reported source reduction activities: these three categories showed greater percentages of forms reporting source reduction activities in 1992 than the other chemical classes and groups. More than 40 percent of the forms for ozone depleters, halo-organics, and chloro-organics report undertaking source reduction activities in 1992. The average for all TRI chemicals was 25 percent.
- The greatest percentage reduction in production-related waste projected between 1992 and 1994 is for chemicals in groups with lesser percentages of reduction or increases in production-related waste reported between 1991 and 1992.
  - Non-metallic inorganics showed a 12 percent increase in production-related waste between 1991 and 1992; a reduction of 14 percent is projected for 1992-1994.
  - Halo-organics showed a decrease of less than one-half of 1 percent in production-related waste between 1991 and 1992; a reduction of 9 percent is projected for 1992-1994.
- Some of the biggest changes in production-related waste between 1991 and 1992 for individual chemicals represent changes in methods of calculating amounts of on-site waste management and, to a lesser degree, reporting errors. (See Chapter 4.)

TRI Waste, 1992

Chemical Composition of TRI Waste

Facilities reported waste for 272 of the 336 TRI chemicals and chemical categories[b] in 1992. Facilities must submit the following information on TRI chemicals on TRI Form R (see Chapter 4, Box 4-A, and Appendix A):

- quantity released to the environment on site and disposed of on and off site (Section 8.1 of TRI Form R);
- quantity used for energy recovery on and off site (Sections 8.2 and 8.3);
- quantity recycled on and off site (Sections 8.4 and 8.5);
- quantity treated on and off site (Sections 8.6 and 8.7); and
- quantity released to the environment due to one-time events (Section 8.8).

[b] Some of the chemicals on the TRI list have been phased out of production for a variety of reasons and are no longer used; therefore, there would be no reporting to TRI. In other cases, some use of the chemicals may continue, but in a particular reporting year no facilities meet the threshold reporting requirements for these chemicals.

The total amount of TRI chemicals in production-related waste (as reported in Section 8) was 37.3 billion pounds. While 272 TRI chemicals were reported in waste, relatively few chemicals dominate the data: the 25 chemicals with the largest amounts of total production-related waste account for 84 percent of all such waste. (See Table 5-1.)

Sulfuric acid ranked as the chemical with the largest total amount of production-related waste, 10.3 billion pounds or more than one-fourth (28 percent) of all production-related waste. Of the 10.3 billion pounds, 4.0 billion pounds (39 percent) is attributable to one facility, First Chemical in Pascagoula, Mississippi. First Chemical seems to have significantly overestimated the true amount of its production-related waste, however, as the result of the way in which it calculated its on-site recycling of sulfuric acid. Sulfuric acid, which is one of the most widely used chemicals in a variety of manufacturing processes, would nevertheless remain the top chemical even if First Chemical had reported zero sulfuric acid waste. (See Chapter 4 for more information about this facility and Appendix B for a discussion of problems associated with the methodology used by facilities to calculate on-site recycling.)

Acetonitrile ranked second with 2.6 billion pounds (7 percent) as the result of the methodology used by one facility, Goodyear Tire and Rubber Company in Beaumont, Texas, to calculate its on-site recycling. In 1994, after the TRI database was "frozen" for use in this report, Goodyear revised the amount of on-site recycling of acetonitrile in 1992 from 2.5 billion pounds to zero. (See Chapter 4.) Hydrochloric acid ranked third with 2.5 billion pounds (7 percent), methanol fourth with 2.2 billion pounds (6 percent), and propylene fifth with 1.6 billion pounds (4 percent).

Facilities manage different TRI chemicals in waste in different ways. The differences are often the result of five factors: the physical-chemical properties of chemicals, the costs of different ways to manage waste, the costs of the chemicals themselves, the availability of different waste management options for each facility, and regulatory restrictions for certain chemicals. It is not surprising, therefore, that chemicals dominating one category of waste management methods do not necessarily dominate in another.

Starting with the second most environmentally beneficial strategy, after source reduction, the five chemicals *recycled* in the greatest quantities were sulfuric acid, acetonitrile, lead compounds, toluene, and copper. The five chemicals used for *energy recovery* in the largest quantities were propylene, ethylene, methanol, toluene, and xylene (mixed isomers). For the *treatment* category, the top five chemicals were sulfuric acid, hydrochloric acid, methanol, ammonia, and propylene. Finally, the five chemicals managed most in the least environmentally desirable way — *released* on site or sent off site for *disposal* — were ammonia, hydrochloric acid, methanol, phosphoric acid, and sulfuric acid. (See Appendix J, Tables J-5 through J-8.)

Table 5-1. The 25 TRI Chemicals with the Largest Total Production-related Waste, 1992

CAS Number	Chemical	Total Recycled Pounds	Total Energy Recovery Pounds	Total Treated Pounds	Quantity Released/ Disposed of Pounds	Total Production-related Waste Pounds	Non-Production-related Waste Pounds
7664-93-9	Sulfuric acid	7,068,452,870	103,428	3,013,392,332	187,976,508	10,269,925,138	3,522,137
75-05-8	Acetonitrile	2,511,466,278	34,186,005	14,241,043	21,429,372	2,581,322,698	12,758
7647-01-0	Hydrochloric acid	189,945,296	57,973	1,986,648,874	298,900,276	2,475,552,419	221,897
67-56-1	Methanol	490,776,751	399,689,097	1,089,038,799	259,001,005	2,238,505,652	639,753
115-07-1	Propylene	343,447,371	744,713,119	505,918,496	21,295,605	1,615,374,591	183,465
7664-41-7	Ammonia	229,573,826	53,556,096	645,124,226	455,599,635	1,383,853,783	1,366,277
108-88-3	Toluene	654,476,356	338,027,884	143,976,640	186,681,857	1,323,162,737	479,129
74-85-1	Ethylene	197,286,622	497,793,629	449,291,528	35,854,137	1,180,225,916	687,169
	Lead compounds	1,042,138,350	41,842	38,181,148	26,999,354	1,107,360,694	1,287,095
7664-38-2	Phosphoric acid	90,922,816	8,898	394,383,391	196,807,410	682,122,515	12,122,137
7440-50-8	Copper	639,505,240	20,819	6,100,296	29,512,497	675,138,852	491,213
67-64-1	Acetone	231,073,609	173,458,645	128,496,339	139,039,676	672,068,269	257,235
107-21-1	Ethylene glycol	448,479,915	13,602,675	78,952,509	20,109,179	561,144,278	198,170
1330-20-7	Xylene (mixed isomers)	149,455,573	238,887,500	52,760,158	108,789,871	549,893,102	661,016
	Copper compounds	311,575,763	52,758	144,365,940	46,462,501	502,456,962	930,700
	Zinc compounds	313,101,884	272,899	36,305,445	120,490,959	470,171,187	1,374,675
78-93-3	Methyl ethyl ketone	196,269,075	123,915,256	56,738,035	88,491,478	465,413,844	121,088
106-99-0	1,3-Butadiene	322,753,595	77,256,906	49,570,205	4,046,531	453,627,237	137,163
7782-50-5	Chlorine	108,816,142	77,503	250,787,204	71,168,030	430,848,879	35,581
108-10-1	Methyl isobutyl ketone	243,664,202	68,661,970	12,797,024	25,840,592	350,963,788	27,958
71-55-6	1,1,1-Trichloroethane	194,945,111	9,517,631	5,964,106	112,587,880	323,014,728	103,973
98-82-8	Cumene	308,424,694	5,631,601	2,619,448	3,715,939	320,391,682	12,065
7697-37-2	Nitric acid	44,113,139	538	237,177,534	29,559,498	310,850,709	56,138
50-00-0	Formaldehyde	169,362,610	10,794,444	101,599,699	16,913,837	298,670,590	29,434
76-13-1	Freon 113	33,838,374	338,224	231,579,359	23,906,231	289,662,188	20,170
	Subtotal	16,533,865,462	2,790,667,340	9,676,009,778	2,531,179,858	31,531,722,438	24,978,396
	Percent of Total	85.41	78.19	87.92	74.42	84.46	73.53
	All Others	2,824,223,935	778,509,373	1,329,113,566	870,206,312	5,802,053,186	8,991,427
	Total	19,358,089,397	3,569,176,713	11,005,123,344	3,401,386,170	37,333,775,624	33,969,823

Beyond the *production-related waste* and its management, discussed above, facilities often generate other waste resulting from one-time events not associated with routine production practices. This *non-production-related waste* includes accidental releases as well as remedial actions to clean up past contamination. The waste may be released on site or sent off site for recycling, energy recovery, treatment, or disposal. One chemical alone, phosphoric acid, accounted for over one-third of all non-production-related waste in 1992; overall, the top 25 chemicals were responsible for 90 percent of the total. In many, but not all, cases the 25 chemicals with the largest quantities of non-production-related waste are also those with some of the largest quantities of production-related waste. Exceptions include, for example, nickel compounds which rank 3rd for non-production-related waste, but 55th in quantity of production-related waste. (See Table 5-1 and Appendix J, Table J-9.)

Release and Disposal of TRI Chemicals in Waste

It is important to identify those TRI chemicals managed in the least desirable way — release/disposal — because these chemicals might be most likely to be found in the environment, and humans and ecosystems might be most exposed to them. The 25 chemicals with the largest quantities released/disposed of (as indicated in Section 8 of TRI Form R) account for more than 84 percent of the releases/disposal of for all TRI chemicals (2.8 billion pounds out of 3.4 billion pounds). (See Appendix J, Table 8.)

The TRI chemicals with the largest quantities of total production-related waste are often the same ones associated with the largest amounts of releases and disposal. Hydrochloric acid, for example, ranks third in total production-related waste and second for release/disposal amounts. This is not always the case, however. Carbon disulfide, which is highly volatile, predominantly released to air, and relatively inexpensive, ranks 11th in quantity of waste released but is not even among the top 25 chemicals for total production-related waste. (See Table 5-1 and Appendix J, Table J-8.)

Knowing the environmental distribution of chemicals that are released or disposed of is also important, because it can indicate the potential environmental pathways by which humans and ecosystems might be exposed to particular pollutants. Sections 5 and 6 of TRI Form R provide data on the amounts of chemical releases to air, water, land, and underground injection and off-site transfers to recycling, energy recovery, treatment, and disposal.[c]

Chemicals display patterns of environmental distribution that are often driven by their physical-chemical properties. For example, almost all of the toluene (98 percent) that is released/disposed of is emitted to air. This is not surprising, given the highly volatile nature of this chemical. Releases and transfers of sulfuric acid, a chemical less volatile than toluene and easily diluted, are more diverse: 52 percent is injected to underground wells, 18 percent is transferred off site for disposal, 17 percent is discharged to surface water, 12 percent is emitted to air, and 1 percent is disposed of on site to land. (See Table 5-2.)

[c] The environmental distribution of the quantities of waste reported as released/disposed of in Section 8.1 of TRI Form R cannot be determined from the information given in Section 8, but rather in data reported for Sections 5 and 6. The amount of waste reported in Section 8.1 as released/disposed of should be approximately equal to the total amount of releases (air, water, underground injection, and land) reported in Section 5 plus the amount of transfers off site for "disposal" as reported in Section 6. Any difference between these sums should be due to the amount of waste released as a result of one-time events as reported in Section 8.8. As noted in Chapter 4, there are inconsistencies in the data reported in various sections of Form R. These are difficult to evaluate or assess quantitatively, but may decrease as facilities gain more experience in reporting Section 8 data. (See Appendix A.)

Table 5-2. Environmental Distribution of the 25 TRI Chemicals with the Largest Quantities of Waste Released/Disposed of (Section 8 of TRI Form R), 1992

CAS Number	Chemical	Total Air Emissions Sec. 5 Pounds	Surface Water Discharges Sec. 5 Pounds	Underground Injection Sec. 5 Pounds	Releases to Land Sec. 5 Pounds
7664-41-7	Ammonia	162,084,835	40,824,196	251,783,103	9,165,277
7647-01-0	Hydrochloric acid	77,109,030	1,927,193	207,817,749	432,770
67-56-1	Methanol	194,790,687	16,422,600	27,084,182	3,328,541
7664-38-2	Phosphoric acid	1,195,609	158,674,836	35,230	46,725,635
7664-93-9	Sulfuric acid	23,721,453	32,719,526	98,631,395	1,737,032
108-88-3	Toluene	190,997,161	84,024	1,573,901	708,278
67-64-1	Acetone	133,953,501	999,584	3,180,700	559,265
	Zinc compounds	4,184,792	1,009,739	126,947	76,540,392
71-55-6	1,1,1-Trichloroethane	114,944,386	13,132	561	76,381
1330-20-7	Xylene (mixed isomers)	109,712,311	41,504	219,270	1,434,430
75-15-0	Carbon disulfide	92,877,037	45,087	2,704	21
78-93-3	Methyl ethyl ketone	90,504,641	153,249	365,395	241,794
75-09-2	Dichloromethane	73,963,205	221,192	1,183,867	79,313
	Manganese compounds	1,798,144	733,225	22,569	61,485,334
7782-50-5	Chlorine	69,912,882	1,217,091	48,252	46,171
	Glycol ethers	45,528,605	350,489	194,386	140,595
6484-52-2	Ammonium nitrate (solution)	1,330,918	6,762,487	37,531,805	2,624,432
	Copper compounds	6,329,997	72,413	201,431	34,489,362
74-85-1	Ethylene	36,606,826	13,413	0	0
	Chromium compounds	463,685	269,667	32,137	23,165,988
100-42-5	Styrene	32,334,616	23,502	83,170	304,179
71-36-3	n-Butyl alcohol	29,723,327	35,369	2,324,731	57,220
7697-37-2	Nitric acid	3,030,928	53,725	22,081,766	664,849
7440-50-8	Copper	1,495,369	41,474	16,736	12,647,313
7783-20-2	Ammonium sulfate (solution)	234,900	4,429,219	5,705,957	4,069,490
	Subtotal	1,498,828,845	267,137,936	660,247,944	280,724,062
	Percent of Total	81.24	97.88	90.95	83.10
	All Others	346,129,491	5,795,017	65,698,471	57,084,991
	Total	1,844,958,336	272,932,953	725,946,415	337,809,053

Transfers to Disposal Sec. 6 Pounds	Total Releases Plus Transfers to Disposal Sec. 5 & 6 Pounds	Quantity Released/ Disposed of Sec. 8 Pounds
3,613,161	467,470,572	455,599,635
12,981,133	300,267,875	298,900,276
2,900,199	244,526,209	259,001,005
1,173,331	207,804,641	196,807,410
34,202,633	191,012,039	187,976,508
936,544	194,299,908	186,681,857
524,172	139,217,222	139,039,676
42,506,449	124,368,319	120,490,959
611,054	115,645,514	112,587,880
1,240,922	112,648,437	108,789,871
1,717	92,926,566	93,554,822
620,881	91,885,960	88,491,478
189,299	75,636,876	75,729,079
12,897,077	76,936,349	75,565,406
27,300	71,251,696	71,168,030
674,074	46,888,149	49,847,660
2,394,025	50,643,667	49,700,242
6,427,267	47,520,470	46,462,501
329	36,620,568	35,854,137
9,880,041	33,811,518	35,745,584
2,624,009	35,369,476	33,687,236
500,583	32,641,230	32,300,656
3,986,437	29,817,705	29,559,498
13,139,578	27,340,470	29,512,497
7,590,648	22,030,214	29,261,313
161,642,863	2,868,581,650	2,842,315,216
62.50	83.38	83.56
96,999,714	571,707,684	559,070,954
258,642,577	3,440,289,334	3,401,386,170

Box 5-A. Carcinogens

EPA developed threshold and release reporting requirements for TRI chemicals when it established the Section 313 rule in February 1988, under the Emergency Planning and Community Right-to-Know Act (EPCRA). The Agency also set limits for determining whether TRI chemicals in mixtures and in trade-name products need to be factored into these threshold and release determinations. A TRI chemical does not have to be considered if its concentration in a mixture or trade name product is below a *de minimis* level.

At the time that the Section 313 rule was promulgated, EPA decided to use *de minimis* concentrations that had already been established by the Occupational Safety and Health Administration (OSHA) for determining whether a Material Safety Data Sheet (MSDS) must be prepared for a chemical in a mixture. The two concentrations established by OSHA and adopted by EPA were 0.1 percent for known or suspect human carcinogens and 1.0 percent for other chemicals.

EPA also chose, at the time of the final rule, to accept OSHA's definition of a carcinogen and apply this definition to the TRI list of chemicals. A chemical is considered by OSHA to be a carcinogen or potential carcinogen if any of the following sources list it as such:

1) National Toxicology Program, *Annual Report on Carcinogens* (latest edition);
2) International Agency for Research on Cancer (IARC), *Monographs* (latest edition); or
3) 29 Code of Federal Regulations Part 1910, Subpart Z, Toxic and Hazardous Substances, Occupational Safety and Health Administration.

While EPA has continued since 1988 to use OSHA's definition for identifying chemicals on the TRI list as carcinogens, the Agency itself has become more involved in evaluating the toxic hazards, including carcinogenic effects, of a variety of chemicals. EPA has developed a more systematic and formal process for performing such evaluations and making them public. The two predominant sources of information on EPA's evaluation of carcinogenic effects of chemicals are the Integrated Risk Information System (IRIS) and the Health Effects Assessment Summary Tables (HEAST). For this *Toxics Watch* report, the list of TRI chemicals considered to be carcinogenic is expanded to include chemicals designated carcinogenic in IRIS or HEAST.

IRIS is a database that contains evaluations, made by multi-Office EPA workgroups, which have undergone a peer review process. Evaluations in this database have Agency-wide authority and represent EPA consensus. In addition, EPA has developed a set of hazard assessments that are less authoritative than those in IRIS because the review process is not so extensive, but widely used to meet the needs of the Superfund program for hazard assessments of chemicals found at hazardous waste sites that do not have evaluations in IRIS. The Agency publishes these additional evaluations in HEAST.

Chemical Classes and Chemical Groups of Special Concern

Basis for Chemical Classes and Groups of Special Concern

In this chapter, TRI chemicals have been grouped two ways. The first grouping of all TRI chemicals and chemical categories is into five classes, based on certain common physical and chemical characteristics:

- organics (non-halogenated),
- acids/bases/salts,
- metals,
- halo-organics, and
- non-metallic inorganics.

EPA assigns a weight-of-evidence classification to a chemical regarding the likelihood of its being a human carcinogen based upon evaluating both human and animal studies. The Agency's system of classification was adapted from IARC's approach to assessing chemicals and includes:

A - Human Carcinogen
B1 or B2 - Probable Human Carcinogen
  B1 indicates that limited human data are available.
  B2 indicates sufficient evidence in animals and inadequate or no evidence in humans.
C - Possible Human Carcinogen
D - Not Classifiable as to human carcinogenicity
E - Evidence of noncarcinogenicity for humans

Chemicals identified as carcinogens in this report include those chemicals that EPA has rated as probable human carcinogens (B1 or B2) or as human carcinogens (A) in IRIS or HEAST. This adds 17 chemicals to the list defined by EPA using OSHA's definition of a carcinogen.

The list of TRI carcinogens that appears in EPA's *1992 Toxics Release Inventory Public Data Release*, however, does not include all the chemicals listed as such in the 1992 TRI Form R instructions. EPA dropped 11 chemicals for a variety of reasons. This *Toxics Watch* report includes the 118 chemicals in the data release and the additional 17 chemicals identified by EPA in IRIS and HEAST. (See Appendix I.)

Using this expanded list of 135 carcinogens, *Toxics Watch* identified a total of 3.0 billion pounds of carcinogenic production-related waste in 1992. This is 93.1 million pounds above the 2.9 billion pounds of waste associated with the list of carcinogens used by EPA in the TRI data release report. *Toxic Watch*'s expanded list also accounted for an increase (compared to the data release) of 2.8 million pounds in the amount of waste considered carcinogenic that was released/disposed of to the environment.

As illustrated above, there is no definitive list of carcinogens, and existing lists are subject to change as new evaluations and re-evaluations are performed. An example of this involves the chemical trichloroethylene (TCE). Prior to July 1989, TCE appeared in the IRIS database as a B2 carcinogen. However, in July 1989, EPA withdrew TCE's carcinogenicity assessment from IRIS as the chemical underwent further review. As of September 1994, the Agency had yet to complete the re-evaluation; therefore, TCE's carcinogenicity assessment still does not appear in IRIS. If TCE were still to be rated as a B2 carcinogen after undergoing the re-evaluation, it would add 271.9 million pounds of production-related waste to the carcinogenic total for 1992 and 28.2 million pounds to the amount of waste of carcinogens released/disposed of to the environment.

Each class contains chemicals that differ chemically from other classes of chemicals. Hence, they tend to have both different industrial applications and different environmental consequences than chemicals of the other classes. For example, industrial uses and environmental concerns with acids and bases tend to relate to their acidity or caustic nature, respectively. While an acid may make a good metal cleaner in an industrial facility, the same acidity in a water effluent may make the receiving waters too acidic to support fish and other aquatic life. In contrast, metals have many well recognized common properties (e.g., their ability to conduct electricity and heat), but as elements they are by definition environmentally persistent. Therefore, to the extent that they are toxic, their environmental

Box 5-B. Ozone Depleters

Increasing attention has focused in the last two decades on depletion of the ozone layer in the earth's upper atmosphere (stratosphere) and on the chemicals involved in causing the depletion, i.e., chlorofluorocarbons (CFCs), halons, 1,1,1-trichloroethane, carbon tetrachloride, and bromomethane. (See Appendix I.) Stratospheric ozone screens out harmful ultraviolet-B radiation from reaching the earth's surface. As the protective ozone layer decreases, the level of this radiation that reaches the earth increases. Ultraviolet-B radiation has been associated with a number of human health and environmental effects including skin cancer (including malignant melanoma), cataracts, and reduction of crop yield.

The conversion of ozone to oxygen is catalyzed by chlorine and bromine, which are known to be released by ozone depleters in the stratosphere, thus resulting in a chain reaction that reduces the ozone concentration. Because ozone depleters remain in the upper atmosphere for many decades, their emission today will impact the levels of stratospheric ozone well into the future.

The 1987 Montreal Protocol on Substances that Deplete the Ozone Layer focused worldwide attention on ozone depleters, and the United States, among the other nations signing the Protocol, agreed on a timetable for phasing out and eliminating use of ozone depleters. (See Chapter 2.) A subsequent meeting in June 1990 broadened the scope of chemicals to be phased out. The Clean Air Act Amendments of 1990 codified the Montreal Protocol agreements for U.S. industry, with some more stringent interim reductions before the 2000 deadline. With the intense focus on ozone depleters, and mounting evidence that ozone depletion was progressing faster than previously predicted, President Bush ordered an accelerated phase-out of certain ozone depleters with a deadline of December 31, 1995. The President's February 1992 order also mandated a priority review of substitutes for ozone depleters that would do less damage to the ozone layer.[1]

[1] 58FR28094, May 12, 1993.

release is of concern. Mixtures and trade-secret chemicals are treated separately because they cannot be combined with other TRI chemicals in any way. These five classes thus cover all TRI chemicals. (See Appendix I.)

The second manner in which TRI chemicals have been classified in this chapter is by a characteristic of the group that makes them of particular concern because of their effects on human health and the environment. The three special groups discussed in this report are:

- carcinogens (see Box 5-A),
- ozone depleters (see Box 5-B), and
- chloro-organics (see Box 5-C).

Many TRI chemicals do not fall into any of these three special groupings, but some fall into more than one of the groups (e.g., 1,1,1-trichloroethane and Freon 113 are both chloro-organic and ozone depleters.) (See Appendix I.)

Another toxic chemical class of environmental importance includes chemicals that bioaccumulate in humans and wildlife. These are not analyzed as a class in this report simply because there is no authoritative list of which TRI chemicals are bioaccumulators. However, this issue will be explored in greater detail in future *Toxics Watch* reports.

Box 5-C. Chloro-organics

Over the last two decades, there has been an increasing focus on chlorine and individual (or closely related) chloro-organic compounds. Chloro-organics include compounds such as chlorofluorocarbons (CFCs), chlorinated pesticides, polyvinyl chloride (PVC), and chlorinated solvents. (See Appendix I.) The adverse health and environmental effects of greatest concern that have been linked to chloro-organics are cancer, reproductive effects, and stratospheric ozone depletion. (See Box 5-B.) Many chloro-organics persist in the environment; thus, exposure to these compounds may continue to occur long after their initial release.

Some chlorinated organics are unwanted byproducts resulting from various manufacturing processes. For example, use of chlorine for bleaching purposes in the Paper industry, as well as its use in the production of chloro-organics, can result in the production of 2,3,7,8-tetrachlorodibenzo-p-dioxin (dioxin), an unwanted byproduct. (Dioxin was an unwanted byproduct in the defoliant Agent Orange.)

As evidence has mounted concerning the potential adverse human health and environmental effects associated with many of these chemicals, the focus has broadened to encompass chloro-organics as a class. Some chloro-organics have been suggested as endocrine-system disrupters, but this is not a characteristic of the class as a whole. (See Box 5-D.)

Concern over chloro-organics has resulted in numerous actions taken or proposed to restrict their use, production, and discharge. For example, EPA has proposed a "cluster" rule that would reduce water discharges and air emissions of chlorinated organics by the Paper industry, under both the Clean Water and Clean Air Acts. This "cluster" rule illustrates not only the broader focus on chloro-organics as a class, but also the multimedia approach (e.g., air and water) being used to deal with pollution that results from the use and production of these chemicals.

Disposition of Production-related Waste by Five Chemical Classes and Three Groups of Special Concern

Analyzing TRI data by chemical class or special group helps identify the effects of various factors that influence management of particular chemical waste and amounts of production-related waste. Of the total production-related waste of 37.3 billion pounds reported under TRI Section 8 in 1992, non-halogenated organics account for 39 percent, acids/bases/salts for 38 percent, metals for 11 percent, halo-organics for 6 percent, and non-metallic inorganics for 5 percent. (See Figure 5-1.)

Particular industries generate more of the production-related waste of the chemical classes and special groups than others, depending on products and manufacturing processes. (See Box 5-E.) Decisions about waste management methods to be applied for chemicals in these classes depend largely on the chemical and physical properties of the chemicals in that class, as well as on their cost. In the case of metals, for example, 81 percent (3.4 billion pounds) of the waste is recycled. Recycling is often a logical waste management option for metals for several reasons. Metals are often costly; they are less amenable to treatment than other types of chemicals (because as elements they cannot be destroyed,

Box 5-D. Endocrine Disrupters in the Environment

In the last several years, increased attention has been focused on chemicals in the environment to which disruptions of endocrine systems both in animals and humans have been attributed. While studies have been going on in this field for many years, only recently have the scientific community, regulatory agencies, industry, and the media come to focus on this issue. Specifically, the greatest attention has been on chemicals that mimic or block the action of the hormone estrogen. Many of the chemicals of concern are man-made and have been introduced into the environment either deliberately (e.g., various pesticides) or accidentally (e.g., spills), but there are also natural environmental chemicals (e.g., plant hormones) that appear to mimic estrogen.

Estrogen, which is often thought of as only a female hormone, is actually present in and serves a variety of important functions in both females and males. In the female, for example, this hormone is involved in pregnancy and lactation. It has also been associated with reducing the risk of heart attacks and osteoporosis. In the male, estrogen can inhibit the production of sperm if it is present in too large an amount. During prenatal and postnatal development of males and females, estrogen plays a role in sexual differentiation as well as in the proper development of the reproductive system.

One of the first man-made endocrine-modulating chemicals to come to the scientific community's attention as one that could have adverse effects in humans was diethylstilbestrol (DES), a synthetic estrogen that was used to prevent miscarriages in women. In 1971 DES was banned based upon evidence that it potentially caused vaginal cancer in the daughters of women who had taken the drug. Since that time, other adverse effects have been discovered, principally in the reproductive systems of both daughters and sons of women who took the drug.

Man-made chemicals that are believed to have an endocrine-modulating ability include such toxic chemicals as DDT, PCBs, dioxin, and kepone. Effects linked to exposure to these types of compounds include abnormal sexual development, dysfunctional reproductive systems, and cancer. The majority of evidence linking endocrine-modulating chemicals in the environment to such adverse effects —and the strongest such evidence — has come from wildlife studies, although there have also been studies suggesting similar adverse effects in humans.

Concern over potential endocrine disrupters has continued to grow, but not without dissent. Some in the scientific community believe that the issue has been blown well out of proportion. Significant disagreements continue, but almost all would agree that further study is warranted. Concern over the matter has reached such a level that in September 1994, the National Research Council announced plans to launch a two-year study financed by EPA and the Department of the Interior to examine critically the literature on hormone-related toxicants that are potentially producing a wide array of adverse effects.

Figure 5-1.

Total TRI Production-related Waste by Chemical Class, 1992

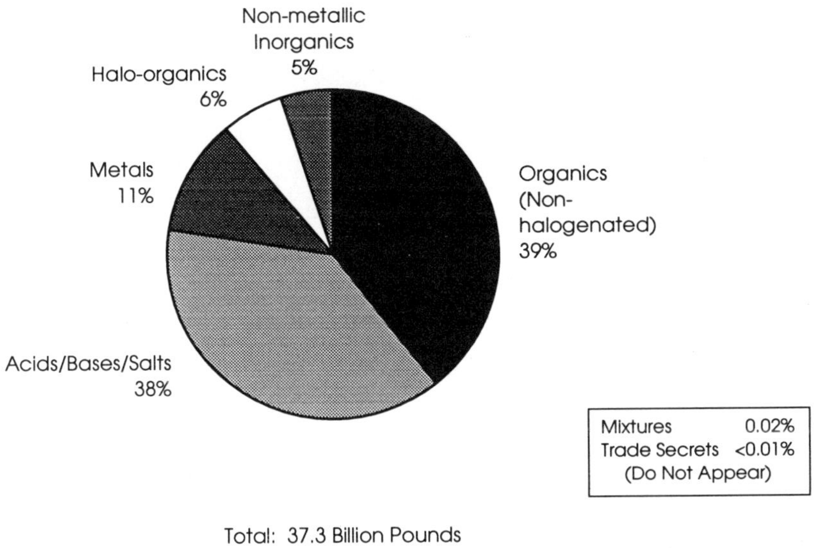

only converted into different metal-containing compounds); they do not burn (so cannot be used for energy recovery); and finally, regulatory restrictions control their release to the environment.

Acids/bases/salts, by contrast, are relatively cheap and easily recycled or treated, but they have little fuel value and restrictions apply to their release to the environment. Such considerations are reflected in how facilities manage this waste: 53 percent is recycled, 0.2 percent is used for energy recovery, 41 percent is treated, and 6 percent is released to the environment. Organic chemicals generally burn, and some are volatile, and so more air releases or use for energy recovery would be expected for organics as a class. (See Figure 5-2 and Table 5-4; see Appendix J, Table J-10, for the chemicals in each class with the largest amount of production-related waste.)

In the case of the three special groupings by health and environmental effects, 8 percent (3.0 billion pounds) of total production-related waste is composed of chemicals considered carcinogenic. Ozone depleters represent 2 percent (738.1 million pounds) of production-related waste, and chloro-organics 6 percent (2.3 billion pounds). Recycling is the waste management option associated with the largest percentage of waste of all three special groups: carcinogens, 65 percent; ozone depleters, 41 percent; and chloro-organics, 54 percent. Treatment is the next most practiced waste management option for these groups. Despite the focus on the health and environmental concerns as well as the regulatory

Table 5-3. TRI Production-related Waste of Special Chemical Groups and Selected Chemical Classes, by Industry, 1992

SIC Code	Industry	All TRI Chemicals		Carcinogens		Ozone Depleters	
		Pounds	Percent	Pounds	Percent	Pounds	Percent
20	Food	389,637,145	1.04	2,004,102	0.07	1,141,494	0.15
21	Tobacco	60,185,440	0.16	0	0.00	56,544,743	7.66
22	Textiles	100,223,930	0.27	2,387,176	0.08	1,727,390	0.23
23	Apparel	3,146,914	0.01	341,782	0.01	354,974	0.05
24	Lumber	63,091,614	0.17	24,277,415	0.82	792,589	0.11
25	Furniture	66,227,908	0.18	1,311,081	0.04	3,574,437	0.48
26	Paper	2,537,521,812	6.80	26,012,567	0.88	1,085,758	0.15
27	Printing	274,812,686	0.74	949,106	0.03	3,475,254	0.47
28	Chemicals	19,897,327,333	53.30	2,025,855,111	68.56	293,828,498	39.81
29	Petroleum	2,945,379,328	7.89	47,503,164	1.61	925,789	0.13
30	Plastics	567,294,382	1.52	60,744,615	2.06	24,705,907	3.35
31	Leather	52,480,219	0.14	567,290	0.02	315,016	0.04
32	Stone/Clay	935,576,617	2.51	38,208,260	1.29	7,958,026	1.08
33	Primary Metals	4,044,002,976	10.83	254,905,265	8.63	20,473,548	2.77
34	Fabr. Metals	962,656,507	2.58	47,019,162	1.59	107,690,937	14.59
35	Machinery	207,000,051	0.55	27,189,438	0.92	59,626,428	8.08
36	Electrical	963,576,363	2.58	62,889,640	2.13	50,749,648	6.88
37	Transportation	471,959,721	1.26	58,346,397	1.97	51,026,163	6.91
38	Measure./Photo.	125,739,677	0.34	25,222,958	0.85	20,143,780	2.73
39	Miscellaneous	55,014,507	0.15	6,283,617	0.21	3,558,952	0.48
	Multiple codes 20-39	2,412,177,342	6.46	240,432,348	8.14	27,539,480	3.73
	No codes 20-39	198,743,152	0.53	2,617,343	0.09	895,221	0.12
	Total	37,333,775,624	100.00	2,955,067,837	100.00	738,134,032	100.00

Box 5-E. Distribution of Production-related Waste of Chemical Classes and Groups of Special Concern, among Industries

The Chemical and Primary Metals industries dominated 1992 production-related waste of carcinogens. Together, these two industries accounted for over three-quarters of all carcinogens in TRI production-related waste reported in 1992. The Chemical industry reported 2.0 million pounds of production-related waste of carcinogens, over two-thirds (69 percent) of the carcinogens reported by all industries. (See Table 5-3.)

The Chemical industry also topped the list of production-related waste by industry for the other two special groups in this *Toxics Watch* report, accounting for 40 percent of the production-related waste of ozone depleters and 59 percent of such waste for chloro-organics. The Fabricated Metals industry ranked second for both chemical groups, with 15 percent of production-related waste of ozone depleters and 11 percent for chloro-organics. This industry shapes metal products such as cans, tools, and automobile parts from sheet metal. Ozone depleters and chloro-organics are used to coat and clean the metal products. (See Table 5-3.)

The Primary Metals industry reported over half (52 percent) of the production-related waste for the chemical class of metals, with the Electrical industry reporting the next largest amount of waste of metals, 12 percent. Because halo-organics include chloro-organics, their domination by the Chemical industry is the same as for chloro-organics (59 percent of production-related waste). (See Table 5-3.)

Chloro-organics		Metals		Halo-organics	
Pounds	Percent	Pounds	Percent	Pounds	Percent
942,818	0.04	1,909,191	0.05	1,439,795	0.06
56,544,743	2.45	6,826	0.00	56,544,743	2.44
7,580,873	0.33	1,339,066	0.03	7,798,625	0.34
548,267	0.02	116,897	0.00	548,267	0.02
1,608,686	0.07	610,651	0.01	1,608,686	0.07
4,362,920	0.19	1,041,725	0.02	4,362,920	0.19
21,005,011	0.91	5,373,492	0.13	21,029,095	0.91
4,484,150	0.19	968,350	0.02	4,484,150	0.19
1,368,191,432	59.29	147,576,757	3.53	1,375,083,971	59.34
1,486,136	0.06	8,327,454	0.20	1,497,781	0.06
66,419,787	2.88	238,049,575	5.70	66,915,432	2.89
514,628	0.02	8,082,478	0.19	514,628	0.02
28,706,049	1.24	106,170,657	2.54	28,714,049	1.24
40,301,025	1.75	2,172,137,413	52.03	40,367,207	1.74
257,421,043	11.16	263,253,688	6.31	257,427,703	11.11
112,659,974	4.88	45,804,309	1.10	112,659,974	4.86
107,094,552	4.64	480,164,916	11.50	108,321,355	4.67
93,943,894	4.07	130,068,832	3.12	93,985,394	4.06
43,562,915	1.89	6,879,680	0.16	43,577,607	1.88
6,962,007	0.30	12,848,514	0.31	6,970,872	0.30
81,234,176	3.52	389,958,948	9.34	81,387,526	3.51
1,918,074	0.08	154,192,463	3.69	1,962,569	0.08
2,307,493,160	100.00	4,174,881,882	100.00	2,317,202,349	100.00

activities associated with these special groups of chemicals, notable release/disposal to the environment of these chemicals still occurs: for carcinogens, 8 percent of the waste is released/disposed of; for ozone depleters, 22 percent; and for chloro-organics, 14 percent. As more regulations take effect regarding these chemicals, relative amounts of the various management methods of these wastes may change. (See Figure 5-2 and Table 5-5; see Appendix J, Tables J-11 through J-13, for the chemicals in each special category with the largest amount of production-related waste, e.g., the top 25 carcinogens.)

As is typical of TRI overall, relatively few facilities generate most of the production-related waste of carcinogens and ozone depleters. The waste management practices reported by the top facilities differ notably from the majority of facilities reporting carcinogenic and ozone-depleting waste. (See Box 5-F.)

Figure 5-2.

Distribution of Percent TRI Production-related Waste by Chemical Class and Group of Special Concern, 1992

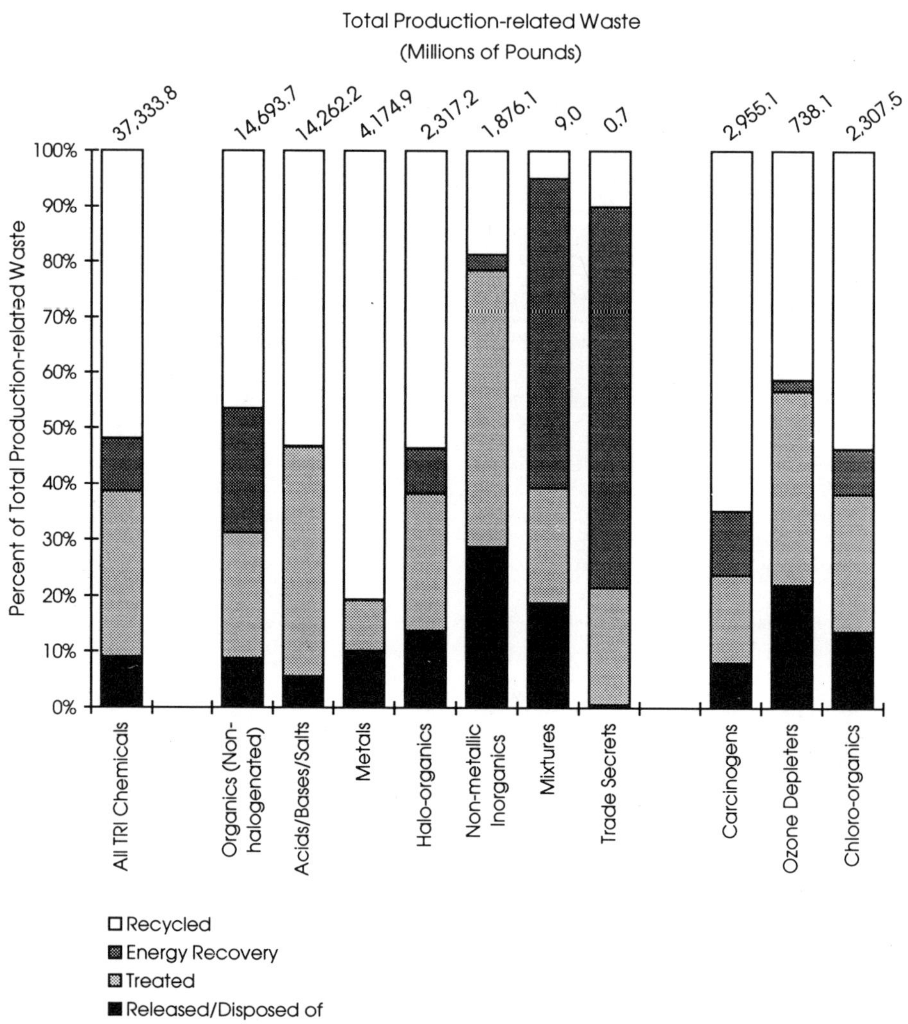

Table 5-4. TRI Production-related Waste by Chemical Class, 1992

Chemical Class	**Total Recycled** Pounds	**Total Energy Recovery** Pounds	**Total Treated** Pounds	**Quantity Released/ Disposed of** Pounds	**Total Production-related Waste** Pounds
Organics (Non-halogenated)	6,815,399,071	3,291,670,114	3,285,596,495	1,301,048,144	14,693,713,824
Acids/Bases/Salts	7,588,016,487	24,718,641	5,838,950,440	810,551,077	14,262,236,645
Metals	3,363,585,794	4,350,318	380,742,365	426,203,405	4,174,881,882
Halo-organics	1,241,493,116	189,317,231	565,856,670	320,535,332	2,317,202,349
Non-metallic Inorganics	349,085,115	53,635,155	931,996,683	541,349,159	1,876,066,112
Mixtures	440,667	5,011,254	1,835,627	1,694,943	8,982,491
Trade Secrets	69,147	474,000	145,064	4,110	692,321
Total for All TRI Chemicals	19,358,089,397	3,569,176,713	11,005,123,344	3,401,386,170	37,333,775,624

Table 5-5. *TRI Production-related Waste by Special Chemical Group Related to Health/Environmental Effects, 1992*

Chemical Group	Total Recycled Pounds	Total Energy Recovery Pounds	Total Treated Pounds	Quantity Released/ Disposed of Pounds	Total Production-related Waste Pounds
Carcinogens	1,913,253,682	337,823,560	464,227,493	239,763,102	2,955,067,837
Ozone Depleters	304,227,698	15,357,041	254,989,818	163,559,475	738,134,032
Chloro-organics	1,236,959,099	189,273,878	565,154,298	316,105,885	2,307,493,160

Box 5-F. Facilities' Waste and Waste Management of Carcinogens and Ozone Depleters

A few facilities generate most of the *carcinogenic waste* reported to TRI. Although 7,662 facilities reported the use of carcinogens in 1992, the top 50 facilities (ranked on total production-related waste in 1991) were responsible for nearly two-thirds of the total production related-waste of carcinogens in both 1991 and 1992. They reported 1.9 billion pounds total production-related waste of carcinogens in 1992. That total represented a 2 percent *decrease* from 1991, compared to a 1 percent *increase* for all TRI facilities reporting carcinogens. (See Tables 5-6 and 5-7.)

A striking difference marks the waste management options reported by these facilities. They reported releases/disposal of less than 1 percent of their production-related waste in 1992, compared to more than 8 percent for all facilities. Recycling is the leading type of waste management reported for carcinogens, and it is more prevalent among the top facilities: 76 percent of their carcinogenic waste, compared to 65 percent for all facilities. Also, the amount of carcinogenic waste recycled reported by the top 50 facilities remained about the same, whereas the amount recycled decreased by 20 percent for all facilities reporting carcinogenic wastes. (See Tables 5-6 and 5-7.)

In contrast to total production-related waste data, the 50 facilities reporting the largest amount of carcinogens released or disposed of in 1991 accounted for less than one-third (30 percent) of all release/disposal of carcinogens reported in 1991 (76.9 million pounds). They reported a 19 percent reduction from 1991 to 1992. By 1994 they project a decrease of 35 percent. These decreases are more than twice that of all facilities reporting on carcinogens. (See Table 5-8.)

Among 4,149 facilities reporting to TRI on *ozone depleters* in 1991 and 1992, the top 50 (ranked on 1991 data) accounted for 70 percent of total production-related waste of ozone depleters in 1992. Their production-related waste of these chemicals totaled 517.0 million that year. These facilities managed their ozone-depleting chemical waste quite differently from the majority. While all facilities released or disposed of 22 percent of production-related waste, the top 50 released or disposed of only 3 percent. Recycling and treatment account about equally for the difference. The top 50 facilities recycled 48 percent of their ozone-depleting waste and treated 47 percent. In comparison, all facilities recycled 41 percent and treated 35 percent. Although responsible for most of the production-related waste reported for these chemicals, these facilities accounted for only 20 percent of the quantity released and disposed of, 36.4 million of a total of 188.7 million pounds released/disposed of in 1992. (See Tables 5-9 and 5-10.)

Although these data indicate that the top facilities manage their ozone-depleting waste better, in terms of the environmental management hierarchy, than facilities with smaller quantities of waste, they did not reduce their production-related waste from 1991 to 1992. Such waste reported by all facilities decreased 1 percent from 1991 to 1992, but waste reported by the top 50 increased 2 percent. (See Table 5-11.)

Data from the leading parent companies reporting carcinogenic waste and ozone-depleting waste reveal similar patterns. (See Appendix O, Tables O-5 through O-12.)

Table 5-6. 1992 Production-related Waste for the 50 TRI Facilities with Largest Total Production-related Waste of Carcinogens in 1991

Total Production-related Waste Rank* 1991 Rank	1992 Rank	Facility	City	State	1992 Total Production-related Waste Pounds
1	1	Goodyear Tire & Rubber Co.	Houston	TX	319,211,600
2	3	Shintech Inc.	Freeport	TX	169,862,100
3	2	Celanese Engineering Resins	Bishop	TX	171,681,660
4	143	Reilly Ind. Inc.	Indianapolis	IN	2,299,033
5	5	East Penn Manufacturing Co.	Lyon Station	PA	110,496,839
6	4	Dow Chemical Co.	Freeport	TX	117,846,723
7	7	Gopher Smelting & Refining Co.	Eagan	MN	67,425,425
8	18	Occidental Chemical Corp.	Gregory	TX	22,135,032
9	8	Dynagen Inc.	Odessa	TX	67,082,745
10	11	Novacor Chemicals Inc.	Decatur	AL	43,362,050
11	12	Dow Chemical Co.	Plaquemine	LA	42,186,281
12	9	PPG Industries Inc.	Lake Charles	LA	64,914,134
13	13	Neste Resins Corp.	Winnfield	LA	38,202,796
14	6	Upjohn Co.	Portage	MI	76,961,805
15	15	Novacor	Indian Orchard	MA	30,227,000
16	17	IBM Corp.	Endicott	NY	22,718,830
17	10	Westlake Petrochemicals Corp.	Sulphur	LA	63,720,234
18	14	Ferro Corp.	Hammond	IN	36,100,340
19	26	Westlake Monomers Corp.	Calvert City	KY	16,352,821
20	16	Shell Oil Co.	Norco	LA	23,415,525
21	39	Dover Electronics Co.	Conklin	NY	10,734,991
22	24	Formosa Plastics Corp.	Point Comfort	TX	17,779,752
23	5260	GNB Battery Tech. Inc.	Frisco	TX	2,402
24	22	Georgia Gulf Corp.	Plaquemine	LA	18,848,658
25	19	Formosa Plastics Corp.	Baton Rouge	LA	21,358,706
26	25	Moore Business Forms	Stillwater	OK	17,086,166
27	27	Lyondell Petrochemical Co.	Channelview	TX	16,265,600
28	21	First Chemical Corp.	Pascagoula	MS	19,965,747
29	20	Goodyear Tire & Rubber Co.	Cheek	TX	20,256,328
30	45	Arco Chemical Co.	Channelview	TX	9,320,570
31	23	Monsanto Co.	Decatur	AL	18,247,712
32	82	Borden Chemicals & Plastics	Geismar	LA	5,461,878
33	35	Hoechst-Celanese Chemical	Pasadena	TX	12,304,828
34	33	Zollner Pistons	Fort Wayne	IN	12,488,413
35	41	Squibb Manufacturing Inc.	Humacao	PR	10,525,230
36	43	Rhone-Poulenc Ag Co.	Kingsland	GA	10,175,002
37	32	Occidental Chemical Corp.	Deer Park	TX	12,575,467
38	34	Pfizer Inc.	Groton	CT	12,336,510
39	28	Sybron Chemicals Inc.	Birmingham	NJ	15,655,442
40	48	Monsanto Co.	Addyston	OH	8,790,200
41	38	Ametek Inc.	Wurtland	KY	10,956,000
42	42	Du Pont	Washington	WV	10,399,500
43	50	Sterling Chemicals Inc.	Texas City	TX	8,363,475
44	60	Vista Chemical Co.	Baltimore	MD	7,287,502
45	85	Bristol-Myers Barceloneta Inc.	Barceloneta	PR	5,148,780
46	58	Blairsville Machine Products	Blairsville	PA	7,585,880
47	47	Geon Co.	La Porte	TX	8,916,597
48	37	Eli Lilly & Co.	Shadeland	IN	11,349,000
49	56	National Starch & Chemical Co.	Salisbury	NC	7,741,487
50	76	Refined Metals Corp.	Memphis	TN	5,820,930
		Subtotal			1,859,951,726
		Percent of Total			62.94
		Total			2,955,067,837

* Rank among total of 7,662 facilities, for total production-related waste of carcinogens.

Type of Waste Management as Percent of Total Production-related Waste			
Recycling Percent	Energy Recovery Percent	Treated Percent	Released/ Disposed of Percent
99.59	0.09	0.18	0.14
99.95	0.00	0.00	0.05
93.20	0.42	5.42	0.96
61.77	37.32	0.20	0.72
99.90	0.00	0.00	0.10
51.86	16.47	30.39	1.28
99.81	0.00	0.00	0.19
0.00	51.29	48.16	0.54
99.45	0.01	0.00	0.54
92.25	7.61	0.05	0.10
0.00	38.09	59.26	2.65
68.74	6.40	24.16	0.69
0.30	0.00	99.68	0.02
93.55	0.02	3.88	2.55
94.29	5.64	0.01	0.07
94.23	0.69	4.45	0.63
0.00	99.49	0.51	0.00
96.95	0.00	0.00	3.05
11.91	87.40	0.43	0.26
0.00	90.88	8.96	0.16
97.20	0.00	0.00	2.80
80.52	19.09	0.05	0.34
0.00	0.00	0.08	99.92
0.00	60.00	39.80	0.19
34.44	47.99	17.28	0.30
99.32	0.07	0.02	0.59
0.00	14.76	82.21	3.03
95.16	4.66	0.00	0.18
96.27	1.21	2.28	0.24
0.00	85.26	10.39	4.35
82.65	0.01	16.97	0.37
0.00	0.00	98.91	1.09
40.63	54.78	2.07	2.52
99.99	0.00	0.00	0.01
75.21	0.00	23.66	1.13
98.60	0.00	0.04	1.36
0.00	0.00	99.80	0.20
96.34	0.63	1.20	1.83
99.33	0.00	0.23	0.44
0.00	28.61	68.47	2.92
98.58	0.00	0.00	1.42
0.00	0.00	98.23	1.77
0.02	68.71	7.66	23.61
93.31	0.05	6.09	0.55
83.77	0.00	14.95	1.28
100.00	0.00	0.00	0.00
0.00	0.00	98.70	1.30
0.00	0.00	80.17	19.83
96.80	0.00	2.34	0.86
94.49	0.00	0.00	5.51
75.61	11.21	12.25	0.93
64.74	11.43	15.71	8.11

Table 5-7. Change in Waste from 1991 to 1992 for the 50 TRI Facilities with Largest Total Production-related Waste of Carcinogens in 1991

Total Production-related Waste Rank*						
1991 Rank	**1992** Rank	**Facility**	**City**	**State**	**TRI Forms** Number	**Change in Total Production-related Waste 1991 to 1992** Percent
1	1	Goodyear Tire & Rubber Co.	Houston	TX	4	17.63
2	3	Shintech Inc.	Freeport	TX	1	10.96
3	2	Celanese Engineering Resins	Bishop	TX	4	14.28
4	143	Reilly Ind. Inc.	Indianapolis	IN	5	-98.09
5	5	East Penn Manufacturing Co.	Lyon Station	PA	5	14.91
6	4	Dow Chemical Co.	Freeport	TX	25	32.59
7	7	Gopher Smelting & Refining Co.	Eagan	MN	2	2.98
8	18	Occidental Chemical Corp.	Gregory	TX	8	-65.45
9	8	Dynagen Inc.	Odessa	TX	2	15.16
10	11	Novacor Chemicals Inc.	Decatur	AL	1	-23.20
11	12	Dow Chemical Co.	Plaquemine	LA	19	-15.47
12	9	PPG Industries Inc.	Lake Charles	LA	10	32.24
13	13	Neste Resins Corp.	Winnfield	LA	1	-0.30
14	6	Upjohn Co.	Portage	MI	4	129.83
15	15	Novacor	Indian Orchard	MA	1	-3.82
16	17	IBM Corp.	Endicott	NY	3	-27.01
17	10	Westlake Petrochemicals Corp.	Sulphur	LA	3	119.65
18	14	Ferro Corp.	Hammond	IN	1	34.25
19	26	Westlake Monomers Corp.	Calvert City	KY	7	-38.70
20	16	Shell Oil Co.	Norco	LA	4	-10.78
21	39	Dover Electronics Co.	Conklin	NY	1	-58.88
22	24	Formosa Plastics Corp.	Point Comfort	TX	6	-24.39
23	5260	GNB Battery Tech. Inc.	Frisco	TX	1	-99.99
24	22	Georgia Gulf Corp.	Plaquemine	LA	6	-15.60
25	19	Formosa Plastics Corp.	Baton Rouge	LA	7	-0.31
26	25	Moore Business Forms	Stillwater	OK	3	-19.59
27	27	Lyondell Petrochemical Co.	Channelview	TX	6	-21.90
28	21	First Chemical Corp.	Pascagoula	MS	4	4.47
29	20	Goodyear Tire & Rubber Co.	Cheek	TX	3	11.49
30	45	Arco Chemical Co.	Channelview	TX	6	-44.22
31	23	Monsanto Co.	Decatur	AL	6	10.00
32	82	Borden Chemicals & Plastics	Geismar	LA	7	-62.86
33	35	Hoechst-Celanese Chemical	Pasadena	TX	6	-11.58
34	33	Zollner Pistons	Fort Wayne	IN	3	0.00
35	41	Squibb Manufacturing Inc.	Humacao	PR	3	-14.18
36	43	Rhone-Poulenc Ag Co.	Kingsland	GA	2	-15.76
37	32	Occidental Chemical Corp.	Deer Park	TX	5	5.60
38	34	Pfizer Inc.	Groton	CT	5	3.72
39	28	Sybron Chemicals Inc.	Birmingham	NJ	11	35.98
40	48	Monsanto Co.	Addyston	OH	4	-15.60
41	38	Ametek Inc.	Wurtland	KY	1	6.40
42	42	Du Pont	Washington	WV	3	1.15
43	50	Sterling Chemicals Inc.	Texas City	TX	7	-18.39
44	60	Vista Chemical Co.	Baltimore	MD	1	-21.68
45	85	Bristol-Myers Barceloneta Inc.	Barceloneta	PR	1	-44.28
46	58	Blairsville Machine Products	Blairsville	PA	2	-16.67
47	47	Geon Co.	La Porte	TX	5	-0.70
48	37	Eli Lilly & Co.	Shadeland	IN	3	30.10
49	56	National Starch & Chemical Co.	Salisbury	NC	5	-10.03
50	76	Refined Metals Corp.	Memphis	TN	2	-32.16
		Subtotal			235	-2.10
		Percent of Total			1.98	
		Total			11,855	1.00

* Rank among total of 7,662 facilities, for total production-related waste of carcinogens.

Total Production-related Waste		Change from 1991 to 1992			
1991 Pounds	**1992** Pounds	**Energy Recycling** Percent	**Recovery** Percent	**Released/ Treated** Percent	**Disposed of** Percent
271,379,600	319,211,600	17.65	87.92	4.77	-5.27
153,078,000	169,862,100	10.97	—	—	5.26
150,224,802	171,681,660	14.29	3.12	28.62	-27.83
120,202,672	2,299,033	-98.82	1,028.95	317.27	5.59
96,157,109	110,496,839	14.92	—	—	8.31
88,880,257	117,846,723	58.72	31.32	4.34	18.79
65,477,036	67,425,425	3.08	—	-30.56	-32.94
64,070,964	22,135,032	—	595.09	-82.89	-10.76
58,250,859	67,082,745	15.34	-94.68	-100.00	16.05
56,458,000	43,362,050	-23.08	-24.31	-52.26	-25.00
49,906,101	42,186,281	—	-29.55	-2.12	-28.15
49,088,615	64,914,134	35.90	1.15	38.30	-44.01
38,319,610	38,202,796	12.91	—	-0.29	-74.16
33,487,092	76,961,805	166.67	-89.41	21.29	-49.18
31,428,300	30,227,000	-5.00	21.71	-83.74	31.25
31,126,170	22,718,830	-27.82	42.64	-16.49	-3.44
29,009,890	63,720,234	—	119.87	87.85	-58.73
26,890,500	36,100,340	34.62	—	-32.00	23.60
26,677,165	16,352,821	-19.51	-40.61	90.74	-72.55
26,245,962	23,415,525	—	-16.61	232.56	-61.20
26,107,124	10,734,991	-59.44	-70.54	-100.00	-20.68
23,515,513	17,779,752	-33.44	76.38	-28.74	-12.00
23,003,315	2,402	-100.00	—	-86.67	-27.27
22,331,320	18,848,658	—	-20.85	-5.06	-73.98
21,424,566	21,358,706	56.80	-34.81	293.40	-13.91
21,248,459	17,086,166	-18.91	140.61	66.78	-68.10
20,826,340	16,265,600	—	0.00	-25.67	13.07
19,112,227	19,965,747	5.56	-14.52	—	47.41
18,169,331	20,256,328	10.80	-12.68	84.89	25.90
16,709,448	9,320,570	—	-46.64	-25.59	-21.28
16,589,504	18,247,712	24.89	2,596.63	-30.11	-19.30
14,705,043	5,461,878	—	—	-63.12	8.33
13,916,690	12,304,828	-29.58	6.98	209.93	-28.63
12,488,413	12,488,413	0.00	—	—	0.00
12,264,850	10,525,230	-13.15	—	-17.83	-0.58
12,079,240	10,175,002	-15.61	—	-70.89	-21.92
11,908,834	12,575,467	—	—	5.57	22.04
11,894,100	12,336,510	6.35	—	-76.01	121.59
11,512,879	15,655,442	36.65	—	-30.06	-15.70
10,415,230	8,790,200	—	-37.28	-0.59	-26.95
10,297,000	10,956,000	6.93	—	—	-20.81
10,281,100	10,399,500	—	—	2.08	-32.81
10,248,630	8,363,475	-93.29	-25.05	11.92	-0.57
9,305,002	7,287,502	-26.09	55.96	1,185.80	-41.18
9,240,800	5,148,780	-43.73	—	-41.98	-73.55
9,103,056	7,585,880	-16.67	—	—	—
8,979,100	8,916,597	—	—	0.08	-37.40
8,723,217	11,349,000	-100.00	—	36.15	66.67
8,604,480	7,741,487	-10.27	—	21.14	-35.79
8,580,381	5,820,930	-35.29	—	-26.83	299.43
1,899,943,896	1,859,951,726	0.35	5.66	-18.89	-14.92
64.94	62.94				
2,925,828,260	2,955,067,837	-19.59	-14.40	-17.27	-7.78

Table 5-8. *The 50 TRI Facilities with the Largest Amount of Carcinogens Released/Disposed of in 1991: Actual and Projected Change 1991-1994*

Released/ Disposed of Rank* 1991 Rank	1992 Rank	Facility	City	State	1991 Released/ Disposed of Pounds
1	1	Eastman Kodak Co.	Rochester	NY	5,212,202
2	2	Magma Copper Co.	San Manuel	AZ	4,200,000
3	11	Upjohn Co.	Portage	MI	3,857,000
4	9	Monsanto Co.	Alvin	TX	3,502,000
5	6	Glenbrook Nickel Co.	Riddle	OR	2,651,259
6	32	General Electric Co.	Mount Vernon	IN	2,398,105
7	8	Cytec Industries Inc.	Westwego	LA	2,307,400
8	12	Abbott Chemicals Inc.	Barceloneta	PR	2,289,692
9	16	Celanese Engineering Resins	Bishop	TX	2,285,300
10	14	BP Chemicals Inc.	Port Lavaca	TX	2,142,672
11	10	Sterling Chemicals Inc.	Texas City	TX	1,985,960
12	255	Yaffe Iron & Metal Co. Inc.	Muskogee	OK	1,965,218
13	15	Arcadian Ohio LP	Lima	OH	1,906,570
14	3	Eli Lilly & Co.	Clinton	IN	1,600,000
15	24	Dow Chemical Co.	Plaquemine	LA	1,553,813
16	159	ISK Biosciences Corp.	Houston	TX	1,516,437
17	21	Du Pont Towanda Plant	Towanda	PA	1,500,000
18	5	Monsanto Co.	Luling	LA	1,407,800
19	4	Eli Lilly & Co.	Shadeland	IN	1,350,000
20	13	Upjohn Manufacturing Co.	Arecibo	PR	1,313,340
21	18	Dow Chemical Co.	Freeport	TX	1,270,190
22	42	Hickory Springs Manufacturing	Conover	NC	1,261,733
23	36	Rubicon Inc.	Geismar	LA	1,220,341
24	19	Hoechst-Celanese Chemical	Bay City	TX	1,191,762
25	20	Hercules Inc.	Magna	UT	1,180,939
26	30	Hickory Springs Manufacturing	Verona	MS	1,143,964
27	27	Monsanto Co.	Muscatine	IA	1,124,460
28	7	Angus Chemical Co.	Sterlington	LA	1,104,800
29	25	Champion International Corp.	Canton	NC	1,100,000
30	69	Xerox Corp.	Oklahoma City	OK	1,090,109
31	58	Boeing Wichita	Wichita	KS	1,078,900
32	37	Ameripol Synpol Corp.	Port Neches	TX	1,061,232
33	162	Wheeling-Pittsburgh Steel Corp	Follansbee	WV	1,000,000
34	44	Ferodo America	Smithville	TN	1,000,000
35	47	General Electric Chemicals Inc.	Washington	WV	994,005
36	23	E. R. Carpenter Co. Inc.	Verona	MS	986,400
37	29	Flexible Foam Products Inc.	Elkhart	IN	982,306
38	222	Merck & Co. Inc.	Albany	GA	960,424
39	65	Shell Oil Co.	Deer Park	TX	952,930
40	110	AK Steel Corp.	Middletown	OH	941,190
41	143	3M Co.	Kearneysville	WV	937,000
42	26	Ferro Corp.	Hammond	IN	890,000
43	100	Du Pont	Victoria	TX	879,989
44	64	Cytec Industries Inc.	Compton	CA	871,380
45	43	Foamex LP	Milan	TN	826,382
46	94	PPG Industries Inc.	Lake Charles	LA	802,498
47	46	Federal Paper Board Co. Inc.	Riegelwood	NC	790,000
48	104	Vulcan Chemicals	Wichita	KS	756,980
49	35	Carolina Eastman	Columbia	SC	756,900
50	338	Du Pont	Orange	TX	750,167
		Subtotal			76,851,749
		Percent of Total			29.56
		Total			259,989,125

* Rank among total of 7,662 facilities, for total production-related waste of carcinogens.

Change in Amount Released/Disposed of 1991 to 1992		Change in Amount Released/Disposed of 1991 to 1994	
Pounds	Percent	Pounds	Percent
-293,014	-5.62	-1,887,531	-36.21
-663,200	-15.79	-1,400,000	-33.33
-1,897,000	-49.18	-2,683,400	-69.57
-1,462,000	-41.75	-1,785,400	-50.98
-565,537	-21.33	613,241	23.13
-1,479,500	-61.69	-1,589,500	-66.28
-241,000	-10.44	-273,600	-11.86
-356,087	-15.55	-1,285,192	-56.13
-636,000	-27.83	-974,000	-42.62
-468,323	-21.86	-326,596	-15.24
-11,235	-0.57	-70,705	-3.56
-1,778,033	-90.48	-1,770,474	-90.09
-241,720	-12.68	-210,670	-11.05
900,000	56.25	-600,000	-37.50
-437,369	-28.15	-865,889	-55.73
-1,220,856	-80.51	-1,245,139	-82.11
-300,000	-20.00	-1,100,000	-73.33
694,900	49.36	794,600	56.44
900,000	66.67	-630,000	-46.67
435,770	33.18	661,360	50.36
238,643	18.79	2,733,643	215.22
-469,042	-37.17	-953,200	-75.55
-357,019	-29.26	-376,521	-30.85
149,711	12.56	-139,903	-11.74
100,237	8.49	-565,239	-47.86
-138,469	-12.10	-730,890	-63.89
-37,990	-3.38	-884,500	-78.66
968,200	87.64	1,436,200	130.00
0	0.00	-1,085,000	-98.64
-524,909	-48.15	-884,909	-81.18
-426,036	-39.49	-441,600	-40.93
-198,232	-18.68	-227,232	-21.41
-710,000	-71.00	-971,000	-97.10
-230,000	-23.00	0	0.00
-261,003	-26.26	-94,000	-9.46
152,100	15.42	391,400	39.68
31,918	3.25	-170,928	-17.40
-742,624	-77.32	-834,024	-86.84
-373,920	-39.24	-494,920	-51.94
-536,790	-57.03	-827,190	-87.89
-613,000	-65.42	-937,000	-100.00
210,000	23.60	-841,000	-94.49
-449,981	-51.13	-449,981	-51.13
-280,015	-32.13	-869,970	-99.84
-39,477	-4.78	-126,162	-15.27
-353,177	-44.01	-628,303	-78.29
-50,000	-6.33	-600,000	-75.95
-341,403	-45.10	-384,580	-50.80
113,100	14.94	203,100	26.83
-602,258	-80.28	-583,367	-77.76
-14,891,640	-19.38	-26,965,971	-35.09
-20,226,023	-7.78	-42,704,084	-16.43

Table 5-9. 1992 Production-related Waste for the 50 TRI Facilities with Largest Total Production-related Waste of Ozone-depleting Chemicals in 1991

Total Production-related Waste Rank*					
1991 Rank	1992 Rank	Facility	City	State	1992 Total Production-related Waste Pounds
1	1	Allied-Signal Inc.	Chesterfield	VA	230,178,000
2	2	Uniform Tubes Inc.	Trappe	PA	72,592,526
3	3	R. J. Reynolds Tobacco Co.	Winston-Salem	NC	55,480,275
4	5	IBM Corp.	Endicott	NY	14,813,840
5	4	Thermo King De Puerto Rico	Arecibo	PR	17,230,000
6	6	Dow Chemical Co.	Freeport	TX	14,615,703
7	7	Thermo King Corp.	Louisville	GA	10,229,100
8	262	Electronic Assembly Plant	College Station	TX	206,600
9	9	Delta Faucet Co.	Greensburg	IN	7,683,176
10	10	Modine Manufacturing Co.	Logansport	IN	6,255,177
11	14	Modine Heat Transfer Inc.	Camdenton	MO	4,696,583
12	13	Modine Manufacturing Co.	Lawrenceburg	TN	4,707,450
13	8	Dow Chemical Co.	Plaquemine	LA	8,062,000
14	11	Kwikset Corp.	Bristow	OK	5,043,442
15	24	TRW	Union Springs	NY	2,323,200
16	22	Textron Aerospace Products	Columbus	GA	2,748,810
17	15	Holnam Inc.	Clarksville	MO	4,200,290
18	19	AG Communication Systems	Northlake	IL	3,439,600
19	16	CF & I Steel Corp.	Pueblo	CO	3,962,920
20	20	Ferodo America	Smithville	TN	3,091,000
21	91	Formosa Plastics Corp.	Baton Rouge	LA	531,673
22	43	U.S. Department of Energy	Piketon	OH	1,070,000
23	25	Acustar Dayton Thermal	Dayton	OH	2,196,460
24	17	AG Communication Systems Corp.	Genoa	IL	3,860,200
25	23	Hughes Georgia Inc.	La Grange	GA	2,362,146
26	18	Zimmer Inc.	Warsaw	IN	3,851,445
27	26	National Machine Co.	Stow	OH	2,011,694
28	12	Olin Corp.	Rochester	NY	5,018,642
29	35	Foamex LP	Orange	CA	1,195,155
30	29	United Tech. Automotive Inc.	Zanesville	OH	1,700,056
31	31	Honda of America Manufacturing Inc.	Marysville	OH	1,631,494
32	45	Du Pont	Deepwater	NJ	872,003
33	27	Cerro Copper Prods. Co.	Sauget	IL	1,730,009
34	96	Matsushita Electric Corp.	Franklin Park	IL	501,179
35	30	Great Dane Trailers Inc.	Brazil	IN	1,694,320
36	28	Dow Chemical Co.	Pittsburg	CA	1,710,550
37	32	AVX Corp.	Myrtle Beach	SC	1,518,000
38	40	ISK Biosciences Corp.	Houston	TX	1,165,667
39	99	U.S. Surgical Corp.	North Haven	CT	495,718
40	38	Filmtec Corp.	Minneapolis	MN	1,189,700
41	36	Du Pont	Antioch	CA	1,190,300
42	34	Thermo King Corp.	Bloomington	MN	1,325,500
43	37	Franklin Steel Co.	Franklin	PA	1,190,100
44	59	Dalton Fndy. Inc.	Warsaw	IN	672,839
45	39	Hercules Inc.	Magna	UT	1,187,824
46	93	Pratt & Whitney	East Hartford	CT	524,750
47	44	BG Automotive Motors	Hendersonville	TN	914,600
48	42	NSK Corp.	Clarinda	IA	1,116,678
49	49	General Dynamics Corp.	San Diego	CA	800,608
50	265	Lockheed Aeronautical Sys. Co.	Marietta	GA	205,400
		Subtotal			516,994,402
		Percent of Total			70.04
		Total			738,134,032

* Rank among total of 4,149 facilities, for total production-related waste of ozone depleters.

Type of Waste Management as Percent of Total Production-related Waste			
Recycling Percent	**Energy Recovery** Percent	**Treated** Percent	**Released/ Disposed of** Percent
0.00	0.00	99.92	0.08
98.93	0.00	0.03	1.05
99.00	0.00	0.00	1.00
98.31	0.16	0.02	1.52
98.75	0.59	0.00	0.67
41.74	0.00	53.33	4.93
98.03	0.00	0.00	1.97
79.67	0.00	0.00	20.33
98.21	0.00	0.00	1.79
97.51	0.00	0.00	2.49
97.60	0.03	0.00	2.37
99.16	0.04	0.00	0.81
0.00	47.13	49.15	3.71
99.39	0.00	0.00	0.61
98.53	0.00	0.00	1.47
98.98	0.00	0.29	0.74
0.00	99.99	0.00	0.01
96.08	0.00	0.00	3.92
95.91	0.00	0.06	4.04
94.66	0.00	0.00	5.34
0.00	92.32	1.89	5.79
76.64	0.00	0.00	23.36
86.96	1.73	0.02	11.29
98.73	0.00	0.00	1.27
97.50	0.00	0.49	2.01
97.54	0.00	0.00	2.46
99.57	0.00	0.00	0.43
98.93	0.00	1.00	0.07
7.22	0.00	0.00	92.78
98.69	0.00	0.00	1.31
20.06	5.75	0.00	74.20
1.15	0.00	64.86	34.00
69.94	1.16	0.00	28.90
94.13	0.00	0.00	5.87
24.79	24.79	24.79	25.63
91.17	0.00	4.60	4.23
36.89	0.00	1.19	61.92
0.00	0.00	90.31	9.69
42.15	0.00	11.92	45.92
92.46	0.00	0.14	7.40
7.07	0.00	0.50	92.42
90.83	0.00	0.11	9.05
0.00	0.00	0.43	99.57
0.00	0.00	0.00	100.00
1.93	0.00	0.00	98.07
78.28	4.38	0.56	16.77
97.42	0.00	0.00	2.58
46.21	0.00	8.22	45.57
84.30	2.93	0.00	12.77
25.56	0.00	0.00	74.44
48.09	1.79	47.23	2.90
41.22	2.08	34.55	22.16

Table 5-10. The 50 TRI Facilities with the Largest Amount of Ozone-depleting Chemicals Released/Disposed of in 1991: Actual and Projected Change 1991-1994

Released/ Disposed of Rank* 1991 Rank	1992 Rank	Facility	City	State	1991 Released/ Disposed of Pounds
1	4	Foamex LP	Orange	CA	1,784,903
2	1	Honda of America Manufacturing Inc.	Marysville	OH	1,327,398
3	5	Du Pont	Antioch	CA	1,327,300
4	2	Franklin Steel Co.	Franklin	PA	1,243,000
5	14	Dalton Foundry Inc.	Warsaw	IN	1,075,281
6	3	Hercules Inc.	Magna	UT	1,028,964
7	6	AVX Corp.	Myrtle Beach	SC	930,000
8	8	Chem-Tech Rubber Inc.	West Haven	CT	915,400
9	212	Lockheed Aeronautical Systems Co.	Marietta	GA	900,000
10	33	Keystone Steel & Wire Co.	Peoria	IL	900,000
11	86	Du Pont	Deepwater	NJ	898,398
12	10	E. R. Carpenter Co. Inc.	Riverside	CA	883,400
13	11	Dow Chemical Co.	Freeport	TX	783,000
14	7	Du Pont	Leland	NC	774,000
15	118	U.S. Surgical Corp.	North Haven	CT	768,442
16	339	Wheeling-Pittsburgh Steel Corp	Yorkville	OH	760,000
17	16	Vought Aircraft Co.	Dallas	TX	745,000
18	31	Teledyne Casting Service	La Porte	IN	720,000
19	9	Uniform Tubes Inc.	Trappe	PA	712,242
20	80	Starcraft Automotive Corp.	Goshen	IN	697,372
21	28	Jones & Vining Inc.	Lewiston	ME	691,500
22	51	Allied-Signal Inc.	Baton Rouge	LA	675,953
23	48	Douglas Aircraft Co.	Long Beach	CA	661,000
24	35	Thiokol Corp.	Clearfield	UT	660,000
25	29	Future Foam Inc.	Fullerton	CA	652,000
26	23	Boeing Wichita	Wichita	KS	641,600
27	42	Du Pont	Washington	WV	641,000
28	41	Thiokol Corp.	Promontory	UT	640,000
29	103	U.S. Department of Energy	Piketon	OH	630,000
30	104	Acustar Dayton Thermal	Dayton	OH	610,000
31	34	Cerro Copper Products Co.	Sauget	IL	610,000
32	43	Elf Atochem N.A. Inc.	Wichita	KS	602,800
33	44	Boeing Commercial Airplane	Everett	WA	590,000
34	144	Boeing Co.	Auburn	WA	589,000
35	32	NSK Corp.	Clarinda	IA	575,459
36	66	Rockwell Graphic Systems	Cedar Rapids	IA	564,695
37	18	American Brass & Iron Foundry	Oakland	CA	554,200
38	197	Briggs & Stratton Corp.	Glendale	WI	536,773
39	30	Briggs & Stratton Corp.	Wauwatosa	WI	536,773
40	17	General Electric Appliances	Louisville	KY	536,050
41	191	E. R. Carpenter Co. Inc.	Temple	TX	513,704
42	26	Ig-Lo Inc.	Hernando	MS	511,000
43	56	Northrop Corp.	Hawthorne	CA	509,000
44	50	Texas Fibers	Brenham	TX	505,252
45	25	R. J. Reynolds Tobacco Co.	Winston-Salem	NC	501,811
46	148	UC Industries Inc.	Tallmadge	OH	500,000
47	217	Carpenter Co.	Elkhart	IN	500,000
48	21	Liggett Group Inc.	Durham	NC	498,919
49	40	Prestige Fabricators Inc.	Asheboro	NC	486,016
50	57	U.S. Enrichment Corp.	Paducah	KY	485,000
		Subtotal			36,383,605
		Percent of Total			19.28
		Total			188,720,991

* Rank among total of 4,149 facilities, for total production-related waste of ozone depleters.

Change in Amount Released/Disposed of 1991 to 1992		Change in Amount Released/Disposed of 1991 to 1994	
Pounds	Percent	Pounds	Percent
-675,988	-37.87	-1,784,903	-100.00
-116,886	-8.81	-116,886	-8.81
-227,200	-17.12	-515,200	-38.82
-58,000	-4.67	-763,000	-61.38
-402,442	-37.43	-1,075,281	-100.00
135,876	13.21	-453,964	-44.12
10,000	1.08	-930,000	-100.00
-152,800	-16.69	-651,400	-71.16
-747,100	-83.01	-650,000	-72.22
-400,000	-44.44	-900,000	-100.00
-601,943	-67.00	-736,398	-81.97
-137,500	-15.56	-33,400	-3.78
-63,100	-8.06	-73,100	-9.34
45,000	5.81	-210,000	-27.13
-540,801	-70.38	-768,442	-100.00
-660,000	-86.84	-760,000	-100.00
-89,000	-11.95	-217,000	-29.13
-191,200	-26.56	-720,000	-100.00
46,810	6.57	164,463	23.09
-398,248	-57.11	-386,163	-55.37
-144,700	-20.93	-366,500	-53.00
-276,091	-40.84	-290,953	-43.04
-241,000	-36.46	-471,000	-71.26
-160,000	-24.24	-210,000	-31.82
-108,000	-16.56	-57,735	-8.86
-83,270	-12.98	-458,600	-71.48
-200,000	-31.20	-248,000	-38.69
-190,000	-29.69	-230,000	-35.94
-380,000	-60.32	-280,000	-44.44
-362,000	-59.34	-362,000	-59.34
-110,000	-18.03	-110,000	-18.03
-162,300	-26.92	-401,800	-66.66
-150,000	-25.42	-452,000	-76.61
-386,000	-65.53	-489,000	-83.02
-66,585	-11.57	-575,459	-100.00
-239,501	-42.41	-564,695	-100.00
63,180	11.40	-276,379	-49.87
-372,484	-69.39	-536,773	-100.00
-617	-0.11	-536,773	-100.00
90,370	16.86	114,030	21.27
-345,994	-67.35	-306,584	-59.68
39,000	7.63	-11,000	-2.15
-133,000	-26.13	-159,000	-31.24
-97,496	-19.30	-505,252	-100.00
52,991	10.56	-501,811	-100.00
-300,000	-60.00	-500,000	-100.00
-350,000	-70.00	-400,000	-80.00
65,800	13.19	-498,919	-100.00
-26,566	-5.47	-36,016	-7.41
-109,000	-22.47	-165,000	-34.02
-9,907,785	-27.23	-21,467,893	-59.00
-25,161,516	-13.33	-129,765,490	-68.76

Table 5-11. Change in Waste from 1991 to 1992 for the 50 TRI Facilities with Largest Total Production-related Waste of Ozone-depleting Chemicals in 1991

Total Production-related Waste Rank* 1991 Rank	1992 Rank	Facility	City	State	TRI Forms Number	Change in Total Production-related Waste 1991 to 1992 Percent
1	1	Allied-Signal Inc.	Chesterfield	VA	1	19.04
2	2	Uniform Tubes Inc.	Trappe	PA	1	0.06
3	3	R. J. Reynolds Tobacco Co.	Winston-Salem	NC	1	10.45
4	5	IBM Corp.	Endicott	NY	2	-40.98
5	4	Thermo King De Puerto Rico	Arecibo	PR	3	-0.39
6	6	Dow Chemical Co.	Freeport	TX	5	-10.12
7	7	Thermo King Corp.	Louisville	GA	2	0.45
8	262	Electronic Assembly Plant	College Station	TX	1	-97.95
9	9	Delta Faucet Co.	Greensburg	IN	1	0.49
10	10	Modine Manufacturing Co.	Logansport	IN	1	-16.95
11	14	Modine Heat Transfer Inc.	Camdenton	MO	1	-32.56
12	13	Modine Manufacturing Co.	Lawrenceburg	TN	1	-16.78
13	8	Dow Chemical Co.	Plaquemine	LA	4	49.15
14	11	Kwikset Corp.	Bristow	OK	1	-0.62
15	24	TRW	Union Springs	NY	1	-49.98
16	22	Textron Aerospace Products	Columbus	GA	1	-33.17
17	15	Holnam Inc.	Clarksville	MO	1	20.01
18	19	AG Communication Systems	Northlake	IL	2	-0.95
19	16	CF & I Steel Corp.	Pueblo	CO	1	15.11
20	20	Ferodo America	Smithville	TN	1	-0.93
21	91	Formosa Plastics Corp.	Baton Rouge	LA	3	-81.34
22	43	U.S. Department of Energy	Piketon	OH	1	-62.19
23	25	Acustar Dayton Thermal	Dayton	OH	2	-20.13
24	17	AG Communication Systems Corp.	Genoa	IL	1	40.63
25	23	Hughes Georgia Inc.	La Grange	GA	2	-4.37
26	18	Zimmer Inc.	Warsaw	IN	2	71.18
27	26	National Machine Co.	Stow	OH	1	0.05
28	12	Olin Corp.	Rochester	NY	1	152.26
29	35	Foamex LP	Orange	CA	1	-37.29
30	29	United Tech. Automotive Inc.	Zanesville	OH	1	-7.61
31	31	Honda of America Manufacturing Inc.	Marysville	OH	2	-7.40
32	45	Du Pont	Deepwater	NJ	6	-50.02
33	27	Cerro Copper Prods. Co.	Sauget	IL	1	1.94
34	96	Matsushita Electric Corp.	Franklin Park	IL	1	-68.85
35	30	Great Dane Trailers Inc.	Brazil	IN	2	6.62
36	28	Dow Chemical Co.	Pittsburg	CA	3	9.03
37	32	AVX Corp.	Myrtle Beach	SC	1	-0.13
38	40	ISK Biosciences Corp.	Houston	TX	2	-19.08
39	99	U.S. Surgical Corp.	North Haven	CT	2	-64.37
40	38	Filmtec Corp.	Minneapolis	MN	1	-11.79
41	36	Du Pont	Antioch	CA	7	-10.97
42	34	Thermo King Corp.	Bloomington	MN	2	1.35
43	37	Franklin Steel Co.	Franklin	PA	1	-4.63
44	59	Dalton Fndy. Inc.	Warsaw	IN	1	-37.43
45	39	Hercules Inc.	Magna	UT	1	13.67
46	93	Pratt & Whitney	East Hartford	CT	2	-48.33
47	44	BG Automotive Motors	Hendersonville	TN	1	-6.96
48	42	NSK Corp.	Clarinda	IA	1	14.26
49	49	General Dynamics Corp.	San Diego	CA	2	-17.56
50	265	Lockheed Aeronautical Sys. Co.	Marietta	GA	1	-78.69
		Subtotal			87	2.20
		Percent of Total			2.10	
		Total			4,149	-1.19

* Rank among total of 4,149 facilities, for total production-related waste of ozone depleters.

Total Production-related Waste		Change from 1991 to 1992			
1991 Pounds	1992 Pounds	Energy Recycling Percent	Recovery Percent	Released/ Treated Percent	Disposed of Percent
193,370,000	230,178,000	—	—	19.17	-51.89
72,551,945	72,592,526	0.00	—	-24.81	6.57
50,231,281	55,480,275	10.45	—	—	10.56
25,099,890	14,813,840	-41.11	-23.55	-96.07	-19.91
17,297,400	17,230,000	0.04	18.82	—	-43.90
16,260,980	14,615,703	-11.15	-93.61	-9.48	-8.06
10,183,700	10,229,100	0.19	—	—	14.77
10,056,000	206,600	-98.36	—	—	0.00
7,646,080	7,683,176	0.00	—	2.50	36.95
7,532,102	6,255,177	-17.31	—	—	0.00
6,963,957	4,696,583	-32.94	8.55	—	-12.20
5,656,307	4,707,450	-16.69	—	—	-29.16
5,405,314	8,062,000	—	137.50	17.71	-31.78
5,075,025	5,043,442	-0.59	—	—	-5.43
4,645,000	2,323,200	-50.27	—	—	-18.57
4,113,200	2,748,810	-33.33	—	-39.81	6.45
3,500,088	4,200,290	—	20.00	—	229.55
3,472,675	3,439,600	-0.36	—	—	-13.56
3,442,670	3,962,920	15.15	—	10.00	14.29
3,120,000	3,091,000	0.90	—	-100.00	-21.43
2,848,671	531,673	—	-82.60	40.73	53.79
2,830,000	1,070,000	-62.73	—	—	-60.32
2,750,000	2,196,460	-7.01	-55.81	—	-59.34
2,745,000	3,860,200	40.43	—	—	58.06
2,470,160	2,362,146	-3.44	—	805.57	-43.20
2,249,900	3,851,445	74.01	—	—	4.04
2,010,700	2,011,694	0.01	—	—	11.12
1,989,465	5,018,642	152.62	—	152.97	-18.79
1,905,903	1,195,155	-28.73	—	—	-37.87
1,840,062	1,700,056	-7.10	—	—	-34.55
1,761,808	1,631,494	-6.25	9.81	0.00	-8.81
1,744,710	872,003	-98.72	—	810.13	-67.00
1,697,055	1,730,009	13.08	17.65	-83.64	-18.03
1,608,992	501,179	-70.25	—	—	27.12
1,589,081	1,694,320	5.40	5.40	5.40	10.32
1,568,909	1,710,550	8.99	—	16.86	2.26
1,520,000	1,518,000	1.82	—	-55.00	1.08
1,440,472	1,165,667	—	—	-15.59	-41.56
1,391,322	495,718	-65.03	—	132.73	-70.38
1,348,700	1,189,700	-8.33	—	-80.46	-37.14
1,336,900	1,190,300	1,085.92	—	140.00	-17.12
1,307,900	1,325,500	0.08	—	-48.28	17.65
1,247,900	1,190,100	—	—	4.08	-4.67
1,075,281	672,839	—	—	—	-37.43
1,044,947	1,187,824	—	—	-99.77	13.21
1,015,640	524,750	-38.82	—	-75.70	-73.49
983,000	914,600	-1.00	—	—	-71.57
977,339	1,116,678	35.43	—	340.55	-11.57
971,085	800,608	-0.75	369.89	-85.00	-64.26
963,900	205,400	-17.84	—	—	-83.01
505,858,416	516,994,402	-7.94	7.02	17.94	-25.68
67.72	70.04				
747,030,073	738,134,032	-6.72	10.03	16.85	-13.33

Figure 5-3.

Environmental Distribution by Percent of TRI Waste Released (Sec. 5) or Transferred to Disposal (Sec. 6) by Chemical Class and Group of Chemical Concern, 1992

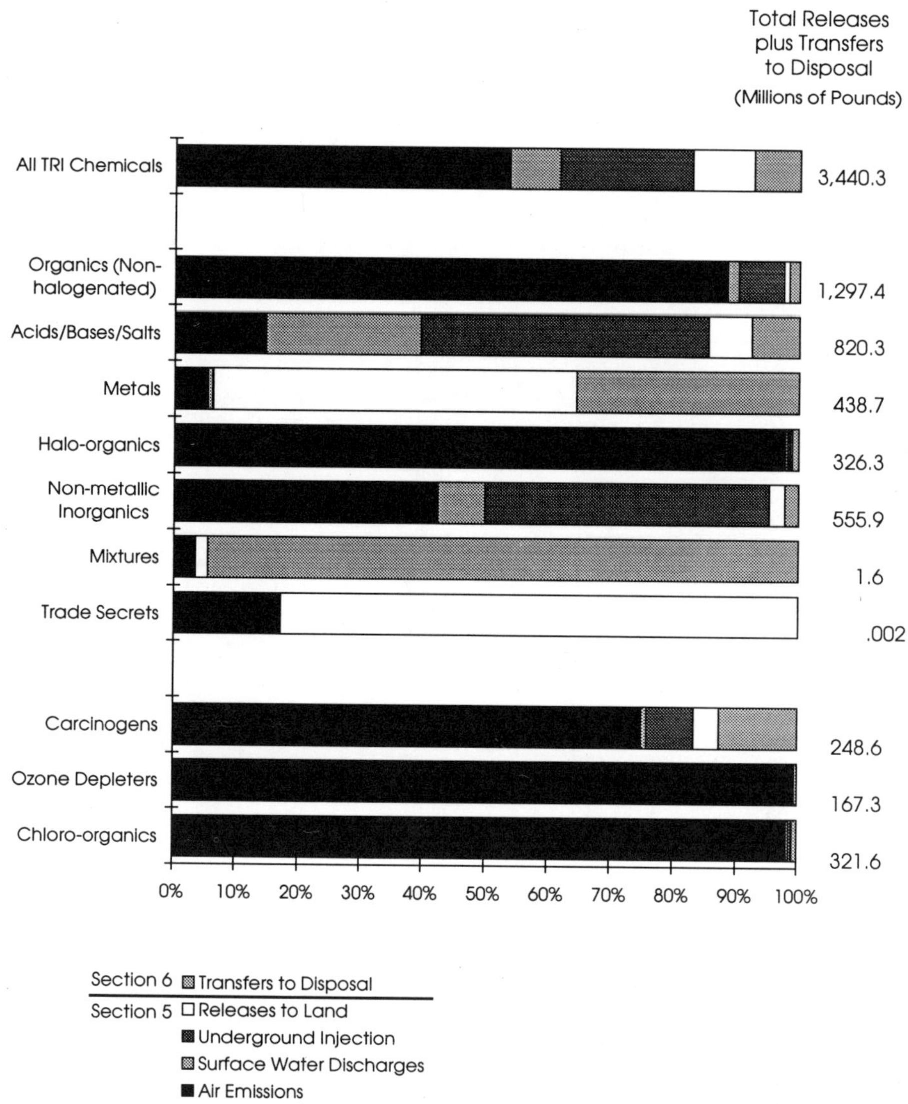

Release and Disposal of TRI Waste by Chemical Class and Group of Special Concern

Fifty-four percent of the total waste of all TRI chemicals released or transferred to disposal in 1992 was emitted to air, 8 percent was discharged to surface water, 21 percent was discharged to underground injection, 10 percent was released to land, and 8 percent was transferred off site for disposal. The environmental distribution of waste in each of the five chemical classes and three groups of special concern, however, varied from the pattern seen for TRI waste overall.

Table 5-12. Environmental Distribution of TRI Waste Released (Sec. 5) or Transferred to Disposal (Sec. 6) by Chemical Class, 1992

Chemical Class	Total Air Emissions Sec. 5 Pounds	Surface Water Discharges Sec. 5 Pounds	Underground Injection Sec. 5 Pounds	Releases to Land Sec. 5 Pounds	Transfers to Disposal Sec. 6 Pounds	Total Releases plus Transfers to Disposal Sec. 5 & 6 Pounds
Organics (Non-halogenated)	1,146,566,764	22,148,423	95,691,029	11,870,384	21,131,483	1,297,408,083
Acids/Bases/Salts	119,777,318	204,656,507	375,689,128	56,295,048	63,851,657	820,269,658
Metals	23,881,957	3,050,313	1,009,243	254,626,846	156,159,210	438,727,569
Halo-organics	319,340,268	1,017,913	1,688,955	822,676	3,464,393	326,334,205
Non-metallic Inorganics	235,329,808	42,059,797	251,868,060	14,141,149	12,483,227	555,882,041
Mixtures	58,086	0	0	32,950	1,552,607	1,643,643
Trade Secrets	4,135	0	0	20,000	0	24,135
Total for All TRI Chemicals	1,844,958,336	272,932,953	725,946,415	337,809,053	258,642,577	3,440,289,334

Distribution patterns, like waste management methods, were greatly affected by the physical-chemical properties common to the various classes. For example, some chemical classes or groups have a much higher percentage of chemicals that tend to evaporate. For these one might expect the percent of air emissions to be higher. This is the case for halo-organics and non-halogenated organics, whose air emissions account for 98 percent and 88 percent, respectively, of their waste released or disposed of. These relatively high percentages of air emissions result mainly from the widespread use of organic chemicals as solvents. Unlike halo-organics and non-halogenated organics, metals are not particularly volatile as a class. Only 5 percent of waste in this group is emitted to air. Most metals in waste are disposed of on land, either on site (58 percent) or off site (36 percent). (See Figure 5-3 and Table 5-12.)

Turning to the three chemical groups of special concern, ozone depleters mostly are released to the air, either during industrial manufacture and processing or during or after use. In fact, direct releases to the air on site at TRI facilities accounted for 99 percent of the production-related waste of ozone depleters and for 98 percent of the waste associated with chloro-organics. (Note that the top two chemicals for amount of production-related waste in the special groups of ozone depleters, chloro-organics, and halo-organics are the same — 1,1,1,-trichloroethane and Freon 113.) Many carcinogens are also highly volatile; air emissions accounted for 75 percent of their production-related waste. (See Figure 5-3 and Table 5-13.)

Source Reduction

The Pollution Prevention Act of 1990 required facilities to begin reporting source reduction activities on TRI Form R, starting with the 1991 reporting year. Although facilities must indicate whether any source reduction activities have been undertaken for a particular chemical and the type of activities undertaken, the form does not ask

Table 5-13. Environmental Distribution of TRI Waste Released (Sec. 5) or Transferred to Disposal (Sec. 6) by Chemical Group of Special Concern, 1992

Chemical Group	Total Air Emissions Sec. 5 Pounds	Surface Water Discharges Sec. 5 Pounds	Underground Injection Sec. 5 Pounds	Releases to Land Sec. 5 Pounds	Transfers to Disposal Sec. 6 Pounds	Total Releases plus Transfers to Disposal Sec. 5 & 6 Pounds
Carcinogens	186,308,301	2,135,443	18,721,875	9,877,082	31,601,620	248,644,321
Ozone Depleters	166,257,508	21,822	49,490	105,526	857,776	167,292,122
Chloro-organics	316,050,569	1,013,528	1,671,597	291,625	2,553,249	321,580,568

for an estimate of the pounds of reductions in waste attributable to these activities. Analysis of the source reduction data from TRI can nevertheless yield some valuable perspective on the extent of forms, facilities, and chemicals involved in any consideration of source reduction. (See Chapter 4 for more information about source reduction nationwide and Chapter 10 for *Toxics Watch* findings on how little change in waste seems to be resulting from source reduction activities in New Jersey, whose expanded toxics reporting system includes amounts of waste reduced due to source reduction.)

Top Chemicals for Source Reduction

Despite the priority status of source reduction as an environmental management strategy and the growing evidence that source reduction can both cut waste and save companies money, only 25 percent of all TRI forms reported any source reduction activities at all. The chemicals with the largest number of forms reporting source reduction activities were 1,1,1-trichloroethane (1,477 forms), toluene (1,430 forms), xylene (mixed isomers) (1,231 forms), acetone (930 forms), and — tied for fifth place — methyl ethyl ketone and sulfuric acid (907 forms each). (See Table 5-14.)

Many of the chemicals with the largest *number* of forms reporting source reduction also had higher-than-average *percentages* of forms reporting such activities (e.g., 47 percent of forms for 1,1,1-trichloroethane reported source reduction and 60 percent for Freon 113). However, this was not always the case. For example, sulfuric acid, tied for fifth in number of forms reporting source reduction activities, had only 16 percent of its forms indicating such activities. (See Table 5-14.)

Table 5-14. The 25 Chemicals with the Largest Number of Forms Reporting Source Reduction, 1992

CAS Number	Chemical	Forms Reporting Source Reduction		Forms Not Reporting Source Reduction		Total Forms Reporting
		Number	Percent	Number	Percent	Number
71-55-6	1,1,1-Trichloroethane	1,477	47.17	1,654	52.83	3,131
108-88-3	Toluene	1,430	38.76	2,259	61.24	3,689
1330-20-7	Xylene (mixed isomers)	1,231	36.48	2,143	63.52	3,374
67-64-1	Acetone	930	36.61	1,610	63.39	2,540
78-93-3	Methyl ethyl ketone	907	37.07	1,540	62.93	2,447
7664-93-9	Sulfuric acid	907	16.07	4,736	83.93	5,643
7664-41-7	Ammonia	666	21.08	2,494	78.92	3,160
67-56-1	Methanol	642	26.34	1,795	73.66	2,437
	Glycol ethers	610	28.69	1,516	71.31	2,126
7647-01-0	Hydrochloric acid	574	17.53	2,700	82.47	3,274
76-13-1	Freon 113	517	60.47	338	39.53	855
	Zinc compounds	478	20.07	1,904	79.93	2,382
75-09-2	Dichloromethane	419	37.61	695	62.39	1,114
7664-38-2	Phosphoric acid	408	15.36	2,249	84.64	2,657
	Chromium compounds	366	25.03	1,096	74.97	1,462
108-10-1	Methyl isobutyl ketone	360	35.50	654	64.50	1,014
71-36-3	n-Butyl alcohol	359	30.79	807	69.21	1,166
100-42-5	Styrene	337	24.14	1,059	75.86	1,396
7697-37-2	Nitric acid	325	17.96	1,485	82.04	1,810
7440-50-8	Copper	323	14.17	1,956	85.83	2,279
100-41-4	Ethylbenzene	315	35.47	573	64.53	888
	Lead compounds	292	33.41	582	66.59	874
107-21-1	Ethylene glycol	286	21.58	1,039	78.42	1,325
	Copper compounds	250	17.37	1,189	82.63	1,439
79-01-6	Trichloroethylene	248	37.41	415	62.59	663
	Subtotal	14,657	27.58	38,488	72.42	53,145
	All Others	5,851	20.99	22,020	79.01	27,871
	Total	20,508	25.31	60,508	74.69	81,016

Source Reduction within the Five Chemical Classes and Three Groups of Special Concern

Source reduction activities were more prevalent within certain chemical groups than within others. Among the chemical classes, halo-organics (most of those on the TRI list are chloro-organics) had the largest percentage of forms reporting source reduction activities (41 percent). The increased scrutiny and regulatory focus on chloro-organics has most likely influenced the level of effort by industry to reduce the use of these compounds. (See Box 5-C.)

Metals and acids/bases/salts had the least number of forms reporting source reduction activity with 17 and 18 percent, respectively. Source reduction may take more time to implement for metals than for some other chemical classes, because metals are often essential components in product formulation. In those cases, source reduction would require either product

Figure 5-4.

TRI Forms Reporting Source Reduction Activity by Chemical Class and Group of Special Concern, 1992

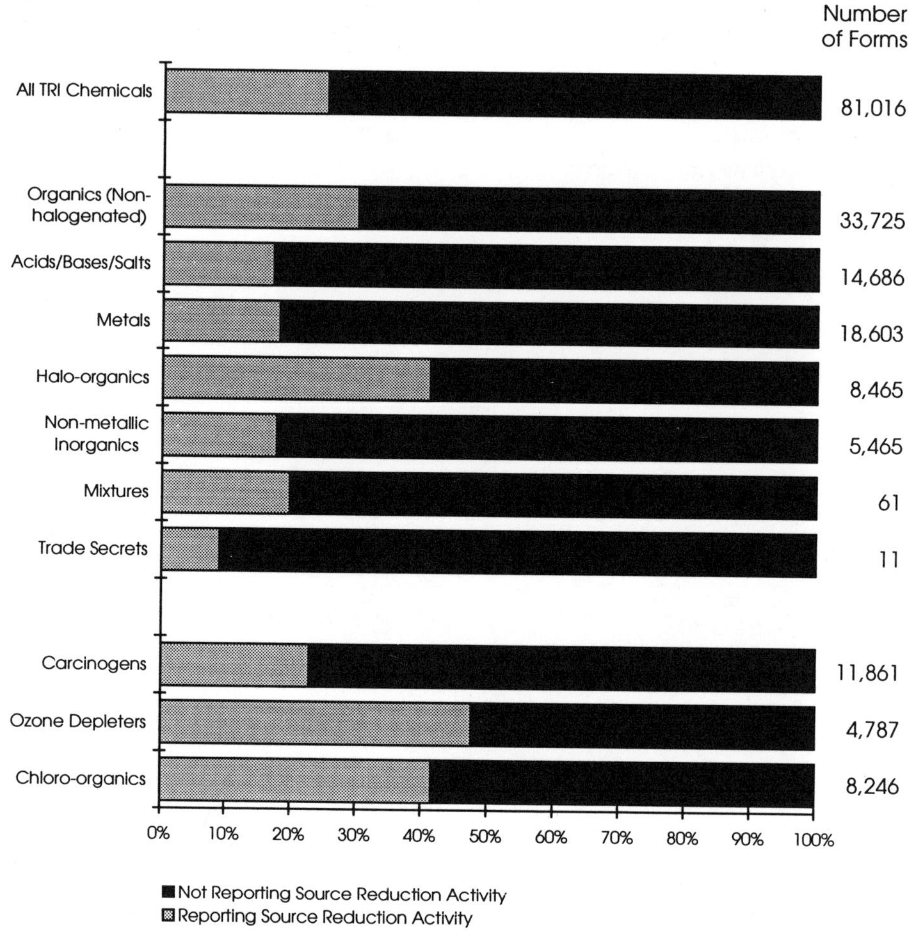

change or major production processes alterations. Acids/bases/salts are relatively inexpensive to buy and are easy to recycle and treat, so the incentives for source reduction would also not be as great for this class.

Ozone depleters and chloro-organics had the largest percentage of forms reporting source reduction among the special chemical groups, with 48 percent and 42 percent, respectively. Given the regulatory focus on these two groups, their source reduction initiatives are not surprising. (See Figure 5-4 and Boxes 5-B and 5-C.)

Changes in Production-related Waste, 1991-1992

1992 was the second year of reporting the waste generation and source reduction information required in Section 8 of TRI Form R.

Because facilities must report not only current data but also the previous year's waste information and projections of the waste expected to be generated in the following two years, 1992 is the first reporting year that allows a full range of comparisons of multi-year data.

TRI Chemicals with Largest Changes in Total Production-related Waste

The five chemicals with largest reported decreases in total TRI production-related waste from 1991 to 1992 were benzene with a reduction of 117.7 million pounds (45 percent), followed by cyclohexane, copper, chlorine, and 1,1,1-trichloroethane with decreases of 111.8 million pounds (54 percent), 45.8 million pounds (6 percent), 34.2 million pounds (7 percent), and 33.6 million pounds (9 percent), respectively. (See Table 5-15.)

Toxics Watch research found, however, that caution is required before accepting large chemical-specific changes in waste at face value. For example, much of the large decrease for benzene is attributable to one facility, Reilly Industries in Indianapolis, Indiana, whose 118.0-million-pound decrease turned out not to be real. The facility had only reclassified benzene-containing waste that it reported in 1991 as "on-site recycling" (reportable to TRI) to "in-process recovery" (not reportable) in 1992. (See Table 5-15.) With regard to the decrease for copper, one facility, AT&T Network Cable Systems of Atlanta, Georgia, significantly influenced this decrease by reporting 89.0 million pounds of total production-related waste of copper in 1991 and 6.4 million in 1992. The amount reported for 1991 was a reporting error; it should have been 8.9 million pounds.

Regulatory focus on chlorine, chloro-organics, and ozone depleters was undoubtedly a strong motivational force behind the decreases in chlorine and 1,1,1-trichloroethane. (See Boxes 5-B and 5-C.) Without being able to normalize the data to level of production activity, it is unclear whether such decreases are related to decreases in production or to source reduction.

Turning to waste increases, the top five chemicals reported were ammonia, showing the largest increase between 1991 and 1992, with 264.3 million pounds (24 percent), followed by hydrochloric acid, an increase of 222.9 million pounds (10 percent); copper compounds, 169.1 million pounds (51 percent); acetonitrile, 98.5 million pounds (4 percent); and manganese compounds, 97 million pounds (69 percent). Of these, only one proved to be "real" in environmental terms: the increase in hydrochloric acid, a widely used chemical reported by 14 percent of TRI facilities. (See Table 5-16.)

Toxics Watch interviews with the facilities reporting the largest changes turned up the following: the number one ammonia increase was due primarily to Star Enterprises in Union, Louisiana, which reported on-site treatment of 9.3 million pounds of ammonia in

Table 5-15. The 25 TRI Chemicals with the Largest Decreases in Total Production-related Waste, 1991-1992

		Total Production-related Waste			
CAS Number	**Chemical**	**1991** Pounds	**1992** Pounds	**1991-1992 Net Difference** Pounds	**1991-1992 Percent Change** Percent
71-43-2	Benzene	262,822,660	145,101,986	-117,720,674	-44.79
110-82-7	Cyclohexane	206,535,537	94,716,569	-111,818,968	-54.14
7440-50-8	Copper	720,952,763	675,138,852	-45,813,911	-6.35
7782-50-5	Chlorine	464,999,928	430,848,879	-34,151,049	-7.34
71-55-6	1,1,1-Trichloroethane	356,623,272	323,014,728	-33,608,544	-9.42
75-00-3	Chloroethane	74,573,103	44,803,130	-29,769,973	-39.92
67-64-1	Acetone	700,607,607	672,068,269	-28,539,338	-4.07
107-21-1	Ethylene glycol	589,066,620	561,144,278	-27,922,342	-4.74
7440-36-0	Antimony	28,870,488	5,268,714	-23,601,774	-81.75
7440-38-2	Arsenic	25,403,181	2,348,508	-23,054,673	-90.76
7664-93-9	Sulfuric acid	10,289,832,954	10,269,925,138	-19,907,816	-0.19
	Antimony compounds	37,692,503	22,690,828	-15,001,675	-39.80
127-18-4	Tetrachloroethylene	145,625,193	132,195,977	-13,429,216	-9.22
100-41-4	Ethylbenzene	109,707,080	96,538,764	-13,168,316	-12.00
108-95-2	Phenol	187,951,700	176,366,012	-11,585,688	-6.16
79-10-7	Acrylic acid	72,265,961	61,790,567	-10,475,394	-14.50
7439-96-5	Manganese	101,360,514	92,712,389	-8,648,125	-8.53
80-62-6	Methyl methacrylate	20,381,980	13,704,586	-6,677,394	-32.76
75-56-9	Propylene oxide ether	22,791,194	16,373,703	-6,417,491	-28.16
108-60-1	Bis(2-chloro-1-methylethyl)	18,084,800	12,859,300	-5,225,500	-28.89
67-66-3	Chloroform	60,034,145	56,079,423	-3,954,722	-6.59
67-72-1	Hexachloroethane	6,755,583	3,232,680	-3,522,903	-52.15
6484-52-2	Ammonium nitrate (solution)	154,371,969	150,857,399	-3,514,570	-2.28
71-36-3	n-Butyl alcohol	156,302,561	152,896,118	-3,406,443	-2.18
75-71-8	Dichlorodifluoromethane (CFC-12)	16,288,900	13,168,673	-3,120,227	-19.16

1991 and 180.0 million pounds in 1992. The amount for 1992 was in error and should be 18.0 million pounds. The third, fourth, and fifth largest increases all resulted in part from facility errors or changes in calculation methods:

- The copper compounds increase of 169.1 million pounds is primarily because of a change in calculation methods by Revere Copper Products in Rome, New York. That facility reported no on-site recycling of copper compounds in 1991, but changed calculation methods and reported 87.6 million pounds in 1992.
- The acetonitrile increase of 98.5 million pounds is largely the result of the 500.0 million-pound increase reported by Goodyear Tire and Rubber Company in Beaumont, Texas, for its on-site recycling of that chemical. In 1994 the facility revised its 1991 and 1992 recycling amounts to

Table 5-16. The 25 TRI Chemicals with the Largest Increases in Total Production-related Waste, 1991-1992

CAS Number	Chemical	Total Production-related Waste 1991 Pounds	1992 Pounds	1991-1992 Net Difference Pounds	1991-1992 Percent Change Percent
7664-41-7	Ammonia	1,119,514,284	1,383,853,783	264,339,499	23.61
7647-01-0	Hydrochloric acid	2,252,607,074	2,475,552,419	222,945,345	9.90
	Copper compounds	333,371,700	502,456,962	169,085,262	50.72
75-05-8	Acetonitrile	2,482,839,851	2,581,322,698	98,482,847	3.97
	Manganese compounds	140,917,370	237,882,578	96,965,208	68.81
106-99-0	1,3-Butadiene	360,546,388	453,627,237	93,080,849	25.82
7664-38-2	Phosphoric acid	603,067,696	682,122,515	79,054,819	13.11
	Lead compounds	1,048,888,834	1,107,360,694	58,471,860	5.57
7429-90-5	Aluminum (fume or dust)	81,108,271	131,824,600	50,716,329	62.53
108-88-3	Toluene	1,279,580,712	1,323,162,737	43,582,025	3.41
	Zinc compounds	427,226,586	470,171,187	42,944,601	10.05
115-07-1	Propylene	1,588,694,983	1,615,374,591	26,679,608	1.68
98-82-8	Cumene	295,188,164	320,391,682	25,203,518	8.54
	Chromium compounds	146,729,962	171,072,379	24,342,417	16.59
78-87-5	1,2-Dichloropropane	45,455,270	68,342,373	22,887,103	50.35
107-06-2	1,2-Dichloroethane	199,646,012	221,813,665	22,167,653	11.10
74-85-1	Ethylene	1,160,221,358	1,180,225,916	20,004,558	1.72
76-13-1	Freon 113	270,240,491	289,662,188	19,421,697	7.19
108-10-1	Methyl isobutyl ketone	332,827,112	350,963,788	18,136,676	5.45
7439-92-1	Lead	242,858,210	260,778,713	17,920,503	7.38
50-00-0	Formaldehyde	282,764,848	298,670,590	15,905,742	5.63
78-93-3	Methyl ethyl ketone	450,131,409	465,413,844	15,282,435	3.40
95-63-6	1,2,4-Trimethylbenzene	30,677,914	45,193,640	14,515,726	47.32
91-20-3	Naphthalene	47,522,801	60,045,613	12,522,812	26.35
7697-37-2	Nitric acid	300,703,408	310,850,709	10,147,301	3.37

zero, based on its changed interpretation of TRI reporting requirements, but these revisions were made after the database was "frozen" for purposes of this report.

- The increase of 97.0 million pounds in manganese compounds is largely attributable to Elkem Metals Company in Marietta, Ohio, which reported zero on-site recycling of manganese compounds in 1991, but changed calculation methods and reported 102.0 million pounds in 1992. (See Table 5-16, Chapter 4, and Appendix B.)

Overall, *Toxics Watch* research found that two of the top five waste decreases and four of the top five waste increases were not "as they appeared." These represented reporting errors and three changes in waste-calculation methods. Depending upon the type of analy-

Table 5-17. TRI Waste by Chemical Class, 1991-1992

	Total Recycling 1991 - 1992		Total Energy Recovery 1991 - 1992	
Chemical Class	**Net Difference** Pounds	**Percent Change** Percent	**Net Difference** Pounds	**Percent Change** Percent
Organics (Non-halogenated)	10,061,746	0.15	151,343,334	4.82
Acids/Bases/Salts	118,342,143	1.58	2,152,672	9.54
Metals	375,299,876	12.56	291,599	7.18
Halo-organics	34,702,483	2.88	-6,729,709	-3.43
Non-metallic Inorganics	-9,774,388	-2.72	-156,411	-0.29
Mixtures	-76,326	-14.76	-974,982	-16.29
Trade Secrets	39,147	130.49	82,000	20.92
Total for All TRI Chemicals	528,594,681	2.81	146,008,503	4.27

Table 5-18. TRI Waste by Chemical Group of Special Concern, 1991-1992

	Total Recycling 1991 - 1992		Total Energy Recovery 1991 - 1992	
Chemical Group	**Net Difference** Pounds	**Percent Change** Percent	**Net Difference** Pounds	**Percent Change** Percent
Carcinogens	48,380,042	2.59	31,480,710	10.28
Ozone Depleters	-21,901,796	-6.72	1,399,752	10.03
Chloro-organics	33,805,856	2.81	-6,760,560	-3.45

sis sought, this makes verification of data with reporting facilities most important.

Chapter 4 discusses in detail examples of reporting errors and reclassifications that affect TRI Section 8 data. Chapter 4 also indicates that the biases of such changes do not tend in one direction. Thus, in the aggregate, the national trends are little affected, but changes in waste generation for any individual chemical can be distorted to a greater degree. Improvements EPA is making in data verification and the experience facilities are gaining in reporting such data should result in greatly improved data for Section 8 in the near future, similar to that which occurred over the first few years that Sections 5 and 6 data were reported to TRI.

Changes in Waste by Five Chemical Classes and Three Groups of Special Concern

The overall reported increase in TRI chemicals in waste between 1991 and 1992 (1.0 billion pounds, or 3 percent) came from many types of chemicals: total production-

Total Treatment 1991 - 1992		Released/Disposed of 1991 - 1992		Total Production-related Waste 1991 - 1992	
Net Difference Pounds	Percent Change Percent	Net Difference Pounds	Percent Change Percent	Net Difference Pounds	Percent Change Percent
28,184,584	0.87	-76,329,135	-5.54	113,260,529	0.78
120,807,940	2.11	61,659,136	8.23	302,961,891	2.17
66,440,627	21.14	-39,818,749	-8.54	402,213,353	10.66
2,227,834	0.40	-41,036,789	-11.35	-10,836,181	-0.47
237,545,528	34.21	-20,154,085	-3.59	207,460,644	12.43
1,522,294	485.84	1,278,142	306.66	1,749,128	24.18
-120,464	-45.37	2,500	155.28	3,183	0.46
456,608,343	4.33	-114,398,980	-3.25	1,016,812,547	2.80

Total Treatment 1991 - 1992		Released/Disposed of 1991 - 1992		Total Production-related Waste 1991 - 1992	
Net Difference Pounds	Percent Change Percent	Net Difference Pounds	Percent Change Percent	Net Difference Pounds	Percent Change Percent
-30,395,152	-6.15	-20,226,023	-7.78	29,239,577	1.00
36,767,519	16.85	-25,161,516	-13.33	-8,896,041	-1.19
2,719,365	0.48	-41,309,962	-11.56	-11,545,301	-0.50

related waste in every chemical class except halo-organics increased. The decrease in halo-organics amounted to 10.8 million pounds (less than one-half of 1 percent). Metals had the largest absolute increase in total production-related waste of 402.2 million pounds (11 percent), and acids/bases/salts had the second largest, with 303.0 million pounds (2 percent). (See Table 5-17.)

Of the three chemical groups of special concern, two decreased slightly in total production-related waste between 1991 and 1992. Ozone depleters decreased by 8.9 million pounds (1 percent), and chloro-organics by 11.5 million pounds (0.5 percent). Only carcinogens increased, by 29.2 million pounds (1 percent). (See Table 5-18.)

TRI Chemicals with Largest Changes in Releases/Disposal

While there is agreement that release/disposal of waste is environmentally the least desirable option, no consistent pattern emerges in whether individual types of chemical waste are being managed by better methods. The chemicals that increased in waste

Figure 5-5.

The TRI Chemicals with the Largest Changes in Waste Released/ Disposed of, 1991 to 1992

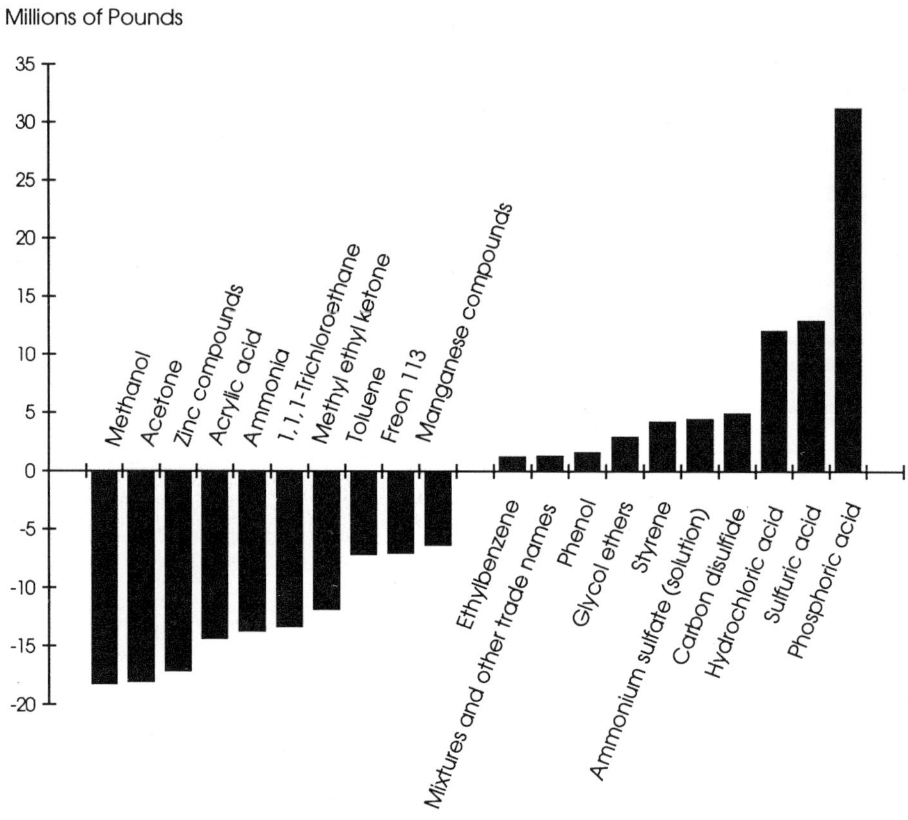

The 10 chemicals with the largest projected decreases and the 10 with the largest projected increases in waste released/ disposed of

released/disposed of (as reported in Section 8) between 1991 and 1992 did increase by somewhat smaller absolute amounts than the decreases reported for chemicals that had the largest decreases, with the exception of phosphoric acid. Phosphoric acid showed the largest change, with an increase of 31.1 million pounds (19 percent). Other large increases were sulfuric acid with 12.9 million pounds (7 percent), hydrochloric acid with 12.0 million pounds (4 percent), carbon disulfide with 4.9 million pounds (6 percent), and ammonium sulfate (solution) with 4.4 million pounds (18 percent). (See Figure 5-5 and Appendix J, Table J-1.)

Methanol had the largest decrease in waste released/ disposed of between 1991 and 1992 , with 18.2 million pounds (7 percent). The next four were acetone with 18.0 million pounds (an 11 percent decrease), zinc compounds with 17.1 million pounds (12 percent decrease), acrylic acid with 14.3 million pounds (74 percent decrease), and ammonia with 13.7 million pounds (3 percent decrease). (See Figure 5-5 and Appendix J, Table J-2.)

Many increases or decreases in the amount of waste released/ disposed of are associated with corresponding changes in the amount of total production-related waste. In some cases, the amount of waste released/disposed of *decreased* despite an *increase* in total production-related waste, indicating at least a movement away from less desirable waste management despite the increase in total waste. For example, the amount of total production-related waste of zinc compounds increased 42.9 million pounds in 1992 from 1991, during the same period that waste of zinc compounds released/disposed of to the environment decreased by 17.1 million pounds. (See Appendix J, Table J-2.)

Changes in Waste Associated with Source Reduction

The actual effects on waste resulting from source reduction would be easier to determine if actual pounds of such waste reduction had to be reported, rather than only the existence of source reduction activities. Chapter 4 describes the problem with normalizing production-related waste data by using the production index, and the reasons that normalization is not attempted in this report. Even without accounting for changes in production, one way to view the data is to compare the changes in data reported between 1991 and 1992 for those forms reporting source reduction activities versus those forms not reporting such activities. Not only can changes in total production-related waste be examined, but differences in the various waste management options can also be evaluated between the two groups of forms.

One reasonable starting assumption is that between 1991 and 1992 the total amount of production-related waste associated with forms reporting source reduction activities would be affected in a positive manner by such activities. It would also be reasonable to expect that the way in which waste is managed would be favorably affected. Facilities that practice source reduction might be more likely to be aware of the environmental management hierarchy and thus more likely to manage their waste accordingly.

Analysis of TRI production-related waste supports both assumptions. Total production-related waste for all TRI chemicals increased overall by 3 percent (1.0 billion pounds) from 1991 to 1992. However, waste associated with forms not reporting source reduction activities increased 4 percent (1.0 billion pounds), while waste associated with forms reporting source reduction activities decreased by 0.3 percent (32.5-million-pounds). (See Table 5-19.)

Changes in production-related waste by chemical class reveal the same type of difference between waste associated with forms reporting and not reporting source reduction. For three of the five chemical classes (acids/bases/salts, halo-organics, and non-metallic inorganics), the change between 1991 and 1992 in total production-related waste associated with forms reporting source reduction was a decrease in quantity, while the change in such waste associated with forms not reporting source reduction was an increase.

Table 5-19. TRI Waste Associated with Forms Reporting and Not Reporting Source Reduction Activity, by Chemical Class, 1991-1992

Chemical Class	Source Reduction Activity	Total Recycled 1991 - 1992		Total Energy Recovery 1991 - 1992	
		Net Difference Pounds	Percent Change Percent	Net Difference Pounds	Percent Change Percent
Organics (Non-halogenated)	with	33,791,064	2.04	125,936,174	11.88
	without	-23,729,318	-0.46	25,407,160	1.22
Acids/Bases/Salts	with	-32,839,007	-4.22	1,431,930	6.81
	without	151,181,15 0	2.26	720,742	47.11
Metals	with	112,833,522	12.90	591,422	19.21
	without	262,466,354	12.42	-299,823	-30.61
Halo-organics	with	-21,837,735	-3.15	-4,139,490	-5.63
	without	56,540,218	11.01	-2,590,219	-2.11
Non-metallic Inorganics	with	-1,353,076	-1.29	-2,669,156	-7.70
	without	-8,421,312	-3.32	2,512,745	13.13
Mixtures	with	-48,557	-15.70	0	-106.00
	without	-27,769	-13.37	-974,982	-16.29
Trade Secrets	with	38,000	126.67	82,000	20.92
	without	1,147	0.00	12,536	41.06
Total for All TRI Chemicals	with	90,584,211	2.20	121,232,880	10.17
	without	438,010,470	2.98	24,775,623	1.11

In the case of metals, while total waste associated with both types of forms increased, the increase for waste associated with source reduction activities was less than that associated with no source reduction — an increase of 86.4 million pounds (8 percent) versus an increase of 315.8 million pounds (12 percent).

Non-halogenated organics presented an apparent contradiction, however: total production-related waste associated with forms reporting source reduction activities for those chemicals increased more than such waste associated with forms not reporting source reduction (a 2 percent increase of 71.5 million pounds versus a 0.4 percent increase of 41.8 million pounds, respectively). Such a difference could be accounted for by differences in production changes between the two groups, but that cannot be determined from the data. (See Table 5-19.)

Similar results appear in analyses of the data for the three chemical groups of special concern. For each group, the total production-related waste associated with forms reporting source reduction decreased between 1991 and 1992, but the waste associated with forms not reporting source reduction increased. Chloro-organics showed the most dramatic difference. Total production-related waste associated with forms reporting source reduction for chloro-organics decreased 85.7 million pounds (6 percent), while such waste associated with forms not reporting source reduction increased 74.2 million pounds (8 percent). (See Table 5-20.)

Total Treated 1991 - 1992		Quantity Released 1991 - 1992		Total Production-Related Waste 1991 - 1992	
Net Difference Pounds	**Percent Change** Percent	**Net Difference** Pounds	**Percent Change** Percent	**Net Difference** Pounds	**Percent Change** Percent
-14,501,781	-1.17	-73,764,251	-12.40	71,461,206	1.57
42,686,365	2.11	-2,564,884	-0.33	41,799,323	0.42
-29,122,324	-1.83	1,335,413	0.44	-59,193,988	-2.20
149,930,264	3.63	60,323,723	13.50	362,155,879	3.21
-1,098,890	-5.82	-25,937,945	-19.30	86,388,109	8.38
67,539,517	22.86	-13,880,804	-4.19	315,825,244	11.52
-21,387,029	-5.91	-38,626,681	-18.42	-85,990,935	-6.43
23,614,863	11.69	-2,410,108	-1.59	75,154,754	7.59
-22,720,802	-10.35	-18,342,133	-5.99	-45,085,167	-6.77
260,266,330	54.81	-1,811,952	-0.71	252,545,811	25.18
-50.96	57.00	1.11	-48,606	-15.45	
1,522,400	486.20	1,278,085	310.46	1,797,734	25.98
-133,000	-56.60	2,500	178.57	-10,500	-1.59
0	0.00	13,683	44.51		
-88,963,932	-2.59	-155,333,040	-10.04	-32,479,881	-0.32
545,572,275	7.66	40,934,060	2.08	1,049,292,428	4.03

A look at the changes between 1991 and 1992 in use of the different waste management options indicates a movement toward more environmentally desirable options for the waste associated with source reduction. Where source reduction was practiced, there was an increase in the quantity of waste recycled or used for energy recovery and a decrease in waste treated or released/disposed of. Total release/disposal of waste associated with forms reporting source reduction *decreased* by 155.3 million pounds (10 percent) between 1991 and 1992. This contrasts with an *increase* of 40.9 million pounds (2 percent) in waste released/disposed of associated with forms reporting no source reduction. Those forms showing no source reduction activity reflected increases in every type of waste management option. The treatment option increased both by the largest absolute amount (545.6 million pounds) and by the largest percentage (8 percent). (See Table 5-19.)

Movement away from the least desirable waste management options for those practicing source reduction can also be seen within various chemical classes and special groups, especially in regard to changes in the amount of waste released/disposed of. In every case except for mixtures and trade secrets, there was either 1) a larger decrease in waste released/disposed of associated with forms reporting source reduction or 2) a substantially smaller increase in waste released/disposed of associated with forms reporting source reduction than the amount of increase associated with forms reporting no such activities. This was true even in the case of

Table 5-20. TRI Waste Associated with Forms Reporting and Not Reporting Source Reduction Activity by Special Chemical Group, 1991-1992

Chemical Class	Source Reduction	Total Recycled 1991 - 1992 Net Difference Pounds	Total Recycled 1991 - 1992 Percent Change Percent	Total Energy Recovery 1991 - 1992 Net Difference Pounds	Total Energy Recovery 1991 - 1992 Percent Change Percent
Carcinogens	with	57,282,293	10.23	4,282,377	3.45
	without	-8,902,251	-0.68	27,198,333	14.91
Ozone Depleters	with	-23,020,830	-8.71	-1,425,825	-13.96
	without	1,119,034	1.81	2,825,577	75.45
Chloro-organics	with	-21,944,740	-3.17	-4,170,140	-5.67
	without	55,750,596	10.93	-2,590,420	-2.11

non-halogenated organics. Despite a greater increase for these organics in total production-related waste for forms reporting source reduction activities than for those not reporting source reduction, waste released/disposed of or treated decreased by 73.8 million pounds (12 percent) and 14.5 million pounds (1 percent), respectively. The increase in total waste for this chemical class therefore came from waste that was recycled or used for energy recovery. (See Tables 5-19 and 5-20.)

Changes in Production-related Waste, 1992-1994

The projections of future waste generation (for each of the next two years) that facilities are required to report in Section 8 of the TRI Form R indicate that the amount of total production-related waste is expected to change little between 1992 and 1994. Although projected decreases or increases for certain chemicals are larger, the net change for all forms is a 0.3 percent increase (126.6 million pounds), from 37.3 billion pounds to 37.5 billion pounds. How any anticipated changes in levels of production influence these estimates cannot be determined.

While the small change expected in the total quantity of waste suggests that U.S. manufacturing facilities are by no means optimizing their source reduction potential, there does appear to be a movement toward less undesirable waste management options. The quantity of waste released/disposed of is projected to decrease by 20 percent (685.3 million pounds). Waste that is treated is expected to decrease by 3 percent (308.8 million pounds), while the amount used for energy recovery is projected to increase 3 percent (112.3 million pounds) and the amount recycled to increase by 5 percent (1.0 billion pounds). (See Table 5-21.)

Total Treated 1991 - 1992		Quantity Released 1991 - 1992		Total Production-Related Waste 1991 - 1992	
Net Difference Pounds	Percent Change Percent	Net Difference Pounds	Percent Change Percent	Net Difference Pounds	Percent Change Percent
-45,431,942	-18.60	-20,183,387	-16.22	-4,050,659	-0.38
15,036,790	6.01	-42,636	-0.03	33,290,236	1.78
35,753,320	17.27	-21,718,432	-18.82	-10,411,767	-1.74
1,014,199	9.06	-3,443,084	-4.70	1,515,726	1.01
-21,225,661	-5.87	-38,374,904	-18.48	-85,715,445	-6.42
23,945,026	11.91	-2,935,058	-1.96	74,170,144	7.54

TRI Chemicals with Largest Projected Changes in Total Production-related Waste, 1992-1994

The projections for specific chemicals do reflect substantial expected changes in waste, despite the small net change in quantity for 1994 compared to 1992 that results from the combined projections of all facilities. (See Chapter 4 for discussion of problems associated with future estimates.)

The top five chemicals with the largest projected decreases are ammonia with 266.5 million pounds (a 19 percent decrease), lead compounds with 217.2 million pounds (20 percent), sulfuric acid with 164.2 million pounds (2 percent), 1,1,1-trichloroethane with 141.2 million pounds (44 percent), and propylene with 87.0 million pounds (5 percent). Many of the chemicals with the largest projected decreases are also those chemicals that had the largest total production-related waste in 1992, some of which were influenced by reporting errors or other single-facility anomalies. (Compare Table 5-1 with Table 5-22.)

The five chemicals with the largest projected increases between 1992 to 1994 are acetonitrile with 498.2 million pounds (19 percent), zinc compounds with 177.3 million pounds (38 percent), cyclohexane with 126.0 million pounds (133 percent), copper compounds with 69.5 million pounds (14 percent), and Freon 113 with 67.4 million pounds (23 percent). (See Table 5-23.)

Projected Changes in Waste for the Five Chemical Classes and Three Groups of Special Concern

Although facility projections for total production-related waste between 1992 and 1994 reflect a net increase, projections for certain chemical classes (acids/bases/salts, halo-organics, and non-metallic inorganics, plus the trade secrets category) show a net decrease. Non-metallic inorganics have the largest

Table 5-21. TRI Waste by Chemical Class, Actual 1992 to Projected 1994

	Total Recycling 1992 - 1994		Total Energy Recovery 1992 - 1994	
Chemical Class	**Net Difference** Pounds	**Percent Change** Percent	**Net Difference** Pounds	**Percent Change** Percent
Organics (Non-halogenated)	768,791,311	11.28	104,592,079	3.18
Acids/Bases/Salts	326,233,651	4.30	-1,029,257	-4.16
Metals	74,656,495	2.22	-3,091,166	-71.06
Halo-organics	-182,229,097	-14.68	11,158,339	5.89
Non-metallic Inorganics	21,197,644	6.07	-5,454,053	-10.17
Mixtures	-233,267	-52.93	6,189,883	123.52
Trade Secrets	-1,147	-1.66	-24,000	-5.06
Total for All TRI Chemicals	1,008,415,590	5.21	112,341,825	0.03

projected decrease of 264.8 million pounds (14 percent), compared to a largest estimated increase in waste generation for organics, with an increase of 648.1 million pounds (4 percent). (See Table 5-21.)

All three groups of special concern show an expected decrease in total production-related waste between 1992 and 1994. Ozone depleters have the largest projected decrease on a percentage basis, 20 percent (147.0 million pounds), and chloro-organics have the largest projected decrease on a quantity basis, 212.8 million pounds (9 percent). These results are not surprising, given the phase-out of ozone depleters and the focus on chloro-organics for health and environmental reasons. The largest special group, carcinogens, with 3.0 billion pounds of production-related waste in 1992, shows the smallest projected decrease by 1994 (a decrease of 58.5 million pounds, or 2 percent). (See Table 5-24.)

TRI Chemicals with Largest Projected Changes in Releases/ Disposal

Overall, the TRI waste managed by release/disposal, the least desirable method, is projected to decrease by 685.7 million pounds (20 percent) between 1992 and 1994. The five chemicals slated for the largest move away from release/ disposal between 1992 and 1994 are sulfuric acid with 111.0 million pounds of decrease (a 59 percent decrease), phosphoric acid with 106.2 million pounds (54 percent), hydrochloric acid with 84.0 million pounds (28 percent), ammonia with 73.4 million pounds (16 percent), and 1,1,1-trichloroethane with 72.3 million pounds (64 percent). (See Figure 5-6 and Appendix J, Table J-4.)

Total Treatment 1992 - 1994		Released/Disposed of 1992 - 1994		Total Production-related Waste 1992 - 1994	
Net Difference Pounds	Percent Change Percent	Net Difference Pounds	Percent Change Percent	Net Difference Pounds	Percent Change Percent
-79,883,259	-2.43	-145,376,779	-11.17	648,123,352	4.41
-180,190,760	-3.09	-315,185,286	-38.89	-170,171,652	-1.19
44,391,939	11.66	7,184,816	1.69	123,142,084	2.95
110,537,318	19.53	-152,874,257	-47.69	-213,407,697	-9.21
-202,767,019	-21.76	-77,806,271	-14.37	-264,829,699	-14.12
-942,735	-51.36	-1,214,130	-71.63	3,799,751	42.30
5,816	4.01	-900	-21.90	-20,231	-2.92
-308,848,700	-2.81	-685,272,807	-20.15	126,635,908	0.34

These chemicals are in many cases the same chemicals with the largest projected decreases in total production-related waste. For example, of the top 25 chemicals with projected decreases in waste released/disposed of, 13 are also on the list of 25 TRI chemicals with the largest estimated decreases in total production-related waste. It is encouraging that the projected decreases in total waste are reflected in many large projected decreases in waste released/disposed of, the least favored option for waste management. (See Table 5-22 and Appendix J, Table J-4.)

The top five chemicals with the largest projected increases in amount of waste released/disposed of are manganese with an increase of 24.2 million pounds (119 percent), creosote with 20.2 million pounds (937 percent), copper compounds with 7.8 million pounds (17 percent), propylene oxide with 2.3 million pounds (160 percent), and carbon disulfide with 2.2 million pounds (2 percent). (See Figure 5-6 and Appendix J, Table J-3.)

Projected Changes in Waste Associated with Source Reduction

Looking at waste reported on TRI forms that also indicate source reduction activities are occurring and comparing it to waste reported on forms not indicating any source reduction is helpful for the 1992-1994 projections, as it was for the 1991-1992 actual waste, in evaluating the potential impact that source reduction might have on future generation of waste. Out of the forms for all TRI chemicals, those indicating that source reduction was used in 1992 project a *decrease* of 16.2 million pounds (0.2 percent) in 1992-1994 pounds. The forms indicating no source reduction in

Table 5-22. The 25 TRI Chemicals with the Largest Projected Decreases in Total Production-related Waste, 1992-1994

		Total Production-related Waste			
CAS Number	Chemical	1992 Pounds	Projected 1994 Pounds	1992-1994 Net Difference Pounds	1992-1994 Percent Change Percent
7664-41-7	Ammonia	1,383,853,783	1,117,353,318	-266,500,465	-19.26
	Lead compounds	1,107,360,694	890,193,151	-217,167,543	-19.61
7664-93-9	Sulfuric acid	10,269,925,138	10,105,682,279	-164,242,859	-1.60
71-55-6	1,1,1-Trichloroethane	323,014,728	181,774,090	-141,240,638	-43.73
115-07-1	Propylene	1,615,374,591	1,528,395,048	-86,979,543	-5.38
74-85-1	Ethylene	1,180,225,916	1,101,144,575	-79,081,341	-6.70
75-69-4	Trichlorofluoromethane (CFC-11)	66,695,343	3,296,804	-63,398,539	-95.06
106-99-0	1,3-Butadiene	453,627,237	396,555,055	-57,072,182	-12.58
75-09-2	Dichloromethane	286,593,104	243,432,591	-43,160,513	-15.06
67-56-1	Methanol	2,238,505,652	2,208,777,616	-29,728,036	-1.33
79-01-6	Trichloroethylene	271,892,548	248,825,195	-23,067,353	-8.48
	Manganese compounds	237,882,578	219,001,881	-18,880,697	-7.94
127-18-4	Tetrachloroethylene	132,195,977	115,628,649	-16,567,328	-12.53
71-43-2	Benzene	145,101,986	128,656,672	-16,445,314	-11.33
7697-37-2	Nitric acid	310,850,709	297,250,887	-13,599,822	-4.38
7664-38-2	Phosphoric acid	682,122,515	671,015,987	-11,106,528	-1.63
	Cadmium compounds	13,924,917	7,163,462	-6,761,455	-48.56
75-71-8	Dichlorodifluoromethane (CFC-12)	13,168,673	6,610,680	-6,557,993	-49.80
79-34-5	1,1,2,2-Tetrachloroethane	25,213,478	18,785,254	-6,428,224	-25.50
6484-52-2	Ammonium nitrate (solution)	150,857,399	145,121,720	-5,735,679	-3.80
67-66-3	Chloroform	56,079,423	51,580,787	-4,498,636	-8.02
	Nickel compounds	63,460,089	59,308,203	-4,151,886	-6.54
109-86-4	2-Methoxyethanol	17,941,981	13,946,911	-3,995,070	-22.27
7783-20-2	Ammonium sulfate (solution)	77,217,088	74,534,448	-2,682,640	-3.47
56-23-5	Carbon tetrachloride	39,136,449	36,592,601	-2,543,848	-6.50

1992 project an *increase* of 142.8 million pounds (0.5 percent). (See Table 5-25.)

However, the picture that emerges from the projections for total production-related waste sorted for the five chemical classes and the three groups of special concern is quite mixed. For several chemical classes, forms reporting source reduction activities do not present more environmentally favorable projections than do forms not reporting source reduction activity. For example, metals waste reported on forms indicating that source reduction activities are occurring in 1992 is projected to *increase* 18 percent (197.0 million pounds) by 1994, while metals waste reported on forms indicating no source reduction is projected to *decrease* — by 2 percent (73.9 million pounds). In the case of carcinogens, the amount of waste reported on forms indicating source reduction activity is projected to decrease by 0.4 percent (4.5 million pounds), but waste reported on forms indicating

Table 5-23. The 25 TRI Chemicals with the Largest Projected Increases in Total Production-related Waste, 1992-1994

		Total Production-related Waste			
CAS Number	**Chemical**	**1992** Pounds	**Projected 1994** Pounds	**1992-1994 Net Difference** Pounds	**1992-1994 Percent Change** Percent
75-05-8	Acetonitrile	2,581,322,698	3,079,499,079	498,176,381	19.30
	Zinc compounds	470,171,187	647,445,514	177,274,327	37.70
110-82-7	Cyclohexane	94,716,569	220,680,731	125,964,162	132.99
	Copper compounds	502,456,962	571,914,778	69,457,816	13.82
76-13-1	Freon 113	289,662,188	357,062,513	67,400,325	23.27
1330-20-7	Xylene (mixed isomers)	549,893,102	602,185,559	52,292,457	9.51
91-20-3	Naphthalene	60,045,613	101,673,836	41,628,223	69.33
67-64-1	Acetone	672,068,269	712,213,956	40,145,687	5.97
107-21-1	Ethylene glycol	561,144,278	600,669,210	39,524,932	7.04
108-88-3	Toluene	1,323,162,737	1,352,847,744	29,685,007	2.24
7439-96-5	Manganese	92,712,389	120,121,294	27,408,905	29.56
7647-01-0	Hydrochloric acid	2,475,552,419	2,500,236,268	24,683,849	1.00
7440-50-8	Copper	675,138,852	699,355,443	24,216,591	3.59
7439-92-1	Lead	260,778,713	284,454,552	23,675,839	9.08
8001-58-9	Creosote	17,554,499	36,321,427	18,766,928	106.91
75-01-4	Vinyl chloride	222,432,306	240,307,940	17,875,634	8.04
7429-90-5	Aluminum (fume or dust)	131,824,600	146,523,078	14,698,478	11.15
100-42-5	Styrene	256,580,387	268,681,204	12,100,817	4.72
75-15-0	Carbon disulfide	127,135,361	138,053,167	10,917,806	8.59
7440-66-6	Zinc (fume or dust)	103,631,113	113,768,000	10,136,887	9.78
78-93-3	Methyl ethyl ketone	465,413,844	474,948,294	9,534,450	2.05
79-10-7	Acrylic acid	61,790,567	71,063,574	9,273,007	15.01
95-47-6	o-Xylene	55,564,796	64,281,233	8,716,437	15.69
7440-02-0	Nickel	87,495,571	94,681,819	7,186,248	8.21
7550-45-0	Titanium tetrachloride	39,816,191	46,659,987	6,843,796	17.19

no source reduction activity is expected to decrease by 2.9 percent (54.1 million pounds). (See Tables 5-25 and 5-26.)

Therefore, while source reduction activities appear to have a positive impact on changes in waste generated in the year such activities are reported compared to the previous year, they may have considerably less impact on the generation of waste in the future. This may be due in part to the fact that where source reduction is already being practiced, the easier activities have probably been implemented first, and therefore, future activities would not be done as readily. This would be in contrast to those who have yet to practice such activities, but who might undertake them in the near future and most likely would implement the easier activities first. Other important factors that could account for apparently contradictory results between those forms reporting and not reporting source reduction activities are anticipated production

Table 5-24. TRI Waste by Chemical Group of Special Concern, Actual 1992 to Projected 1994

Chemical Class	Total Recycling 1992 - 1994		Total Energy Recovery 1992 - 1994	
	Net Difference Pounds	**Percent Change** Percent	**Net Difference** Pounds	**Percent Change** Percent
Carcinogens	28,001,084	1.46	-54,163,584	-16.03
Ozone Depleters	-152,521,936	-50.13	-1,664,627	-10.84
Chloro-organics	-182,022,898	-14.72	11,161,930	5.90

changes and the questionable accuracy of some 1992 forms submitted by certain individual facilities. If a 1992 reporting error led to an underestimated 1992 amount for a chemical, but the projected 1994 amounts for the chemical are reasonable, then the data will show a large artificial increase that may not be offset by real decreases anticipated by other facilities reporting source reduction. The pattern that actually emerges in future reporting years will tell much about whether source reduction is being given top priority in accordance with the environmental management hierarchy.

Determining Amounts of Waste Containing Specific Chemicals in BRS and TRI

Facilities report amounts of their toxic waste generated to the Biennial Reporting System (BRS), as mandated under RCRA, by calculating the total amount of individual waste streams. These waste streams contain specific toxic chemicals, but typically also contain carrier materials, such as water or soil. The exact amounts of toxic chemicals contained in BRS waste streams are not reported. (See Appendix K for the 1991 BRS data by waste code.)

Calculating the total volume of waste streams containing a particular chemical is not always possible either. Facilities report the identities of chemicals in waste streams by means of waste codes. (See Appendix E.) These waste codes designate that the waste stream contains a single chemical or one or more combinations of chemicals, in addition to carrier materials. In addition, facilities may describe a waste stream by more than one waste code.[d] Only the single-chemical waste code waste streams are certain to contain the specific chemical.

The process of determining the amount of BRS waste generated for a single chemical begins by adding

[d] This happens when individual waste code waste streams are combined for treatment, for example.

Total Treatment 1992 - 1994		Released/Disposed of 1992 - 1994		Total Production-related Waste 1992 - 1994	
Net Difference Pounds	Percent Change Percent	Net Difference Pounds	Percent Change Percent	Net Difference Pounds	Percent Change Percent
-9,892,214	-2.13	-22,478,061	-9.38	-58,532,775	-1.98
111,797,305	43.84	-104,603,974	-63.95	-146,993,232	-19.91
110,601,902	19.57	-152,491,782	-48.24	-212,750,848	-9.22

together the amounts of waste streams described by single-chemical waste codes for that chemical. (See Table 5-27.) For example, waste code U080 is the only waste code that describes only dichloromethane, therefore, all waste streams listed as waste code U080 will definitely contain dichloromethane. The next step is to add together the amounts of all multiple-chemical waste code waste streams that may contain the chemical. For example, toluene may be a component of waste streams described by waste codes F005 (certain non-halogenated solvents including toluene) and K036, (still bottoms from toluene reclamation distillation in the production of disulfoton). Finally, amounts of waste streams described by more than one waste code are added together. These waste streams are described by waste codes corresponding to single or multiple chemicals, along with other waste codes. For example, some waste stream reports contain waste codes K049 (slop oil emulsion solids from the Petroleum industry) and K052 (leaded tank bottoms from the Petroleum industry). Only K052 may contain lead, but K049 does not, and both are included in the waste stream.

The end result is a range of amounts of waste that may contain a specific chemical. For example, the amount of BRS toxic waste generated in 1991 containing lead and lead compounds was at least 11.3 billion pounds (the amount of single-chemical waste code waste streams containing lead and lead compounds) and could have ranged as high as 72.1 billion pounds (total for all waste streams that may contain lead and lead compounds). Again, the amount of lead contained in these waste streams is not known because even single-chemical waste code waste streams include amounts of carrier materials. (See Table 5-27.)

By contrast, facilities report to TRI amounts of specific chemicals in waste — individual chemicals released to air, land, underground injection, and water, off-site transfers, and amounts of on- and off-site waste management. (Compare Tables 5-27 and 5-28.) Production-related waste in TRI is the sum of on- and off-site recycling, energy recovery, and treatment, plus the "quantity released" — the equivalent of the amounts of the chemical in on-site releases plus the amount in off-site transfers to

Figure 5-6.

The TRI Chemicals with the Largest Projected Changes in Waste Released/ Disposed of, 1992 to 1994

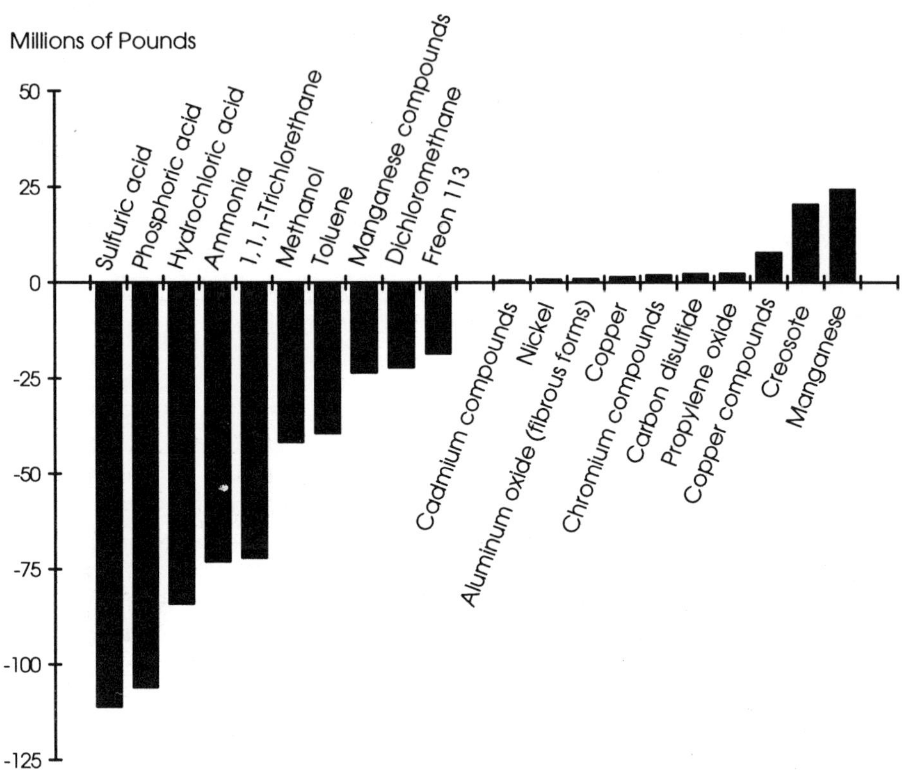

The 10 chemicals with the largest projected decreases and the 10 with the largest projected increases in waste released/ disposed of

disposal. Since data elements in TRI are actual quantities, chemical-specific analyses are possible.

Comparing the data reported to each system for specific chemicals underscores the differences in the consideration of individual toxic chemicals in waste. Subtracting air emissions from TRI production-related waste yields an adjusted waste generation figure similar in coverage of waste media to BRS data, which is limited to liquid and solid hazardous wastes. (See Table 5-29.) It is tempting to compare TRI adjusted production-related waste with the BRS data. However, it is not possible to determine how much of the waste reported to TRI is also reported to BRS for two reasons: facilities may not be required to report to both systems (see Box 4-C), and even BRS single-chemical waste code waste streams containing a specific toxic chemical may not meet RCRA toxicity criteria for reporting and therefore not appear in a facility's BRS reports (see Chapter 6).

Table 5-25. TRI Total Production-related Waste Associated with Forms Reporting and Not Reporting Source Reduction by Chemical Class, Actual 1992 to Projected 1994

		Total Production-related Waste			
Chemical Class	**Source Reduction Activity**	**1992** Pounds	**Projected 1994** Pounds	**1992-1994 Net Difference** Pounds	**1992-1994 Percent Change** Percent
Organics (Non-halogenated)	With	4,623,811,448	4,545,395,393	-78,416,055	-1.70
	Without	10,069,902,376	10,796,441,783	726,539,407	7.21
Acids/Bases/Salts	With	2,632,687,427	2,645,627,887	12,940,460	0.49
	Without	11,629,549,218	11,446,437,106	-183,112,112	-1.57
Metals	With	1,117,109,895	1,314,124,417	197,014,522	17.64
	Without	3,057,771,987	2,983,899,549	-73,872,438	-2.42
Halo-Organics	With	1,252,184,304	1,122,535,893	-129,648,411	-10.35
	Without	1,065,018,045	981,258,759	-83,759,286	-7.86
Non-metallic Inorganics	With	620,458,397	602,557,025	-17,901,372	-2.89
	Without	1,255,607,715	1,008,679,388	-246,928,327	-19.67
Mixtures	With	265,962	108,663	-157,299	-59.14
	Without	8,716,529	12,673,579	3,957,050	45.40
Trade Secrets	With	647,900	623,000	-24,900	-3.84
	Without	44,421	49,090	4,669	10.51
Total for All TRI Chemicals	With	10,247,165,333	10,230,972,278	-16,193,055	-0.16
	Without	27,086,610,291	27,229,439,254	142,828,963	0.53

Table 5-26. TRI Total Production-related Waste Associated with Forms Reporting and Not Reporting Source Reduction by Special Chemical Group, Actual 1992 to Projected 1994

		Total Production-related Waste			
Chemical Class	**Source Reduction Activity**	**1992** Pounds	**Projected 1994** Pounds	**1992-1994 Net Difference** Pounds	**1992-1994 Percent Change** Percent
Carcinogens	With	1,048,726,184	1,044,270,568	-4,455,616	-0.42
	Without	1,906,341,653	1,852,264,494	-54,077,159	-2.84
Ozone Depleters	With	586,536,180	506,622,353	-79,913,827	-13.62
	Without	151,597,852	84,518,447	-67,079,405	-44.25
Chloro-organics	With	1,250,057,014	1,120,689,451	-129,367,563	-10.35
	Without	1,057,436,146	974,052,861	-83,383,285	-7.89

Table 5-27. Quantities of Four Chemicals in BRS Waste Streams, 1991

		Dichloromethane			Lead and Lead Compounds		
		Waste Code(s)	**BRS Reports** Number	**Toxic Waste Generated** Pounds	**Waste Code(s)**	**BRS Reports** Number	**Toxic Waste Generated** Pounds
Single-Chemical Waste Code Waste Streams	Waste code definitely contains chemical of interest as sole toxic constituent.	U080	234	1,561,140	D008	7,462	11,282,068,080
					P110	7	3,600
					U144	31	40,880
					U145	3	860
					U146	6	40
		Subtotal	234	1,561,140	Subtotal	7,509	11,282,113,460
Multiple-Chemical Waste Code Waste Streams	Waste stream may contain chemical of interest. May also contain other chemicals.	F001	10,915	380,666,820	K046	9	1,615,660
		F002	9,188	549,783,860	K052	34	1,586,900
					K065	0	0
					K069	7	5,545,000
					K086	54	1,766,440
					K100	0	0
		Subtotal	20,103	930,450,680	Subtotal	104	10,514,000
Multiple Waste Code Waste Streams*	Waste stream contains at least one single- or multiple-chemical waste code waste stream listed above and may contain the chemical of interest.	DF	19,547	19,097,526,580	D	17,432	45,178,276,220
		DFK	68	61,159,042,280	DF	8,477	6,270,285,080
		DFL**	37	44,140	DFK	111	915,798,980
		DFP	89	4,660,672,100	DFL	28	18,480
		DFPK	3	5,428,600	DFP	37	4,659,795,400
		DFPU	162	3,543,800	DFPK	3	4,967,740
		DFPUK	13	48,397,440	DFPU	100	2,331,600
		DFU	1,192	858,567,620	DFPUK	13	51,676,440
		DFUK	74	10,261,544,000	DFU	514	659,351,860
		DFUL	14	2,670,880	DFUK	51	94,156,900
		DPU	24	778,360	DFUL	12	2,665,700
		DU	258	4,007,560	DK	163	1,138,167,120
		DUK	5	117,360	DL	44	20,920
		F	4,630	99,050,092,340	DP	219	43,438,800
		FK	17	37,728,340	DPU	300	44,502,320
		FL	1	0	DPUK	6	241,492,920
		FP	9	460,060	DU	580	9,723,940
		FPU	22	10,134,660	DUK	2	74,200
		FPUK	11	1,767,373,520	DUL	6	4,180
		FU	351	620,744,520	FK	18	2,216,440
		FUK	16	174,996,960	FP	1	20
		PU	7	5,180	FPUK	9	1,292,155,400
		U	177	38,602,180	FUK	9	103,375,580
		UL	1	40	K	10	62,210,360
					P	1	280
					PU	16	440
					U	14	7,220
		Subtotal	26,728	197,802,478,520	Subtotal	28,176	60,776,714,540
Total for All Waste Streams	Upper bound for waste streams containing chemical of interest.	Total	47,065	198,734,490,340	Total	35,789	72,069,342,000

* "D" indicates that all waste streams are described by at least two "D" waste codes. "DF" indicates that the waste stream is described by at least one "D" and one "F" waste code, etc.

** "L" denotes laboratory waste

Sulfuric Acid			Toluene		
Waste Code(s)	**BRS Reports** Number	**Toxic Waste Generated** Pounds	**Waste Code(s)**	**BRS Reports** Number	**Toxic Waste Generated** Pounds
Chemical is not classified under any single chemical waste code			U220	153	15,626,980
Subtotal	0	0	Subtotal	153	15,626,980
D002	2,048	57,440,625,620	F005	3,527	323,763,060
K131	0	0	K036	0	0
Subtotal	2,048	57,440,625,620	Subtotal	3,527	323,763,060
D	13,668	62,719,734,900	DF	31,170	12,040,987,220
DF	3,921	21,559,132,840	DFK	87	1,178,358,480
DFK	20	61,131,472,280	DFL	23	8,720
DFL	11	36,260	DFP	80	4,660,630,920
DFP	73	4,668,322,040	DFPK	5	75,329,740
DFPK	3	70,383,740	DFPU	141	6,116,200
DFPU	106	3,498,860	DFPUK	12	36,982,040
DFPUK	16	104,221,780	DFU	1,126	586,841,240
DFU	505	778,043,640	DFUK	64	10,163,846,640
DFUK	31	10,230,567,580	DFUL	10	2,665,900
DFUL	3	27,720	DPU	30	4,836,800
DK	159	12,585,244,720	DPUK	1	12,000
DL	20	25,400	DU	426	35,627,780
DP	497	66,158,920	DUK	5	36,643,740
DPL	3	260	DUL	2	14,500
DPU	176	46,284,340	F	6,513	101,372,653,680
DPUK	10	4,729,409,960	FK	21	762,130,060
DU	1,128	605,340,020	FL	2	840
DUL	5	6,320	FP	10	472,720
K	3	1,239,145,560	FPU	22	9,975,940
			FPUK	10	1,638,136,220
			FU	147	606,938,620
			FUK	15	174,883,540
			K	1	3,420
			PU	7	100,652,200
			PUK	1	80
			U	127	250,794,480
			UK	6	3,740,820
Subtotal	20,358	180,537,057,140	Subtotal	40,064	133,749,284,540
Total	22,406	237,977,682,760	Total	43,744	134,088,674,580

Table 5-28. Quantities of Four Chemicals Reported to TRI, 1991

	Dichloro-methane	Lead and Lead Compounds*	Sulfuric Acid	Toluene
Number of Forms, 1991	1,278	1,773	5,685	3,879
Releases	Pounds	Pounds	Pounds	Pounds
Fugitive or Nonpoint Air Emissions	31,896,963	556,138	1,443,842	75,638,113
Stack or Point Air Emissions	48,227,792	1,309,076	20,281,499	130,598,817
Surface Water Discharges	98,924	139,781	37,001,838	105,120
Underground Injection	1,317,706	928	94,720,218	1,373,957
Releases to Land	118,560	17,025,678	7,679,146	179,941
Total Releases	81,659,945	19,031,601	161,126,543	207,895,948
Off-site Transfers	Pounds	Pounds	Pounds	Pounds
Transfers to Recycling	28,453,488	220,243,568	718,934,821	26,155,482
Transfers to Energy Recovery	3,728,253	69,357	94,156	80,504,551
Transfers to Treatment	11,988,448	4,444,637	43,570,440	20,383,839
Transfers to POTWs**	1,302,759	335,240	33,289,571	1,294,467
Transfers to Disposal	495,784	17,211,252	31,389,905	1,693,546
Other Off-site Transfers	164,918	103,218	128,357	174,107
Total Off-site Transfers	46,133,650	242,407,272	827,407,250	130,205,992
Production-related Waste	Pounds	Pounds	Pounds	Pounds
Recycled On Site	159,314,271	753,521,856	5,754,741,182	634,334,232
Recycled Off Site	26,592,944	282,539,196	1,151,390,500	25,108,400
Energy Recovery On Site	14,270,049	116,475	63,405	255,099,437
Energy Recovery Off Site	6,115,207	62,899	27,466	87,368,972
Treated On Site	33,986,328	42,357,633	2,950,965,541	127,941,491
Treated Off Site	10,741,232	5,607,300	78,524,834	15,487,586
Quantity Released	81,070,815	36,775,939	185,170,184	202,322,584
Total Production-related Waste	332,090,846	1,120,981,298	10,120,883,112	1,347,662,702

* Amounts of lead and lead compounds are reported separately to TRI, but are combined in this table.
** Publicly owned treatment works.

Table 5-29. Comparison of Quantities of Four Chemicals in Waste Reported to BRS and TRI, 1991

	Dichloro-methane Pounds	**Lead and Lead Compounds** Pounds	**Sulfuric Acid** Pounds	**Toluene** Pounds
1991 BRS Data				
Waste Generation for Single-Chemical Waste Code Waste Streams	1,561,140	11,282,113,460	0	15,626,980
Waste Generation for Multiple-Chemical Waste Code Waste Streams	930,450,680	10,514,000	57,440,625,620	323,763,060
Waste Generation for Multiple Waste Code Waste Streams	197,802,478,520	60,776,714,540	180,537,057,140	133,749,284,540
Total Waste Generation for All Waste Streams	198,734,490,340	72,069,342,000	237,977,682,760	134,088,674,580
1991 TRI Data				
Production-related Waste	332,090,846	1,120,981,298	10,120,883,112	1,347,662,702
Total Air Emissions (Fugitive air emissions plus point source air emissions)	80,124,755	1,865,214	21,725,341	206,236,930
Adjusted Production-related Waste (Production-related waste minus air emissions)	251,966,091	1,119,116,084	10,099,157,771	1,141,425,772

Chapter 6

Toxics in Waste by Industry

Introduction

While the chemical and physical properties of toxic chemicals and government policies toward those chemicals significantly influence toxic waste generation and environmental release and disposal, ultimately it is the facilities, parent companies, and industries that create and use toxic chemicals that are accountable for them. A number of highly publicized company and industry initiatives have declared this accountability by creating programs to limit waste generation as well as to reduce environmental release and disposal going well beyond compliance with environmental regulations. For example:

- In 1986 the Dow Chemical Company announced its Waste Reduction Always Pays (WRAP) Program, committing to multimedia waste reduction through source reduction and recycling.[1]
- After assembling its company-wide 1987 TRI data, Monsanto announced a goal of reducing toxic air emissions worldwide 90 percent by the end of 1992, with an ultimate goal of zero air emissions.[2]
- DuPont has established pollution prevention goals aimed at reducing toxic air emissions 60 percent by 1993 and carcinogenic air emissions 90 percent by 2000 from 1987 levels. In addition, the company has pledged to reduce total hazardous waste 35 percent by 2000 and eliminate toxic releases to land by that same year, through elimination of discharges and other waste management activities.[3]
- In 1988 the Chemical Manufacturers Association (CMA) began its Responsible Care program, which requires member companies to establish and maintain priorities, goals, and plans for waste and release reduction. Responsible Care also requires that preference be given first to source reduction, second to recycling and reuse, and third to treatment as means of accomplishing these reductions.[4]

Such initiatives, if successful, should over time have an important impact in reducing toxics in waste. In addition to company and industry publications reporting on their programs (see Box 6-A), the data reported to EPA's two major toxic waste reporting systems, the Toxics Release Inventory (TRI) and

Box 6-A. Corporate Environmental Reporting: Supplementing State and National Inventory Data

In the 1990s, corporate environmental reports have emerged as a source of data on pollution prevention activities at companies. The reports allow corporations to present and discuss their environmental data in a form that integrates data with their corporate environmental policy.

Corporate environmental reports are not mandatory, nor are companies required to include all of the data that they submit to states or the federal government. In the United States, two organizations have developed guidelines for companies seeking to produce corporate environmental reports. The Public Environmental Reporting Initiative, or PERI, is an organization of environmental executives of U.S. corporations designed to provide companies with a framework for developing reports and guidelines for the types of data that should be included. CERES (Coalition for Environmentally Responsible Economies) is a Boston-based public interest organization which seeks to gain explicit agreements from companies on social and environmental issues. CERES asks companies to report in a different format: CERES reports are answers to specific qualitative and quantitative environmental questions. Neither PERI nor CERES guidelines asks for the full range of data that U.S. companies provide to TRI, although companies can go beyond the guidelines and provide additional data.

For companies located in European Union countries, the European chemical industrial trade organization, CEFIC, has also developed a set of guidelines for corporate environmental reporting. These guidelines ask for reporting on very few specific chemicals, mostly chemical groups such as volatile organic chemicals (VOCs), sulfur oxides, and nitrous oxides because of their role in ground-level ozone production, as well as discharges of some metals to surface water.

How useful are these corporate environmental reports for providing data on pollution prevention and product stewardship? Hampshire Research Institute (HRI) and World Wildlife Fund (WWF) have studied over 85 corporate environmental reports containing quantitative environmental data to determine the range of data provided and the possible analyses that can be performed using the reports.[1] (See Appendix F for a table from the report that compares reporting

the Biennial Reporting System (BRS) can often provide the means of measuring progress toward these goals and, in some cases, determining whether reductions in releases and disposal have been accompanied by actual reductions in the generation of waste. (See Chapter 4.)

Amounts and types of waste generation and environmental management options differ for different industries, in large part, based on the characteristics of the industries. One national approach that explicitly recognizes these differences is that of the Netherlands, where source reduction commitments are being negotiated industry by industry. (See Box 6-B.)

Companies that manufacture chemicals as products have different waste profiles and ways of addressing their waste problems than companies that use chemicals in the manufacture of other materials. This chapter provides an overview of the status of industrial waste generation and environmental management as of 1991 and 1992 and projected changes in generation and management from 1992 to 1994.

systems and corporate reports to a reporting benchmark based on a range of environmental questions encountered by WWF in its pollution prevention work.)

No corporate environmental report provides as much data as can be acquired from the various national reporting inventories such as TRI, although the study concludes that as companies evolve in the process of creating these reports, they are starting to include more of this type of data. Facility-level presentation of data is rare. In particular, U.S. companies that have facilities in other countries are beginning to assemble TRI-like data for those facilities and present these data in their reports. No U.S. reports provide data on amounts of specific chemicals going into products, and while most provide qualitative descriptions of source reduction progress, even the qualitative source reduction data reported to TRI for each chemical is not included in the reports.

Many countries have developed or are in the process of developing mandatory or voluntary national Pollutant Release and Transfer Registers (PRTRs), although companies located in those countries do not include the full range of their country's PRTR data in their corporate reports. Many of the reports from companies in European Union countries include the data from the CEFIC guidelines, and some are beginning to include limited amounts of data on chemicals in products.

Often companies writing environmental reports do not consider them to be independent sources of data, but rather as supplements to data from reporting systems such as TRI, compiled on a company-wide basis and presented in an appealing and understandable format. At their best, corporate environmental reports provide such compilations plus descriptions of source reduction achievements to supplement quantitative environmental data. The reports can also provide information on conservation activities that can be of local interest. For companies located in countries without publicly available PRTR data, however, the reports can serve as an important source of data not easily available by other means.

[1] Frances H. Irwin, *et al.*, *A Proposed Benchmark for Industrial Pollutant Release and Transfer Reporting*, World Wildlife Fund, January 1995.

Summary of Findings

According to the most recently available reports by industrial facilities to TRI and (under the Resource Conservation and Recovery Act) to BRS, relatively few industries and facilities dominate toxic waste generation. Some facilities, companies, and smaller industries are achieving significant reductions, but their reductions between 1991 and 1992 are more than offset by the lack of accomplishments of the others. The bottom line: in the aggregate no net reduction occurred in waste generation of TRI chemicals from 1991 to 1992, nor is any projected in the next two years. The 1992 TRI data and the 1991 BRS data reveal the following on an industry-by-industry[a] basis:

- The Chemical industry's toxic waste volumes are so large compared to the other manufacturing industries reporting to TRI, that this industry dominates nearly all TRI statistics on the generation of production-related

[a] Industry groups, as defined by their Standard Industrial Classification (SIC) codes, are listed with the full names of the industries in Appendix L.

Box 6-B. Government and Chemical Industry Sign Far-reaching Pollution Reduction Agreement in the Netherlands

The second National Environmental Policy Plan (NEPP) of the Netherlands, which is a comprehensive plan to strengthen the implementation of environmental policy, calls for the country to achieve sustainable development[1] by the year 2010. One objective of the NEPP is to reduce pollution at the source, rather than at the end of pipe.

The Government of the Netherlands believes that polluters, in collaboration with the government, should have a greater opportunity to formulate and implement their environmental policy. In cooperation with industry, agriculture, energy, construction, and consumers, the government has signed several "covenants" or voluntary agreements, which are binding under civil law. In establishing a covenant, the government is not required to write legislation, which can sometimes be difficult to draft and costly to enforce, but can still monitor the industrial sectors' environmental practices. Covenants are used in collaboration with legislation that already exists and do not replace existing law.

The industrial sector is heavily regulated, but the regulations do not always specify how the goals will be achieved. The covenants, on the other hand, specify how different industries will meet the targets for emission reduction set by the National Environmental Policy Plan. The following industrial sectors, which include 12,000 companies that produce 90 percent of the industrial pollution, have signed covenants or will have done so by 1995: printing and packaging printers, base metals, chemicals, dairy, metal products and electronics, textiles, abattoirs/meat industry, paper and paper products, leather, rubber and plastic products, brick and roofing tiles, concrete and cement products, and other mineral products.

The environmental targets for the covenants are addressed in a formal document for each industrial sector called the "Declaration of Intent." This document specifies the required percentage reduction for emissions of a given chemical to land, air, and water by the years 1995, 2000, and 2010, using 1985 as a base year. For example, the chemical industry's goals call for aggregate emissions to land, air, and water to be reduced by about 90 percent by the year 2010, varying somewhat among particular chemicals. The Declaration of Intent also addresses climate

waste.[b] The Chemical industry generated 53 percent (19.9 billion pounds) of TRI waste in 1992 — over half of the 37.3-billion-pound total. It also generated 69 percent of all carcinogens in TRI waste. Its recycling alone accounts for almost a third of all TRI production-related waste. Two chemical plants reported a third of the industry's and 18 percent of the nation's total production-related toxic waste. The Primary Metals industry reported the second largest amount of production-related waste to TRI (4.0 billion pounds).

- In the 1991 BRS, the Chemical industry also reported more RCRA toxic waste[c] generation (388.6 billion pounds) than any

[b] "Production-related" waste excludes waste associated with one-time events, such as accidents or spills, or waste from clean-up activities, or other waste not related to ongoing production at the reporting facility. This chapter is concerned exclusively with production-related waste. (See Chapter 4.)

[c] In this report, RCRA toxic waste is any waste that exhibits the characteristic of toxicity designated by the July 1,1993, Federal Code of Regulations (40 CFR Parts 261.24 through 261.33), or that contains TRI constituents. This excludes RCRA hazardous waste that is corrosive, ignitable, or reactive unless the waste contained toxic constituents as defined above. (See Appendix E.)

change, acidification, diffusion, eutrophication, waste disposal, noise, odor, safety, storage, cleanup, and management systems.

The goals of a specific industry for the years 1995, 2000, and 2010 are termed the sector's Integrated Environmental Target Plan (IETP). Individual companies that sign an agreement to conform with the Declaration of Intent are required to formulate their own specific environmental compliance plans that will collectively achieve the industry's goals. The company environmental plan, which is the equivalent to a company's permit, is prepared in collaboration with the central, provincial, and municipal governments, which are the licensing authorities. Company environmental policy plans must extend over a period of four years, and they must also provide a four-year projection plan.

Best available technology will be used to achieve company goals. As technology changes and improves, the goals of individual companies will be renegotiated, while still achieving the overall goals of the Declaration of Intent. Companies must also monitor their progress to determine if they are meeting their planned goals and report their findings to the licensing/regulatory authorities. These reports are aggregated for a particular industrial sector, and the aggregate is compared to the target environmental levels for each chemical covered in the IETP. The reporting system allows the government to track compliance, figure out where problems occur, and study the long-term effects and changes to a particular industry. The annual reports and environmental plans are publicly available, except for confidential business information.

One of the indirect outcomes of the Dutch covenants is that some industries that are not regulated at present have been encouraged to explore and implement environmental policies that may affect them in the future. For example, the 1991 covenant on packaging waste helped influence the imminent European Union Directive on Packaging Waste.

[1] Sustainable development, as defined in the Netherlands' National Environmental Policy Plan, is that which satisfies the needs of the present generation without compromising the ability of future generations to meet their own needs.

other industry. The Petroleum industry reported the second largest amount (270.9 billion pounds) to BRS.

- Although 23,630 facilities reported on production-related waste to TRI in 1992, waste generation is concentrated within relatively few facilities for most industries. The five facilities with the largest amount of production-related waste within each industry group together contribute 36 percent of the total production-related waste for all industries. A single R. J. Reynolds facility in Winston-Salem, North Carolina, reported 92 percent of the entire Tobacco industry's production-related waste to TRI in 1992.
- The waste generation reported to BRS was even more concentrated in a few facilities than the production-related waste reported to TRI. In 1991 just 17 out of 22,344 facilities reported more than 50 percent of all the RCRA toxic waste generated.
- Half of the RCRA toxic waste reported to BRS is managed in units exempt from RCRA regulation (e.g., water treatment plants covered by the Clean Water Act), and eight industries manage over 99 percent of their toxic waste in

such units. EPA's required biennial report to Congress on hazardous waste accounts only for waste managed in RCRA-regulated units and not for RCRA hazardous wastes that were managed in exempt units, even though facilities must report exempt wastes if they report to BRS.

- According to TRI, which provides the most recent and reliable measure of year-to-year toxic waste generation, only 5 of the 22 industry groups[d] showed net decreases in production-related waste from 1991 to 1992. These were the "Multiple Codes in 20-39 range" (118.4-million-pound reduction), Stone/Clay/Glass (64.4-million-pound reduction), Electrical (30.9-million-pound reduction), Lumber (4.7-million-pound reduction) and Machinery (4.3-million-pound reduction) industries. The industries with the largest amounts of waste reported to TRI showed net increases from 1991 to 1992: the Chemical industry increased 1 percent (224.9 million pounds), the Primary Metals industry increased 11 percent (389.1 million pounds), the Petroleum industry increased 15 percent (382.5 million pounds), and the Paper industry increased 2 percent (46.1 million pounds).
- TRI facilities in most industries project progress in reducing toxic waste generation between 1992 and 1994, but not enough to offset increases in a few of the larger industries. Out of the 22 industry groups, 16 project decreases, but increases in the Primary Metals, Stone/Clay/Glass, and Chemicals industries more than offset these decreases resulting in a net projected increase of 0.3 percent.
- Source reduction activity was not widely reported to TRI. In 1992, 72 percent of TRI production-related waste was reported on forms showing no source reduction activity at the facility for the chemical reported. This was true for most industry groups. Only four industries (Tobacco, Printing, Machinery, and Measuring/Photographic) reported more than half of their production-related waste on forms showing source reduction activity.
- The BRS data show that industry reduced its toxic waste generation by less than 1 percent through source reduction activities from 1991 to 1992. The Textiles and Tobacco industries reported the greatest percent reductions due to source reduction: 26 percent and 23 percent, respectively.
- There is some evidence of movement away from the least environmentally desirable waste management methods to more desirable options. TRI projections by facilities for 1992-1994 show a projected 20 percent decrease in releases and disposal of TRI chemicals, which is the least desirable option. This projected decrease is broadly based across industries, except for the Primary Metals industry, which projects an increase in releases and disposal of just over 1 percent.

[d] The 20 industry groups represented by SIC codes 20 through 39, plus all facilities that report more than one SIC code ("Multiple Codes") and those that report none ("No Codes"). (See Box 6-C.)

Figure 6-1.

Top Five Industries for Total Production-related Waste Reported to TRI, 1992

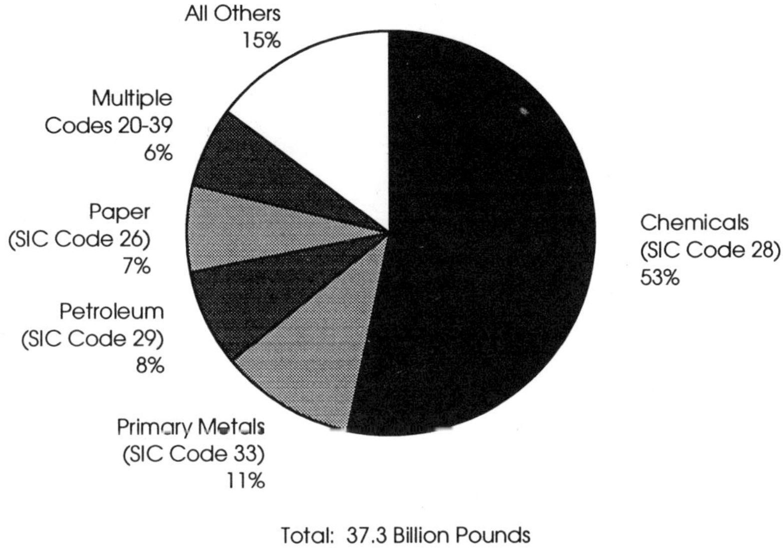

Overall Industry Toxic Waste Generation

The Chemical industry, as producer and user of toxic chemicals for production of other chemicals and chemical products, dominates both reporting systems, TRI and BRS, that collect data on toxic waste generation from industrial facilities. Both reporting systems cover manufacturing industries, but they collect data on fundamentally different types of toxic wastes, so the distribution among the manufacturing industries is different in the two databases. While BRS collects information on the total material in waste streams, TRI more directly measures the amount of toxic chemicals in waste. (See Appendices A and D.)

TRI Distribution of Total Production-related Waste by Industry, 1992

Of the 22 industry groups reporting to TRI, 5 account for 85 percent of all TRI production-related waste. By far the largest waste generator is the Chemical industry, which generated 19.9 billion pounds of production-related waste in 1992, more than half (53 percent) of the 37.3 billion pounds of such waste reported to TRI. This is almost five times more waste than the 4.0 billion pounds generated by the next largest generator of TRI waste, the Primary Metals industry, almost seven times more than the 2.9 billion pounds generated by the Petroleum industry, and almost eight times more than the 2.5 billion pounds generated by the Paper industry. (See Figure 6-1 and Table 6-1.)

Table 6-1. TRI Production-related Waste by Industry, 1992

SIC Code	Industry	Total Production-related Waste: Pounds	Percent	Rank
20	Food	389,637,145	1.04	11
21	Tobacco	60,185,440	0.16	19
22	Textiles	100,223,930	0.27	16
23	Apparel	3,146,914	0.01	22
24	Lumber	63,091,614	0.17	18
25	Furniture	66,227,908	0.18	17
26	Paper	2,537,521,812	6.80	4
27	Printing	274,812,686	0.74	12
28	Chemicals	19,897,327,333	53.30	1
29	Petroleum	2,945,379,328	7.89	3
30	Plastics	567,294,382	1.52	9
31	Leather	52,480,219	0.14	21
32	Stone/Clay	935,576,617	2.51	8
33	Primary Metals	4,044,002,976	10.83	2
34	Fabr. Metals	962,656,507	2.58	7
35	Machinery	207,000,051	0.55	13
36	Electrical	963,576,363	2.58	6
37	Transportation	471,959,721	1.26	10
38	Measure./Photo.	125,739,677	0.34	15
39	Miscellaneous	55,014,507	0.15	20
	Multiple codes 20-39	2,412,177,342	6.46	5
	No codes 20-39	198,743,152	0.53	14
	Total	37,333,775,624	100.00	

The next largest generator of TRI waste is the category of facilities reporting multiple SIC codes, which accounts for 6 percent of production-related waste. Much of the toxic waste reported by facilities with multiple SIC codes is associated with the four industries generating the most TRI production-related waste. More than 40 percent of the multiple-codes waste is accounted for by combined SIC codes 28 and 29, the Chemical and Petroleum industries. The Chemical industry is combined with other industries for roughly two-thirds of the production-related waste reported as Multiple Codes 20-39. (See Figure 6-2 and Box 6-C.)

Waste Management Components of TRI Production-related Waste

Industries manage their waste in widely varying ways. After source reduction, the most environmentally desirable of the four waste management components of production-related waste is recycling (reported in Section 8 of TRI Form R), fol-

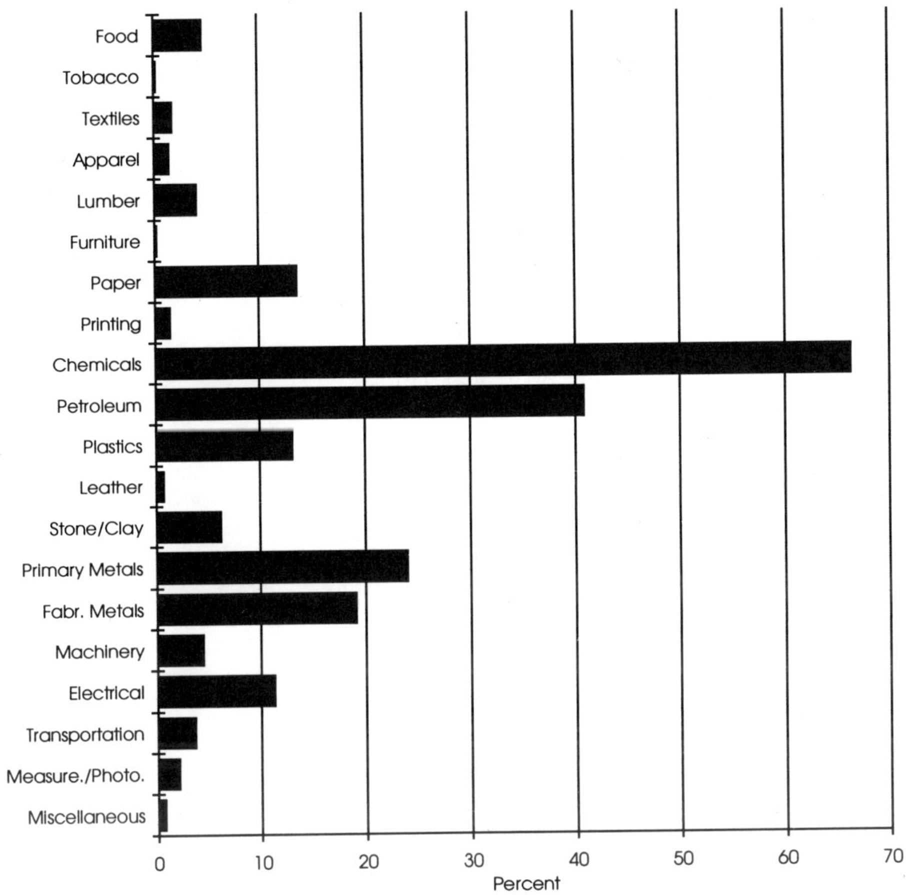

Figure 6-2.

Percent of Production-related Waste Reported with Multiple Codes (SIC Codes 20-39) for Which Industry is Among Those Reported, 1992

Percentages add to more than 100 percent because pounds for facilities with multiple industries have been assigned to all applicable industries.

lowed by energy recovery, treatment, and finally the least desirable waste management option, releases and disposal.

Industry as a whole recycled 52 percent of its production-related waste in 1992, but several industries recycled a considerably larger share. The Tobacco industry recycled 92 percent of its waste. The Printing, Machinery, Electrical, and Primary Metals industries recycled about two-thirds of their waste. With the exception of the Primary Metals industry, these are mostly smaller industries whose recycled amounts are dwarfed by recycling in the Chemical industry. (See Table 6-2.)

Although the Chemical industry ranks sixth in the percentage of its waste that is recycled, its 11.8 billion pounds of TRI chemicals recycled accounted for 61 percent of all recycling and 32 percent of all production-related waste for industries reported in 1992. Primary Metals facilities reported the next highest absolute amount of recycling, 2.7 billion pounds, which is less than a fourth of the Chemical industry's total. (See Appendix N, Table N-2.)

Box 6-C. SIC Code Reporting

The Office of Management and Budget publishes the Standard Industrial Classification (SIC) Manual which by its own description is "the statistical classification standard underlying all establishment-based Federal economic statistics classified by industry." Both the TRI and BRS forms collect SIC code data on toxic waste generators and management facilities for use in industry-specific analyses.

TRI SIC Code Reporting

The SIC designation is especially important to TRI because it defines who must report their toxic waste information. Only a facility that otherwise meets reporting requirements and whose total value of products falling within SIC Ccodes 20-39 (the manufacturing sector of the economy) is greater than 50 percent of the entire value of products at the facility is required to file TRI reports. The first two digits of a facility's SIC code determine whether it falls in the range. Facilities outside of this SIC range are not required to file these reports, but sometimes they "volunteer" reports. (See Appendix L for a listing of SIC codes covered by TRI.)

TRI collects SIC information on the facility for as many manufacturing SIC codes as apply to the operations at the facility, in Section 4.5 of Form R. (See Appendix A for a copy of Form R.) The "No codes 20-39" category in this report includes forms that reported only SIC codes outside the 20-39 range or reported no SIC code information. These forms account for only 0.5 percent of the TRI production-related waste in 1992.

There is no provision on the Form R for a facility with multiple SIC codes to relate the amount of TRI chemicals generated as waste, or any other chemical-specific information, to each individual SIC code within the facility. A breakdown of the quantities of production-related waste for each combination of 2-digit SIC codes reported reveals, however, that a few combinations of large industry codes account for most of this waste:

SIC Codes	Pounds	Percent
28 / 29	973,939,642	40
33 / 34	183,865,867	8
26 / 28	157,414,694	7
30 / 33 / 34 / 36	127,434,250	5
28 / 30	100,345,145	4
28 / 33	90,183,813	4
20 / 28	85,163,249	4
All other combinations	1,718,346,660	28
Total	2,412,177,342	100

Energy recovery, the next most environmentally desirable management method, accounted for 10 percent of all TRI production-related waste in 1992. The Stone/Clay/Glass industry, where blending waste as fuel for cement kilns is a common practice, reported that 65 percent of its production-related waste (608.3 million pounds) went to energy recovery. Even greater volumes of production-related waste were managed through energy recovery in the Chemical industry (1.5 billion pounds) and the Petroleum industry (832.8 million pounds). Both of these industries have large amounts of production-related waste made up of hydrocarbons and other chemicals with high fuel value. Energy recovery accounts for a larger share of the Petroleum industry's production-related waste (28 percent) than the Chemical industry's production-related waste (7 percent) because many petroleum-related waste products are not

BRS SIC Code Reporting

The BRS obtains reports of up to four 4-digit SIC codes from each facility. (See Appendix D for BRS Form IC.) Reporting to BRS is not limited to the manufacturing sectors. Instead, BRS requires each facility meeting the criteria to report unless all the wastes it generates are exempt from reporting. (See Chapter 4.) Like TRI, where 7 percent of all facilities report multiple SIC codes in the 20-39 range, 10 percent of all facilities reporting toxic waste to BRS give multiple SIC codes (of any 2-digit SIC codes). The primary SIC code cannot be determined from the BRS Form IC for facilities reporting more than one SIC code.

SIC codes are also reported on BRS Form GM. Each Form GM has only one SIC code, and that SIC code applies to the product or service whose waste stream is reported on the Form GM. While Form IC gives all SIC codes applicable to operations at the facility, each Form GM has only the one SIC code applicable to the specific operation which has generated the waste stream. Thus, the amounts of waste generation are tied to single SIC codes under the BRS.

This is in contrast to TRI, where the set of SIC codes applicable to the facility operations as a whole is reported on each chemical form. Amounts of production-related waste for individual chemicals are generally not separated by the different SIC code operations at facilities falling under multiple SIC code classifications, as they are under BRS for separate waste streams.

easily recycled. The Petroleum and Stone/Clay/Glass industries manage about three-quarters of their production-related waste by either recycling or energy recovery. (See Table 6-2 and Appendix N, Table N-2.)

Treatment (11.0 billion pounds) and releases and disposal (3.4 billion pounds), the least desirable management option, accounted for 29 percent and 9 percent of production-related waste, respectively. Industries that largely invested in these methods include the Food and Paper industries, which each treated over 70 percent of its total production-related wastes. Three other industries, Furniture, Lumber, and Apparel, had relatively small amounts of total waste, but reported over half of their production-related waste as releases and disposal. Indeed, the Furniture industry reported 76 percent of its total production-related waste returned

Table 6-2. Waste Management Components as Percent of TRI Production-related Waste by Industry, 1992

SIC Code	Industry	1992 Total Production-related Waste Pounds	Waste Management Component of Total: Recycled Percent	Energy Recovery Percent	Treated Percent	Releases and Off-site Disposal Percent	Total Production-related Waste Percent
20	Food	389,637,145	8.48	0.07	80.08	11.37	100.00
21	Tobacco	60,185,440	91.91	0.01	2.10	5.97	100.00
22	Textiles	100,223,930	12.49	6.07	56.82	24.63	100.00
23	Apparel	3,146,914	15.33	12.87	18.63	53.17	100.00
24	Lumber	63,091,614	31.12	7.03	8.56	53.29	100.00
25	Furniture	66,227,908	8.15	10.78	4.82	76.25	100.00
26	Paper	2,537,521,812	6.81	10.18	73.66	9.35	100.00
27	Printing	274,812,686	70.80	1.99	14.23	12.98	100.00
28	Chemicals	19,897,327,333	59.29	7.31	25.48	7.92	100.00
29	Petroleum	2,945,379,328	44.23	28.27	25.07	2.42	100.00
30	Plastics	567,294,382	56.30	4.70	12.80	26.20	100.00
31	Leather	52,480,219	5.66	1.84	57.63	34.86	100.00
32	Stone/Clay	935,576,617	10.64	65.02	21.54	2.79	100.00
33	Primary Metals	4,044,002,976	65.95	1.66	21.20	11.19	100.00
34	Fabr. Metals	962,656,507	52.87	10.00	24.77	12.36	100.00
35	Machinery	207,000,051	68.88	1.79	11.72	17.62	100.00
36	Electrical	963,576,363	66.60	1.87	24.30	7.23	100.00
37	Transportation	471,959,721	48.32	5.25	15.99	30.44	100.00
38	Measure./Photo.	125,739,677	21.19	4.76	45.81	28.24	100.00
39	Miscellaneous	55,014,507	43.42	4.87	15.75	35.96	100.00
	Multiple codes 20-39	2,412,177,342	45.22	6.00	38.90	9.88	100.00
	No codes 20-39	198,743,152	6.13	0.69	85.38	7.79	100.00
	Total	37,333,775,624	51.85	9.56	29.48	9.11	100.00

to the environment as releases and disposal. (See Table 6-2 and Appendix N, Table N-2.)

In terms of quantities of production-related waste treated, the Chemical industry treated the most (5.1 billion pounds), followed by the Paper industry (1.9 billion pounds). The Chemical industry also had the greatest quantity released/disposed of (1.6 billion pounds), nearly three and a half times more than the second-ranked Primary Metals industry (452.6 million pounds). (See Appendix N, Table N-2.)

Impact of Major Facilities on TRI Industry Data

Just as two industries, Chemicals and Primary Metals, dominate the national data for TRI production-related waste, so do a handful of facilities sometimes overwhelm the statistics for a particular industry or even for national production-related waste profiles. In fact, the top five generators of production-related waste in each industry group

Table 6-3. Top Five Facilities as a Percentage of Facilities and TRI Production-related Waste within Each Industry, 1992

SIC Code	Industry	Facilities Number	1992 Total TRI Production-related Waste Pounds	1992 Total TRI Production-related Waste Percent	Top Five Facilities: 1992 Total TRI Production-related Waste Pounds	Top Five Facilities: Percent of All Facilities in SIC Percent	Top Five Facilities: Percent of Total Quantity in SIC Percent
20	Food	2,036	389,637,145	1.04	162,180,906	0.25	41.62
21	Tobacco	21	60,185,440	0.16	58,670,289	23.81	97.48
22	Textiles	471	100,223,930	0.27	35,671,904	1.06	35.59
23	Apparel	48	3,146,914	0.01	1,980,982	10.42	62.95
24	Lumber	722	63,091,614	0.17	14,757,234	0.69	23.39
25	Furniture	547	66,227,908	0.18	8,710,829	0.91	13.15
26	Paper	583	2,537,521,812	6.80	287,418,220	0.86	11.33
27	Printing	374	274,812,686	0.74	115,910,183	1.34	42.18
28	Chemicals	4,193	19,897,327,333	53.30	7,622,185,386	0.12	38.31
29	Petroleum	425	2,945,379,328	7.89	1,378,577,357	1.18	46.80
30	Plastics	1,868	567,294,382	1.52	297,821,762	0.27	52.50
31	Leather	155	52,480,219	0.14	28,439,343	3.23	54.19
32	Stone/Clay	634	935,576,617	2.51	365,837,262	0.79	39.10
33	Primary Metals	1,886	4,044,002,976	10.83	959,573,050	0.27	23.73
34	Fabr. Metals	3,141	962,656,507	2.58	283,326,172	0.16	29.43
35	Machinery	1,094	207,000,051	0.55	75,587,733	0.46	36.52
36	Electrical	1,554	963,576,363	2.58	195,630,961	0.32	20.30
37	Transportation	1,251	471,959,721	1.26	82,013,479	0.40	17.38
38	Measure./Photo.	414	125,739,677	0.34	75,796,995	1.21	60.28
39	Miscellaneous	376	55,014,507	0.15	16,073,967	1.33	29.22
	Multiple codes 20-39	1,630	2,412,177,342	6.46	1,105,518,832	0.31	45.83
	No codes 20-39	207	198,743,152	0.53	174,210,662	2.42	87.66
	Total	23,630	37,333,775,624	100.00	13,345,893,508	0.02	35.75

together account for 36 percent of the national TRI total for such waste. In the case of the Tobacco, Apparel, Plastics, Leather, and Measuring/Photographic industries, the five facilities in each industry with the largest amount of production-related waste in 1992 account for over half the total for their industry. (See Table 6-3.) The aggregated data for these highly concentrated industries are heavily influenced by the waste management practices and reporting calculations of their largest facilities.

Two Chemical facilities (First Chemical Corporation in Pascagoula, Mississippi, and Goodyear Tire and Rubber Company in Beaumont, Texas) together accounted for a third of the Chemical industry's production-related waste in 1992. The waste generated by just these two facilities is 18 percent of the nation's total. Chapter 4 explains that these facilities report large amounts of recycled waste, and the ways they calculate the amounts make them the largest reporters of production-related waste.

The Tobacco industry exhibits a dramatic concentration of production-related waste. The R. J. Reynolds Tobacco Company facility in Winston-Salem, North Carolina, 1 of only 21 TRI facilities in this relatively small industry, reported 92 percent of that industry's production-related waste.[e] Other dominating facilities within their industries include Eastman Kodak Company in Rochester, New York, which accounts for 41 percent of the production-related waste of the Measuring/Photographic industry; Gates Rubber Company in Iola, Kansas (39 percent of the Plastics industry); and Forbo Industries Inc. in Hazelton, Pennsylvania (25 percent of the Apparel industry). (See Appendix M.)

Distribution of BRS Toxic Waste Generation by Industry, 1991

The Chemical industry strongly dominates toxic waste generation as reported to the BRS under RCRA. The 388.6 billion pounds of toxic waste generated by the Chemical industry accounts for 41 percent of the 948.2 billion pounds of total toxic waste generation reported under RCRA in 1991. The Petroleum industry is the second largest generator of RCRA toxic waste, with a share of 29 percent (270.9 billion pounds). This yields a significantly different BRS distribution of waste generation among industries than indicated by TRI, in which the Primary Metals facilities report the second largest amount.

The two top BRS industries, Chemicals and Petroleum, account for over two-thirds of all toxic waste reported to BRS. The Primary Metals industry, the second largest TRI generator, was only the seventh largest RCRA toxic waste generator, accounting for 3 percent of all such BRS waste. (See Figures 6-1 and 6-3 and Tables 6-1 and 6-4.)

Exempt Toxic Waste Management by Industry, 1991 BRS

To keep the focus on the *generation* of toxic waste, whose reduction is the objective of pollution prevention programs, this *Toxics Watch* report includes all reported waste that contains toxic constituents. This includes toxic waste managed in units exempt from RCRA regulation (e.g., toxic waste that is put into a sewer and sent to a water treatment plant covered by the Clean Water Act) that are not included in EPA's reports to Congress summarizing BRS data. Facilities reporting to BRS must report these exempt wastes, and they account for half of the generated waste containing toxic constituents reported to BRS. (See Appendix E.)

Exempt units include enclosed wastewater treatment tanks, which typically discharge their treated wastes to surface waters or POTWs, and closed-loop recycling units. According to the 1991 BRS report, industry managed 481.5 billion pounds of waste containing toxic constituents in such units. This amount does not cover all toxic waste managed in exempt units, because facilities do not have to file

[e] According to Carl Martin of R. J. Reynolds, this facility, although reporting under SIC code 21 to TRI, also maintains other operations, including a packaging plant.

Figure 6-3.

Top Five Industries for Toxic Waste Reported to BRS, 1991

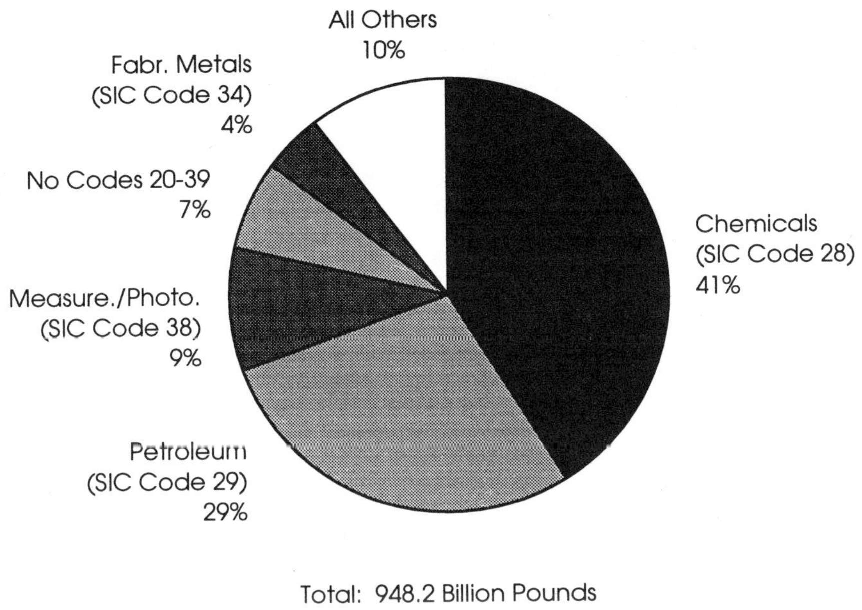

a BRS report unless they have RCRA-regulated generation or management units.[f] (See Table 6-5.)

The 1991 BRS data show an even split between RCRA-regulated and exempt toxic waste managed on site. Three industries, the Food, Tobacco, and Leather industries, reported managing all of their waste containing toxic constituents in the exempt category. Five other industries — Textiles, Furniture, Paper, Printing, and Measuring/ Photographic industries — manage virtually all (over 99 percent) in exempt units. The Apparel industry is alone at the other end of the range, managing only 4 percent of its toxic waste in exempt units. These industries significantly contrast with the two largest generating industries, the Chemical and Petroleum industries, which managed 32 and 38 percent, respectively, of their toxic waste in exempt units. (See Table 6-5.)

Impact of Major Facilities on BRS Industry Data

As in TRI, a few facilities account for a large percentage of the BRS-reported RCRA toxic waste generated in 1991. Only 17 facilities out of the 22,344 facilities reporting accounted for over 50 percent of all RCRA toxic waste generated, and all but 2 of the 17 are in the Chemical or Petroleum industries. These two are both Eastman Kodak facilities, one in New York and one in Texas. The Eastman Kodak

[f] The amount of RCRA toxic waste managed is, in some cases, larger than the amount reported as generated in Table 6-5 because the "managed" category includes wastes that may have been generated in a prior year but transferred off-site for treatment or disposal in the current year. The amount managed may be less if the waste is sent off-site for treatment or stored on-site.

Table 6-4. BRS Quantities of Toxic Waste Generated by Industry, 1991

SIC Code	Industry	1991 Total Quantity of Toxic Waste Generated	
		Pounds	Percent
20	Food	88,710,920	0.01
21	Tobacco	343,200	0.00
22	Textiles	1,079,880,480	0.11
23	Apparel	68,752,020	0.01
24	Lumber	335,354,620	0.04
25	Furniture	199,752,520	0.02
26	Paper	3,993,351,820	0.42
27	Printing	217,093,120	0.02
28	Chemicals	388,570,517,800	40.98
29	Petroleum	270,856,101,200	28.56
30	Plastics	376,091,940	0.04
31	Leather	203,725,540	0.02
32	Stone/Clay	362,430,800	0.04
33	Primary Metals	30,608,272,760	3.23
34	Fabr. Metals	40,687,820,920	4.29
35	Machinery	2,910,808,380	0.31
36	Electrical	33,679,602,720	3.55
37	Transportation	18,618,250,440	1.96
38	Measure./Photo.	85,061,296,940	8.97
39	Miscellaneous	6,002,867,540	0.63
	No Codes 20-39	64,322,724,440	6.78
	Total	948,243,750,120	100.00

facility in New York reported the largest amount of RCRA toxic waste of any BRS facility, 83.2 billion pounds, which is 9 percent of the total. This facility managed all but 33,000 tons of toxic waste in exempt management units. Dow Chemical in Midland, Michigan, reported the second largest amount, 60.2 billion pounds or 6 percent of the national total, all in non-exempt units. (See Table 6-6.)

Impact of Differences Between TRI and BRS on Industry Data

Only 3 of the 25 BRS facilities with the largest quantities of toxic waste generation in 1991 also rank among the top 25 TRI facilities for total production-related waste in 1992. (See Table 6-6.) This highlights the fact that the two reporting systems measure very different things, and their data are not easily reconcilable. BRS has different sets of criteria for reporting, covers different chemicals, and seeks data on the total waste stream, including water, soil, and other nontoxic constituents. TRI focuses on the specific toxic constituents in waste. The BRS system also contains about 7 percent of its waste from outside the manufacturing sector and does not track air emissions, but these data can be subtracted from BRS and TRI, respectively, to make them more comparable. The amount of nontoxic constituents included in the BRS data but not collected by TRI cannot be subtracted, however.

Table 6-5. Percent of BRS Toxic Waste Managed in Units Exempt from RCRA, 1991

SIC Code	Industry	1991 Quantity Managed Pounds	Quantity Managed in RCRA Units Pounds	Quantity Managed in Exempt Units Pounds	Quantity Managed in Storage Pounds	Quantity Managed in Exempt Units of Total Percent
20	Food	84,464,740	0	84,464,740	0	100.00
21	Tobacco	83,620	0	83,620	0	100.00
22	Textiles	1,005,915,220	1,745,260	1,004,169,960	0	99.83
23	Apparel	75,523,860	72,801,000	2,695,340	27,520	3.57
24	Lumber	790,909,060	51,985,440	738,921,280	2,340	93.43
25	Furniture	158,429,480	1,172,000	157,222,840	34,640	99.24
26	Paper	3,997,803,120	481,200	3,997,302,160	19,760	99.99
27	Printing	148,441,420	48,780	148,358,820	33,820	99.94
28	Chemicals	394,541,671,380	268,143,047,400	124,948,856,560	1,449,767,420	31.67
29	Petroleum	270,572,809,260	168,245,998,880	101,687,373,240	639,437,140	37.58
30	Plastics	287,544,520	20,650,440	266,852,300	41,780	92.80
31	Leather	107,292,040	0	107,292,040	0	100.00
32	Stone/Clay	530,886,640	274,910,880	255,930,760	45,000	48.21
33	Primary Metals	35,580,830,500	9,482,239,300	23,992,220,980	2,106,370,220	67.43
34	Fabr. Metals	43,218,253,160	5,208,907,320	38,008,697,500	648,340	87.95
35	Machinery	5,948,417,800	1,352,821,940	4,595,555,860	40,000	77.26
36	Electrical	33,687,080,540	5,580,123,240	28,102,515,360	4,441,940	83.42
37	Transportation	18,410,419,940	6,028,988,160	12,380,889,800	541,980	67.25
38	Measure./Photo.	84,840,104,060	74,366,400	84,765,671,740	65,920	99.91
39	Miscellaneous	5,969,123,300	5,329,741,500	639,375,400	6,400	10.71
	No Codes 20-39	63,961,562,620	8,240,717,420	55,633,913,860	86,931,340	86.98
	Total	963,917,566,280	478,110,746,560	481,518,364,160	4,288,455,560	49.95

Because BRS requires reporting every two years, and its most recent year is 1991, the two databases are more comparable using TRI data from 1991 and subtracting air emissions, which are not reported to BRS, from TRI. These modified TRI waste generation data are more similar to BRS data in coverage of on-site and off-site waste management options and releases to water and land after these adjustments. Because of the remaining differences mentioned above and in Chapter 4, however, especially that TRI data are chemical-specific and do not contain nontoxic components of the waste stream that BRS includes, the BRS figures are 28 times larger than the "adjusted" TRI data for the same set of manufacturing industries, although this factor varies widely by facility and industry. Examination of the top five manufacturing industries in each system points out the differences in the wastes reported to BRS and TRI. (See Table 6-7.)

The Chemical industry ranks highest in both reporting systems, although its percentage of total adjusted TRI waste is greater than for BRS wastes (60 percent and 44 percent, respectively). On the other hand, the Petroleum industry ranks second in BRS waste and fourth for adjusted TRI wastes and constitutes a much higher percentage of BRS wastes (31 percent for BRS and 8 percent for adjusted TRI). (See Table 6-7.)

Table 6-6. The 25 BRS Facilities with Largest Quantity of Toxic Waste Generated, 1991

1992 TRI Rank*	1991 BRS Rank	Facility	City
107	1	Kodak Park	Rochester
117	2	The Dow Chemical Company	Midland
240	3	Amoco Oil Company Refinery	Texas City
71	4	E.I. Dupont-Chambers Works	Deepwater
119	5	Shell Oil Company	Deer Park
13	6	Citgo Petroleum Corporation	Lake Charles
698	7	Chevron USA Products Company	Philadelphia
800	8	Shell Oil Co/Martinez Mfg Comp	Martinez
389	9	Shell Oil Co	Roxana
583	10	Amoco Chemical Company - Chocolate Bayou	Alvin
296	11	Phillips Petroleum Sweeny Complex	Old Ocean
505	12	Chevron	Pascagoula
215	13	Union Carbide Chemicals & Plastics Comp.	Taft
970	14	Sun Company, Inc. Marcus Hook Refinery	Marcus Hook
193	15	Texas Eastman Division, Eastman Chemical	Longview
135	16	Hercules,Incorporated	Radford
272	17	BP Oil Company - Alliance Refinery	Belle Chasse
48	18	ARCO Products Co	Ferndale
295	19	Sun Refining & Mktg. Co. - Tulsa Ref.	Tulsa
2209	20	Coastal Refining & Marketing, Inc.	Corpus Christi
97	21	Dupont De Nemours & Co.	Victoria
10	22	Dow Chemical U.S.A.	Freeport
**	23	Robins AFB	Warner Robins
189	24	Mobil Chemical Co O/A Plant	Beaumont
8	25	Kemira Inc	Savannah
		Subtotal	
		Total	

* TRI Rank is for total production-related waste, including any air emissions.
** The Robins Air Force Base, as a government facility, is not required to report to TRI.

County	State	1991 Quantity of Toxic Waste Generated Pounds	Percent of Total Percent	Cumulative Percent of Total Percent
Monroe	NY	83,225,844,980	8.78	8.78
Midland	MI	60,274,801,720	6.36	15.13
Galveston	TX	52,275,053,600	5.51	20.65
Salem	NJ	48,843,789,760	5.15	25.80
Harris	TX	38,738,555,340	4.09	29.88
Calcasieu	LA	27,121,056,040	2.86	32.74
Philadelphia	PA	24,434,042,460	2.58	35.32
Contra Costa	CA	21,547,852,000	2.27	37.59
Dixon	IL	18,882,321,460	1.99	39.58
Brazoria	TX	16,503,998,360	1.74	41.32
Brazoria	TX	15,005,072,500	1.58	42.91
Jackson	MS	13,528,679,760	1.43	44.33
St Charles	LA	13,021,427,200	1.37	45.71
Delaware	PA	12,000,230,120	1.27	46.97
Harrison	TX	11,348,671,660	1.20	48.17
Montgomery	VA	11,241,373,400	1.19	49.35
Plaquemines	LA	10,681,891,800	1.13	50.48
Whatcom	WA	10,220,819,820	1.08	51.56
Tulsa	OK	8,717,414,960	0.92	52.48
Nueces	TX	8,441,243,760	0.89	53.37
Victoria	TX	7,890,537,600	0.83	54.20
Brazoria	TX	7,486,554,200	0.79	54.99
Houston	GA	7,379,602,300	0.78	55.77
Jefferson	TX	6,846,048,420	0.72	56.49
Chatham	GA	6,716,824,000	0.71	57.20
		542,373,707,220	57.20	57.20
		948,243,750,120	100.00	100.00

Table 6-7. Comparison of TRI Production-related Waste and BRS Toxic Waste Generation, 1991

SIC Code	Industry	1991 BRS Toxic Waste Generation			1991 TRI Production-related Waste
		Pounds	**Percent**	**Rank**	
		Pounds	Percent		Pounds
20	Food	88,710,920	0.01	18	380,691,966
21	Tobacco	343,200	0.00	20	55,046,792
22	Textiles	1,079,880,480	0.12	11	98,220,702
23	Apparel	68,752,020	0.01	19	2,883,172
24	Lumber	335,354,620	0.04	14	67,834,787
25	Furniture	199,752,520	0.02	17	62,729,636
26	Paper	3,993,351,820	0.45	9	2,491,445,311
27	Printing	217,093,120	0.02	15	266,876,401
28	Chemicals	388,570,517,800	43.96	1	19,672,469,407
29	Petroleum	270,856,101,200	30.64	2	2,562,915,297
30	Plastics	376,091,940	0.04	12	508,051,776
31	Leather	203,725,540	0.02	16	44,987,787
32	Stone/Clay	362,430,800	0.04	13	999,977,077
33	Primary Metals	30,608,272,760	3.46	6	3,654,952,230
34	Fabr. Metals	40,687,820,920	4.60	4	919,137,839
35	Machinery	2,910,808,380	0.33	10	211,347,793
36	Electrical	33,679,602,720	3.81	5	994,456,225
37	Transportation	18,618,250,440	2.11	7	459,765,222
38	Measure./Photo.	85,061,296,940	9.62	3	122,969,517
39	Miscellaneous	6,002,867,540	0.68	10	51,696,646
	Subtotal	883,921,025,680	100.00		33,628,455,583
	Multiple Codes 20-39**	N/A			2,530,599,122
	No Codes 20-39	64,322,724,440			157,908,372
	Total	948,243,750,120			36,316,963,077

* Adjusted production-related waste is total production-related waste minus total air emissions.

** Each waste stream form from BRS has just one SIC code, so no multiple codes exist in BRS.

1991 TRI Total Air Emissions Pounds	**1991 Adjusted Production-related Waste*** Pounds	**BRS:TRI Ratio After Adjustment**	**1991 Adjusted TRI Production-related Waste** Percent	**Adjusted TRI Rank 1991**
27,901,738	352,790,228	0.25	1.11	8
2,274,774	52,772,018	0.01	0.17	18
24,663,645	73,557,057	14.68	0.23	13
1,372,527	1,510,645	45.51	0.00	19
32,387,483	35,447,304	9.46	0.11	17
55,593,104	7,136,532	27.99	0.02	20
211,325,277	2,280,120,034	1.75	7.17	3
47,024,834	219,851,567	0.99	0.69	11
607,402,595	19,065,066,812	20.38	59.97	1
59,589,969	2,503,325,328	108.20	7.87	4
148,866,049	359,185,727	1.05	1.13	9
9,653,883	35,333,904	5.77	0.11	14
19,496,128	980,480,949	0.37	3.08	5
154,019,367	3,500,932,863	8.74	11.01	2
109,173,160	809,964,679	50.23	2.55	7
38,422,011	172,925,782	16.83	0.54	12
84,223,249	910,232,976	37.00	2.86	6
147,461,683	312,303,539	59.62	0.98	10
38,843,384	84,126,133	1,011.12	0.26	16
20,242,784	31,453,862	190.85	0.10	15
1,839,937,644	31,788,517,939	27.81	100.00	
172,424,522	2,358,174,600			
13,043,420	144,864,952			
2,025,405,586	34,291,557,491			

These two industries point out some of the major differences in reporting to BRS and TRI. Chemical industry facilities, obviously, produce and use large amounts of chemicals. However, some of the individual waste streams at these facilities, although containing chemicals reportable under TRI and RCRA, do not meet RCRA criteria for toxicity levels and so are not subject to BRS reporting. Reporting to TRI, on the other hand, is based solely on production or use levels of a TRI chemical. If the threshold reporting amounts for production or use of a chemical are met, all amounts of the chemical in any kind of waste stream are reportable to TRI. Therefore, the percentage of total waste in the adjusted TRI figures for the Chemical industry is relatively high compared to the BRS waste for the same industry. A similar situation occurs in the Primary Metals industry, which also uses a large amount of TRI- and BRS-reportable chemicals, but whose waste streams do not all meet RCRA toxicity criteria. Thus, this industry shows a higher percentage of adjusted TRI waste (11 percent) compared to BRS waste (3 percent). (See Table 6-7.)

The reverse occurs in the Petroleum industry. That industry uses a relatively large amount of wastewater treatment, due to the volume of liquid waste it generates that contains chemicals that can be handled by industrial or municipal wastewater treatment facilities. Since the entire amount of the wastewater stream is reported under RCRA, while only the chemical constituent portions are reported to TRI, the Petroleum industry's percentage of BRS waste is higher than its share of adjusted TRI.

Other industry groups show even greater differences between their relative share of BRS waste versus TRI waste. The Measuring/Photographic industry ranks 3rd for BRS waste but 16th out of the 20 manufacturing industries for adjusted TRI waste. The high BRS ranking is due to the large amounts of wastewater generated by Eastman Kodak's Kodak Park facility in Rochester, New York. This facility reports large amounts of dilute wastewater streams to BRS and significant air emissions to TRI. When air emissions are removed from TRI data for comparison with BRS, the adjusted TRI figure for the Kodak facility diminishes considerably. The amount of discharges to water is considerably lower in the facility's TRI data, since the water volume and nontoxic constituents are not counted, than it is in the amounts reported to BRS.

Conversely, the Paper and Stone/Clay/Glass industries rank third and fifth, respectively, for adjusted TRI, and ninth and thirteenth for BRS wastes. In these industries, the actual amounts of TRI chemicals managed on and off site are high (and are reported to TRI), yet because of the varying toxicity of individual waste streams, portions of the chemical-containing waste do not meet RCRA reporting criteria (and are not reported to BRS). In the Stone/Clay/Glass industry, for example, the manufacture of television picture tubes entails large amounts of on- and off- site recycling of lead compounds used to manufacture the tube components. Wastes from the picture tube plates and funnels are managed separately, and the waste streams generated from the funnel components are reported to BRS while the plate waste streams, where the lead content is more dilute, are not. Nonetheless, the lead content of both types of streams must be reported to TRI, boosting the percentage of adjusted TRI versus RCRA toxic waste.

Changes in TRI Waste Generation and Management by Industry, 1991-1992

Production-related toxic waste generation as reported to TRI in 1992 for all industry increased slightly (3 percent) between 1991 and 1992.[g] The Chemical industry's 1 percent increase heavily influenced the overall industry change, however, because that industry reports the majority of the total in any year. (See Appendix N, Table N-2.) The picture is different for many other industries that have less influence on the overall national trends, but that may play a significant role in certain geographic areas or for certain chemicals, environmental media, or methods of waste management and pollution prevention. (See Figure 6-4 and Appendix M for national and individual industry profiles.)

Reductions in the quantity of waste released/disposed of between 1991 and 1992 for all but a few of the smaller industries indicate that less waste is being handled by these least desirable methods. Between 1991 and 1992, releases and disposal decreased 3 percent over all industries. This decrease ran counter to the trend in all other waste management categories. Treatment and energy recovery each increased 4 percent, and recycling increased 3 percent.

Because changes in TRI data cannot be compared to changes in BRS data, this chapter's analysis of year-to-year changes relies solely on TRI data. Also, although BRS data were collected in 1989 as well as in 1991, changes in the scope, coverage, and implementation of the BRS between those two years had impacts that can only be partially identified. In particular, a more stringent Toxicity Characteristic Leachate Procedure (TCLP) went into effect in 1991 lowering the concentrations of toxic constituents that would require facilities to report to BRS. EPA also brought several previously unregulated wastes and boilers and industrial furnaces (BIFs) under RCRA regulation and reporting requirements in mid 1991. In addition, EPA clarified its BRS report instructions and conducted training and outreach efforts to capture previously unreported data, and convinced more states to use the standardized federal form to report their data in 1991.

[g] This section compares 1991 with 1992 data for facilities reporting in 1992. There were 2,401 facilities in 1991 that did not report for 1992. Total production-related waste in 1991 for these facilities was 422.0 million pounds. If this amount is added to the 1991 figure, then the increase would be 2 percent instead of 3 percent. The impact of these facilities that did not report for 1992 in the various industries is not significant and, of course, there are no projections for these facilities.

Figure 6-4.

Industry Profile: National Summary

Reported Production-related Toxic Waste Generation

Reporting Year/Source	Pounds	Rank**
1991 BRS	948,243,750,120	
1991 TRI	36,316,963,077	
1992 TRI	37,333,775,624	
1993 TRI*	37,445,906,395	
1994 TRI*	37,460,411,532	

Special Groups, 1992 TRI	
Carcinogens	2,955,067,837
Ozone depleters	738,134,032
Chloro-organics	2,307,493,160
Metals	4,174,881,882
Halo-organics	2,317,202,349

Top 5 Chemicals, 1992 TRI		Pounds
7664-93-9	Sulfuric acid	10,269,925,138
75-05-8	Acetonitrile	2,581,322,698
7647-01-0	Hydrochloric acid	2,475,552,419
67-56-1	Methanol	2,238,505,652
115-07-1	Propylene	1,615,374,591

Top 5 Facilities, 1992 TRI	
First Chemical Corp., Pascagoula, MS	4,046,638,711
Goodyear Tire & Rubber Co., Beaumont, TX	2,526,855,525
Uno-Ven Co., Lemont, IL	488,229,292
Solvay Polymers Inc., Deer Park, TX	412,262,000
Cyprus Miami Mining Corp., Claypool, AZ	394,955,000

Top 5 Facilities, 1991 BRS	
Kodak Park, Rochester, NY	83,225,844,980
Dow Chemical Company, Midland, MI	60,274,801,720
Amoco Oil Company Refinery, Texas City, TX	52,275,053,600
DuPont-Chambers Works, Deepwater, NJ	48,843,789,760
Shell Oil Company, Deer Park, TX	38,738,555,340

TRI Production-related Waste, 1991-1994*

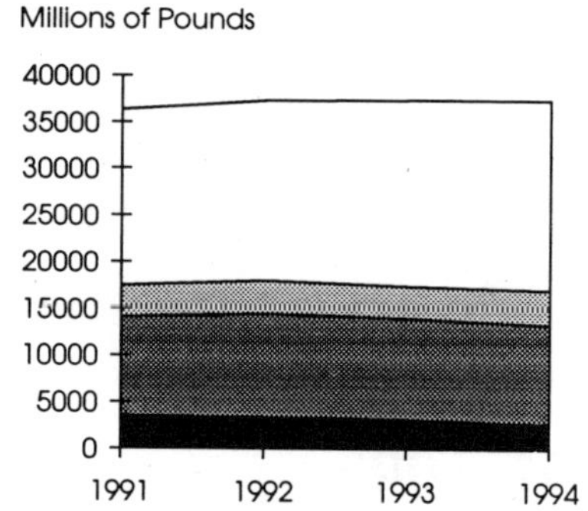

Total TRI Releases, 1992

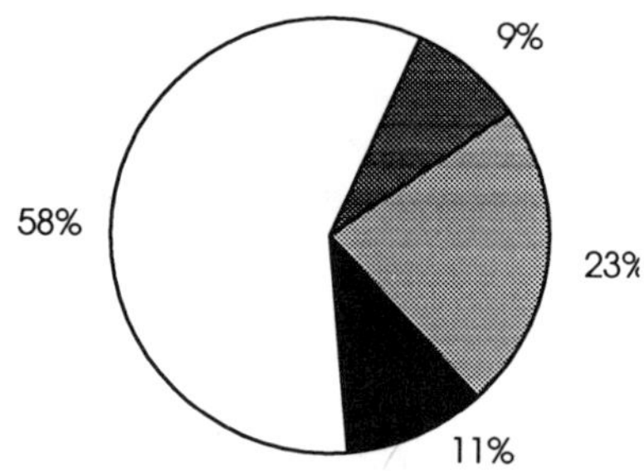

Total: 3,181.6 Million Pounds

Total Air Emissions	58%
Surface Water Discharges	9%
Underground Injection	23%
Releases to Land	11%

	Pounds	Pounds	Pounds
Facility with Largest Reported TRI Increase	**1991**	**1992**	**Increase**
Doe Run Co., Boss, MO	50,358,284	231,500,858	181,142,574
Facility with Largest Reported TRI Decrease	**1991**	**1992**	**Decrease**
DuPont Chambers Works, Deepwater, NJ	243,531,644	69,782,276	-173,749,368
Facility with Largest Projected TRI Increase	**1992**	**1994***	**Increase**
Goodyear Tire & Rubber Co., Beaumont, TX	2,526,855,525	3,027,332,113	500,476,588
Facility with Largest Projected TRI Decrease	**1992**	**1994***	**Decrease**
SCM Chemicals, Baltimore, MD	287,807,796	36,808,552	-250,999,244

*Projected ** Rankings appear in individual Industry Profiles in Appendix M.

Large Industry Domination of TRI Changes, 1991-1992

Industry-wide changes in the levels of total production-related waste and its management components (recycling, energy recovery, treatment, and releases and disposal) principally reflect the trends in a few large industries. Despite any changes in other industries' waste generation or source reduction, the Chemical and Primary Metals industries exert the greatest influence, because together they generated 64 percent of total production-related waste in 1992.

The primary reason for the 3 percent increase in total production-related waste between 1991 and 1992 was that the Chemical industry experienced a 1 percent increase. If the Chemical industry amounts were removed from the 1991 and 1992 TRI data, the overall increase for the remaining industries would have been 5 percent. The 1 percent increase for the Chemical industry would have had an even greater influence on the overall figures were it not for the 11 percent increase for Primary Metals. If the Chemical industry data were included in the 1991 and 1992 amounts, but the Primary Metals data were removed, the change for the remaining industries would have been only a 2 percent increase. (See Table 6-8.)

Similar effects can be seen in the changes for the least desirable waste management option, releases and disposal, when comparing the variety of increases and decreases among industries to the overall change. Quantities released/disposed of decreased overall by 3 percent between 1991 and 1992, whereas the Chemical industry made less progress, experiencing only a decrease of 0.04 percent. Were the Chemical industry amounts excluded entirely from the 1991 and 1992 figures, the decrease for the remaining industries would have been 6 percent rather than 3 percent.

Looking at the individual smaller industries reveals an interesting variation of increases and decreases in different waste management categories and shows mixed progress in pollution prevention. Facilities in the Printing industry were most successful of all TRI facilities in decreasing their releases and disposal. They achieved a 14 percent reduction in these wastes. However, the gains did not reflect pollution prevention progress. The Printing industry increased the waste it reported by 3 percent. The TRI numbers reveal that the industry coped with its larger waste generation by an increased reliance on waste treatment, which rose 15 percent. The Leather industry reported an overall increase of 17 percent in production-related waste, including a 25 percent increase in releases and disposal. The Plastics industry, while showing an overall increase of 12 percent, reported a 2 percent decrease in releases and disposal offset by a 19 percent increase in recycling and an 18 percent increase in treated wastes. Only five industries (Lumber, Stone/Clay/Glass, Machinery, Electrical, and Multiple Codes) show any decrease in total production-related waste, and those industries with decreases account for only 12 percent of such waste in 1992. (See Appendix N, Table N-2.)

Table 6-8. Change in TRI Total Production-related Waste by Industry, 1991-1992

SIC Code	Industry	Total Production-related Waste 1991 Pounds	1992 Pounds	Change 1991 to 1992 Pounds	Rank	Percent	Rank
20	Food	380,691,966	389,637,145	8,945,179	14	2.35	10
21	Tobacco	55,046,792	60,185,440	5,138,648	11	9.34	17
22	Textiles	98,220,702	100,223,930	2,003,228	7	2.04	8
23	Apparel	2,883,172	3,146,914	263,742	6	9.15	16
24	Lumber	67,834,787	63,091,614	-4,743,173	4	-6.99	1
25	Furniture	62,729,636	66,227,908	3,498,272	10	5.58	14
26	Paper	2,491,445,311	2,537,521,812	46,076,501	18	1.85	7
27	Printing	266,876,401	274,812,686	7,936,285	13	2.97	12
28	Chemicals	19,672,469,407	19,897,327,333	224,857,926	20	1.14	6
29	Petroleum	2,562,915,297	2,945,379,328	382,464,031	21	14.92	20
30	Plastics	508,051,776	567,294,382	59,242,606	19	11.66	19
31	Leather	44,987,787	52,480,219	7,492,432	12	16.65	21
32	Stone/Clay	999,977,077	935,576,617	-64,400,460	2	-6.44	2
33	Primary Metals	3,654,952,230	4,044,002,976	389,050,746	22	10.64	18
34	Fabr. Metals	919,137,839	962,656,507	43,518,668	17	4.73	13
35	Machinery	211,347,793	207,000,051	-4,347,742	5	-2.06	5
36	Electrical	994,456,225	963,576,363	-30,879,862	3	-3.11	4
37	Transportation	459,765,222	471,959,721	12,194,499	15	2.65	11
38	Measure./Photo.	122,969,517	125,739,677	2,770,160	8	2.25	9
39	Miscellaneous	51,696,646	55,014,507	3,317,861	9	6.42	15
	Multiple codes 20-39	2,530,599,122	2,412,177,342	-118,421,780	1	-4.68	3
	No codes 20-39	157,908,372	198,743,152	40,834,780	16	25.86	22
	Total	36,316,963,077	37,333,775,624	1,016,812,547		2.80	

Impact of Major Facility Changes

As in any single year, reports from a few facilities dominate changes in TRI production-related waste from year to year. The Primary Metals industry showed the largest absolute change from 1991 to 1992, an increase of 389.1 million pounds (11 percent). (See Table 6-8.) This resulted in large part from reports by three facilities: Doe Run Company in Boss, Missouri; Elkem Metals in Marietta, Ohio; and Revere Copper Products in Rome, New York, which together reported an increase of 385.4 million pounds. For the Doe Run facility, operations began in the middle of 1991, so the 1992 figure reflects a full year's operations for the first time. The other two facilities decided to count the reincorporation of scrap metal as recycling, which makes their increases apparent rather than a reflection of any actual changes. (See Chapter 4, Table 4-7.)

It is important to verify facility data for TRI waste generation and waste generation changes, as described in Chapter 4. Chapter 4 also indicates why TRI Section 8 data are likely to improve significantly over the next few years.

The Petroleum industry had the second largest absolute change, an increase of 382.5 million pounds (15 percent). The five facilities in this industry with the largest increases had a combined increase of 290.5 million pounds in production-related waste: ARCO Cherry Point Refinery in Ferndale, Washington (81.4 million pounds),[h] Chevron USA in Port Arthur, Texas (63.0 million pounds), Uno-Ven in Lemont, Illinois (57.3 million pounds), Texaco's Star Enterprises also in Port Arthur, Texas (44.4 million pounds), and El Paso Refinery in El Paso, Texas (44.4 million pounds).

Even though Chemical industry facilities reported a total net increase of 224.9 million pounds, three of the five facilities in the nation reporting the largest decreases in production-related waste are Chemical facilities: DuPont Chambers Works plant in Deepwater, New Jersey; Reilly Industries in Indianapolis, Indiana; and Carolina Eastman in Columbia, South Carolina. Together these three facilities reported a total decrease of 509.4 million pounds. However, these decreases were offset by the Goodyear Tire and Rubber plant in Beaumont, Texas, also a Chemical facility, with an increase of 103.2 million pounds, and by many smaller chemical facilities with increases.[i] (See Chapter 4 for an explanation of these changes in relation to changes in how recycling amounts were calculated.)

TRI facilities that report multiple codes together reported the largest amount of decrease (118.4 million pounds) for any industry category. One facility, the Phillips 66 Company in Sweeny, Texas, reported a decrease of 132.6 million pounds, but it does not expect to achieve that low level of waste in future years. (See Chapter 4.)

TRI Production-related Waste Projections, 1992-1994

TRI, unlike BRS, requires facilities to project how much waste will be generated during the next two years. Industry projections from facilities reporting to TRI in 1992 project production-related waste leveling off to a 0.3 percent increase between 1992 and 1994, after increasing 3 percent from 1991 to 1992. The projections do not include any facilities which may in the future come under TRI reporting that do not now.[j] The projections do include facilities now reporting to TRI that expect to either close or reduce their use of TRI chemicals sufficiently so that they will not be required to report then. (See Table 6-9.)

The Primary Metals industry, the industry with the largest *increase* in production-related waste from 1991 to 1992 (389.1 million pounds), is

[h] In a conversation on September 13, 1994, Daisy Wong stated that the 1991 amounts in the TRI database for ARCO Cherry Point are in error, and that there was no increase between 1991 and 1992.

[i] Goodyear Tire and Rubber has subsequently revised its data, eliminating the increase.

[j] Of the 23,630 facilities that reported in 1992, 1,737 (7 percent) had not reported in 1991. These facilities account for 0.7 percent (275.6 million pounds) of total production-related waste in 1992.

Table 6-9. Projected Change in TRI Production-related Waste by Industry, 1992-1994

SIC Code	Industry	Total Production-related Waste: Actual 1992 Pounds	Total Production-related Waste: Projected 1994 Pounds	Projected Change 1992 to 1994: Pounds (Pounds)	Rank	Percent (Percent)	Rank
20	Food	389,637,145	382,807,750	-6,829,395	13	-1.75	13
21	Tobacco	60,185,440	3,754,369	-56,431,071	4	-93.76	1
22	Textiles	100,223,930	84,499,332	-15,724,598	10	-15.69	7
23	Apparel	3,146,914	2,020,519	-1,126,395	15	-35.79	2
24	Lumber	63,091,614	75,824,342	12,732,728	18	20.18	20
25	Furniture	66,227,908	62,853,431	-3,374,477	14	-5.10	10
26	Paper	2,537,521,812	2,445,343,962	-92,177,850	3	-3.63	12
27	Printing	274,812,686	264,199,957	-10,612,729	12	-3.86	11
28	Chemicals	19,897,327,333	20,058,858,183	161,530,850	20	0.81	17
29	Petroleum	2,945,379,328	2,900,069,882	-45,309,446	5	-1.54	15
30	Plastics	567,294,382	422,046,257	-145,248,125	1	-25.60	3
31	Leather	52,480,219	52,167,105	-313,114	16	-0.60	16
32	Stone/Clay	935,576,617	1,165,083,734	229,507,117	21	24.53	21
33	Primary Metals	4,044,002,976	4,345,464,739	301,461,763	22	7.45	19
34	Fabr. Metals	962,656,507	971,522,127	8,865,620	17	0.92	18
35	Machinery	207,000,051	174,373,640	-32,626,411	8	-15.76	6
36	Electrical	963,576,363	850,486,153	-113,090,210	2	-11.74	8
37	Transportation	471,959,721	435,593,168	-36,366,553	7	-7.71	9
38	Measure./Photo.	125,739,677	103,299,566	-22,440,111	9	-17.85	5
39	Miscellaneous	55,014,507	41,498,672	-13,515,835	11	-24.57	4
	Multiple codes 20-39	2,412,177,342	2,370,238,092	-41,939,250	6	-1.74	14
	No codes 20-39	198,743,152	248,406,552	49,663,400	19	24.99	22
	Total	37,333,775,624	37,460,411,532	126,635,908		0.34	

projecting a somewhat smaller increase from 1992 to 1994 (301.5 million pounds). Likewise, the Chemical industry, with an increase of 224.9 million pounds from 1991 to 1992, is also projecting a smaller increase (161.5 million pounds) from 1992 to 1994. The Stone/Clay/Glass, Lumber, and Fabricated Metals industries, plus those facilities not reporting any 20-39 SIC codes, are the other industry groups projecting increases. Indeed, the Stone/Clay/Glass industry expects to reverse its 1991-1992 decrease. (See Figure 6-5 and Table 6-9.)

The Petroleum industry, on the other hand, with the second largest absolute increase from 1991 to 1992 (of 382.5 million pounds) is projecting a *decrease* from 1992 to 1994 of 45.3 million pounds (a 2 percent decrease). The Plastics industry is also planning to reverse direction, going from a 12 percent increase in 1991-1992 to a projected 26 percent decrease (of 145.2 million pounds) between 1992 and 1994. The Paper industry, which had a 2 percent increase between 1991 and 1992, is projecting a 4 percent decrease between 1992 and 1994, which amounts to 92.2 million pounds. (See Figure 6-5 and Appendix N, Table N-2.)

Figure 6-5.

Change in TRI Production-related Waste, by Industry, Actual 1991 to 1992 and Projected 1992 to 1994

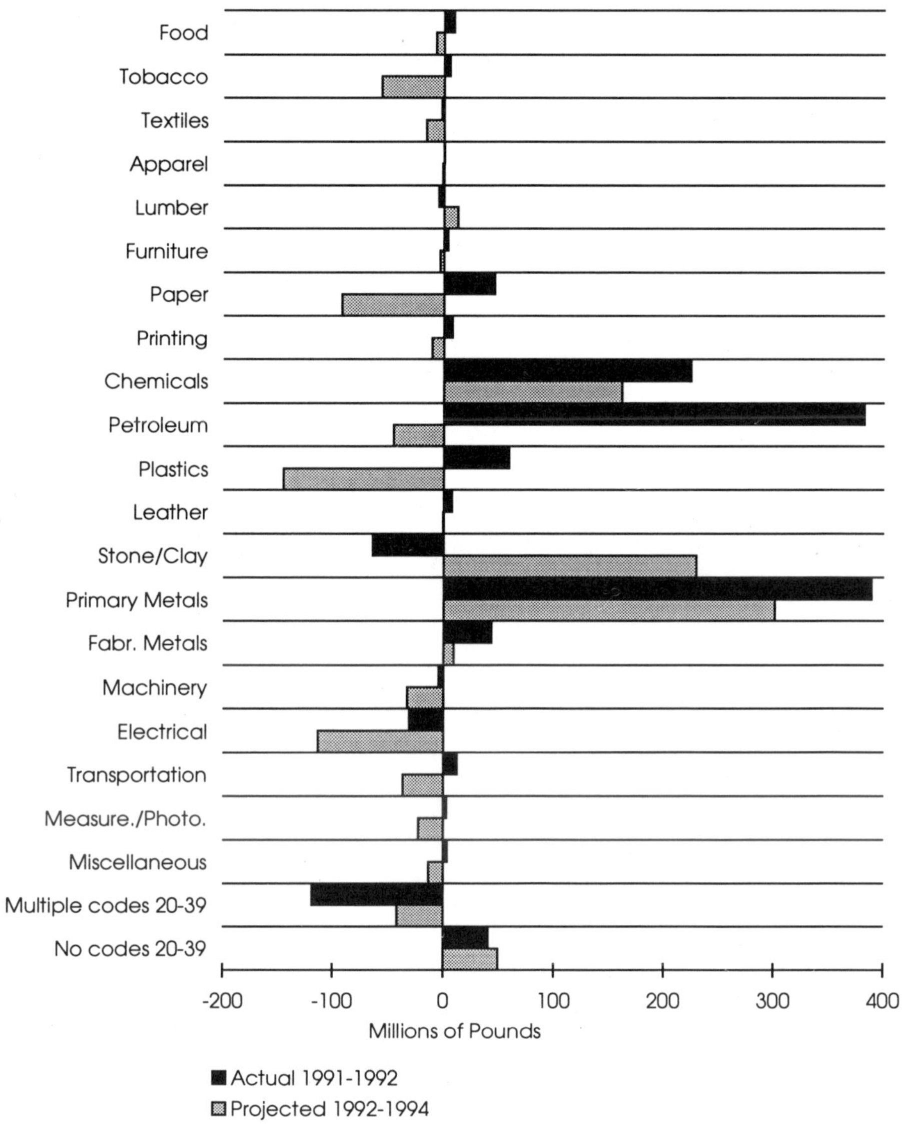

The Tobacco and Apparel industries project the largest expected *percentage decreases* from 1992 to 1994, amounting to 94 percent and 36 percent, respectively. The R. J. Reynolds Tobacco Company in Winston-Salem, North Carolina, reported total production-related waste of 55.5 million pounds in 1992, but expected zero TRI chemicals in waste in 1993 and beyond. The company expects to achieve this in 1994 with the complete elimination of two ozone depleters on the TRI list, by finding substitutes for trichlorofluoromethane and 1,1,1-trichloroethane.

Projections for 1992-1994 for the separate components of production-related waste show that TRI facilities as a whole expect to move away from less desirable waste management options in the coming years. The slight overall increase in total production-related waste is the result principally of more waste being recycled (the most favorable waste management option other than source reduction); less desirable waste management options are forecast by the reporting facilities to decrease for many industries. TRI facilities expect to reduce releases and disposal of TRI chemicals to a much greater extent in future years, by 20 percent from 1992 to 1994, compared with the 3 percent reduction achieved from 1991 to 1992.

The other types of waste management show varying degrees of projected change. On-site recycling is projected to increase by 7 percent, while off-site recycling is projected to decrease by 1 percent, for a net increase of 5 percent. A 5 percent increase in on-site energy recovery and a 6 percent decrease in off-site energy recovery combine for a projected 3 percent increase. Treatment of wastes is projected to decrease, by 2 percent for on-site treatment and by 12 percent for off-site treatment, for a net decrease of 3 percent.

The projected reduction for releases and disposal of waste is broadly based across all industries except for the Lumber and Primary Metals industries. The Lumber industry projects an increase of 47 percent in releases and disposal (15.9 million pounds) which more than offsets projected decreases in treatment, energy recovery, and recycling, resulting in a net increase of 20 percent in total production-related waste for that industry. However, in verifying the data, *Toxics Watch* found that more than three-quarters of this increase is accounted for by a reporting error made by one Kerr-McGee facility, the Forest Products Division, in Columbus, Mississippi. This facility, which reports the use of creosote as an article component at its facility, projects an increase from 5.8 million pounds in 1992 to 26.0 million pounds of total production-related waste in 1994. The error Kerr-McGee made was to forecast an increase in release and disposal of creosote from 24.7 *thousand* pounds in 1992 to 20.0 *million* pounds in 1994, instead of a decrease to 20.0 *thousand* pounds (and 6.0 million pounds of total production-related waste) in 1994.[5] The Primary Metals industry is the only other industry to project an increase in quantities released/disposed of: a 1 percent increase amounting to 6.5 million pounds. (See Appendix N, Table N-2.)

In contrast to the Lumber and Primary Metals industries' releases and disposal projections, some industries are projecting decreases of various waste management components that exceed the projected national averages. For example, the Apparel industry's projected overall decrease of 36 percent is to be accomplished by decreasing each of the different types of waste management. The Plastics industry's projected 26 percent reduction in total production-related waste is based on expected decreases in recycling of 36 percent and in releases and disposal of 21 percent.

TRI Changes by Parent Company, 1991-1994

The five parent companies owning TRI facilities with the largest amounts of production-related waste in both 1991 and 1992 were First Mississippi Corporation, DuPont, and Hoechst Celanese, with TRI facilities in the Chemical industry; Goodyear Tire and Rubber, with TRI facilities in the Rubber and Plastics industry and in the Chemical industry (which includes the manufacture of synthetic rubber); and Texaco, a petroleum refining company.[k] The top 10 parent companies for 1991 remained in the top 10 for 1992, with the exception of the Occidental Petroleum Corporation which ranked 10th in 1991 and 17th in 1992. Occidental Petroleum's TRI facilities reported an overall reduction of 18 percent from 1991 to 1992. Allied-Signal Company's TRI facilities, which make transportation, electrical, and fabricated metal equipment, reported an overall increase in production-related waste from 1991 to 1992 of 20 percent, which raised its rank from 15th to 10th. (See Table 6-10.)

The 50 parent companies with facilities reporting the greatest aggregate amount of total production-related waste in 1991 account for 57 percent (20.6 billion pounds) of that waste but only 6 percent of all TRI facilities. For four of these companies, only one facility reports to TRI so that the one facility accounts for the large amount of production-related waste. On the other hand, the General Motors Corporation, the automobile manufacturer, has among the largest number of facilities reporting to TRI, a total of 131. (See Table 6-10.)

While TRI facilities belonging to these 50 parent companies reported a small decrease in total production-related waste from 1991 to 1992 (less than 0.3 percent), the decrease was primarily in recycling. As reported in Chapter 4 and earlier in this chapter, several of these facilities changed their definition of recycling from on-site recycling to in-process recovery without making any operational changes to account for the apparent decrease. Indeed, these 50 companies show a somewhat smaller percentage decrease in waste released or disposed of (2.7 percent decrease) than do TRI facilities as a whole (3.3 percent decrease). These companies also increased energy recovery more rapidly from 1991 to 1992 than all TRI facilities.

[k] TRI data in this report were aggregated for parent companies by using the parent company identifiers reported by facilities to TRI and information in the Dun and Bradstreet database. (See Appendix O.)

*Table 6-10. Change in Waste from 1991 to 1992 for the 50 TRI Parent Companies with Largest Total Production-related Waste in 1991**

Total Production-related Waste Rank* 1991 Rank	1992 Rank	Parent Company	TRI Facilities Number	Change in Total Production-related Waste 1991 to 1992 Percent	Total Production-related Waste 1991 Pounds	1992 Pounds
1	1	First Mississippi Corporation	7	0.04	4,052,567,255	4,054,298,758
2	2	Goodyear Tire & Rubber Co	37	5.64	2,711,678,031	2,864,512,848
3	4	DuPont	82	-10.30	871,763,023	781,956,864
4	3	Texaco Inc	23	25.15	679,817,476	850,779,190
5	5	Hoechst Celanese Corporation	32	4.63	664,260,025	695,043,839
6	8	Solvay America Inc	11	-11.00	464,330,610	413,270,803
7	9	Cyprus Minerals Company	8	-9.57	449,838,157	406,802,516
8	7	Uno-Ven Company	1	13.30	430,919,553	488,229,292
9	6	Dow Chemical Company	26	29.32	400,178,093	517,495,767
10	17	Occidental Petroleum Corp	37	-18.06	378,978,357	310,551,333
11	34	Eastman Kodak Company	22	-41.02	374,792,471	221,067,151
12	18	Elf Aquitaine Inc	29	-13.95	360,822,594	310,500,972
13	11	International Paper Company	75	9.85	357,861,789	393,119,070
14	15	Kemira Holdings Inc	1	-5.93	336,468,720	316,522,270
15	10	Allied-Signal Inc	82	20.19	327,224,403	393,304,084
16	16	National Cooperative Refinery	1	-3.22	323,281,992	312,856,711
17	19	Monsanto Company	29	-4.18	318,539,891	305,224,967
18	14	Amoco Corporation	42	9.93	302,200,939	332,195,627
19	21	PPG Industries Inc	41	-2.51	294,347,709	286,962,296
20	12	HM Anglo-American Ltd	45	22.06	286,415,645	349,598,460
21	13	Atlantic Richfield Company	11	21.98	286,073,412	348,950,397
22	24	Coulton Chemical Corp.	1	0.32	272,609,056	273,469,050
23	22	Georgia-Pacific Corporation	68	5.36	271,657,667	286,216,696
24	20	American Cyanamid	31	8.88	268,790,236	292,663,520
25	28	Bristol-Myers Squibb Company	15	-3.64	264,382,024	254,755,612
26	65	American Petrofina Holding Co	7	-55.66	263,065,287	116,650,527
27	26	Lafarge Corporation	12	10.48	246,731,180	272,588,945
28	23	Asarco Incorporated	12	18.91	230,912,617	274,577,841
29	27	Citgo Petroleum Corporation	3	11.73	230,374,230	257,398,721
30	25	Zeneca Holdings Inc	59	21.04	225,500,012	272,952,202
31	53	EC Acquisition Inc	14	-33.04	211,416,430	141,554,974
32	42	Weyerhaeuser Company	25	-8.51	202,608,033	185,370,540
33	37	General Motors Corporation	131	1.69	201,885,284	205,303,728
34	99	Phillips Petroleum Company	16	-62.33	201,285,528	75,822,794
35	36	Shell Petroleum Inc	20	3.54	200,444,529	207,535,270
36	38	Quaker State Corporation	4	0.01	200,427,416	200,443,094
37	94	Reilly Industries Inc	6	-60.65	197,345,362	77,653,080
38	29	Johnson Controls Inc	28	26.30	197,001,615	248,804,407
39	39	Courtaulds United States Inc	13	1.26	196,889,648	1 99,372,005
40	33	Gates Corporation	19	23.44	186,119,501	229,743,060
41	41	Timken Co	17	9.97	172,795,626	190,028,461
42	191	Corning Inc	23	-80.77	171,656,190	33,013,240
43	51	Mobil Corporation	30	-15.39	169,661,117	143,543,010
44	46	Freeport-Mcmoran Inc	4	-1.52	169,503,206	166,929,776
45	31	Union Carbide Corporation	21	37.90	167,547,040	231,052,269
46	35	Upjohn Company	4	33.77	160,474,577	214,667,954
47	157	Pacific Dunlop Holdings Inc	21	-70.82	157,758,502	46,030,080
48	71	Champion International Corp	19	-29.09	157,177,353	111,459,868
49	45	Stone Container Corporation	15	7.43	156,939,166	168,606,473
50	40	Ford Motor Company	52	23.18	156,762,332	193,092,838
		Subtotal	1,332	-0.28	20,582,080,909	20,524,543,250
		Percent of Total	5.64		56.67	54.98
		Total	23,630	2.80	36,316,963,077	37,333,775,624

* Rank is among total of 10,840 parent companies.

Change from 1991 to 1992 in:			
Recycling Percent	**Energy Recovery** Percent	**Treated** Percent	**Released/ Disposed of** Percent
0.08	-1.08	—	-25.24
5.58	41.31	13.06	4.52
-68.12	24.27	0.70	3.69
11.31	-45.03	514.00	-10.41
4.64	1.42	13.73	-2.06
-10.18	1.71	-29.39	-4.72
-9.52	—	—	-14.62
4639.78	30.97	5.03	-58.54
34.40	-3.55	44.54	-5.33
0.69	93.22	-30.30	-10.10
-96.87	20.18	-9.35	-16.80
7.75	27.49	-16.87	5.76
3.00	11.88	13.83	-8.09
-7.14	—	-0.38	36.63
27.08	16.22	19.20	-10.43
—	-3.25	12.52	1.57
-23.06	-34.07	8.92	0.53
12.74	-15.59	9.77	-18.14
7.87	-21.61	-15.29	3.70
-23.93	18.17	22.20	140.02
36.99	30.63	-32.68	-4.32
-0.03	0.00	71.67	-0.01
-6.65	23.12	5.72	-5.60
8.87	12.04	38.33	2.85
-2.18	-51.38	-8.46	-24.62
-75.98	-23.27	-55.13	23.61
—	10.40	116.82	-2.69
32.29	—	143.15	-9.62
10.65	-78.54	70.10	-44.53
9.96	36.91	26.33	-11.58
-9.88	—	-44.65	29.90
35.10	-3.45	-10.36	-9.57
14.87	-25.93	-3.29	-16.57
-76.91	4.03	31.51	-0.53
55.57	-5.07	-3.69	9.61
-0.01	65.63	0.00	6.31
-63.77	467.92	7.98	-81.87
27.41	36.99	-48.36	-7.31
0.48	-5.87	7.89	1.84
23.07	192.83	227.82	4.55
13.90	-37.27	6.66	-2.98
-84.18	54.25	5.81	-3.91
25.89	-33.62	-21.75	-19.91
-19.63	-20.28	-48.48	3.82
789.94	-26.55	14.15	-12.53
42.22	25.01	-10.86	-14.65
-76.95	21.11	3.20	-6.50
440.11	41.02	-36.15	-0.85
-2.50	131.29	0.82	2.51
19.04	-3.31	122.83	-2.73
-1.87	6.07	2.46	-2.70
2.81	4.27	4.33	-3.25

Comparing the changes in production-related waste for the top ranked parent companies shows that, while their ranks did not change in most cases, there were substantial increases and decreases. DuPont facilities reported an overall decrease in production-related waste of 10 percent, which was due to a decrease in recycling only (of 68 percent), with much of that due to redefinition of recycling activities or cessation of production. (See Chapter 4.) DuPont TRI facilities reported increases in all other categories of waste management. On the other hand, Texaco facilities reported an overall increase of 25 percent, due to the amount treated and recycled, while they reported decreases in amounts of releases and disposal and in energy recovery. Other substantial changes occurred at Dow Chemical facilities, which reported an increase in total production-related waste of 29 percent, due to increased recycling and treatment. Eastman Kodak facilities reported an overall decrease of 41 percent, due to the virtual elimination of recycling (a 97 percent decrease) and a decrease of 17 percent in releases and disposal of wastes. (See Figure 6-6.)

The 50 parent companies with the largest amount of production-related waste in 1991 reported a total of 20.5 billion pounds of production-related waste in 1992, 55 percent of the 1992 total. Even though these companies reported a decrease in recycling from 1991 to 1992, 62 percent of their waste still was recycled in 1992. This is higher than the 52 percent for all TRI facilities and, consequently, energy recovery, treatment, and disposal represent a lower portion of total waste for the top 50 companies than is true for the average of other TRI facilities. (See Table 6-11.)

The companies with TRI facilities reporting the largest amounts of releases and disposal of production-related waste are not the same companies reporting largest total production-related waste. The five companies that reported the largest amounts of waste released or disposed of in both 1991 and 1992 are DuPont, Freeport-McMoran, American Cyanamid, Asarco, and Monsanto. The DuPont, American Cyanamid, and Monsanto TRI facilities manufacture a variety of chemicals. The Freeport-McMoran TRI facilities manufacture agricultural fertilizers. Asarco owns TRI facilities that are primary metal smelters and refiners and chemical manufacturing facilities. Four of these five companies reported increases in the amount of waste released/disposed of from 1991 to 1992. However, all except Monsanto projected decreases in releases and disposal of wastes by 1994. (See Figure 6-7 and Table 6-12.)

The next five companies with the largest amount of waste released/disposed of in 1991 are Eastman Kodak (chemicals), Renco Group (primary metals), BP America (oil refining, chemicals, plastics, electrical, and other machinery), General Motors (automobiles), and 3M Company (chemicals, paper products, photographic equipment, abrasives). While all five of these companies reported a decrease in chemicals released/disposed of from 1991 to 1992 and project additional decreases from 1992 to 1994, decreases from 1991 to 1992 led to General Motors' and 3M Company's no longer ranking among the top 10 in 1992. General Motors' facilities reported a

Figure 6-6.

Change in Waste from 1991 to 1992 for TRI Parent Companies with Large Total Production-related Waste in 1991

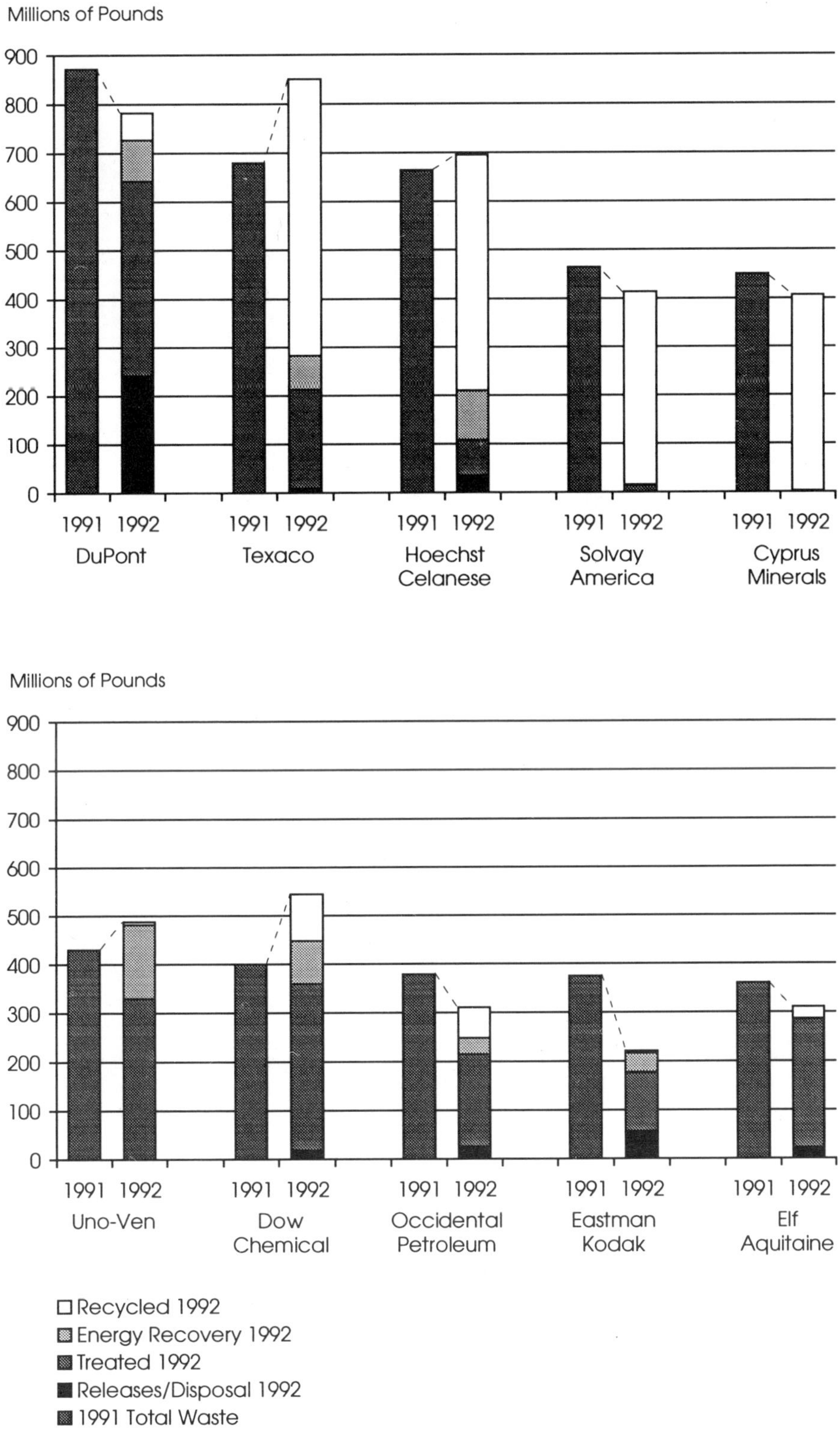

*Table 6-11. 1992 Production-related Waste for the 50 TRI Parent Companies with Largest Total Production-related Waste in 1991**

Total Production-related Waste Rank*				Type of Waste Management as Percent of Total Production-related Waste			
1991 Rank	1992 Rank	Parent Company	1992 Total Production-related Waste Pounds	Recycling Percent	Energy Recovery Percent	Treated Percent	Released/ Disposed of Percent
1	1	First Mississippi Corporation	4,054,298,758	99.71	0.18	0.00	0.11
2	2	Goodyear Tire & Rubber Co	2,864,512,848	99.42	0.17	0.15	0.26
3	4	DuPont	781,956,864	7.05	10.85	51.29	30.81
4	3	Texaco Inc	850,779,190	66.75	8.22	24.07	0.96
5	5	Hoechst Celanese Corporation	695,043,839	69.72	14.87	10.27	5.14
6	8	Solvay America Inc	413,270,803	96.18	0.14	3.49	0.18
7	9	Cyprus Minerals Company	406,802,516	99.16	0.00	0.00	0.84
8	7	Uno-Ven Company	488,229,292	1.17	31.23	67.58	0.02
9	6	Dow Chemical Company	517,495,767	18.54	17.21	60.85	3.40
10	17	Occidental Petroleum Corp	310,551,333	19.97	10.77	60.75	8.52
11	34	Eastman Kodak Company	221,067,151	2.00	17.73	54.87	25.4
12	18	Elf Aquitaine Inc	310,500,972	7.64	0.33	84.83	7.20
13	11	International Paper Company	393,119,070	18.02	10.37	65.12	6.49
14	15	Kemira Holdings Inc	316,522,270	82.14	0.00	17.55	0.31
15	10	Allied-Signal Inc	393,304,084	30.96	2.13	63.77	3.13
16	16	National Cooperative Refinery	312,856,711	0.00	99.75	0.10	0.15
17	19	Monsanto Company	305,224,967	13.36	9.24	52.35	25.04
18	14	Amoco Corporation	332,195,627	77.73	1.75	16.47	4.06
19	21	PPG Industries Inc	286,962,296	61.64	6.21	30.09	2.06
20	12	HM Anglo-American Ltd	349,598,460	2.15	0.21	95.20	2.44
21	13	Atlantic Richfield Company	348,950,397	1.53	89.34	6.66	2.47
22	24	Coulton Chemical Corp.	273,469,050	99.10	0.05	0.83	0.02
23	22	Georgia-Pacific Corporation	286,216,696	3.94	8.00	80.15	7.91
24	20	American Cyanamid	292,663,520	30.14	4.58	13.64	51.64
25	28	Bristol-Myers Squibb Company	254,755,612	89.81	0.42	7.93	1.84
26	65	American Petrofina Holding Co	116,650,527	9.32	13.09	75.29	2.31
27	26	Lafarge Corporation	272,588,945	0.00	99.74	0.18	0.09
28	23	Asarco Incorporated	274,577,841	71.85	0.00	1.96	26.19
29	27	Citgo Petroleum Corporation	257,398,721	88.20	0.00	9.45	2.34
30	25	Zeneca Holdings Inc	272,952,202	2.64	1.72	86.07	9.57
31	53	EC Acquisition Inc	141,554,974	42.94	0.00	55.72	1.34
32	42	Weyerhaeuser Company	185,370,540	5.03	4.06	86.60	4.31
33	37	General Motors Corporation	205,303,728	59.34	3.29	15.54	21.83
34	99	Phillips Petroleum Company	75,822,794	51.83	11.45	28.38	8.34
35	36	Shell Petroleum Inc	207,535,270	16.33	16.38	59.04	8.25
36	38	Quaker State Corporation	200,443,094	99.78	0.01	0.02	0.19
37	94	Reilly Industries Inc	77,653,080	90.14	7.71	1.72	0.43
38	29	Johnson Controls Inc	248,804,407	99.07	0.17	0.56	0.20
39	39	Courtaulds United States Inc	199,372,005	69.69	0.66	7.57	22.08
40	33	Gates Corporation	229,743,060	98.86	0.19	0.44	0.51
41	41	Timken Co	190,028,461	48.09	0.00	51.46	0.45
42	191	Corning Inc	33,013,240	78.95	0.36	7.56	13.13
43	51	Mobil Corporation	143,543,010	20.86	3.12	68.27	7.75
44	46	Freeport-Mcmoran Inc	166,929,776	0.11	2.13	4.67	93.09
45	31	Union Carbide Corporation	231,052,269	26.58	7.86	60.34	5.21
46	35	Upjohn Company	214,667,954	82.21	9.97	3.83	3.99
47	157	Pacific Dunlop Holdings Inc	46,030,080	72.84	0.05	23.52	3.59
48	71	Champion International Corp	111,459,868	0.06	11.98	78.55	9.41
49	45	Stone Container Corporation	168,606,473	3.47	10.93	78.64	6.96
50	40	Ford Motor Company	193,092,838	67.90	1.40	15.30	15.40
		Subtotal	20,524,543,250	61.77	8.71	23.52	6.00
		Percent of Total	54.98				
		Total	37,333,775,624	51.85	9.56	29.48	9.11

* Rank is among total of 10,840 parent companies.

Figure 6-7.

Projected Change in Waste and Releases/Disposal from 1991 to 1994 for TRI Parent Companies with Large Releases/ Disposal in 1991

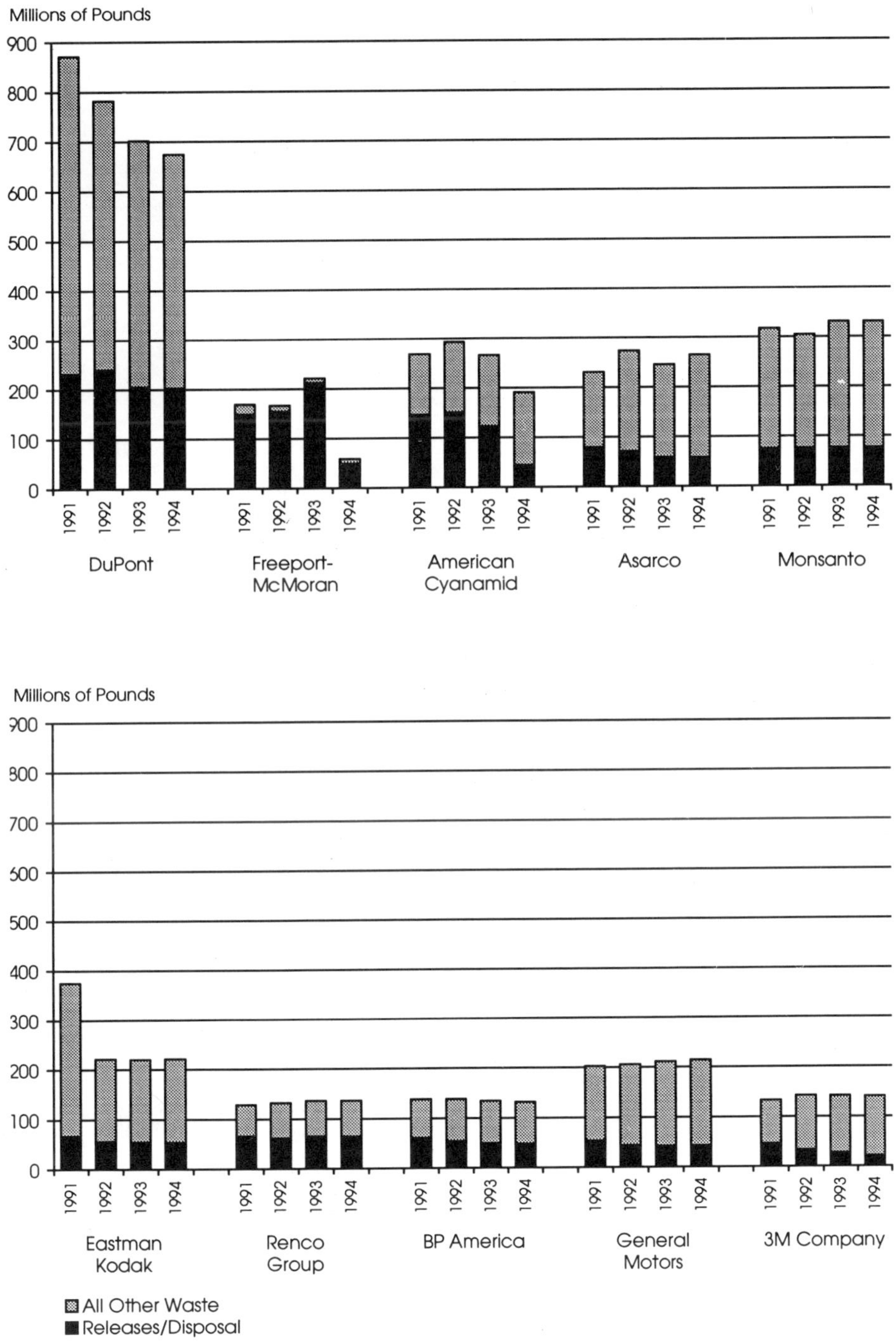

Table 6-12. The 50 TRI Parent Companies with Largest Amount Released/Disposed of in 1991: Actual and Projected Change 1991-1994*

Released/ Disposed of Rank* 1991 Rank	1992 Rank	Parent Company	1991 Released/ Disposed of Pounds	Change in Amount Released/Disposed of 1991 to 1992 Pounds	Percent	Change in Projected Amount Released/Disposed of 1992 to 1994 Pounds	Percent
1	1	DuPont	232,304,835	8,583,353	3.69	-37,813,922	-15.70
2	2	Freeport-McMoran Inc	149,683,106	5,714,466	3.82	-105,264,967	-67.74
3	3	American Cyanamid	146,937,759	4,186,326	2.85	-106,373,108	-70.39
4	5	Asarco Incorporated	79,567,915	-7,654,308	-9.62	-13,515,804	-18.79
5	4	Monsanto Company	76,030,994	401,415	0.53	876,771	1.15
6	8	Eastman Kodak Company	67,501,537	-11,342,928	-16.8	-2,280,544	-4.06
7	6	Renco Group Inc	66,465,019	-4,259,219	-6.41	2,946,801	4.74
8	10	BP America Inc	61,096,520	-6,718,822	-11.00	-6,140,850	-11.29
9	11	General Motors Corporation	53,713,427	-8,900,894	-16.57	-1,038,522	-2.32
10	15	3M Minnesota Mining & Mfg Co	46,918,373	-12,788,372	-27.26	-13,615,757	-39.89
11	12	Courtaulds United States Inc	43,231,126	794,365	1.84	-3,149,679	-7.15
12	7	Vulcan Materials Company	41,457,797	19,152,444	46.20	-52,661,201	-86.88
13	13	Sterling Chemicals Inc	36,751,872	441,078	1.20	-1,132,635	-3.05
14	14	Hoechst Celanese Corporation	36,448,835	-751,100	-2.06	-6,046,523	-16.94
15	9	Arcadian Corporation	36,187,699	18,377,871	50.78	-9,016,778	-16.52
16	17	Inland Steel Industries Inc	33,194,154	-1,656,302	-4.99	-27,052,312	-85.78
17	18	Ford Motor Company	30,569,399	-834,913	-2.73	390,314	1.31
18	20	Zeneca Holdings Inc	29,548,944	-3,422,948	-11.58	-9,117,141	-34.90
19	19	Occidental Petroleum Corp	29,419,283	-2,972,316	-10.10	-5,769,526	-21.82
20	21	International Paper Company	27,743,313	-2,244,765	-8.09	126,420	0.50
21	22	Phelps Dodge Corporation	26,621,209	-3,381,707	-12.70	5,507,022	23.70
22	23	Georgia-Pacific Corporation	23,986,125	-1,344,255	-5.60	-2,975,121	-13.14
23	16	Cabot Corporation	23,839,689	9,184,513	38.53	-4,761,013	-14.42
24	24	Magma Copper Company	23,680,400	-1,109,300	-4.68	-196,600	-0.87
25	25	Elf Aquitaine Inc	21,133,862	1,216,728	5.76	-8,700,471	-38.93
26	26	Lenzing Fibers Corp	21,022,210	499,905	2.38	3,500,000	16.26
27	32	General Electric Company	20,370,488	-5,241,980	-25.73	-3,460,312	-22.87
28	41	Unocal Corporation	20,311,967	-8,002,818	-39.40	-2,335,312	-18.97
29	27	Dow Chemical Company	18,601,720	-990,822	-5.33	351,462	2.00
30	28	Westvaco Corporation	17,712,365	-544,855	-3.08	-2,443,669	-14.23
31	30	Elkem Metals Company	17,599,964	-819,623	-4.66	-130,000	-0.77
32	96	Doe Run Company	16,988,973	-10,376,507	-61.08	3,094,594	46.80
33	36	Amoco Corporation	16,462,547	-2,987,013	-18.14	-485,998	-3.61
34	131	BASF Corporation	16,126,029	-11,718,316	-72.67	-1,327,042	-30.11
35	29	Shell Petroleum Inc	15,615,362	1,500,302	9.61	-5,267,775	-30.78
36	38	Exxon Corporation	14,950,399	-1,976,636	-13.22	-2,009,439	-15.49
37	45	Farmland Industries Inc	14,536,546	-2,535,517	-17.44	151,400	1.26
38	49	Mobil Corporation	13,887,719	-2,765,075	-19.91	-1,241,079	-11.16
39	44	Union Carbide Corporation	13,770,629	-1,725,275	-12.53	48,550	0.40
40	42	Allied-Signal Inc	13,740,395	-1,433,390	-10.43	-4,087,589	-33.21
41	221	Ahlstrom Filtration Inc	13,719,000	-11,490,400	-83.76	-1,000	-0.04
42	31	MGF Industries	13,336,400	2,533,600	19.00	-11,853,000	-74.69
43	56	NKK USA Corporation	13,304,860	-2,961,445	-22.26	1,644,442	15.90
44	58	Reynolds Metals Company	13,056,853	-3,296,586	-25.25	-384,027	-3.93
45	57	R R Donnelley & Sons Company	12,900,090	-2,804,616	-21.74	-890,537	-8.82
46	37	Harrisons & Crosfield America	12,749,394	647,274	5.08	8,296	0.06
47	39	Northwestern Steel & Wire Co	11,900,590	1,045,340	8.78	402,220	3.11
48	63	Wheeling-Pittsburgh Corp	11,889,180	-3,101,265	-26.08	-948,873	-10.8
49	47	Mississippi Chemical Corp	11,882,272	-479,703	-4.04	-6,433,536	-56.42
50	52	Maxwell Communication Corp	11,833,506	-1,046,914	-8.85	1,269,217	11.77
		Subtotal	1,822,302,650	-71,401,925	-3.92	-511,006,078	-29.19
		Percent of Total	51.83				
		Total	3,515,785,150	-114,398,980	-3.25	-685,272,807	-20.15

* Rank is among total of 10,840 parent companies.

decrease of 17 percent in chemicals released/disposed of from 1991 to 1992, resulting in a drop to 11th position. (Projections indicate that it will rise again to the 10th position in 1994.) The 3M company reported a 27 percent decrease, with further decreases projected for 1994. (See Figure 6-7 and Table 6-12.)

The 50 parent companies with the largest amount of waste released or disposed of in 1991 reported overall decreases of 4 percent from 1991 to 1992 and projected decreases of 29 percent from 1992 to 1994. These are somewhat larger than the average decrease for all TRI facilities from 1991 to 1992 (3 percent) and half again as large as the average projected decreases from 1992 to 1994 (20 percent for all TRI facilities). (See Table 6-12.)

For similar information about the 100 parent companies reporting the largest amounts of production-related waste to TRI in 1992, see Appendix O, Tables O-1 through O-4.

Source Reduction and Waste Minimization

Both TRI and BRS collect some information on source reduction, but neither includes specific data on the amount of a toxic constituent reduced at the source. The TRI Form R requires a facility only to report what *type* of source reduction activity, if any, it undertook during the reporting year. The BRS forms ask if source reduction activity was undertaken on a facility-wide basis and how much total waste was reduced at the source on a waste-stream basis. For TRI, 36 percent of the facilities reported some type of source reduction activity. For BRS, 47 percent of the facilities indicated they had begun or expanded some type of source reduction activity during the reporting period. For BRS facilities reporting manufacturing operations, that is, one or more SIC code from 20 to 39, the percent that reported undertaking source reduction activity was 54 percent. However, as described below, the amount of source reduction of waste accomplished was considerably smaller — less than 2 percent of the amount of BRS toxic waste was not generated due to source reduction.

Source Reduction Activities in TRI

While the TRI Form R asks whether or not a facility undertook source reduction activities for the TRI chemical during the year, it does not ask for the amount of pounds that waste was reduced due to the activities, so there is no way to quantify source reduction or to know what impact the activities actually had. Instead, what can be said about source reduction activity is 1) how many facilities are undertaking some source reduction and 2) whether those facilities reporting source reduction activity are decreasing production-related waste to a greater extent than facilities not reporting source reduction activity.

Environmental reports published by individual companies present another potential source of information on corporate source reduction activity. In the United States, these tend to illustrate and publicize company-wide data such as is

Figure 6-8.

Source Reduction Activity by Industry, Percent of TRI Production-related Waste on Forms with and without Source Reduction Activity Reported, 1992

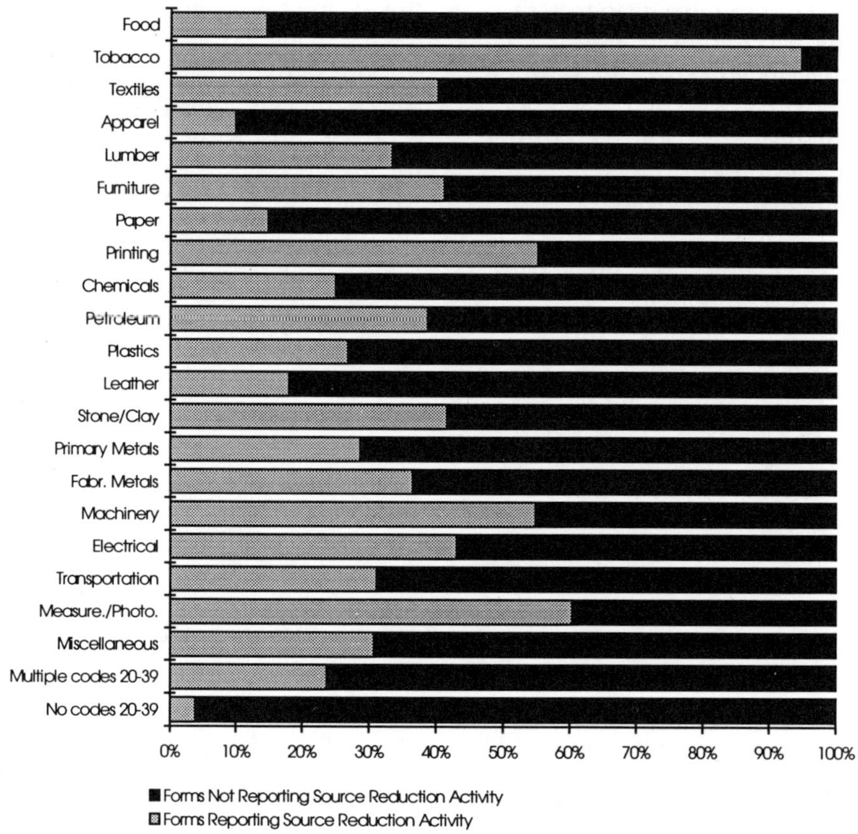

reported to TRI; none provides sufficient quantitative data to permit actual measurement of source reduction. (See Box 6-A.)

Source Reduction Activity by Industry

Overall, 27 percent of the 1992 production-related waste was reported on TRI forms that indicated some source reduction activity and 73 percent on forms without an indication of source reduction. However, facilities in the Tobacco, Measuring/Photographic, Printing, and Machinery industries each reported more than half of their production-related waste subject to source reduction activities, while facilities in the Apparel, Paper, and Leather industries reported less than a quarter of their production-related waste subject to source reduction activities. (See Figure 6-8 and Appendix N, Table N-1.)

Source Reduction Activity and Waste Generation by Industry

One might assume that source reduction activity would result in decreased waste generation, although that is not always the case for a variety of reasons.[1] Overall, the forms reporting source reduction activity in 1992 were associated with a small decrease (0.3 percent) in the generation of production-related waste between 1991 and 1992, and those forms projected another small decrease (0.16 percent) between 1992 and 1994. On the other hand, the forms reporting no source reduction activity in 1992 were associated with a 4 percent increase in 1991-1992 waste generation and projected a further 1 percent increase between 1992 and 1994. In 16 of the 22 industry groups, forms reporting no source reduction activity reported a smaller decrease in their production-related waste from 1991 to 1992 (or a larger increase in their waste) than forms indicating some source reduction activity. (See Figure 6-9 and Appendix N, Table N-1.)

Facilities of the Lumber and Paper industries reporting source reduction activity achieved the largest percentage reductions in waste in this period among industry groups (reductions of 36 percent and 23 percent, respectively). The Medite Company (a Lumber industry facility) in Las Vegas, New Mexico, reported decreases in total production-related waste from 6.8 million pounds to 578,000 pounds and reported undertaking source reduction activities to improve operating practices and finish-application techniques and change product specifications in its use of formaldehyde. Two Paper industry facilities together account for 119.9 million pounds of decrease in total production-related waste from 1991 to 1992. ITT Rayonier Company in Jesup, Georgia, installed new chlorine dioxide production equipment, enabling it to reduce its on-site recycling of sulfuric acid. Champion International Corporation in Courtland, Alabama, reduced both chlorine and chloroform waste through process modifications.

A similar picture emerges for projected waste generation. Forms with source reduction activity reported for 1992 are projecting greater reductions in production-related wastes from 1992 to 1994, compared to forms not reporting source reduction activity, in 16 of the 22 industry groups. Overall, a *decrease* in production-related waste of 0.2 percent is projected on forms reporting source reduction activity, compared to an *increase* of 0.5 percent on forms not reporting source reduction activity. The industry groups whose forms reporting source reduction activity in 1992 project the largest 1992-1994 *percentage decreases* in production-related waste are the Tobacco, Leather, and Apparel industries. (See Figure 6-10.) A Leather industry facility, Garden State Tanning in Fleetwood, Pennsylvania, projects that its total production-related waste will decrease from 3.6 million pounds to 401,000 pounds from 1992 to 1994. This facility reports using substitute coating materials as its source reduction activity.

[1] If overall production at a facility were increasing, for example, with a related increase in waste generation, source reduction activities might keep the increase from being potentially higher, yet waste generation could still increase.

Figure 6-9.

Percent Change in TRI Production-related Waste by Industry, 1991-1992

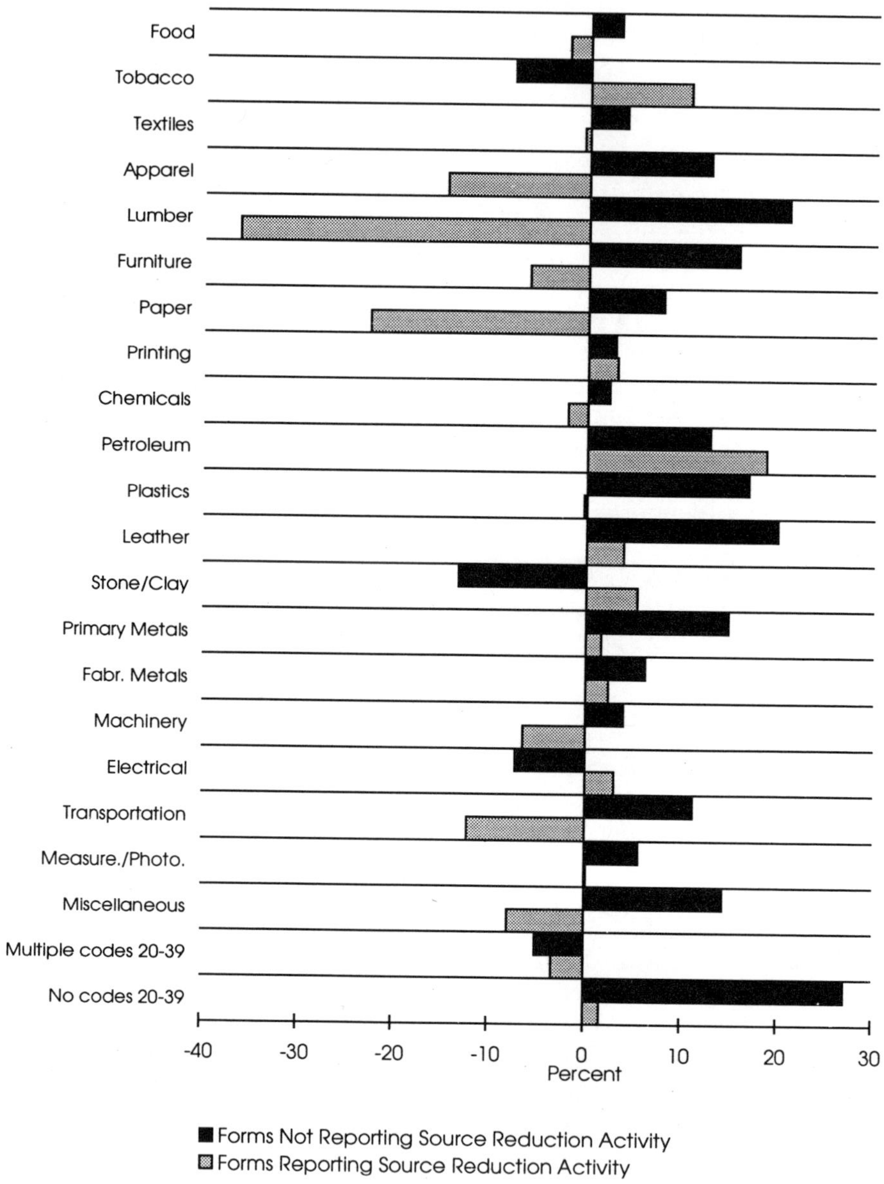

Figure 6-10.

Percent Change in TRI Production-related Waste by Industry, Projected, 1992-1994

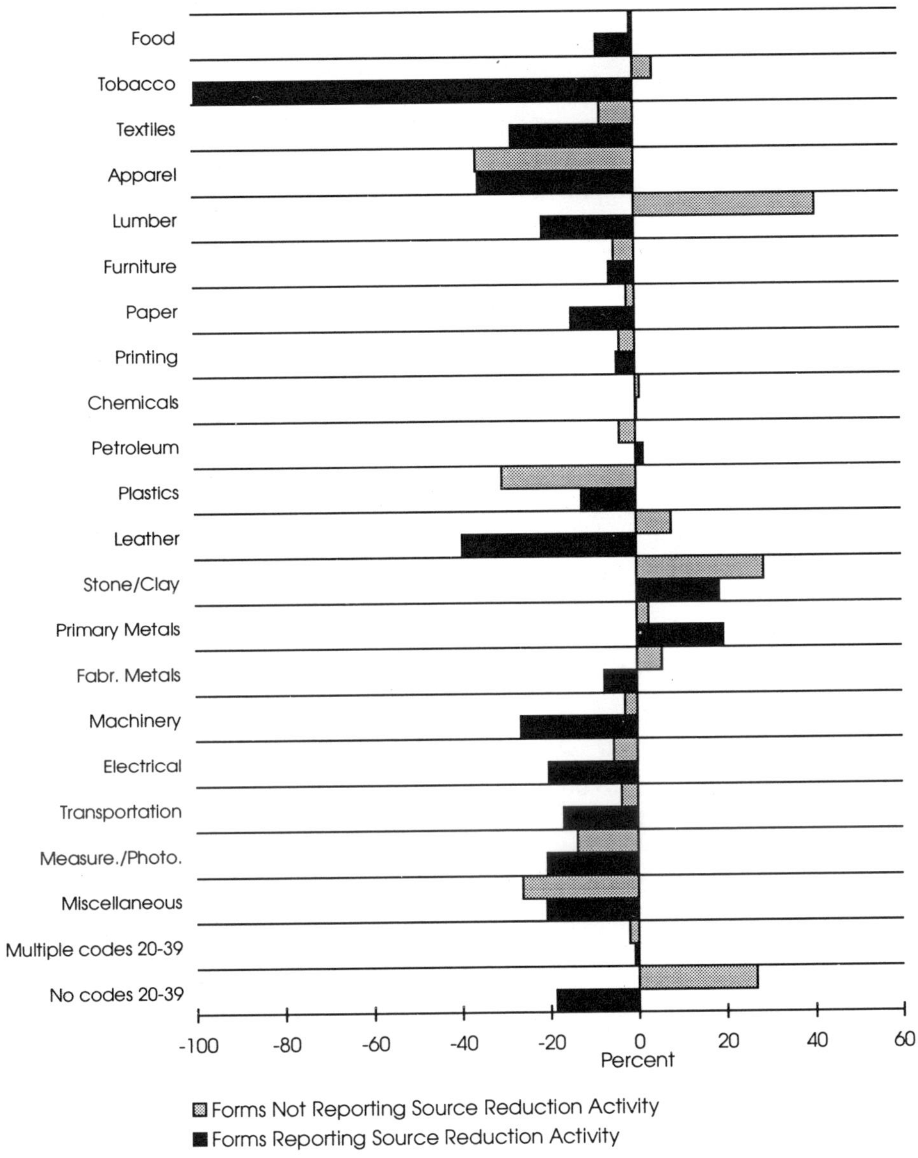

RCRA Waste Minimization Reporting

Unlike TRI, the BRS Form GM requires each facility to report directly on the reporting form how much it reduced each of its waste streams by new source reduction and on-site recycling activities during the report year.[m] Both types of activities fall under the heading of "waste minimization" on the reporting form. (See Appendix D.) The reports for 1991 show very little impact, on a percentage basis, on waste generation by source reduction or new recycling activities.

Reporting of Source Reduction to BRS

In 1991 facilities reported on the BRS forms that they had reduced waste generation by 11.8 billion pounds through source reduction. This was just 1 percent of all reported waste generation. Only the Textile and Tobacco industries reported substantial source reduction on a percentage basis: 26 percent and 23 percent, respectively. In absolute terms, however, these two industries combined had less than a 10th of the source reduction reported by the Chemical industry. Its 3.3 billion pounds of source reduction represented less than 1 percent of its waste generation. Only three other industries reported over a billion pounds of source reduction: the Electrical industry, the Fabricated Metals industry, and the Waste Management industry (which is included in the "No codes SIC 20-39" category). (See Table 6-13.)

Reporting of Waste Minimization Due to New Recycling Activity

The Primary Metals industry reported the largest absolute amount of toxic waste recycled due to new waste minimization activities, 95.3 million pounds, or 31 percent of the total amount reported by all industries. The only industry reporting new waste minimization activities that amounted to more than 1 percent of its waste generation was the Tobacco industry, whose facilities reported 42,000 pounds of recycled waste due to waste minimization, or 12 percent of its total quantity of toxic waste generated. (See Table 6-13.)

[m] See Appendix D for BRS definitions of source reduction, recycling, and waste minimization.

Table 6-13. BRS Quantities of Toxic Waste Generated, Source Reduction, and Recycling, by Industry, 1991

SIC Code	Industry	1991 Total Quantity of Toxic Waste Generated	Reductions due to New Source Reduction Activity		Reductions due to New Recycling Activity	
		Pounds	Pounds	Percent	Pounds	Percent
20	Food	88,710,920	43,260	0.05	1,700	0.00
21	Tobacco	343,200	79,360	23.12	41,800	12.18
22	Textiles	1,079,880,480	279,298,120	25.86	164,400	0.02
23	Apparel	68,752,020	1,846,620	2.69	1,360	0.00
24	Lumber	335,354,620	2,126,940	0.63	735,620	0.22
25	Furniture	199,752,520	1,460,320	0.73	365,860	0.18
26	Paper	3,993,351,820	1,625,180	0.04	390,580	0.01
27	Printing	217,093,120	8,814,580	4.06	1,452,140	0.67
28	Chemicals	388,570,517,800	3,283,166,640	0.84	66,715,140	0.02
29	Petroleum	270,856,101,200	506,544,660	0.19	58,947,880	0.02
30	Plastics	376,091,940	8,362,120	2.22	1,306,380	0.35
31	Leather	203,725,540	1,035,660	0.51	8,760	0.00
32	Stone/Clay	362,430,800	17,192,340	4.74	2,801,120	0.77
33	Primary Metals	30,608,272,760	700,729,060	2.29	95,334,920	0.31
34	Fabr. Metals	40,687,820,920	1,285,503,060	3.16	34,734,940	0.09
35	Machinery	2,910,808,380	29,412,460	1.01	1,726,880	0.06
36	Electrical	33,679,602,720	1,416,287,900	4.21	12,242,280	0.04
37	Transportation	18,618,250,440	623,525,220	3.35	11,501,200	0.06
38	Measure./Photo.	85,061,296,940	28,794,520	0.03	1,505,960	0.00
39	Miscellaneous	6,002,867,540	2,217,740	0.04	294,960	0.00
	No Codes 20-39	64,322,724,440	3,582,439,740	5.57	21,913,640	0.03
	Total	948,243,750,120	11,780,505,500	1.24	312,187,520	0.03

1 Dow Chemical Company, *1993 Environment, Health, and Safety Report;* Letter from J. B. Martin, Director of Environmental Affairs to EPA's 33/50 Program, DCN 33-50-91001569, August 21, 1994,

2 Monsanto Company, *1993 Environmental Annual Review.*

3 Letter from E. P. Blanchard, Jr., Vice Chairman of the Board, DuPont, to EPA's 33/50 Program, DCN 33-50-91000118, April 26, 1991.

4 U.S. Environmental Protection Agency, *Pollution Prevention 1991: Progress on Reducing Industrial Pollutants,* EPA 21P-3003, October 1991, 40-41.

5 Conversation with Nick Bock, Kerr McGee Corporation, September 15, 1994.

Chapter 7

Geography and Waste

Introduction

Geographical analyses of waste generation and management are important nationally, regionally, and locally. Federal officials are interested in learning which states or regions have the greatest toxic waste problem. Meanwhile, residents of communities or officials in cities, counties, or states, concerned about toxic chemical exposures must consider the regional or local concentration of industries, the types of chemical wastes they generate, and how those wastes are managed.

There are many more geographical representations of the data than can be covered in this edition of *Toxics Watch*. This chapter examines waste generation and their environmental management nationally, by state and county, to provide examples of the types of geography-driven analyses that can be done at this level with data from the Toxics Release Inventory (TRI) and from the Biennial Reporting System (BRS) under the Resource Conservation and Recovery Act (RCRA). Other types of analyses, which are likely subjects of future *Toxics Watch* reports or which readers can pursue themselves, include: analyses on a watershed or air-shed basis, co-analyses with demographic data (e.g., toxic chemical releases per capita or on the basis of population density), and analyses of facilities upwind or upstream of political jurisdictions. With facility data in conjunction with good locational coordinates (e.g., latitude and longitude), as is the case for TRI and BRS, the possibilities are very broad for geographical analyses.

Summary of Findings

- Although every state has both TRI and BRS facilities within its borders, facilities generating the largest amounts of toxic chemicals are concentrated in only a few states. TRI reports for 1992 and BRS reports for 1991, the latest years for which data are publicly available, document clearly that Texas and Louisiana continue to be the states with the largest amounts of toxic waste.
- For TRI chemicals in waste released on site and transferred off site, the least desirable environmental management methods, Louisiana, with one-quarter the number of facilities of Texas had 84 percent of the

amount of Texas' releases and transfers. For both states, total releases and transfers increased between 1991 and 1992.

- Releases and transfers of TRI chemicals remain concentrated in relatively few of the approximately 3,000 counties in the nation. The 100 counties with the largest amount of releases and transfers accounted for 60 percent of the national total in 1992.
- Texas, Mississippi, and Louisiana are the states generating the largest amounts of TRI chemicals as production-related waste. In 1992 Texas is first-ranked because of the large number of facilities (1,238) located there, as well as the large amounts of waste they generated. Mississippi ranks second mainly because one of its 191 facilities (First Chemical in Pascagoula) had very large amounts of waste generation. Louisiana is third-ranked because its 326 facilities generated, on average, large amounts of waste per facility.
- Facilities in Texas and Louisiana reported the largest increases in total TRI production-related waste from 1991 to 1992, while facilities in Georgia and New Jersey reported the largest decreases.
- Facilities in Texas projected the largest increase in total TRI production-related waste from 1992 to 1994, and facilities in Louisiana projected the largest decrease. These projections are expected to have only a slight effect on the future ranking of states for production-related waste.
- Source reduction activity was reported on TRI chemical forms with the largest percentage of production-related waste in Connecticut (81 percent) and Nevada (73 percent). However, only 11 states had more than half of their waste amounts associated with forms that reported some source reduction activities.
- Facilities in Texas reported the largest amount of toxic waste generated under RCRA (as well as TRI). New York had the second largest amount of RCRA toxic waste, because of one facility (Eastman Kodak's Kodak Park facility in Rochester).
- Generally, rankings and changes in the RCRA waste generation data are due to single facilities, because the 50 facilities reporting the largest amounts of toxic waste generated to BRS accounted for 72 percent of all BRS toxic waste. Sixteen of these facilities are located in Texas.

TRI Releases and Transfers, 1988-1992

As shown in Chapter 4, there has been a steady decrease in on-site releases from facilities reporting to TRI every year since 1987. A similar decrease in off-site transfers of toxic chemicals in waste has ceased, however, and an increase was reported between 1991 and 1992. This increase comes primarily from increases in transfers of waste off site to treatment locations. From 1988 to 1992, for those chemicals and reporting categories required in both those years, total releases and transfers decreased by 35 percent. (Releases decreased just slightly more than transfers, on a percentage basis.) From 1991 to 1992, releases decreased by 6 percent, but off-site transfers increased by 2 percent.[a] (See Chapter 4, Table 4-1.)

The success of facilities in a particular state in reducing releases and transfers of TRI chemicals in waste from 1988 to 1992 varies. Fifty of the 54 states and other jurisdictions reported decreases to TRI, and among those, Texas and Louisiana have decreased their totals by the largest amount — Texas by 375.0 million pounds and Louisiana by 273.4 million pounds. Yet they remain the states with the largest amounts of releases and transfers. (See Table 7-1.)

The state with the greatest percentage decrease from 1988 to 1992 is Wyoming, whose facilities reported an overall decrease of 67 percent (30.4 million pounds). Hawaii and American Samoa reported large percentage decreases of 64 and 62 percent, respectively; because these states have few TRI facilities, however, the reduction in pounds was small.

Four more reporting jurisdictions (South Carolina, Alabama, Mississippi, and the Virgin Islands) reported decreases of less than 10 percent. The slim progress of facilities in Alabama and Missouri in decreasing their waste has moved these states up in rank to among the top 10 in 1992, from 16th and 12th, respectively, in 1988. They took the places of California and Virginia, which have moved out of the top 10 by 1992. (See Map 7-1 and Table 7-1.)

Four states in all (Montana, North Dakota, Nevada, and South Dakota) reported increases from 1988 to 1992. Montana reported the largest increase, 8.6 million pounds (24 percent).

TRI Releases and Transfers, 1991-1992

Starting in 1991, TRI required reporting on recycling and energy recovery in addition to the original categories of releases and transfers. (See Chapter 4.) Looking at the expanded categories of releases and transfers and including chemicals added to the original TRI list, total releases decreased 7 percent from 1991 to 1992, while off-site transfers of chemicals in waste increased by 17 percent, mainly due to addition of transfers to off-site recycling, treatment, and energy recovery. The net result of these changes is that total releases and transfers increased by 6 percent. (See Chapter 4, Table 4-2.)

Total releases and transfers, including transfers to off-site recycling, treatment, and energy recovery, increased between 1991

[a] Because these data include only those chemicals and reporting categories required in both 1988 and 1992, these 1991-1992 comparisons do not include the additional categories of transfers for recycling and energy recovery added to TRI reporting in 1991. See next section for the full data for 1991 and 1992.

*Table 7-1. TRI Releases and Transfers by State, 1988 and 1992**

	1988 Total Releases and Transfers		1992 Total Releases and Transfers		Change 1988-1992	
State	**Pounds**	**Rank**	**Pounds**	**Rank**	**Pounds**	**Percent**
	Pounds		Pounds		Pounds	Percent
Alabama	140,594,548	16	132,492,913	10	-8,101,635	-5.76
Alaska	27,517,867	39	14,857,319	41	-12,660,548	-46.01
American Samoa	29,500	53	11,240	53	-18,260	-61.90
Arizona	76,448,298	25	48,896,473	25	-27,551,825	-36.04
Arkansas	77,648,091	24	50,327,955	24	-27,320,136	-35.18
California	203,833,344	9	102,664,914	14	-101,168,430	-49.63
Colorado	20,680,147	42	9,085,695	43	-11,594,452	-56.07
Connecticut	54,414,977	31	25,323,183	34	-29,091,794	-53.46
Delaware	15,816,523	45	8,615,059	44	-7,201,464	-45.53
District of Columbia	1,000	54	0	54	-1,000	-100.00
Florida	158,180,687	14	102,560,364	15	-55,620,323	-35.16
Georgia	134,163,264	18	70,611,752	23	-63,551,512	-47.37
Hawaii	2,990,331	49	1,067,482	52	-1,922,849	-64.30
Idaho	18,072,755	43	10,413,867	42	-7,658,888	-42.38
Illinois	258,359,897	6	220,995,601	5	-37,364,296	-14.46
Indiana	281,927,004	4	183,337,251	6	-98,589,753	-34.97
Iowa	60,669,085	29	48,154,851	26	-12,514,234	-20.63
Kansas	131,484,061	19	103,393,048	13	-28,091,013	-21.36
Kentucky	122,067,986	21	83,978,629	19	-38,089,357	-31.20
Louisiana	745,371,846	2	471,971,271	2	-273,400,575	-36.68
Maine	22,912,230	41	16,829,975	39	-6,082,255	-26.55
Maryland	34,371,956	36	19,768,853	38	-14,603,103	-42.49
Massachusetts	67,086,855	27	26,925,231	33	-40,161,624	-59.87
Michigan	209,962,258	8	139,528,386	8	-70,433,872	-33.55
Minnesota	73,090,960	26	39,843,506	28	-33,247,454	-45.49
Mississippi	128,571,388	20	121,013,357	11	-7,558,031	-5.88
Missouri	171,572,238	12	152,173,327	7	-19,398,911	-11.31
Montana	35,472,080	35	44,080,246	27	8,608,166	24.27
Nebraska	24,414,305	40	21,666,136	36	-2,748,169	-11.26
Nevada	3,239,020	47	3,739,733	47	500,713	15.46
New Hampshire	15,959,164	44	7,448,838	45	-8,510,326	-53.33
New Jersey	168,276,631	13	78,813,635	21	-89,462,996	-53.16
New Mexico	31,262,176	37	20,573,558	37	-10,688,618	-34.19
New York	178,286,359	11	81,705,267	20	-96,581,092	-54.17
North Carolina	143,232,323	15	117,284,616	12	-25,947,707	-18.12
North Dakota	1,523,223	52	2,219,507	49	696,284	45.71
Ohio	374,440,810	3	223,626,418	4	-150,814,392	-40.28
Oklahoma	56,600,658	30	36,832,978	29	-19,767,680	-34.92
Oregon	35,484,204	34	27,625,720	32	-7,858,484	-22.15
Pennsylvania	217,355,284	7	136,234,640	9	-81,120,644	-37.32
Puerto Rico	27,799,443	38	22,964,425	35	-4,835,018	-17.39
Rhode Island	15,003,246	46	6,496,509	46	-8,506,737	-56.70
South Carolina	86,585,072	23	84,038,807	18	-2,546,265	-2.94
South Dakota	3,132,696	48	3,250,049	48	117,353	3.75
Tennessee	263,086,028	5	234,686,506	3	-28,399,522	-10.79
Texas	892,454,679	1	517,441,011	1	-375,013,668	-42.02
Utah	138,867,853	17	84,363,708	17	-54,504,145	-39.25
Vermont	2,573,605	50	1,112,390	51	-1,461,215	-56.78
Virgin Islands	1,850,198	51	1,724,133	50	-126,065	-6.81
Virginia	203,649,727	10	90,760,008	16	-112,889,719	-55.43
Washington	52,554,800	32	29,000,572	31	-23,554,228	-44.82
West Virginia	66,195,927	28	31,115,622	30	-35,080,305	-52.99
Wisconsin	103,274,748	22	71,836,745	22	-31,438,003	-30.44
Wyoming	45,459,973	33	15,064,207	40	-30,395,766	-66.86
Total	6,425,873,328		4,200,547,486		-2,225,325,842	-34.63

* Excludes delisted chemicals and aluminum oxide and excludes off-site transfers to recycling and energy recovery.

Map 7-1.

TRI Releases and Transfers by State, Percent Change, 1988 to 1992

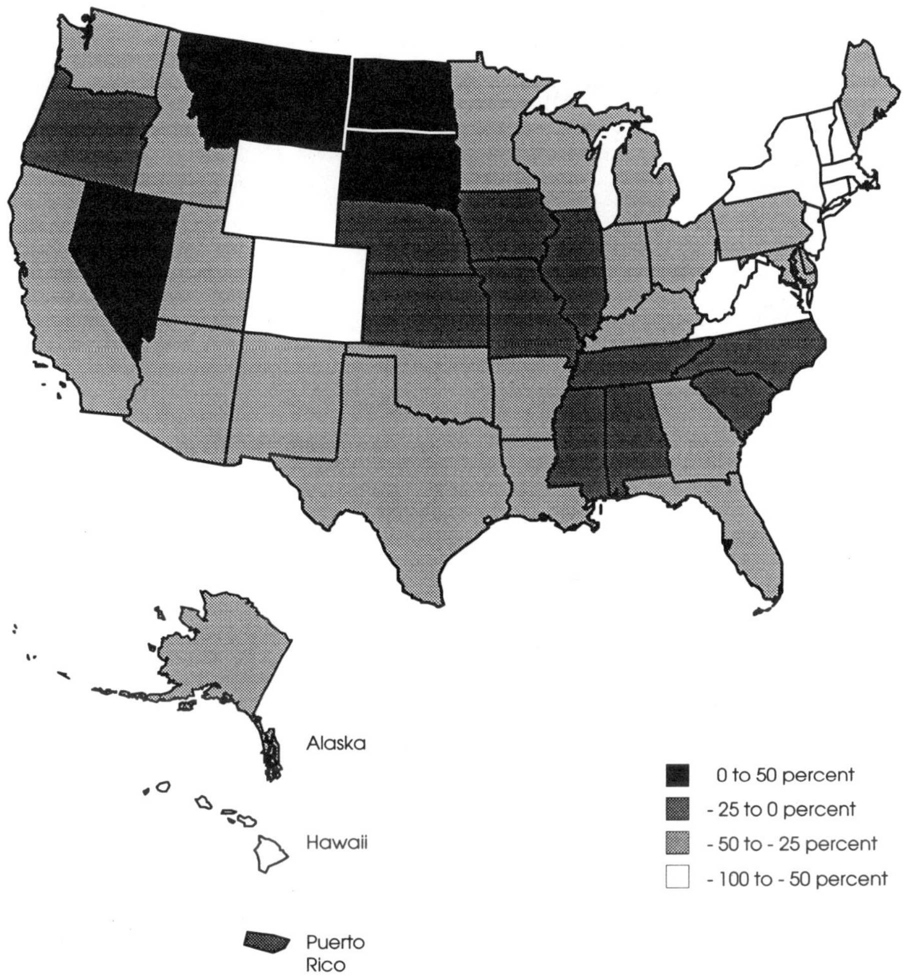

Excludes delisted chemicals and aluminum oxide. Excludes off-site transfers to recycling and energy recovery.

and 1992 in 25 of the 54 states and other reporting jurisdictions. Missouri facilities reported the largest overall increase of 141 percent (203.3 million pounds) and Vermont facilities reported the second highest increase of 47 percent (2.0 million pounds). The large increase in Missouri put it into the top 10 for total releases and transfers. Missouri ranked 6th in 1992, up from 18th in 1991.

In 28 reporting jurisdictions, total releases and transfers decreased, with American Samoa's two facilities reporting the largest combined decrease of 49 percent (11,000 pounds) and New Mexico facilities reporting a total decrease of 48 percent (19.3 million pounds). Ohio's lesser percentage decrease (13 percent) resulted in the largest absolute change, a decrease of 64.4 million pounds. (See Map 7-2 and Table 7-2.)

Map 7-2.

TRI Releases and Transfers by State, Percent Change, 1991 to 1992

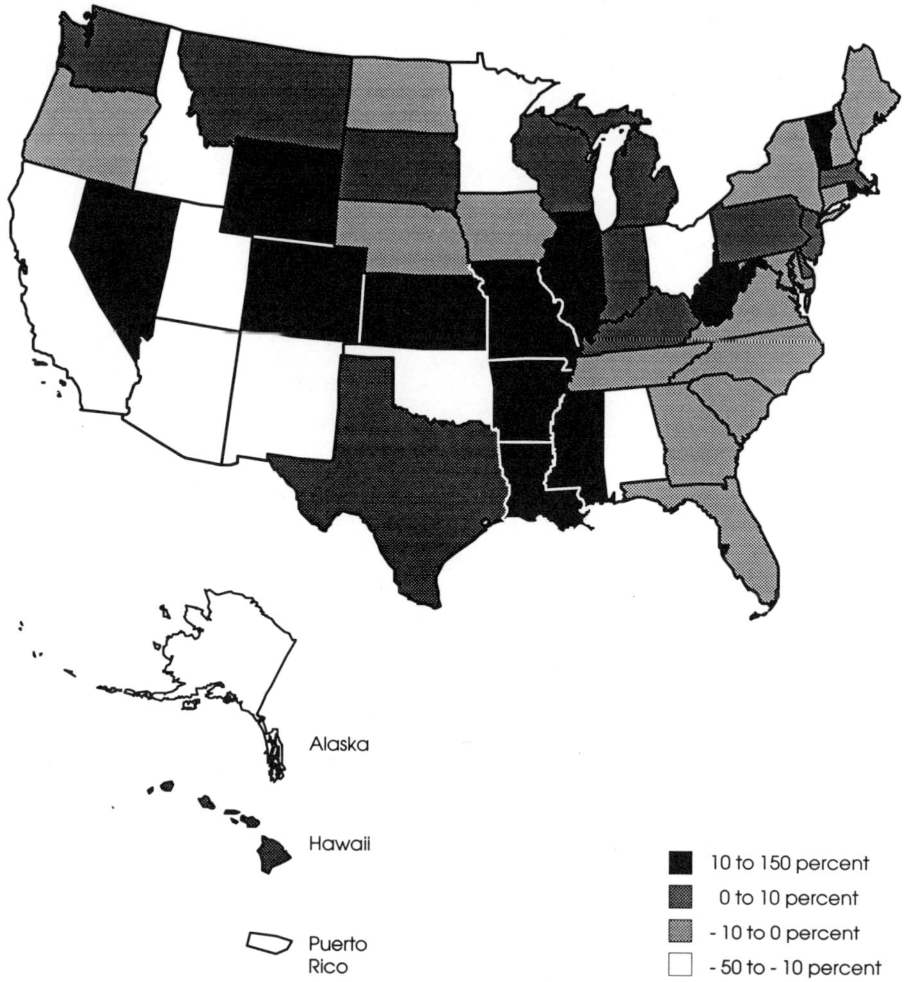

Lake County, Indiana, ranked number one in the nation for total releases and transfers in 1992; Texas' Harris County was the second-ranked county; and Missouri's Iron County was third. For Indiana and Missouri, the one county is the major contributor to the state's overall high ranking. For Louisiana, second only to Texas for total TRI releases and transfers, four of its parishes rank among the top 10 counties. The 100 counties with the largest reported releases and transfers accounted for almost 60 percent of the total for the nation. (See Map 7-3 and Table 7-3.)

Table 7-2. TRI Releases and Transfers by State, 1991-1992

	1991 Total Releases and Transfers		1992 Total Releases and Transfers		Change 1991-1992	
State	**Pounds** Pounds	**Rank**	**Pounds** Pounds	**Rank**	**Pounds** Pounds	**Percent** Percent
Alabama	219,836,692	11	182,021,950	14	-37,814,742	-17.20
Alaska	18,028,754	41	15,099,692	43	-2,929,062	-16.25
American Samoa	22,000	53	11,240	53	-10,760	-48.91
Arizona	89,376,241	26	75,494,091	27	-13,882,150	-15.53
Arkansas	90,179,373	25	108,640,278	24	18,460,905	20.47
California	279,230,949	8	241,006,792	10	-38,224,157	-13.69
Colorado	18,467,863	40	20,465,888	39	1,998,025	10.82
Connecticut	55,723,437	31	51,380,196	32	-4,343,241	-7.79
Delaware	17,791,447	42	17,813,460	41	22,013	0.12
Florida	132,286,712	20	127,869,613	20	-4,417,099	-3.34
Georgia	145,732,831	17	132,744,795	19	-12,988,036	-8.91
Hawaii	999,710	52	1,094,231	52	94,521	9.45
Idaho	12,702,261	45	11,062,997	46	-1,639,264	-12.91
Illinois	322,851,273	6	416,136,327	5	93,285,054	28.89
Indiana	508,704,088	4	544,443,897	3	35,739,809	7.03
Iowa	72,290,084	28	68,828,241	28	-3,461,843	-4.79
Kansas	123,626,195	22	150,645,445	17	27,019,250	21.86
Kentucky	146,713,636	16	159,485,621	16	12,771,985	8.71
Louisiana	540,230,123	2	712,459,678	2	172,229,555	31.88
Maine	21,645,140	39	20,074,168	40	-1,570,972	-7.26
Maryland	47,635,653	34	45,057,859	34	-2,577,794	-5.41
Massachusetts	54,294,607	32	55,568,138	30	1,273,531	2.35
Michigan	324,944,461	5	336,313,020	7	11,368,559	3.50
Minnesota	72,716,478	27	63,618,226	29	-9,098,252	-12.51
Mississippi	166,168,075	14	188,540,173	13	22,372,098	13.46
Missouri	143,949,537	18	347,267,089	6	203,317,552	141.24
Montana	44,395,302	35	46,679,134	33	2,283,832	5.14
Nebraska	39,518,788	38	37,025,619	37	-2,493,169	-6.31
Nevada	3,788,858	48	4,218,621	48	429,763	11.34
New Hampshire	15,833,684	43	14,906,296	45	-927,388	-5.86
New Jersey	203,843,408	12	212,891,242	12	9,047,834	4.44
New Mexico	40,567,768	37	21,223,540	38	-19,344,228	-47.68
New York	150,807,625	15	146,729,231	18	-4,078,394	-2.70
North Carolina	246,032,765	10	239,608,345	11	-6,424,420	-2.61
North Dakota	2,435,353	50	2,394,911	50	-40,442	-1.66
Ohio	514,856,078	3	450,431,768	4	-64,424,310	-12.51
Oklahoma	63,514,589	30	51,718,647	31	-11,795,942	-18.57
Oregon	41,360,778	36	41,010,160	36	-350,618	-0.85
Pennsylvania	268,932,059	9	275,285,244	9	6,353,185	2.36
Puerto Rico	51,901,179	33	44,895,917	35	-7,005,262	-13.50
Rhode Island	14,965,828	44	17,609,483	42	2,643,655	17.66
South Carolina	169,847,372	13	166,897,836	15	-2,949,536	-1.74
South Dakota	3,507,832	49	3,774,525	49	266,693	7.60
Tennessee	308,462,012	7	298,770,598	8	-9,691,414	-3.14
Texas	763,514,590	1	814,283,272	1	50,768,682	6.65
Utah	131,694,935	21	117,076,656	23	-14,618,279	-11.10
Vermont	4,077,760	47	5,981,678	47	1,903,918	46.69
Virgin Islands	1,897,077	51	1,724,836	51	-172,241	-9.08
Virginia	134,725,148	19	124,129,832	21	-10,595,316	-7.86
Washington	102,069,400	24	103,446,127	25	1,376,727	1.35
West Virginia	70,125,685	29	78,649,224	26	8,523,539	12.15
Wisconsin	111,188,114	23	119,673,563	22	8,485,449	7.63
Wyoming	11,983,948	46	15,071,960	44	3,088,012	25.77
Total	7,141,995,555		7,549,251,370		407,255,815	5.70

Map 7-3.

The 100 Counties with Largest Total TRI Releases and Transfers, 1992

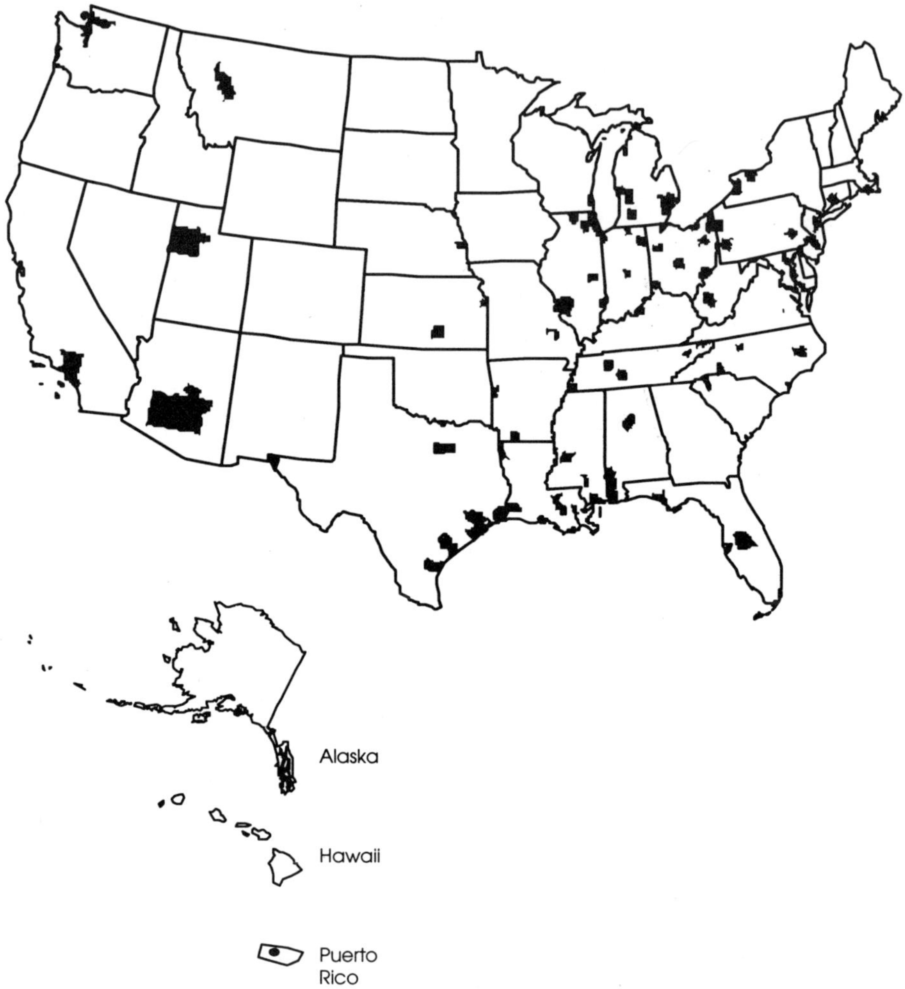

Table 7-3. The 100 Counties with Largest Total TRI Releases and Transfers, 1992

Rank	State	County	Total Releases and Transfers Pounds	Rank	State	County	Total Releases and Transfers Pounds
1	IN	Lake	299,225,360	51	OH	Allen	26,505,148
2	TX	Harris	237,171,889	52	OH	Hamilton	26,504,837
3	MO	Iron	219,431,309	53	CA	Orange	26,107,525
4	LA	Jefferson	188,045,711	54	AL	Jefferson	26,060,851
5	LA	Calcasieu	182,567,916	55	OH	Trumbull	25,711,374
6	LA	St James	149,872,790	56	NJ	Burlington	25,589,498
7	CA	Los Angeles	124,572,665	57	IL	Douglas	24,826,421
8	MI	Wayne	97,986,894	58	OH	Washington	24,697,782
9	TX	El Paso	81,021,487	59	TN	Hamblen	24,475,398
10	LA	Ascension	79,279,996	60	TX	Orange	24,005,135
11	IL	Cook	78,284,018	61	AZ	Pinal	23,820,018
12	KS	Sedgwick	75,744,711	62	MO	Saint Louis City	23,277,421
13	TX	Brazoria	75,284,586	63	IL	Winnebago	23,249,772
14	TX	Jefferson	71,754,092	64	TX	Tarrant	22,565,804
15	NJ	Middlesex	71,537,183	65	NJ	Essex	22,446,611
16	AL	Mobile	69,890,831	66	NJ	Bergen	22,409,688
17	TX	Galveston	67,815,768	67	IN	Marion	22,196,051
18	WA	Skagit	63,739,374	68	OH	Franklin	21,306,174
19	UT	Tooele	60,992,587	69	CT	New Haven	21,074,389
20	KY	Jefferson	59,955,006	70	AR	Columbia	20,983,334
21	MS	Harrison	56,506,094	71	IL	Madison	20,655,376
22	TN	Humphreys	53,919,080	72	PA	Mercer	19,648,290
23	OH	Stark	50,913,419	73	NY	Monroe	19,396,746
24	IL	Lawrence	50,138,465	74	IL	Lake	19,351,269
25	UT	Salt Lake	48,118,087	75	AZ	Maricopa	18,662,488
26	TX	Calhoun	45,123,517	76	NJ	Union	18,453,792
27	SC	Greenville	44,813,622	77	KY	Carroll	18,397,598
28	IL	St Clair	43,885,666	78	MI	Muskegon	18,138,147
29	MT	Lewis and Clark	43,474,013	79	NE	Douglas	17,897,525
30	OH	Cuyahoga	40,774,532	80	PR	Barceloneta	17,626,616
31	TN	Shelby	40,028,791	81	MI	Kent	17,472,485
32	NC	Forsyth	39,241,721	82	TX	Dallas	17,181,574
33	TN	Maury	38,492,258	83	OH	Ashtabula	17,132,406
34	TN	Sullivan	37,932,725	84	KS	Johnson	16,866,310
35	WV	Kanawha	37,855,518	85	MI	Macomb	16,481,335
36	IL	Kane	36,829,957	86	DE	New Castle	16,461,444
37	MI	Kalamazoo	34,616,360	87	FL	Bay	16,337,958
38	PA	Allegheny	34,302,010	88	PA	Philadelphia	16,150,773
39	FL	Polk	34,134,427	89	MD	Baltimore	16,137,084
40	MS	Lamar	33,757,792	90	IN	Elkhart	16,075,925
41	TX	Victoria	33,506,441	91	TX	Nueces	16,065,283
42	NC	Cleveland	32,460,998	92	NC	New Hanover	15,951,895
43	WI	Milwaukee	29,010,759	93	AL	Washington	15,645,410
44	AZ	Gila	28,879,900	94	AR	Sebastian	15,590,734
45	PA	Berks	28,725,590	95	MD	Baltimore City	15,323,812
46	LA	East Baton Rouge	28,194,764	96	NC	Beaufort	15,211,131
47	IN	Allen	28,084,510	97	MS	Hinds	15,018,615
48	VA	Hopewell City	27,768,283	98	NY	Erie	14,998,248
49	MO	St Louis	26,637,281	99	OH	Lucas	14,612,346
50	MI	Oakland	26,550,368	100	LA	Caddo	14,568,752
						Subtotal	4,474,175,719
						Percent of Total	59.27
						Total	7,549,251,370

Pollution Prevention Act Data in TRI

Also beginning in 1991, expanded reporting requirements have obligated facilities to report, in addition to how much of the toxic chemical is being released on site or transferred off site in waste, how much of the chemical they generate as waste. Seven types of waste can be added up to give the total production-related waste generated by a facility: the quantity recycled on and off site, used for energy recovery on and off site, treated on and off site, and released on site or disposed of off site. Each year the facility must report how much production-related waste was generated the year before as well as the current year; it must also provide projections for the following two years. (See Chapter 4.)

TRI Production-related Waste, 1992

Texas facilities reported the largest total amount of production-related waste in 1992, 7.5 billion pounds, as they had reported the largest total amount of releases and transfers. Except for Mississippi, the five states with the largest production-related waste are also the five with the largest releases and transfers. Indiana ranked third for total releases and transfers but ranked ninth for total production-related waste. (See Tables 7-2 and 7-4.)

Mississippi is in the top five for production-related waste because of one facility, First Chemical in Pascagoula, that reported 4.0 billion pounds of production-related waste, which amounted to 88 percent of that state's total. (Since most of the facility's waste was reported as on-site recycling, Mississippi was not among the top five states for total releases and off-site transfers.) First Chemical reported 60 percent more than the amount of waste of any other facility in the nation. (See Chapter 4 for an explanation of how First Chemical's method of calculating on-site recycling makes the facility the largest TRI waste generator in the nation.)

Kansas and Alabama also rank within the top 10 for total production-related waste, but not for releases and transfers. (See Tables 7-2 and 7-4.) Each of these states have just a few facilities reporting a large percentage of the state's total. In Kansas three facilities account for 71 percent of all production-related waste in the state: the Texaco Refinery in El Dorado with 357.3 million pounds, the National Cooperative Refinery in McPherson with 312.9 million pounds, and Gates Rubber Company in Iola with 219.5 million pounds. Together these facilities reported 3.2 million pounds of releases and transfers, which represent 21 percent of the total for Kansas.

In Alabama two facilities account for 35 percent of the state's total production-related waste: the Zeneca Inc. facility in Bucks with 215.3 million pounds and Courtaulds Fibers Inc. in Axis with 194.2 million pounds. Zeneca and Courtaulds Fibers reported 6.9 million and 42.8 million pounds of releases and transfers, respectively, which together represent 27 percent of the state's total releases and transfers.

Table 7-4. Total TRI Production-related Waste by State, 1992

State	**Facilities** Number	**Forms** Number	**1992 Total Production-related Waste** **Pounds** Pounds	**Rank**	**Average Pounds per Facility** Pounds	**Rank for Average Pounds per Facility**
Alabama	504	1,905	1,181,195,139	8	2,343,641	11
Alaska	6	50	19,970,768	49	3,328,461	7
American Samoa	2	2	22,000	53	11,000	53
Arizona	181	538	581,526,987	21	3,212,856	8
Arkansas	394	1,232	383,577,198	26	973,546	29
California	1,830	5,400	782,627,050	14	427,665	44
Colorado	192	540	72,547,663	41	377,852	49
Connecticut	416	1,215	295,194,518	29	709,602	37
Delaware	68	274	108,397,639	38	1,594,083	15
Florida	525	1,462	389,964,008	25	742,789	34
Georgia	739	2,395	890,212,189	13	1,204,617	20
Hawaii	21	76	8,346,391	50	397,447	47
Idaho	53	172	36,015,107	46	679,530	39
Illinois	1,401	4,915	1,542,619,277	5	1,101,084	26
Indiana	1,033	3,637	1,155,887,370	9	1,118,962	24
Iowa	423	1,304	223,260,324	31	527,802	41
Kansas	278	1,012	1,260,461,656	6	4,534,035	5
Kentucky	449	1,653	529,159,067	22	1,178,528	21
Louisiana	326	2,063	2,600,889,361	3	7,978,188	2
Maine	110	367	125,223,336	37	1,138,394	23
Maryland	229	724	437,042,093	24	1,908,481	14
Massachusetts	615	1,744	172,621,095	33	280,685	51
Michigan	969	3,747	1,133,090,235	10	1,169,340	22
Minnesota	539	1,570	229,006,955	30	424,874	45
Mississippi	319	1,072	4,593,256,982	2	14,398,925	1
Missouri	596	2,024	746,677,384	15	1,252,814	19
Montana	23	140	136,507,431	36	5,935,106	4
Nebraska	180	540	86,921,381	39	482,897	42
Nevada	44	111	31,119,125	47	707,253	38
New Hampshire	129	362	55,852,711	43	432,967	43
New Jersey	751	2,678	647,720,786	18	862,478	32
New Mexico	44	156	84,324,430	40	1,916,464	13
New York	907	2,741	939,417,690	11	1,035,742	27
North Carolina	978	2,970	913,342,671	12	933,888	31
North Dakota	36	97	4,626,739	52	128,521	52
Ohio	1,679	6,070	1,738,211,020	4	1,035,266	28
Oklahoma	260	858	159,334,475	34	612,825	40
Oregon	251	782	180,891,224	32	720,682	36
Pennsylvania	1,291	4,310	1,229,906,732	7	952,678	30
Puerto Rico	178	566	140,958,043	35	791,899	33
Rhode Island	169	440	47,980,693	44	283,909	50
South Carolina	501	1,904	712,164,731	17	1,421,486	17
South Dakota	56	111	40,913,138	45	730,592	35
Tennessee	667	2,245	743,078,240	16	1,114,060	25
Texas	1,238	5,927	7,504,039,760	1	6,061,421	3
Utah	130	489	305,071,736	28	2,346,706	10
Vermont	50	117	20,088,624	48	401,772	46
Virgin Islands	3	27	6,549,139	51	2,183,046	12
Virginia	474	1,626	608,341,254	19	1,283,420	18
Washington	332	1,035	506,780,869	23	1,526,448	16
West Virginia	148	724	596,560,885	20	4,030,817	6
Wisconsin	868	2,765	329,788,029	27	379,940	48
Wyoming	25	132	64,492,276	42	2,579,691	9
Total	23,630	81,016	37,333,775,624		1,579,931	

Map 7-4.

The 100 Counties with Largest Total TRI Production-related Waste, 1992

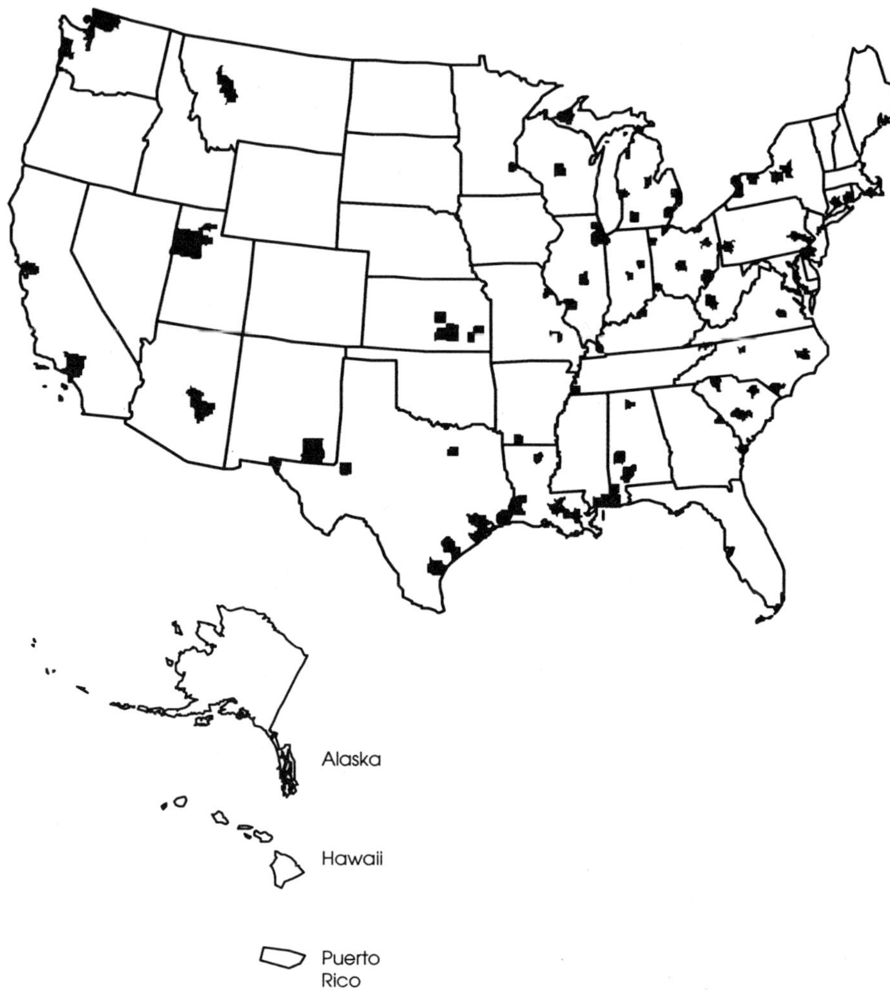

Texas is the state with the largest reported production-related waste because it has a large number of facilities that generate relatively large amounts of waste. Louisiana, however, is ranked second because it has a relatively small number of facilities that generate even larger amounts of waste. Texas has 1,238 facilities that generated, on average, 6.1 million pounds per facility of production-related waste in 1992. Louisiana has one-fourth as many facilities (326), but these facilities generated, on average, 8.0 million pounds of waste, one-third more than Texas facilities. On the other hand, California has the most TRI facilities (1,830), but they generated, on average, 428,000 pounds of waste, making that state rank as low as 14th in total production-related waste. Only nine other state or other reporting jurisdictions have as low an average generation of waste per facility as California facilities. (See Table 7-4.)

Table 7-5. The 100 Counties with Largest Total TRI Production-related Waste, 1992

Rank	State	County	1992 Total Production-related Waste Pounds	Rank	State	County	1992 Total Production-related Waste Pounds
1	MS	Jackson	4,170,829,845	51	IN	Marion	114,473,708
2	TX	Jefferson	3,115,561,515	52	MO	Pike	113,039,170
3	TX	Harris	1,882,465,091	53	UT	Salt Lake	107,418,152
4	LA	Calcasieu	691,409,255	54	NC	Forsyth	106,898,164
5	TX	Brazoria	654,627,407	55	NJ	Gloucester	106,481,954
6	AL	Mobile	564,334,220	56	TN	Sullivan	106,387,837
7	IL	Will	537,169,677	57	OH	Hamilton	105,010,399
8	AZ	Gila	479,734,256	58	TX	Victoria	103,919,898
9	IN	Lake	392,567,610	59	NY	Oneida	101,975,313
10	LA	St James	386,546,476	60	PA	Philadelphia	101,328,880
11	MD	Baltimore City	380,796,905	61	CT	New London	94,765,643
12	GA	Chatham	379,107,731	62	CA	Contra Costa	91,419,518
13	IL	Cook	378,042,390	63	PA	Montgomery	91,324,796
14	CA	Los Angeles	374,883,963	64	DE	New Castle	90,328,720
15	KS	Butler	361,378,139	65	MT	Lewis and Clark	88,958,172
16	OH	Lucas	327,784,020	66	OH	Cuyahoga	86,342,963
17	LA	Iberville	321,166,564	67	KS	Sedgwick	86,254,952
18	KS	Mc Pherson	313,137,909	68	MN	Dakota	85,680,489
19	MO	Iron	290,186,066	69	GS	Richmond	84,999,963
20	OH	Stark	279,274,998	70	TX	Dallas	79,749,929
21	NC	Beaufort	255,948,961	71	MI	St Clair	78,426,945
22	PA	Berks	249,053,887	72	NJ	Salem	77,146,936
23	TX	Nueces	249,015,241	73	TX	Ector	75,570,500
24	VA	Chesterfield	240,866,096	74	AL	Monroe	75,376,964
25	NY	Onondaga	221,518,872	75	MI	Muskegon	75,168,960
26	KS	Allen	219,623,344	76	TX	San Patricio	74,132,285
27	LA	Jefferson	214,220,761	77	OH	Paulding	73,670,196
28	TX	Galveston	212,156,284	78	MI	Midland	72,367,853
29	MI	Wayne	210,738,112	79	IL	Macon	72,063,411
30	MI	Kalamazoo	207,881,631	80	SC	Orangeburg	70,300,911
31	WV	Hancock	203,228,311	81	AR	Columbia	68,629,179
32	LA	St Charles	201,872,552	82	NY	Niagara	68,172,499
33	LA	Ascension	200,527,659	83	NY	Monroe	67,698,639
34	SC	Spartanburg	197,463,696	84	AL	Marengo	67,089,454
35	TX	Orange	180,978,343	85	WI	Wood	65,831,954
36	OH	Washington	174,671,257	86	KY	Marshall	65,572,715
37	TX	El Paso	168,745,888	87	WA	Skagit	65,401,156
38	CT	New Haven	157,604,051	88	KS	Wilson	64,581,221
39	TX	Calhoun	154,238,242	89	LA	Ouachita	64,510,418
40	WV	Kanawha	150,456,853	90	IN	Delaware	64,050,743
41	MI	Ontonagon	149,802,824	91	MS	Harrison	63,522,706
42	NY	Erie	146,835,487	92	OH	Franklin	62,561,712
43	WA	Whatcom	143,383,083	93	WV	Wood	62,005,055
44	NJ	Middlesex	141,566,602	94	UT	Weber	61,462,000
45	LA	East Baton Rouge	140,877,464	95	WA	Grays Harbor	61,072,391
46	KY	Jefferson	127,206,428	96	IL	Madison	61,071,565
47	TN	Shelby	125,739,094	97	SC	Darlington	60,971,111
48	AL	Morgan	120,316,947	98	NC	Columbus	60,277,684
49	PA	Allegheny	117,722,319	99	LA	Beauregard	60,165,752
50	UT	Tooele	117,606,925	100	NM	Eddy	59,942,703
						Subtotal	25,648,449,978
						Percent of Total	68.7
						Total	37,333,775,624

Table 7-6. Change in Total TRI Production-related Waste by State, 1991-1992

State	Facilities Number	Forms Number	1991 Total Production-related Waste: Pounds	Rank
Texas	1,238	5,927	7,279,744,704	1
Mississippi	319	1,072	4,508,188,519	2
Louisiana	326	2,063	2,332,099,101	3
Ohio	1,679	6,070	1,555,678,575	4
Illinois	1,401	4,915	1,391,883,455	5
Kansas	278	1,012	1,270,148,375	7
Pennsylvania	1,291	4,310	1,314,761,669	6
Alabama	504	1,905	1,121,986,862	9
Indiana	1,033	3,637	1,211,772,213	8
Michigan	969	3,747	1,011,819,512	11
New York	907	2,741	854,751,340	12
North Carolina	978	2,970	839,856,944	13
Georgia	739	2,395	1,081,002,287	10
California	1,830	5,400	837,390,781	14
Missouri	596	2,024	571,091,377	21
Tennessee	667	2,245	743,218,186	17
South Carolina	501	1,904	811,845,671	15
New Jersey	751	2,678	757,816,503	16
Virginia	474	1,626	592,371,759	20
West Virginia	148	724	517,278,408	22
Arizona	181	538	610,780,041	18
Kentucky	449	1,653	597,426,687	19
Washington	332	1,035	406,886,782	24
Maryland	229	724	428,539,135	23
Florida	525	1,462	405,282,187	25
Arkansas	394	1,232	346,036,260	26
Wisconsin	868	2,765	299,316,058	27
Utah	130	489	295,426,641	29
Connecticut	416	1,215	297,779,999	28
Minnesota	539	1,570	218,541,450	31
Iowa	423	1,304	285,762,912	30
Oregon	251	782	184,815,831	32
Massachusetts	615	1,744	175,924,953	33
Oklahoma	260	858	169,174,821	34
Puerto Rico	178	566	155,421,415	35
Montana	23	140	104,784,465	38
Maine	110	367	111,347,611	36
Delaware	68	274	110,881,778	37
Nebraska	180	540	84,752,501	39
New Mexico	44	156	72,207,431	40
Colorado	192	540	53,944,610	41
Wyoming	25	132	52,337,005	43
New Hampshire	129	362	53,644,495	42
Rhode Island	169	440	44,144,753	44
South Dakota	56	111	28,891,744	46
Idaho	53	172	38,121,423	45
Nevada	44	111	22,415,988	48
Vermont	50	117	20,091,338	49
Alaska	6	50	23,329,176	47
Hawaii	21	76	8,163,678	50
Virgin Islands	3	27	1,580,911	52
North Dakota	36	97	4,484,907	51
American Samoa	2	2	17,850	53
Total	23,630	81,016	36,316,963,077	

1992 Total Production-related Waste		Change 1991-1992		1992 Total Releases and Transfers
Pounds	Rank	Pounds	Percent	Rank
7,504,039,760	1	224,295,056	3.08	1
4,593,256,982	2	85,068,463	1.89	13
2,600,889,361	3	268,790,260	11.53	2
1,738,211,020	4	182,532,445	11.73	4
1,542,619,277	5	150,735,822	10.83	5
1,260,461,656	6	-9,686,719	-0.76	17
1,229,906,732	7	-84,854,937	-6.45	9
1,181,195,139	8	59,208,277	5.28	14
1,155,887,370	9	-55,884,843	-4.61	3
1,133,090,235	10	121,270,723	11.99	7
939,417,690	11	84,666,350	9.91	18
913,342,671	12	73,485,727	8.75	11
890,212,189	13	-190,790,098	-17.65	19
782,627,050	14	-54,763,731	-6.54	10
746,677,384	15	175,586,007	30.75	6
743,078,240	16	-139,946	-0.02	8
712,164,731	17	-99,680,940	-12.28	15
647,720,786	18	-110,095,717	-14.53	12
608,341,254	19	15,969,495	2.70	21
596,560,885	20	79,282,477	15.33	26
581,526,987	21	-29,253,054	-4.79	27
529,159,067	22	-68,267,620	-11.43	16
506,780,869	23	99,894,087	24.55	25
437,042,093	24	8,502,958	1.98	34
389,964,008	25	-15,318,179	-3.78	20
383,577,198	26	37,540,938	10.85	24
329,788,029	27	30,471,971	10.18	22
305,071,736	28	9,645,095	3.26	23
295,194,518	29	-2,585,481	-0.87	32
229,006,955	30	10,465,505	4.79	29
223,260,324	31	-62,502,588	-21.87	28
180,891,224	32	-3,924,607	-2.12	36
172,621,095	33	-3,303,858	-1.88	30
159,334,475	34	-9,840,346	-5.82	31
140,958,043	35	-14,463,372	-9.31	35
136,507,431	36	31,722,966	30.27	33
125,223,336	37	13,875,725	12.46	40
108,397,639	38	-2,484,139	-2.24	41
86,921,381	39	2,168,880	2.56	37
84,324,430	40	12,116,999	16.78	38
72,547,663	41	18,603,053	34.49	39
64,492,276	42	12,155,271	23.23	44
55,852,711	43	2,208,216	4.12	45
47,980,693	44	3,835,940	8.69	42
40,913,138	45	12,021,394	41.61	49
36,015,107	46	-2,106,316	-5.53	46
31,119,125	47	8,703,137	38.83	48
20,088,624	48	-2,714	-0.01	47
19,970,768	49	-3,358,408	-14.40	43
8,346,391	50	182,713	2.24	52
6,549,139	51	4,968,228	314.26	51
4,626,739	52	141,832	3.16	50
22,000	53	4,150	23.25	53
37,333,775,624		1,016,812,547	2.80	

The geographic pattern of the 100 counties in the nation whose facilities report the largest total production-related waste is fairly similar to the pattern of top counties for total releases and transfers. In both cases the largest concentrations are the Gulf Coast and Great Lakes regions, with others along the Atlantic Coast, but few in the middle of the country. Harris County, Texas, and Lake County, Indiana, are among the top 10 in production-related waste, as they are for total releases and transfers. Texas and Louisiana together are responsible for half of the top 10 spots in both categories. (See Maps 7-3 and 7-4 and Tables 7-3 and 7-5.)

TRI Production-related Waste, 1991-1992

The state breakdown of total TRI production-related waste changed little between 1991 and 1992. Nine of the top 10 states remained the top-ranked states. The exception was Michigan, which rose from 11th to 10th displacing Georgia, which dropped from 10th to 13th. (See Table 7-6.) In Michigan, the Upjohn Company in Portage increased its total production-related waste by 53.4 million pounds.

Among these top-ranked states all but Kansas, Pennsylvania, and Indiana showed increases in total production-related waste, with Louisiana, Ohio, and Illinois all reporting increases greater than 10 percent. Overall, 21 reporting jurisdictions reported decreases and 32 reported increases. (See Table 7-6.)

Just a few facilities account for a large portion of the 1991-1992 increases and decreases in production-related waste reported in some states. Facilities with the five largest increases and five largest decreases in production-related waste are listed in Table 7-7. Chapter 4 describes these facilities in greater detail and explains how changes in calculation of on-site waste management, reporting errors, and production anomalies, identified by *Toxics Watch* in interviews with companies, are responsible for the 10 largest changes in waste generation. All in all, the 10 facilities reported a total of 693.1 million pounds of decreases and 643.5 million pounds of increases in production-related waste not attributable to any waste management actions taken at the facilities.

Only 1 of the top 10 facilities, DuPont Chambers Works in Deepwater, New Jersey, could attribute a large part of its change in production-related waste management to changes in activities — in this case, phase-out of chloroethane production and replacement of on-site treatment of hydrochloric acid with a regeneration process, converting the waste hydrochloric acid into a marketable product.

This should alert *Toxics Watch* readers to the importance of verifying 1992 data with companies. Any ranking of states for change in production-related waste should be viewed with these facts in mind. (See Chapter 4 for a more detailed discussion of the need for verification of facility data and expected improvements in future TRI data.)

*Table 7-7. Facilities with Largest Change in Total TRI Production-related Waste, 1991-1992**

Facility	**City, County**	**State**	**Change in Total Production-related Waste 1991 to 1992** Pounds	**Reason for Change**
Largest Decreases				
DuPont Chambers Works	Deepwater, Salem	NJ	-173,749,368	Phase-out of production and change in calculation method
Corning Asahi Video Products	State College, Centre	PA	-141,973,140	Reporting error
Phillips 66 Co.	Sweeny, Brazoria	TX	-132,582,243	Unexplained increase in process efficiency
Reilly Industries Inc.	Indianapolis, Marion	IN	-123,744,885	Change in calculation method
Carolina Eastman Co.	Columbia, Calhoun	SC	-121,020,100	Change in calculation method
Largest Increases				
Doe Run Co.	Boss, Iron	MO	181,142,574	Increase in production/start-up
Star Enterprises Inc.	Union, St James	LA	170,652,814	Reporting error
Goodyear Tire & Rubber Co.	Beaumont, Jefferson	TX	103,176,783	Change in calculation method
Elkem Metals Co.	Marietta, Washington	OH	101,058,821	Change in calculation method
Revere Copper Prods. Inc.	Rome, Oneida	NY	87,507,113	Change in calculation method

* See Chapter 4 for explanation of changes.

Figure 7-1.

Largest Changes in Total TRI Production-related Waste by State, 1991-1992

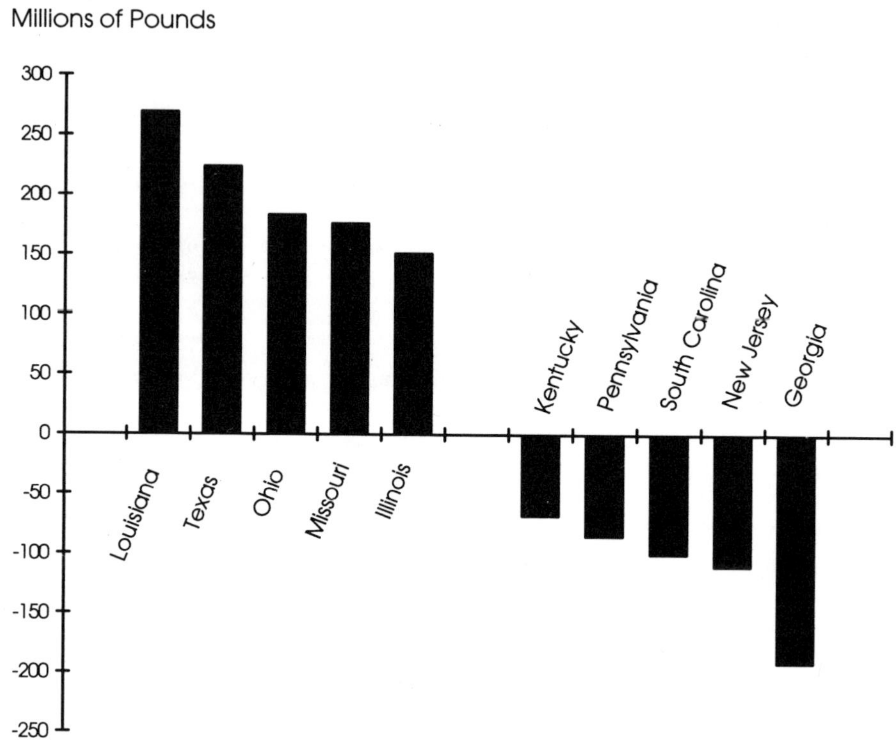

The five states with the largest increases and the five with the largest decreases in total TRI production-related waste

Sixty percent of the states and other reporting jurisdictions (32 out of 53) reported an increase in total production-related waste from 1991 to 1992. Louisiana led the increases with an increase of 268.8 million pounds (a 12 percent increase), and Texas followed with a 224.3-million-pound increase (3 percent). These increases dominated decreases, where the largest were in Georgia, with 190.8 million pounds of decrease (an 18 percent decrease) and New Jersey, whose facilities reported 110.1 million pounds of decrease (15 percent). (See Table 7-6.)

In Georgia, DSM Chemical Company in Augusta showed the largest decrease from 1991 to 1992, a decrease in total production-related waste of 48.0 million pounds. In New Jersey, the DuPont Chambers Works plant reported a total decrease of 173.7 million pounds. (See Chapter 4 for explanation of changes at the DuPont facility.) (See Figure 7-1.)

The Virgin Islands reported the largest percentage increase, where the Hess Oil Virgin Islands Corp. in Kingshill, St. Croix, reported an increase of 5.0 million pounds,

Map 7-5.

Total TRI Production-related Waste by State, Percent Change, 1991 to 1992

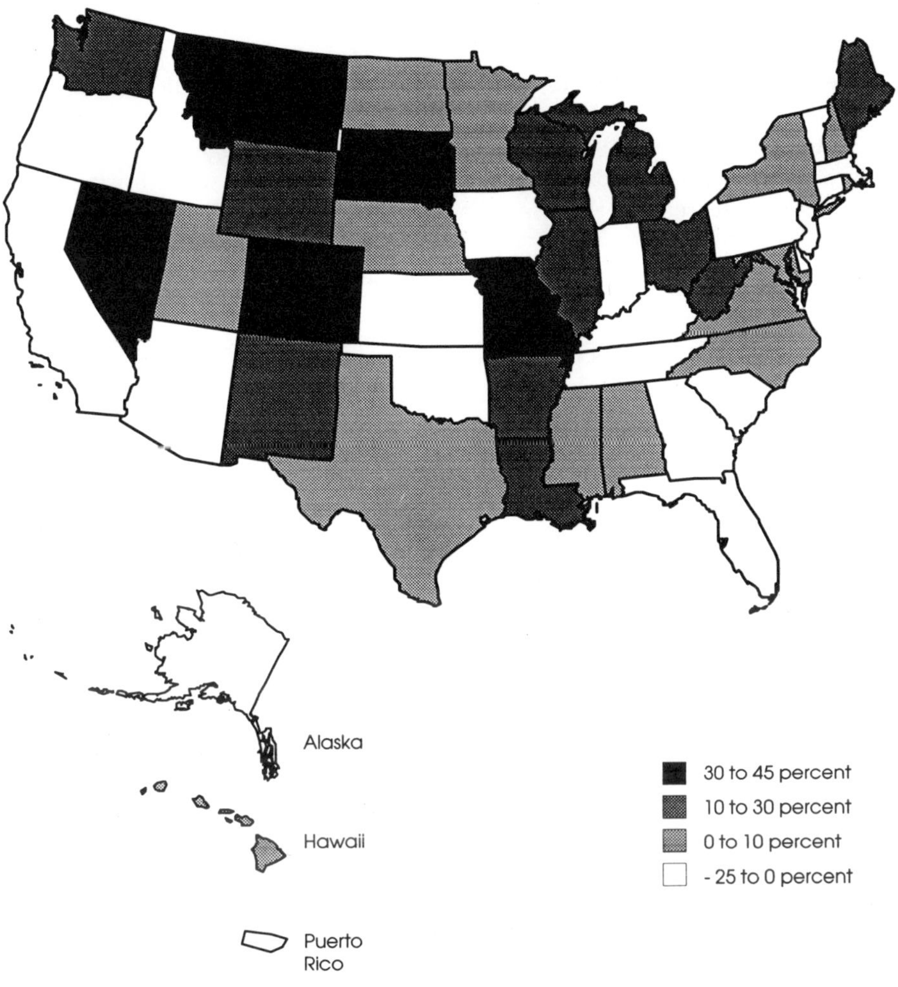

which led to more than a 300 percent increase for the Island's facilities.[b] The next largest percent increase was in South Dakota, a 42 percent increase of 12.0 million pounds. Only one state, Iowa, reported more than a 20 percent decrease (22 percent and 62.5 million pounds decrease). (See Map 7-5 and Table 7-6.)

TRI Production-related Waste, 1992-1994

While facility projections show the overall total staying approximately the same between 1992 and 1994 (a 0.3 percent increase), decreases of 20 percent are expected in quantity released on site or disposed of off site and smaller decreases in recycling, energy recovery, and treatment off site. The increases are expected in on-site recycling and on-site energy recovery. (See Chapter 4, Table 4-15.)

While more states had increases from 1991 to 1992, the opposite is projected for the 1992-1994 period. Facilities in 30 states and other reporting jurisdictions have projected net total decreases in production-related waste from 1992 to 1994, compared to projected increases in 23 jurisdictions. However, the ranking of states is not expected to change significantly by 1994. The top 10 states for largest amounts of production-related waste would remain the same. (See Table 7-8.)

Texas and Louisiana, the top states in 1992 for reported amounts of total releases and transfers and total production-related waste, also project much larger changes than the other states. Texas expects the largest increase in production-related waste (609.2 million pounds, an 8 percent increase). On the other hand, facilities in Louisiana (the second-ranked state in 1992 for waste amount) project the largest decrease by 1994 (479.3 million pounds, an 18 percent decrease). (See Figure 7-2 and Table 7-8.)

The state with the largest expected percentage decrease is Maryland, with a 60 percent decrease. Rhode Island facilities project a 53-percent increase, although all other projected increases are below 20 percent. (See Map 7-6 and Table 7-8.)

[b] This facility has since revised its TRI forms so that the increase is 2.1 million pounds after the revisions. The increase for all facilities in the Virgin Islands then becomes 135 percent, which is still the largest percentage increase.

Table 7-8. Total TRI Production-related Waste by State, Actual 1992 and Projected 1994

State	Facilities	1992 Actual Production-related Waste		1994 Projected Production-related Waste		Projected Change 1992 to 1994	
	Number	Pounds	Rank	Pounds	Rank	Pounds	Percent
Texas	1,238	7,504,039,760	1	8,113,193,969	1	609,154,209	8.12
Mississippi	319	4,593,256,982	2	4,668,855,567	2	75,598,585	1.65
Louisiana	326	2,600,889,361	3	2,121,570,175	3	-479,319,186	-18.43
Ohio	1,679	1,738,211,020	4	1,833,009,221	4	94,798,201	5.45
Illinois	1,401	1,542,619,277	5	1,496,181,565	5	-46,437,712	-3.01
Pennsylvania	1,291	1,229,906,732	7	1,468,202,734	6	238,296,002	19.38
Alabama	504	1,181,195,139	8	1,333,081,102	7	151,885,963	12.86
Michigan	969	1,133,090,235	10	1,248,303,803	8	115,213,568	10.17
Indiana	1,033	1,155,887,370	9	1,112,195,510	9	-43,691,860	-3.78
Kansas	278	1,260,461,656	6	1,097,281,421	10	-163,180,235	-12.95
North Carolina	978	913,342,671	12	881,058,283	11	-32,284,388	-3.53
Georgia	739	890,212,189	13	854,955,690	12	-35,256,499	-3.96
New York	907	939,417,690	11	852,321,115	13	-87,096,575	-9.27
Tennessee	667	743,078,240	16	748,692,705	14	5,614,465	0.76
California	1,830	782,627,050	14	740,611,228	15	-42,015,822	-5.37
Virginia	474	608,341,254	19	709,560,370	16	101,219,116	16.64
South Carolina	501	712,164,731	17	708,240,569	17	-3,924,162	-0.55
Missouri	596	746,677,384	15	656,780,267	18	-89,897,117	-12.04
Arizona	181	581,526,987	21	651,215,041	19	69,688,054	11.98
West Virginia	148	596,560,885	20	608,487,506	20	11,926,621	2.00
New Jersey	751	647,720,786	18	579,243,745	21	-68,477,041	-10.57
Kentucky	449	529,159,067	22	548,612,140	22	19,453,073	3.68
Washington	332	506,780,869	23	500,147,585	23	-6,633,284	-1.31
Arkansas	394	383,577,198	26	390,380,982	24	6,803,784	1.77
Florida	525	389,964,008	25	380,816,643	25	-9,147,365	-2.35
Utah	130	305,071,736	28	348,117,692	26	43,045,956	14.11
Wisconsin	868	329,788,029	27	322,650,016	27	-7,138,013	-2.16
Connecticut	416	295,194,518	29	291,816,162	28	-3,378,356	-1.14
Minnesota	539	229,006,955	30	237,739,441	29	8,732,486	3.81
Iowa	423	223,260,324	31	222,283,490	30	-976,834	-0.44
Oregon	251	180,891,224	32	189,650,244	31	8,759,020	4.84
Maryland	229	437,042,093	24	176,697,992	32	-260,344,101	-59.57
Massachusetts	615	172,621,095	33	157,872,632	33	-14,748,463	-8.54
Oklahoma	260	159,334,475	34	142,308,148	34	-17,026,327	-10.69
Maine	110	125,223,336	37	131,180,526	35	5,957,190	4.76
Puerto Rico	178	140,958,043	35	124,321,858	36	-16,636,185	-11.80
Delaware	68	108,397,639	38	120,908,883	37	12,511,244	11.54
Montana	23	136,507,431	36	119,078,315	38	-17,429,116	-12.77
New Mexico	44	84,324,430	40	93,231,723	39	8,907,293	10.56
Nebraska	180	86,921,381	39	81,736,646	40	-5,184,735	-5.96
Colorado	192	72,547,663	41	79,232,660	41	6,684,997	9.21
Rhode Island	169	47,980,693	44	73,507,855	42	25,527,162	53.20
Wyoming	25	64,492,276	42	54,144,394	43	-10,347,882	-16.05
New Hampshire	129	55,852,711	43	47,290,631	44	-8,562,080	-15.33
South Dakota	56	40,913,138	45	43,929,071	45	3,015,933	7.37
Idaho	53	36,015,107	46	37,318,176	46	1,303,069	3.62
Nevada	44	31,119,125	47	17,954,073	47	-13,165,052	-42.31
Alaska	6	19,970,768	49	14,586,430	48	-5,384,338	-26.96
Vermont	50	20,088,624	48	12,239,322	49	-7,849,302	-39.07
Hawaii	21	8,346,391	50	8,599,092	50	252,701	3.03
Virgin Islands	3	6,549,139	51	4,597,583	51	-1,951,556	-29.80
North Dakota	36	4,626,739	52	4,409,541	52	-217,198	-4.69
American Samoa	2	22,000	53	10,000	53	-12,000	-54.55
Total	23,630	37,333,775,624		37,460,411,532		126,635,908	0.34

Figure 7-2.

Largest Projected Changes in Total TRI Production-related Waste by State, 1992-1994

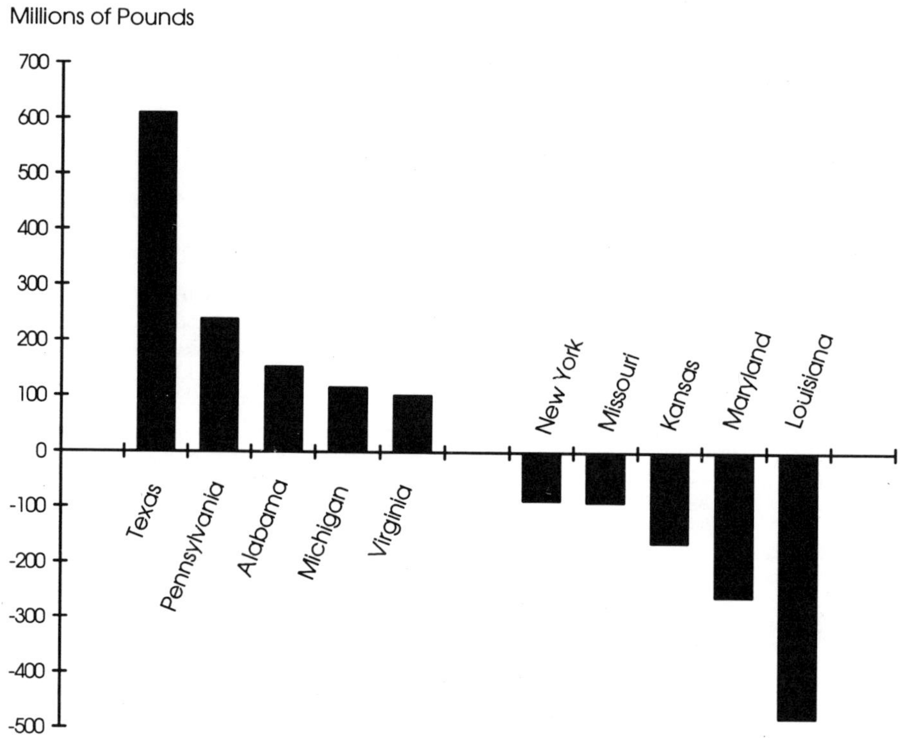

The five states with the largest projected increases and the five with the largest projected decreases in total TRI production-related waste

Map 7-6.

Total TRI Production-related Waste by State, Percent Change, Actual 1992 to Projected 1994

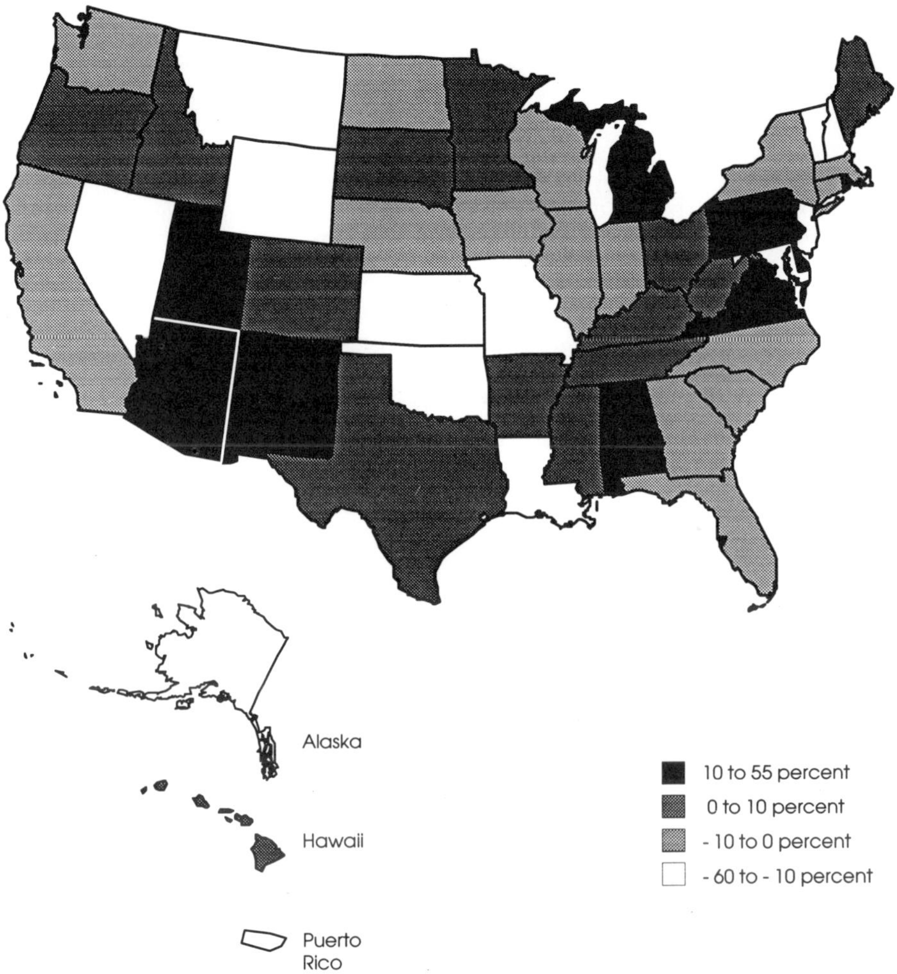

TRI Source Reduction Activity, 1992

Facilities report to TRI whether or not they undertook source reduction activities during the year. The reports on source reduction activity are for each chemical at the facility and show only what type of activity, but not how much waste might have been reduced because of the activity. For 1992, 27 percent of total production-related waste was associated with forms in which some source reduction activity was reported.

By state, the percent of waste reported on forms showing some source reduction activity varied from none to over 80 percent. Connecticut had the highest percent of its total production-related waste (81 percent) on forms indicating source reduction activities. Nevada had the second highest, with 73 percent of its production-related waste reported on forms indicating source reduction activities. However, only 11 states had more than half of their waste reported on forms showing any source reduction activity during 1992. (See Map 7-7 and Table 7-9.)

RCRA Biennial Reporting System Data

Every two years, facilities that generate hazardous waste (as defined under the Resource Conservation and Recovery Act) must report on the quantity and management of this waste. The 1991 RCRA Biennial Reporting System (BRS) contains reports from 24,378 facilities, of which 92 percent (22,344 facilities) reported on "toxic" waste. While the BRS does not make this distinction, for the purposes of this report a RCRA "toxic" waste is a waste stream that contains one or more toxic chemicals specified under either RCRA or TRI or that is otherwise designated "toxic" under RCRA. It excludes waste streams that are *solely* ignitable, corrosive, or reactive. (See Chapter 4 and Appendix E.)

RCRA Biennial Reporting System Data, 1991

As in the case of facilities reporting to TRI, facilities in Texas reported the largest amount of toxic RCRA waste generated, over twice as much as the next state, New York. Although New York has almost three times as many facilities reporting to RCRA as Texas, it does not have as many facilities generating large amounts of waste as Texas. One New York facility, Kodak Park in Rochester, reported 80 percent of the New York state total. Michigan, ranked fourth for RCRA toxic waste generated in 1991, is a similar case. It has fewer facilities than third-ranked Pennsylvania; but one facility, the Dow Chemical plant in Midland, accounted for over 75 percent of all RCRA toxic waste generated in Michigan in 1991. (See Table 7-10 and Table 4-17.)

There is some correlation among geographic areas ranking high in RCRA toxic waste and TRI waste,

Map 7-7.

Percent of States' Total Production-related Waste Reported on Forms that Report Source Reduction Activity, 1992

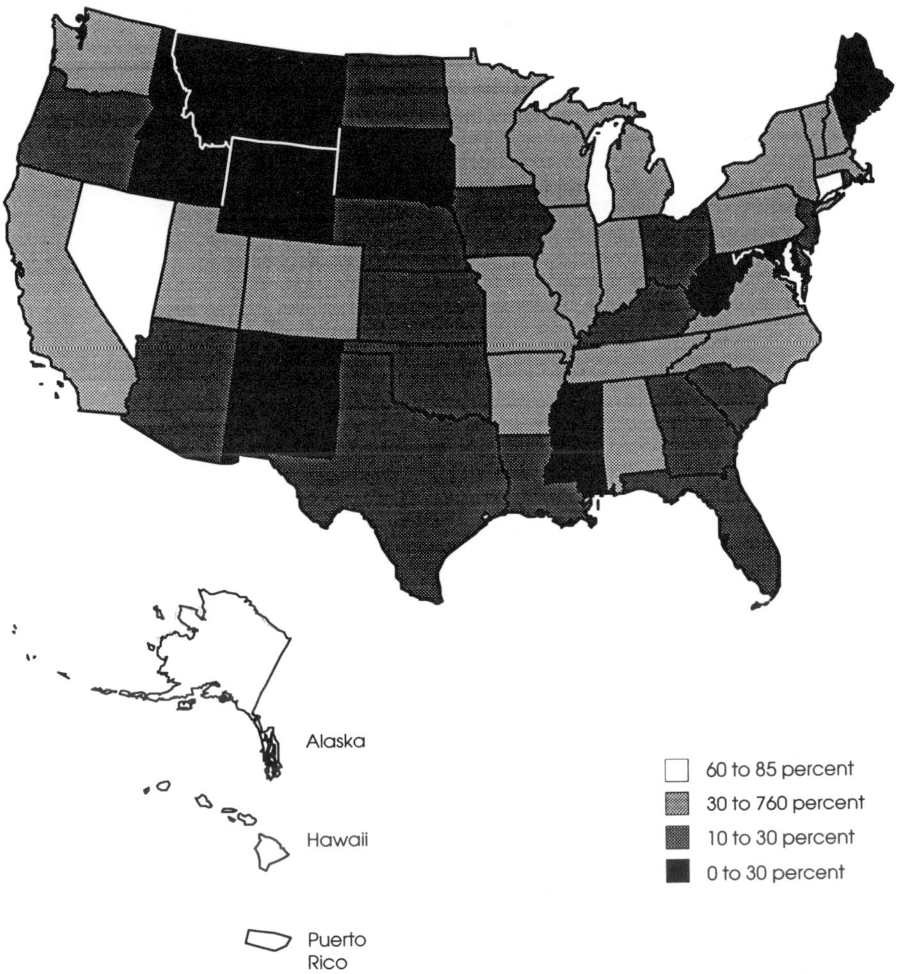

Table 7-9. Total TRI Production-related Waste by State, With and Without Source Reduction Activity, 1992

State	Total Production-related Waste			Percent of Total With Source Reduction Activity
	With Source Reduction Activity Pounds	No Source Reduction Activity Pounds	Total Pounds	Percent
Alabama	392,244,376	788,950,763	1,181,195,139	33.21
Alaska	13,030,039	6,940,729	19,970,768	65.25
American Samoa	0	22,000	22,000	0.00
Arizona	133,806,650	447,720,337	581,526,987	23.01
Arkansas	118,617,216	264,959,982	383,577,198	30.92
California	308,313,261	474,313,789	782,627,050	39.39
Colorado	37,799,718	34,747,945	72,547,663	52.10
Connecticut	239,926,352	55,268,166	295,194,518	81.28
Delaware	22,924,815	85,472,824	108,397,639	21.15
Florida	74,247,346	315,716,662	389,964,008	19.04
Georgia	149,580,859	740,631,330	890,212,189	16.80
Hawaii	5,928,010	2,418,381	8,346,391	71.02
Idaho	3,183,756	32,831,351	36,015,107	8.84
Illinois	761,321,143	781,298,134	1,542,619,277	49.35
Indiana	562,007,260	593,880,110	1,155,887,370	48.62
Iowa	48,993,727	174,266,597	223,260,324	21.94
Kansas	188,308,261	1,072,153,395	1,260,461,656	14.94
Kentucky	126,301,613	402,857,454	529,159,067	23.87
Louisiana	746,557,928	1,854,331,433	2,600,889,361	28.70
Maine	9,857,977	115,365,359	125,223,336	7.87
Maryland	19,605,038	417,437,055	437,042,093	4.49
Massachusetts	84,035,563	88,585,532	172,621,095	48.68
Michigan	517,155,561	615,934,674	1,133,090,235	45.64
Minnesota	127,050,413	101,956,542	229,006,955	55.48
Mississippi	107,004,521	4,486,252,461	4,593,256,982	2.33
Missouri	302,440,471	444,236,913	746,677,384	40.50
Montana	1,361,239	135,146,192	136,507,431	1.00
Nebraska	18,148,519	68,772,862	86,921,381	20.88
Nevada	22,807,224	8,311,901	31,119,125	73.29
New Hampshire	26,221,183	29,631,528	55,852,711	46.95
New Jersey	112,197,094	535,523,692	647,720,786	17.32
New Mexico	1,998,010	82,326,420	84,324,430	2.37
New York	528,973,282	410,444,408	939,417,690	56.31
North Carolina	447,174,807	466,167,864	913,342,671	48.96
North Dakota	1,178,533	3,448,206	4,626,739	25.47
Ohio	410,007,785	1,328,203,235	1,738,211,020	23.59
Oklahoma	41,593,989	117,740,486	159,334,475	26.10
Oregon	39,486,510	141,404,714	180,891,224	21.83
Pennsylvania	494,316,864	735,589,868	1,229,906,732	40.19
Puerto Rico	85,389,515	55,568,528	140,958,043	60.58
Rhode Island	10,214,624	37,766,069	47,980,693	21.29
South Carolina	137,058,840	575,105,891	712,164,731	19.25
South Dakota	1,784,778	39,128,360	40,913,138	4.36
Tennessee	280,624,079	462,454,161	743,078,240	37.77
Texas	1,621,776,845	5,882,262,915	7,504,039,760	21.61
Utah	168,375,621	136,696,115	305,071,736	55.19
Vermont	11,280,035	8,808,589	20,088,624	56.15
Virgin Islands	252,500	6,296,639	6,549,139	3.86
Virginia	335,450,638	272,890,616	608,341,254	55.14
Washington	188,164,827	318,616,042	506,780,869	37.13
West Virginia	49,459,640	547,101,245	596,560,885	8.29
Wisconsin	109,946,870	219,841,159	329,788,029	33.34
Wyoming	1,679,608	62,812,668	64,492,276	2.60
Total	10,247,165,333	27,086,610,291	37,333,775,624	27.45

Table 7-10. RCRA Biennial Report Data by State, 1991

State	Facilities	Reports	1991 Toxic Waste Generated		1991 Total Production-Related Waste
			Pounds	Rank	Rank
	Number	Number	Pounds		
Alabama	278	2,506	3,455,740,400	24	9
Alaska	70	668	117,746,060	46	47
Arizona	235	1,911	1,725,437,400	33	18
Arkansas	145	677	1,524,662,940	35	26
California	2,058	14,261	52,920,910,880	7	14
Colorado	143	1,339	1,048,319,000	39	41
Connecticut	469	4,543	10,448,447,660	17	28
Delaware	62	559	2,020,240,000	30	37
District of Columbia	10	329	2,190,000	52	—
Florida	404	6,517	805,418,180	41	25
Georgia	384	2,682	28,186,487,340	9	10
Guam	9	204	322,800	55	—
Hawaii	34	693	3,278,940	51	50
Idaho	43	611	9,558,941,640	18	45
Illinois	1,160	5,583	26,880,698,480	10	5
Indiana	651	3,110	13,640,476,740	14	8
Iowa	156	1,222	1,549,987,460	34	30
Kansas	170	1,194	6,964,357,740	20	7
Kentucky	434	2,048	7,176,562,440	19	19
Louisiana	287	1,825	69,358,465,800	5	3
Maine	170	903	36,821,800	47	36
Maryland	424	4,022	3,162,351,780	26	23
Massachusetts	510	38,970	4,224,546,780	23	33
Michigan	725	3,656	78,119,380,140	4	11
Minnesota	271	2,124	12,658,130,500	15	31
Mississippi	191	731	16,662,737,460	13	2
Missouri	378	2,479	1,461,323,780	36	21
Montana	54	193	25,555,120	49	38
Nebraska	83	556	2,014,259,640	31	39
Nevada	69	409	28,290,660	48	48
New Hampshire	160	1,083	1,021,579,400	40	42
New Jersey	1,965	8,939	53,041,140,060	6	16
New Mexico	68	1,047	316,356,220	45	40
New York	2,433	9,643	102,873,489,000	2	12
North Carolina	575	6,793	2,737,664,260	28	13
North Dakota	16	148	1,371,779,960	38	51
Ohio	1,454	8,345	3,290,044,280	25	4
Oklahoma	158	786	10,819,614,640	16	34
Oregon	181	872	703,094,020	43	32
Pennsylvania	1,231	7,861	83,286,677,140	3	6
Puerto Rico	99	774	6,805,784,340	21	35
Rhode Island	106	752	684,094,300	44	44
South Carolina	326	1,710	1,774,303,900	32	15
South Dakota	20	80	1,630,700	53	46
Tennessee	629	3,119	2,598,577,440	29	17
Texas	867	2,982	242,694,883,840	1	1
Trust Territories	3	70	4,771,880	50	—
Utah	103	1,381	6,381,960,920	22	29
Vermont	59	573	770,535,800	42	49
Virgin Islands	1	6	1,622,000	54	52
Virginia	263	2,450	18,970,526,520	11	20
Washington	889	32,554	29,556,279,740	8	24
West Virginia	117	787	18,226,336,300	12	22
Wisconsin	516	2,202	1,387,648,040	37	27
Wyoming	28	84	3,141,265,960	27	43
Total	22,344	201,566	948,243,750,220		

Table 7-11. States Ranked among Top 10 in TRI and BRS, 1991

State	1991 TRI Total Releases and Transfers Rank	1991 TRI Total Production-related Waste Rank	1991 RCRA Toxic Waste Generated Rank
Texas	1	1	1
New York	15	12	2
Pennsylvania	9	6	3
Michigan	5	11	4
Louisiana	2	3	5
California	8	14	6
New Jersey	12	16	7
Georgia	17	10	8
Washington	24	24	9
Illinois	6	5	10
Mississippi	14	2	13
Indiana	4	8	14
Kansas	22	7	20
North Carolina	10	13	26
Alabama	11	9	28
Missouri	18	21	29
Tennessee	7	17	30
Ohio	3	4	31

but also considerable variation.[c] Louisiana, which ranked third in TRI production-related waste and second in TRI total releases and transfers in 1991, ranked fifth for BRS waste generated in that same reporting year.[d] Ohio ranked 4th in 1991 in TRI total production-related waste, yet only 31st in generation of BRS toxic waste. While Texas facilities reported the largest amounts in all three categories, only Louisiana facilities also ranked in the top five for each category. Three other states, Pennsylvania, Michigan, and Illinois, ranked in the top 10 for each category. (See Table 7-11.)

Generally, these rankings are dependent on the location of individual facilities with large reported waste generation. In 1991 the top 50 facilities in the nation accounted for 72 percent of all BRS toxic waste generated. (See Map 7-8 for the counties where they are located and Table 4-17.)

[c] TRI data contain information on releases to air, while BRS data are limited to solid and liquid wastes. Other difficulties arise in comparing TRI and BRS data; see discussion in Chapter 6.

[d] This chapter uses 1991 TRI data for purposes of comparison with 1991 BRS data, the latest available. When analyzing TRI data alone, the chapter uses 1992 TRI data, the latest available for that reporting system.

Map 7-8.

Counties in which the 50 RCRA Facilities with Largest Total Toxic Waste Generated are Located, 1991

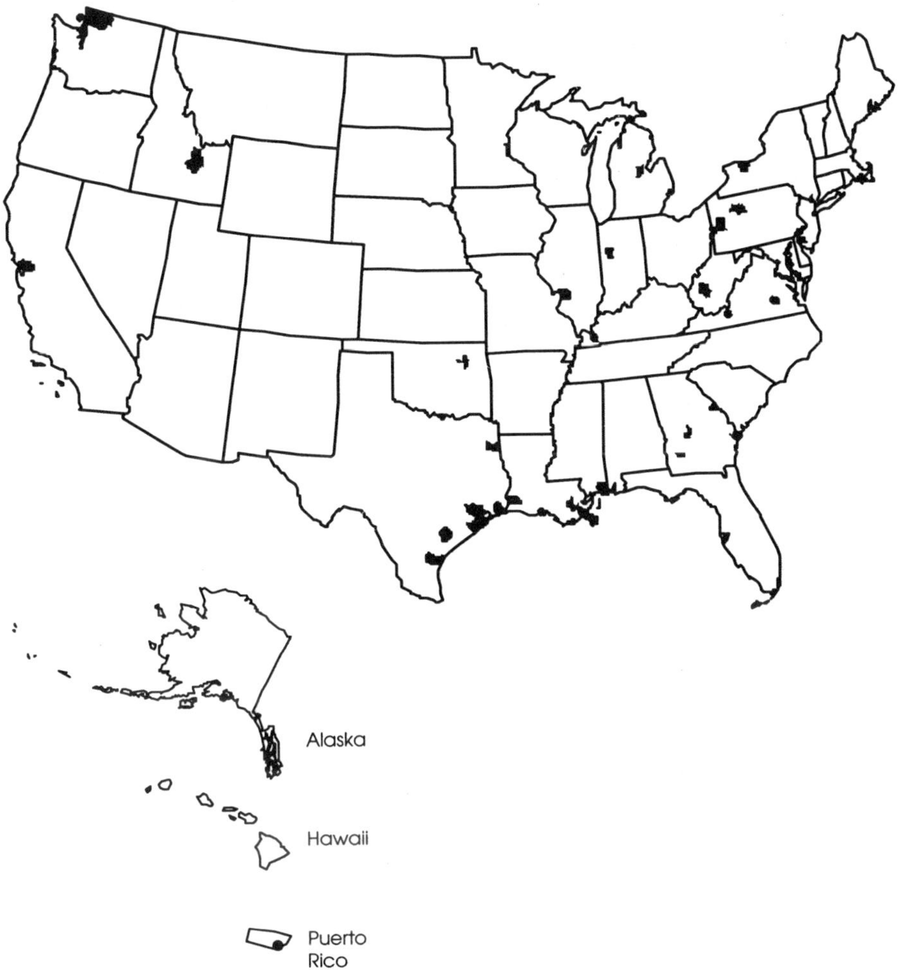

The top 50 RCRA waste generators are located in a total of 37 counties. Several counties host more than one.

RCRA Biennial Report Data, 1989-1991

As discussed in Chapter 4, the specific types of data reported to BRS vary for each state, especially for 1987. Even the 1989 data are incomplete with regard to SIC codes and other elements. State comparisons can be made on the amount of waste generated. However, since new waste codes were added for 1991 reporting, comparing the BRS data for 1989 with that for 1991 requires limiting the data to those waste codes common to both 1989 and 1991.

Although 8 of the states in the top 10 for toxic waste generated in 1989 remained in the top 10 in 1991, New York rose from 32nd place to 1st and Tennessee fell from 3rd to 24th. These changes in rank were due to one facility belonging to the same company in each state. In New York, Eastman Kodak's Kodak Park facility increased the amount of toxic waste generated by 83.2 billion pounds, and its Tennessee Eastman facility reported a decrease of 65.0 billion pounds. Connecticut also shifted its position, from 9th to 12th place. New Jersey dropped from first place in 1989 to fourth because DuPont's Chambers Works plant decreased its toxic waste generation by 44.5 billion pounds. As with production-related waste generation in TRI, a single facility can determine the rank of its entire state for BRS toxic waste. (See Table 7-12.)

Table 7-12. RCRA Biennial Report Data by State, Toxic Reports, 1989 and 1991

State	1989 Toxic Waste Generated Pounds	1991 Toxic Waste Generated Pounds	Change in Toxic Waste Generated 1989 to 1991 Pounds	Toxic Waste Generated 1989 Rank	Toxic Waste Generated 1991 Rank
New York	709,756,600	101,422,431,800	100,712,675,200	32	1
Michigan	83,569,520,020	77,982,740,940	-5,586,779,080	2	2
Texas	64,980,417,400	67,936,398,540	2,955,981,140	4	3
New Jersey	93,933,099,880	46,623,310,260	-47,309,789,620	1	4
Pennsylvania	41,296,143,220	36,824,053,740	-4,472,089,480	5	5
California	18,738,865,420	30,847,885,800	12,109,020,380	6	6
Georgia	12,990,241,140	22,918,297,800	9,928,056,660	7	7
Virginia	12,736,670,640	16,465,049,580	3,728,378,940	8	8
Louisiana	9,175,251,400	12,908,534,000	3,733,282,600	10	9
Indiana	3,397,738,440	11,298,637,380	7,900,898,940	16	10
Washington	7,127,401,340	10,528,674,940	3,401,273,600	12	11
Connecticut	11,231,612,100	10,447,124,860	-784,487,240	9	12
Idaho	2,126,542,020	9,551,200,480	7,424,658,460	19	13
Minnesota	7,348,099,980	7,378,249,780	30,149,800	11	14
Illinois	1,065,153,100	7,129,726,020	6,064,572,920	28	15
Utah	6,023,914,780	5,789,237,960	-234,676,820	13	16
Massachusetts	54,292,540	4,216,711,800	4,162,419,260	41	17
West Virginia	24,365,520	4,137,459,440	4,113,093,920	44	18
Kentucky	1,243,022,680	3,767,264,660	2,524,241,980	26	19
Mississippi	577,552,760	3,483,781,540	2,906,228,780	34	20
Kansas	3,634,751,080	3,310,747,640	-324,003,440	15	21
Ohio	4,810,871,080	3,043,719,720	-1,767,151,360	14	22
North Carolina	2,145,757,340	2,595,084,000	449,326,660	18	23
Tennessee	75,914,176,260	2,561,252,720	-73,352,923,540	3	24
Alabama	1,441,982,100	2,340,057,500	898,075,400	24	25
Maryland	1,154,179,980	2,319,508,480	1,165,328,500	27	26
Oklahoma	750,242,260	2,065,606,800	1,315,364,540	31	27
Nebraska	270,432,020	2,006,710,460	1,736,278,440	36	28
Arizona	820,117,360	1,632,294,780	812,177,420	29	29
Iowa	1,548,568,760	1,548,999,520	430,760	23	30
Arkansas	1,790,632,440	1,488,322,960	-302,309,480	20	31
Missouri	1,664,135,100	1,450,576,900	-213,558,200	22	32
South Carolina	201,315,600	1,314,164,500	1,112,848,900	37	33
New Hampshire	704,178,540	1,021,349,040	317,170,500	33	34
Wisconsin	816,886,780	911,317,580	94,430,800	30	35
Puerto Rico	543,859,080	891,317,580	347,458,500	35	36
Delaware	32,414,060	789,455,400	757,041,340	42	37
Vermont	24,642,000	769,659,600	745,017,600	43	38
Florida	72,120,500	768,031,040	695,910,540	39	39
Rhode Island	5,969,940	683,942,540	677,972,600	49	40
Oregon	2,569,953,300	634,820,720	-1,935,132,580	17	41
Colorado	1,706,792,000	310,492,360	-1,396,299,640	21	42
Alaska	10,732,660	76,348,840	65,616,180	48	43
Maine	103,055,060	36,697,840	-66,357,220	38	44
Nevada	15,088,800	28,038,800	12,950,000	46	45
Montana	15,150,920	20,898,460	5,747,540	45	46
New Mexico	1,355,166,460	18,241,960	-1,336,924,500	25	47
Trust Territories	23,580	4,769,140	4,745,560	55	48
North Dakota	57,685,640	4,333,900	-53,351,740	40	49
Wyoming	2,372,160	3,739,360	1,367,200	52	50
Hawaii	3,584,960	2,401,360	-1,183,600	51	51
District of Columbia	4,688,400	2,188,380	-2,500,020	50	52
South Dakota	1,207,660	1,630,700	423,040	53	53
Virgin Islands	11,514,000	1,183,400	-10,330,600	47	54
Guam	542,280	320,000	-222,280	54	55
Total	482,554,451,140	526,314,995,300	43,760,544,160		

Chapter 8

Toxics in the Environment

Introduction

What can be said about the conditions and trends of contamination of our environment by toxic chemicals on a nationwide basis using currently available databases? What can be said of national relevance by analyzing data on a subset of chemicals, chosen as representative of the list of chemicals of concern in this report? And what specific databases are available on the concentration of chemicals monitored or measured in air, water, soil, and biological tissue, as opposed to the release of toxic chemicals to the environment or to the presence of toxic chemicals in waste?

This chapter sought to address these three questions, to gain insight on how clearly the national toxics challenge can be understood. Answers are vital. Knowing the ambient concentrations of chemicals in our air, water, soils, or biological species provides important clues to identifying which chemicals are most likely to be a problem for the environment or for general human health outside of occupational settings. For harm to result from toxic chemicals, there must be exposures, and chemical concentrations in the environment provide a relatively direct measure of ecosystem exposure and an important, although imperfect, predictor of human exposure.

While local measurements that document local conditions are needed to characterize local pollution problems and find remedial or preventive responses, national analyses have key purposes as well. They are essential if policymakers are to identify problems that are national in scope and the chemicals and environmental settings that should receive priority attention for research, control and prevention programs, technical assistance, or other appropriate actions. If a few lakes and rivers are contaminated with a certain chemical, the problem may be best addressed locally. If, however, a large number of waterways show high levels or increasing levels of a certain toxic chemical, then a closer look for a pattern of proximity of a certain type of industry or geographic patterns of product use (such as agricultural pesticides) may be warranted.

Equally importantly, national databases help supply the information needed to determine whether environmental contamination by toxics is improving or getting worse. National databases are useful not just to national public and private organizations, but also to people wishing to compare the environmental contamination and trends in a particular community or region to that of other areas.

After six months of searching out chemical concentration databases, *Toxics Watch* found that the central questions posed here could not be answered. This research did yield some insights on air, water, and soil concentrations and an overview of the databases that do exist. The summary of findings below is followed by a discussion in some detail of the databases that were located and that may be useful to *Toxics Watch* readers in addressing particular problems.

Summary of Findings

- Measurements of toxics in the environment are more closely associated with human and ecosystem exposure and risk than are data on environmental releases of chemicals in waste. Databases on chemical releases, while valuable for understanding waste released from manufacturing facilities, are of little use for predicting national or regional environmental concentrations — the environmental transport and reactions that occur after chemicals are released are too complex. For example, some toxic chemicals released to the air from factories in large quantities may be almost immediately broken down or neutralized into less harmful substances, whereas other toxic chemicals may travel long distances from their point of origin, some to accumulate in certain parts of the environment (e.g., sediment on lake bottoms) or in plant or animal tissue. The presence of toxic chemicals as measured in the environment is difficult (if not impossible) to trace back to a source, but is one indication of what types of contamination are likely to be problems in what situations and which pollutants are increasing or decreasing in frequency of detection or amount under certain circumstances.
- While there are hundreds or perhaps thousands of databases that contain information on toxic chemicals in the environment, research for this report identified fewer than a score that are both national in scope and broad in coverage of toxic chemicals. Few of those are current and non-duplicative. The preponderance of information on toxic chemicals in the environment is collected under the authority of state and local governments and maintained either by them or by the entities that they regulate. These databases may serve the needs of those groups very well. Their content, however, is not sufficiently uniform or well-defined to permit combination for analysis on a larger geographic area as large as the entire country. Other databases, while national in scope, are narrowly focused on a small set of chemicals, reflecting the information needs of specific regulatory programs.
- The few databases that both are national in scope and cover a large set of toxic chemicals generally contain comparatively few measurements on many of those chemicals. Although some of these databases are described

as containing information on several hundred chemicals and information from tens of thousands of sampling sites, *Toxics Watch* found particular chemicals too often have been measured at only a tiny fraction of the sites and/or on a few occasions.

- An important opportunity for collecting nationwide data on toxics contamination at comparatively low cost and effort, however, is provided by the existence of large, national monitoring networks that collect data on a limited set of air and surface water contaminants using well-described and consistent protocols. Much of the expense involved in environmental monitoring reflects the collection of samples and is ongoing. Expanding the set of chemicals for which analyses are conducted may greatly magnify the utility of these data collection networks, with a comparatively minor increase in marginal costs.

- At present, a relatively small fraction of information in the few databases with broad coverage is suitable for assessing trends or making comparisons on a national level. Most of these databases contain information that was collected and submitted by dozens of independent agencies and organizations for different purposes. The lack of consistency in monitoring methods and conditions for the different data sources results in uncertainty about any particular portion of the data. Problems of quality control and consistency in reporting and maintaining data have different impacts. When data are aggregated from so many data sources, the relative importance of each problem becomes moot; the net result is that making comparisons is difficult and long-term trend analysis is unreliable.[a]

- The limitations of the databases described in the chapter greatly decrease the confidence that can be placed in any *nationwide* conclusions that can be drawn about contamination of the ambient environment by toxic chemicals. This clearly does not mean to suggest that such contamination does not exist or cannot be characterized in more limited geographic areas or for a more limited group of contaminants, but only that it cannot be adequately characterized in broad national assessments.

Air

- A huge amount of information is available on the six chemical substances for which National Ambient Air Quality Standards (NAAQS) have been set.[b] Hundreds of stations across the country routinely measure concentrations of these contaminants in air, using standardized methodology, so that detailed

[a] For example, if comparing one measurement with known accuracy to the nearest 1 part per billion to another measurement with unknown accuracy that may only be to the nearest 1,000 parts per million, the combination of the two results might be an accurate representation of the data but of limited usefulness. If comparing one measurement that is recorded in parts per million and another in frequency of occurrence, the two results could not be combined at all. But if both of these situations are mixed together with thousands of other unknowns and peculiarities, overall conclusions can only be educated guesses.

[b] Carbon monoxide, nitrogen oxide, reactive volatile organic compounds (VOCs), sulfur dioxide, lead, and ozone. Data are also collected on particulates.

time-trend data are available on a local, regional, and national basis. Publications and computer tools make these data readily accessible.

- No such consistent data collection goes on with regard to other toxic chemicals in air. Several hundred stations in the Aerometric Information Retrieval System (AIRS) maintained by EPA do monitor toxic organics and heavy metals, but far fewer data are available on far fewer chemicals than the theoretical coverage of the database indicates. For a majority of stations the type of monitoring is unknown, and the methods of measurement and reporting and the meaning of the reported data are inconsistent or unknown. The data that have been collected do not support any national conclusions for chemicals other than those that are the subject of NAAQS.

Water

- EPA's STORET database contains a Water Quality System (WQS), with information reported by 800,000 sampling sites on approximately 14,000 water quality parameters. Data on approximately 2,500 discrete chemicals are reported. Similarly to the air data, most of these data that were collected to meet local needs are of uneven or unknown quality and consistency; thus they are not useful for making reliable assessments of broad regional or national water quality.

- The U.S. Geological Survey (USGS) maintains a nationwide system of several hundred stations that monitor water quality, with nationally consistent measurement and reporting; these data are available in WQS.[c] This very small subset of WQS data is suitable for evaluating water conditions on a nationwide basis. Only one of the toxic chemicals on the search list for this report (see Table 8-1), phosphorus, was reported by most of these stations. A small subset of the search list chemicals (primarily heavy metals and pesticides) was reported over a 10-year period by more than 20 of these stations. A slightly larger subset (including a number of toxic organics) was reported by several stations between 1988 and 1991, but not thereafter.

Especially in the case of water, any comparison of data among stations is greatly complicated by the site-specific nature of water pollution. A given concentration of a chemical in one location may be very dangerous, while the same concentration may not be considered a problem at another location, depending on the characteristics of the flow, temperature and acidity of the water, uses of the water body, and many other factors. Matched-stations analysis, necessary for accurate conclusions about trends, further restricts the number of sampling stations and chemicals. In fact, only six stations consistently report data on any of these chemicals for the full 10-year period.

[c] They are also available in the National Water Data Exchange system (NAWDEX), maintained by USGS.

Analyses of the available data for all stations, covering five heavy metals and three organics, suggests that average concentrations of heavy metals are decreasing, while those of organic chemicals are not. Data from the matched stations are generally similar to those from the whole set of stations, although for cadmium and lead the trend of decreasing concentrations is less pronounced.

Land

- There is no national database on contaminants in soil comparable to those for air and water. The most complete, consistent database on soil contamination comes from investigations of the highly contaminated soil found at Superfund sites. This CARD database[d] contains information from hundreds of sites on the majority of the toxic chemicals in the search set. Because of the nature of site selection and sampling strategy, these data are not broadly representative of national conditions and cannot be used to investigate temporal trends. They do, however, indicate the chemicals that are most frequently found at contaminated sites and those found in the highest concentrations. These are chemicals that, in at least one sense, represent significant environmental problems. The chemicals in the search set that were found at the largest number of contaminated sites are dichloromethane, di-(2-ethylhexyl) phthalate, toluene, trichloroethylene, benzene, chlorobenzene, 1,4-dichlorobenzene, 1,2,4-trichlorobenzene, dieldrin, and anthracene. Six of these are carcinogens.

Criteria for Selecting Databases for This Study

Toxics Watch's survey of databases on toxic contamination of the environment is by no means exhaustive; it focuses specifically on the type of databases that are required for the broad national analyses of ambient conditions — i.e., databases that are current and actively maintained, national in scope, broad in chemical coverage, and publicly accessible. Databases of chemical contamination of human tissue, food, or other plants and animals were not included. A number of databases were rejected for this study that are useful for other purposes, and most of the databases that are described were developed for other applications.

The task of looking at every database for contamination information on every toxic chemical would be practically impossible, because there are hundreds of databases that include information on some aspect of chemicals in the environment. Most are designed to meet specific program needs or regulatory requirements, not for assessing national trends. In some cases, the problem is one of content coverage; in other cases, organization of the data does not readily permit retrieval for purposes other than the original one. For example,

[d] Contract Laboratory Program Analytical Results Database. It is maintained by EPA's Office of Solid Waste and Remedial Response

a system that is designed to be searched on the basis of monitoring station location is difficult to use when looking for aggregate data on a set of chemicals for a wide geographic area. Criteria used for selecting databases to be searched for this report include currency, geographic scope, chemical scope, and accessibility.

To assess present conditions and trends, the database should be *active and current*, with continuing data entry and accessibility. A purely historical analysis could, by contrast, make use of some discontinued databases, if they were still accessible. Some historical data (covering 1970 to 1987) are available on chemical contaminants in human fat and on contamination of ambient air by volatile organic compounds.

Many data on environmental contamination by chemicals have been collected in the context of local, state, and regional investigations. These data are not generally maintained in any central national location, but may be found at the decentralized level in specialized databases developed for each specific project. These specialized data collections do not offer the *geographic scope* needed for a national examination. Such a broad look at ambient environmental contamination as is attempted in this report requires data that are reasonably comparable for different locations and have been combined in an accessible national database. It would not be feasible to contact each locality, state, and regional organization that maintains a database to ascertain what data they have, what they represent, and what are the characteristics that would determine which of the data could be compared to those in another database.

Some databases contain data on environmental contamination and are national in scope, but the data were collected by many methods for many different purposes. Although such databases were used in this report, their data are difficult to combine and compare for national assessments because of different methods used in collecting and reporting the data, in establishing quality controls, and in maintaining the data. Some of the data in such databases are extremely valuable; some are almost useless. Even when the data from one source are of high quality and are internally consistent, a difference in sampling methods or analytical procedures from data in another source may preclude meaningful comparison. The total concentration of a chemical in water and its dissolved concentration cannot be directly compared, for example, nor can the average annual concentration of a chemical in ambient air for 10 monitoring stations in a community and the peak one-time concentration at a single monitoring station.

Many databases are designed to capture data on relatively narrowly specified sets of chemicals; they do not meet the criterion of this report for *chemical scope.* While such "tailored" databases may contain a great deal of generally useful information, the pre-selection process for chemical coverage limits their applicability for broader analyses of the sources of environmental contamination. A database devoted to pesticides, for example, can provide little information on the relative contributions of pesticides and of other commercial chemicals to measured contamination.

The purpose of *Toxics Watch* is to inform the general public, making *public accessibility* the final criterion. Accordingly, this chapter addresses only those databases for which information is publicly available from government sources; it does not include data that are proprietary, confidential, "sensitive," or otherwise publicly unavailable.[e] (See Appendix Q for information on access to the databases discussed in this chapter.)

National Databases Relevant to Environmental Toxics Contamination

Databases on Air Contamination

The Air Quality Subsystem (AQS) of EPA's Aerometric Information Retrieval System (AIRS) contains measurements of ambient concentrations of air pollutants at 120,000 sites, with associated meteorological data.[f] The system primarily addresses the air pollutants for which National Ambient Air Quality Standards (NAAQS) have been set and for which data must be reported to EPA,[g] but some data on toxic pollutants are also available, with a total of 139 chemicals covered. Air quality data must be reported quarterly and emissions data annually. The AQS subsystem has been in operation since 1987, but it includes data from as early as the mid-1950s. EPA has collected nationwide data since the early 1970s. Raw data are available online for the past 10 years, with older data archived.

A useful source of information on data concerning toxic chemicals in air is NATICH (the National Air Toxics Information Clearinghouse). This is not a database of measurements, but an electronic information clearinghouse, used to distribute publications and communicate information. While it does not contain or provide access to any monitoring data, it does include a guide to information on air toxics data collected by various state authorities. For any specified pollutant, the states that monitor that pollutant and the analytical methods they employ can be retrieved electronically. Currently the clearinghouse addresses monitoring of 228 chemicals. Data are also available on the regulatory levels for toxic air contaminants set by state and local authorities.

[e] It should be noted, however, that many of the data reported here may not be as readily available to the reader as they have been to the authors of this report, who worked closely for long hours with government officials and contractors who maintain the databases.

[f] Other components are the AFS - Air Facility Subsystem, and AMS - Area/Mobile Source Subsystem. All are linked via GCS - Geo-Common System.

[g] As stated above: carbon monoxide, nitrogen oxide, reactive volatile organic compounds (VOCs), sulfur dioxide, lead, and ozone; data are also collected on particulates.

Databases on Water Contamination

The Water Quality System (WQS), a part of STORET,[h] contains information on approximately 2,500 chemicals,[i] based on approximately 200 million observations measured at 800,000 locations in freshwater surface water bodies across the United States. Data collected since 1965 cover the entire nation, but the system includes more limited reports from as far back as 1901. This WQS data set includes information from the nationwide system of *NA*tional *S*tream *QU*ality *A*ccounting *N*etwork (NASQUAN) stations maintained by USGS, which are also stored in the USGS WATSTORE database.

The Federal Reporting Data System (FRDS-II) database contains information on violations of the Safe Drinking Water Act at regulated public drinking water supply systems, including the concentrations of contaminants *in excess* of National Primary Drinking Water Standards. For small public water supply systems, all measurements are reported, not just violations.

The Ocean Data Evaluation System (ODES) contains data on 1,100 chemicals measured at 500 sites in coastal and estuarine water, beginning in the 1970s. This database was not addressed for this report because of its limited focus, but will be considered in future editions.

Databases on Soil Contamination and with Multimedia Data

Contacts with a range of government agencies revealed no nationwide database of general soil contamination data comparable to either WQS or AQS. Data on chemicals found in soil at certain contaminated sites can be obtained from CARD (the Contract Laboratory Program Analytical Results Database), which also contains data on water contamination[j] at those sites. This system contains the results of analyses of environmental samples from 33,000 locations, primarily sites being investigated under Superfund.[k] CARD includes all data developed by analytical laboratories working under EPA Superfund contracts.

The CARD data primarily include 167 chemicals on the "Target Compound List" developed under Section 110 of the Superfund Amendments and Reauthorization

[h] STORET (Storage and Retrieval of U.S. Waterways Parametric Data), one of the oldest environmental computer databases still in active use, was originally developed in 1964 by the Public Health Service, but for most of its existence has been maintained by EPA. It consists of 11 linked databases covering a broad range of information on surface water, including chemical discharges, water flow, hydrological linkages, and fish kills.

[i] System personnel indicate that coverage is between 3,000 and 4,000 discrete chemicals; staff conducting this study were able to document approximately 2,500 discrete CAS numbers. Some chemical parameter codes may not have corresponding CAS numbers.

[j] The system contains data on both groundwater and surface water. Because the focus of the database is on chemical analyses, water samples are not reliably coded as to whether they represent surface water or groundwater. Personnel supervising site studies would have independent access to this information.

[k] This is a much larger number of sites than those that are actually designated for the Superfund National Priorities List.

Act (SARA). Data are also available on "Tentatively Identified Compounds"; these chemicals are not on the Target Compound List and are not specifically analyzed, but have been identified in samples submitted for analysis.[1] Data on inorganic chemicals were temporarily unavailable from the CARD database during preparation of this report, except for hydrochloric acid, because of upgrades to the database being implemented at that time. These data should be available for future reports.

Data on Biological Contamination

Evaluations of the risks posed by toxic chemicals in the environment have typically focused on four environmental compartments or media. In addition to air, water, and soil, it is important to consider the *biological* environment, both in terms of chemicals in plants and animals and in terms of the load of environmental contaminants that is present in each human body. There are not as yet any national databases of plant and animal contamination comparable to the ambient environmental quality databases discussed in this chapter. Some of the more important, but more narrowly focused, biological contamination databases will be discussed in the next *Toxics Watch*.

Limitations on Conclusions That Can be Drawn from Available Data

All of the databases discussed here were designed to be broad in both geographic and chemical focus; all proved to be limited in their ability to support analyses of conditions and trends in contamination by toxics. A typical database might be described as containing observations on 140 chemicals and observations from 120,000 measurement sites, but most of the sites have measurements on only half a dozen chemicals, while only a handful of sites have measurements on more than a dozen chemicals, and none may have measurements on all of the 140 chemicals. To a large extent, this reflects the specific, limited, programmatic needs that the databases were designed to meet; they were not designed, nor funded, to be comprehensive.

Even in the rare cases where much nationwide information is available on a given chemical, national conclusions have their limitations, because pollution is so dependent on local conditions. If a certain chemical is hardly ever detected in water, it is reasonable to conclude that it does not pose a serious water pollution threat (unless it is a strong bioaccumulator or such a potent toxicant that it is

[1] These are generally identified by comparing chromatographic spectra to libraries of known compounds.

dangerous at levels that are barely detectable by commonly used monitoring methods). But if it is frequently detected in water, the extent of the problem may be difficult to determine. High readings in some locations may be offset by low readings in others, so that the average seems acceptable despite a serious problem at some sites. As mentioned above, a concentration that is considered dangerous in one location may be perfectly safe in another. The national conclusions that can be drawn may be just qualitative indications of where to look more carefully.

Selecting a Core Set of Chemicals to Search

Constraints of staff time, both for the study team and those maintaining the databases, limited the number of chemicals for which *Toxics Watch* could seek to retrieve data. Resources were simply not available to search all chemicals reported to the Toxics Release Inventory (TRI) or the RCRA Biennial Reporting System (BRS), for example. A small set of chemicals was selected that would be more or less representative of the universe of toxic chemicals covered by this report. The initial list was developed without regard to the chemical coverage of the databases that had been selected to search:

- the 10 chemicals with the largest quantity of production-related waste reported to TRI in each of four groups distinguished on the basis of special environmental concerns: carcinogens, bioaccumulating[m] chemicals, chloro-organics, and ozone-depleting substances, and
- the 10 Hazardous Air Pollutants with the largest reported air *emissions* (as opposed to total quantities of waste) in TRI.

These 5 groups generated a list of 35 chemicals, because of the overlap in group definitions. The following chemicals were then added to the list:

- five chemicals (not included in any of the preceding groups) covered by the 33/50 Program[n] for voluntary reductions in environmental releases: three heavy metals (cadmium, chromium,[o] and nickel) and two organic chemicals (chloroform and methyl isobutyl ketone);
- six chemicals that are generally well represented in databases of environmental contamination; and
- one chemical that is known to be a potent carcinogen (dieldrin, a pesticide) and six chemicals that produce other (non-cancer) toxic effects at low doses — that are represented in at least two databases on environmental contamination.

[m] As defined by EPA in *1992 Toxics Release Inventory Public Data Release.*

[n] This voluntary program administered by EPA solicits agreements by firms to decrease releases and off-site transfers of 17 toxic chemicals 33 percent by 1992 and 50 percent by 1995, relative to 1988 amounts.

[o] Because EPA uses separate CAS registry numbers to distinguish trivalent and hexavalent chromium, both numbers were used.

Table 8-1. Chemicals in Toxics Watch *Search Set*

CAS Number	Chemical Name
Carcinogens, Bioaccumulators, Chlorine Compounds, and Ozone Depleters Produced as Waste in Large Quantities, and Hazardous Air Pollutants with Large Emissions	
50-00-0	Formaldehyde
56-23-5	Carbon tetrachloride
67-56-1	Methanol
67-72-1	Hexachloroethane
71-43-2	Benzene
71-55-6	1,1,1-Trichloroethane
75-01-4	Vinyl chloride
75-05-8	Acetonitrile
75-09-2	Dichloromethane
75-15-0	Carbon disulfide
75-69-4	Trichlorofluoromethane (CFC-11)
75-71-8	Dichlorodifluoromethane (CFC-12)
76-13-1	Freon 113
78-87-5	1,2-Dichloropropane
78-93-3	Methyl ethyl ketone
79-00-5	1,1,2-Trichloroethane
79-01-6	Trichloroethylene
87-68-3	Hexachloro-1,3-butadiene
95-50-1	1,2-Dichlorobenzene
100-42-5	Styrene
106-46-7	1,4-Dichlorobenzene
106-99-0	1,3-Butadiene
107-06-2	1,2-Dichloroethane
107-21-1	Ethylene glycol
108-88-3	Toluene
117-81-7	Di-(2-ethylhexyl) phthalate
118-74-1	Hexachlorobenzene
120-12-7	Anthracene
120-82-1	1,2,4-Trichlorobenzene
127-18-4	Tetrachloroethylene
1330-20-7	Xylene (mixed isomers)
7439-92-1	Lead
7439-97-6	Mercury
7647-01-0	Hydrochloric acid
7782-50-5	Chlorine
Additional Chemicals from the 33/50 Program	
67-66-3	Chloroform
108-10-1	Methyl isobutyl ketone
7440-02-0	Nickel
7440-43-9	Cadmium
7440-47-3	Chromium
Chemicals with Good Coverage in Environmental Databases	
74-87-3	Chloromethane
75-00-3	Chloroethane
75-25-2	Bromoform
79-34-5	1,1,2,2-Tetrachloroethane
100-41-4	Ethylbenzene
108-90-7	Chlorobenzene
Potent Carcinogens and Particularly Toxic Chemicals, Found in Two or More Databases	
60-57-1	Dieldrin
88-74-4	ortho-Nitroaniline
106-93-4	1,2-Dibromoethane
107-02-8	Acrolein
1024-57-3	Epoxyheptachlor
7439-96-5	Manganese
7723-14-0	Phosphorus (yellow or white)

The final *Toxics Watch* search set therefore consisted of 53 chemicals for which attempts were made to retrieve data on environmental concentrations. (See Table 8-1.) Success in retrieving data on the various chemicals varied considerably, both because only those sampling stations with consistent nationwide reporting were examined in each database, and because many of these chemicals have only been measured at a very small subset of the sampling stations contained in any given database. (See Table 8-2.)

Table 8-2. Coverage of Chemicals in Toxics Watch *Search Set in Databases**

CAS Number	Chemical	NAMS	SLAMS	AQS** Unknown	AQS** Other	AQS** Industrial
50-00-0	Formaldehyde				32	7
56-23-5	Carbon tetrachloride					
60-57-1	Dieldrin					
67-56-1	Methanol					4
67-66-3	Chloroform					
67-72-1	Hexachloroethane					
71-43-2	Benzene			34	92	16
71-55-6	1,1,1-Trichloroethane					
74-87-3	Chloromethane					
75-00-3	Chloroethane			36	19	2
75-01-4	Vinyl chloride			36	27	
75-05-8	Acetonitrile					
75-09-2	Dichloromethane			36	63	14
75-15-0	Carbon disulfide					
75-25-2	Bromoform					
75-69-4	Trichlorofluoromethane (CFC-11)			8	8	
75-71-8	Dichlorodifluoromethane (CFC-12)			8	7	
76-13-1	Freon 113				5	
78-87-5	1,2-Dichloropropane			36	25	
78-93-3	Methyl ethyl ketone					
79-00-5	1,1,2-Trichloroethane			36	24	
79-01-6	Trichloroethylene			35	54	
79-34-5	1,1,2,2-Tetrachloroethane					
87-68-3	Hexachloro-1,3-butadiene			8	7	
88-74-4	ortho-Nitroaniline					
95-50-1	1,2-Dichlorobenzene			36	25	5
100-41-4	Ethylbenzene			34	66	16
100-42-5	Styrene			8	41	11
106-46-7	1,4-Dichlorobenzene			36	24	9
106-93-4	1,2-Dibromoethane			8	36	
106-99-0	1,3-Butadiene					7
107-02-8	Acrolein				26	2
107-06-2	1,2-Dichloroethane			36	46	14
107-21-1	Ethylene glycol					
108-10-1	Methyl isobutyl ketone					
108-88-3	Toluene			34	80	16
108-90-7	Chlorobenzene					
117-81-7	Di-(2-ethylhexyl) phthalate					
118-74-1	Hexachlorobenzene					
120-12-7	Anthracene				1	
120-82-1	1,2,4-Trichlorobenzene			8	8	
127-18-4	Tetrachloroethylene			36	57	12
1024-57-3	Epoxyheptachlor					
1330-20-7	Xylene (mixed isomers)				5	
7439-92-1	Lead	145	444	339	541	48
7439-96-5	Manganese		3	279	102	
7439-97-6	Mercury		2		23	
7440-02-0	Nickel		3	255	95	
7440-43-9	Cadmium		3	285	117	23
7440-47-3	Chromium		3	275	117	14
7647-01-0	Hydrochloric acid					8
7723-14-0	Phosphorus (yellow or white)					
7782-50-5	Chlorine					
	Number of Stations Reporting Any Chemical in Search Set	145	444	464	650	63

* Acronyms appear at end of glossary.

WQS	CARD				
	TCL		TIC		
NSQUAN	Soil	Water	Soil	Water	FRDS-II
			1		
14	86	327			
31	1,617	1,282			240
14	675	1,096			1,136
5	40	120			
5	1,772	1,485			
14	506	678			
12	148	430			1,131
14	80	379			1,130
16	118	466			
			31	32	
14	2,314	1,840			
	670	688			
14	61	286			1,130
51			142	117	1,134
6			49	28	1,134
			384	184	
15	61	326			
	1,387	684			
14	116	329			
15	1,784	1,594			
14	218	424			1,130
5	27	36			1,134
	25	16			
16	166	175			
5	770	515			
4	266	201			
16	1,648	1,331			
3			3	8	
2					
5	167	489			
	501	342			
6	2,240	1,630			
14	1,695	1,469			
5	2,264	1,626			
7	123	59			
5	1,433	223			
5	1,622	1,313			
14	750	736			
29	605	247			
4	1,070	707			
74					
68					
61					
75					
69					
			1	1	
462					
465	2,647	2,270	531	328	1,159

Toxics in Air

The AQS database was developed primarily to address those pollutants for which National Ambient Air Quality Standards (NAAQS) have been set (carbon monoxide, lead, nitrogen dioxide, ozone, and sulfur dioxide),[p] of which only lead is among those toxic chemicals that are the focus of this report. The database developers have provided systems for presenting current information, on both ambient concentrations and emissions of these criteria pollutants, that are quite sophisticated and easy to use, with instantaneous presentation of maps, charts, and graphs of data that are updated monthly. EPA annually issues the *National Air Quality and Emissions Trends Report,*[1] which presents detailed data on trends in concentrations of these six NAAQS contaminants. Data on other toxic pollutants are less available.

In addition to the data from the National Air Monitoring System (NAMS) stations that are its primary focus, AQS contains concentration data reported by a variety of monitoring systems or types. (See Appendix G, Table G-6.) These monitor types vary with respect to the degree of quality assurance and quality control that can be assumed for reported data. According to technical support personnel, NAMS, SLAMS (State and Local Air Monitoring System), and PAMS (Photochemical Air Monitoring System) monitors have consistent, high quality data. The nature, quality, and consistency of data reported for other monitor types is generally unknown to AQS support staff or system users.

Some data are available in AQS for almost two-thirds (33 of 53) of the chemicals in the search set described above. Most of these data, however, come from monitor types described as "Other" or "Unknown." Of the 33 chemicals, NAMS data were available only for lead, the one chemical on the list for which a NAAQS has been set. SLAMS data were available for lead, with a few observations for five additional heavy metals associated with suspended particulates. The other 28 chemicals had data reported only from less authoritative sources. The largest number of chemicals (30) was reported for "other" monitor types, and the largest percentage (46 percent) of individual observations was from "unknown" monitor types. (See Figure 8-1 and Table 8-2.)

The SLAMS data represent a small fraction of the observations reported in AQS on the chemicals in the search set (14 percent). These data address only heavy metals, so none of the organic chemicals or non-metallic inorganics in the data set are represented. Although a few of these stations did monitor for these heavy metals, the actual number of measurements taken was insufficient to support an analysis for any chemical other than lead. The number of stations reporting a measurement for any one of the five other metals is extremely small, and none of the reporting stations had a continuous record of measurements for more than two consecutive years. It is therefore not possible to

[p] Reactive volatile organic compounds (VOCs) and particulate matter are also covered, but these are not discrete, identifiable chemicals.

Figure 8-1.

Chemicals in Toxics Watch *Search Set Found in Air Quality Subsystem, by Type of Station*

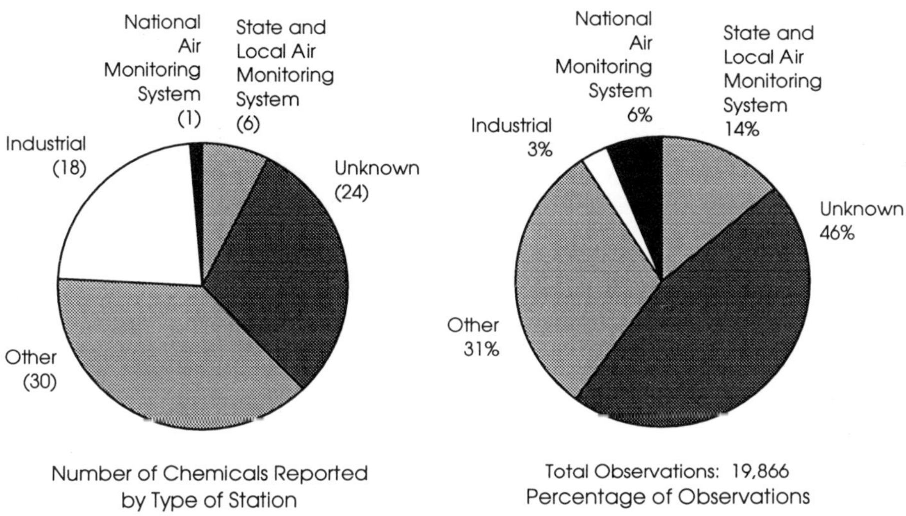

See list of chemicals, Table 3-1

make any meaningful statement on spatial or temporal patterns of air contamination from this limited data set. In general, SLAMS data expand the geographic range of NAMS data, but do not significantly expand chemical coverage. (See Table 8-3.)

It might be possible to obtain useful information on trends by studying those stations classified as "Other" and "Unknown," if one selected only those stations that reported data on a set of chemicals in each of several consecutive years. Aggregations across different stations, however, would be unreliable. For stations classified "Other," only six stations reported on one or more chemicals in the search set in eight consecutive years. Because these stations covered only three states, with four stations in a single state, no further analyses were pursued. For the chemicals in the search set, 402 monitors of "Unknown" type reported data between 1984 and 1993. Only 20 of these reported data in ten consecutive years, with an additional 11 reporting data in nine consecutive years. Again, the geographic scope of the data was limited: of these 31 stations, 14 were located in Illinois, 16 in Kansas, and one in Nebraska.

Toxics in Water

Using and Interpreting WQS Data on Contaminants in Surface Waters

STORET and its WQS subsystem have evolved considerably over the past 30 years, incorporating many types of data that were not envisioned when the system was

Table 8-3. State and Local Air Monitoring System (SLAMS) Stations Reporting Metals from 1983 through 1993

	Number of Stations Reporting Each Chemical					
Year	**Cadmium**	**Chromium**	**Lead**	**Manganese**	**Mercury**	**Nickel**
1983	0	0	266	0	0	0
1984	0	0	304	0	0	0
1985	0	0	303	0	0	0
1986	0	0	307	0	0	0
1987	0	0	266	0	0	0
1988	1	1	252	1	0	1
1989	0	0	201	0	0	0
1990	0	0	204	0	0	0
1991	0	0	192	0	0	0
1992	2	2	197	2	2	2
1993	2	1	186	1	2	2

Source: Aerometric Information Retrieval System (AIRS)

originally designed.[q] The creative adaptations have made the system able to accommodate information of more recent concern, but make comparisons over time very difficult. Another difficulty results from the nature of the sources of STORET data. STORET is maintained as a convenience for roughly 1,000 federal, state, and local agencies, and its data are contributed not only by those but also by universities, contractors, and even individuals. Each individual or agency reporting data to WQS is independently responsible for the nature and quality of the data.[r] Multiple agencies may also submit similar, but not identical, data to the system, so that data on any single chemical may be represented by several distinct water quality parameters, some of which appear to be redundant.

For any assessment of surface water quality, it is critical to bear in mind that each local water body has distinctive characteristics of setting, flow regime, and fundamental chemistry that will influence the behavior of toxic contaminants. Accordingly, it is even more important than in air monitoring to ensure that trend data reflect samples from a consistent set of stations. Otherwise, different characteristics of the set of monitoring stations used to derive data for different years may induce spurious temporal trends.

[q] The system was originally intended to maintain data on surface water samples (ranging from the concentrations of chemical contaminants to ratings of the severity of floating garbage), but now also includes information on groundwater, sediments, and fish tissue samples. Data fields have been creatively adapted to accommodate new information, such that the meaning of a particular data field is not necessarily constant, but depends upon the contents of other fields. For example, time code fields are used instead for species designations, when fish tissue data, rather than water data, are reported.

[r] While the system does provide some checks to ensure that entered data are valid, any of these limitations may be overridden by the agency submitting data.

Selection of Monitoring Stations to Search

Because of the practical impossibility of ascertaining the quality of STORET data from the dozens of agencies supplying it, investigations for this report used only data from the National Stream Quality Accounting Network (NASQUAN) stations maintained by USGS. These are the only stations in the database that offer consistent reporting on a nationwide basis. For specific local studies, in contrast, it may be possible or desirable to make effective use of state and local data as well.[s]

Coverage of the Chemical Search Set

STORET parameter codes for the chemicals searched for in this study are presented in Appendix G, Table G-7.[t] Eventually all but 2 of the 53 chemicals in the search set were found in WQS; no parameter codes were located for Freon 113 (1,1,2-trichloro-1,2,2-trifluoroethane) or for ortho-nitroaniline. Of the remaining 51 chemicals, 40 have data from at least one NASQUAN station; the others are presumably reported by other agencies.

For many of the chemicals, the number of stations that report concentration data or any specific type of information is few. No more than 10 stations were found to report 15 of the chemicals, and 20 or fewer stations reported 31 chemicals. Only 7 of the chemicals are reported by more than 50 stations, and only phosphorus is reported by more than 100 stations,[u] out of the 605 stations that were searched. Of the 605 stations, 462 have data on at least one of the chemicals in the search set. The pattern appears to be that most stations report concentration data for very few of the chemicals searched for, while a very few stations report such data for many chemicals. Accordingly, any conclusions drawn from these data for most of these chemicals may not truly represent national trends.

Temporal trends are difficult to discern from this database, because reporting over time is sporadic. Eight chemicals (cadmium, lead, chromium, manganese, nickel, trichlorofluoromethane [CFC-11], dieldrin, and epoxyheptachlor) were consistently reported by several stations in each of the 10 years from 1984 through 1993. Another 16 chemicals were reported by at least eight stations between 1988 and 1991, with reporting by a slightly smaller number of stations in 1987. The remaining 15 chemicals of the 40 with any data are reported sporadically by a small number of stations. (See Figure 8-2.)

Unfortunately, however, the number of stations that consistently report data on a chemical over time is much smaller. Only 10 stations consistently report data on

[s] The data retrieval routines for STORET are principally oriented toward the user seeking data about a specific, limited, geographic area.

[t] There are multiple parameters for most chemicals; the selected ones represent total water concentrations, rather than dissolved or suspended fractions.

[u] The widespread reporting of phosphorus is probably related to concerns over its contribution to eutrophication, rather than to its toxicity.

Figure 8-2.

Number of NASQUAN Stations Reporting Chemicals in Toxics Watch *Search Set, 1984 -1993*

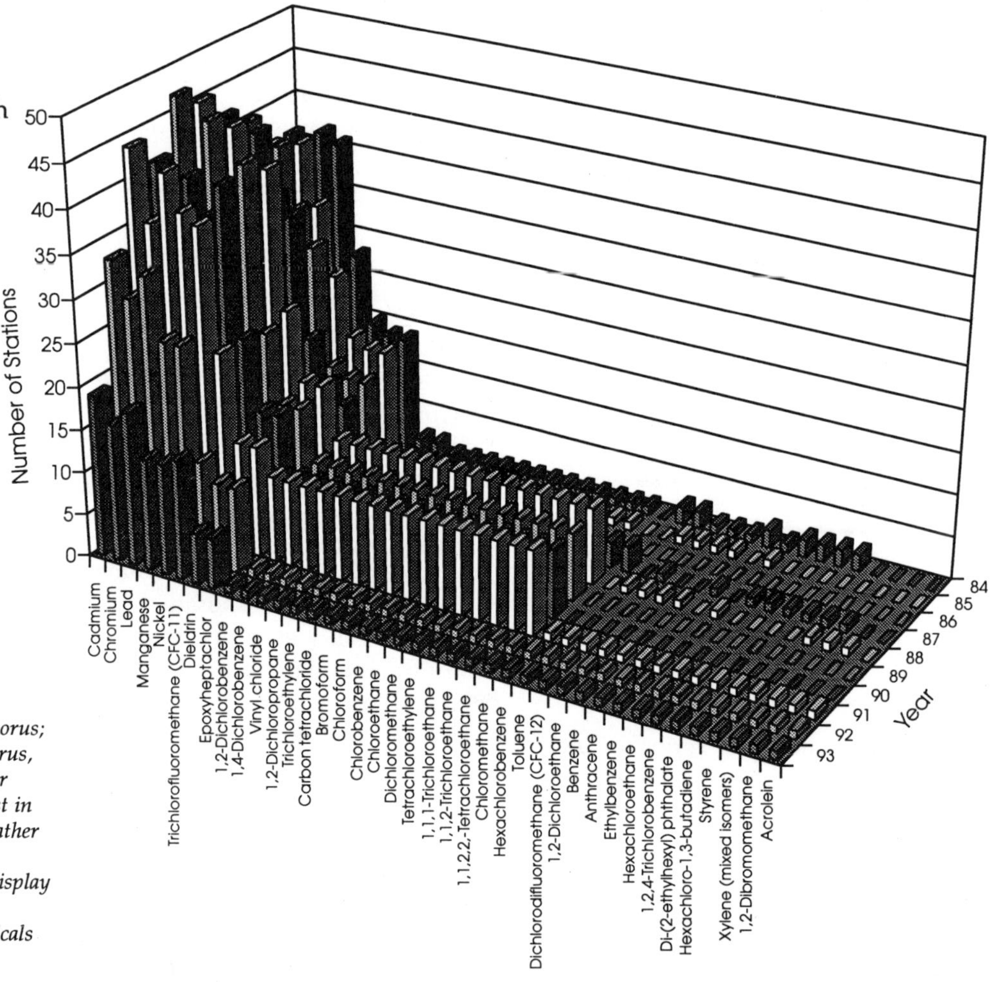

Excludes phosphorus; data for phosphorus, collected for other purposes (interest in eutrophication rather than toxicity), overwhelm the display of data for the remaining chemicals

chemicals other than phosphorus for the full 10-year period, and these data cover only three chemicals (cadmium, chromium, lead). Six of these stations have data on manganese and six have data on nickel (only two stations have data on both metals). A larger number of stations present data in each of the four years 1988-1991, ranging from 34 stations with data on lead to 24 stations for chromium. In general, the data from the matched stations are similar to those for the full set of reporting stations (Figure 8-3), although the decreases seen in average concentrations of cadmium and lead are less pronounced. No significant trends were observed in the four-year data series from matched stations, which substantially resemble the data from all stations for those years.

Figure 8-3.

Number of NASQUAN Stations Reporting Chemicals in Toxics Watch *Search Set over Four- and Ten-Year Periods ("Matched Stations"), 1984-1993*

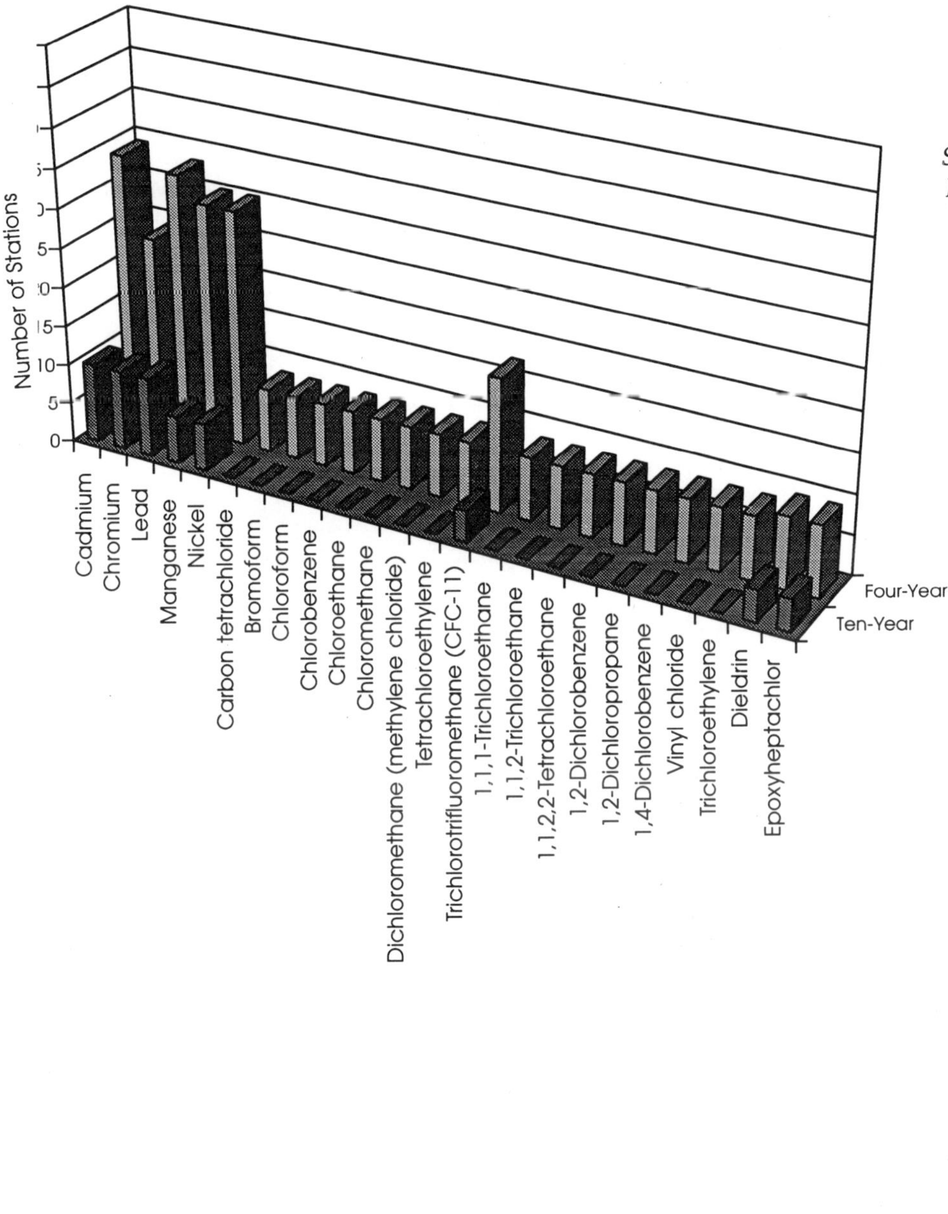

Figure 8-4.

Concentrations of Water Contaminants Reported in Water Quality System of STORET, 1984-1993

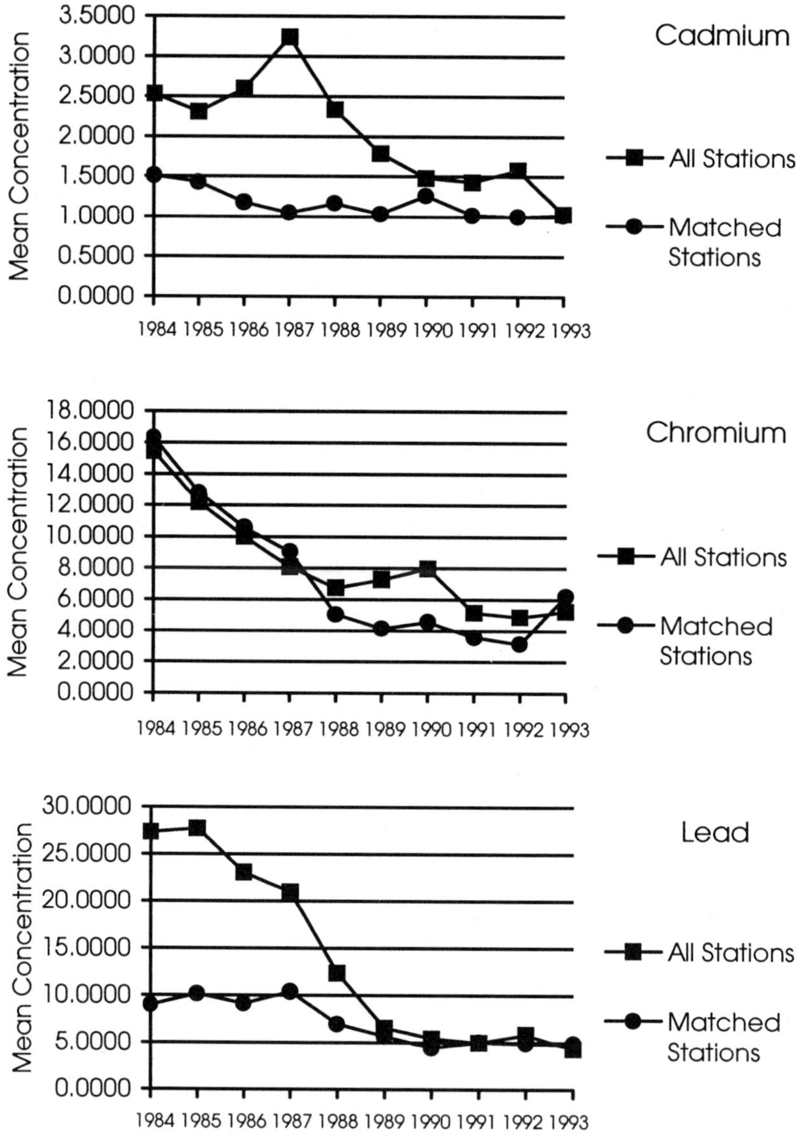

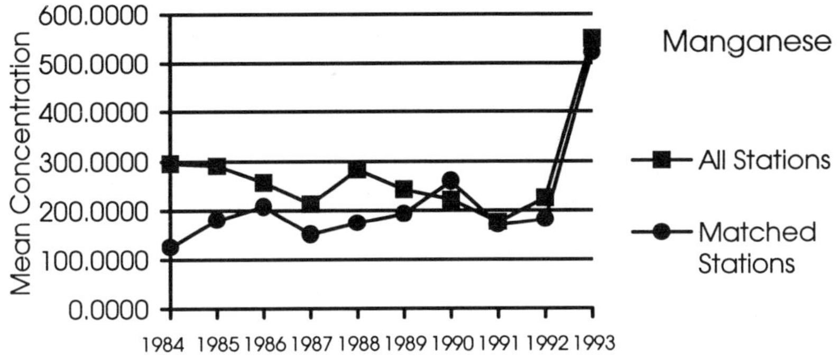

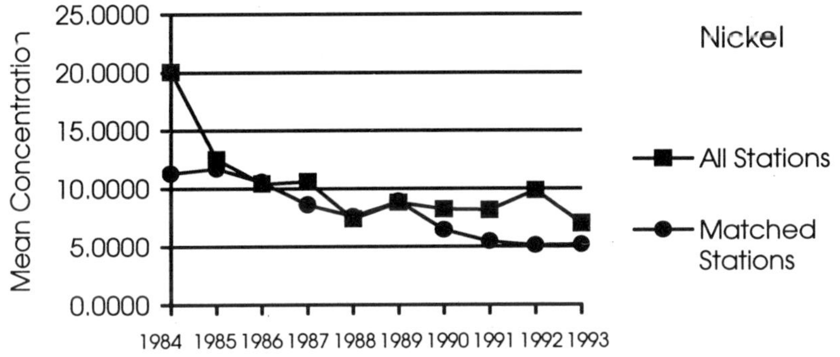

National Trends in Contaminant Concentrations in Surface Waters

Of the five heavy metals for which reporting is consistently available over the past decade, three (cadmium, lead, and chromium) show a marked, continuing decline in mean concentration reported by NASQUAN stations, while one (nickel) shows a decline occurring principally in the first two years of the decade. Only manganese concentrations in surface water do not appear to be decreasing, with a slight decline between 1984 and 1991 offset by a marked increase in 1993. (See Figure 8-4.)

In contrast, none of the three organic compounds (trichloro-trifluoromethane [CFC-11], dieldrin, and epoxyheptachlor) for which data are available for the entire decade shows any evidence of decreasing concentrations. These data suggest that, while in some respects the quality of the nation's surface water is improving, other aspects of toxic contamination are not being ameliorated. With such a limited sample set, however, one would not wish to place too much reliance on these trends.

Contaminants in Drinking Water Supplies

Some data were available in FRDS-II for nine of the chemicals in the *Toxics Watch* search set: eight halogenated organics, many of which are byproducts of water chlorination, and the pesticide dieldrin. For the subset of stations (small public water supply systems) that report data on all measured concentrations of a chemical, and not only those in excess of standards, there were 235 that reported data on all nine chemicals, 880 that reported on eight chemicals,[v] and 44 that reported on fewer than eight chemicals.

This represents a rich data set. Unfortunately, it has little utility for assessing national trends, as the station identifiers indicate that only three states are represented by reporting stations, and that more than three-quarters of these are located in Missouri.

Contaminated Sites — The CARD Database

CARD contains data on almost all of the organic chemicals in the search set. For soil measurements, data were available for 41 chemicals; only 4 of the organic chemicals did not have CARD data (methanol, 1,3-butadiene, acrolein, and ethylene glycol). Of the 41 chemicals, 34 were Target Compound List chemicals that were explicitly analyzed for in samples. The remaining seven were Tentatively Identified Compounds for which specific analysis had not been conducted. For water measurements, CARD data were available for 40 organic chemicals (all but the 4 listed above and formaldehyde). (See Figure 8-5.)

For the compounds in the search set, usable data were available for many more sites in CARD than was the case for either AQS or WQS. CARD data were available on one or more Target Compound List compounds in soil for 2,647 sites and in water for 2,270 sites. Tentatively Identified Compounds on the search list were reported for 531 sites and 328 sites in soil and water, respectively. (See Table 8-2.)

In contrast to SLAMS monitors in AQS, which are almost exclusively dedicated to monitoring NAAQS chemicals, or the slightly broader scope of NASQUAN stations, the majority of CARD sites appear to include explicit analysis for a broad range of chemicals. The higher proportion of usable data obtained from CARD reflects the purpose and design of the database. Not only does CARD contain more data useful to national assessment purposes, but the data it includes are of higher quality, because quality assurance control procedures (QA/QC) are an explicit focus of this database and all data are collected under EPA-specified protocols.

[v] Whenever eight of the nine chemicals were reported, dieldrin was the missing chemical.

Figure 8-5.

Chemicals in Toxics Watch *Search Set Found at Hazardous Waste Sites, Reported to CARD*

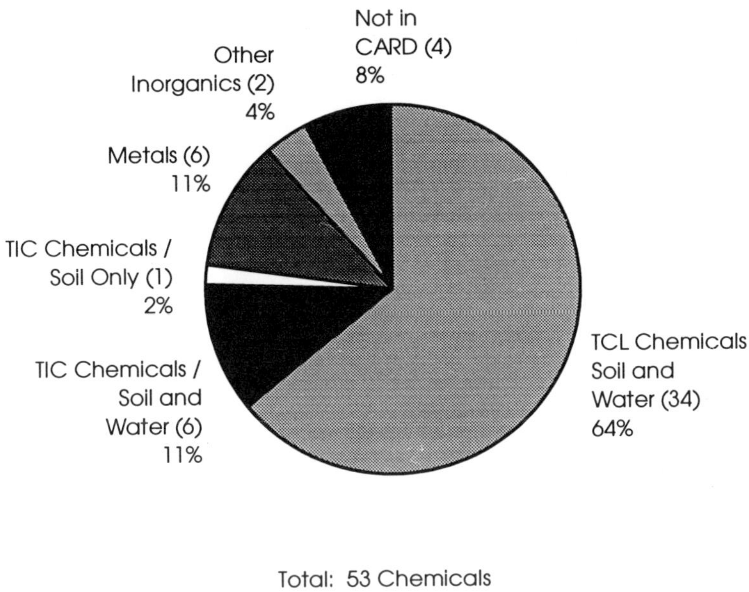

CARD: Contract Laboratory Program Analytical Results Database

TIC: Tentatively Identified Compounds;

TCL: Target Compound List

The greatest drawback of CARD data is imposed by the nature of the contaminated-site investigations for which these data are gathered. The data do not represent soil and water conditions generally, because they are collected only at sites where there is strong reason to expect contamination. Also, data are gathered during a certain (usually brief) time period for each site; no meaningful time series data are collected.

Chemicals Found at Contaminated Sites

Because the coverage of chemicals in the search set is so complete and the sampling sites are by definition environmental problems (Superfund sites), the data in CARD *are* useful as an indicator of which of these chemicals represent the most significant *known* problems of soil and water contamination at such sites. For the Target Compound List compounds at least, which are explicitly analyzed at most sites, *frequency of detection* either within or across sites provides an indication of the pervasiveness of the problem represented by the chemical. Contaminant *concentrations* indicate the severity of the problem posed by the chemical.

Chemicals in Soil at Contaminated Sites

Of the 34 Target Compound List chemicals in the search set that were detected in soil (which excludes the metals and other inorganic chemicals temporarily unavailable from the database), 12 were detected at more than 1,000 sites, 9 at more than 1,500 sites, and 3 at more than 2,000

Figure 8-6.

Frequency of Detection and Average Concentrations of TCL Contaminants of CARD Sites: Soil

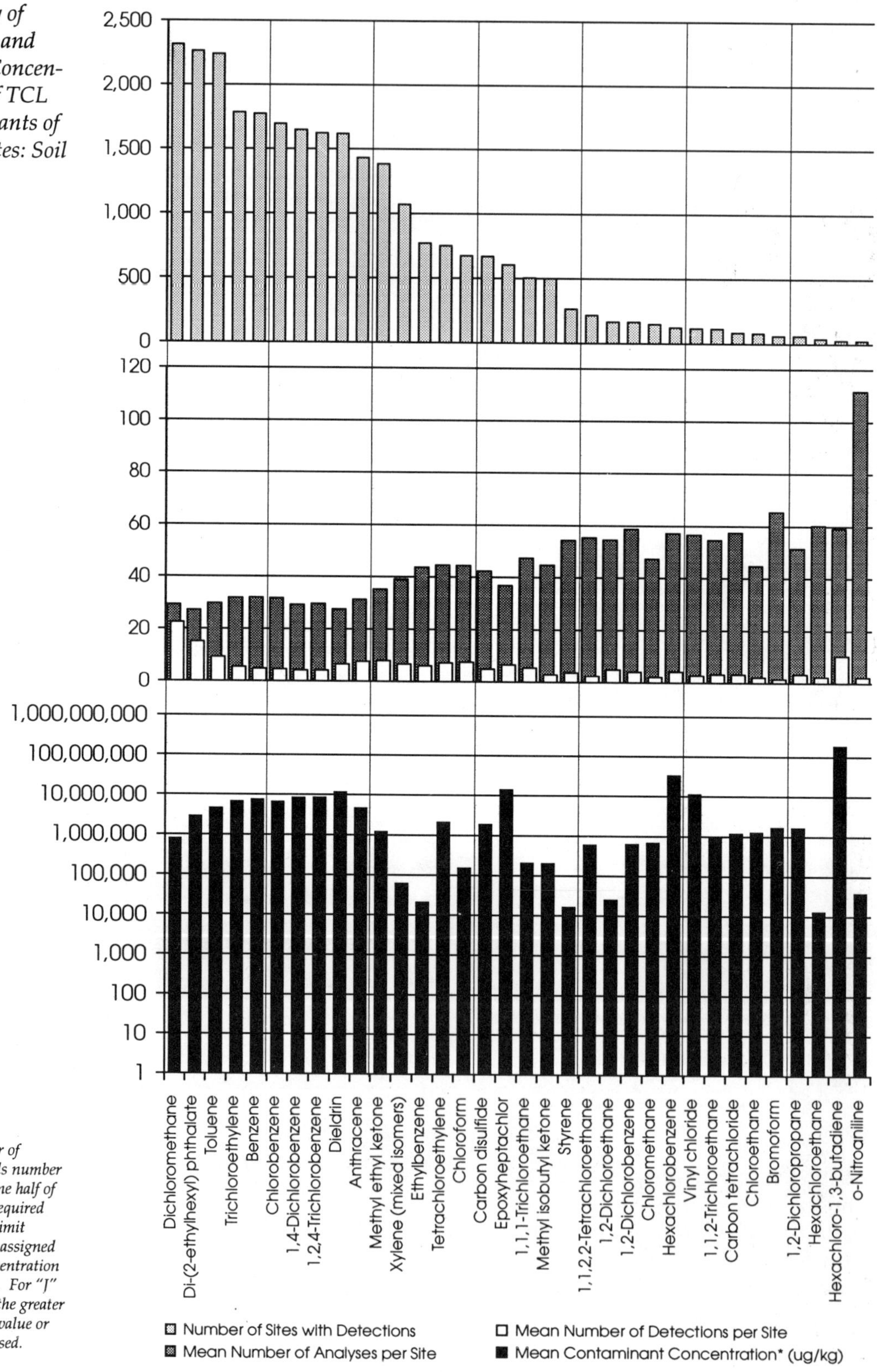

**Where number of analyses exceeds number of detections, one half of the Contract Required Quantitation Limit (CRQL/2) was assigned as a proxy concentration for non-detects. For "J" qualified data, the greater of the reported value or CRQL/2 was used.*

*Table 8-4. Target Compound List Chemicals Most Frequently Detected in Soil**

CAS Number	Chemical	Detections	Carcinogen	Halo-organic
75-09-2	Dichloromethane	2,314	✖	✖
117-81-7	Di-(2-ethylhexyl) phthalate	2,264	✖	
108-88-3	Toluene	2,240		
79-01-6	Trichloroethylene	1,784	✖	✖
71-43-2	Benzene	1,772	✖	
108-90-7	Chlorobenzene	1,695		✖
106-46-7	1,4-Dichlorobenzene	1,648	✖	✖
120-82-1	1,2,4-Trichlorobenzene	1,622		✖
60-57-1	Dieldrin	1,617	✖	✖
120-12-7	Anthracene	1,433		

* Excludes metals

sites. The three chemicals found at the largest number of sites (dichloromethane, di-[2-ethylhexyl] phthalate, and toluene) were also the three that were found in the highest proportion of soil samples at each site.

The average *concentrations* of Target Compound List chemicals in soil at a site varied over four orders of magnitude.[W] In general, the average detection concentration bore little relationship to the number of sites at which the chemical was detected, indicating that some chemicals are found in high concentrations at a limited number of sites. Of the five organic chemicals with the highest average concentrations (hexachloro-1,3-butadiene, hexachlorobenzene, epoxyheptachlor, dieldrin, and vinyl chloride), none was among the five most frequently detected; only one was among the ten most frequently detected or detected at more than 1,000 sites (dieldrin). Because many of the chemicals with the highest average concentrations were detected at relatively few sites, they will not be discussed further. (See Figure 8-6.)

Of the 10 most frequently detected Target Compound List chemicals in soil (again, excluding metals) at these sites, six are carcinogens and six are halo-organics (chloro-organics). (See Table 8-4.)

Because the identification of Tentatively Identified Compounds is not definite, greater care is appropriate in describing findings concerning them. Of the seven Tentatively Identified Compounds detected in soil samples, only two (both halogenated organics) were detected at more than 100 sites (Freon 113 and trichlorotrifluoro-

[W]Non-detections were assigned a proxy value of one-half of the contract-required quantitation limit. This is a standard practice for dealing with the failure to detect a chemical in all samples at a given site. A failure to detect may reflect either the true absence of the chemical or simply the insensitivity of the analytical methodology. The proxy value assumes that either cause is equally likely.

Figure 8-7.

Frequency of Detection and Average Concentrations of TIC Contaminants of CARD Sites: Soil

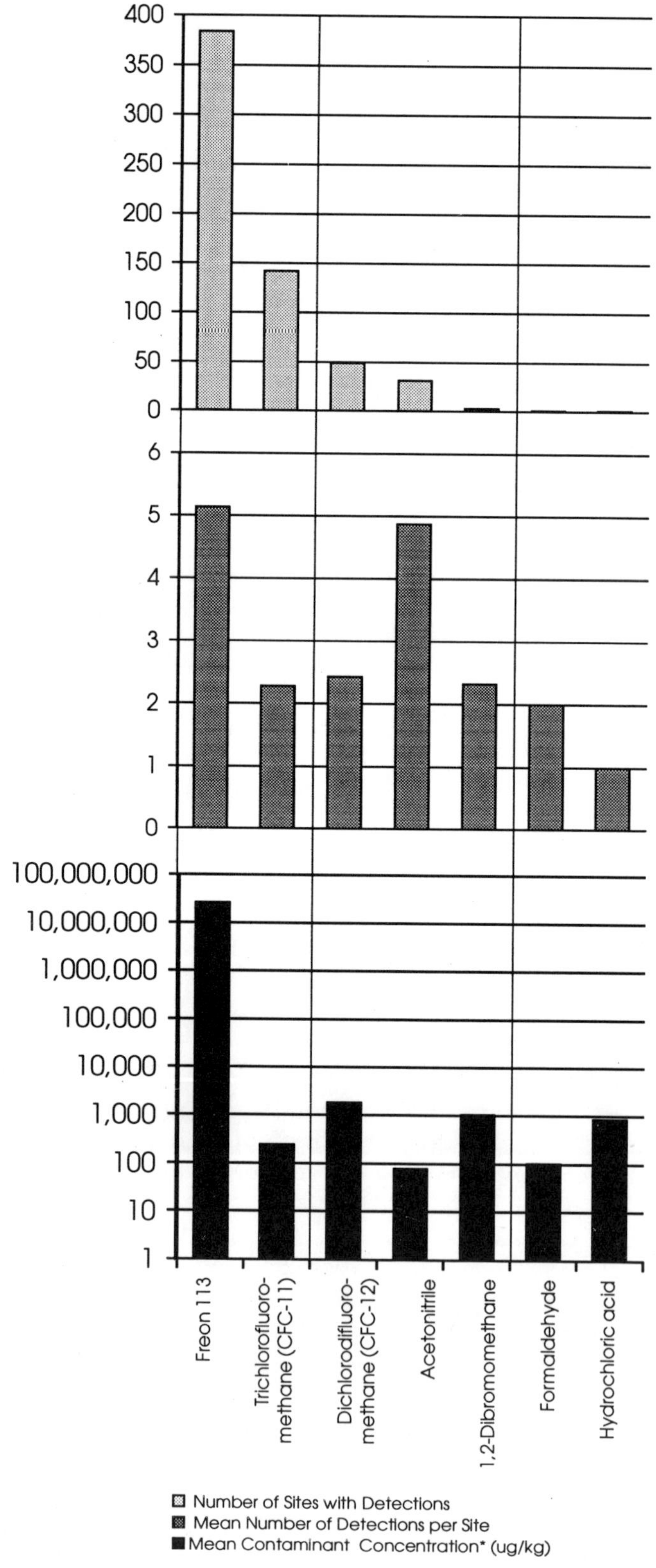

**Where number of analyses exceeds number of detections, one half of the Contract Required Quantitation Limit (CRQL/2) was assigned as a proxy concentration for non-detects. For "J" qualified data, the greater of the reported value or CRQL/2 was used.*

methane [CFC-11]). (See Figure 8-7.) Both chemicals are common laboratory contaminants.

Chemicals in Water at Contaminated Sites

Data for water samples at these contaminated sites show a close similarity to data for soil samples.[x] Ten of the search chemicals were detected in surface or groundwater samples at more than 1,000 sites; with a single exception, these are the same chemicals listed above as most frequently found in soil samples As expected, anthracene was rarely found in water samples, since it has a very low water solubility (0.04 milligrams per liter). Chloroform, a carcinogen and chloro-organic, was found in water at 1,096 sites. This is a common byproduct of water chlorination, although it is not clear whether this is relevant to its detection at contaminated sites. (See Figure 8-8.)

As in the case of the soil data, average frequency of detection at each site was correlated with the number of sites at which a chemical was detected, but average concentration was not. Rather, as was the case for soil data, the most frequently detected chemicals had concentrations that were higher than the median concentration, but not the highest detected concentrations.

The same two Tentatively Identified Compounds that were found in soil samples at more than 100 sites (Freon 113 and trichlorotrifluoromethane [CFC-11]) were found in water samples at more than 100 sites. As noted, these are common laboratory contaminants. (See Figure 8-9.)

[x] Water in this case may represent either surface water or groundwater (data fields distinguishing these two media in CARD are not deemed reliable by database staff, as they are not part of mandatory reporting).

Figure 8-8.

Frequency of Detection and Average Concentrations of TCL Contaminants of CARD Sites: Water

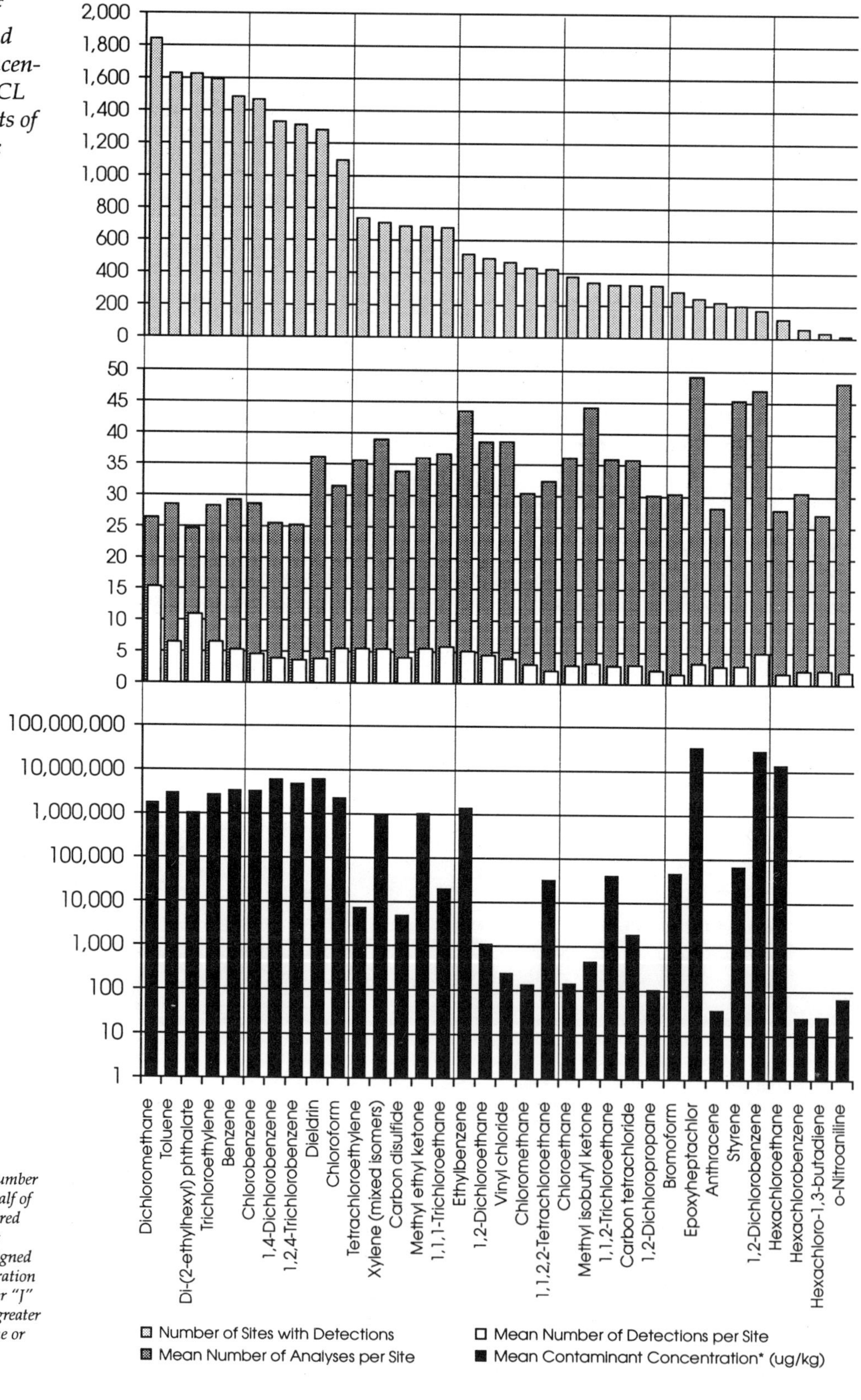

**Where number of analyses exceeds number of detections, one half of the Contract Required Quantitation Limit (CRQL/2) was assigned as a proxy concentration for non-detects. For "J" qualified data, the greater of the reported value or CRQL/2 was used.*

Figure 8-9.

Frequency of Detection and Average Concentrations of TIC Contaminants of CARD Sites: Water

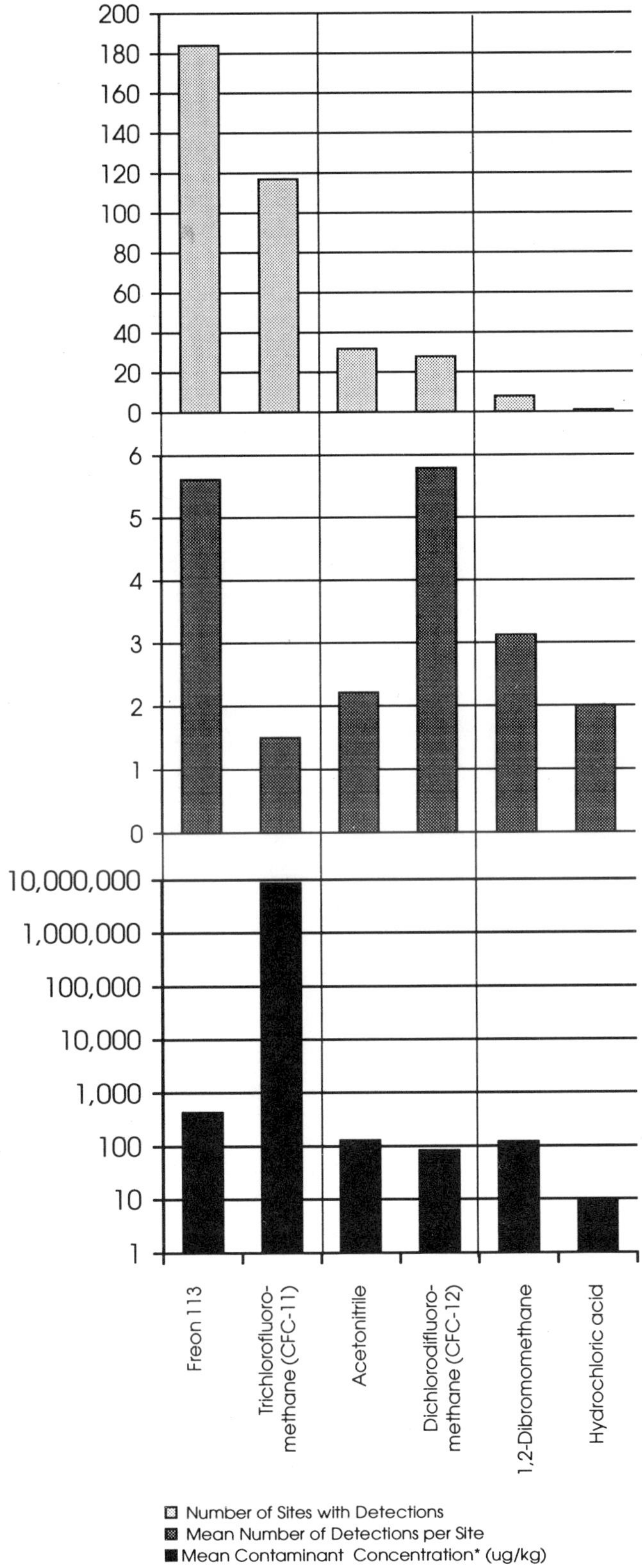

**Where number of analyses exceeds number of detections, one half of the Contract Required Quantitation Limit (CRQL/2) was assigned as a proxy concentration for non-detects. For "J" qualified data, the greater of the reported value or CRQL/2 was used.*

Analyses in Future Editions of *Toxics Watch*

Currently available data provide little basis for meaningful description of the current status or trends in contamination of the environment by toxic chemicals on a national basis. The data that are available, however, do provide for alternative analyses that may have great utility. In addition, new data systems under development may open opportunities for future study of questions that could not be successfully addressed in this volume. Future reports may include the following further analyses:

- Examinations of databases with narrower focus, including the Ocean Data Evaluation System (ODES) and Pesticide Monitoring Inventory (PMI). Although restricted in geographic and/or chemical focus, these systems still may provide critical information on contamination conditions and trends for the particular chemicals and locations they cover.
- Evaluation of databases that contain information on contaminant levels in human tissues, other animals, and plants.
- Evaluation of newly developed databases, and extensions of current databases.
- A series of specific area studies, which may also guide readers in those and other locations in obtaining information available to them. For example, a specific community might be identified, and all data sources with relevant local information on contaminant concentrations (and environmental releases) for that community identified and evaluated.
- A review of developments in the techniques for collecting, storing, and retrieving environmental data, such as the analysis of these data using Geographic Information Systems (GIS), which allow users to relate many different types of data related to a particular location.

---

1 U.S. Environmental Protection Agency, *National Air Quality and Emissions Trends Report, 1992*. EPA 454/R-93-031, October 1993.

Chapter 9

Environmental Justice

Introduction

Almost from the awakening of the modern environmental movement in the 1960s, fairness and equality have emerged as concerns for minority and low income groups. The "environmental justice" movement has grown from local controversies and isolated studies to a matter of national attention for environmental groups, government, industry, grassroots organizations, and academia. Environmental justice refers to the principle of *equal* protection from environmental hazards for all races, ethnicities, and socioeconomic groups. The ideal goal of the environmental justice movement is *adequate* protection for all.[1] (See Box 9-A.)

Most people agree with the general concept of environmental justice, but many aspects of the issue are highly controversial. There is little consensus on the answers to many of the important questions: To what extent are certain groups of people disproportionately and unfairly affected by environmental pollution? To the extent that they are, is this the result of racism or other factors working alone or in combination? How can minority groups be better represented in environmental decision making? What are appropriate remedies for inequities that do exist? Regardless of the answer to any of these questions, it is clear that environmental justice is an important issue to understand.

The purpose of this chapter is to familiarize policymakers, legislators, industry officials, environmental groups, journalists, and the general public with the background and current status of the environmental justice movement so that they will be better prepared to participate in the issues it raises. This review presents information and viewpoints put forward by various sides in the debate, but does not seek to judge the relative merit of all the views described. In keeping with the purposes of this book, toxics issues have been emphasized throughout.

Summary of Findings

- The environmental justice movement, which emerged in the late 1960s, has steadily evolved and broadened. The movement began with a few isolated instances of activism against

Box 9-A. Definition of Terms in Environmental Justice Movement

Three terms are used by activists, scholars, and government officials to discuss the issues involved in the environmental justice movement: *environmental racism, environmental equity,* and *environmental justice.*

The term *environmental racism* refers to the *causes* of perceived disproportionate environmental impacts on racial and ethnic minorities. The phrase was originally coined in 1982 by Dr. Benjamin Chavis, who at that time was Executive Director of the United Church of Christ's Commission for Racial Justice.[1] Dr. Chavis elaborated on his definition in March 1993 while testifying before Congress:

> Environmental racism is defined as racial discrimination in environmental policy making and the unequal enforcement of environmental laws and regulations. It is the deliberate targeting of people of color communities for toxic waste facilities and the official sanctioning of a life threatening presence of poisons and pollutants in people of color communities. It is also manifested in the history of excluding people of color from the leadership of the environmental movement.[2]

Dr. Chavis's definition of environmental racism describes intentional discrimination against racial and ethnic minorities. Other activists and scholars use the term to include racist outcomes that are not the result of individual intent, but rather an unintended result of institutional structure. Professor Robert D. Bullard, a sociologist at the University of California at Riverside refers to environmental racism as "any policy, practice, or directive that differentially affects or disadvantages (whether intended or unintended) individuals, groups, or communities based on race or color."[3] Under this definition, a practice can be labeled environmentally racist if the predicted or actual distribution results in disproportionate adverse impacts on minorities. Failure to take considerations of racial impact into account can thereby be construed as racist.[4]

The term *environmental equity* was the term originally used by EPA when the agency responded to the concerns of the environmental justice movement. The term originates from the assumption

perceived environmental injustice; in the 1990s, a strong network of organizations shares information nationwide. Currently thousands of multiracial, grassroots organizations serve as advocates for the environmental, economic, social, and public health interests of African Americans, Hispanic Americans, Native Americans, Asian Americans, Native Hawaiians, Pacific Islanders, and others.

- Environmental justice issues are broad. Environmental justice issues related to toxic chemicals to date focus on the siting of hazardous waste treatment, disposal, and storage facilities, chemical manufacturing plants, and all other polluting facilities; the enforcement of environmental protection legislation; the demographics of air pollution and of lead poisoning; consumption patterns of contaminated fish; occupational safety regarding toxic chemicals; and protection against pesticide poisoning for farm workers. (The environmental justice movement also addresses issues related to land use, energy development, and other matters not within the scope of this report.)

within risk assessment that human exposures to environmental hazards can be measured. From this perspective, environmental equity refers to the possibility of objectively measuring exposure levels and that ideal in which no one group is burdened with higher exposures to environmental hazards than others. Some members of the environmental justice movement have objected to the EPA phrasing. Charles Lee, Director of the Special Project on Toxic Injustice for the United Church of Christ, objects to the implication that the problem of exposure to environmental hazards is acceptable if it is equally shared by everyone. Ideally, "we'd like to see no community impacted by hazardous pollution."[5]

The broadest and the most widely used and accepted term is *environmental justice.* There is consensus among all those involved in environmental justice issues that fairness and equality should be the underlying principles in efforts to protect individuals and communities from negative environmental impacts. Environmental justice refers to the ideal of equal protection from environmental hazards for all races, ethnicities, and socioeconomic groups. It also refers to the goal of providing adequate environmental health protection for these groups.[6]

1 Benjamin F. Chavis, Jr., Testimony submitted to the U.S. House of Representatives, Committee on the Judiciary, Subcommittee on Civil and Constitutional Rights, March 3, 1993.
2 Chavis, Testimony, House Subcommittee on Civil and Constitutional Rights, March 3, 1993.
3 Robert D. Bullard, Testimony submitted to the U.S. House of Representatives, Committee on the Judiciary, Subcommittee on Civil and Constitutional Rights, March 3, 1993, 2.
4 Gerald Torres, "Introduction: Understanding Environmental Racism,"*University of Colorado Law Review,* Natural Resources Issue: Race, Class and Environmental Regulation, 63, no. 4 (1992): 840.
5 Charles Lee as quoted in Marianne Lavalle, "Residents Want 'Justice,' The EPA Offers 'Equity,'" *National Law Journal,* September 21, 1992, 12.
6 Ken Sexton and Yolanda Banks Anderson, Foreword, *Toxicology and Industrial Health,* Special Issue, 9, no. 5 (September-October 1993): vi.

- Of the numerous studies reviewed and cited in this chapter, most present evidence that support claims of disproportionate impact on minorities of environmental pollutants or in the siting of hazardous waste facilities. Several studies conclude that correlations between residing near a facility and being a member of a racial or ethnic minority group are statistically significant independent of other factors such as income, while other studies fail to find statistically significant correlations and challenge the findings of inequities. The challenges neither refute nor validate the original claims of inequities, as significant differences in study methodology and basic definitions prevent the studies from being compared. For example the studies often have a different geographical scope (two in cities, one in the southeastern United States, and five national); a different minority study population (one African-American only, three African-American and Hispanic, one African-American and Hispanic separately, and three total minorities); or different environmental concerns (one studied 202 waste-to-energy plants, one studied 800 hazardous waste disposal sites, and three studied 400-500 hazardous waste treatment, storage, or disposal facilities).

- No courts have yet found intent to discriminate in lawsuits concerned with the siting of facilities. The Equal Protection Clause of the 14th Amendment has been invoked in efforts to stop the siting of new facilities in minority neighborhoods. However, in the three cases to date, the courts have ruled against the plaintiffs for lack of evidence of intent to discriminate on the basis of race. Evidence of disproportionate impact alone is insufficient to prove such intent. EPA has received complaints under Title VI of the Civil Rights Act of 1964 regarding environmental justice issues.
- Research has found that minorities are disproportionately exposed to air pollution and lead. Minorities, low income groups, and urban dwellers all suffer disproportionately from exposure to air pollutants (e.g., 57 percent of whites, 65 percent of African Americans, and 80 percent of Hispanic Americans live in cities or counties failing to meet EPA air quality standards). In addition, African American children have the highest blood lead levels of all groups and blood lead levels are higher among Hispanics, urban dwellers, and low income groups when compared to the national average.
- A 1988 survey of 11 national environmental organizations found only six members of minorities serving on boards and less than 2% of minority staff serving in professional positions.
- Minorities are becoming more involved in environmental activities, not only through organizations dedicated to the interests of racial or ethnic populations, but also through the activities of national environmental groups. The momentum has come from the protests by minorities at their perceived exclusion from environmental organizations and by the positive initiatives to be more inclusive.
- Recent Executive Branch actions have produced federal-level attention to environmental justice issues. EPA established an Office of Environmental Justice in 1992, and President Clinton signed the Executive Order on Environmental Justice in 1994. This order requires integration of environmental justice into the missions and strategies of all federal agencies.
- State and federal legislators are developing proposed environmental justice legislation. Arkansas passed the first environmental justice statute in 1993 and since then four other states have proposed laws, initiated programs, or set up commissions, including Tennessee, Louisiana, and Florida. Actions often include requiring public hearings, data collection on the health impacts of environmental hazards, and restrictions on siting new facilities within communities with existing facilities.
- Industry has begun responding to environmental justice concerns through initiatives within the past two years that include increasing community participation in their safety planning, establishing new avenues of communications with local

communities, planning ways that facilities might provide greater local employment and other benefits, holding industry workshops on environmental justice issues, and participating in dialogues about these issues. In the next several years, federal and state activities and legislation relating to environmental justice are likely to greatly affect the way industry involves outside groups in making environmental decisions.

African Americans and the Environmental Justice Movement

"This is the cutting edge of a new civil rights struggle."

Wade Hendersen, Director, Washington, D.C., Office of the National Association for the Advancement of Colored People[2]

Historically, the roots of the environmental justice movement lie not in the mainstream environmental movement, but rather in the civil rights movement of the 1950s and 1960s, as well as in the social justice activism of the 1970s and 1980s. Today, the environmental justice movement in the United States consists of thousands of grassroots groups, many organized around specific issues that affect local communities. Sixty-five percent of these multiracial groups are estimated to have been formed during the 1980s and 1990s, 24 percent during the 1970s, and 11 percent during the late 1960s.[3]

Emergence of the Issue in the 1960s and 1970s

Activism and research related to environmental justice issues began in the late 1960s. In 1967, African American students gathered in Houston to protest, among other things, the existence of a city-owned garbage dump in a predominantly African American neighborhood.[4] That same year, a study documented levels of pesticides in human fat to vary according to race.[5] In 1971, the annual report of the President's Council on Environmental Quality discussed air pollution studies from 1966, 1969, and 1971 that reported higher concentrations of pollutants in low income and minority urban areas.[6]

In 1979, the first environmental justice challenge to the siting of a waste facility was filed against the State of Texas, the City of Houston, and Browning Ferris Industries. Residents of a middle-class, predominantly African American community slated for a sanitary landfill organized themselves into the Northeast Community Action Group (NECAG) and filed suit based on racial discrimination.[7] Robert D. Bullard, then a sociologist at Texas Southern University,[a] collected data on the siting of municipal landfills and incinerators in Houston in connection with the suit. Although Bullard concluded that waste facilities were disproportionately located in African American neighborhoods, the lawsuit was unsuccessful.[8]

[a] Bullard is now Ware Professor of Sociology and Director of the Environmental Justice Resource Center at Clark Atlanta University.

Increased Research and Activism in the 1980s

In 1982 residents of Warren County, North Carolina, and the national organization of the United Church of Christ staged a demonstration against the siting of a PCB landfill in the Warren County community, which was 60 percent African American.[b] The demonstration consisted of a nonviolent civil disobedience campaign that resulted in over 500 arrests, including that of Benjamin Chavis (see Box 9-A) and Walter E. Fauntroy, congressman from the District of Columbia. The National Association for the Advancement of Colored People (NAACP) requested a preliminary injunction against the PCB landfill on the basis of racial discrimination.[9] Although the request for an injunction was denied and the landfill was built, protest activities received extensive media coverage and focused national attention on environmental justice issues for the first time. In addition, Walter Fauntroy requested that the U.S. General Accounting Office (GAO) report on the demographic characteristics of landfill sites in the South.

In 1983, the GAO undertook a study of hazardous waste landfills in the southeastern region of the United States. The study, focused on four hazardous waste sites in Alabama, North Carolina, and South Carolina (including the Warren County landfill), and concluded that three out of the four were located in areas with a higher African American population than the state in which they were located.[10]

The United Church of Christ Commission for Racial Justice (UCCCRJ) was the first organization to analyze environmental justice issues at the national level. In 1987, the UCCCRJ published a landmark report on the demographics of communities containing hazardous waste facilities. The report claimed that there was a consistent national pattern of communities hosting hazardous waste facilities having higher minority populations and that communities with the greatest number of facilities had the highest percentage of minorities. The report also concluded that race was more likely to determine residence near a facility than low income.[11]

Environmental Justice Comes of Age in the 1990s

In January 1990, environmental justice activists and scholars gathered together for the first time at a Conference on Race and the Incidence of Environmental Hazards, organized by Associate Professor Bunyan Bryant and Assistant Professor Paul Mohai of the University of Michigan School of Natural Resources. The majority of those who presented scholarly papers were people of color, while participant observers from federal and state agencies contributed to discussions of strategies for change and follow up. Several of the scholar-activists organized themselves into a group called the

[b] The county's population was comprised of 60% African Americans and the census area in which the landfill was to be located contained a 66% African American population.

Michigan Coalition. After the conference the Michigan Coalition arranged a meeting with EPA Administrator William Reilly to discuss their environmental justice concerns, which provided some of the impetus for the changes at that agency described below.[12]

The UCCCRJ organized the First National People of Color Environmental Leadership Summit in October 1991 to bring together leaders of grassroots, civil rights, and environmental groups from around the country. Over 600 individuals from almost every state and territory attended as participants or participant observers. One of the most influential outcomes of the event was the creation of a set of 17 Principles of Environmental Justice, which were adopted by the movement leaders attending the summit.[13] These principles codified the philosophy of the environmental justice movement and allowed outsiders an increased understanding of its goals.

In September 1992, *The National Law Journal* published an award-winning special issue that described the results of a staff study of community demographics and enforcement actions. The study alleged that penalties against polluters were lower for facilities in minority neighborhoods than for facilities in white communities and that it took longer for abandoned toxic waste sites discovered in minority communities to be placed on the National Priorities List (NPL) as compared to sites discovered in white neighborhoods. Finally, *The National Law Journal* reported that its study showed that white communities were more likely to receive more extensive cleanup for sites than minority communities.[14]

By the early 1990s environmental justice issues had already reached the agenda of industry management, national environmental groups, federal agencies, and the White House itself. As these groups struggled to frame their responses, debate continued on the meaning and validity of studies presenting evidence for and against the existence of environmental injustice.

Questions of Evidence

Scope of Environmental Justice Study Issues

Equity can be taken to mean outcome equity or process equity.[15] Environmental justice advocates claim a lack of equity in both senses. They claim that *outcome inequity*, in the form of disproportionate impact from environmental hazards, exists in that hazardous waste treatment, storage, disposal, and producing facilities are located in minority neighborhoods to a greater extent than in non-minority neighborhoods;[16] in that air pollution and lead poisoning negatively affect minorities to a greater extent than the rest of the population;[17] and in that minorities are more likely to be exposed to occupational health hazards.[18]

Environmental justice activists and scholars argue that *process inequity*, in the form of racism, exists in the facility siting decisions made by developers and government officials, who they claim are more likely to target minority communities;[19] because residents of these communities are excluded from participation in the decision-making processes relevant to facility sitings;[20] and because minorities are under-represented in the organizational bodies that develop and implement environmental policy, including federal agencies, local planning boards, and national environmental organizations.[21]

Between 1967 and 1994, more than 65 empirical studies have attempted to measure differences in exposure to chemical environmental hazards according to race/ethnicity or income.[22] Although many of these studies were undertaken independently of the environmental justice movement, all address crucial issues of concern to the movement. Some address the question of outcome equity; others the question of process equity. The topics examined include the siting of solid and hazardous waste facilities; levels of air pollution in different regions of the country; human exposures to lead; occupational exposure to toxic chemicals and pesticides; circumstances surrounding facility expansion plans; and the distribution of regulatory actions taken by EPA.

Many of the studies have been concerned with solid and hazardous waste treatment, storage, and disposal facilities (TSDFs), the impact of these facilities on the surrounding communities, and the question of whether or not racism exists in the siting and regulation of these facilities. Sitings of such facilities have historically provided important rallying points for the environmental justice movement. Much of the early grassroots activism arose in communities targeted as sites for waste facilities.

As discussed below, some of the studies support claims that minorities are disproportionately impacted by waste facility siting; others suggest that factors other than racial/ethnic composition of neighborhoods are more important.

Studies of Racial/Ethnic Factors in Siting of Waste Facilities

Since the early 1980s, a number of studies have focused on the question of whether or not solid and hazardous waste facilities tend to be located in communities that have higher percentages of racial minorities and the poor than non-host communities. Eight studies whose methodology and findings are analyzed here portray the problems involved in establishing or disproving evidence of disproportionate impact in siting and convey the nature of the controversy surrounding such studies. Although many of the studies examine both issues of race and income, this analysis will focus predominantly on the issue of race.

GAO and Bullard Studies

Two of the important early studies on the racial composition of communities that contain solid and hazardous waste, mentioned above, were published in 1983 and prepared by the GAO and Robert Bullard. Both made straightforward comparisons between the number of facilities located in areas with predominantly minority versus predominantly non-minority populations.

The GAO study examined the racial and socio-economic characteristics of the communities surrounding four hazardous waste landfills in EPA's Region IV. The study, using 1980 U.S. Census data, found that three of the four landfills were located in U.S. Census areas[c] with African American populations ranging from 52 to 90 percent, while the African American populations of the host states ranged from 26 to 42 percent. The study has frequently been cited as providing evidence of disproportionate impact in the siting of landfills in this region of the United States.[23]

Robert Bullard looked at the location of solid waste landfills and incinerators in the City of Houston and used information from interviews and field notes to define "neighborhoods" as being either African American, Hispanic, or white. Bullard found that four out of five incinerators that the city operated between 1920 and the early 1970s were located in African American neighborhoods. The fifth was located in a Hispanic neighborhood. Two out of three mini-incinerators in operation between 1972 and 1975 were located in African American neighborhoods, with the third being located in a white neighborhood. All five municipal landfills operated between 1920 and the early 1970s were located in African American neighborhoods. In addition, from 1970 to 1978, the Texas Department of Health permitted 21 solid waste sites in the Houston area. Eleven of these (54 percent) were located in neighborhoods that Bullard defined as African American. Based on an African American population in Houston of 26 percent in 1970 and 28 percent in 1980, Bullard concluded that African Americans were disproportionately impacted by these sites.[24]

United Church of Christ Study

The first study to focus specifically on the racial composition of communities with hazardous waste facilities on the *national* level was the 1987 report by the United Church of Christ Commission for Racial Justice (UCCCRJ).[25] This report looked at zip code areas throughout the nation containing 415 commercial hazardous waste facilities that received off-site waste. 1980 Census data was used to determine the combined minority (African American, Hispanic, and all other non-white categories) population of these zip code areas and of zip code areas that did not contain facilities. The study found that the zip code areas that contained two or more such hazardous waste facilities *or* that contained one of the five largest hazardous waste landfills contained a higher percentage minority population (38 percent) than zip code areas containing one facility (24 percent) or those containing none of the hazardous waste facilities included in the study (12 percent). The study also reported that minorities are slightly more likely than non-minorities to live in areas with waste sites. The percentage of the entire minority population that lives in a host zip code is 56 percent, slightly higher than the percentage for non-minorities (53.6 percent) or the total population (54.2 percent). This

[c] The GAO report defines a census area as an area within a county such as a township or a subdivision.

study had a profound impact on the environmental justice movement. It galvanized increased activism and research and has frequently been cited as evidence of the nationwide disproportionate impact of environmental hazards on minorities. The first three studies described above represent the early work on facility siting that helped bring the issues of environmental justice to national attention.

Mohai and Bryant Study

In 1990, Paul Mohai and Bunyan Bryant of the School of Natural Resources at the University of Michigan examined the relationship between race, income, and the location of 16 commercial hazardous waste facilities in the three-county area surrounding Detroit.[26] Their work represented a new approach to the study of environmental inequity in that they looked at the minority population in the area within concentric circles of a facility. This method, although time-consuming and not suitable for national analysis, avoids the problems associated with using areas delineated for different purposes. Using interviews of a random sample of residents, they determined the combined minority (African American and other non-white) population and the population below the poverty line of the areas within 1 mile of the facilities, between 1 and 1.5 miles away, and more than 1.5 miles away. Within 1 mile of the facilities, the minority population was found to be 48 percent with 29 percent of the population having household incomes below the poverty line. Between 1 and 1.5 miles from the facilities, the minority population was 39 percent, with 18 percent having household incomes below the poverty line. More than 1.5 miles beyond the facilities, the minority population was 18 percent with 10 percent having household incomes below the poverty line.

The study by Mohai and Bryant added to the evidence that supported claims of disproportionate impact in Houston, in Detroit, in the Southeastern region of the United States, and in the nation as a whole. In the early 1990s, however, several studies were completed which highlighted the difficulties of drawing conclusions from work of this type.

Greenberg Study

Michael Greenberg, professor of urban studies and community health at Rutgers University, undertook a study in 1993 on whether the location of 202 waste-to-energy facilities in the United States disproportionately impacts minorities and the poor.[27] This study and the Zimmerman study discussed below have contributed greatly to the environmental justice debate by directly addressing the problems associated with measuring environmental equity. The two authors explore the varying results obtained from using different statistical techniques and different geographic areas for comparison. Neither Greenberg nor Zimmerman comes to concrete conclusions regarding the existence of environmental inequities. Rather their work focuses on delineating the problems inherent in this type of study.

Greenberg chose the town in which the facility was located as his geographical unit and found that environmental equity results depend on the choice of facilities, areas compared, and statistical methods used. Greenberg first looked at the minority (African American plus Hispanic) population and per capita income of people living in small towns (less than 25,000 population) that contain facilities with small capacities (less than 1,000 tons/day). He compared these to the minority population and income of people living in the "service areas" of the facilities (as obtained from the 1991 Resource Recovery Handbook). Greenberg reasoned that the minority population of the area adversely affected by a facility (the host town) should be compared to the minority population of the area that benefited from the facility (the service area). The data showed that the small town residents had a somewhat greater minority population and a slightly higher per capita income than the service area for their facility. Next, Greenberg made the same comparisons for facilities with large capacities (greater than 1,000 tons/day) located in large towns (greater than 100,000 population). In this case, he found that the large town residents had a significantly greater minority population and lower per capita income than their service areas. Greenberg concluded from these comparisons that different results regarding the existence of environmental inequity could be obtained by varying the choice of facilities.

Greenberg next examined whether he would arrive at different results in terms of inequity if he varied the area with which the host community was compared. To do this, he compared the minority population and per capita income of towns with waste-to-energy facilities to both their service areas and the United States as a whole. He found that income results were not affected by the choice of comparison area: towns with facilities had lower per capita incomes than both their service areas and the United States as a whole. Results for minority populations, however, depended on the comparison: the minority composition of facility towns was 4 percent *less* than the United States as a whole, but 45 percent more than their service areas.

Finally, Greenberg examined whether or not the choice of evaluation statistic affected the results of comparisons between the minority population and per capita income of facility towns and those of the United States. He compared (1) the arithmetic mean value,[d] (2) the proportions value,[e] and (3) the population-weighted value.[f] According to his results, the per capita income comparison was not significantly affected by the choice of statistical method. All three values indicated that towns with facilities had lower per capita income than the United States. The question of disproportionate impact

[d] The arithmetic mean value is calculated, for example, by summing the percentage minority populations of each host town and dividing this sum by the number of host towns to obtain the average minority population of host towns.

[e] The proportions value is calculated, for example, by comparing individual host towns to their service areas to see if they have higher or lower minority populations. A proportions value of 30 percent would indicate that 30 percent of the host towns had higher minority populations than their service areas.

[f] The population-weighted value is calculated, for example, by taking the minority population of each host town and multiplying it by the total population of the host town, then summing all the multiplied totals and dividing them by the sum of the populations of all the towns to get the population-weighted average minority population of host towns.

for minorities was dependent upon the statistics, however. The arithmetic mean and proportions value did not support claims of environmental inequity, but the population-weighted value did. The arithmetic mean indicated that the minority population of facility towns was about the same as in the United States as a whole (actually, 4 percent less). The comparison of proportions indicated that 38 percent of facility towns had a higher percentage of African and Hispanic Americans than the United States. In order to support claims of environmental inequity, this number would have to be greater than 50 percent. However, the population-weighted value indicated that environmental inequity exists. The minority population of facility towns was 65 percent higher than in the general population. These results prove Greenberg's point that outcomes in environmental equity studies can vary depending on choices made in designing studies.

Zimmerman Study

Rae Zimmerman, from the Robert F. Wagner School of Public Service at New York University examined the race, ethnicity, income, and political activism of communities surrounding more than 800 Superfund sites.[27] Like Greenberg, she used different types of statistics to evaluate the validity of her results. She chose U.S. Census designated places[g] as her geographical unit and used 1990 U.S. Census population data. Zimmerman compared the arithmetic mean value and population-weighted value of African American and Hispanic populations in communities with Superfund sites to the total population of these minority groups in the United States.

As in Greenberg's research, different statistical methods used produced different results. When the arithmetic mean value was used, the percentage of African Americans and Hispanics in Superfund communities was comparable to the national as well as to the regional averages. When the population-weighted value was used, Zimmerman found that African American populations were approximately 50 percent higher in communities with Superfund sites than in the nation as a whole. Using the population-weighted value, Hispanics are also relatively more prevalent in communities with Superfund sites than in the nation as a whole. Zimmerman found that Superfund site locations were correlated more closely with race and ethnicity than with poverty. The Greenberg and Zimmerman studies both examine the methodology of facility siting surveys and how different methodologies affect outcomes without coming to concrete conclusions about the existence of inequities.

Anderton and Revised United Church of Christ Studies

Most recently, in 1994, two new studies were published which revisit the findings of the influential 1987 UCCCRJ report. Douglas Anderton and his colleagues at the

[g] Census designated places are defined as densely populated areas without legally defined corporate limits or corporate powers, defined in cooperation with state officials and local data users.

Social and Demographic Research Institute at the University of Massachusetts-Amherst did a national study of the differences in demographic characteristics, including minority population, of U.S. Census tracts with and without hazardous waste facilities.[29] The UCCCRJ, the Center for Policy Alternatives (CPA), and the National Association for the Advancement of Colored People (NAACP) cosponsored the second report updating the 1987 UCCCRJ findings with 1993 data.[30]

The Anderton study focused on 400 commercial TSD facilities that accepted waste produced off-site. The authors used 1980 U.S. Census data and chose census tracts as their geographical unit, citing the relatively homogenous populations of these approximately 4,000 person units and the fact that they are delimited by local individuals.[h] Using an arithmetic mean, their results indicated that there was no significant difference between the African American or Hispanic populations of census tracts with or without hazardous waste facilities. In order to examine more closely the reason why their results differed from the UCCCRJ study of zip codes (which are larger than census tracts, and which vary greatly in population and size), the authors calculated the minority populations of all tracts located within a 2.5 mile radius of each facility tract and compared these to the minority populations within the facility tracts and the tracts lying adjacent to them. Their results indicated that the percentage of African Americans in tracts adjacent to those with facilities was not significantly different from that in tracts with facilities (16 percent versus 12 percent). However, the African American population within the 2.5 mile area was significantly higher (33 percent). The Hispanic population within these three geographical areas remained the same (15 percent, 14 percent, and 15 percent). Anderton and his colleagues concluded that there was no nationally consistent and statistically significant differences between the racial and ethnic composition of census tracts with and without facilities.

The 1994 UCCCRJ study utilized 1990 census data that had been updated to 1993 and, much like the earlier study, calculated the combined minority population of zip code areas with and without the 50 commercial hazardous waste facilities included in the study. The updated study found that the concentration of minorities living in all zip code areas with commercial hazardous waste facilities had increased from 25 percent in 1980 to 31 percent in 1993 and concluded that there are even greater racial disparities in the placement of toxic waste sites today than in the 1980s.

Comparison of Waste Facility Siting Studies

The studies described above have had a great deal of influence on the environmental justice debate. The early studies were used to support claims that minorities were burdened to a disproportionate extent by environmental hazards. Later studies have been used in efforts to clarify or refute these

[h] Census tracts are defined as small locally defined areas which are characterized by stable boundaries and relatively homogeneous demographic characteristics.

claims. Unfortunately, there are a number of difficulties involved in comparing the work done and evaluating the relevance of each study. The studies vary in many respects, including the following:

General geographic region. Two of the studies look at cities (Houston and Detroit), one looks at an EPA region (the Southeastern United States), and five look at characteristics of sites on the national level.

Types of facilities. Of the five studies at the national level, one looks at 200 waste-to-energy incinerators, one looks at 800 Superfund sites, and three look at similar groups of 400-500 commercial hazardous waste treatment, storage and disposal facilities. Anderton and his colleagues stress that the facilities they studied constitute only 11 percent of those regulated by RCRA, which in turn are only a fraction of the larger set of known public and private hazardous waste facilities. Moreover, very little data exist on illegal hazardous waste dump sites.[31]

Definition of "surrounding community." Authors have used towns, census tracts, census designated places, block numbering areas, zip codes, sociologically-defined "neighborhoods," and the concentric area within 1 and 1.5 miles of a facility.

Basis of comparison. Studies compare the minority population of the "surrounding community" to that of the nation, to that of communities without facilities, and to that of the "service area" of the facility.

Minority population. One study looks only at African Americans, three separately examine both the African American and Hispanic American populations, one looks at the combined African American and Hispanic populations, and three look at the total combined minority population (including African Americans, Hispanic Americans, Asian Americans, Native Americans, and others).

Time period of data used. Four studies use Census data from 1980, one utilizes 1990 data, one uses 1990 data updated to 1993, and two fail to specify their population information sources. The choice of data on populations is important as a great deal will change in the course of a decade.

Statistical method. Different statistical methods are used to compute the "average minority population" in areas studied.

As the more recent studies described above have shown, the level of disproportionate impact found is dependent on the methods used to compute averages, on the geographical areas used to signify "surrounding communities," and on which comparisons are made. Because of the use of different variables and different statistical methods, the accumulated results of these studies serve to broaden the debate on environmental justice rather than progressing towards consensus on conclusions.

The work by Anderton *et al.* of the University of Massachusetts-Amherst has received a great deal of media attention and has been described as effectively refuting claims of environmental racism by refuting studies indicating disproportionate impact.[32] This impression is incorrect. Although none of the studies undertaken can be said to have conclusively proved that environmental injustice exists, Anderton and his colleagues caution against interpreting their work to mean that it does *not* exist.

Study of Other Factors in Siting of Waste Facilities

Discrimination against racial or ethnic minorities in the siting of hazardous waste facilities is a particularly serious charge if any such discrimination occurred deliberately. A number of researchers and legal scholars are accepting the premise that minorities are inequitably burdened by environmental hazards, but are working to understand whether or not the causes of these inequities are actually racist.

Several theories discussed below, provide alternative explanations. One argues that income, not race, is the relevant factor, and that minorities are disproportionately impacted because they are disproportionately represented in low income brackets. Another theory suggests that the level of political opposition in a community is the deciding factor in siting questions. Minorities and low income groups might be targeted more frequently for facility siting because they have less information and fewer resources with which to express their opposition. A third theory suggests that a complex set of market factors influence the creation of minority communities around facilities.

Income

Looking to income rather than race as a deciding factor in siting inequities, if low income communities were systematically targeted for the siting of hazardous waste facilities, minorities would also be disproportionately impacted because of the high poverty rate in minority groups. Several of the studies described above included income as one of the characteristics examined in communities containing hazardous waste treatment, storage and disposal facilities. They looked at whether there was disproportionate impact of environmental hazards according to income and whether income was a better predictor of location than race.

Two of the studies found both race and income to be indicators of the existence of a facility in the community. The GAO study found that three out of the four landfill census areas had majority African American populations and that all four areas had populations with at least 26 percent living below the poverty level.[33] Bryant and Mohai found that in the Detroit area both the percentage of the population that was minority and the percentage of the population living below the poverty line was greater in areas closer to facilities.[34] One study, by Anderton et al., found that neither race nor income varied with the existence of a facility; there were no significant differences either in the mean percentage of families living below the poverty line, the mean percentage of households receiving public assistance, or the mean percentage African American population.[35] Three studies found that race and income varied differently. The 1987 UCCCRJ study found income to be a weaker indicator than race when using the arithmetic mean.[36] Zimmerman found that income in census places with Superfund sites was comparable to the national level, while race varied to different degrees, depending on the method used to calculate the comparison value.[37] Finally, Greenberg found that inequities for race and income each depend on the size of the community and the comparison made.[38]

The studies described above arrive at varying results and fail to provide conclusive evidence that low income communities either are or are not disproportionately impacted by the siting of hazardous waste facilities. Although low income may still be a factor in disproportionate impact, little evidence exists that it is the only explanation for inequities that may be faced by racial or ethnic minorities or that income is a better predictor of facility location than race.

Potential for Political Opposition

"I've heard industry's explanation, that they look for cheap water and land. But I also think the political and economic strength of the neighborhood to oppose or interfere with the company's plans goes into its decision."

Professor Robert Kuehn, Tulane Environmental Law Clinic[39]

A second explanation for inequities in the siting of hazardous waste facilities revolves around the ability of different communities to politically resist such a siting. Scholars point out that middle and upper income areas currently have a political climate that is hostile towards facilities.[40] Minority and low income neighborhoods possess, on average, fewer resources, such as time, money, contacts and knowledge of the political system, with which to express their opposition.[41] Two studies have looked at the potential for political action within a community and the effect this has on siting and regulatory action.

James Hamilton, an economist at Duke University, studied whether or not the potential for collective action within a community affected decisions to expand existing facilities or to shut down capacity.[42] Hamilton looked at capacity expansion plans of 250 commercial hazardous waste treatment, storage and disposal facilities reported to EPA in 1987. He used the percentage of a county's voting-age population that voted in the 1980 presidential election as an indicator of the potential for collective political action in that community. Hamilton compared counties where facilities had expansion plans to those where facilities did not have expansion plans. He found no significant differences in household income or minority population. However, voter turnout was lower in counties with expansion plans as compared to counties without expansion plans (52 versus 56 percent), which could suggest that the potential for collective action in a community has an effect on siting decisions. In addition, Hamilton looked at 18 counties with plans for capacity *reductions* and found that counties with higher voter turnout were more likely to have such plans.

Rae Zimmerman looked at the effect of controversy on the cleanup process for Superfund sites.[43] This issue is relevant to the siting issue because it speaks to the question of whether political controversy affects environmental decision making at the local level. The existence of a Record of Decision (ROD) is used as a measure of cleanup status. A ROD, a publicly reviewed decision made by state and federal officials on a course and schedule for cleanup, is signed toward the end of the cleanup planning process prior to remedial action. A community would want a ROD to be signed, therefore, so that the remedial action could commence. Zimmerman devised an index of controversy from the combination of news media entries and a survey of opinions of Federal Superfund site managers. She found that 66 percent of controversial sites had RODs signed as compared to 46 percent for non-controversial sites, thus indicating that controversy prompts a faster cleanup process.

In further work, Zimmerman looked at the role of controversy in minority communities. She found more, rather than less, controversy in minority communities, but also found that controversy in a minority community was less likely to result in the signing of a ROD than controversy in non-minority communities. In analyzing 867 Superfund sites, she found controversy in 54 to 75 percent of those surrounded by minority communities as compared to 45 percent of all sites combined. However, only 38 to 47 percent of minority communities with controversial sites had RODs signed compared to 66 percent of all controversial sites in general. Zimmerman notes that RODs take a long time to prepare, that sites designated as Superfund sites longer may be more likely to have RODs signed, and that Superfund sites in minority communities have been designated for a relatively shorter period of time than those in non-minority communities. She concludes that if there is an inequity issue, it is more likely to have occurred in the site selection process than with respect to the preparation of the ROD.

Market Dynamics

> *[T]heoretically, even if the current distribution of LULUs ["locally undesirable land uses"] could be rearranged to yield an unquestionably fair distribution, the interaction of poverty, racial discrimination in housing markets, and the normal forces of residential mobility might soon recreate a situation where those living next to LULUs were predominantly poor and people of color.*
>
> Vicki Been, New York University School of Law[44]

Finally, some researchers suggest that a complex set of market dynamics causes communities surrounding hazardous waste facilities to become increasingly populated by minority and low income groups after siting has taken place.[45] Families with low incomes may be attracted to lower property values surrounding facilities or, alternatively, may not have the financial resources to move out of neighborhoods where a facility has been sited. In addition, it is well documented that racial discrimination in the sale and rental of housing exists and may result in minorities living in less desirable neighborhoods, regardless of their income level. These two trends, combined with the fact that 17 to 20 percent of households in the United States move to a new home every year, could plausibly lead to increased minority and low income populations in communities surrounding hazardous waste facilities.[46]

One way to test this hypothesis is to look at the median value of houses in communities with facilities. Although several authors have included this variable in their studies, no clear pattern emerges. Anderton et al. found that, for the 25 largest metropolitan areas in the United States, the value of housing was significantly lower in census tracts with, as compared to without, hazardous waste facilities. However, the Hamilton and Zimmerman studies found no significant differences in housing value.

Another way to test the market dynamics hypothesis is to look at the racial composition of communities before and after a facility has been sited. This type of study was undertaken by Vicki Been of the New York University School of Law, who revised and extended the work of Robert Bullard and the General Accounting Office. She compared the racial composition of these communities at the time that siting decisions were made to their minority populations in subsequent years using 1970, 1980 and 1990 Census data.[47]

Of the four landfills studied by GAO, Been found that one became operational in 1972, two in 1977, and one in 1979. Assuming that the siting decision was made several years before the landfills became operational, she used 1970 census data for the first three and 1980 census data for the fourth. Been found that, at the time of the siting decisions, all four communities had African American populations 1.6 to 3.3 times that of their state, a finding that serves to support the claim that the siting process was racially discriminatory. In addition, she found that each of the four communities experienced a decrease in African American population following the siting. The decline was insignificant in two communities, but constituted 32 and 36 percent of the African American population of the remaining two. These data provide no support for the theory that market dynamics cause host neighborhoods to become increasingly populated with minorities.

Vicki Been revised Bullard's study of 25 incinerators and landfills in the Houston area by eliminating several that were sited too early to obtain meaningful data and several that were double-counted. In addition, she utilized census tracts as communities rather than Bullard's "neighborhoods," which were impossible to replicate. The final subgroup contained three mini-incinerators and seven landfills. All three mini-incinerators and four landfills were sited in the early 1970s, two landfills were sited in the 1950s, and one landfill was sited in 1978. Data from 1970, 1960, and 1980 were used respectively. Been found that, at the time of siting, one landfill had an African American population comparable to Houston's (26 percent), three had African American populations lower than Houston's (4, 7, and 7 percent), and three had higher percentages (68, 79, and 87 percent). One mini-incinerator was sited in an almost 100-percent white neighborhood, and the remaining two were sited in census tracts with 64 and 90 percent African American populations. In total, five facilities were located in neighborhoods with predominantly African American populations, and five were located in neighborhoods with African American populations less than or equal to that of Houston. Been reasoned that these results indicate disproportionate effect in the siting process since only one-quarter of Houston's population was African American.

In looking at demographic data for the years following the original sitings, Been found support for the theory that market dynamics plays a role in creating environmental inequity. Between 1970 and 1990, the African American percentage of the population increased in six landfill communities and in one community with a mini-incinerator. By 1990, nine out of the ten facilities studied had African American populations considerably higher than that of Houston as a whole (between 33 and 91 percent as compared to Houston's overall 27 percent).

In summary, Been found significant support for the market dynamics theory in her revision of Robert Bullard's urban study, while finding no support in her revision of the GAO rural study. She suggests that the results may be attributable to the different rates of residential mobility in rural and urban areas and the differences in size and nature of the facilities studied.

Influence of These Other Factors

The alternative explanations described above are intuitively appealing and are supported to some extent by established research done for other purposes than determining environmental injustice. For example, demographic research indicates that minorities are disproportionately represented among low income groups, and racial discrimination in the housing market has been well documented for decades. However, efforts to distinguish among the effects of income, political activity, or market dynamics as opposed to race/ethnicity have produced no conclusive results. In any case, it does not appear that these three potential explanations, singly or in combination, have been shown to account for all cases in which minority groups may bear an unequal share of exposure to potential environmental hazards.

Court Responses to Allegations of Environmental Racism

Studies that examine whether or not race/ethnicity is a determining factor in siting decisions or look at the statistical distribution of facilities within communities can have significant legal implications. By affecting the course of lawsuits, they can profoundly influence the lives of residents in communities targeted for facilities.

Since 1979, several communities protesting the planned location of solid waste facilities in their midst have commenced environmental racism lawsuits based on the Equal Protection Clause of the 14th Amendment. Prior to 1976, some federal courts allowed plaintiffs to prevail on equal protection claims if they could establish that the challenged practice had a statistically discriminatory impact. However, in a landmark case, *Washington v. Davis,*[48] the Supreme Court ruled that it was not sufficient to prove discriminatory impact; it was necessary to show intent to discriminate.[49] The following year, in *Arlington Heights v. Metropolitan Housing Development Corp.,*[50] the Supreme Court identified five factors, without claiming to be exhaustive, that would constitute evidence of discriminatory intent: (1) the disparate impact of the official action; (2) the historical background of the decision; (3) the sequence of events leading up to the challenged decision; (4) any departures, substantive or procedural, from the normal decision-making process; and (5) the legislative or administrative history of the challenged decision.[51]

Bean v. Southwestern Waste Management Corporation

In 1979 residents of the East Houston-Dyersdale Road area of Harris County, Texas challenged a decision by the Texas Department of Health granting Southwestern Waste Management Corporation permission to operate a solid waste facility in their neighborhood.[52] Residents claimed that approval of the landfill constituted racial discrimination. They argued (1) that this decision was part of a pattern of discrimination on the part of the Texas Department of Health and (2) that the location of the landfill constituted discrimination because of the location of other landfills.

The court examined the statistics for the first allegation and disagreed with the plaintiffs. Of the 17 sites approved by the Department of Health as of 1978, the court found that 10 landfills were located in census tracts with a minority population of less than 25 percent. The court also disagreed with the data sets provided in support of the second allegation. For example, residents pointed out that the eastern half of Houston, where 62 percent of the minority population lived, contained 68 percent of the city's solid waste facilities. The western half of Houston, where 73 percent of the city's white population lived, accommodated only 32 percent of these sites. By focusing on census tracts rather than city halves, the court determined that white census tracts bore their share of the burden. In addition, the court found that the location of many waste sites could be explained by their proximity to Houston's industrial center in the eastern part of the city. The district court ruled against the plaintiffs and the 5th Circuit affirmed.[53]

Despite ruling in favor of the state health department, the court described as "illogical" the decision to permit a solid waste facility within 1700 feet of a predominantly African American high school and a little farther from a predominantly African American residential neighborhood. The court noted that the decision was both "unfortunate and insensitive," and that residents had successfully established that the facility would pose a threat of irreparable injury to the nature of their community.[54]

East Bibb Twiggs Neighborhood Association v. Macon-Bibb County Planning and Zoning Commission (Georgia)

Ten years later, in 1989, the East Bibb Twiggs Neighborhood Association, comprised of residents of Macon-Bibb county in Georgia, brought a lawsuit against the county's planning and zoning commission because of the association's opposition to a planned private landfill in its community.[55] Residents alleged that the siting decision (1) had a discriminatory impact and (2) exemplified a pattern of locating undesirable land uses in African American communities. The plaintiff's claim of discriminatory impact was based on the fact that the census tract in which the landfill was to be built was 60 percent African American. Moreover, the governmental district in which this and the only other Commission-approved landfill were located was 70 percent African American.

The court, however, noted that the other Commission-approved landfill was located in a census tract with a 76 percent white population and concluded that discriminatory impact had not been established.[56] The court also noted that the historical evidence of racially motivated decision making presented by the plaintiffs pertained to decisions made by agencies other than the planning and zoning commission. The district court ruled against the plaintiffs and the 11th Circuit Court affirmed the opinion.[57]

R.I.S.E., Inc. v. Kay (Virginia)

Officials in King and Queen County, Virginia, incurred substantial community protest in 1987 by approving a new solid waste landfill. A nonprofit, bi-racial community organization, Residents Involved in Saving the Environment (R.I.S.E.), filed suit in opposition to the siting.[58] R.I.S.E. contended that approval of the new facility constituted discrimination on the basis of race. The plaintiffs pointed out that the African American population within one half-mile of the proposed landfill was 64 percent, while the African American population of the county was only 42 percent. The three existing landfills in the county, which had been sited in 1969, 1971, and 1977, were all located in communities where the African American population was 95 percent or greater. In addition, a landfill located in a white neighborhood in 1986 had been closed after a few months because geological conditions did not meet necessary standards.[59]

The district court agreed that the placement of landfills in King and Queen County from 1969 onwards had resulted in a disproportionate impact on African American residents. However, it ruled that "official action will not be held unconstitutional solely because it results in a racially disproportionate impact. Such action violates the Fourteenth Amendment's Equal Protection Clause only if it is intentionally discriminatory."[60] The Fourth Circuit affirmed.

Title VI of the Civil Rights Act of 1964

Although the Equal Protection Clause has had little success in remedying environmental justice problems, Title VI of the Civil Rights Act of 1964 is receiving increased attention as a legal strategy. EPA's Office of Civil Rights has already accepted for processing two complaints alleging racial discrimination under Title VI, which prohibits discrimination on the grounds of race, color, or national origin in programs or activities receiving federal financial assistance. The Title VI regulations and environmental statutes themselves provide EPA with the authority to promote environmental justice policies. This strategy offers advantages and disadvantages when compared to the Equal Protection Clause. The burden of proof is much lower, as Title VI does not require a finding of intent. However, jurisdiction is limited to entities receiving federal funding.[61]

Other Groups and Environmental Justice Issues

Although the environmental justice movement originally sprang from the civil rights activism of African Americans, other racial and ethnic minorities in the United States have faced similar problems. Today, the movement encompasses environmental justice issues of Hispanic Americans, Native Americans, Asian Americans, and Pacific Islanders, as well as issues that are specifically urban.

Hispanic Americans

Americans of Hispanic ethnicity[i] constituted nine percent of the population in 1990.[62] Hispanic Americans are most highly concentrated in the Southwest although there are also large populations in New York and Florida.[63] These Hispanic Americans face a number of environmental justice issues including toxic chemical storage or manufacturing facilities in their communities, pesticide-related health problems of migrant farm workers, and urban air pollution. Related areas of concern for the Hispanic American environmental justice community that are not covered in this chapter include the high levels of industrial pollution in Puerto Rico and the poor living and working conditions in Mexican factories along the United States/Mexico border.

Hispanic Activism in the American Southwest

Although Hispanic communities throughout the United States are raising questions about environmental justice, the majority of grassroots organizing has taken place in the Southwest. The Southwest Organizing Project (SWOP) was organized in New Mexico in 1981. Although Chicanos[j] and Native Americans make up over 50 percent of the state's population,

[i] "Hispanic" is used here to refer to individuals of Spanish, Portuguese, Latin or Central American descent. Individuals of Hispanic ethnicity may be of any race.
[j] "Chicano" refers to Mexican-American individuals.

SWOP's founders felt that their concerns were not being addressed. SWOP engages in direct organizing with the goal of empowering communities of color in the Southwest to campaign for safe working conditions, clean drinking water, and proper sewage and to oppose the siting of facilities that emit toxics.[64] In 1990 SWOP initiated a dialogue among different racial and ethnic minority groups that resulted in the formation of the Southwest Network for Environmental and Economic Justice (SNEEJ). SNEEJ enables southwestern activists and organizations from eight states to work together on issues of social, racial, economic, and environmental justice.[65]

In 1991 a community group called El Pueblo para el Aire y Agua Limpio (People for Clean Air and Water) won an important environmental justice victory in Kettleman City, California. The County of Kings board had approved a permit to build a hazardous waste incinerator in the low income and predominantly Hispanic community. With the aid of the California Rural Legal Assistance Foundation, the community group filed a civil rights lawsuit against the county and won. The court found that the county's environmental impact report did not satisfy California Environmental Quality Act (CEQA) provisions. More importantly, from an environmental justice perspective, the court ruled that the county's failure to supply a Spanish translation of the environmental analysis violated CEQA's requirement for public participation. Since 40 percent of the residents of Kettleman City were monolingual in Spanish, the absence of a translation deprived these citizens of meaningful involvement in the decision making process.[66]

Pesticides and Farm Workers

Minorities tend to be over represented in occupations with high health hazards and to suffer more frequently from job-related illnesses. Data compiled in the early 1980s showed that African Americans had a 37 percent higher risk of occupationally induced disease and a 20 percent higher death rate from occupationally related diseases than whites.[67] A 1990 study of California workers showed that Hispanic American men faced a 33 percent greater chance of suffering from occupational injury or illness, and Hispanic American women, a 19 percent greater chance, than non-Hispanic whites.[68]

Farm work is an occupation with a high risk of injury and a high percentage of minority workers. The National Safety Council has calculated that the death rate in agriculture is 66 per 100,000 as compared to the industrial average of 18 per 100,000. These high risks are associated with exposure to pesticides, heat, mechanical hazards, noise, and dust.[69]

The U.S. Department of Agriculture estimates that 2 million hired farm workers and 3 million farm owners and their families work on farms in the United States. A 1990 national survey of hired farm workers by the U.S. Department of Labor found that 77 percent identify themselves as part of a minority group. Of the two-thirds who were foreign born, 92 percent were Mexican and 4 percent were of another Hispanic ethnicity. Of those who were born in the United States, 34 percent were Hispanic Americans and 60 percent were non-

Hispanic whites. A separate survey found that over 90 percent of California farm workers were of Mexican descent.[70]

According to the U.S. Department of Labor, the nation's farm workers have the highest rate of exposure to toxic poisoning of any occupational group in the United States.[71] The source of the poisoning is pesticides, but no reliable data exist on the extent of pesticide-related illness. Reported poisonings of farm workers range from 10,000 to 20,000 annually, but EPA estimates that between 200,000 and 300,000 farm workers are actually injured or become acutely ill every year.[72] Currently, there is no nationwide mandatory reporting system for pesticide poisonings.[73]

Migrant farm workers may be especially susceptible to pesticide-related illnesses due to substandard living and working conditions, lack of proper health care, and a reluctance to lose work due to illness.[74] Studies of migrant farm workers have found a number of health problems potentially related to pesticides, including abnormal liver and kidney functions and skin rashes. A health survey of migrant farm workers in the Rio Grande Valley in Texas found that over 50 percent had experienced dizziness, 40 percent chronic headaches, and 23 percent blurred vision.[75] In 1986, Evergreen Legal Services surveyed 460 migrant farm workers who regularly applied pesticides and found that two-thirds had never received any safety instruction. This is important because many migrant minority farm workers cannot read safety instructions on their own. Of the survey respondents, 43 percent reported that pesticides had been directly sprayed on them or had drifted on them while they were working.[76]

Farm workers are for the most part excluded from the National Labor Relations Act, the Fair Labor Standards Act, and the Occupational Safety and Health Act. The Occupational Safety and Health Act as passed in 1970 required basic sanitation facilities for all workers, but in 1971 OSHA exempted agricultural employers from the sanitation rule. The National Congress of Hispanic American Citizens challenged the action in 1973, but it was not until 1988 that OSHA's field sanitation standard was expanded to include agriculture. The field sanitation standard, which requires that toilets, hand-washing facilities, and clean drinking water be provided, protects workers from several types of health problems, including pesticide injuries from dermal exposure, which can be greatly mitigated if soap and water are available.[77] In August 1992, EPA published new standards for the protection of farm workers from pesticides.[78]

Native Americans

In 1990, Native Americans, including Eskimos and Aleuts, numbered 2 million and comprised 1 percent of the population of the United States. Native Americans are concentrated in the West with Eskimos and Aleuts heavily concentrated in Alaska and the Pacific Coast States. There are currently over 500 tribes and approximately one third of the Native American population lives on reservations or other Indian lands.[79] Native American environmental justice issues regarding toxics include the siting of hazardous waste facilities, tribal difficulties in managing their own municipal landfills, and the ingestion of toxics through fish consumption. Environmental justice concerns are part of a complex effort to maintain jurisdiction over tribal territories and to protect indigenous rights and cultures. Other issues outside the scope of this report include government uranium mine tailings on Navajo and Laguna Pueblo lands, radioactive waste from nuclear testing at the Nevada test site, military overflights of Indian reservations, and energy development in the Arctic National Wildlife Refuge near the Gwich'in tribe of Alaska.

Landfills and Incinerators

The independent status of Native American governments has resulted in questions regarding whether or not state and federal environmental laws apply to Native lands. In recent years, tribes have negotiated with energy and hazardous waste companies offering financial incentives and employment in exchange for allowing hazardous waste facilities to be located on their land. The socio-economic conditions of the tribes and their lack of information regarding dangers to human health and the environment have led some tribes to accept such offers. More than three dozen reservations have hazardous waste landfills and incinerators currently pending.[80]

Some tribes are now organizing to oppose the siting of landfills and incinerators on Indian lands. In 1991 a proposed 6,000-acre municipal landfill on the Rosebud Sioux reservation in South Dakota was successfully blocked by a Native grassroots organization called the Good Road Coalition. In the same year, the Choctaws of Mississippi defeated a plan to locate a 466-acre hazardous waste landfill in their midst.[81]

Current environmental laws are presenting problems for Indian tribes which lack the funds or the expertise to comply. Of the 650 solid waste disposal sites on Indian lands, 108 are tribally owned landfills that were constructed before Congress established the standards for RCRA. As a result, only two are in compliance, and it would take at least $68 million to upgrade the others to current requirements.[82] In March 1993, an Amendment to the Solid Waste Disposal Act (H.R.1267) was introduced which would grant state status to Indian tribes for purposes of enforcement of that act. In 1994, Congress passed the Indian Lands Open Dump Clean-Up Act (S. 720) which provides the Indian Health Service with technical and financial support to assess and close open waste dumps on Native American lands.[83]

Fish Contamination

Some Native American tribes eat more fish and other wildlife than the general population and therefore may be at greater risk from toxic chemicals that bioaccumulate in nature. EPA originally based water quality standards and fish consumption advisories on the assumption that the average person eats 6.5 grams of fish per day. It was later found that many minority groups, including some Native Americans, may eat as much as 250 grams of fish per day.[84] A study of the impact of a mercury spill on the Grassy Narrows band of Ojibwa in

Ontario, Canada, indicated that they were exposed to higher levels of mercury than the surrounding white community, because of their high fish consumption.[85]

Activism and Tribal Capacity Building among Native Americans

Native Americans today have developed a large number of grassroots organizations that work with environmental, civil rights, and environmental justice issues. There is an increasing amount of cooperation among tribes. The Indigenous People's Network promotes the interests of the tribes and shares information and assistance.

Efforts are being made to increase the ability of Native Americans to protect the natural environment on their lands. In May 1992, the First National Tribal Conference on Environmental Management brought together tribal government representatives and federal government agencies to discuss issues of solid waste management. EPA's Office of Solid Waste and Emergency Response (OSWER) sponsored a series of Indian Lands Forums in April 1992 and an Indian law seminar for EPA employees. OSWER is providing funding for circuit riders to Indian tribes to provide training and technical assistance in the implementation of RCRA regulations as well as guidance concerning underground storage tanks on Indian lands.

Asian American and Pacific Islander Environmental Justice Issues

Asian Americans and Pacific Islanders comprised 3 percent of the U.S. population (7.3 million) in 1990. This minority group is composed of Chinese, Filipino, Japanese, Asian Indian, Korean, Vietnamese, Hawaiian, Samoan and other nationalities and ethnicities. Asian Americans and Pacific Islanders are also concentrated in the West and are the fastest growing racial group in the country.[86]

Environmental justice issues for Asian Americans include occupational exposures to toxic chemicals. In the San Francisco Bay area, 53 percent of all textile and apparel workers are Asian women and 28 percent are Asian men. These workers are exposed to chemical dyes and often work with poor ventilation. In California, Cambodian and Vietnamese farm workers are hindered, through lack of English language skills, from receiving information on pesticide hazards.[87]

Pacific Islanders are an indigenous population of the United States with their own unique environmental justice concerns. Native Hawaiians have organized to oppose the development of a geothermal plant using an active volcano on the island of Hawaii.[88] Inhabitants of the Marshall Islands in the Pacific are still facing the environmental after-effects of 66 nuclear tests in the region in the 1940s and 1950s.[89]

After the First National People of Color Environmental Leadership Summit in 1991, the Asian Pacific Islanders Network was established to improve information-sharing among Asian Americans, Native Hawaiians, and Pacific Islanders and to work with environmental justice issues at the national level.[90]

Urban Environmental Justice Issues

Minorities are more likely to live in urban than in rural areas and are more likely to live in urban areas when compared to non-minorities. In 1990, well over half the population of each minority group, excluding Native Americans, lived in urban areas. Of the total minority population, 86 percent lived in cities compared to 75 percent of non-Hispanic whites.[91] These minority groups are particularly exposed to urban environmental problems. The environmental justice dimension of these problems is exacerbated by factors such as high population density, large traffic volume, and decaying infrastructure. Air pollution and lead poisoning are two of the most important environmental health concerns for minority and low income groups in cities.

Air Pollution

Under the Clean Air Act, EPA established standards for a number of air pollutants, including ozone, carbon monoxide, sulfur dioxide, lead, and particulate matter. Areas that have a higher concentration of these substances than the EPA ambient air quality standard are determined to have poor air quality. A study at Argonne National Laboratory examined the percentages of different racial and ethnic groups living in areas with high concentrations of these air pollutants.[92]

The study found that minorities are more likely to live in areas with poor air quality than whites or the poor. In 1990, 437 of the 3,109 counties and independent cities in the United States failed to meet at least one of the EPA standards. Researchers found that 57 percent of all whites, 65 percent of all African Americans, and 80 percent of all Hispanic Americans live in these 437 counties. They also found that 5 percent of whites, 10 percent of African Americans, and 15 percent of Hispanics live in the seven most polluted counties, those where four or more pollutants exceeded air quality standards. The study found that the percentages of African Americans and Hispanic Americans potentially exposed to air pollution were higher than percentages of low income people drawn from all population groups who were potentially exposed.

The results were consistent when looking at individual air pollutants and the different regions of the country. Counties with high ozone concentrations are home to 52 percent of the white population, 62 percent of the African American population, and 71 percent of the nation's Hispanic American population. Similar distributions were found for all pollutants studied. Although air polluting facilities are not evenly distributed over the United States, each of the four census regions had greater percentages of minority populations living in polluted areas. For the Northeast census region, 50 percent of whites, 85 percent of African Americans, and 88 percent of Hispanic Americans live in areas with excessive carbon monoxide.

Lead Poisoning

> *"While everyone is exposed to some lead, lead has a very skewed profile of exposure and uptake by race and social class."*
>
> Joel Schwartz and Ronnie Levin, U.S. EPA[93]

Although everyone is exposed to lead to some extent, minorities and low income groups appear to be exposed at greater rates. Minorities are over represented in occupations with high exposure to lead, such as construction, primary and secondary smelting, automobile repair, welding, and salvage work. Minorities and low income groups are more likely to be exposed to lead because they live in older homes. The risk of exposure is increased in houses where old paint is likely to have higher concentrations of lead and may be in poor condition and where leaded dust from renovation work may pose a serious hazard. The concentration of minorities in urban areas also makes them more vulnerable to contamination resulting from decades of emissions from leaded gasoline. Finally, the calcium and iron deficiencies that are common among low income groups heighten lead absorption.[94]

Lead exposure is especially dangerous for children because it interferes with their development. Lead poisoning in children can lead to lowered intelligence, erratic behavior, and learning impairment. In the late 1970s, the Second National Health and Nutrition Examination Survey (NHANES II) found that minority and low income children had higher blood lead levels than white children. The study was conducted between 1976 and 1980 and found that the average blood lead level for children six years old and under was 16 micrograms of lead per deciliter of blood (ug/dl). For low income children, the average level was 20 ug/dl; for African American children, the average level was 21 ug/dl; and for low income African American children living in an urban setting, the level was 23 ug/dl.[95] NHANES II found that 8 million urban children were at risk for low-level lead damage.[96]

The phasing out of lead in gasoline brought national blood lead levels down dramatically, as lead in gasoline accounted for more than half of the blood lead levels of children in the 1970s. Lead in household paint was limited to 0.06 percent in 1978, and lead solder, which was present in 47 percent of food and soft drink cans in 1980, has not been used in the production of cans in the United States since 1991.[97]

A dramatic drop in mean blood lead levels of all population groups was found in Phase 1 of the Third National Health and Nutrition Examination Survey (NHANES III) which was completed between 1988 and 1991. For persons of all ages, the overall blood lead level dropped from 12.8 ug/dl to 2.8 ug/dl. In 1991, only 9 percent of American children aged 1-5 had blood lead levels greater than or equal to 10 ug/dl, as compared to 88 percent in the late 1970s.

While mean blood lead levels had dropped for all population groups by the late 1980s, minority, urban, and low income groups still retained higher levels. Overall blood lead levels were found to be 3.5 ug/dl for African Americans, 3.0 ug/dl for Mexican Americans, and 2.7 ug/dl for non-Hispanic whites. African American children aged 1-5 averaged blood lead levels of 5.7 ug/dl, while Mexican American children averaged 4.1 ug/dl, and non-Hispanic white children averaged 3.2 ug/dl. Urban dwellers ranged from 2.9 to 3.9 ug/dl and low income groups averaged 3.4 ug/dl as compared to the national average of 2.8 ug/dl.[k 98] (See also Chapter 2.)

Minorities and the Environmental Movement

Charges of Racism in the Mainstream Environmental Movement

> *"Last summer, a railway-car herbicide spill in the Sacramento River, which killed several thousand fish, received more attention than the estimated 300,000 farm workers, most of whom are people of color, who may be poisoned every year by pesticides."*
>
> Deeohn Ferris, Director, Washington Center on Environmental Justice[l,99]

As the environmental justice movement developed, minority groups protesting environmental hazards in their neighborhoods began to question the absence of minorities in the mainstream environmental movement. Environmental and social justice organizations have criticized established environmental organizations for their inadequate efforts to attract minority participation, hire minority staff, or address issues that especially affect minority communities.

Historically, the environmental movement in the United States has been composed primarily of white, middle-class, well-educated individuals. In 1988, the Human Environment Center conducted an informal survey regarding minority staff at 11 national environmental organizations. The survey found only six members of minority groups serving on boards and 17 percent minority staff. Less than 2 percent of the minority staff members consisted of professionals.[100] A 1992

[k] The average blood lead level for African American children aged one to five years was caculated from the following data: non-Hispanic black males age one to two, 6.3 ug/dl; non-Hispanic black males age three to five, 5.9 ug/dl; non-Hispanic black females age one to two, 5.8 ug/dl; and non-Hispanic black females age three to five; 5.0 ug/dl. The average blood lead level for Mexican American children aged one to five years was calculated from the following data: Mexican American males age one to two, 4.2 ug/dl; Mexican American males age three to five, 4.0 ug/dl; Mexican American females age one to two, 4.8 ug/dl; and Mexican American femals age three to five, 3.6 ug/dl. The average blood lead level for non-Hispanic white children aged one to five years was calculated from the following data: non-Hispanic white males age one to two, 3.5 ug/dl; non-Hispanic white males age three to five, 2.9 ug/dl; non-Hispanic white females age one to two, 3.6 ug/dl; and non-Hispanic white females age three to five, 3.0 ug/dl. Group sizes varied. Data source was Brody *et al.*

[l] At the time of this quote, Ferris was Director of Environmental Quality for the National Wildlife Federation.

report by the Environmental Career Organization (ECO) found that minority participation was much lower in traditional environmental groups than in social justice and environmental justice organizations.[101]

In 1990, charges of environmental racism were levied against the largest national environmental organizations, known as the "Group of Ten."[m] Two grassroots environmental justice organizations led by African Americans and Hispanics initiated the charges. On January 16, 1990, the Gulf Coast Tenants Leadership Development Project sent a letter to members of the Group of Ten pointing out the "whiteness" of the environmental movement and calling for an end to racist hiring practices. The letter requested that these organizations cease operations in minority communities until their staffs were 35 to 40 percent minority. On March 16, 1990, a second letter sent by the Southwest Organizing Project (SWOP) criticized the Group of Ten for disrupting minority communities with their activities and for not being accountable to these communities. The letter stated that corporate funding from known polluters made it impossible for these organizations to adequately represent minority issues. SWOP's letter decried the lack of minorities in decision making positions within the environmental organizations' executive staff and boards and reiterated the request for a steep increase in minority employees.[102]

The letters seriously shook the environmental establishment and received national media coverage.[103] As a result, discussions took place between mainstream and grassroots groups that addressed questions such as how environmental issues could fit within a social, racial, and economic framework and what role environmental organizations might play in the social and racial justice movement in the United States.[104]

Response of the Mainstream Environmental Movement

Established environmental organizations are responding to the challenge of the environmental justice movement by working to increase the number of minorities among their staffs, boards, and membership and by finding ways to increase the number of minorities entering the environmental professions. They are also seeking ways to collaborate with grassroots environmental and social justice organizations and are preparing to broaden the range of issues they define as environmental.

According to Robert Bullard, tremendous changes have occurred within the mainstream environmental organizations. He cites the Sierra Club, the Natural Resources Defense Council, and the Environmental Defense Fund as leaders in the move to diversify their staffs

[m] The "Group of Ten" consisted of the Sierra Club, the Sierra Club Legal Defense Fund, the National Audubon Society, the National Wildlife Federation, the Environmental Defense Fund, the Environmental Policy Institute/Friends of the Earth, the Izaak Walton League, The Wilderness Society, the National Parks and Conservation Association, and the Natural Resources Defense Council.

and boards.[105] The National Audubon Society (NAS) has pushed to diversify its 600,000 member organization and has increased the number of political issues, such as urban problems, that the organization confronts. In addition, a Washington, DC chapter of NAS was recently created. This group has an ethnically diverse board of directors and seeks to recruit more minorities to NAS and the environmental movement in general.[106]

Environmental organizations with a national scope seek to collaborate with minority-led grassroots environmental justice organizations. Greenpeace has increased its level of collaboration, as has the Natural Resources Defense Council (NRDC). NRDC has collaborated with Mothers of East Los Angeles and Concerned Citizens of South Central Los Angeles to oppose plans for a toxic waste incinerator in a low income, Hispanic community and has worked with West Harlem Environmental Action on a project involving a sewage plant in the area.[107] NRDC and the Sierra Club have each hired minority professionals to build links with rural minority communities and local environmental justice organizations.[108]

In 1989, the Group of Ten formed The Environmental Consortium for Minority Outreach (TEC) to increase the number of minorities in the environmental professions.[109] That same year, the Environmental Career Organization (ECO) prepared a study on minorities in the environmental professions and reached the following conclusions:

- Most employers are seeking minority candidates but are unsuccessful in finding them;
- There is a lack of exposure to environmental issues and career opportunities within minority communities;
- There is no educational or career pipeline in place to encourage minorities to enter the environmental field;
- The supply of minority environmental professionals and minority graduates in science and engineering is limited;
- When provided with opportunities, minorities are interested and competent in entering the environmental field; and
- Extensive networks exist in both the environmental and minority communities but with little overlap between the two.

As a result of this report, the Diversity Initiative, originally called the Minority Opportunities Program, was created to increase the numbers and presence of people of color in the environmental field. In 1993, the program placed 167 minority students in a variety of paid internships and developed, managed, and evaluated environmental career development programs with budgets totaling $1.5 million.[110] Another program, the Conservation Career Development Program, was founded in 1991 in cooperation with the Student Conservation Association to increase the diversity of employees in conservation.[111]

Environmental Activism among Minorities

Lack of minority participation in the traditional environmental movement in the United States has been the source of much speculation. Historians have argued that the movements' roots in nineteenth century natural science created an elitist orientation in terms of class and racial/ethnic background. According to some environmental justice scholars, this initial elitist orientation was perpetuated by a system of internal networking that resulted in institutional racism. Other scholars postulate that minorities have been too preoccupied with providing for basic necessities to spend time on environmental issues. Minority activists assert, however, that they have now redefined environmental issues to include the survival issues they have been involved with all along.

Large numbers of minorities have become active in the environmental movement, via environmental justice issues, since the late 1980s. Minority activism has been galvanized by increased awareness of the existence of toxics in minority communities and by the publication of research linking race, class, and disproportionate exposures to toxics. This activism has been aided by the organization of conferences and workshops on the issues of environmental and social justice and the emergence of committed activists and leaders.[112] The Congressional Black Caucus and the Congressional Hispanic Caucus have recently received high scores from the League of Conservation Voters for their voting records on environmental issues.[113]

One of the few minority initiatives created as a national environmental organization is the Center for Environment, Commerce, and Energy (CE)^2). This Washington, DC-based nonprofit organization was founded in 1985 for the purpose of mobilizing African Americans to participate in environmental issues and to make environmental organizations aware of the need for minority involvement. (CE)^2 monitors national environmental policy while taking an active role in the local community. In 1990, the African American Environmentalist Association (AAEA) was founded as the membership arm of (CE)^2. AAEA publishes a quarterly newsletter and strives to increase awareness and promote environmental activism within the African American community.[114]

Government and Environmental Justice

Actions at the Environmental Protection Agency

In 1971, shortly after its formation, EPA interpreted the limitations on what it could do as a regulatory agency. The agency took a narrow view of its role under the Civil Rights Act of 1964.[115] William Ruckelshaus, EPA's first administrator, testified before the U.S. Commission on Civil Rights that EPA was a technical and scientific agency and that it was not equipped to judge the disparate impacts on minority communities from pollution.[116] In 1975, the Commission on Civil Rights criticized EPA for not recognizing its responsibility to ensure that minorities were included in EPA assistance.[117]

Environmental Equity Report

EPA did not officially take on environmental equity as an issue until 1991, after Administrator Reilly met with a group of environmental justice scholars and activists and created the Environmental Equity Workgroup to address their concerns. The workgroup consisted of staff members from each EPA office and region and was charged with assessing the evidence that racial minority and low income communities were faced with greater environmental risks than the general population. In June 1992, the workgroup submitted its report, "Environmental Equity: Reducing Risk For All Communities."

The EPA staff who participated in the workgroup concluded, based upon an extensive literature review, that racial minorities and low income populations experienced higher than average exposures to air pollutants, hazardous waste facilities, contaminated fish, and agricultural pesticides in the workplace. In addition, they found that there were clear differences between racial groups in terms of disease and death rates. However, data was too limited to explain the relationships among environmental hazards, health effects, race, and income. Only lead poisoning and air pollution data could be analyzed for exposure by race.[118]

The workgroup recommended that EPA give environmental justice issues increased priority. EPA was urged to develop a research plan and to start collecting data that could provide a basis for assessing environmental risks by income and race. The report concluded that EPA should identify and target areas with high risk concentrations and improve its communications with minority and low income communities. In addition, the workgroup recommended that EPA incorporate environmental equity considerations into all areas of its work, including risk assessment processes; major rule makings; and permit, grant, monitoring, and enforcement procedures.[119]

Although the report confirmed many claims of the environmental justice movement, it was heavily criticized when submitted for review to environmental justice activists, scholars, and community groups: 1) for not providing a timetable and strategies for implementing its recommendations, 2) for overstating the lack of data on environmental risks to low income and minority communities and the complexity of defining environmental equity, 3) for not attempting to discover the causes of environmental inequity.[120]

Creation of the Office of Environmental Justice

The Office of Environmental Equity was established in 1992 in response to the Environmental Equity Workgroup's recommendations. In March 1994, it was renamed the Office of Environmental Justice in accordance with the preferences of environmental justice activists and of EPA Administrator Carol Browner, who has made environmental justice one of her top four priorities.[121] The Office of Environmental Justice has responsibility for coordinating communications and for educating the public on environmental justice issues. The office will also serve as a central repository of environmental equity information and provide institutional access to groups concerned with environmental justice. Programs are being developed to provide technical and financial assistance to minority and low income communities.[122]

The Office of Environmental Justice also administers the Minority Academic Institutions Project, which is designed to build links between EPA and Historically Black Colleges and Universities (HBCUs), the Hispanic Association of Colleges and Universities (HACU), and Tribal Colleges in an effort to increase the participation of minorities in the environmental professions.

Other Environmental Justice Projects at EPA

Since taking on the issue, EPA has initiated a number of environmental justice projects at the national and local levels. These activities remain fairly decentralized, despite the coordinating role of the Office of Environmental Justice. The Environmental Justice Hotline (1-800-962-6215), established in 1992, receives calls from citizens concerned about toxics in their communities and assists in the resolution of environmental justice issues. A database is under development that will integrate health data from the third National Health and Nutrition Examination Survey (NHANES-III), demographic data from the 1990 Census, and environmental data from air monitoring stations and the TRI database. The Office of Water has produced a pamphlet in English, Spanish, and Vietnamese that explains various aspects of fish contamination and suggests ways to minimize possible impacts.[123] At the local level, EPA has undertaken a project to clean up the Anacostia River in Washington, DC, and to economically revitalize the predominantly African American and low income Anacostia community. EPA also initiated a project to enforce Safe Drinking Water Standards in California migrant farm worker camps.

The Office of Solid Waste and Emergency Response (OSWER) received extensive recommendations from its environmental justice task force in 1994. The task force recommended that OSWER attempt to mediate, and consider alternative sites, when complaints arise in siting new hazardous waste facilities. If communities perceive they are being treated unfairly, OSWER must respond, even if empirical evidence of environmental discrimination is sparse.[124] OSWER initiated a study on RCRA enforcement and a pilot study of the demographics of the populations living within 4 miles of 300 National Priorities List (NPL) sites. The study is to be expanded to include all 1,200 NPL sites.[125]

Most recently, EPA has created the Environmental Justice Federal Advisory Council to advise the Administrator on environmental justice policy and issues. The Council consists of representatives from community groups, industry and business, and federal, state, tribal, and local governmental organizations.

Executive Order on Environmental Justice

"All Americans have the right to be protected from pollution, not just those who can afford to live in the cleanest, safest communities."
President Bill Clinton[126]

On February 11, 1994, President Clinton signed Executive Order 12898, entitled "Federal Actions To Address Environmental Justice in Minority Populations and Low income Populations." The executive order requires each federal agency to make environmental justice part of its mission and to develop, within one year, a strategy for addressing the health and environmental impacts of its programs on minority and low income populations. Several sections also direct agencies to collect and analyze data that specifically look at human health and environmental effects according to race, national origin, and income. This information is to be made available to minority and low income populations and these populations are to have the opportunity to comment on research design.[127]

President Clinton also signed a memorandum to all federal departments and agencies underscoring the fact that existing environmental and civil rights statutes provide many opportunities to address environmental hazards in minority and low income communities. The memorandum cited in particular the following legislation: Title VI of the Civil Rights Act of 1964, which states that all programs receiving federal funding shall not discriminate on the basis or race, color, or national origin; the National Environmental Policy Act of 1969 (NEPA), which requires agencies to analyze the environmental, human health, economic, and social effects of federal actions; and Section 309 of the Clean Air Act, which requires EPA to review the environmental effects of proposed actions of federal agencies.[128]

The Federal Working Group on Environmental Justice is responsible for working out the details of the executive order. The working group is headed by the EPA Administrator and consists of the heads of federal agencies. The Administration appears to be targeting all use of federal funds, not just direct federal spending, and industry may or may not face additional reporting requirements.[129]

Proposed Federal Environmental Justice Legislation

Numerous bills addressing aspects of environmental justice were unsuccessfully introduced to the 103rd Congress. A proposed amendment to the Solid Waste Disposal Act would have required a community information statement as part of the permitting process for any new off-site hazardous waste treatment or disposal facility. The community information statement would have identified the economic effects of the proposed facility, potential human health impacts associated with waste and releases, the demographic characteristics of the community, and whether or not there is an existing facility in the community.[130]

The Environmental Health Equity Information Act of 1993 would have amended the Comprehensive Environmental Response, Compensation, and Liability Act of 1980 (CERCLA) to require the collection of data on the race, gender, ethnic origin, income level, and educational level of persons living in communities adjacent to toxic substances contamination.[131] The Environmental Equal Rights Act of 1993 sought to amend the Solid Waste Disposal Act by granting the right to petition to prevent the siting of a solid or hazardous waste facility in an environmentally disadvantaged community. An environmentally disadvantaged community was defined in this proposed legislation as an area within two miles of the borders of a proposed facility site where (1) the percentage minority population is greater than that of the state or the United States *or* 20 percent or more of the population lives below the poverty line *or* the per capita income is 80 percent of the national average or less; *and* (2) the area already contains a solid or hazardous waste facility, a Superfund site, or a TRI facility reporting toxics that are likely to have adverse health impacts.[132]

The most comprehensive bill, however, was the Environmental Justice Act of 1992, which was originally introduced by Congressman John Lewis and then-Senator Al Gore. This bill would have required EPA to identify Environmental High Impact Areas (EHIAs), defined as the 100 areas nationwide with the highest total weight of toxic chemicals released. EPA would then be required to conduct mandatory inspections of facilities in these areas to ensure compliance with environmental health and safety standards and to collect information on the health effects of emissions.[133]

State Environmental Justice Legislation

In April 1993, Arkansas became the first state to pass environmental justice legislation. Arkansas' Act 1263 prohibits the construction or operation of any high-impact, solid waste management facility within twelve miles of an existing facility. The Governor of Tennessee signed a resolution (HRJ 146) in May 1993 which paves the way for a hypothetical "Environmental Justice Act." In June 1993, Louisiana passed Act 767 which directs the state environmental agency to hold hearings on environmental justice issues and make recommendations to the legislature. In addition, Virginia passed a resolution ordering a study of the impact of solid and hazardous waste facilities on minority communities.[134]

In 1994, Florida enacted Act 1369 which created the Environmental Equity and Justice Commission to examine the magnitude of minority disproportionate impact. The commission will present a report to the Florida legislature and will hold five public hearings. The commission will also prepare model legislation to be considered by the Florida legislature in 1996.[135]

The state environmental justice laws vary widely in their approaches, containing one or more of the following elements: a requirement to hold public hearings on environmental justice issues; a requirement to study the location of existing facilities, or the history of enforcement in the state, or the impact of facilities on surrounding communities; a requirement for providing demographic data and/ or community economic development plans as part of the permitting process for new facilities; an authorization for the state to establish a toxics release inventory; a requirement to identify 20 EHIAs in the state; or an authorization to place a moratorium on new facilities in the vicinity of existing ones.[136]

Industry and Environmental Justice

The industrial sector, especially the chemical industry, is becoming increasingly concerned with addressing charges of environmental racism. Industry representatives categorically deny any intentional targeting of minority communities for the placement of facilities. They state that the suitability of sites, such as deep river ports and access to raw materials, is the defining criterion. However, many in industry are voicing the opinion that environmental justice is a legitimate issue and that prudence dictates working out a strategy to address concerns.[137]

The Chemical Manufacturer's Association (CMA) has created its own task force to deal with environmental justice issues and has participated in the National Association of Manufacturers (NAM) task force that was created in 1993. The NAM task force has developed an environmental justice policy, approved by the Board of Directors in September 1994, that members can use for guidance. In addition, NAM has presented the business point of view in debates and workshops on environmental justice issues. According to its environmental justice policy, NAM supports compliance with environmental laws and regulations, maintaining economic viability in an environmentally responsible manner, open and informed dialogue with citizens, nondiscriminatory enforcement of environmental laws and regulations, continued scientific research into the potential link between health effects and exposure to pollutants, use of risk assessment to evaluate and prioritize health and environmental risks, and the development of additional measures to protect human health where scientific research evidence exists to confirm that existing laws and regulations do not provide adequate protection.[138]

Environmental justice activists have made a number of requests to industry regarding participation, benefits, safety, and equity. Activists have expressed a desire for increased community participation in decision making and for improved links between industry and local schools and organizations. Activists have also encouraged industry to hire local residents and provide training programs in order to increase benefits to the immediate community. In terms of safety, community residents request that industry assure them of the safety of chemicals in use, limit emissions via pollution prevention activities, and clean up contaminated areas. Finally, emissions in highly impacted communities should not be increased and each plant should be operated "as if it were in Beverly Hills or Kennebunkport."[139]

Although environmental justice is still an emerging issue for the business community, some change has already occurred. Companies are becoming increasingly aware that communicating with communities is good business practice.[140] Among some companies, there is now more emphasis on training and hiring local residents, as well as developing local procurement. Industry representatives agree that community residents should benefit from facilities in their midst.[141]

Through new requirements, the environmental justice movement may have a significant impact on business and industry. EPA's environmental justice initiatives and proposed federal and state legislation could increase enforcement activities, restrict the siting of hazardous waste and chemical manufacturing facilities, and impose increased permitting costs in the form of community compensation, community development activities, and mandatory community training programs. New laws and regulations might delay and increase the costs of siting industrial facilities and hazardous waste treatment, storage, and disposal facilities. Government authority to inspect operations in highly impacted communities may be increased and higher fines may be imposed. New legislation may change the legal bases of environmental justice claims and expand the rights of community residents. Cleanup activities under RCRA and CERCLA may be affected, as well as implementation of Clean Air Act programs.[142]

Although the precise nature and extent of the effects on industry practices of environmental justice initiatives and legislation that may develop over the next several years is not known, the most positive conceivable effect would be a spur to greater pollution prevention activities. To the extent that environmental justice activists raise legitimate local and national concerns about toxic pollution, their efforts may have an important spin-off effect that would benefit all Americans:

> *Communities of color and low income Americans seek not to redistribute pollution, from dirtier and overexposed areas to cleaner and underexposed areas. They, instead, seek to prevent pollution at the source so that all Americans can breathe clean air, drink clean water and eat clean food.*

Representative John Conyers, Jr.,
Chairman, Subcommittee on
Legislation and National Security,
Committee on Government Operations,
U.S. House of Representatives[143]

---

1 Ken Sexton and Yolanda Banks Anderson, Foreword, *Toxicology and Industrial Health,* Special Issue, 9, no.5 (September-October 1993): vi.

2 Marianne Lavalle, "The Minorities Equation," *National Law Journal*, September 21, 1992, 6.

3 Dorceta E. Taylor, "Environmentalism and the Politics of Inclusion," in Robert D. Bullard, ed., *Confronting Environmental Racism: Voices from the Grassroots*, Boston, MA: Southend Press, 1993, 56. *The People of Color Environmental Groups 1994-1995 Directory*, edited by Robert Bullard, is available from the Charles Stewart Mott Foundation.

4 Robert D. Bullard, "Grassroots Flowering: The Environmental Justice Movement Comes of Age," *Amicus Journal*, Spring 1994, 32.

5 William S. Hoffman *et al.*, "Relation of Pesticide Concentration in Fat to Pathological Changes in Tissues," *Archives of Environmental Health*, 15 (1967): 758-765.

6 Council on Environmental Quality, *Environmental Quality: The Second Annual Report*, Washington, DC, August 1971, 191-193.

7 Robert D. Bullard, "Dumping in Black and White," in *We Speak for Ourselves: Social Justice, Race, and Environment*, Dana Alston, ed., Washington, DC: Panos Institute, 1990, 4.

8 NAACP vs. *Gorsuch*, No. 82-768-5 (E.D. N.C. August 10, 1982). Described in Thomas J. Henderson and W. Lawrence Wallace, *Environmental Justice Cases: Cases Involving Challenges to Environmental Decisions That Raise Claims of Race or National Origin Discrimination*, Environmental Justice Project of the Lawyers' Committee on Civil Rights Under Law, March 1993, 8-10; Office of Environmental Equity, U.S. Environmental Protection Agency, *Environmental Justice Initiatives: 1993*, February 1994, 2.

9 For information on the Warren County protest, see Stephanie Pollack and JoAnn Grozuczak, *Reagan, Toxics and Minorities*, Washington, DC: Urban Environment Conference, Inc., September 1984, 23-24, and Ken Geiser and Gerry Waneck, "PCBs and Warren County," in *Unequal Protection: Environmental Justice and Communities of Color*, Robert D. Bullard, ed., San Francisco, CA: Sierra Club Books, 1994, 43-52.

10 U.S. General Accounting Office, *Siting of Hazardous Waste Landfills and Their Correlation with Racial and Economic Status of Surrounding Communities*, Washington, DC, June 1, 1983.

11 United Church of Christ Commission for Racial Justice, *Toxic Wastes and Race in the United States: A National Report on the Racial and Socio-Economic Characteristics of Communities with Hazardous Waste Sites,*, New York, NY, 1987, xiii.

12 Bunyan Bryant and Paul Mohai, "Introduction," in *Race and the Incidence of Environmental Hazards*, Bryant and Mohai, eds., Boulder, CO: Westview Press, 1992, 1-9.

13 Proceedings of the First National People of Color Environmental Leadership Summit, New York, NY: United Church of Christ Commission for Racial Justice, 1992.

14 Marcia Coyle and Marianne Lavalle, "Unequal Protection: The Racial Divide in Environmental Law," Special Issue, *National Law Journal*, September 21, 1992.

15 Michael Greenberg, "Proving Environmental Inequity in Siting Locally Unwanted Land Uses," *Risk: Issues in Health and Safety*, 4, no. 3 (Summer 1993): 236.

16 For claims of outcome inequity regarding siting of facilities that treat, store, or produce hazardous waste, see U.S. General Accounting Office, *Siting of Hazardous Waste Landfills*; United Church of Christ Commission for Racial Justice, *Toxic Wastes and Race in the United States*; Paul Mohai and Bunyan Bryant, "Environmental Racism: Reviewing the Evidence," in *Race and the Incidence of Environmental Hazards*, 163-176.

17 For claims of outcome inequity regarding air pollution, see Brian J.L. Berry, *The Social Burdens of Environmental Pollution: A Comparative Metropolitan Data Source*, Cambridge, MA: Ballinger Publishing Company, 1977; D.R. Wernette and L.A. Nieves, "Breathing Polluted Air," *EPA Journal*, 18, no. 1 (March/April 1992): 16-17; Ken Sexton *et al.*, "Air Pollution Health Risks: Do Class and Race Matter?" *Toxicology and Industrial Health*, 9, no. 5 (September/October 1993): 843-878. For claims of outcome inequity regarding lead poisoning, see Joel Schwartz and Ronnie Levin, "Lead: Example of the Task Ahead," *EPA Journal*, 18, no. 1 (March/April 1992): 42-44; U. S. Environmental Protection Agency, *Environmental Equity: Reducing Risk for All Communities*, Vol. II., Washington, DC, June 1992, 9-10; Laura E. Montgomery and Olivia Carter-Pokras, "Health Status by Social Class and/or Minority Status: Implications for Environmental Equity Research," *Toxicology and Industrial Health*, 9, no. 5 (September/October 1993): 729-773.

18 For claims of outcome inequity regarding exposure to occupational health hazards, see Pollack and Grozuczak, *Reagan, Toxics and Minorities*, 29-39; Beverly Hendrix Wright, "Effects of Occupational Injury, Illness, and Disease on the Health Status of Black Americans: A Review," in *Race and the Incidence of Environmental Hazards*, 114-125; Marion Moses, "Farm Workers and Pesticides," in *Confronting Environmental Racism*, 161-178; Marion Moses *et al.*, "Environmental Equity and Pesticide Exposure," *Toxicology and Industrial Health*, 9, no. 5 (September/October 1993): 913-959.

19 For claims of process inequity due to siting decision-making practices, see Robert D. Bullard, *Dumping in Dixie: Race, Class, and Environmental Quality*, Boulder, CO: Westview Press, 1990; discussion of legal cases in Rachel D. Godsil, "Remedying Environmental Racism," *Michigan Law Review*, 90, no. 2 (November 1991) : 394-427; Naiking Tsao, "Ameliorating Environmental Racism: A Citizen's Guide to Combating the Discriminatory Siting of Toxic Waste Dumps," *New York University Law Review*, 67, no. 2 (May 1992): 366-418.

20 For claims of process inequity due to exclusion of community residents from decision-making processes, see Michael Guerrero and Louis Head, "Informed Collective Action — A Powerful Weapon" in *We Speak for Ourselves: Social Justice, Race and Environment;* Katherine L. Ratcliffe, "Fusing Civil, Environmental Rights," *Christian Science Monitor*, May 24, 1991, 12.

21 For claims of process inequity due to underrepresentation of minorities in policymaking bodies, see letters from Gulf Coast Tenant Leadership Development Project (January 16, 1990) and Southwest Organizing Project (March 15, 1990) to the 10 largest national environmental organizations; Benjamin F. Chavis, Jr., Testimony, House Subcommittee on Civil and Constitutional Rights, March 3, 1993; Robert D. Bullard, "Solid Waste Sites and the Black Houston Community," *Sociological Inquiry*, 53, no. 2/3 (Spring 1983): 273-288.

22 Benjamin Goldman compiled a list of 64 empirical studies undertaken between 1967 and 1993, published in Benjamin A. Goldman, *Not Just Prosperity: Achieving Sustainability with Environmental Justice*, Washington, DC: National Wildlife Federation, December 1993, 5-6. Since that time, additional studies have been published.

23 U.S. General Accounting Office, *Siting of Hazardous Waste Landfills.*

24 Bullard, "Solid Waste Sites and the Black Houston Community," 273-288.

25 United Church of Christ Commission for Racial Justice, *Toxic Wastes and Race in the United States.*

26 Mohai and Bryant, "Environmental Racism: Reviewing the Evidence," in *Race and the Incidence of Environmental Hazards*, 161-176.

27 Greenberg, "Proving Environmental Inequity," 235-252.

28 Rae Zimmerman, "Social Equity and Environmental Risk," *Rick Analysis*, 13, no. 6 (1993): 649-666.

29 Douglas Anderton *et al.*, "Environmental Equity: The Demographics of Dumping," *Demography*, 31, no. 2 (May 1994): 229-248.

30 Benjamin A. Goldman and Laura Fitton, *Toxic Wastes and Race Revisited*, Washington, DC: Center for Policy Alternatives, 1994.

31 Anderton *et al.*, "Environmental Equity," 244.

32 See, for example, Ronald Begley, "Environmental Justice: Racism Questioned in Two Studies," *Chemical Week*, April 20, 1994, 8; "Reality of Environmental Racism Questioned," *Pesticide and Toxic Chemical News*, April 13, 1994, 4; "Two New Reports Challenge Claims of Race-Based Industry Siting Decisions," *Daily Environment Report*, April 11, 1994, AA-1-2.

33 U.S. General Accounting Office, *Siting of Hazardous Waste Landfills*, 1.

34 Mohai and Bryant, "Environmental Racism: Reviewing the Evidence," in *Race and the Incidence of Environmental Hazards*, 174.

35 Anderton *et al.*, "Environmental Equity," 235-236.

36 United Church of Christ Commission for Racial Justice, *Toxic Wastes and Race in the United States*, 41.

37 Rae Zimmerman, "Social Equity and Environmental Risk," 649-666.

38 Greenberg, "Proving Environmental Inequity," 243-247.

39 Quoted in Marcia Coyle, "Saying No to Cancer Alley," *National Law Journal*, September 21, 1993, 5.

40 Rachel Godsil, "Remedying Environmental Racism," 400.

41 See Paul Mohai and Bunyan Bryant, "Race, Poverty, and the Environment: The Disadvantaged Face Greater Risks," *EPA Journal*, 18, no. 1 (March/April 1992): 7; Cerrell Associates, Inc., *Political Difficulties Facing Waste to Energy Conversion Plant Siting,* Report to the California Waste Management Board, Los Angeles, CA, 1984 as cited in James T. Hamilton, "Politics and Social Costs: Estimating the Impact of Collective Action on Hazardous Waste Facilities," *RAND Journal of Economics*, 24, no. 1 (Spring 1993): 106.

42 Hamilton, "Politics and Social Costs," 101-125.

43 Rae Zimmerman, "Risk and Public Controversy at Hazardous Waste Sites," Final Report to U.S. Environmental Protection Agency, Office of Solid Waste and Emergency Response, January 15, 1992 as cited in Zimmerman, "Social Equity and Environmental Risk," 661-663.

44 Vicki Been, "What's Fairness Got to Do With It? Environmental Justice and the Siting of Locally Undesirable Land Uses," *Cornell Law Review*, 78, no. 6 (September 1993): 1007.

45 See Been, Godsil, Hamilton, and Mohai and Bryant, among others.

46 Vicki Been, "Locally Undesirable Land Uses in Minority Neighborhoods: Disproportionate Siting or Market Dynamics," *Yale Law Journal*, 103, no. 6 (April 1994): 1388.

47 Been, "Locally Undesirable Land Uses," *Yale Law Journal*, 1383-1422.

48 *Washington v. Davis*, 426 U.S. 229 (1976) as cited in Richard J. Lazarus, "Pursuing 'Environmental Justice': The Distributional Effects of Environmental Protection," *Northwestern University Law Review*, 87, no. 3 (Spring 1993): 833.

49 Tsao, "Ameliorating Environmental Racism," 406.

50 *Arlington Heights v. Metropolitan Housing Development Corp.*, 429 U.S. 252 (1977) as cited in Lazarus, "Pursuing 'Environmental Justice':The Distributional Effects of Environmental Protection," 832-833.

51 Tsao, "Ameliorating Environmental Racism," 407.

52 *Bean v. Southwestern Waste Management*, S.D. Texas (1979), 5th Circuit (1986). The lawsuit was filed by Linda McKeever Bullard who was married to Robert D. Bullard.

53 Robert W. Collin, "Environmental Equity: A Law and Planning Approach to Environmental Racism," *Virginia Environmental Law Journal,* 11, no. 4 (Summer 1992): 521-523.

54 Collin, "Environmental Equity," 523.

55 *East Bibb Twiggs Neighborhood Association. v. Macon-Bibb County Planning and Zoning Commission*, M.D. Georgia (1989), 11th Circuit (1989).

56 Anthony R. Chase, "Assessing and Addressing Problems Posed by Environmental Racism," *Rutgers Law Review*, 45, no. 2 (Winter 1993): 356.

57 Godsil, "Remedying Environmental Racism," 411; Chase, "Assessing and Addressing Problems," 356.

58 *R.I.S.E., Inc. v. Kay*, E.D. Virginia (1991) and 4th Circuit (1992) as cited in Lazarus, "Pursuing 'Environmental Justice':The Distributional Effects of Environmental Protection," 833.

59 Collin, "Environmental Equity," 527-533; Tsao, "Ameliorating Environmental Racism," 411; Chase, "Assessing and Addressing Problems," 356-357.

60 As quoted in Chase, "Assessing and Addressing Problems," 357-358.

61 U.S. Environmental Protection Agency, *Environmental Justice Initiatives 1993.*

62 Laura E. Montgomery and Olivia Carter-Pokras, "Health Status by Social Class and/or Minority Status: Implications for Environmental Equity Research," *Toxicology and Industrial Health*, 9, no. 5 (September/October 1993): 737.

63 William P. O'Hare, "America's Minorities: The Demographics of Diversity," *Population Bulletin*, 47, no. 4 (December 1992): 21.

64 "Southwest Organizing Project," *Ms.*, July/August 1994, 51.

65 Richard Moore and Louis Head, "Building a Network That Works: SWOP," in *Unequal Protection: Environmental Justice and Communities of Color*, 191-206.

66 Lazarus, "Pursuing 'Environmental Justice': The Distributional Effects of Environmental Protection," 787-857.

67 *Taking Back Our Health: A Training Manual on Job Safety and Health for Black and Latino Workers,* Washington, DC: Urban Environment Conference, Inc., November 1981, 1.

68 The First National People of Color Environmental Leadership Summit Program Guide, New York, NY: United Church of Christ Commission for Racial Justice, 1991, 35.

69 Pollack and Grozuczak, *Reagan, Toxics and Minorities,* 41-42.

70 Moses, "Farm Workers and Pesticides," in *Confronting Environmental Racism,* 161-162.

71 Hawley Truax, "Minorities at Risk," *Environmental Action,* January/February 1990, 20.

72 Bureau of National Affairs, "Final Farm Worker Protection Rule Issued After Six Years of Wrangling," *Daily Environment Report,* August 14, 1992, AA-1.

73 Ivette Perfecto, "Pesticide Exposure of Farm Workers and the International Connection" in *Race and the Incidence of Environmental Hazards,* 180; Moses, "Farm Workers and Pesticides," in *Confronting Environmental Racism,* 174.

74 Perfecto, "Pesticide Exposure of Farm Workers," 183-184.

75 Pollack and Grozuczak, *Reagan, Toxics and Minorities,* 43.

76 Truax, "Minorities at Risk," 20.

77 Pollack and Grozuczak, *Reagan, Toxics and Minorities,* 43; Moses, "Farm Workers and Pesticides," in *Confronting Environmental Racism,* 172.

78 U.S. Environmental Protection Agency, *Environmental Justice Initiatives 1993.*

79 O'Hare, "America's Minorities," 10,12-13,23.

80 Robert D. Bullard, "In Our Backyards," *EPA Journal,* 18, no. 1 (March/April 1992): 11-12.

81 Bullard, "In Our Backyards," 11-12.

82 "Expanding the Dialogue," *EPA Journal,* 18, no. 1 (March/April 1992): 35.

83 Environmental and Energy Study Institute, *Environment, Energy, and Natural Resources Status Report for the 103rd Congress,* October 13, 1994, 25.

84 Bureau of National Affairs, "Tougher Permitting, Enforcement May Grow From EPA 'Equity' Report," *Daily Environment Report,* July 24, 1992, A-12.

85 Patrick C. West, "Health Concerns for Fish-Eating Tribes?" *EPA Journal,* 18, no. 1 (March/April 1992): 15-16.

86 1990 Bureau of the Census statistics as reported in *The World Almanac and Book of Facts 1994,* Mahwah, NJ: Funk and Wagnalls Corp., 1993, 362, and O'Hare, "America's Minorities," 9.

87 Office of Environmental Equity, U.S. Environmental Protection Agency, "Environmental Justice Issues of Asian and Pacific Americans," *Environmental Equity Update,* July 1993, 15.

88 Rick Carroll, "The Pele Defense Fund," *EPA Journal,* 18, no. 1 (March/April 1992): 49-51.

89 Gary Lee, "Postwar Pacific Fallout Wider than Thought," *Washington, Post,* February 24, 1994, A20.

90 "Panel Outlines Strategies to Fight Racial Justice," *Environmental Forum,* January/February 1994, 53.

91 O'Hare, "America's Minorities," 23.

92 D.R. Wernette and L.A. Nieves, "Breathing Polluted Air: Minorities are Disproportionately Exposed," *EPA Journal,* 18, no. 1 (March/April 1992): 16-17.

93 Schwartz and Levin, "Lead: Example of the Job Ahead," 42.

94 Schwartz and Levin, "Lead: Example of the Job Ahead," 44.

95 Schwartz and Levin, "Lead: Example of the Job Ahead," 42.

96 Pollack and Grozuczak, *Reagan, Toxics and Minorities,* 6.

97 David Brown, "Lead Level in Americans' Blood Has Fallen 75 Percent Since Late 1970s," *Washington Post,* July 27, 1994, A2; Debra J. Brody *et al.,* "Blood Lead Levels in the U.S. Population," *Journal of the American Medical Association,* 272, no. 4 (July 27, 1994): 277-283; James L. Pirkle *et al.,* "The Decline in Blood Lead Levels in the United States," *Journal of the American Medical Association,* 272, no. 4 (July 27, 1994): 284-291.

98 Pirkle *et al.,* "The Decline in Blood Lead Levels," 284-291.

[99] Deeohn Ferris, "A Challenge to EPA: An Environmental Justice Office is Needed," *EPA Journal,* 18, no. 1 (March/April 1992): 28-29.

[100] As reported in Marcia T. Chen, *The Minority Opportunities Study,* Boston, MA: CEIP Fund, Inc., August 1989, 6.

[101] *Beyond the Green: Redefining and Diversifying the Environmental Movement,* Boston, MA: Environmental Careers Organization, 1992.

[102] Richard Moore and Louis Head, "Building a Net that Works: SWOP," in *Unequal Protection: Environmental Justice and Communities of Color,* 201; Letter to Jay D. Hair, President, National Wildlife Federation, from the Gulf Coast Tenant Leadership Development Project, January 16, 1990; Letter to Jay D. Hair, President, National Wildlife Federation, from the Southwest Organizing Project, March 16, 1990.

[103] Claudia MacLachlan, "Tension Underlies Rapport with Grassroots Groups," *National Law Journal,* September 21, 1992, 10.

[104] Michael Guerrero and Louis Head, "The Environment: Redefining the Issue" in *We Speak for Ourselves: Social Justice, Race and Environment,* Washington, DC: The Panos Institute, December 1990, 11.

[105] Robert D. Bullard as quoted in MacLachlan, "Tension Underlies Rapport with Grassroots Groups," 10.

[106] "Audubon Broadens Sights: DC Chapter Seeks More Minorities, Targets City's Environment," *Washington Post,* January 7, 1993, DC6.

[107] John H. Adams, "The Mainstream Environmental Movement: Predominantly White Memberships Are Not Defensible," *EPA Journal,*18, no. 1 (March/April 1992): 25-17.

[108] David Hahn-Baker, "Rocky Roads to Consensus: Traditional Environmentalism Meets Environmental Justice," *Amicus,* Spring 1994, 41-42; Timothy Noah, "Sierra Club Takes an Edifying Tour of Black America," *Wall Street Journal,* June 24, 1993, A1.

[109] "Status Statement," The Environmental Consortium for Minority Outreach, January 1990; Environmental Careers Organization 1993 Annual Report.

[110] Chen, *The Minority Opportunities Study.* The Center for Environmental Intern Programs became the Environmental Career Organization in 1992.

[111] Charles Jordan, "Minorities in Conservation: An Uphill Battle," *Earth Work,* April 1991, 5 and 30.

[112] Dorceta Taylor, "The Environmental Justice Movement: No Shortage of Minority Volunteers," *EPA Journal,* 18, no. 1 (March/April 1992): 23-24.

[113] Telephone conversation with Patricia Williams, Counsel and Legislative Representative, Solid and Hazardous Waste Issues, National Wildlife Federation, December 12, 1994.

[114] *African American Environmentalist,* 1, no. 1 (1990) and 1, no. 2 (September 1990).

[115] Richard J. Lazarus, "Pursuing 'Environmental Justice': The Distributional Effects of Environmental Protection," *Northwestern University Law Review,* 87, no. 3 (Spring 1993): 837.

[116] Marianne Lavalle, "Residents Want 'Justice,' The EPA Offers 'Equity,'" *National Law Journal,* September 21, 1992, 12.

[117] Lazarus, "Pursuing 'Environmental Justice,'" 837.

[118] U.S. Environmental Protection Agency, *Environmental Equity: Reducing Risk For All Communities,* Washington, DC, June 1992, Vol. 1, 3.

[119] U.S. Environmental Protection Agency, *Environmental Equity: Reducing Risk For All Communities,* Vol. 1, 4.

[120] U.S. Environmental Protection Agency, *Environmental Equity: Reducing Risk For All Communities,* Vol. 2, 72-79.

[121] Lois R. Ember, "EPA Giving Increased Priority to Environmental Equity Issues," *Chemical and Engineering News,* January 24, 1994, 22-23.

[122] Office of Environmental Equity, U.S. Environmental Protection Agency, *Environmental Equity Update,* October 27, 1992, 3.

[123] Office of Environmental Equity, U.S. Environmental Protection Agency, *Environmental Equity Update,* December 30, 1992, 3, 9.

124 "Environmental Justice to be Included in All Hazardous Waste Decisions," *Pesticide and Toxic Chemical News*, May 4, 1994, 4.

125 "EPA to Expand Environmental Equity Study to Include all NPL Sites," *Environmental Policy Alert*, April 27, 1994, 10.

126 As quoted in "Clinton Seeks 'Environmental Justice,'" *Washington Post*, February 12, 1994, A6.

127 Executive Order 12898 of February 11, 1994 (59FR7629, February 16, 1994).

128 "Clinton Signs Executive Order, Browner Criticized by Community Groups," *Daily Environment Report*, February 2, 1994, AA-1, AA-2.

129 "Order to be Issued on Civil Rights, Pollution Link," *Wall Street Journal*, February 11, 1994, A14.

130 S. 533, 103rd Congress, 1st Session (1993), March 9, 1993.

131 H.R. 1925, 103rd Congress, 1st Session (1993), April 29, 1993.

132 H.R. 1924, 103rd Congress, 1st Session (1993), April 29, 1993.

133 S. 1161, 103rd Congress, 1st Session (1993), June 22, 1993.

134 Center for Policy Alternatives, "States Take on Environmental Racism," *Alternatives*, 1, no. 4 (September/October 1993): 2.

135 Barton Hacker, *Environmental Justice: Legislation in the States*, Washington, DC: Center for Policy Alternatives, September 1994.

136 Center for Policy Alternatives, news release, July 30, 1993.

137 Ronald Begley and Elisabeth Kirschner, "The Demand for Environmental Justice: Industry Faces a Nationwide Campaign," *Chemical Week*, September 15, 1993, 27; National Association of Manufacturers, "Policy on Environmental Justice," September 24, 1994.

137 Telephone conversation with John Kyte, Director, Environmental Quality Committee, National Association of Manufacturers, September 8, 1994.

139 Begley and Kirschner, "The Demand for Environmental Justice," 27.

140 Telephone conversation with John Kyte, Director, Environmental Quality Committee, National Association of Manufacturers, September 8, 1994.

141 Begley and Kirschner, "The Demand for Environmental Justice," 27.

142 Stephen C. Jones, "Inequities of Industrial Siting Addressed," *National Law Journal*, August 16, 1993, 20.

143 John Conyers, Jr., Statement, United States House of Representatives, Committee on Government Operations, Subcommittee on Legislation and National Security, April 28, 1993, 1.

Chapter 10

State Databases

Use, Materials Accounting, and Pollution Prevention in New Jersey and Massachusetts

Introduction

Massachusetts and New Jersey collect information from facilities in their states that goes beyond the data required for the federal Toxics Release Inventory (TRI). The databases in these two states provide an opportunity to explore the usefulness of such additional information in understanding more fully the risks of a toxic chemical at a facility, how toxic chemicals are used, the amount of toxic chemicals in commerce, and the amount of source reduction of toxic chemicals in industrial waste. The profiles of activities involving toxic chemicals in New Jersey and Massachusetts are different in that the type of information collected differs between the two states and because there is a very different mix of industry in New Jersey as compared to Massachusetts. (See Figures 10-1 through 10-3 for a pictorial comparison of the reporting systems in these two states with the federal TRI.)

Summary of Findings

- While the data collected by New Jersey and Massachusetts are different, both permit a much clearer picture of toxic chemical *use* than does the data collected for TRI. In both states, chemical, industrial, and geographical distribution is revealed to be very different with respect to *use of chemicals* than it is for either *waste generation* or *environmental releases and transfers*.
- New Jersey offers the most complete picture of the flow of a chemical into a facility, through its processes, and into its waste and product outputs. This picture can provide perspectives completely lacking from the TRI data for the same facility.
- Massachusetts offers the most complete picture of the conditions of use of the chemical at a

Figure 10-1.

Toxics Release Inventory (TRI) Data

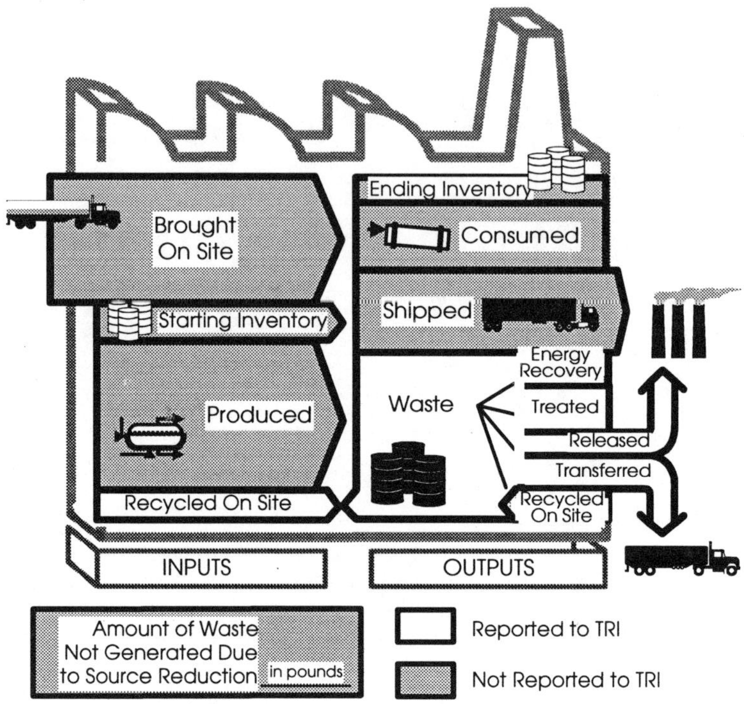

facility, obtaining a description of each process (production unit), the range of amount of chemical use, and the percent change in waste by process, instead of facility-wide as in New Jersey.

- Both New Jersey and Massachusetts data reveal how much of a toxic chemical is shipped as or in the products from the facilities. In New Jersey, 54 percent of the toxic chemical inputs to the manufacturing process ended up in products (a total of 10.7 billion pounds in 1992), and in Massachusetts 42 percent did (a total of 424.9 million pounds in 1992). Such data are valuable because toxics in commerce pose as large or larger environmental threats than industrial wastes, but ones with much less information about them. (See Chapters 2 and 3.)

- Only in New Jersey are the pounds of source reduction reported. The reasons for changes in waste generation from one year to the next are much clearer in the New Jersey data than in TRI, because New Jersey requires facilities to report the specific amount of waste reduced due to source reduction activities, the amount of change due to discontinuation of use or export of the use to another facility, and changes in production level.

- The New Jersey data, which yield the clearest picture of how much source reduction is actually occurring, reveal that, despite much fanfare by government and

Figure 10-2.

New Jersey Materials Accounting Data

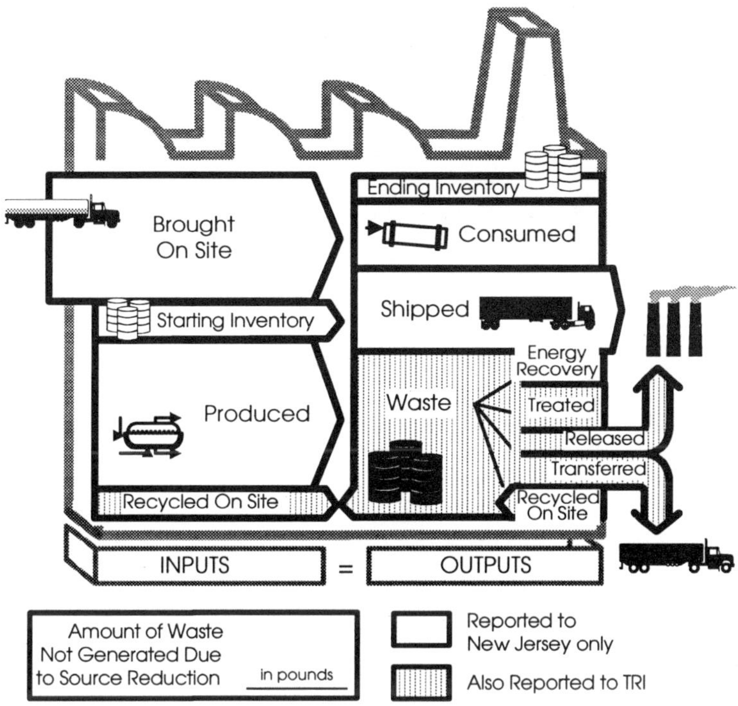

Figure 10-3.

Massachusetts Materials Accounting Data

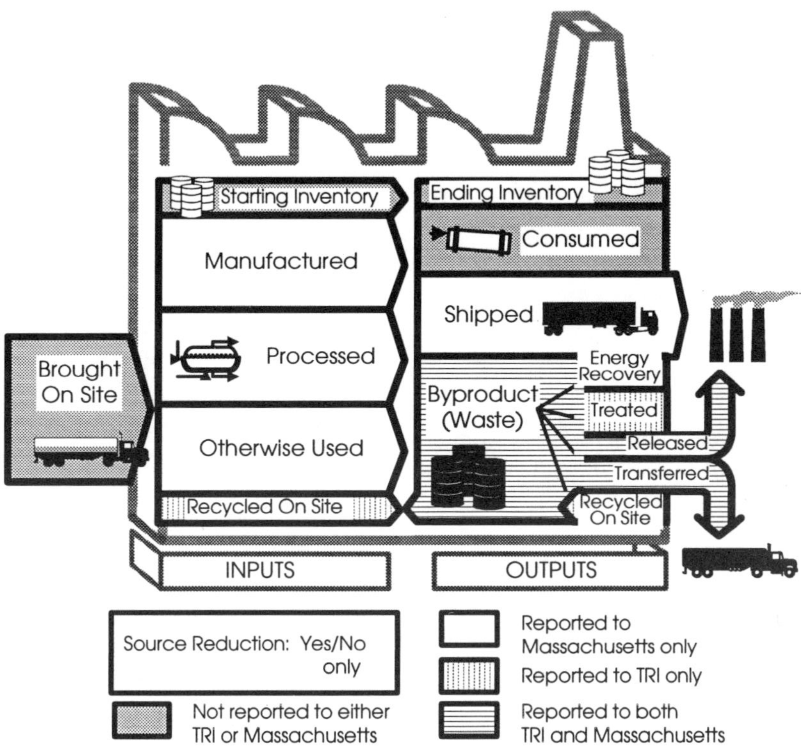

industry over a new emphasis on source reduction, source reduction of industrial toxic waste is not occurring to any appreciable extent (at least in New Jersey). Furthermore, in New Jersey the trend is in the wrong direction: fewer facilities reported any source reduction activity in 1992 than in 1991, and the amount of source reduction they reported was both a smaller amount and a smaller percentage of waste generation.

- In Massachusetts, a higher percentage of facilities (52 percent compared to 44 percent) reported *some* source reduction activity in 1992 than in 1991. Since source reduction activity is reported for a single chemical at a single production unit, some facilities included in the group reporting source reduction activity may engage in such activity only in one section of the facility's operations. In 1991, 37 percent of production units had source reduction activities reported for at least one chemical associated with the production unit, while in 1992 that figure was 39 percent. TRI collects the same information about type of source reduction activity, but does so for each chemical facility-wide without indicating how widespread the activity may be in the facility.

- Source reduction progress in New Jersey for special chemical groups of health or environmental concern was extremely modest or nonexistent. For example, source reduction for carcinogens reduced the amount of carcinogen-containing waste generated only by about 0.1 percent, and some of the facilities releasing the most carcinogens reported no source reduction.

- In New Jersey and Massachusetts, as in the nation as a whole, a relatively few large facilities dominate the data. In New Jersey, for example, facilities reporting greater than 3 million pounds of toxic chemical use in 1992 represented only 11 percent of all forms, but they reported 96 percent of the use, 73 percent of the waste generated, and 51 percent of total releases and transfers. These data exclude one facility, whose reported amounts in 1992 are so large, and so inconsistent with what the facility reported in 1991, that they must be excluded from the data when analyzing what is going on at other facilities.

- In New Jersey, the facilities using the largest amounts of chemicals tend to report relatively smaller percentages of waste generated, and much smaller source reduction accomplished, than do facilities using smaller amounts of the same chemicals, with proportionately higher waste generation and much greater source reduction.

- Massachusetts includes in its reporting system some non-manufacturing industries that are not covered by TRI. The non-manufacturing industries reporting in 1992 accounted for 7 percent of use and 1 percent of total releases and transfers in Massachusetts. Massachusetts has also phased in reporting on additional chemicals not currently covered by TRI. Because the phase-in was completed in reporting year 1993, it is too early to evaluate the ramifications of this expansion.

Information Collected by New Jersey and Massachusetts

The TRI database is particularly valuable for tracking toxic chemical releases and transfers nationally. While TRI data give an overall picture of toxic chemicals in waste at reporting facilities, the database has limits in its usefulness, particularly for pollution prevention planning and measurement. TRI also has no information on the amount of chemicals used or manufactured at a facility nor the amount produced or shipped from the facility.

New Jersey's and Massachusetts' state programs supplement the federal TRI with publicly available information[a] that provides the means to evaluate more of toxic chemical flows at reporting facilities. New Jersey's database has the expanded data from 1979, 1984, and 1987-1992, whereas Massachusetts has been collecting its expanded data since 1990. The two programs differ from TRI in their coverage of chemicals and facilities, the extent to which they require detailed accounting of amounts of chemicals used in particular ways, and the way that their information can be used to relate waste generation to source reduction. Both states, in their next reporting cycle, will be collecting information on pollution prevention planning and progress, which will help to increase public understanding of and public accountability for progress in pollution prevention.

New Jersey has led the learning curve on facility-specific data collection; in fact, its original New Jersey Industrial Survey of 1979 inspired development of the federal TRI. The original concept was to have a full "materials accounting" of chemical inputs to and outputs from the manufacturing process. These data have been collected continuously in New Jersey since 1987. Since then, the state's new requirements for pollution prevention data, discussed below, have gone beyond both TRI and other state reporting requirements.

Although the Massachusetts program does not require quantitative data for a full materials accounting of chemical inputs and outputs to the same extent as New Jersey's, the Massachusetts database tracks amounts associated with chemical uses in more detail than TRI or New Jersey. The Massachusetts program also includes some details on each chemical at the production unit or process level within a facility, rather than just facility-wide. It further includes facilities and chemicals not covered by TRI.

Understanding how the New Jersey and Massachusetts reporting requirements and databases differ from TRI and from each other makes it possible to evaluate the usefulness of these states' approaches and to interpret what is happening there with regard to toxics in waste and pollution prevention. The brief explanation of

[a] The databases are available to the public free or at cost. (See Appendix Q.)

these reporting systems below is followed by a toxics chemical profile for each of these states.

Another state that has more recently expanded its collection of data on toxic chemicals to include throughput data and pollution prevention planning is Maine. This state has also instituted mandatory reduction goals. (See Box 10-A.)

Materials Accounting Data

To fully understand or evaluate the flow of toxic chemicals within an industrial facility, a materials accounting of the amounts of toxic chemical is needed. A complete materials accounting profile at a facility includes the following, where the sum of the amounts on the left equals the sum of the amounts on the right:

Inputs	Outputs
Brought on site	Consumed
Produced on site	Shipped as or in product
Starting inventory	Ending inventory
Recycled on site	Waste (also called byproduct or nonproduct output)

Waste, called "nonproduct output" in the New Jersey program and "byproduct" in the Massachusetts program, is the amount of the toxic chemical that remains after the production process is completed — that was not used up during production (consumed), not sold as or in a product, and not put into inventory for future use. The amount of waste is reported to both TRI and New Jersey according to how it is managed; in Massachusetts, the total amount is reported. (See Box 10-B.)

The objective of materials accounting is to identify the elements of the chemical flows within a facility such that all are accounted for. When inputs equal outputs in a materials accounting, it is likely that important flows have been identified and that no major mistakes have been made in estimating their magnitude. A materials accounting of a chemical can provide perspectives on the risks at different stages of production that the uses of a toxic chemical pose, on the efficiency with which the reporting facility uses the chemical, and on the opportunities for pollution prevention.

Knowing the amounts of a chemical being brought on site and shipped in product provides insights into the possibility for storage, transfer, and transportation risks. These data also are useful in providing insights into product stewardship and in learning about toxics in commerce. The inventory amounts give perspectives on the possibility for industrial accidents and the need for precautions in storage and on-site transfers.

The condition of use of the chemical has important implications for the ease of adopting source reduction initiatives. For example, substitution for a toxic chemical produced or consumed on site is often more difficult than for one just used on site (e.g., as a solvent). Therefore, the produced and consumed on site figures, in conjunction with the other materials accounting data, provide a valuable perspective on the pollution

Box 10-A. Maine: Facility Planning and Mandatory Reductions in Releases and Transfers

Maine is another state that has initiated pollution prevention planning, process-specific reporting, and throughput data collection. Maine has also gone farther, by making *mandatory* a 30 percent reduction in releases and transfers for each facility by 1998, compared to a base year of 1990 or 1991. Interim goals are 10 percent by 1994 and 20 percent by 1995.

Mandatory pollution prevention planning took effect in 1992, and staff of Maine's Department of Environmental Protection (DEP) report that many facilities found both significant cost savings and effective opportunities for source reduction.[1] Maine facilities prepared their first revised plans in 1994. Pollution prevention plans remain at the facility, but the Maine DEP will receive plan summaries for those that fail to meet the 10 percent reduction in releases and transfers in 1994.

Maine invited reporting facilities to submit throughput data for the 1993 reporting year, and from conversations with submitters, DEP staff expected many to do so.

[1] Telephone conversation with Ann Pistell, Office of Pollution Prevention, Maine Department of Environmental Protection, August 30, 1994.

Box 10-B. Elements of Materials Accounting Reported to TRI, New Jersey, and Massachusetts

	TRI	New Jersey	Massachusetts	
Inputs				
Brought on site		✓	Processed	✓
Produced on site		✓	Manufactured	✓
Starting inventory		✓	Otherwise used	✓
Recycled on site	✓	✓		
Outputs				
Consumed		✓		
Shipped as/in product		✓	✓	
Ending inventory		✓		
Waste			✓**	
Treated on site	✓	✓		
Released on site	✓	✓	✓	
Recycled on site	✓	✓		
Energy recovery on site	✓	✓*		
Transferred off site for			✓***	
Treatment	✓	✓		
Disposal	✓	✓		
Energy recovery	✓	✓*		
Recycling	✓	✓		

* Included in "other" category until 1993.
** One total waste figure reported, called byproduct.
*** One figure for all off-site transfers.

prevention potential and progress of facilities. (See Chapter 3 for a discussion of conditions of use.)

One broad measure of efficiency compares how much of the toxic chemical input into the production process (called "use" in this report) is consumed in the process or is included in the shipped product and, therefore, does not end up as waste. The less that is generated as waste the more efficient the facility's production process is.

Facilities are required to report differently to New Jersey and Massachusetts. New Jersey collects data on use in the form of:

Use = brought on site
+ produced on site
+ recycled on site
+ starting inventory
- ending inventory

Massachusetts requires data on use in the form of:

Use = processed
+ manufactured
+ otherwise used

New Jersey included information on the use and production of each reportable chemical (called "throughput" data) in its pre-TRI survey, in order to track each chemical through the manufacturing process and thus provide facility-specific information on all of its uses at the facility. Throughput information includes:

- starting and ending inventory,
- amount of chemical brought on site,
- amount produced (manufactured),
- amount consumed during the production process,
- amount shipped off site (as or in the product), and
- amount recycled on site.

(See Figure 10-2.)

Although TRI does not include throughput information (only waste data) in its reporting requirements, New Jersey's Department of Environmental Protection (DEP) chose to continue collecting these data by using a state supplement to the federal TRI Form R.[b] (See Figure 10-4.)

The Massachusetts Department of Environmental Protection (DEP) also collects some of this information, although in a different format and not a complete materials accounting. (See Figure 10-5.) The information required includes the amounts of the chemical manufactured, processed, or otherwise used, and balances these data with the amounts of the chemical shipped as or in product and generated as byproduct.[c] What's missing for a materials accounting are the amounts brought on site, recycled, consumed, and held in inventory. (See Figure 10-3.)

[b] The additional survey was called New Jersey Community Right-to-Know Supplemental Information. Modified to include pollution prevention information, this survey is now the Pollution Prevention and Release Report, Form DEQ-114. (See Figure 10-4.)

[c] The sum of the two types of data (the left and right side of question 1.2, Figure 10-5) will often be equal. However, the reported quantities may not balance because the chemical is recycled on site, was consumed or transformed, or was held in inventory. The Massachusetts form invites facilities to explain discrepancies, although not by quantity. The quantities of these items are required by New Jersey, as part of its throughput information.

Figure 10-4.

New Jersey Materials Accounting Information, 1992

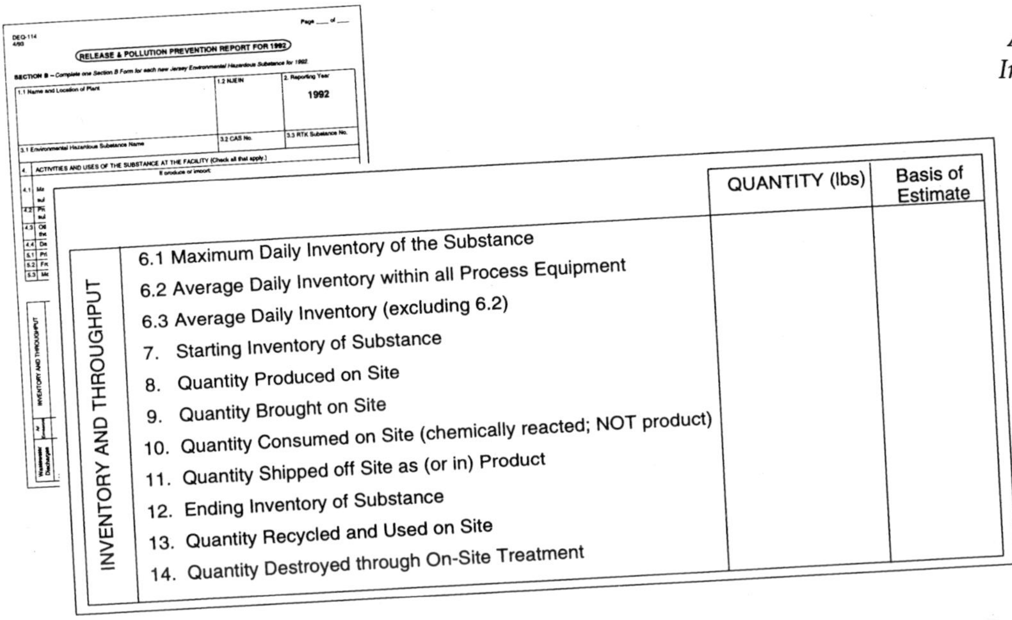
DEQ-114

RELEASE & POLLUTION PREVENTION REPORT FOR 1992

1992

INVENTORY AND THROUGHPUT	QUANTITY (lbs)	Basis of Estimate
6.1 Maximum Daily Inventory of the Substance		
6.2 Average Daily Inventory within all Process Equipment		
6.3 Average Daily Inventory (excluding 6.2)		
7. Starting Inventory of Substance		
8. Quantity Produced on Site		
9. Quantity Brought on Site		
10. Quantity Consumed on Site (chemically reacted; NOT product)		
11. Quantity Shipped off Site as (or in) Product		
12. Ending Inventory of Substance		
13. Quantity Recycled and Used on Site		
14. Quantity Destroyed through On-Site Treatment		

From New Jersey Department of Environmental Protection, Form DEQ-114

Massachusetts also requires a description of each production unit that uses the chemical and the amount (in ranges) of the chemical used. These data help explain how the chemical is used at the facility and help identify opportunities for source reduction.

Source Reduction Data

Both New Jersey and Massachusetts require facilities in the state to report on their pollution prevention planning and progress (which TRI does not).

The number of pounds of chemical waste reduced at source has been reported at the facility level to New Jersey since 1988. In addition, facilities have reported the amount of pounds of chemical waste reduced due to discontinuation of the product or export of use of the product, to further explain changes in waste from year to year. (See Figure 10-6.) New Jersey's Pollution Prevention Act of 1991[1] requires still more information from facilities on their pollution prevention progress. Facilities must begin reporting the percent of waste reduced due to source reduction activities, for both processes and the whole facility — data similar to Massachusetts', but not collected by the federal TRI.

Because New Jersey collects data on the number of pounds of chemicals in waste reduced due to source reduction or the other causes listed

Figure 10-5.

Massachusetts Materials Accounting Information, 1992, 1993

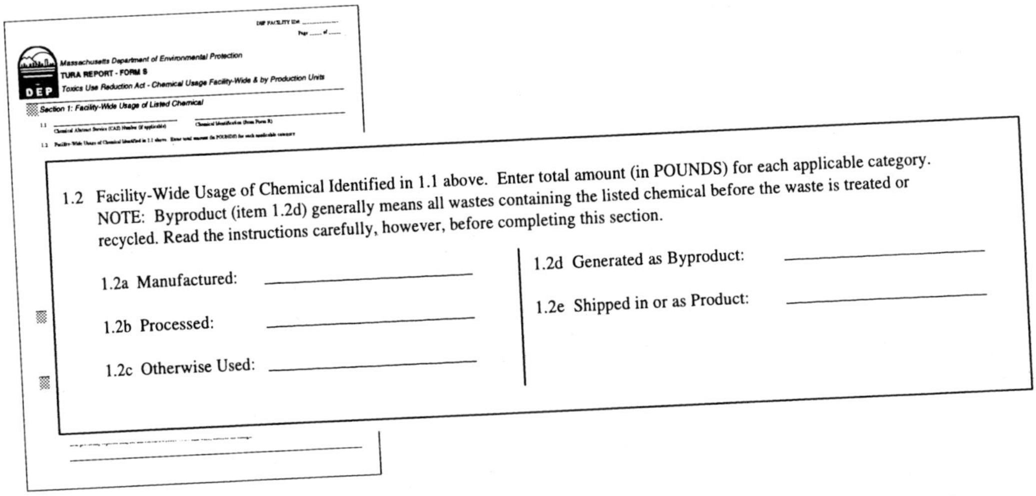
DEP FACILITY ID#: ______
Page ___ of ___

DEP

Massachusetts Department of Environmental Protection
TURA REPORT - FORM S
Toxics Use Reduction Act - Chemical Usage Facility-Wide & by Production Units

Section 1: Facility-Wide Usage of Listed Chemical

1.1 Chemical Abstract Service (CAS) Number (if applicable) ______ Chemical Identification (from Form R) ______

1.2 Facility-Wide Usage of Chemical Identified in 1.1 above. Enter total amount (in POUNDS) for each applicable category.
NOTE: Byproduct (item 1.2d) generally means all wastes containing the listed chemical before the waste is treated or recycled. Read the instructions carefully, however, before completing this section.

1.2a Manufactured: ______
1.2b Processed: ______
1.2c Otherwise Used: ______
1.2d Generated as Byproduct: ______
1.2e Shipped in or as Product: ______

From Massachusetts Department of Environmental Protection, Form S

above, the state can directly measure facility successes and failures in source reduction. Both TRI and Massachusetts require a facility to report *whether* it is undertaking any source reduction activities, but not the amounts associated with those activities. Forty-four percent of Massachusetts facilities reported source reduction activities in 1992 (as did 36 percent of TRI facilities nationally). The New Jersey data show, however, that, when facilities have had to quantify the amounts of waste reduction achieved through source reduction, no appreciable amount of source reduction is occurring.

The Massachusetts system includes information on source reduction activities[d] that is more detailed than TRI. When Massachusetts facilities report on source reduction activities, they must calculate for each production unit two numbers representing the percentage change per unit of product in the waste they generate and in releases and transfers, which indicates the progress being made in reducing waste and releases and transfers due to source reduction. They also must report the source reduction techniques used to achieve these results.

[d] Massachusetts uses the term "toxics use reduction" to denote the types of activities that are included in the term "source reduction" in this report.

Figure 10-6.

New Jersey Pollution Prevention Information, 1992

24. Has any pollution prevention method been employed to reduce the quantity of this Substance during 1992 relative to 1991 levels? Yes ☐ No ☐ If "Yes," fill in the table below:

POLLUTION PREVENTION METHODOLOGY (Complete all appropriate sections)	Quantity of Substance Reduced (lbs) (1991 to 1992)	Basis of Estimate
24.1 Material-Related Change (changes in the amount of Substance used due to substitution of other substance)		

Name and Quantity of Substitute Substance

CAS NUMBER	SUBSTANCE	QUANTITY (lbs.)
a)		
b)		
c)		

	Quantity of Substance Reduced (pounds) (1991 to 1992)	Basis of Estimate
24.2 Reformulation or Redesign of Product (resulting in the reduction of Substance generated)		
24.3 Process or Procedure Modiifications (using existing equipment to reduce Substance generated)		
24.4 Equipment or Technology Modifications (using new equipment or technology to reduce Substance generated)		
24.5 Improved Operations (due to housekeeping, training, material handling or inventory control to reduce Substance generated)		
24.6 Discontinuance of Operations, excluding operations transferred to or undertaken by another facility		
24.7 Export of Use		
24.8 Miscellaneous		

25. Does your facility anticipate reducing the generation of the Substance (as a waste) in the future due to pollution prevention? Yes ☐ No ☐ If "Yes," indicate your projections in the table below:

PROJECTION	YEAR	
	1994	1997
Quantity of Substance Reduced per Year due to Pollution Prevention (pounds)		

From New Jersey Department of Environmental Protection, Form DEQ-114

Massachusetts data do not reveal how much waste was reduced through source reduction at the production unit or facility level because only a percent reduction is reported. To know the amount of source reduction achieved, it would be necessary to know how much waste was generated from that production unit during the base year to which the percent change applies. However, the amount of waste is only reported on a facility-wide basis not a production-unit basis, and the base year may be before 1990 when waste reporting became mandatory. These data, however, do indicate where source reduction activities have and have not been undertaken and, therefore possibly, where source reduction opportunities still lie. They enable comparisons of source reduction activity among facilities where the conditions of use of a chemical are the same, even if the facilities themselves manufacture different products.

Pollution Prevention Planning and Progress Reporting

Beyond reporting the types of source reduction activities a facility has implemented and, as a result, how much waste was reduced (in New Jersey) or what percent of waste per unit of product from a production unit was reduced (in Massachusetts), both states require their facilities to prepare pollution prevention plans. The facilities must look at each of their processes or products and identify changes that can lead to either reductions in use of the chemical per unit of product manufactured or reductions in waste of the chemical per unit of product manufactured.

New Jersey requires its facilities to provide:

- a five-year pollution prevention goal, with explanations of the facility's progress and, if appropriate, of why pollution prevention is less than anticipated, and
- a description of process-level pollution prevention techniques planned for the coming year.

New Jersey facilities filed their first pollution prevention plan summaries in July 1994. Five industries were required to submit these summaries: Paper (SIC code 26), Chemicals (28), Plastics (30), Primary Metals (33), and Fabricated Metals (34). Other industries will have to file plan summaries for the first time on July 1, 1996.

The Massachusetts DEP, under its Toxics Use Reduction Act (TURA), also requires toxics use reduction planning. Facilities must provide:

- an inventory of chemicals flowing in and out of each production unit;
- a toxics use reduction plan for each production unit;
- a projection of the percentage reduction in waste (byproduct) per unit of product for each chemical from each production unit expected over the next two and five years;.
- similar two- and five-year projections of percentage reduction in use; and

- the techniques they will apply to achieve these reductions.

Both the New Jersey[2] and the Massachusetts[3] state environmental departments consider these planning requirements as tools for "self-help" pollution prevention, because facilities that work though such a planning process will discover opportunities to reduce waste and use of toxic chemicals. The process is intended to help facilities identify more efficient production methods that will both prevent pollution and save money, while enabling the public to track the progress facilities are making. It can also help the states identify facilities that have not implemented source reduction efforts for chemicals and particular uses of chemicals that other facilities are reporting success in reducing.

Both New Jersey's and Massachusetts' planning requirements are too new to evaluate their impacts. These will be covered in a future *Toxics Watch* report.

Additional Chemicals

New Jersey requires reporting on the same list of chemicals as the federal TRI, which includes 316 chemicals and 20 chemical categories for 1992. Massachusetts requires broader reporting — in addition to the TRI chemicals, facilities in the state must report on all chemicals specified as hazardous substances under the Comprehensive Environmental Response, Compensation, and Liability Act of 1980 (CERCLA). This adds about 550 more chemicals to the reporting list. Massachusetts phased in the CERCLA chemicals over a three-year period (reporting years 1991-1993).[e]

Not all TRI or CERCLA chemicals appear in reports submitted by facilities in these two states, presumably because some chemicals are not used over the threshold amount by any of the reporting facilities. New Jersey facilities reported using 189 TRI chemicals in 1992, and the Massachusetts database includes forms on 117 TRI chemicals and 42 non-TRI chemicals for that reporting year.

Additional Industries

Massachusetts, unlike New Jersey and TRI, collects data from some non-manufacturing industries. Starting with reporting year 1992, TURA requires reporting, in addition to manufacturing SIC codes 20 through 39, by facilities in the following categories:

- Mining (SIC codes 10-14);
- certain industries in Transportation, Communications, Electric, Gas, and Sanitary Services (40, 44-49);
- Wholesale Trade (50-51); and
- selected Services, specifically Personal Services (72), such as dry cleaners and beauty shops, Business Services (73), Automotive Repair and Services, (75), and Miscellaneous Repair Services (76).

[e] U.S. EPA has added 286 chemicals to the federal TRI list, to be reported for the year 1995 and beyond, which include some chemicals already on the Massachusetts list. (See Appendix C.)

In 1994 EPA announced a pre-proposal to expand TRI industry coverage. EPA's initial review similarly identified Mining (SIC codes 10-14), a number of Transportation and related industries (40, 42, 46, 49), Wholesale Trade (50-51), and others.[4] If such an expansion is put into regulations, it will not apply before the 1996 reporting year.

Unlike TRI, Massachusetts requires facilities with *any* business activity in one of the covered SIC codes to report. TRI limits reporting to facilities with more than 50 percent of their business in manufacturing (SIC codes 20-39).

Usefulness of Expanded Databases

With chemical use data, such as is collected in Massachusetts, it is possible to see how facilities produce very different amounts of waste and releases and transfers with the same amount of the chemical used. For example, two polystyrene manufacturers in Massachusetts reported the same amount of releases and transfers of styrene, but one reported twice as much use of the chemical as the other. Thus, if only TRI data on releases and transfers were available, these two facilities would appear to be the same. However, with the expanded data a great difference in their use is evident.

With the full picture of throughput data as reported in New Jersey, however, it is possible to go further. Because New Jersey facilities must also report how much of each chemical is brought on site, how much is consumed in the manufacturing process, and how much of the waste is reduced through source reduction efforts, further possible differences in the facilities emerge.

New Jersey facilities using large amounts of reportable chemicals report relatively smaller percentages of waste generated and very little source reduction accomplished. The facilities with smaller use of the chemicals report relatively higher amounts of waste generated and more source reduction. With New Jersey's chemical use data, the two types of facilities can be distinguished and their efforts recognized. Without the use data, the patterns of the larger facilities overwhelm the data.

Both Massachusetts and New Jersey also require facilities to report how much of a toxic chemical goes into the products shipped off site by the facility, unlike TRI. This additional data allow analyses of how different types of facilities use and release toxic chemicals, how much of the chemical is in the products manufactured and in waste, and how that might affect the opportunities for source reduction.

The additional data that New Jersey requires (noted above) reveal a much more detailed picture of the reasons for changes from year to year. New Jersey requires facilities to report on:

- the amount of waste reduced due to source reduction activities,
- the amount of change due to discontinuation of use or export of the use to another facility, and
- changes in production level.

Such information not only helps explain the performance of a specific facility, but also permits the grouping of facilities to detect patterns of change (e.g., to determine whether facilities reporting increases in production level have corresponding increases in waste generation, compared to facilities reporting no change or decreases in production). In the same vein, Massachusetts data allow grouping of the different uses of chemicals at different facilities, by means of production unit descriptions, and comparisons of whether or not source reduction has taken place and what percentage changes have occurred at the production-unit level.

Aside from the opportunities that these expanded toxics reporting systems present for conducting more useful statewide analyses of what is happening to toxics in waste, the reporting facilities themselves may benefit. Having to report detailed use information, quantities of source reduction, and materials accounting information may in time lead to environmental, technological, and economic benefits at the facility level. It is too early to tell whether this will in fact occur. Environmental groups and industry and governmental officials will no doubt be observing closely whether any significant differences can be discerned between facilities that are and are not included under expanded reporting systems.

Toxic Chemical Profile for New Jersey, 1992

The magnitude and complexity of chemical use and chemical waste[f] in New Jersey make the additional data the New Jersey DEP collects particularly useful. In 1992 a total of 751 New Jersey facilities submitted forms to TRI, reporting a total of 212.9 million pounds of releases and transfers. The state ranked 12th (among 53 states and other TRI reporting jurisdictions) for total releases and transfers. For total transfers off site, however, the state ranked eighth. Off-site transfers totaled 191.4 million pounds or 90 percent of New Jersey's total releases and transfers, whereas off-site transfers represented 56 percent of total releases and transfers for the nation as a whole.

In the same year, 686 facilities submitted 2,515 forms for 189 chemicals to New Jersey's Right-to-Know Program. This is 65 fewer facilities than reported to TRI; they reported 159.5 million pounds of total releases and transfers to the 1992 New Jersey database.[g] This latter database, created by the state, is used for the remaining New Jersey data analyses in this chapter.

[f] "Use" and "waste" as used in this chapter in regard to New Jersey data are calculated from separate numbers reported on the New Jersey form. Use is calculated as the starting inventory of a chemical, minus the ending inventory, plus the amount produced, plus the amount brought on site, plus the amount recycled on-site. Waste is calculated as use minus amount consumed in the production process minus amount shipped as product or contained in product, but it can also be calculated as amounts treated, released, transferred and recycled on site. While the components are reported, the reporters are not required to add the numbers and identify inconsistencies. The data as given in this chapter are as reported to New Jersey by the facility and may not always add exactly. For specific examples, see Figures 10-7 through 10-13, which examine chemical flow through facilities.

[g] The New Jersey data for 1992 were obtained from the New Jersey Department of Environmental Protection in August 1994. The federal TRI data are from the public data release in April 1994. The reporting base is the same, and discrepancies come about because of the different times the data were obtained.

New Jersey Use, Waste Generated, and Releases and Transfers

Releases and transfers of toxic chemicals in waste was the original emphasis of federal analyses of TRI data and is a subject of continued primary interest. Clearly, the amount of chemicals that a facility releases directly to the environment or transfers to another facility, whether across the street or across state boundaries, is of great importance in assessing the potential for harmful ecological and health effects.

In 1991 TRI added items to be reported concerning the *waste generated;* it also required reporting on *source reduction* activities, though not on the amount of waste reduced due to those activities. This additional federally mandated data collection did not result in any further changes to New Jersey required reporting.

Releases and transfers are often an order of magnitude or more smaller than uses of the same chemical. In 1992, for example, 686 New Jersey facilities reported releases and transfers of 159.5 million pounds of 189 toxic chemicals. The facilities reported that these releases and transfers resulted from 6.7 billion pounds of waste and 20.0 billion pounds of use of toxic chemicals. Thus, on average, one-third of the amount of toxic chemicals used in New Jersey ends up as waste, and the releases and transfers represent less than 1 percent of the actual amount of toxic chemicals used in the state. This means on the one hand that little of the toxic chemicals present at manufacturing facilities is lost to the environment. On the other hand, it implies that there may be significant risks at facilities and in commerce that are not at all reflected in industrial toxics release and transfer data presentations. (See Table 10-1.)

Toxic Chemicals in Products, New Jersey

Reporting to New Jersey also includes how much of the toxic chemical is shipped off site in the products manufactured at the facility. These data are of growing importance as concerns grow about the risks of toxics in products, in use, when recycled, or when disposed of. Overall, New Jersey data show that over half (54 percent) of the chemicals used as inputs to the manufacturing process goes into product that is shipped off site. (See Table 10-1.) This is much more than the amount consumed during the manufacturing process (14 percent) and much more than the amount left in waste (34 percent).

The New Jersey data also show that the industries that ship the largest percentage of their use of toxic chemicals in products are Lumber (SIC 24) and Primary Metals (SIC 33). Many primary metals are on the toxic chemical list, so that their products would be counted as "shipped as product." The report of the lumber company, Atlantic Wood Industries in Savannah, New Jersey, states that 6.8 of the 7.6 million pounds of toxic chemicals it uses are shipped off site in product. The company reports shipping lumber treated with creosote, a wood preservative. (See Table 10-2.)

Table 10-1. Materials Accounting and Source Reduction Data, New Jersey, 1992

	1992 Number		
Facilities	686		
Forms	2,515		
	Pounds	**Percent of Use** Percent	**Percent of Waste** Percent
Inputs			
Use *	20,034,716,490		
Net Inventory	-53,156,979		
Starting Inventory	913,428,894		
Ending Inventory	966,585,873		
Produced On site	10,380,497,232		
Brought On site	9,472,156,885		
Recycled On site	234,774,996		
Outputs			
Consumed	2,798,344,099	13.97	
Shipped as/in Product	10,732,269,042	53.57	
Waste *	6,726,089,975	33.57	
Destroyed through Treatment	176,020,369		
Release and Transfer Data			
Total Releases and Transfers	159,527,216	0.80	2.37
Total Releases	19,099,459		
Total Air Emissions	18,789,771		
Surface Water Discharges	193,644		
Land Releases	115,437		
Groundwater Discharges	607		
Total Transfers	140,427,757		
Transfers to POTWs	45,326,325		
Off-site Transfers by Mgt. Technique			
Incineration	13,679,853		
Water Treatment	0		
Groundwater Disposal	54,986		
Land Disposal	2,174,644		
Recycled	59,175,136		
Other	20,016,813		
Data on Reduction in Waste			
Quantity of Source Reduction	4,969,849		
Reformulation of Product	1,216,191		
Process Modifications	1,304,985		
Technology/Equipment Modifications	518,418		
Improved Operations	1,930,255		
Discontinued Operations	108,273,514		
Export of Use	77,106		
Miscellaneous Decreases	1,550,926		
Projected Reduction in Two Years	77,908,892		
Projected Reduction in Five Years	24,915,207		

* For individual forms, if the calculation of use or waste resulted in a negative number, then the value was set to zero. Therefore, "Use" is not exactly equal to net inventory + produced + brought on site + recycled, and" Waste" is not exactly equal to use - consumed - shipped + recycled on site.

Table 10-2. Use, Chemicals in Product, and Chemicals in Waste by Industry, New Jersey, 1992

SIC Code	Industry	Use Pounds	Shipped as/ in Product Pounds	Percent of Use Percent	Waste Pounds	Percent of Use Percent
20	Food	11,318,879	1,348,054	11.91	3,503,370	30.95
22	Textiles	1,477,479	64,661	4.38	1,171,705	79.30
24	Lumber	8,680,675	7,649,129	88.12	100,748	1.16
25	Furniture	67,035	0	0.00	67,035	100.00
26	Paper	14,106,775	1,706,002	12.09	11,154,552	79.07
27	Printing	1,017,461	16,223	1.59	997,272	98.02
28	Chemicals	4,345,778,445	1,804,313,025	41.52	359,324,162	8.27
29	Petroleum	14,987,836,225	8,433,511,934	56.27	6,271,258,822	41.84
30	Plastics	88,576,081	46,389,166	52.37	11,235,096	12.68
31	Leather	2,415,319	193,598	8.02	974,671	40.35
32	Stone/Clay	7,301,570	1,950,643	26.72	2,080,215	28.49
33	Primary Metals	352,486,503	291,138,893	82.60	29,668,275	8.42
34	Fabr. Metals	44,066,029	27,242,523	61.82	16,908,321	38.37
35	Machinery	16,589,367	13,259,072	79.93	2,663,117	16.05
36	Electrical	111,024,240	75,660,237	68.15	4,622,145	4.16
37	Transportation	7,830,164	4,154,457	53.06	2,722,262	34.77
38	Measure./Photo.	11,222,800	7,144,316	63.66	2,497,075	22.25
39	Miscellaneous	22,587,672	16,405,494	72.63	5,099,863	22.58
50	Wholesale, durable	193,732	0	0.00	22,751	11.74
51	Wholesale, non-durable	140,039	121,615	86.84	18,518	13.22
	Total	20,034,716,490	10,732,269,042	53.57	6,726,089,975	33.57

While the 25 chemicals with the largest reported use have a similar overall percentage shipped as product as do the total of all chemicals, several chemicals have a larger percent. For example, methyl tert-butyl ether has 89 percent of its use shipped in products, all of which is reported by Petroleum industry facilities as a formulation component in their refined oil products. The Exxon Company's chemical plant in Linden, New Jersey, manufactures naphthalene, all of which is shipped as product. (See Table 10-3.)

New Jersey Chemicals

The identity of the "top" chemicals differs for use, waste generation, and releases and transfers. For example, although methanol ("wood alcohol") was the chemical with the largest releases and transfers (37.7 million pounds) in New Jersey in 1992, toluene led in use (4.6 billion pounds) and amount of waste generated (2.3 billion pounds). Toluene is not only toxic, but also flammable, so large amounts of its use raise the need for industrial precautions to avoid not only spills, but also fires and explosions. (See Table 10-3.)

The 25 chemicals with the largest reported use accounted for 94 percent of New Jersey's total use and 98 percent of total waste generated, but 64 percent of total releases and transfers. Of the five chemicals with the largest total releases and transfers — methanol (37.7 million pounds), sulfuric acid (24.5 million pounds), toluene (11.3 million pounds), ammonium sulfate (9.2 million pounds), and acetone (9.1 million pounds) — only the first three appear on the list of top 25 for total use. (See Table 10-3.)

The chemical with the greatest use in New Jersey, toluene, is also generated as waste in the highest amount (at a rate of 51 percent of its use) and released or transferred in amounts behind only methanol and sulfuric acid. On the other hand, methanol has the highest amount of releases and transfers, but ranks 21st for total use. This occurs because a large proportion of the use and waste generated of methanol is subsequently released or transferred. In New Jersey, chemical companies use methanol as a solvent or processing aid in their manufacture of other chemicals. Used in this way, none of the methanol ends up in the product or transformed, and relatively large amounts of the chemical used are then generated as waste. The amount of methanol generated as waste is 41 percent of the amount of the chemical used, and the amount of methanol released or transferred is 25 percent of the use and 61 percent of the waste generated.

New Jersey facilities must report the amount of waste that is not generated, as the result of source reduction activities. Only 100 facilities out of 682 (15 percent) reported any source reduction quantities in 1992. Furthermore, the total amount they reported was 5.0 million pounds, a very small amount of source reduction in relation to the waste generated — only a 0.07 percent reduction in waste due to source reduction. With many studies demonstrating that industrial toxic wastes can be reduced significantly, this showing is discouraging. (See Table 10-3.)

The 25 chemicals used in the largest amounts in New Jersey (constituting 94 percent of chemical use) accounted for a smaller percentage (69 percent) of the amount of source reduction reported. Individual chemicals show wide variation in the amount of source reduction reported. For example, New Jersey facilities reported 547,000 pounds of source reduction for toluene (the chemical with the largest amounts of use and waste generation) and 324,000 pounds for methanol (the chemical with the largest amounts of releases and transfers). Because of the lower use and related waste generation associated with methanol compared to toluene, source reduction for methanol is at a rate 26 times greater in relation to waste generated for methanol than for toluene, a source reduction of 0.5 percent of waste generated for methanol, compared to 0.02 percent for toluene.

Table 10-3. Use, Waste, and Releases and Transfers by Chemical, New Jersey, 1992: The 25 Chemicals with Largest Use

Use Rank	Waste Rank	Releases and Transfers Rank	Chemical	Use Pounds	Shipped as/in Product Pounds	Shipped as Percentage of Use Percent
1	1	3	Toluene	4,557,756,909	2,166,263,123	47.53
2	2	8	Xylene (mixed isomers)	4,456,813,396	2,399,341,332	53.84
3	9	2	Sulfuric acid	1,085,470,070	792,940,092	73.05
4	3	26	Ethylbenzene	996,399,791	496,999,971	49.88
5	22	53	Propylene	957,987,958	519,820,400	54.26
6	8	46	Methyl tert-butyl ether	906,649,503	811,000,043	89.45
7	5	49	1,2,4-Trimethylbenzene	903,697,986	566,237,947	62.66
8	6	31	Benzene	839,443,394	503,500,072	59.98
9	4	35	tert-Butyl alcohol	588,726,575	222,593,480	37.81
10	49	64	Vinyl chloride	415,352,129	890	0.00
11	14	21	Nitric acid	354,084,755	183,710,560	51.88
12	7	37	Cumene	350,905,593	164,357,617	46.84
13	11	55	Cyclohexane	297,880,204	148,585,103	49.88
14	15	6	Copper	292,703,342	250,752,816	85.67
15	65	43	Vinyl acetate	209,192,432	83,032,962	39.69
16	38	74	Ethylene	208,440,462	83,152,700	39.89
17	21	12	Ammonia	202,726,689	100,258,469	49.45
18	12	36	Hydrochloric acid	183,511,737	84,295,740	45.93
19	74	72	Naphthalene	171,650,683	172,123,692	100.28
20	19	71	Chlorine	166,654,915	13,101,338	7.86
21	10	1	Methanol	152,639,614	35,173,070	23.04
22	30	14	Ethylene glycol	144,315,348	134,867,992	93.45
23	28	10	Lead compounds	115,804,210	81,584,684	70.45
24	70	87	Phthalic anhydride	109,558,563	67,500	0.06
25	25	28	Butyl benzyl phthalate	104,778,849	99,425,254	94.89
			Subtotal	18,773,145,107	10,113,186,847	53.87
			Percent of Total	93.70	94.23	
			Total	20,034,716,490	10,732,269,042	53.57

Waste Pounds	**Waste as Percent-age of Use** Percent	**Total Releases and Transfers** Pounds	**Releases and Transfers as Percent-age of Use** Percent	**Source Reduction Quantity** Pounds
2,323,397,324	50.98	11,261,602	0.25	547,434
2,202,520,951	49.42	5,468,684	0.12	515,685
92,792,282	8.55	24,453,199	2.25	32,090
498,509,328	50.03	700,892	0.07	36,563
6,300,593	0.66	154,014	0.02	0
95,645,274	10.55	205,354	0.02	0
341,021,221	37.74	189,424	0.02	693
261,314,044	31.13	348,098	0.04	105,200
366,036,116	62.17	332,789	0.06	0
796,469	0.19	71,613	0.02	1,100
25,490,013	7.20	1,129,337	0.32	0
156,799,075	44.68	302,678	0.09	2,130
59,532,411	19.99	122,778	0.04	230
13,512,887	4.62	7,484,522	2.56	1,232,918
298,940	0.14	231,771	0.11	0
1,365,231	0.65	47,667	0.02	0
6,531,369	3.22	3,453,705	1.70	218,985
57,702,989	31.44	315,754	0.17	162,905
144,867	0.08	53,134	0.03	40
8,255,215	4.95	55,837	0.03	50,000
61,933,009	40.57	37,716,237	24.71	323,662
2,351,888	1.63	2,699,043	1.87	80,000
3,860,359	3.33	4,226,629	3.65	103,339
219,695	0.20	27,521	0.03	3,015
4,045,595	3.86	451,289	0.43	310
6,590,377,145	35.11	101,503,571	0.54	3,416,299
97.98		63.63		68.74
6,726,089,975	33.57	159,527,216	0.80	4,969,849

Use, Waste, and Releases/Transfers of New Jersey Chemicals of Special Concern

Overall the percentage of toxic chemicals used that ends up as waste in New Jersey is 34 percent. For certain chemical classes of concern, the halo-organics, and other special groups of chemicals based on potential health and environmental effects — carcinogens, ozone depleters, and chloro-organics — however, this percentage is smaller, ranging from 17 percent for carcinogens to 2 percent for halo-organics and chloro-organics. For the class of metals and their compounds, the amount of waste as a percentage of use is 7 percent, and for ozone depleters, it is 3 percent. (See Table 10-4.)

The percentage of use ending up as releases and transfers is relatively low for the carcinogens, as it is for all the toxic chemicals, while the metals group is much higher at 4 percent because metals are sent off-site for recycling in larger amounts. Releases and transfers are 3 percent of use for ozone depleters, primarily because of their volatility, which leads to relatively large amounts of air emissions. Releases and transfers as a percent of waste range from 97 percent for the volatile ozone depleters to 3 percent for carcinogens, or just a little higher than that for all toxic chemicals. Releases and transfers of chloro-organics and halo-organics as a percent of waste is 79 percent, with the largest proportion being sent off-site for recycling. (See Table 10-4.)

Source Reduction of New Jersey Chemicals of Special Concern

Carcinogens

New Jersey facilities reported little progress in reducing carcinogenic wastes by source reduction activities. As for all of the toxic chemicals, source reduction of carcinogens reduced the amount of total waste generated by only about 0.1 percent. (See Table 10-4.) The best efforts at source reduction of carcinogens were modest, and some of the facilities shown to be releasing the most carcinogens reported *no* source reduction.

While 92 percent of all forms for carcinogens (these forms representing 93 percent of the total releases and transfers of carcinogens) had no report of source reduction, Sybron Chemicals, Inc. (SIC 28) in Birmingham reported the largest amount of source reduction, 104,000 pounds of styrene waste reduced by process modifications. The facility's total waste generation in 1992 was 12,000 pounds. The New Jersey facility reporting the largest single amount of releases and transfers of a carcinogen in 1992, Merck & Company in Rahway, a pharmaceutical facility (SIC 28), reported using 1.3 million pounds of dichloromethane and releasing and transferring all of that amount, with no source reduction.

Ozone Depleters

For ozone-depleting chemicals, which are being phased out under various deadlines mandated by the Clean Air Act and the Montreal

Table 10-4. Use, Waste, and Releases and Transfers by Chemical Groups, New Jersey, 1992

	Total TRI Chemicals	Carcinogens	Ozone Depleters	Chloro-Organics	Metals	Halo-Organics
Number of Forms	2,515	327	131	233	469	241
	Pounds	Pounds	Pounds	Pounds	Pounds	Pounds
Inputs						
Use *	20,034,716,490	1,684,932,166	124,179,299	716,983,600	588,037,396	719,274,635
Net Inventory	-53,156,979	-14,531,794	2,656,057	2,951,342	33,845,977	3,984,641
Starting Inventory	913,428,894	77,042,880	7,728,307	22,012,755	84,502,140	23,735,305
Ending Inventory	966,585,873	91,574,674	5,072,250	19,061,413	50,656,163	19,750,664
Produced on Site	10,380,497,232	714,023,876	11,212,718	122,518,892	73,695,925	122,518,892
Brought on Site	9,472,156,885	975,791,497	110,008,122	588,948,804	355,984,588	590,205,448
Recycled on Site	234,774,996	9,648,587	302,402	2,564,562	124,163,650	2,565,654
Outputs						
Consumed	2,798,344,099	718,776,419	48,775,431	587,230,511	67,209,701	587,231,425
Shipped as/in Product	10,732,269,042	694,622,711	71,571,546	115,600,537	521,307,300	117,774,159
Shipped as Percent of Use	53.57	41.23	57.64	16.12	88.65	16.37
Waste *	6,726,089,975	280,109,749	3,835,893	14,992,792	39,510,035	15,113,475
Waste as Percent of Use	33.57	16.62	3.09	2.09	6.72	2.10
Destroyed through Treatment	176,020,369	1,942,692	27,925	1,524,360	1,937,080	1,524,360
Release and Transfer Data						
Total Releases and Transfers	159,527,216	7,537,823	3,730,755	11,872,623	24,303,916	11,923,854
Total Releases	19,099,459	1,354,217	1,919,333	3,362,940	409,369	3,379,652
Total Air Emissions	18,789,771	1,342,751	1,918,376	3,353,348	286,987	3,370,023
Surface Water Discharges	193,644	6,607	957	3,123	16,127	3,156
Land Releases	115,437	4,853	0	6,469	106,227	6,469
Groundwater Discharges	607	6	0	0	28	4
Total Transfers	140,427,757	6,183,606	1,811,422	8,509,683	23,894,547	8,544,202
Transfers to POTWs	45,326,325	538,842	20,788	390,331	1,294,955	390,331
Off-site Transfers by Mgt. Technique						
Incineration	13,679,853	390,591	338,895	1,200,527	246,804	1,200,527
Water Treatment	0	0	0	0	0	0
Groundwater Disposal	54,986	0	0	0	8,000	0
Land Disposal	2,174,644	188,060	589	1,744	1,497,112	36,262
Recycled	59,175,136	4,497,942	1,281,217	5,655,972	20,228,654	5,655,973
Other	20,016,813	568,171	169,933	1,261,109	619,022	1,261,109
Releases/Transfers as Percent of Use	0.80	0.45	3.00	1.66	4.13	1.66
Releases/Transfers as Percent of Waste	2.37	2.69	97.26	79.19	61.51	78.90
Data on Reduction in Waste						
Quantity of Source Reduction	4,969,849	388,911	92,695	495,497	1,415,430	495,637
Reformulation of Product	1,216,191	131,484	764	44,971	137,650	44,971
Process Modifications	1,304,985	243,040	17,609	211,644	26,497	211,784
Technology/Equip. Modif.	518,418	324	20,700	22,890	13	22,890
Improved Operations	1,930,255	14,063	53,622	215,992	1,251,270	215,992
Source Reduction as Percent of Waste **	0.07	0.14	2.36	3.20	3.46	3.18
Discontinued Operations	108,273,514	4,402,572	11,242,728	15,895,804	78,002,978	15,912,524
Export of Use	77,106	0	44,106	44,106	0	44,106
Miscellaneous Decreases	1,550,926	327,747	161,800	261,800	665,923	261,800
Projected Reduction in Two Years	77,908,892	2,383,295	16,413,607	18,526,294	7,137,834	18,685,874
Projected Reduction in Five Years	24,915,207	2,840,683	383,315	2,384,849	2,611,120	2,656,899

* For individual forms, if the calculation of use or waste resulted in a negative number, then the value was set to zero. Therefore, "Use" is not exactly equal to net inventory + produced + brought on site + recycled, and "Waste" is not exactly equal to use - consumed - shipped + recycled on site.

** Percent source reduction is the percent of waste that would have been generated, i.e., source reduction amount divided by the sum of waste plus source reduction amount.

Protocol, facilities reported total source reduction of only 2 percent of waste generated. Allied-Signal Aerospace in Teterboro (SIC 38), which manufactures navigation instruments, reported the largest amount of source reduction for an ozone-depleting chemical. It reported using and generating as waste 29,000 pounds of 1,1,1-trichloroethane, but having reduced the amount almost in half from the previous year by improved operations during 1992.

The DuPont facility in Deepwater, a chemical manufacturer (SIC 28), reported the largest amount of waste and releases and transfers of ozone-depleting chemicals. It reported releasing 298,000 pounds of such chemicals to the air and sending an additional 565,000 pounds off site for recycling, but reported no source reduction activity in relation to these chemicals. (See section on Portraits of Individual Facilities below.)

Chloro-organics

New Jersey facilities achieved source reduction of chloro-organics of 3 percent. The DuPont facility in Deepwater reported the largest amount of releases and transfers of a chloro-organic, but also the largest amount of source reduction, though the amount was 10 percent of its off-site transfers in 1992. This facility reported using 13.9 million pounds of 1,2-dichlorobenzene and transferring 1.5 million pounds of the resulting waste off site, of which one-third was destined for incineration and two-thirds for recycling. It reported 150,000 pounds of source reduction for the chemical through process modifications.

Metals

New Jersey facilities reported amounts of source reduction of metals equal to 3 percent of waste. Almost all of this, however, is attributable to one facility: the Phelps Dodge Specialty Copper facility (SIC 33) in Elizabeth, which reported 1.2 million pounds of source reduction of copper, amounting to a 30 percent reduction of its waste from the previous year. It still reported 2.8 million pounds of releases and transfers of copper in 1992.

Halo-organics

New Jersey facilities achieved source reduction of halo-organics of 3 percent. The facility with the largest amount of releases and transfers and source reduction was the DuPont Deepwater facility, as noted above for chloro-organics since 1,2-dichlorobenzene is also a halo-organic. The Frigidaire Company (SIC 35) in Edison, New Jersey, achieved the second largest amount of source reduction, 120,984 pounds of trichloroethylene. This represents a decrease in waste of 55 percent from 1991.

New Jersey Facilities

Individual facilities account for much of the patterns in use, waste, and releases and transfers of toxic chemicals in New Jersey, as they do for the nation as a whole. Four Petroleum industry (SIC 29) facilities in New Jersey each reported the use of more than 1 billion pounds of toxic chemicals: Coastal Eagle Point Oil Company in Westville, Exxon Company in Linden, Mobil Oil Company in Paulsboro, and Shell

Oil Company in Sewaren. The first three facilities are petroleum refineries, and the fourth stores and distributes petroleum products. Those four facilities (0.6 percent of total reporting facilities) used 14.7 billion pounds of toxic chemicals, which represents 74 percent of the total use for all New Jersey facilities. Of these four, only the Exxon facility reported any source reduction, and that amounted to only 15,000 pounds out of 52.1 million pounds of waste generated. (See Table 10-5. Also see Box 10-C for more information about unusual aspects of the data from Coastal Eagle Point Company.)

The Coastal Eagle Point Oil Company and Exxon Company facilities also ranked first and third, respectively, for amount of waste generated. The DuPont Company (SIC 28) in Deepwater ranked second for waste generated, with 57.7 million pounds of waste generated, which is 15 percent of its reported 379.1 million pounds of toxic chemicals used.

Sybron Chemicals in Birmingham (SIC 28), producer of specialty chemicals, led in releases and transfers, with 19.3 million pounds. This amount represented 85 percent of its 22.7 million pounds of waste generated and 38 percent of its total use of 50.5 million pounds. Merck & Company in Rahway reported the second largest amount of releases and transfers with 9.8 million pounds, which is 87 percent of its 11.3 million pounds of waste generated and 39 percent of its 25.1 million pounds of total use. Both of these facilities reported quantities of source reduction achieved, for a total of 734,000 pounds. For the Merck facility, source reduction amounted to 5.6 percent of its waste generation in 1992; for Sybron the percentage is 0.5 percent.

Box 10-C. Coastal Eagle Point Oil Company Facility

One facility, Coastal Eagle Point Oil Company in Westville, reported very different amounts of toxic chemical use in 1991 and 1992. This facility reported the largest amount of use in 1992 of any New Jersey facility, having increased its use from 1991 to 1992 by 10 times, from 835.5 million pounds to 8.3 billion pounds. Its waste increased from 19.8 million to 6.2 billion pounds. This single facility therefore represents 42 percent of all use and 94 percent of all waste reported by New Jersey facilities in 1992. Despite the huge variation in use and waste, the releases and transfers reported were at about the same level for the two years.

Although overall production levels remained the same, the facility produced different products in the two years. The facility explained that such a large variation is possible because the midpoint ranges from corporate Material Safety Data Sheets are used to estimate use, assays are not performed, and product composition and formulations change from year to year.

The picture of changes for all New Jersey facilities is much clearer without this one facility. Any depiction of change in use that includes the Coastal Eagle Point Oil facility will reflect only that facility's change and not changes of other facilities because it is such a large portion of the total numbers. The discussion in this chapter of changes from 1991 to 1992 therefore makes comparisons based on the New Jersey data without the Coastal Eagle Point Oil Company's 1991 and 1992 data, as do the related tables.

Table 10-5. Top 10 Facilities for Use, Waste, and Releases and Transfers, New Jersey, 1992

Use Rank	Waste Rank	Releases and Transfers Rank	Facility	City	County
Facilities with Largest Use					
1	1	80	Coastal Eagle Point Oil Co	Westville	Gloucester
2	3	67	Exxon Company USA	Linden	Union
3	166	171	Mobil Oil Corporation	Paulsboro	Gloucester
4	118	89	Shell Oil Company	Sewaren	Middlesex
5	28	28	E I DuPont De Nemours & Co	Gibbstown	Gloucester
6	64	224	B F Goodrich Co	Pedricktown	Salem
7	2	3	E I DuPont De Nemours & Co	Deepwater	Salem
8	10	42	Monsanto Company	Bridgeport	Gloucester
9	40	195	Huntsman Polypropylene Corp	Woodbury	Gloucester
10	470	418	Amerada Hess Corp	Woodridge	Middlesex
			Subtotal		
			Percent of Total		
Facilities with Largest Waste					
1	1	80	Coastal Eagle Point Oil Co	Westville	Gloucester
7	2	3	E I DuPont De Nemours & Co	Deepwater	Salem
2	3	67	Exxon Company USA	Linden	Union
14	4	13	Aqualon Company	Parlin	Middlesex
25	5	100	Hoffmann-La Roche Inc	Belvidere	Warren
27	6	1	Sybron Chemicals Inc	Birmingham	Burlington
34	7	4	International Flavors & Fragrances	Union Beach	Monmouth
43	8	9	Miles Inc	Haledon	Passaic
51	9	6	Sun Chemical Corp	Newark	Essex
8	10	42	Monsanto Company	Bridgeport	Gloucester
			Subtotal		
			Percent of Total		
Facilities with Largest Releases and Transfers					
27	6	1	Sybron Chemicals Inc	Birmingham	Burlington
32	11	2	Merck & Co Inc	Rahway	Union
7	2	3	E I DuPont De Nemours & Co	Deepwater	Salem
34	7	4	International Flavors & Fragrances	Union Beach	Monmouth
29	22	5	Old Bridge Chemicals Inc	Old Bridge	Middlesex
51	9	6	Sun Chemical Corp	Newark	Essex
60	29	7	Co-Steel Raritan	Perth Amboy	Middlesex
46	30	8	New Jersey Steel Corporation	Sayreville	Middlesex
43	8	9	Miles Inc	Haledon	Passaic
90	25	10	Hercules Inc	Kenvil	Morris
			Subtotal		
			Percent of Total		
			Total for All New Jersey Facilities		

SIC Code	Business	Use Pounds	Waste Pounds	Waste as Percent-age of Use Percent	Total Releases and Transfers Pounds	Total Releases and Trans-fers as Percent-age of Use Percent	Source Reduc-tion Quantity Pounds
29	Petroleum Refinery	8,309,225,974	6,216,425,774	74.81	334,682	0.00	0
29	Petroleum Refinery	3,477,193,900	52,093,500	1.50	440,904	0.01	14,880
29	Petroleum Refinery	1,939,446,520	219,500	0.01	93,769	0.00	0
29	Storage and Distribution of Petroleum Products	1,007,049,815	464,176	0.05	274,480	0.03	0
28	Chemical Manufacturer	383,503,513	4,246,102	1.11	1,519,792	0.40	0
28	Manufacture Polyvinyl Chloride	379,821,137	1,420,161	0.37	52,092	0.01	0
28	Chemical Manufacturer	379,129,615	57,743,949	15.23	5,572,481	1.47	150,000
28	Chemical Manufacturer	348,313,615	12,000,642	3.45	906,102	0.26	42,901
28	Manufacture of Polypropylene	333,268,461	2,500,955	0.75	76,634	0.02	10,200
29	Bulk Petroleum Storage	238,979,208	5,334	0.00	5,334	0.00	0
		16,795,931,758	6,347,120,093	37.79	9,276,270	0.06	217,981
		83.83	94.37		5.81		4.39
29	Petroleum Refinery	8,309,225,974	6,216,425,774	74.81	334,682	0.00	0
28	Chemical Manufacturer	379,129,615	57,743,949	15.23	5,572,481	1.47	150,000
29	Petroleum Refinery	3,477,193,900	52,093,500	1.50	440,904	0.01	14,880
28	Manufacture of Polymers in Bulk	150,800,923	26,536,557	17.60	2,766,941	1.83	0
28	Manufacture of Fine Chemicals	60,877,270	23,778,908	39.06	223,621	0.37	10,700
28	Production of Batch Speciality Chemicals	50,536,825	22,737,294	44.99	19,331,876	38.25	104,000
28	Manufacture of Fragrance Ingredients	22,675,151	19,571,136	86.31	5,238,076	23.10	297,000
28	Manufacture of Organic Pigments	15,776,720	13,124,890	83.19	3,026,964	19.19	0
28	Manufacture Synthetic Organic Chemicals	12,400,000	12,400,000	100.00	4,048,500	32.65	0
28	Chemical Manufacturer	348,313,615	12,000,642	3.45	906,102	0.26	42,901
		12,826,929,993	6,456,412,650	50.33	41,890,147	0.33	619,481
		64.02	95.99		26.26		12.46
28	Production of Batch Speciality Chemicals	50,536,825	22,737,294	44.99	19,331,876	38.25	104,000
28	Bulk Pharmaceutical Intermediates	25,055,900	11,285,900	45.04	9,773,330	39.01	630,000
28	Chemical Manufacturer	379,129,615	57,743,949	15.23	5,572,481	1.47	150,000
28	Manufacture of Fragrance Ingredients	22,675,151	19,571,136	86.31	5,238,076	23.10	297,000
28	Manufacture of Inorganic Zinc Compounds	48,380,221	5,336,394	11.03	5,024,597	10.39	0
28	Manufacture Synthetic Organic Chemicals	12,400,000	12,400,000	100.00	4,048,500	32.65	0
33	Elec Arc Furnace, Produce Steel	10,402,950	4,031,400	38.75	4,031,090	38.75	0
33	Mini Mill Steel Facility	14,194,157	3,743,669	26.37	3,750,480	26.42	0
28	Manufacture of Organic Pigments	15,776,720	13,124,890	83.19	3,026,964	19.19	0
28	Manufacture of Smokeless Propellents	5,682,980	4,534,505	79.79	3,017,233	53.09	0
		584,234,519	154,509,137	26.45	62,814,627	10.75	1,181,000
		2.92	2.30		39.38		23.76
		20,034,716,490	6,726,089,975		159,527,216		4,969,849

Table 10-6. Use, Waste, and Releases and Transfers, by Industry, New Jersey, 1992

SIC Code	Industry	Use Pounds	Waste Pounds	Waste as Percentage of Use Percent	Total Releases and Transfers Pounds	Total Releases and Transfers as Percentage of Use Percent	Source Reduction Quantity Pounds
20	Food	11,318,879	3,503,370	30.95	1,222,730	10.80	12,300
22	Textiles	1,477,479	1,171,705	79.30	681,500	46.13	1,400
24	Lumber	8,680,675	100,748	1.16	117,533	1.35	0
25	Furniture	67,035	67,035	100.00	78,338	116.86	0
26	Paper	14,106,775	11,154,552	79.07	2,577,816	18.27	36,740
27	Printing	1,017,461	997,272	98.02	268,548	26.39	1,432
28	Chemicals	4,345,778,445	359,324,162	8.27	115,851,366	2.67	2,646,301
29	Petroleum	14,987,836,225	6,271,258,822	41.84	2,399,317	0.02	15,006
30	Plastics	88,576,081	11,235,096	12.68	3,046,544	3.44	74,190
31	Leather	2,415,319	974,671	40.35	555,333	22.99	0
32	Stone/Clay	7,301,570	2,080,215	28.49	729,014	9.98	103,188
33	Primary Metals	352,486,503	29,668,275	8.42	17,058,868	4.84	1,294,318
34	Fabr. Metals	44,066,029	16,908,321	38.37	6,536,254	14.83	318,070
35	Machinery	16,589,367	2,663,117	16.05	2,416,051	14.56	129,310
36	Electrical	111,024,240	4,622,145	4.16	2,627,670	2.37	16,255
37	Transportation	7,830,164	2,722,262	34.77	1,349,583	17.24	87,035
38	Measure./Photo.	11,222,800	2,497,075	22.25	1,181,230	10.53	204,304
39	Miscellaneous	22,587,672	5,099,863	22.58	807,487	3.57	30,000
50	Wholesale, durable	193,732	22,751	11.74	21,551	11.12	0
51	Wholesale, non-durable	140,039	18,518	13.22	483	0.34	0
	Total	20,034,716,490	6,726,089,975	33.57	159,527,216	0.80	4,969,849

New Jersey Industries

Because the four facilities that use the largest amounts of toxic chemicals are all in the Petroleum refining sector (SIC 29) , the Petroleum industry ranks first in toxic chemical use. In the case of the Petroleum industry, the toxic chemicals can be present as contaminants in the crude oil being refined, and the "use" amount includes estimates of these contaminants as part of the inputs to the refining process. The Petroleum industry also ranks first in waste generated, but eighth for total releases and transfers. It used 15.0 billion pounds, which is 75 percent of all toxic chemicals used in New Jersey in 1992. (See Table 10-6.)

The Chemical industry ranks second for total use and for waste generated, but first for total releases and transfers. This industry accounts for 73 percent of all releases and transfers in New Jersey in 1992.

While the Chemical industry facilities reported the largest amount of source reduction (2.6 million pounds or 53 percent of the total source reduction reported by all New Jersey facilities), the Petroleum industry reported almost no source reduction (15,000 pounds out of 6.3 billion pounds of waste generated). Instead, the Primary Metals industry, which ranks third for waste generation, reported the second largest amount of source reduction of all industry groups. This industry reported 1.3 million pounds of source reduction, representing 0.4 percent of its reported waste generation. This amount came in large part from one facility, the Phelps Dodge Specialty Copper Company in Elizabeth, mentioned above for its source reduction of copper.

The differences among the industrial sectors extend to their relative generation of waste and releases and transfers. The five facilities reporting for the Lumber industry had among the smallest percentage of use ending up as waste and releases and transfers, about 1 percent, while the two Furniture facilities reported that all of their use of toxic chemicals ended up as waste and releases and transfers.[h] In between these extremes was the Printing industry, which reported as waste 98 percent of the amount used, but released or transferred 26 percent of the amount used. (See Table 10-6.)

Toxic Chemicals by New Jersey County

Not all areas of New Jersey are equally affected by toxic chemicals, nor are patterns of use, waste, and releases and transfers consistent on a county basis. While Middlesex County had the most facilities reporting and the largest amount of total releases and transfers, Gloucester County had reports totaling the most use and waste generated in 1992. The 6.2 billion pounds of waste generated in Gloucester County represents 90 percent of the state total. Two of the four largest users of toxic chemicals are located in Gloucester County: Coastal Eagle Point Oil Company in Westville and the Mobil Oil Corporation's facility in Paulsboro. The fifth largest user, DuPont's facility in Gibbstown, is also located in Gloucester County. These three facilities reported using 10.6 billion pounds of toxic chemicals, 93 percent of the county's total and 53 percent of the state total. (See Map 10-1, Table 10-7, and Box 10-C.)

While most of the use and waste generation of toxic chemicals is concentrated in Gloucester and Middlesex Counties, the second-ranked county for releases and transfers is Burlington, where Sybron Chemicals is located. Bergen County has the second largest number of facilities, but ranks lower in the other measures, being fifth for releases and transfers, seventh for waste generation, and eighth for use. (See Table 10-7.)

Two facilities mentioned above with source reduction are located in Union County, giving that county the largest amount of source reduction reported. They are Phelps Dodge in Elizabeth with 1.2 million pounds and Merck & Co. in Rahway with a total of 630,000 pounds of source reduction.

[h] One facility, Media-Stack in Vineland, a manufacturer of steel book shelving, reported in error more releases and transfers (32,457 pounds) than use (20,958 pounds) in 1992, so total releases and transfers for the Furniture industry are more than 100 percent of use.

Table 10-7. Use, Waste, and Releases and Transfers by County, New Jersey, 1992

County	Use Pounds	Waste Pounds	Waste as Percentage of Use Percent	Total Releases and Transfers Pounds	Total Releases and Transfers as Percentage of Use Percent	Source Reduction Quantity Pounds
Bergen	131,580,833	40,766,188	30.98	13,514,614	10.27	336,562
Burlington	213,001,624	29,397,540	13.80	21,653,169	10.17	145,660
Camden	47,375,493	3,130,997	6.61	1,384,579	2.92	18,555
Cumberland	2,059,691	1,641,584	79.70	220,867	10.72	77,000
Essex	781,474,921	46,646,879	5.97	21,405,596	2.74	268,965
Gloucester	11,453,647,977	6,242,324,120	54.50	4,787,839	0.04	54,314
Hudson	114,325,421	19,572,059	17.12	4,027,491	3.52	79,773
Hunterdon	16,327,538	10,003,401	61.27	390,757	2.39	106,800
Mercer	24,549,115	4,839,937	19.72	942,830	3.84	17,924
Middlesex	2,247,942,243	94,392,311	4.20	37,161,286	1.65	689,663
Monmouth	126,119,010	21,907,499	17.37	6,616,958	5.25	383,629
Morris	27,611,305	9,147,668	33.13	6,295,952	22.80	11,740
Ocean	1,150,010	604,866	52.60	52,890	4.60	310
Passaic	88,147,871	28,201,998	31.99	10,019,134	11.37	244,198
Salem	776,553,868	65,653,416	8.45	6,392,759	0.82	151,600
Somerset	72,776,022	4,263,630	5.86	2,999,174	4.12	80,105
Sussex	1,204,673	1,095,204	90.91	811,739	67.38	30,200
Union	3,722,761,606	75,097,163	2.02	19,164,730	0.51	2,252,125
Warren	185,710,477	27,229,893	14.66	1,511,926	0.81	12,400
Total	20,034,319,698	6,725,916,353	33.57	159,354,290	0.80	4,961,523

Map 10-1.

New Jersey TRI Releases and Transfers, Use, and Source Reduction, by County, 1992

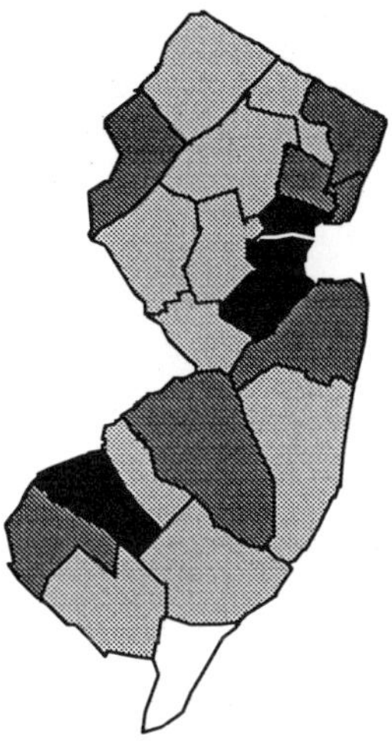

Use

- More than 1,000 million
- 100 to 1,000 million
- 0.1 to 100 million
- 0

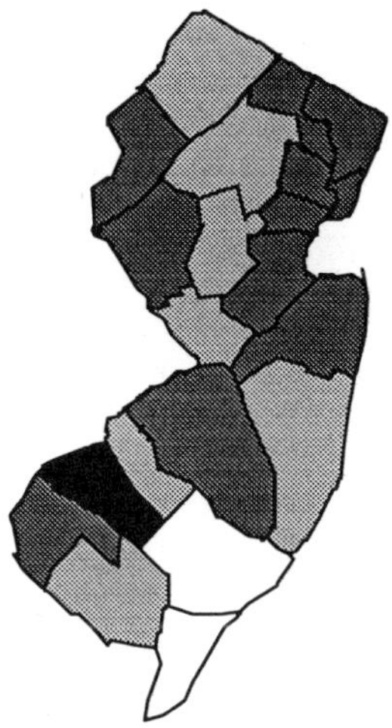

Waste

- More than 100 million
- 10 to 100 million
- 0.1 to 10 million
- 0

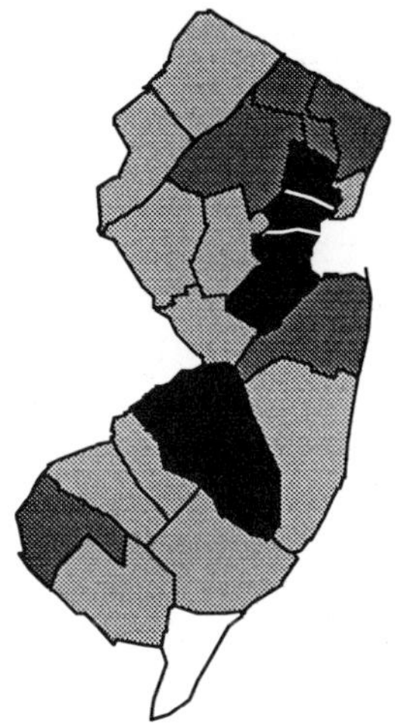

Total Releases and Transfers

- More than 15 million
- 5 to 15 million
- 0.01 to 5 million
- 0

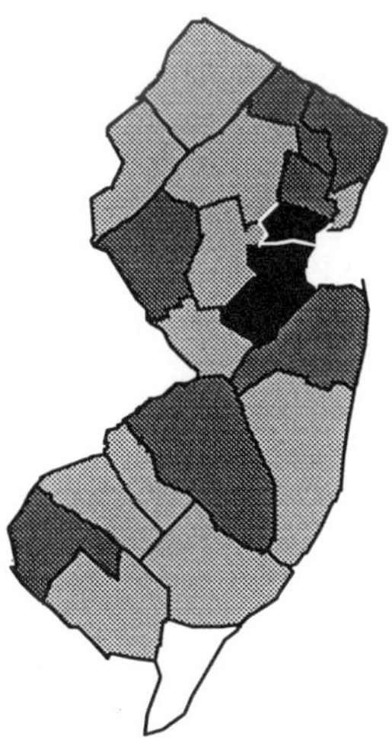

Source Reduction

- More than 500,000
- 100,000 to 500,000
- 100 to 100,000
- 0

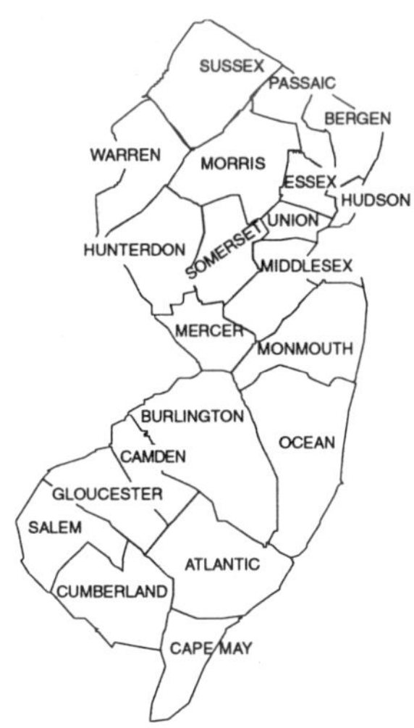

in Pounds

Portraits of Individual Facilities, Using New Jersey Data

The above analysis of the New Jersey data shows ways that the use, waste, and release/transfer data can be used to evaluate progress in reducing toxic chemical pollution by comparing industries and waste management options associated with the different toxic chemicals. This type of comparison is also informative when distinguishing the efforts of individual facilities.

Looking at an individual facility tells how a chemical that is brought on site or manufactured then goes through the various operations at the facility and how much ends up as waste. For example, the DuPont facility in Deepwater uses Freon 113, a chloro-organic that is an ozone-depleting chemical. It brought on site 3.3 million pounds of that chemical in 1992, consumed half of that (1.7 million pounds) in its manufacturing processes, shipped one-quarter (835,000 pounds) in products, and put 2 percent (79,000 pounds) into inventory. The remaining 700,000 pounds, therefore, was waste. DuPont released to the air 129,000 pounds of the waste Freon and sent off site for recycling 565,000 pounds. Thus, 21 percent of the Freon used at DuPont ended up as waste, with 4 percent of this ozone-depleting chemical released to the air from the site. (See Figure 10-7.)

The New Jersey data can be used to compare the difference in waste generation and releases and transfers of toxic chemicals at individual facilities that manufacture the same type of product using the same chemicals. For example, consider the data from two lead-acid battery manufacturers in Paterson, New Jersey. The Atlantic Battery Corporation used 10.8 million pounds of lead compounds in 1992, shipping in its batteries 10.3 million pounds of the lead compounds. The waste generated from the manufacture of the batteries was thus 0.6 million pounds (5 percent of its use), which Atlantic reported was sent off site for recycling. On the other hand, the Power Battery Company, also in Paterson, used slightly over half as much lead compounds (5.7 million pounds) and reported 70,000 pounds of waste generated, which was also sent off site for recycling. This amount of waste is just over 1 percent of its use, or less than one-quarter the rate at which Atlantic Battery is generating waste and releases and transfers of lead compounds. (See Figures 10-8 and 10-9.)

Another example shows use of the same chemical — 1,1,1-trichloroethane, a chloro-organic and ozone-depleting chemical — but in different manufacturing processes, where it can be expected that waste generation rates would vary. The American Gas & Chemical Company in Northvale used 27,580 pounds of 1,1,1-trichloroethane in the manufacture of specialty chemicals. It shipped 24,013 pounds in its products and generated waste of 1,139 pounds with the rest going to inventory. The waste was sent off site, half to be recycled and half to be incinerated. The Allied-Signal Aerospace Company in Teterboro used about the same amount of 1,1,1-trichloroethane, 29,703 pounds

Figure 10-7.

New Jersey Materials Accounting Data: Freon 113 at DuPont Chambers Works, Deepwater

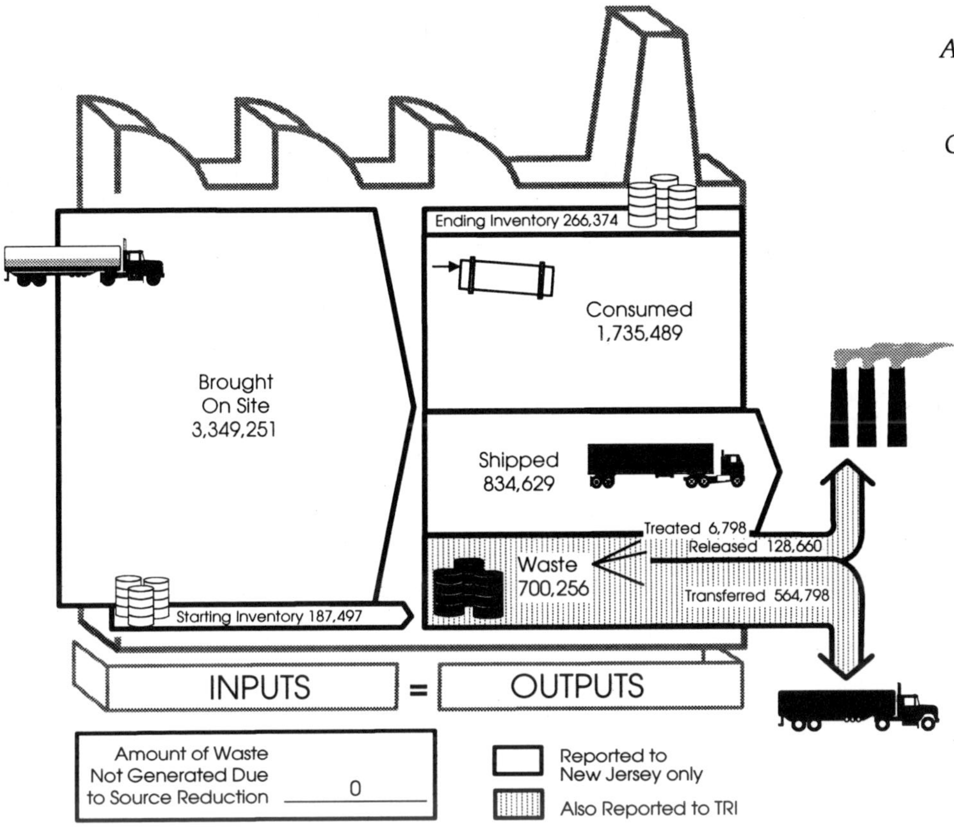

in Pounds (not drawn to scale)

Freon 113 (ozone depleter and chloro-organic)

in 1992 with 849 pounds going to inventory. However, in its manufacture of navigation instruments, none of the chemical is shipped in the product and all is generated as waste. Allied-Signal released to the air 760 pounds and sent the rest of the waste off site to be recycled. American Gas & Chemical reported no source reduction activity for this chemical. However, Allied-Signal Aerospace reported that its waste of 1,1,1-trichloroethane was reduced by 26,686 pounds from 1991 to 1992 due to source reduction activities. Production also decreased from 1991 to 1992, so that the total reduction in waste generated was about 32,900 pounds. Allied-Signal projects that in five years it will have eliminated use of this chemical. (See Figures 10-10 and 10-11.)

The data for Merck & Company in Rahway show the value of having the facility report the quantities of reduction due to different changes in operations. This facility uses ethylene glycol in the manufacture of pharmaceuticals. It used 261,000 pounds in 1991 and 139,000 pounds in 1992. None of the

Figure 10-8.

New Jersey Materials Accounting Data: Lead Compounds at Atlantic Battery Corp., Paterson

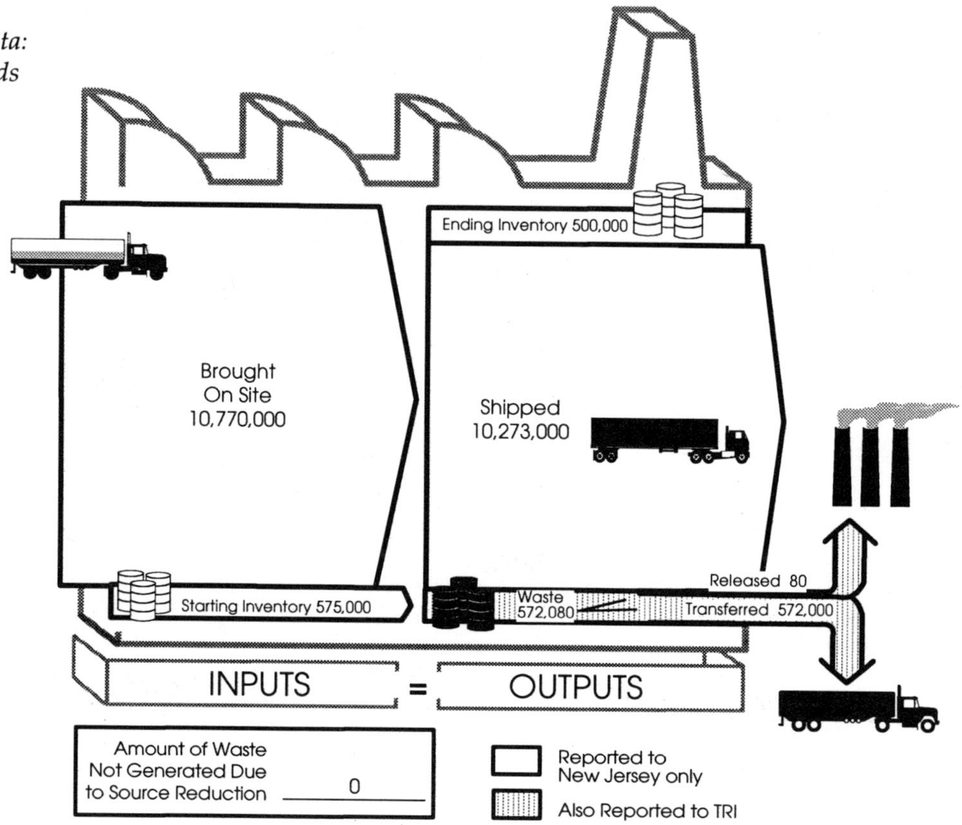

in Pounds (not drawn to scale)

Lead Compounds (metal and carcinogen)

chemical was consumed or shipped in products; all of the amount used was generated as waste and sent off site to the municipal sewage treatment plant. The 261,000 pounds of waste generated in 1991 was reduced to 139,000 pounds in 1992. Merck reported to New Jersey that 20,000 pounds of the reduction was due to discontinuing the product and 80,000 pounds was due to source reduction activities, and Merck expects to eliminate the waste generated within five years. (See Figures 10-12 and 10-13.)

Figure 10-9.

New Jersey Materials Accounting Data: Lead Compounds at Power Battery Co., Paterson

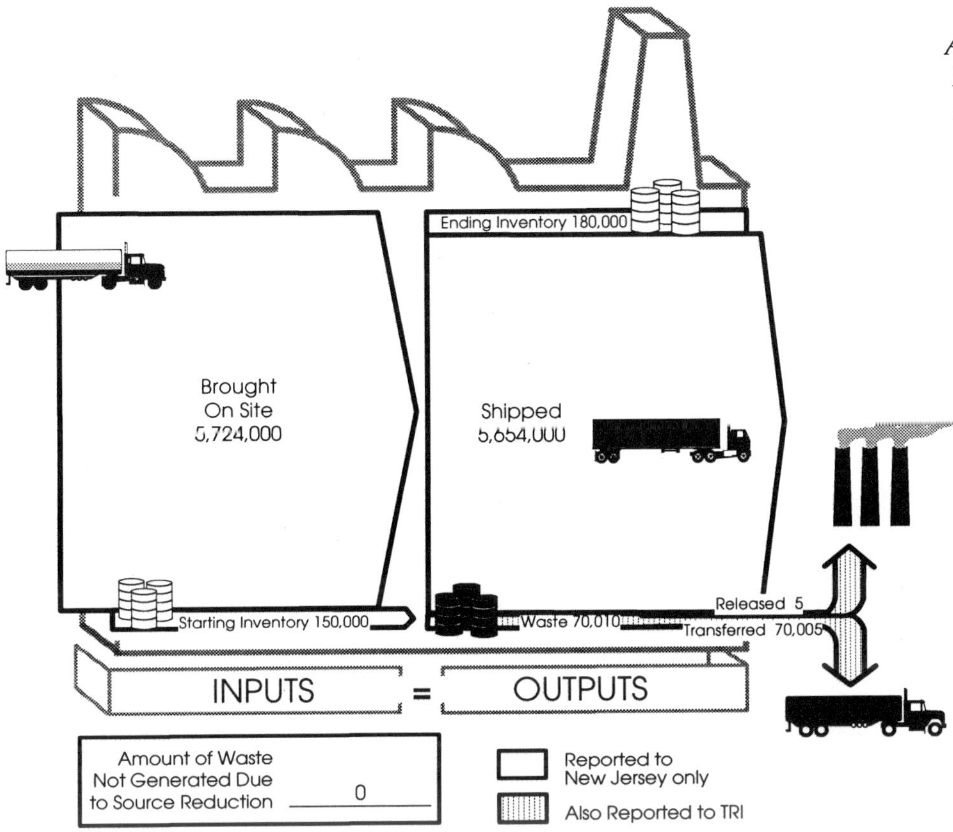

in Pounds (not drawn to scale)

Lead Compounds (metal and carcinogen)

Figure 10-10.

New Jersey Materials Accounting Data: 1,1,1-Trichloroethane at American Gas & Chemical Co., Northvale

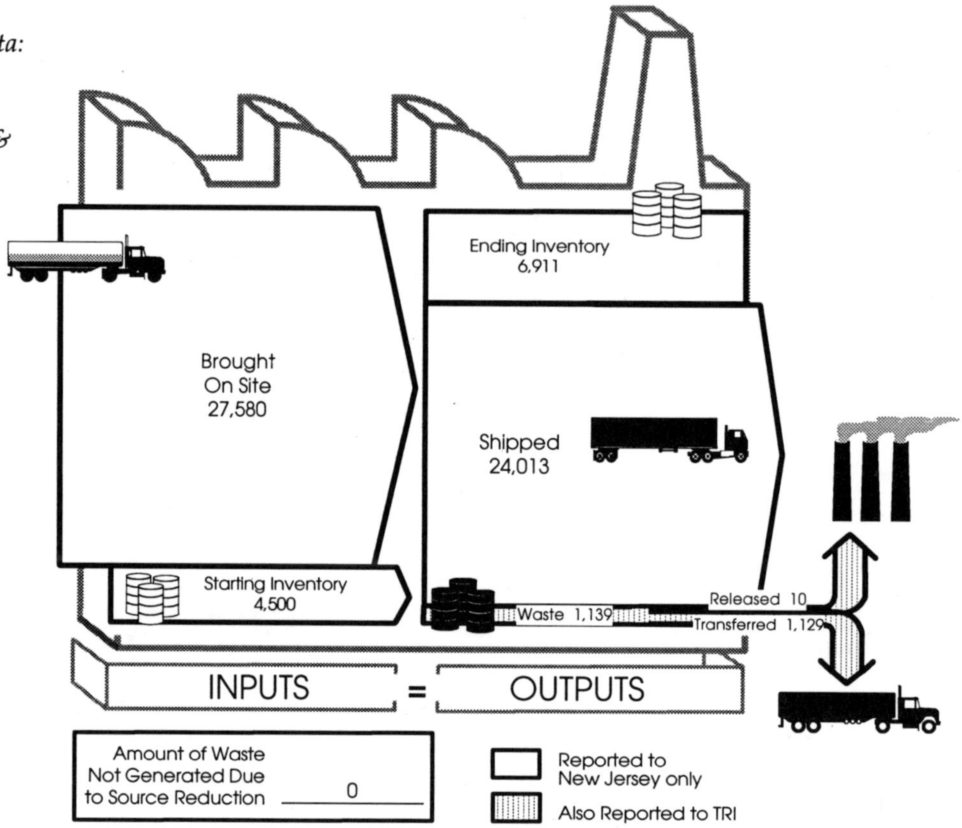

in Pounds (not drawn to scale)

1,1,1-Trichloroethane (chloro-organic and ozone depleter)

Figure 10-11.

New Jersey Materials Accounting Data: 1,1,1-Trichloroethane at Allied-Signal Aerospace Co., Teterboro

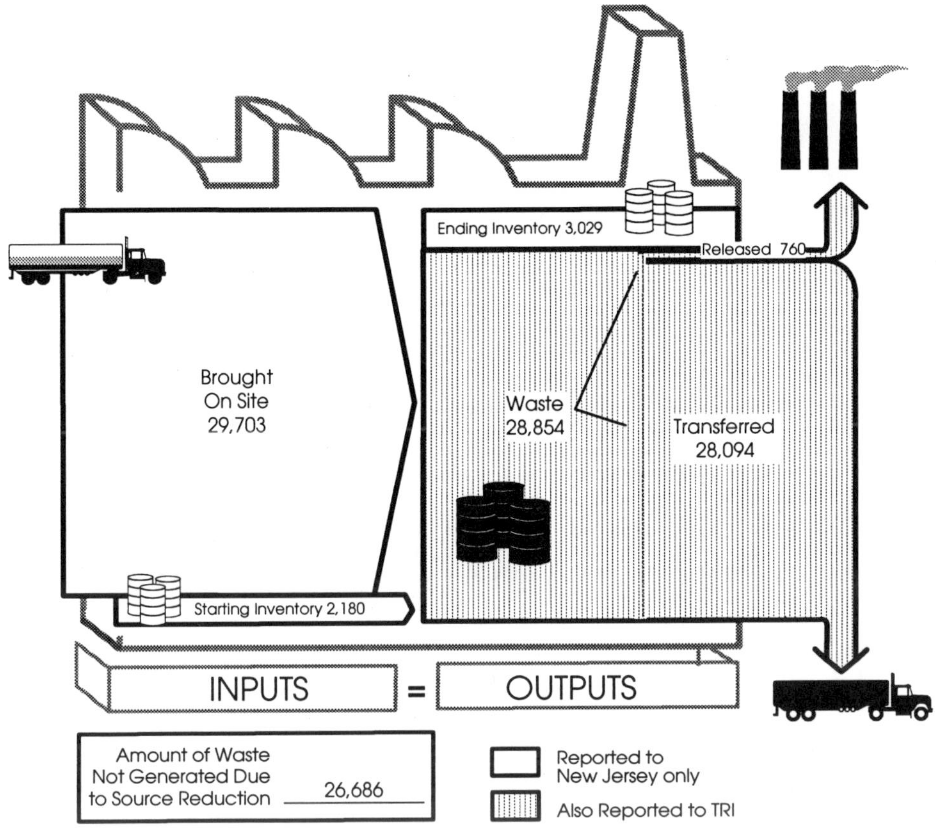

in Pounds (not drawn to scale)

1,1,1-Trichloroethane (chloro-organic and ozone depleter)

Figure 10-12.

New Jersey Materials Accounting Data: Ethylene Glycol at Merck & Co., Rahway, 1991

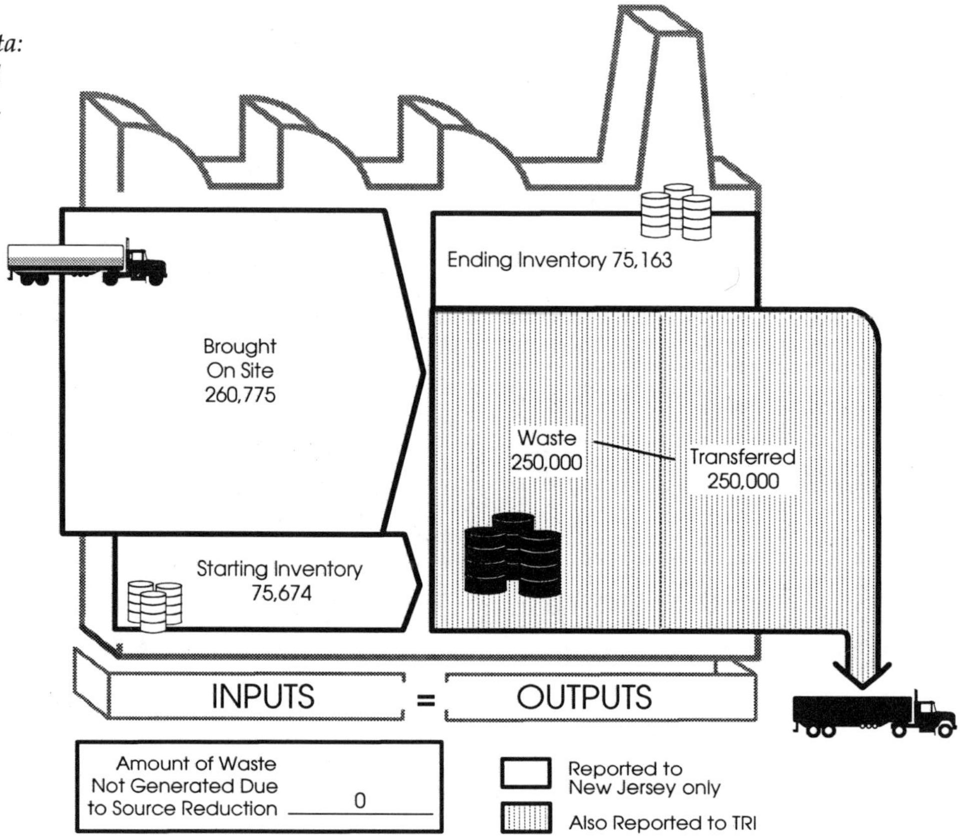

in Pounds (not drawn to scale)

Ethylene Glycol

Figure 10-13.

New Jersey Materials Accounting Data: Ethylene Glycol at Merck & Co., Rahway, 1992

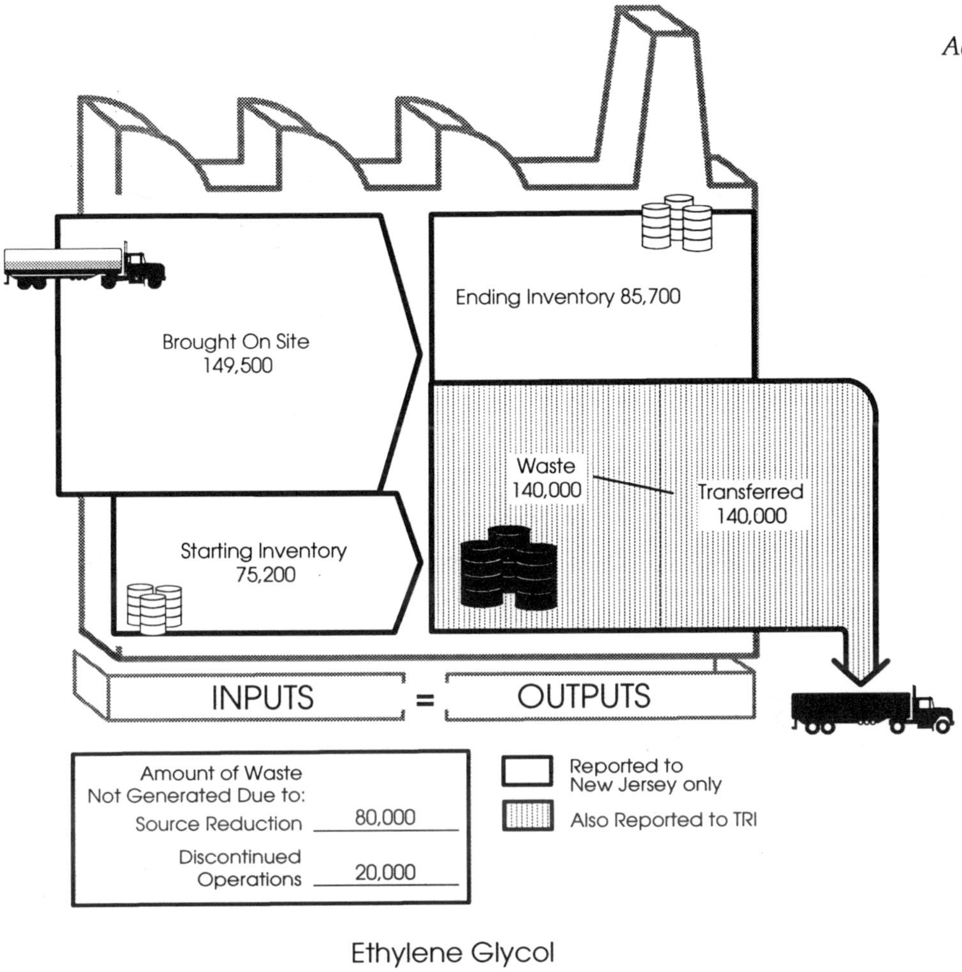

in Pounds (not drawn to scale)

Changes in New Jersey Use, Waste, and Releases / Transfers, 1991-1992

Total *use* of toxic chemicals in New Jersey declined overall by 19 percent from 1991 to 1992. Total waste generated and releases and transfers declined less, waste by 15 percent and total releases and transfers by 4 percent. The smaller decrease in waste occurred because overall the amount of toxic chemicals that was consumed was proportionately less in 1992 than in 1991. The percent decrease in the amount consumed was 14 percent compared to the 19 percent decrease in use so that proportionately more of the toxic chemical ended up in waste than consumed in 1992 compared to 1991. (See Table 10-8.)

In the summary above and the rest of this section, the discussion of changes from 1991 to 1992 makes comparisons based on the New Jersey data without the Coastal Eagle Point Oil Company's 1991 and 1992 data. The reasons for this exclusion are explained in Box 10-C.

Effect of Changes in Source Reduction and Other Reductions

Source reduction activity, small in 1991, was even smaller in 1992. While in 1991, 18 percent of New Jersey facilities (128 out of 699) had reported reductions due to source reduction, 15 percent (100 out of 621) did so in 1992. The amount of waste generation that was reduced fell by 41 percent, from 12.1 million pounds to 5.0 million pounds. In 1992 most source reductions achieved were due to improved operations. (See Table 10-9.)

In 1992 other types of reductions included 108.3 million pounds due to ceased operations, which means that use would have been 108.3 million pounds (0.9 percent) higher in 1992 if the operations had not ceased.

Effect of Absolute Amount of Use and Changes in Use

The New Jersey data show that how much a *change in use* affects the amount of waste generated and the amount of releases and transfers is related to the *absolute amount of use* (as well as to any change in the level of production). Because the patterns of change are different depending on the amount of use of the toxic chemical, the New Jersey forms are divided into three groups: large use is greater than 3 million pounds, medium use falls between 100,000 pounds and 3 million pounds, and small use is 100,000 pounds or less. Forms reporting large use represented only 9 percent of all forms but reported 95 percent of the use, 68 percent of the waste generated, and 42 percent of the total releases and transfers. The forms reporting medium use represented 41 percent of all forms, 5 percent of the use, 28 percent of the waste, and 49 percent of the releases and transfers. Small use forms, representing 51 percent of all forms, reported just 0.4 percent of use, 4 percent of waste, and 8 percent of releases and transfers. (See Figure 10-14 and Table 10-10.)

Table 10-8. Use, Waste, and Releases and Transfers, New Jersey, 1991 and 1992

	1991* Number	**1992*** Number	**Change 1991-1992** Number	**Percent Change 1991-1992** Percent
Facilities	699	681	-18	-2.58
Forms	2,634	2,497	-137	-5.20
	Pounds	Pounds	Pounds	Percent
Inputs				
Use **	14,491,872,285	11,725,490,516	-2,766,381,769	-19.09
Net Inventory	25,731,386	18,231,094	-7,500,292	-29.15
Starting Inventory	817,880,842	673,724,399	-144,156,443	-17.63
Ending Inventory	792,149,456	655,493,305	-136,656,151	-17.25
Produced On-site	6,087,894,401	4,932,787,396	-1,155,107,005	-18.97
Brought On-site	8,201,535,098	6,570,750,976	-1,630,784,122	-19.88
Recycled On-site	175,516,508	203,276,694	27,760,186	15.82
Outputs				
Consumed	3,182,095,675	2,737,764,917	-444,330,758	-13.96
Shipped as/in Product	10,742,925,368	8,700,048,024	-2,042,877,344	-19.02
Waste **	597,214,819	509,664,201	-87,550,618	-14.66
Destroyed through Treatment	216,224,191	175,277,773	-40,946,418	-18.94
Release and Transfer Data				
Total Releases and Transfers	165,375,671	159,192,534	-6,183,137	-3.74
Total Releases	22,080,123	18,803,162	-3,276,961	-14.84
Total Air Emissions	20,741,512	18,510,991	-2,230,521	-10.75
Surface Water Discharges	507,977	176,127	-331,850	-65.33
Land Releases	827,844	115,437	-712,407	-86.06
Groundwater Discharges	2,790	607	-2,183	-78.24
Total Transfers	143,295,548	140,389,372	-2,906,176	-2.03
Transfers to POTWs	42,314,134	45,326,325	3,012,191	7.12
Off-site Transfers by Mgt. Technique				
Incineration	11,810,723	13,656,198	1,845,475	15.63
Water Treatment	0	0	0	
Groundwater Disposal	8,350	54,986	46,636	558.51
Land Disposal	1,799,038	2,174,644	375,606	20.88
Recycled	68,784,240	59,175,136	-9,609,104	-13.97
Other	18,579,063	20,002,083	1,423,020	7.66

* Does not include one facility, Coastal Eagle Point Oil Co., Westville, New Jersey.

** For individual forms, if the calculation of use or waste resulted in a negative number, then the value was set to zero. Therefore, "Use" is not exactly equal to net inventory + produced + brought on site + recycled, and "Waste" is not exactly equal to use - consumed - shipped + recycled on site.

Table 10-9. Source Reduction Data, New Jersey, 1991 and 1992

	1991*	1992*	Change 1991-1992	Percent Change 1991-1992
	Number	Number	Number	Percent
Facilities	699	681	-18	-2.58
Forms	2,634	2,497	-137	-5.20
	Pounds	Pounds	Pounds	Percent
Use	14,491,872,285	11,725,490,516	-2,766,381,769	-19.09
Waste	597,214,819	509,664,201	-87,550,618	14.66
Data on Reductions in Waste				
	Number	Number	Number	Percent
Facilities Reporting Source Reduction	128	100	-28	-21.88
Forms Reporting Source Reduction	364	282	-82	-22.53
	Pounds	Pounds	Pounds	Percent
Quantity of Source Reduction	12,095,551	4,969,849	-7,125,702	-58.91
Reformulation of Product	1,865,843	1,216,191	-649,652	-34.82
Process Modifications	3,550,673	1,304,985	-2,245,688	-63.25
Technology/Equipment Modifications	6,068,244	518,418	-5,549,826	-91.46
Improved operations	610,791	1,930,255	1,319,464	216.03
Source Reduction as Percent of Waste **	1.98%	0.96%		
Discontinued Operations	219,183,275	108,273,514	-110,909,761	-50.60
Export of Use	1,823,629	77,106	-1,746,523	-95.77
Miscellaneous Decreases	666,771	1,550,926	884,155	132.60
Projected Reduction in Two Years	113,685,318	77,850,306	-35,835,012	-31.52
Projected Reduction in Five Years	127,525,733	24,915,207	-102,610,526	-80.46

* Does not include one facility, Coastal Eagle Point Oil Co.

** Source reduction as percent of waste is percent of waste that would have been generated, i.e., source reduction amount divided by the sum of waste plus source reduction amount.

Figure 10-14.

Distribution by Use, of Forms, Use, Waste, Releases and Transfers, New Jersey, 1992

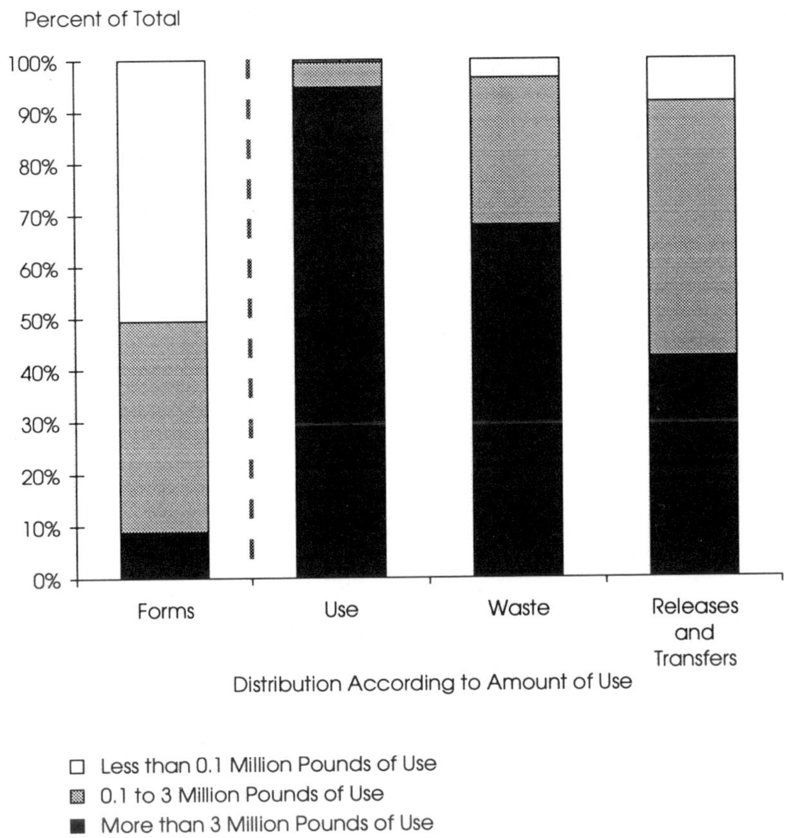

Facilities reporting large amounts of use of toxic chemicals dominate the state totals of waste generation and releases and transfers. However, such facilities report proportionately less releases and transfers of toxic chemicals than do facilities reporting smaller amounts of use. (See Figure 10-15.)

Source reduction is being practiced differently by the facilities associated with the three groups of forms — those reporting large, medium, and small use — as can be seen by looking separately at the data for each group. Although forms with large use accounted for 68 percent of all New Jersey waste generated in 1992, they reported only 43 percent of the amount of source reduction accomplished and this amount was 0.6 percent of the waste reported on the large-use forms. Forms with medium use reported higher rates of source reduction, although still just 1.5 percent of their total waste generated. The small-use forms reported the greatest. Source reduction by the small-use forms represented 3 percent of the waste generated by the small-use group. (See Table 10-11.)

*Table 10-10. Distribution of Forms Based on Use, New Jersey, 1992**

	Forms	Use	Waste	Releases and Transfers
Total Amount				
Range in Pounds of Use	Number	Pounds	Pounds	Pounds
> 20 million	73	9,996,399,031	183,175,509	22,147,322
10 to 20 million	37	491,515,188	35,128,291	8,921,316
5 to 10 million	58	404,322,776	84,085,114	27,136,140
4 to 5 million	23	104,271,712	26,913,076	2,694,812
3 to 4 million	31	107,918,928	17,245,026	6,543,463
2 to 3 million	47	114,286,021	28,011,129	13,862,103
1 to 2 million	133	184,290,125	45,891,248	26,486,777
500,000 to 1 million	183	128,192,153	34,419,232	16,727,655
100,000 to 500,000	649	144,939,538	36,475,422	21,431,192
<= 100,000	1,263	49,355,044	18,320,154	13,241,754
Total	2,497	11,725,490,516	509,664,201	159,192,534
Cumulative Percent of Total				
Range in Pounds of Use	Percent	Percent	Percent	Percent
> 20 million pounds	2.92	85.25	35.94	13.91
10 to 20 million	4.41	89.45	42.83	19.52
5 to 10 million	6.73	92.89	59.33	36.56
4 to 5 million	7.65	93.78	64.61	38.26
3 to 4 million	8.89	94.70	68.00	42.37
2 to 3 million	10.77	95.68	73.49	51.07
1 to 2 million	16.10	97.25	82.50	67.71
500,000 to 1 million	23.43	98.34	89.25	78.22
100,000 to 500,000	49.42	99.58	96.41	91.68
<= 100,000 pounds	100.00	100.00	100.00	100.00

* Does not include one facility, Coastal Eagle Oil Point Co., Westville, New Jersey.

Figure 10-15.

Waste and Releases and Transfers as Percent of Use by Size, New Jersey, 1992

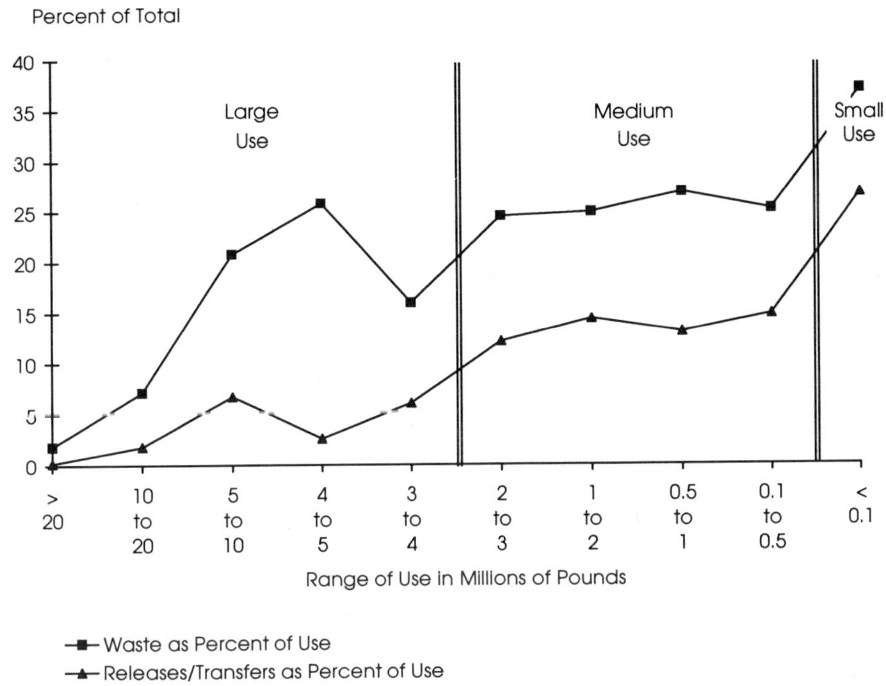

*Table 10-11. Distribution of Source Reduction Based on Use, New Jersey, 1992**

	Large Use **> 3,000,000 lbs** Pounds	**Medium Use** **100,000 to** **3,000,000 lbs** Pounds	**Smaller Use** **<= 100,000 lbs** Pounds	**Total** Pounds
Waste Generated	346,547,016	144,797,031	18,320,154	509,664,201
Source Reduction	2,134,739	2,217,736	617,374	4,969,849
	Percent	Percent	Percent	Percent
Source Reduction as Percent of Waste**	0.61	1.51	3.26	0.97

* Does not include one facility, Coastal Eagle Oil Point Co., Westville, New Jersey.

** Source reduction as percent of waste is percent of waste that would have been generated, i.e., source reduction amount divided by the sum of waste plus source reduction amount.

Figure 10-16.

Percent Change in Use, Waste, Releases and Transfers, New Jersey, 1992

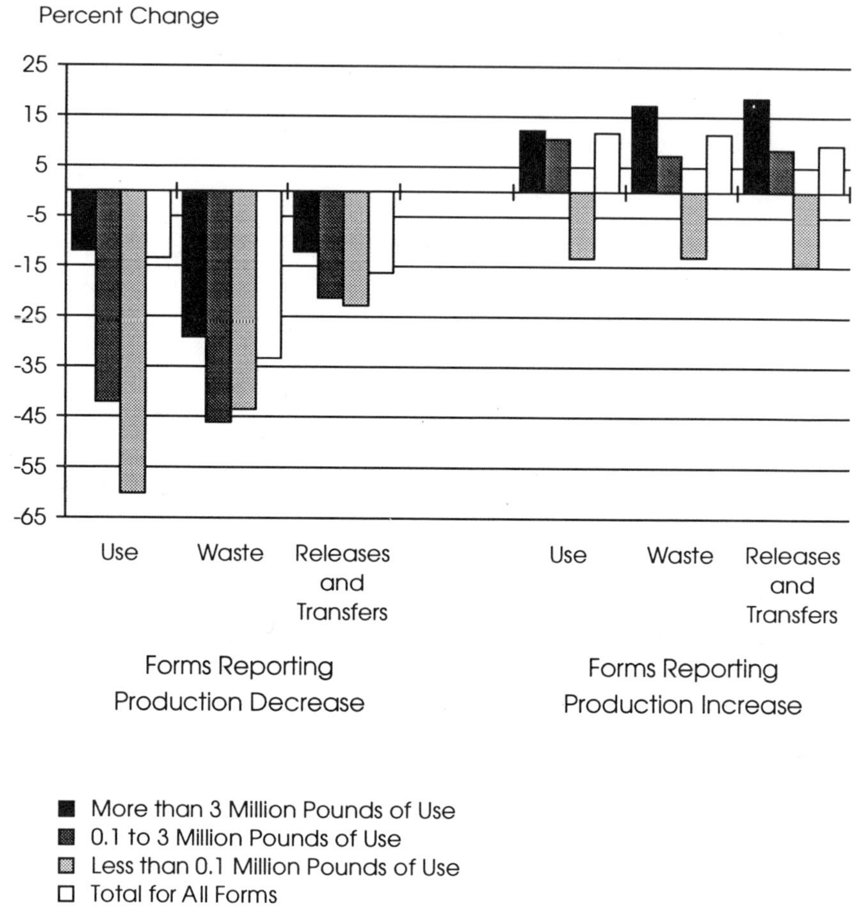

Effect of Changes in Production Level

The production level in units of production for the current year and the previous year is reported on each toxic chemical form. This means of reporting the change in production is generally considered a more reliable indicator than the reporting of a production index or ratio, as in the Massachusetts and TRI reporting systems, because an index involves an additional calculation which is prone to error. However, where there may be several different products using the same chemical at a facility, a ratio which prorates the use or, as in the case of Massachusetts, reporting a percent change ratio for each production unit for each chemical may better reflect such changes. New Jersey allows for reporting more than one set of production levels for a given chemical in these cases.

The pattern of change in production compared to changes in use, waste, and releases and transfers is also different for forms falling into the three "use" groups. For forms reporting a *decrease in production,*

*Table 10-12. Distribution of Change Based on Use, New Jersey, 1991-1992**

	Large Use > 3,000,000 lbs	Medium Use 100,000 lbs to 3,000,000 lbs	Small Use <= 100,000 lbs	Total for All Forms
	Percent Change	Percent Change	Percent Change	Percent Change
Production Decrease				
Percent Change in Use	-12.02	-41.99	-60.09	-13.37
Percent Change in Waste	-29.10	-46.15	-43.50	-33.34
Percent Change in Releases and Transfers	-12.13	-21.30	-22.77	-16.31
No Change in Production				
Percent Change in Use	-15.92	-56.85	-33.44	-18.75
Percent Change in Waste	41.37	-24.44	-21.62	2.20
Percent Change in Releases and Transfers	-7.14	-9.62	-23.92	-9.40
Production Increase				
Percent Change in Use	12.22	10.59	-13.24	11.82
Percent Change in Waste	17.21	7.31	-13.04	11.60
Percent Change in Releases and Transfers	18.72	8.47	-14.84	9.41

* Excludes one facility, Coastal Eagle Point Oil Co., Westville, New Jersey, and includes only forms reported in both years.

forms reporting large use reported a 29 percent decrease in waste and a 12 percent decrease in releases and transfers. These changes resulted from a 12 percent decrease in use. Medium-use forms, with production decrease, reported larger decreases overall, 42 percent decrease in use, 46 percent decrease in waste, and 21 percent decrease in releases and transfers. The small-use forms reported the largest decreases in use (60 percent) and releases and transfers (23 percent). (See Figure 10-16 and Table 10-12.)

The changes on large-use forms mask the different pattern of changes reported by the other forms. The overall state pattern of change in use, waste, and releases and transfers for all forms looks like the change for the large-use forms, even though these represent only 9 percent of the total forms reporting.

For forms reporting *production increases*, only those with small use reported decreases, about 13 percent for each category. Both the large-use and medium-use forms with production increases reported increases in use, waste, and releases and transfers. For the large-use forms, the increases in waste were larger than their increases in use, while for the medium-use forms their increases in waste and releases and transfers were less than their increases in use. (See Figure 10-16 and Table 10-12.)

Table 10-13. Comparison of Source Reduction Reporting, TRI and New Jersey, 1992

SIC Code	Facility	City	Chemical	TRI Total Production-related Waste 1991 Pounds	TRI Production Index
2851	Akzo Coatings	Somerset	Acetone	23,838	0.92
2851	Akzo Coatings	Somerset	Dibutyl phthalate	323	0.92
2851	Akzo Coatings	Somerset	Methanol	8,626	0.92
2851	Akzo Coatings	Somerset	Methyl ethyl ketone	189,523	0.92
2851	Akzo Coatings	Somerset	Methyl isobutyl ketone	5,165	0.92
2851	Akzo Coatings	Somerset	n-Butyl alcohol	5,286	0.92
2851	Akzo Coatings	Somerset	Toluene	20,981	0.92
2851	Akzo Coatings	Somerset	Xylene (mixed isomers)	42,637	0.92
2833	American Cyanamid	Bound Brook	1,2-Dichlorobenzene	251,120	4.24
2833	American Cyanamid	Bound Brook	Dichloromethane	139,200	1.23
2834	Arsynco Inc	Carlstadt	Xylene (mixed isomers)	5,997,358	1.15
3491	Hoke Inc	Cresskill	1,1,1-Trichloroethane	78,764	0.92
2865	Monsanto	Bridgeport	Phenol	79,300	1.03
2865	Monsanto	Bridgeport	Ammonia	48,000	0.98
3861	Polychrome Corp	Clark	Methanol	121,416	1.02
2865	Troy Chemical Corp	Newark	Maleic anhydride	100	1.08
2865	Troy Chemical Corp	Newark	Methanol	657,700	1.13
2865	Troy Chemical Corp	Newark	Styrene	822	0.90
3651	Union Camp Corp	Englewood	Xylene (mixed isomers)	70,470	1.25

* Expected TRI Waste is TRI Waste 1991 times index.

** Calculated source reduction is Expected minus Actual TRI Waste 1992; a negative number means the amount of actual waste increased more than the expected waste, implying no source reduction.

*** A positive number means more source reduction was reported to New Jersey than calculated from the TRI index. A negative number means less source reduction was reported to New Jersey than calculated from the TRI index.

Production Index and Source Reduction

New Jersey forms require facilities to report the amount of waste from the previous year that was reduced because of source reduction activities, as noted above. Neither Massachusetts nor TRI has this data element. TRI requires reporting of a production activity index which indicates how production changed from the previous year. Theoretically, this number could be used to calculate the amount of source reduction by multiplying the waste generated in the previous year by the index to get an expected amount of waste generation. This expected amount takes into account the production change that is reflected in the index number. If the actual waste generated is less than the expected amount, the difference could be ascribed to source reduction.

Expected TRI Waste 1992* Pounds	Actual TRI Waste 1992 Pounds	TRI Calculated Source Reduction** Pounds	Amount of Source Reduction Reported to New Jersey Pounds	Difference Between Amount of Source Reduction Reported to New Jersey and TRI Calculated Source Reduction*** Pounds	Percent
21,931	60,431	-38,500	5,000	43,500	870.0
297	187	110	25	-85	-340.6
7,936	5,526	2,410	1,000	-1,410	-141.0
174,361	146,028	28,333	20,000	-8,333	-41.7
4,752	2,148	2,604	600	-2,004	-334.0
4,863	2,590	2,273	200	-2,073	-1,036.6
19,303	7,148	12,155	9,000	-3,155	-35.1
39,226	1,790	37,436	6,000	-31,436	-523.9
1,064,749	824,770	239,979	13,800	-226,179	-1,639.0
171,216	157,000	14,216	22,825	8,609	37.7
6,896,962	6,231,320	665,642	155,000	-510,642	-329.4
72,463	69,679	2,784	10,880	8,096	74.4
81,679	57,860	23,819	34,901	11,082	31.8
47,040	40,000	7,040	8,000	960	12.0
123,844	102,734	21,110	39,733	18,623	46.9
108	160	-52	5	57	1,140.0
743,201	610,186	133,015	77,558	-55,457	-71.5
740	709	31	121	90	74.5
88,088	100,600	-12,513	30,000	42,513	141.7

However, this assumes a linear relation of waste generation and source reduction with production changes and that the index number reflects all changes in use of the chemical. For this *Toxics Watch* report, a comparison was done for some New Jersey facilities on the forms for which they reported source reduction to New Jersey and which could be matched to TRI data. This comparison of the amount of source reduction as reported to New Jersey with the production index and total production-related waste that these facilities reported to TRI shows that the calculation of source reduction using only TRI data does not match the amount reported to New Jersey. The TRI calculation in some cases overstates the amount and in other cases understates the amount. (See Table 10-13.) While this looks at just a small number of facilities because the TRI and New Jersey databases are not linked and finding the TRI data for each New Jersey facility is not possible, the matches found do represent a variety of industries and chemicals to which the problem applies.

Also, in comparing the index as reported to TRI with the index as calculated from the New Jersey reports of production amounts in the current and previous year, the calculations of the index in the two reporting systems do not match for many forms. This *Toxics Watch* report, therefore, uses the index feature of these reporting systems to group facilities into categories of changes in production rather than using the index to calculate source reduction.

Toxic Chemical Profile for Massachusetts, 1992

Although Massachusetts is the same size in terms of land area as New Jersey (8,000 square miles), it has a smaller population (6.0 million people in 1992 as opposed to 7.8 million people in New Jersey); Massachusetts also does not hold so prominent a position in national toxic chemical statistics as does New Jersey. In 1992 TRI total releases and transfers of 55.6 million pounds were reported on forms from 615 Massachusetts facilities. The state ranks 38th in the nation for total releases (14.5 million pounds) and 26th for total transfers (41.0 million), according to the national TRI database.

The Chemical industry, dominant in New Jersey and nationally, plays a smaller role in the Massachusetts economy and, therefore, in the state's releases and transfers of toxic chemicals. As a percentage of total employment, the chemical industry accounts for 12 percent in New Jersey, 5 percent in the United States, and 3 percent in Massachusetts.[5] In 1992, according to each state's database, the Chemical industry accounted for 10 percent of Massachusetts' total releases and transfers from the manufacturing sector,[i] compared to 37 percent nationwide and 72 percent in New Jersey.[j]

Nearly all of Massachusetts' reported releases — 97 percent — are air emissions, a much higher proportion than is typical nationally, where air emissions are 58 percent of all releases, but the same as New Jersey where air emissions are 98 percent of all releases. In other states, underground injection (not practiced in either New Jersey or Massachusetts) and large surface water discharges (in Louisiana in particular) add significantly to releases, leaving air emissions with a smaller share of the total. (See Chapter 7.)

[i] Although these figures do not include releases and transfers for chemicals at two Monsanto chemical plants that have claimed trade secret status for those chemicals, the TRI releases and transfers from these two plants add 3.0 million pounds of releases and transfers. If these amounts were included, then the Chemical industry would account for about 15 percent of total releases and transfers in Massachusetts, still less than for New Jersey and the nation.

[j] Chemical industry's share of total releases and transfers for Massachusetts calculated from TURA data, excluding non-manufacturing industries; percentage for the United States calculated from federal TRI data.

Box 10-D. Monsanto Facilities in Massachusetts with Trade Secret Claims

The two Monsanto facilities located in Massachusetts, one in Springfield and one in Everett, have submitted data on use and byproduct to Massachusetts but have claimed they are trade secrets for some of the chemicals used at the facilities. Thus only summary numbers are available for some portion of the facilities' data. Both are chemical facilities; the Springfield plant produces polyvinyl resins, and the Everett plant produces polymer resins, according to their Massachusetts' submissions.

Total use and byproduct at the facilities are as follows:

	Use Pounds	**Byproduct** Pounds
Monsanto Springfield	233,338,701	14,105,170
Monsanto Everett	25,800,841	1,127,523

The Monsanto Springfield plant is, therefore, the largest in Massachusetts in terms of both use and byproduct, representing 17 percent of all use reported to Massachusetts and 9 percent of reported byproduct in 1992. The Monsanto Everett plant reported the ninth largest amount of use of toxic chemicals for 1992.

The amounts for those chemicals for which there are trade secret claims from these two Monsanto facilities, as well as all other facilities claiming trade secrets, are not included in the analysis is this chapter because of their trade secret status.

In 1992 Massachusetts DEP received forms from 644 facilities, which reported 16.3 million pounds in releases and 41.2 million pounds in transfers off site, for a total of 57.5 million pounds. As explained above, in addition to TRI chemicals and manufacturing industry sectors, Massachusetts collects data from non-manufacturing sectors and the expanded CERCLA list of chemicals.

In 1992 Massachusetts facilities reported using 1.3 billion pounds of toxic chemicals and generating 157.7 million pounds of toxic chemicals in waste. However, among the facilities claiming trade secrets were two Monsanto facilities representing 17 percent of all reported use and 9 percent of the reported byproduct. (See Box 10-D.) Specific data from facilities with trade secret claims are not included in the database available to the public and are not included in the following analysis.

Therefore, without the trade secret data, in 1992 Massachusetts facilities reported using 1.0 billion pounds of toxic chemicals, with 14 percent (142.7 million pounds) of the amount of use generated as byproduct and 6 percent (57.5 million pounds) as releases and transfers. Thus, 40 percent of the toxic chemicals generated as waste ("byproduct") ended up as releases or transfers.[k] (See Table 10-14.)

[k] The data from Massachusetts were obtained in January 1994. The data on trade secret claims were obtained in November 1994. (See Box 10-D.)

Materials Accounting Data in Massachusetts

The materials accounting data, as reported to Massachusetts, include:

- the amount processed,
- amount produced,
- amount otherwise used,
- amount shipped as/in product, and
- the total byproduct (waste). (See Box 10-B.)

In 1992 Massachusetts facilities reported total use (processed plus produced plus otherwise used) of 1.0 billion pounds, 424.9 million pounds shipped as or in product, and 142.7 million pounds generated as byproduct. Because Massachusetts does not require reporting the full materials accounting data, facilities are invited, but not required, to explain any discrepancies in inputs versus outputs. The total discrepancy for all facilities is 454.8 million pounds, or 44 percent of total use. (See Table 10-14.)

A look at the top 50 forms for largest generated byproduct suggests how, and how well, facilities account for the differences. The top 50 forms report 233.2 million pounds of total use (inputs) and 90.6 million pounds of byproduct and product combined (outputs). The collective discrepancy of 142.6 million pounds means that a higher portion of total use — 61 percent — is unaccounted for by the materials accounting data from these top 50 forms than is true for all forms.

On 17 of the top 50 forms, inputs and outputs balance precisely. On-site recycling is most often cited to explain differences where outputs exceed inputs (16 of 21 forms with net outputs). Forms with inputs greater than outputs most often indicate that the chemical was consumed or transformed (9 of 12 forms with net inputs). Seven forms with differences give no explanation. Overall, 68 percent (1,645 of the 2,355 forms) report inputs and outputs that balance within 2 percent.

Toxic Chemicals in Products, Massachusetts

Reporting to Massachusetts also includes how much of the toxic chemical is shipped off site in the products manufactured at the facility. Overall, 42 percent of the chemicals used as inputs to the manufacturing process is in the product when it is shipped off site. (See Table 10-14.) The industries that ship the largest percentage of their use of toxic chemicals in products are the Petroleum industry (SIC 29) and a non-manufacturing industry, wholesalers of non-durable goods (SIC 51). (See Table 10-15.) The Mobil Oil facility in East Boston distributing petroleum products reported that 1.8 million pounds of zinc compounds were shipped in its lubricating oils and additives in 1992.

Two Lumber facilities, Northeast Treaters and Universal Forest Products both located in Belchertown, reported a total of 1.5 million pounds of copper, chromium, and arsenic compounds used in the form of chromated copper arsenic as a

Table 10-14. Use, Byproduct, and Releases and Transfers, Massachusetts, 1992

	1992 Number			
Facilities	644			
Forms	2,355			
	Pounds	**Percent of Use** Percent	**Percent of Byproduct** Percent	**Total with Trade Secret Claims*** Pounds
Use	1,022,370,068			1,323,622,456
Manufactured	20,501,858			
Processed	814,474,044			
Otherwise Used	187,394,166			
Shipped as/in Product	424,911,092	41.56		
Byproduct (Waste)	142,662,835	13.95		157,720,818
Total Releases and Transfers	57,514,301	5.63	40.31	
Total Releases	16,346,944			
Total Air	15,901,822			
Fugitive Air	5,706,596			
Point Air	10,195,226			
Surface Water	198,494			
Underground Injection	156,393			
On-site Land	90,235			
Total Transfers	41,167,357			
POTW Transfers	4,046,880			
Other Transfers	37,120,477			

* See Box 10-D.

Table 10-15. Use, Chemicals in Product, and Chemicals in Byproduct by Industry, Massachusetts, 1992

SIC Code	Industry	Use Pounds	Shipped as/ in Product Pounds	Percent of Use Percent	Byproduct Pounds	Percent of Use Percent
20	Food	5,506,293	3,348,434	60.81	1,044,446	18.97
22	Textiles	32,606,076	1,903,621	5.84	15,343,796	47.06
24	Lumber	1,670,781	1,647,538	98.61	23,242	1.39
25	Furniture	232,963	24,541	10.53	164,512	70.62
26	Paper	20,340,859	1,264,715	6.22	7,309,292	35.93
27	Printing	919,059	0	0.00	1,028,379	111.89
28	Chemicals	483,685,224	121,294,851	25.08	16,798,514	3.47
29	Petroleum	2,137,237	2,130,541	99.69	6,696	0.31
30	Plastics	31,839,961	18,351,023	57.64	4,664,326	14.65
31	Leather	2,110,640	254,449	12.06	913,123	43.26
32	Stone/Clay	4,392,909	741,856	16.89	417,560	9.51
33	Primary Metals	92,908,219	80,023,302	86.13	10,659,450	11.47
34	Fabr. Metals	29,821,948	17,129,505	57.44	10,163,579	34.08
35	Machinery	3,620,117	2,460,546	67.97	1,126,526	31.12
36	Electrical	29,355,322	9,020,073	30.73	13,084,356	44.57
37	Transportation	1,536,434	812,951	52.91	492,622	32.06
38	Measure./Photo.	15,831,410	1,652,711	10.44	15,199,272	96.01
39	Miscellaneous	18,019,357	13,985,740	77.62	1,287,218	7.14
45	Air Transportation	438,991	0	0.00	438,991	100.00
49	Electric/Gas Services	13,261,692	0	0.00	2,196,791	16.56
51	Wholesale-nondurable	55,738,664	52,703,872	94.56	108,826	0.20
72	Personal Services	234,579	0	0.00	70,190	29.92
76	Repair Services	11,356	0	0.00	11,356	100.00
80	Health Services	38,234	96	0.25	38,138	99.75
	Multiple codes	163,087,447	93,385,918	57.26	25,518,012	15.65
	No SIC code given	13,024,296	2,774,809	21.30	14,553,622	111.74
	Total	1,022,370,068	424,911,092	41.56	142,662,835	13.95

wood preservative in their products. Toxic chemicals in products shipped by food industry facilities are 61 percent of use and include 940,000 pounds of acetic acid (used as a flavoring, to lower pH, and for product safety) in salad dressing from Ken's Foods located in Marlborough and 1.9 million pounds of phosphoric acid (used as a flavoring) in soft drinks shipped from Mid Atlantic Canners Association in Northampton. Acids such as these are toxic in high concentrations but not in the low concentrations found in foods.

Massachusetts Chemicals

Styrene is the chemical used in the largest amount in Massachusetts: facilities reported 292.9 million pounds used in 1992, which is 29 percent of all toxic chemical use in the state. Three polystyrene manufacturers (SIC 28) are responsible for 88 percent of that amount. (See facilities discussion below.) Facilities used copper in the second largest amount, 116.6 million pounds representing 11 percent of total use. Northeast Cable Corporation in Attleboro (SIC 33) reported using 43.8 million pounds of copper (38 percent of all copper use in Massachusetts) in 1992. This facility makes wire cables and rubber and plastic coverings for cable. (See Tables 10-16 and 10-17.)

The chemical with the third largest amount of use was sodium hydroxide; it is also the chemical generated as byproduct in the largest quantity in Massachusetts. Users of this chemical reported 17.2 million pounds of sodium hydroxide byproduct, which represents 15 percent of its total use amount. Sodium hydroxide was dropped from the federal TRI list, but is included on the Massachusetts list beginning in 1992, because it is a CERCLA chemical.

Toluene is the chemical generated as byproduct in the second largest amount, 16.7 million pounds in 1992. Toluene, a volatile organic chemical, has the largest amount of total releases and transfers in Massachusetts, 6.8 million pounds. Half of that amount (3.4 million pounds) is released to air, making toluene the top chemical for air emissions as well. Rexham Graphics of South Hadley (no SIC code reported, but a maker of coated paper and film and specialty chemicals) accounted for 15 percent (2.6 million pounds) of the total byproduct of this chemical generated in the state.

Massachusetts Chemicals of Special Concern

Byproduct as Percentage of Total Use

Use and byproduct generation are most relevant to consideration of pollution prevention goals; byproduct generation is of special interest to those concerned about immediate potential effects from toxic chemicals in waste. Comparing these amounts gives a perspective on efficiency in use. (See Chapter 2 of this report concerning the extent to which incorporation of toxic chemicals in products is often of equal or greater concern compared to toxics in waste.)

Table 10-16. Top 10 Facilities for Use, Byproduct, and Releases and Transfers, Massachusetts, 1992

Use Rank	Waste Rank	Releases and Transfers Rank	Facility	City	County	SIC Code
Facilities with Largest Use*						
1	14	256	Novacor Chemical Inc	Indian Orchard	Hampden	28
2	235	251	BASF Corp	Holyoke	Hampden	28
3	62	18	Novacor Chemical Inc	Leominster	Worcester	28
4	148	105	Northeast Cable Corp	Attleboro	Bristol	33
5	258	198	Boremco Specialty Chemicals	Fall River	Bristol	Mult.
6	428	376	American Polymers	Oxford	Worcester	28
7	6	99	Eastman Gelatin Corp	Peabody	Essex	28
8	336	413	Axton Cross	Holliston	Middlesex	51
9	296	231	Procter & Gamble	Quincy	Norfolk	28
10	372	387	Astro Chemicals Inc	Springfield	Hampden	51
			Subtotal			
			Percent of Total			
Facilities with Largest Byproduct (Waste)						
17	1	4	Rexham Graphics Inc	South Hadley	Hampshire	None
19	2	1	Polaroid Corporation	Waltham	Middlesex	38
15	3	25	Revere Copper Products	New Bedford	Bristol	33
42	4	15	Flexcon Co	Spencer	Worcester	22
16	5	2	ChemDesign Corp	Fitchburg	Worcester	28
7	6	99	Eastman Gelatin Corp	Peabody	Essex	28
28	7	21	Monsanto Chemical Co	Springfield	Hampden	Mult.
11	8	3	Texas Instruments	Attleboro	Bristol	Mult.
57	9	54	Wollaston Alloys Inc	Braintree	Norfolk	33
34	10	19	General Electric Co.	Pittsfield	Berkshire	Mult.
			Subtotal			
			Percent of Total			
Facilities with Largest Releases and Transfers						
19	2	1	Polaroid Corporation	Waltham	Middlesex	38
16	5	2	ChemDesign Corp	Fitchburg	Worcester	28
11	8	3	Texas Instruments	Attleboro	Bristol	Mult.
17	1	4	Rexham Graphics Inc	South Hadley	Hampshire	None
120	66	5	Wyman Gordon Company	North Grafton	Worcester	Mult.
63	22	6	Modern Alum Anodizing	North Adams	Berkshire	34
85	26	7	Malden Mills Industries Inc	Lawrence	Essex	22
31	30	8	Delta Surprenant	Clinton	Worcester	Mult.
100	15	9	AT&T	North Andover	Essex	36
82	13	10	Polaroid Corporation	Assonet	Bristol	38
			Subtotal			
			Percent of Total			
			Total for All Massachusetts Facilities			

* Two Monsanto facilities have claimed trade secret status for some of their chemicals and therefore their entire amounts do not appear on this table. (See Box 10-D.) The two facilities would rank first and ninth in terms of use. The Monsanto Springfield facility would rank second instead of seventh in terms of byproduct.

Use Pounds	Byproduct Pounds	Byproduct as Percentage of Use Percent	Total Releases and Transfers Pounds	Total Releases and Transfers as Percentage of Use Percent	Total Releases and Transfers as Percentage of Byproduct Percent
144,010,100	1,778,015	1.23	29,732	0.02	1.67
71,820,614	58,118	0.08	31,398	0.04	54.02
46,575,078	513,900	1.10	513,653	1.10	99.95
45,391,618	169,126	0.37	110,434	0.24	65.30
43,309,578	46,166	0.11	46,117	0.11	99.89
31,271,474	12,984	0.04	12,894	0.04	99.31
29,344,900	3,028,500	10.32	127,635	0.43	4.21
19,945,036	27,566	0.14	8,453	0.04	30.66
18,070,266	35,223	0.19	35,033	0.19	99.46
14,414,582	20,447	0.14	11,495	0.08	56.22
464,153,246	5,690,045	1.23	926,844	0.2	16.29
45.4	3.99		1.61		
10,363,225	14,507,522	139.99	2,502,111	24.14	17.25
9,811,711	11,258,322	114.74	4,976,227	50.72	44.20
10,970,147	5,598,787	51.04	396,958	3.62	7.09
4,525,015	4,548,495	100.52	603,620	13.34	13.27
10,650,140	4,102,320	38.52	2,872,214	26.97	70.01
29,344,900	3,028,500	10.32	127,635	0.43	4.21
6,951,701	2,927,400	42.11	450,104	6.47	15.38
13,480,200	2,927,100	21.71	2,797,380	20.75	95.57
3,362,479	2,319,273	68.98	224,618	6.68	9.68
5,806,175	2,303,510	39.67	512,235	8.82	22.24
105,265,693	53,521,229	50.84	15,463,102	14.69	28.89
10.3	37.52		26.89		
9,811,711	11,258,322	114.74	4,976,227	50.72	44.20
10,650,140	4,102,320	38.52	2,872,214	26.97	70.01
13,480,200	2,927,100	21.71	2,797,380	20.75	95.57
10,363,225	14,507,522	139.99	2,502,111	24.14	17.25
1,297,646	481,050	37.07	2,024,368	156.00	420.82
3,058,770	1,294,404	42.32	1,768,250	57.81	136.61
1,990,313	1,135,712	57.06	1,132,305	56.89	99.70
6,540,764	948,760	14.51	948,761	14.51	100.00
1,682,000	1,609,120	95.67	802,635	47.72	49.88
2,063,772	1,877,821	90.99	776,048	37.60	41.33
60,938,541	40,142,131	65.87	20,600,299	33.81	51.32
5.96	28.14		35.82		
1,022,370,068	142,662,835	13.95	57,514,301	5.63	40.31

Table 10-17. Top 25 Chemicals for Use, Massachusetts, 1992

Use Rank	By-product Rank	Releases and Trans-fers Rank	Chemical	Forms Number	Use Pounds	Byproduct Pounds	Byproduct as Percentage of Use Percent	Total Releases and Transfers Pounds	Total Releases and Trans-fers as Percent-age of Use Percent	Total Releases and Trans-fers as Percent-age of Byproduct Percent
1	15	27	Styrene	17	292,881,733	2,109,845	0.72	386,439	0.13	18.32
2	10	2	Copper	99	116,577,051	5,047,266	4.33	5,210,798	4.47	103.24
3	1	12	Sodium hydroxide (solution)	174	82,408,109	17,161,231	20.82	1,678,347	2.04	9.78
4	3	25	Sulfuric acid	173	66,106,319	12,473,995	18.87	445,766	0.67	3.57
5	9	33	Hydrochloric acid	81	41,900,946	5,241,277	12.51	284,307	0.68	5.42
6	2	1	Toluene	96	31,042,210	16,704,236	53.81	6,777,185	21.83	40.57
7	7	6	Copper compounds	34	21,951,527	7,613,636	34.68	2,870,774	13.08	37.71
8	4	3	Methyl ethyl ketone	66	18,602,270	11,476,572	61.69	3,541,311	19.04	30.86
9	28	21	Zinc compounds	63	17,325,857	708,715	4.09	645,785	3.73	91.12
10	8	7	Methanol	65	16,067,846	5,768,270	35.90	2,737,894	17.04	47.46
11	11	5	1,1,1-Trichloroethane	93	14,734,385	3,632,631	24.65	2,908,026	19.74	80.05
12	16	11	Ammonia	83	13,778,377	1,945,781	14.12	1,711,600	12.42	87.96
13	19	14	Chromium	50	12,988,179	1,700,650	13.09	1,569,984	12.09	92.32
14	40	38	Formaldehyde	15	12,832,089	261,262	2.04	225,589	1.76	86.35
15	5	4	Acetone	68	12,435,741	10,635,386	85.52	3,442,739	27.68	32.37
16	17	8	Nickel	49	12,161,957	1,826,216	15.02	2,490,714	20.48	136.39
17	13	20	Acetic acid	37	11,272,201	2,785,117	24.71	767,031	6.80	27.54
18	22	10	Phosphoric acid	38	11,176,183	1,530,171	13.69	1,781,297	15.94	116.41
19	47	41	Ammonium hydroxide	14	9,833,752	200,601	2.04	173,734	1.77	86.61
20	6	16	Ethylacetate	31	9,313,688	8,363,691	89.80	1,451,404	15.58	17.35
21	58	67	Methyl methacrylate	10	9,106,974	89,986	0.99	41,786	0.46	46.44
22	25	17	Glycol ethers	52	8,791,318	1,177,554	13.39	985,548	11.21	83.69
23	12	9	Dichloromethane	38	8,349,831	2,913,059	34.89	2,446,481	29.30	83.98
24	39	36	Lead compounds	31	7,818,457	266,492	3.41	270,766	3.46	101.60
25	24	22	Ethylene glycol	34	7,682,814	1,411,451	18.37	624,736	8.13	44.26
			Subtotal	1,511	867,139,814	123,045,091	14.19	45,470,041	5.24	36.95
			Percent of Total	64.16	84.82	86.25		79.06		
			Total	2,355	1,022,370,068	142,662,835	13.95	57,514,301	5.63	40.31

While the overall proportion of byproduct generated as a percentage of total use is 14 percent for the chemicals reported in Massachusetts, for the group of carcinogens the percentage is 3 percent. (See Table 10-18.) For those chemical classes and other groups of chemicals of special interest for their potential health and environmental effects, this is not the case. For ozone-depleting, chloro-organic, and halo-organic chemicals, generated byproduct is 25 percent or more of total use, while for metals the proportion is closer to that for all chemicals, 9 percent. Furthermore, for each of these special groups of chemicals, including carcinogens, a much greater proportion (79 to 84 percent) of byproduct becomes releases and transfers than for all TURA chemicals, for which releases and transfers constitute 40 percent of byproduct generated. (See Table 10-18.)

Carcinogens

Styrene, the chemical used in the largest amount in Massachusetts, is a carcinogen. Other carcinogens among the 25 chemicals used in the largest amounts are chromium, formaldehyde, nickel, and dichloromethane.[l]

It is not the largest generators of carcinogen byproducts that are principally responsible for large carcinogen releases and transfers. The facility ranked 16th for generation of carcinogenic byproducts, Wyman Gordon Company of North Grafton, accounted for more than twice the amount of carcinogen releases and transfers of any other Massachusetts facility. This Fabricated Metals (SIC 34) facility in Worcester County makes stainless steel and other metal alloy forgings and reported 1.6 million pounds of releases and transfers of nickel and chromium, primarily as off-site transfers.[m]

Wollaston Alloys Inc. in Braintree, a steel foundry (SIC 33) making sand-molded metals and metal castings, generated more carcinogens as byproduct (1.9 million pounds) than any other facility in the state, including 899,000 pounds of nickel. Novacor Chemical in Indian Orchard, a Chemical facility (SIC 28) manufacturing polystyrene, generated 1.7 million pounds of styrene byproduct. (See further analysis of Novacor data below under Massachusetts Facilities.) These two facilities generated 34 percent of the state's carcinogenic byproduct in 1992.

Ozone Depleters

The leading facility for generating byproduct of ozone depleters is Northrop Corporation (SIC 38) in Norwood, with 562,200 pounds of byproduct, of which 146,261 pounds are released and transferred. It uses the ozone-depleters 1,1,1-trichloroethane and Freon 113 for cleaning gyroscope parts.[n] The AT&T facility (SIC 36) in North Andover generates the second largest amount of byproduct of ozone depleter, with 377,000 pounds of 1,1,1-trichloroethane byproduct and 323,000 pounds of releases and transfers. This facility uses 1,1,1-trichloroethane in metal plating and etching.

Chloro-organics

The Polaroid facility, which synthesizes and blends photographic chemicals (SIC 38), in Waltham leads the state in generating chloro-organic byproducts, with

l Chromium and nickel form many different compounds, some of which are carcinogenic and others are not.

m The off-site transfers of 1.2 million pounds of nickel were to recycling. The reporting on this facility's form is in error. The amount sent off site to recycling was not included in amount processed nor in amount shipped as product — as it should have been if it was sent directly to a recycler and the material required no further processing before sale — nor in byproduct — as it should have been if it required treatment before resale. Therefore, the total releases and transfers is greater than byproduct and use. (See also Table 10-16.)

n Details about what a Massachusetts facility produces are available from the TURA database in the form of a description of each production unit. This is more detailed information than New Jersey, which includes a short description of the type of business for the whole facility, and than TRI which has only the 4-digit SIC code(s).

Table 10-18. Use, Byproduct, and Releases and Transfers by Chemical Group, Massachusetts, 1992

	All TURA Chemicals	Only TRI Chemicals	Carcinogens	Ozone Depleters	Chloro-Organics	Metals	Halo-organics
Number of Forms	2,355	2,153	280	155	253	527	267
	Pounds	Pounds	Pounds	Pounds	Pounds	Pounds	Pounds
Use	1,022,370,068	958,498,997	368,095,800	22,348,244	41,588,605	220,782,428	42,877,146
Manufactured	20,501,858	17,073,403	847,299	1,917,811	1,900,000	1,961,523	1,917,811
Processed	814,474,044	776,029,801	363,581,372	16,035,826	30,372,989	211,371,448	31,625,519
Otherwise Used	187,394,166	165,395,793	3,667,129	4,394,607	9,315,616	7,449,457	9,333,816
Shipped as/in Product	424,911,092	399,954,257	81,159,684	16,722,605	26,527,735	193,714,036	27,764,461
Byproduct (Waste)	142,662,835	128,662,935	10,775,277	5,557,552	11,512,754	19,809,220	11,566,447
Byproduct as Percent of Use	13.95%	13.42%	2.92%	24.86%	27.68%	8.97%	26.97%
Total Releases and Transfers	57,514,301	54,035,520	8,841,896	4,683,001	9,354,496	15,742,479	9,407,797
Total Releases	16,346,944	14,759,368	1,576,507	3,416,171	5,555,128	156,552	5,579,618
Total Air Emissions	15,901,822	14,320,111	1,529,323	3,401,423	5,540,123	107,547	5,562,908
Water Discharges	198,494	198,064	5,038	260	515	4,364	520
Underground Injection	156,393	156,213	31	0	2	166	2
On-site Land Releases	90,235	84,980	42,115	14,488	14,488	44,475	16,188
Total Transfers	41,167,357	39,276,152	7,265,389	1,266,830	3,799,368	15,585,927	3,828,179
Transfers to POTWs	4,046,880	3,616,746	56,282	7,209	40,311	239,246	41,096
Other Off-site Transfers	37,120,477	35,659,406	7,209,107	1,259,621	3,759,057	15,346,681	3,787,083
Releases/Transfers as Percent of Use	5.62%	5.63%	2.40%	20.95%	22.49%	7.13%	21.94%
Releases/Transfers as Percent of Byproduct	40.31%	41.99%	82.05%	84.26%	81.25%	79.47%	81.33%

1.3 million pounds of dichloromethane, 1,2-dichlorobenzene, and chlorobenzene. Releases and transfers of these chemicals totaled 528,000 pounds. (See Massachusetts Facilities discussion below.) The facility with the second largest byproduct of chloro-organic chemicals is the AT&T facility in North Andover. Its byproduct of 1,1,1-trichloroethane is discussed above in the section on ozone depleters, since this chemical is both a chloro-organic and an ozone depleter.

Halo-organics

1,1,1-Trichloroethane, dichloromethane, trichloroethylene, and Freon 113 are the four halo-organic chemicals that appear among the 25 chemicals with the largest byproduct reported in 1992. All halo-organics represented 8 percent of the total byproduct and 16 percent of the total releases and transfers reported to Massachusetts in that year. Because of the byproduct associated with dichloroethane at the Polaroid plant in

Waltham and the byproduct associated with 1,1,1-trichloroethane at the AT&T plant in North Andover, as mentioned above, these plants also are the two facilities with the largest amount of byproduct of halo-organics reported in 1992.

Metals

Copper, copper compounds, nickel, nickel compounds, and zinc compounds are all among the top 25 chemicals for generated byproduct in Massachusetts. Metals make up 14 percent of generated byproducts and 27 percent of all releases and transfers in the state. Massachusetts facilities generated 19.8 million pounds of metals in byproduct in 1992 and 15.7 million pounds in releases and transfers.

Revere Copper Products (SIC 33) in New Bedford generated 5.4 million pounds of metals as byproduct, nearly all copper compounds. This facility melts copper alloys into ingots and rolls the ingots into plates and sheets. Texas Instruments (Multiple SIC codes) in Attleboro generated 2.4 million pounds, mostly of copper compounds and nickel compounds. Releases and transfers reported by Revere Copper totaled 358,000 pounds, while those reported by Texas Instruments totaled virtually all of its 2.4 million pounds of byproduct. This facility produces a variety of industrial metal products such as precision controls, motor controls, switches, sockets, and steel clad wire products.

Third in the state for total releases and transfers, this Texas Instruments facility also ranks among the top 10 in other categories. Its large quantity of generated byproduct places it second for generated byproduct for metals, third for carcinogens, sixth for TRI chemicals, eighth for chloro-organics, and eighth for all TURA chemicals.

Massachusetts Facilities

As with New Jersey, several individual facilities report a large proportion of use of toxic chemicals in the state. The 10 Massachusetts' facilities with the largest use of toxic chemicals in 1992, of which 6 are Chemical industry facilities, contribute 45 percent (464.2 million pounds) of the state's total use. However, they report just 4 percent of the state's byproduct generated and 2 percent of total releases and transfers. (See Table 10-16.) (See Box 10-D, which explains that the Monsanto plant in Springfield is not included in the table even though it has the largest use reported because of the trade secret claims made by the facility.)

The top three facilities are all polystyrene manufacturers, but they exhibit striking differences in their use and generated waste of toxic chemicals. Novacor Chemical[o] in Indian Orchard (part of the city of Springfield) used 139.0 million pounds of styrene (all of it processed). The plant reported that none of the styrene was shipped in its products and that 1.7 million pounds (1 percent) ended up as byproduct. Of this byproduct, just 0.02 percent was reported as releases and transfers (20,000

[o] The Novacor Chemical plant in Indian Orchard was previously owned by Polysar, Inc., and reported to Massachusetts under that name in 1992.

Figure 10-17.

Massachusetts Materials Accounting Data: Styrene at Novacor Chemical Inc., Indian Orchard

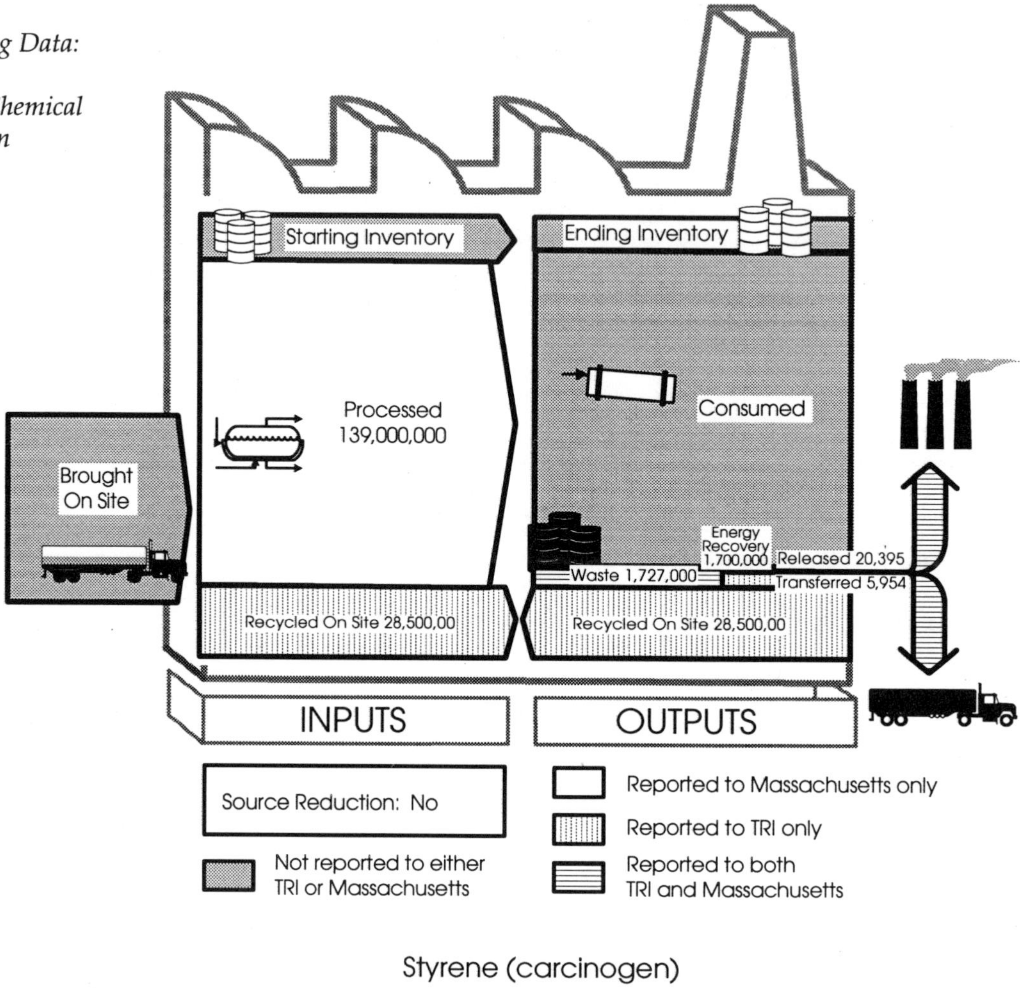

in Pounds (not drawn to scale)

pounds as air emissions and 6,000 pounds as transfers). This facility's federal TRI data show that substantially more was generated as waste and then recycled or used in energy recovery on site. The TRI data show that 28.5 million pounds was recycled on site and that 1.7 million pounds was used for energy recovery.[p] (See Figure 10-17.)

The second-ranked facility, BASF Corporation's plant in nearby Holyoke, reported using 71.8 million pounds of styrene. It shipped 34,400 pounds in its products, and 42,600 pounds ended up as byproduct. The BASF plant reported recycling on site 23,000 pounds but, unlike Novacor, included this amount in byproduct. BASF reported half the amount of

[p] The Massachusetts DEP stated that the TRI reporting is in error because the recycling is in process or "hard-piped" and should not have been reported to TRI. (Suzi Peck, telephone conversation, November 14, 1994.)

Figure 10-18.

Massachusetts Materials Accounting Data: Styrene at BASF Corp., Holyoke

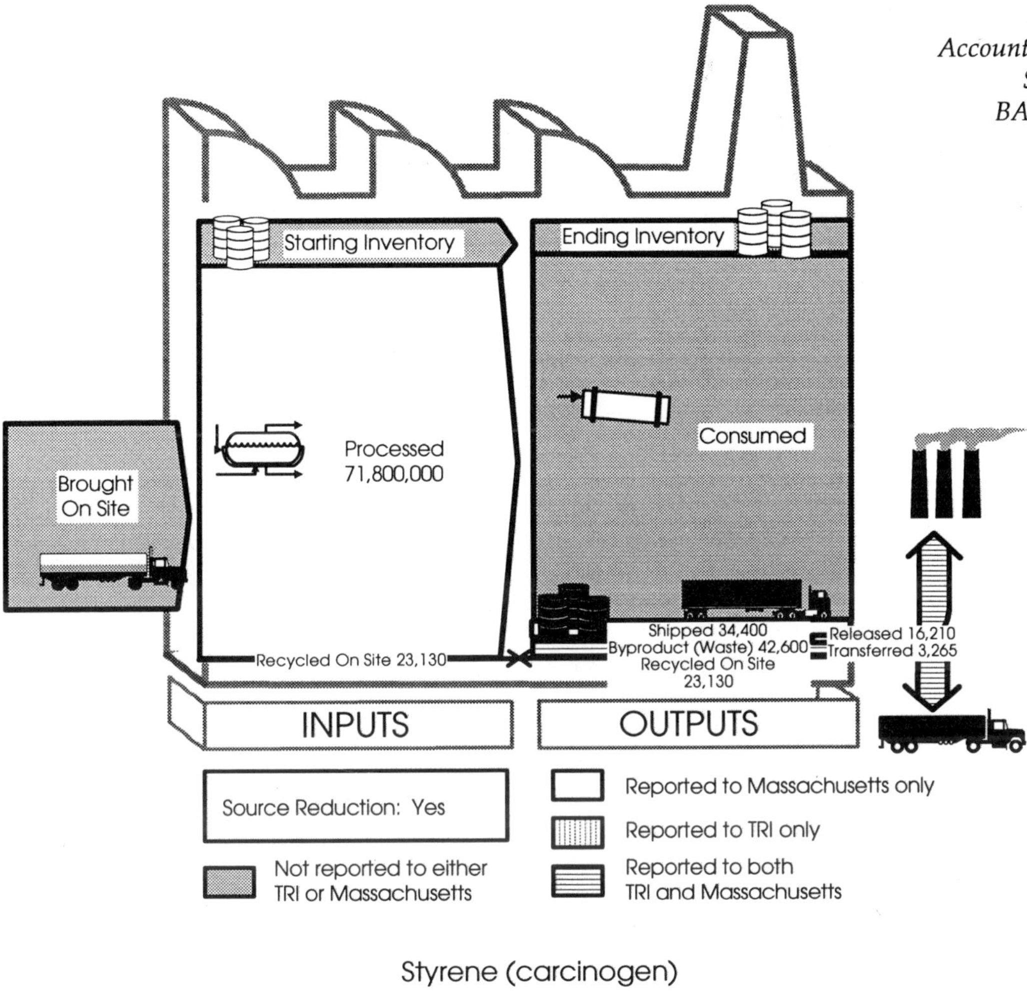

in Pounds (not drawn to scale)

use of styrene of Novacor but more than half of the amount of releases and transfers that Novacor did, releasing 16,200 pounds to the air from the site compared to 20,400 pounds from Novacor. (See Figure 10-18.)

The third-ranked facility, another Novacor Chemical facility, in Leominster, showed about the same rate of byproduct generation as the Novacor plant in Indian Orchard. Its use of styrene was 46.3 million pounds. It reported as byproduct 240,000 pounds, which does not include 1.6 million pounds recycled on site reported to TRI but does include 190,000 pounds of energy recovery on site. All of the byproduct was reported as releases and transfers. This level of use is one-third that of the Indian Orchard Novacor plant. The rate of byproduct generation is 1 percent of use, the same as the Novacor plant in Indian Orchard but 10 times that reported by the BASF plant.

The BASF facility has reported undertaking source reduction activities since 1990; it reported modernizing both materials handling and process operations in 1992. The Novacor Indian Orchard facility reported source reduction in 1991 only, and Novacor in Leominster has never reported using source reduction.

Only one of the facilities with the largest amount of use, Eastman Gelatin in Peabody, ranked among the top 10 for byproduct generated. This chemical facility makes photographic gelatins. The 10 facilities reporting the largest amount of byproduct generated account for 38 percent (53.5 million pounds) of the state's total byproduct. Their portion of Massachusetts' total use is 10 percent (105.3 million pounds), and their proportion of total releases and transfers is 27 percent (15.5 million pounds). Three of the top 10 facilities reported larger amounts of byproduct generated than the amount used; all explained this by reporting that they recycled the chemicals on site. (See Table 10-16.)

The leading facility for byproduct generated, Rexham Graphics, Inc., in South Hadley, produces coated paper and film and specialty chemicals. This facility submitted three of the top four forms for largest generated byproduct in 1992: acetone (5.2 million pounds), methyl ethyl ketone (3.2 million), and toluene (2.6 million). All three were recycled on site, which explains why its byproduct amounts to 140 percent of total use.

The facility with the second largest amount of byproduct generated, Polaroid Corporation's facility in Waltham, produces photographic chemicals. It generated as byproduct 1.7 million pounds of acetone and, after on-site recycling, transferred 1.1 million pounds off site. Of its 5.0 million pounds of total releases and transfers, 1.2 million were acetone.

This same Polaroid facility reported the largest amount of total releases and transfers in Massachusetts in 1992; its 5.0 million pounds represented 9 percent of the state's total. The 10 facilities reporting the largest total releases and transfers accounted for 36 percent of the state's total releases and transfers, but just 6 percent of the total use and 28 percent of the total byproduct generated.

Massachusetts Industries

Industrial Patterns of Use, Byproduct, and Releases and Transfers

The relationships of use, byproduct, and releases and transfers vary strikingly from industry to industry in Massachusetts. Despite the lesser prominence of the Chemical industry in this state than in many others, that industry does have the most TURA-reporting facilities in Massachusetts of all industry sectors and reports almost half of all use of toxic chemicals in the state. However, it ranks second for amount of generated byproduct and third for releases and transfers, with about the same amount of releases and transfers as both the Electrical and the Measuring/ Photographic industries. Since the Chemical industry has the most facilities, its average releases and

Table 10-19. Use, Byproduct, and Releases and Transfers by Industry, Massachusetts, 1992

SIC Code	Industry	Facilities Number	Forms Number	Use Pounds	Byproduct Pounds	Byproduct as Percentage of Use Percent	Total Releases and Transfers Pounds	Total Releases and Transfers as Percentage of Use Percent	Total Releases and Transfers as Percentage of Byproduct Percent
20	Food	15	35	5,506,293	1,044,446	18.97	384,010	6.97	36.77
22	Textiles	34	113	32,606,076	15,343,796	47.06	3,605,885	11.06	23.50
24	Lumber	4	10	1,670,781	23,242	1.39	26,262	1.57	112.99
25	Furniture	6	11	232,963	164,512	70.62	141,054	60.55	85.74
26	Paper	31	89	20,340,859	7,309,292	35.93	1,159,528	5.70	15.86
27	Printing	9	12	919,059	1,028,379	111.89	439,777	47.85	42.76
28	Chemicals	94	505	483,685,224	16,798,514	3.47	6,831,644	1.41	40.67
29	Petroleum	2	3	2,137,237	6,696	0.31	6,560	0.31	97.97
30	Plastics	45	117	31,839,961	4,664,326	14.65	2,280,942	7.16	48.90
31	Leather	9	28	2,110,640	913,123	43.26	565,729	26.80	61.96
32	Stone/Clay	7	23	4,392,909	417,560	9.51	379,894	8.65	90.98
33	Primary Metals	45	121	92,908,219	10,659,450	11.47	2,703,658	2.91	25.36
34	Fabr. Metals	92	276	29,821,948	10,163,579	34.08	5,655,270	18.96	55.64
35	Machinery	18	38	3,620,117	1,126,526	31.12	608,752	16.82	54.04
36	Electrical	61	219	29,355,322	13,084,356	44.57	6,861,314	23.37	52.44
37	Transportation	9	24	1,536,434	492,622	32.06	426,703	27.77	86.62
38	Measure./Photo.	21	90	15,831,410	15,199,272	96.01	6,831,345	43.15	44.95
39	Miscellaneous	19	59	18,019,357	1,287,218	7.14	1,963,613	10.90	152.55
45	Air Transportation	2	2	438,991	438,991	100.00	260,116	59.25	59.25
49	Electric/Gas Services	19	43	13,261,692	2,196,791	16.56	156,603	1.18	7.13
51	Wholesale-Nondurable	6	98	55,738,664	108,826	0.20	81,070	0.15	74.50
72	Personal Services	5	5	234,579	70,190	29.92	94,025	40.08	133.96
76	Repair Services	1	1	11,356	11,356	100.00	11,356	100.00	100.00
80	Health Services	1	1	38,234	38,138	99.75	38	0.10	0.10
	Multiple codes	78	405	163,087,447	25,518,012	15.65	13,383,638	8.21	52.45
	No SIC code given	11	27	13,024,296	14,553,622	111.74	2,655,515	20.39	18.25
	Total	644	2,355	1,022,370,068	142,662,835	13.95	57,514,301	5.63	40.31

transfers per facility (72,700 pounds per facility) are much less than that of the Electrical industry (112,500 pounds per facility) or the Measuring/Photographic industry (330,100 pounds per facility). (See Table 10-19.)

In the Chemical industry, more of the chemical used goes into the chemical product. The Measuring/Photographic industry, makers of instruments and producers of photographic goods, and the Electrical industry, for example, use more solvents, which are far more likely to end up in waste. Relationships between use and releases and transfers characterize differences among industries; they may also suggest prospects for efforts in toxics use reduction. For example, an Electrical industry facility may be able to substitute a less toxic substance or procedure for its solvent use, whereas a polystyrene manufacturer must use styrene but can concentrate on reducing the waste, or lost raw material, from the manufacturing process, thereby reducing inputs.

Industries with similar quantities of byproduct do not necessarily show similar patterns of release and transfer. In 1992 Massachusetts' Primary Metals industry used 92.9 million pounds of reportable chemicals, three and a half times the use reported by Fabricated Metals facilities (29.8 million pounds). The two industries generated approximately equal quantities of byproduct: 10.7 million and 10.2 million pounds, respectively. Releases and transfers of the Primary Metals industry totaled 2.7 million pounds, less than half the 5.7 million pounds that the Fabricated Metals industry released or transferred. Releases and transfers by the Fabricated Metals industry amount to 56 percent of its reported byproduct, while releases and transfers from the Primary Metals industry are 25 percent of its byproduct quantity. Primary Metals manufacturers are more likely to be able to reuse as feedstock portions of their toxic chemical byproduct. This could also account for the difference in byproduct they generate as a percentage of use: 34 percent for Fabricated Metals and 12 percent for Primary Metals. (See Table 10-19.)

Even less consistent is the relationship between byproduct and use from one industry to the next. Massachusetts' Chemical industry generated 16.8 million pounds as byproduct in 1992, or 3 percent of its total use. Among manufacturing industries, only the Lumber (SIC 24) and Petroleum (SIC 29) industries in Massachusetts generated less byproduct as a percentage of use. Byproduct in the Measuring/Photographic industry (SIC 38) amounted to 96 percent of total use, and the Printing industry (SIC 27) reported byproduct in excess of its total use, 112 percent. Of the nine Printing industry facilities in Massachusetts, one reported total use greater than its byproduct due to the chemical being consumed in the production process. Of those reporting byproduct greater than use, three indicated this was due to recycling and one did not indicate why.

Industrial Distribution of Releases and Transfers

The industry category that dominates Massachusetts' releases and transfers is "Multiple Codes," that is, facilities that list more than one SIC code on their forms. This category led in quantities of use, byproduct, and releases and transfers. In 1992, facilities reporting Multiple Codes accounted for 13.4 million pounds of Massachusetts' total releases and transfers (23 percent). (See Table 10-19.)

Among those reporting Multiple Codes, the 11 facilities that reported the combination of Primary Metals (SIC 33) and Fabricated Metals (SIC 34) had the largest amount of releases and transfers of any multiple-code combination, with 3.0 million pounds. The code combination with the second largest amount of releases and transfers was that reported by one facility, Texas Instruments located in Attleboro, which reported 2.8 million pounds. That facility reported under seven SIC codes: Plastics (30), Stone/Clay/Glass (32), Primary

Metals (33), Fabricated Metals (34), Electrical (36), Transportation (37), and Measuring/Photographic (38).

Non-manufacturing Industries

Non-manufacturing industries (i.e., those required to report to TURA although not to TRI) accounted for 603,000 pounds of 1992 releases and transfers, just 1 percent of the total. These industries include Air Transportation (SIC 45), Electric/Gas Services (49), Non-durable Wholesale Trade (51), Personal Services (72), Repair Services (76), and Health Services (80). Among the non-manufacturing industries, facilities in Non-durable Wholesale Trade submitted the most forms (98 forms) in 1992.

Only the Air Transportation industry, among both manufacturing and non-manufacturing sectors, reported releases to media other than air greater than 20,000 pounds. This was entirely due to one facility, the TWA Hangar at Logan Airport, Boston, which reported a total of 260,000 pounds of ethylene glycol (a chemical used to de-ice airplanes) released to surface waters and underground injection wells, 130,000 pounds to each.

Although 22nd among reporting industries for releases and transfers, Non-durable Wholesale Trade ranked 4th in total use (behind Chemicals, Multiple Codes, and Primary Metals) with 55.7 million pounds. These facilities receive industrial chemicals in bulk and repackage them for distribution.

Toxic Chemicals by Massachusetts Counties

Facilities located in 12 of the 14 counties in Massachusetts report the use of toxic chemicals; the exceptions are Dukes and Nantucket Counties, which encompass islands off the southeast coast. One county, Hampden, accounts for 28 percent of total use in the state. Middlesex County, however, has the most facilities reporting, the largest amount of byproduct generated, and the largest amount of releases and transfers. Worcester County has the second largest amounts of all three measures. (See Map 10-2 and Table 10-20.)

Hampden County is first-ranked in total use because the two facilities with the largest total use reported are located there — Novacor in Indian Orchard and BASF in Holyoke, which together account for 71 percent of the county's total reported toxic chemical use. Middlesex County has more facilities contributing to its share of toxic chemical waste, but the Polaroid facility in Waltham does account for 37 percent each of that county's generated byproduct and its total releases and transfers.

Map 10-2.

Massachusetts Releases and Transfers, Byproduct, and Use, by County, 1992

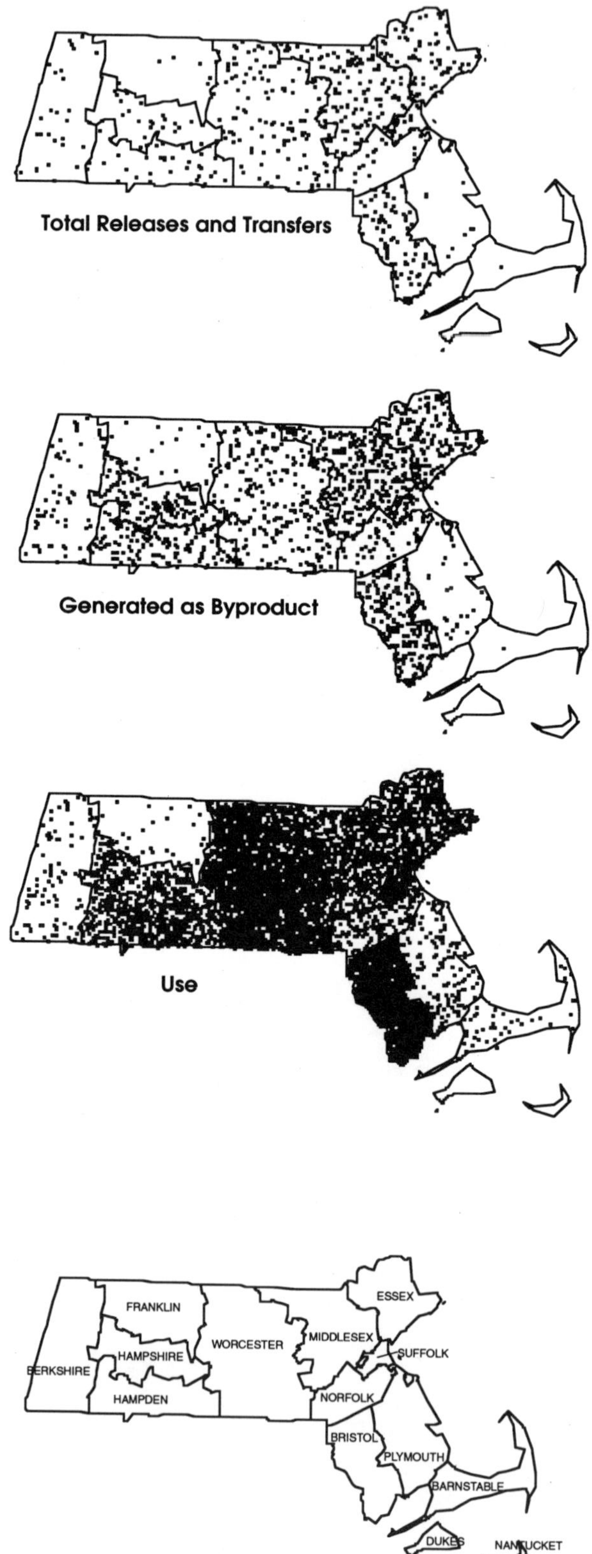

Each dot = 100,000 pounds

Table 10-20. Use, Byproduct, and Releases and Transfers by County, Massachusetts, 1992

County	Facilities	Total Use		Byproduct		Total Releases and Transfers	
	Number	Pounds	Percent	Pounds	Percent	Pounds	Percent
Barnstable	3	9,848,788	0.96	278,242	0.20	283,451	0.49
Berkshire	14	13,490,143	1.32	6,590,726	4.62	2,870,874	4.99
Bristol	87	201,528,687	19.71	21,961,317	15.39	9,415,725	16.37
Dukes	0	0	—	0	—	0	—
Essex	87	100,096,765	9.79	17,903,444	12.55	7,720,906	13.42
Franklin	13	7,954,211	0.78	2,375,643	1.67	658,629	1.15
Hampden	74	289,460,199	28.31	13,174,952	9.24	3,371,080	5.86
Hampshire	16	30,589,966	2.99	15,050,106	10.55	2,752,360	4.79
Middlesex	141	107,614,524	10.53	30,229,302	21.19	13,339,886	23.19
Nantucket	0	0	—	0	—	0	—
Norfolk	52	43,257,866	4.23	5,404,610	3.79	2,369,555	4.12
Plymouth	23	15,109,771	1.48	3,479,079	2.44	990,936	1.72
Suffolk	34	17,892,133	1.75	2,720,867	1.91	1,569,204	2.73
Worcester	100	185,527,015	18.15	23,494,547	16.47	12,171,695	21.16
Total	644	1,022,370,068	100.00	142,662,835	100.00	57,514,301	100.00

Facility Portraits in Massachusetts

While the Massachusetts data do not contain all the component details of the use of the toxic chemical, the data elements do allow for determination of the amount used and the amount of waste generated. Together with data reported to the federal TRI, one can see how the chemical goes from being an input to being used in the facility's operations to being shipped as part of a product (or not) and finally ending up as waste. These data, like their counterparts in New Jersey, allow the comparison of individual facilities and reveal why releases and transfers might differ. This in turn may aid in identifying source reduction opportunities in a way that is not possible when only the amounts of releases and transfers are available.

Individual facilities in different manufacturing sectors use the same toxic chemical but in different ways. The Massachusetts data aid in comparisons of these differences. For example, the Heatbath Corporation in Indian Orchard blends chemicals to make liquid phosphate products and uses zinc compounds in the process. It produced 158,000 pounds of zinc compounds in 1992 and processed an additional 49,500 pounds, shipping in its products 158,000 pounds. The waste generated amounted to 141 pounds, of which (according to the federal TRI data) 119 were recycled, 22 pounds were released to the air, and 1 pound was sent to the municipal sewage treatment plant. (See Figure 10-19.)

In contrast, the New England Plating Company in Worcester, a zinc plater, produced 94,800 pounds of zinc compounds in 1992, processed an additional 74,600

Figure 10-19.

Massachusetts Materials Accounting Data: Zinc Compounds at Heatbath Corp., Indian Orchard

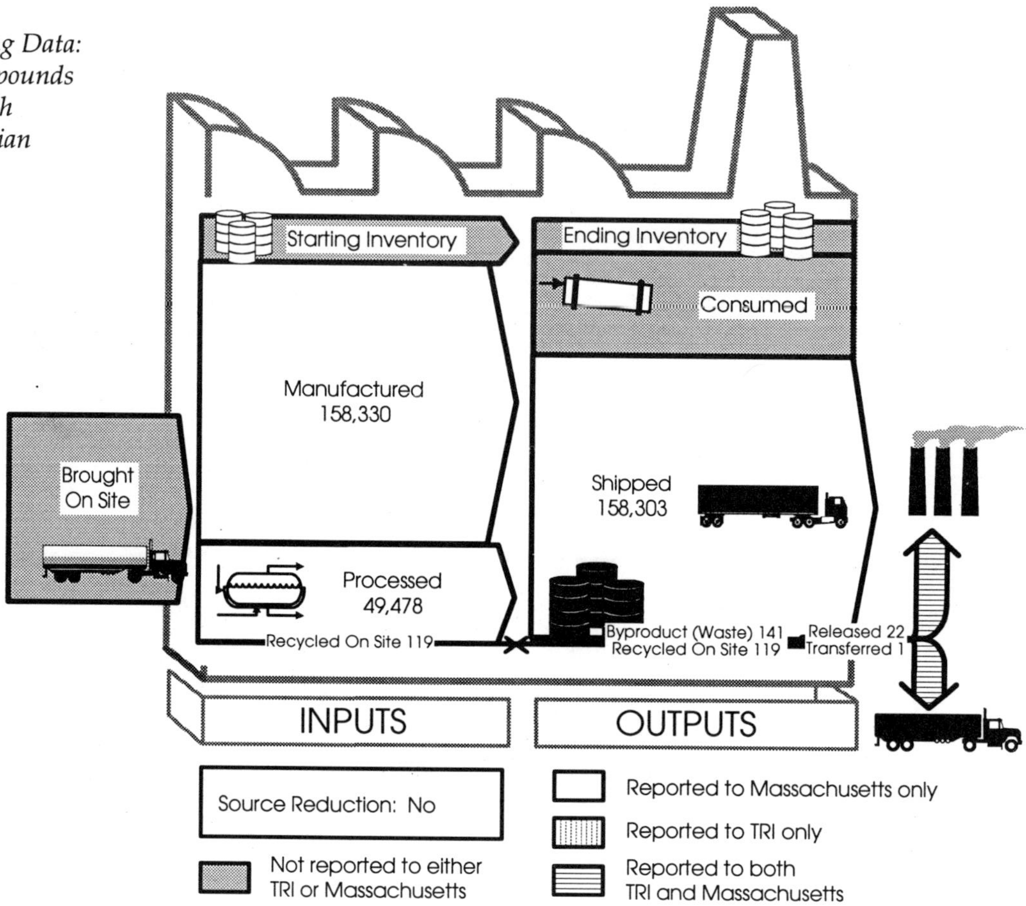

in Pounds (not drawn to scale)

Zinc Compounds (metal)

pounds, and otherwise used 20,200 pounds, for a total use of 189,600 pounds. It shipped in its products 74,600 pounds and generated as byproduct 20,200 pounds, indicating the excess in use was held in inventory. Of the byproduct amount, 15,100 pounds were transferred off site and 300 pounds were discharged to surface waters from the site. Thus, while Heatbath used 208,000 pounds of zinc compounds, it generated less than 0.07 percent as waste (141 pounds) in its blending operations. New England Plating, on the other hand, used 18,400 pounds less of zinc compounds (189,600 pounds) but

Figure 10-20.

Massachusetts Materials Accounting Data: Zinc Compounds at New England Plating, Worcester

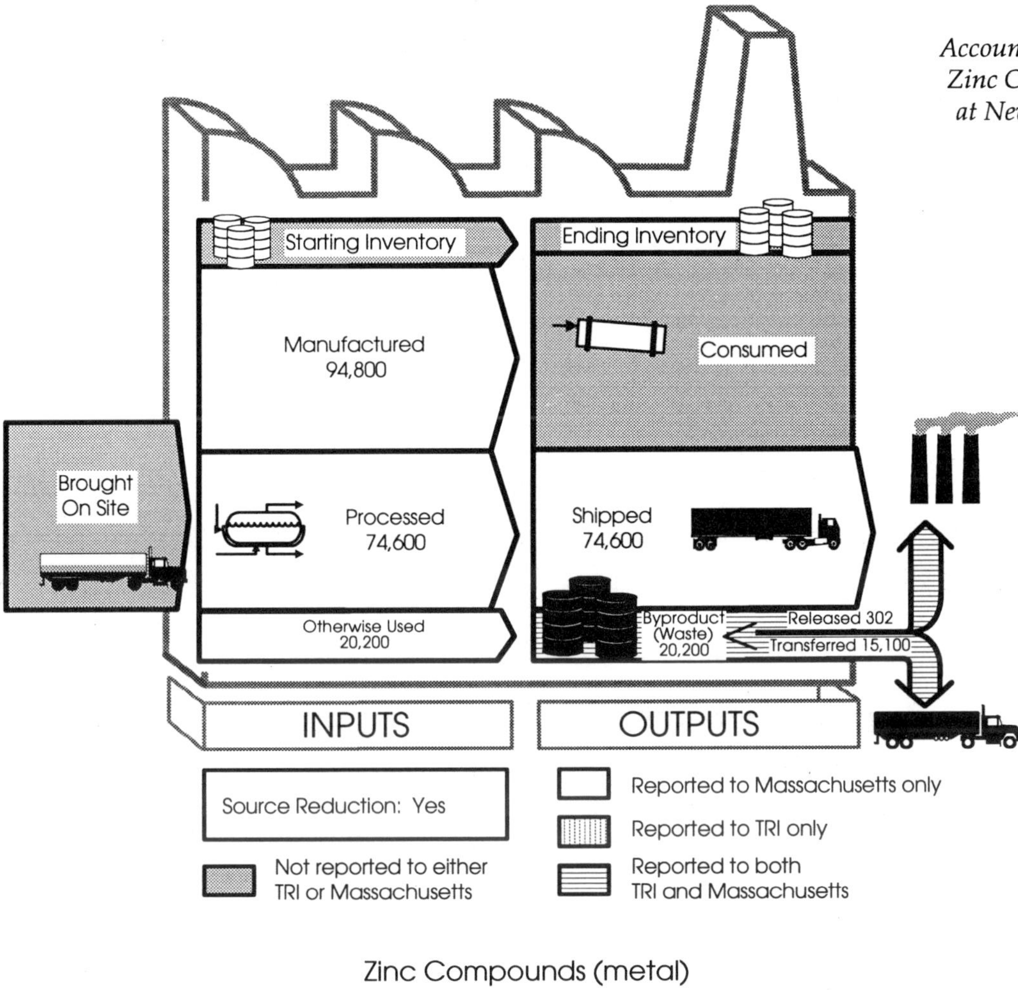

in Pounds (not drawn to scale)

generated 20,200 pounds of waste in its zinc plating operations. These are not surprising differences. Blending operations by definition use all of the raw material to make the product. Any waste is due to poor housekeeping or inefficiency. Plating operations remove a chemical from the plating bath solution and deposit it onto the product, leaving what is not needed in the remainder of the plating solution as waste. Although plating solutions can be reused, they often become contaminated, resulting in waste. (See Figures 10-19 and 10-20.)

Figure 10-21.

Massachusetts Materials Accounting Data: Tetrachloroethylene at Standard Uniform Services, Agawam

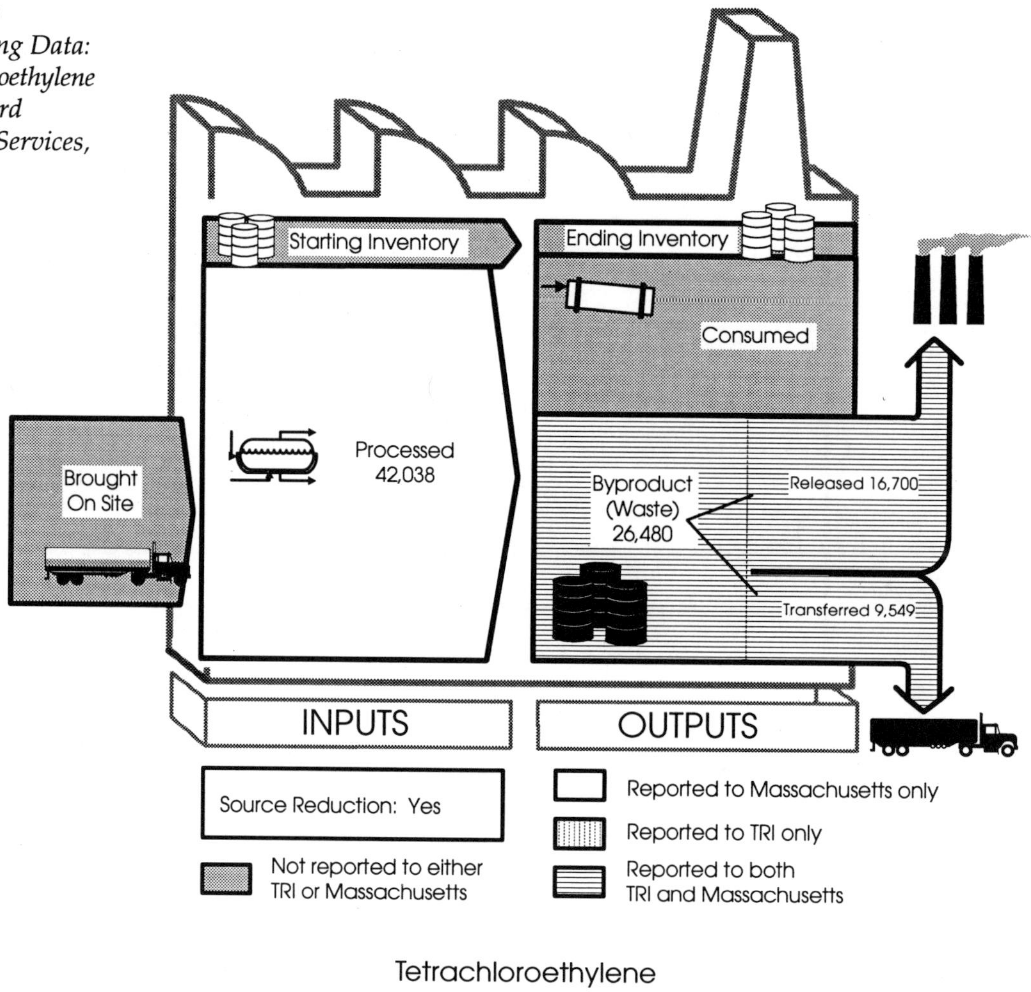

in Pounds (not drawn to scale)

The Massachusetts data from the non-manufacturing facilities that do not report to the federal TRI show that these are not insignificant sources of waste and releases and transfers of toxic chemicals. The Standard Uniform Services Company in Agawam employs tetrachloroethylene, a common dry-cleaning agent that is a carcinogen according to EPA's classification for TRI, to clean uniforms. It used 42,038 pounds of the chemical in 1992 and reported 26,480 pounds of byproduct, indicating that the excess was held in inventory. It released 16,700 pounds to the air from the site and transferred off site 9,549 pounds. (See Figure 10-21.)

Figure 10-22.

Massachusetts Materials Accounting Data: Tetrachloroethylene at ChemiGraphic Inc., Ludlow

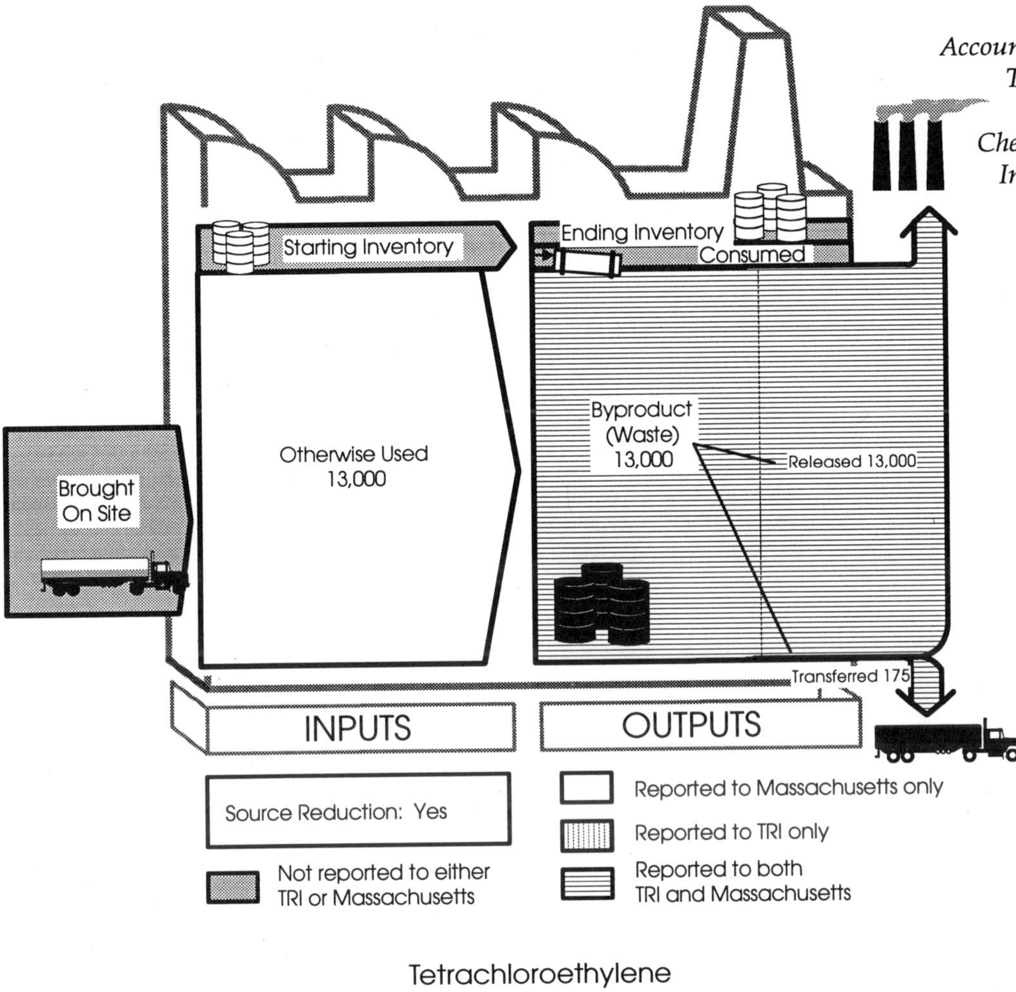

in Pounds (not drawn to scale)

The Chemi-Graphic Inc. facility in Ludlow used 13,000 pounds of tetrachloroethylene in its final cleaning of the printed textiles that it manufactures. All of this amount was generated as byproduct and released to the air from the site. Because Standard Uniform Services Company does not manufacture the clothing it cleans, it does not have to report to the federal TRI, but it releases twice as much tetrachloroethylene as air emissions as the Chemi-Graphic plant, which must report these releases to TRI. These facilities are both located in Hampden County, one on each side of the city of Springfield. (See Figures 10-21 and 10-22.)

Changes in Massachusetts Data, 1991-1992, and Role of Source Reduction

Reports from Massachusetts manufacturing facilities showed a decrease of 9 percent from 1991 to 1992 in the use of TRI toxic chemicals,[q] and the byproduct generated decreased by 7 percent. Total releases and transfers *increased* by 5 percent, however, because of an increase in transfers to POTWs of 35 percent and in other off-site transfers of 20 percent. These large increases were offset by a decrease of 21 percent in releases. (See Table 10-21.)

Unlike New Jersey, no quantity in pounds for source reduction is reported to Massachusetts. The Massachusetts form does provide for reporting on source reduction activities undertaken and the percent change per unit of product in both byproduct and releases and transfers, if any, due to those activities. Although the Massachusetts legislation emphasizes *use* reduction, Form S tracks quantity of byproduct generated and "emissions" as the measure of progress. Byproduct is any chemical leaving the production unit boundary not in a product, and "emissions" are any byproduct leaving the facility, including air emissions, but also releases to water and land and transfers to recycling or disposal facilities, for example. The measure is reported for each production unit for each reportable chemical at the facility.

For each toxic chemical, facilities calculate the amount of byproduct per the quantity of product (i.e., unit of waste per unit of widget) from each production line (process) associated with that chemical. Each year, this is compared to the base year (a year chosen by the facility) for that process. A similar, process-specific index tracks progress for "emissions" or releases and transfers. The measure is reported as the percent that byproduct and the percent that emissions have been reduced, since the base year, due to source reduction. The facility also reports what type of source reduction activity it was.

In this way, Massachusetts' data provide a view of the improvement in the efficiency, or lack thereof, with which each production line handles a particular chemical. The percent change figures will make evident to plant managers, for example, the differences in toxic chemical waste generated by older and newer equipment.

While the Massachusetts reporting at the production-unit level can better reflect changes in chemical use than reporting facility-wide, these measures, as opposed to absolute amounts, have their limitations. The calculation of indices or percentage change may not always be done correctly, with a common error making the change wrong by orders of magnitude

[q] Because chemicals other than TRI chemicals were reported in 1992 but not in 1991, and some non-manufacturing facilities reported for the first time in 1992, only TRI chemicals and only manufacturing facilities are included in any comparisons of reporting years 1991 and 1992 that include quantities in pounds.

Table 10-21. Use, Byproduct, and Releases and Transfers, Massachusetts, 1991 and 1992: For TRI Chemicals and Manufacturing Facilities Only

	1991	1992		Facilities Reporting Source Reduction in 1992*	
Number of Facilities	627	592		320	
Number of Forms	1,971	1,874		1,210	
	Pounds	Pounds	Change from 1991 to 1992 Percent	Pounds	Change from 1991 to 1992 Percent
Use	908,910,973	831,680,216	-8.50	412,414,135	3.77
Manufactured	14,701,579	13,616,315	-7.38	9,205,570	15.96
Processed	763,798,975	695,657,638	-8.92	301,089,032	5.48
Otherwise Used	130,410,419	122,406,263	-6.14	102,119,533	-1.83
Shipped as/in Product	384,842,019	350,137,708	-9.02	174,963,621	-4.44
Byproduct (Waste)	117,972,532	109,491,626	-7.19	84,488,733	-1.74
Byproduct as Percent of Use	13.38%	13.95%		13.95%	
Total Releases and Transfers	49,400,841	51,871,072	5.00	38,534,347	8.97
Total Releases	18,251,532	14,369,707	-21.27	10,520,189	-23.89
Total Air Emissions	17,572,622	14,209,231	-19.14	10,433,258	-22.28
Water Discharges	611,770	49,296	-91.94	40,907	-88.86
Underground Injection	0	26,213	26,207		
On-site Land Releases	67,140	84,967	26.55	19,817	-36.35
Total Transfers	31,149,309	37,501,365	20.39	28,014,158	30.05
Transfers to POTWs	1,710,958	2,316,063	35.37	1,894,896	36.70
Other Off-site Transfers	29,438,351	35,185,302	19.52	26,119,262	29.60
Releases/Transfers as Percent of Use	5.42%	5.62%		5.62%	
Releases/Transfers as Percent of Byproduct	40.50%	40.31%		40.31%	

* Includes new chemicals at these facilities not reported in 1991.

(a percent change of 100 when the true value is 1), which has a large effect on any analysis using the figures.

More Massachusetts facilities, and a greater percentage of reporting facilities, reported source reduction activities in 1992 than in 1991. In 1991, 44 percent of all the Massachusetts manufacturing and non-manufacturing facilities (292 out of 664) reported at least one source reduction technique applied to a production unit. In 1992 that percentage had reached 52 percent (336 out of 644 facilities). Source reduction activity may be reported for only a portion of a facility's operations, since it is reported for a single chemical for a single production unit. In 1991, 37 percent and, in 1992, 39 percent of all production units had reports indicating that source reduction activity accounted for reductions in waste of at least one toxic chemical from that production unit.[r]

For the more limited group of all Massachusetts *manufacturing* facilities reporting on *TRI chemicals* in 1992, 54 percent reported on source reduction activities at their facility associated with those chemicals. These facilities reported overall an *increase* in the use of the TRI chemicals, contrary to the direction reported by all the Massachusetts manufacturing facilities reporting on all chemicals subject to TURA. Even with this increase in use of 4 percent, however, the facilities reporting source reduction had a small *decrease* in byproduct generated of 2 percent. These facilities also reported an increase in transfers (of 30 percent) and a decrease in releases (of 24 percent), as did all manufacturing facilities in Massachusetts. (See Table 10-21.)

[r] Based on a count of the number of production units with at least one source reduction activity code reported for that year.

---

1 N.J.A.C. 7:1K-1 *et seq.*

2 New Jersey Department of Environmental Protection and Energy, *Industrial Pollution Prevention Planning: Meeting Requirements under the New Jersey Pollution Prevention Act*, July 1993, and transmittal letter from Jeanne Herb, Director, Office of Pollution Prevention, New Jersey Department of Environmental Protection and Energy, September 1993.

3 Massachusetts Department of Environmental Protection, *An Overview of the Massachusetts Toxics Use Reduction Act*, Massachusetts Department of Environmental Protection, Boston, February 1989, 3.

4 U.S. Environmental Protection Agency, "EPA Releases 1992 Toxics Release Inventory Data," press release, April 16, 1994; "Potential TRI Universe: Sector Approach to TRI Industry Expansion," handout from EPA press packet, April 16, 1994.

5 U.S. Bureau of the Census, *1991 Survey of Manufactures*.

Chapter 11

Tackling Industrial Toxic Waste Through Voluntary Action

EPA's 33/50 Program and Preliminary Findings of INFORM's Research

In 1991 the U.S. Environmental Protection Agency launched an innovative initiative called the 33/50 Program aimed at reducing toxic chemical pollution through voluntary, direct action by industry. In contrast to the "command-and-control" approaches upon which EPA had largely depended before, the 33/50 Program called upon industry to voluntarily become partners with the Agency in an effort to significantly cut toxic waste and emissions from industrial facilities. The 33/50 Program aimed to demonstrate whether voluntary reduction programs could complement the traditional command and control regulatory approach by achieving targeted reductions more quickly than would regulations alone.[1] Now in its fourth year, the Program has been widely publicized and has sparked a variety of subsequent voluntary programs at federal and state levels to encourage energy conservation and waste reduction.[a] The Program has progressed to a point where some preliminary insights can be gained, since 1991 and 1992 TRI data are available and 1992 is one of the Program's milestone years.

33/50 — Assessing a New Type of Program

While other entities and organizations, including Citizen Action, the General Accounting Office, and Resources for the Future, have been looking at and

[a] Programs such as EPA's Green Lights, and the State of Minnesota's Minnesota 50 Program. In addition, many states have encouraged companies to participate in the 33/50 Program.

writing about the 33/50 Program, INFORM's independent evaluation of EPA's voluntary initiative was sought by EPA to gain a long-term understanding of the dynamics and results of this type of government program. INFORM will again evaluate the Program next year and possibly the year after.

This first INFORM examination of the 33/50 Program — new as it is — is too early to assess the program's impact. However, INFORM has created and lays out in this chapter the framework and design that will be used to track 33/50 Program progress in the years ahead. Our research addresses four basic questions: Have the TRI release and transfer reduction goals of the Program been met? If so, by what means (i.e., pollution prevention, pollution control, plant closings, etc.)? How has participation in the 33/50 Program impacted these reductions? And, what promising features of the Program, if any, might be recommended for use in future voluntary initiatives?

This first report both describes INFORM's framework and discusses some preliminary findings based on the two years of TRI data (1991 and 1992) available since the Program began.

33/50 Program Goals

The name of the program derives from its numerical goals: an interim goal of a 33-percent reduction in 1992 and an ultimate goal of a 50-percent reduction by 1995 in nationwide environmental releases and off-site transfers for treatment and disposal of 17 toxic chemicals using EPA's 1988 Toxics Release Inventory (TRI) reporting as a baseline. (TRI is EPA's annually updated database of the quantity of waste generation, direct releases to air, land, and water, and off-site transfers of more than 320 chemicals from industrial sources). EPA would measure these reduction goals nationwide rather than for each company or facility and for aggregate reductions in releases and transfers of all 17 chemicals rather than for each one. Companies, however, had the latitude to decide what goals to set for the chemicals and types of releases and transfers that pertain to their particular facilities. (See Box 11-A.)

The 33/50 Program's primary goal is to bring about accelerated reductions in the amount of environmental releases and transfers of specified toxic chemicals through voluntary action. Companies had already begun reducing releases and transfers of toxic chemicals in response to having to report the data to TRI. Scrutiny of the 1987 TRI data by the public and by companies themselves revealed previously unimagined amounts of releases, particularly releases to air. EPA states that the central theme of the Program is to encourage pollution prevention rather than "end-of-pipe" treatment technologies as the best means of achieving reductions in toxic chemical emissions[2] — to instill a "pollution prevention ethic" in the leadership of American businesses.[3] The driving force behind the Program is "public expectations of reduced risk through reductions . . . . in the generation of toxic chemical wastes."[4]

Companies were initially invited to reduce releases of the 17 toxic chemicals; the invitation was later amended to include releases and off-site transfers to treatment and disposal, and the Program goals are stated as such. Companies were asked to consider achieving reductions by source reduction of wastes, in preference to recycling, energy recovery, or treatment of the wastes.

Companies committing to the Program have full flexibility not only in selecting the reduction method(s) they will employ, but also in deciding which chemicals to reduce (including chemicals other than the 17 targeted by 33/50) and the amount and pace of reductions. In fact, companies sending a letter of intent to participate in the Program without specifying any numerical reduction goals are counted as participating in the Program.

As stated previously, EPA measures 33/50 Program progress based on year-to-year changes in national aggregate releases and transfers of the 17 Program chemicals for all facilities reporting to TRI regardless of 33/50 Program commitment status. In addition, EPA examines reductions in 33/50 Program chemicals as compared to reductions for all TRI chemicals and compares reductions made by Program participants and non-participants.

Although the 33/50 Program was formally announced in 1991, participating companies can count reductions made since 1988 against the reduction goals they set. For measuring 33/50 reductions, EPA uses only the TRI categories companies were required to report in 1988, namely on-site releases to all environmental media and off-site transfers to treatment and disposal. Elements that were not required reporting in 1988, such as off-site transfers to recycling and energy recovery and on-site waste management data, are not included in 33/50 Program analyses.[b] (See Chapter 4 for details on data elements reported to TRI.)

Box 11-A. 33/50 Program Chemicals

Benzene	Methyl ethyl ketone
Cadmium and compounds	Methyl isobutyl ketone
Carbon tetrachloride	Nickel and compounds
Chloroform	Tetrachloroethylene
Chromium and compounds	Toluene
Cyanides	1,1,1-Trichloroethane
Dichloromethane	Trichloroethylene
Lead and compounds	Xylene (mixed isomers)
Mercury and compounds	

[b] Some facilities did report off-site transfers to recycling or energy recovery in 1998, although not required to do so until 1991. EPA includes these in the 1988 baseline but not in 1991 or later years. For these facilities, reductions will thus be over-reported.

EPA Strategies

In August 1989 EPA's then-Administrator William K. Reilly applied the concept of voluntary action for reducing toxic emissions by negotiating voluntary waste reduction agreements with the nine "ATERIS" (Air Toxics Emissions Reductions Inventory System) companies to reduce emissions of butadiene and other air toxics 83 percent by 1993. The Science Advisory Board's report, *Setting Priorities and Strategies for Environmental Protection,* issued in September 1990, identified toxic chemicals as among the most serious threats to the environment and public health. Emphasizing reduction of chemical wastes at the source as the preferred option for reducing risk, the report significantly influenced development of the 33/50 Program toward promoting Administrator Reilly's broader application of the voluntary action principle. The debate over and eventual passage of the 1990 Pollution Prevention Act was another significant influence. In September 1990 Administrator Reilly informed the Office of Toxic Substances of his decision to implement a voluntary program stressing pollution prevention for "high priority" chemicals.[5]

The 17 toxic chemicals that became 33/50 Program targets were selected through an Agency-wide process which determined that these chemicals:

(a) represent a serious health and environmental concern,

(b) are high-volume industrial chemicals with substantial releases,

(c) can be reduced through pollution prevention,[6] and

(d) are also regulated under the provisions of the 1990 Clean Air Act.

EPA used 1988 TRI data to identify the facilities that reported releases and transfers of one or more of the 17 chemicals (the results revealed 12,000 facilities owned by more than 6,000 parent companies). EPA designated 1988 as the base year for measuring reductions under the 33/50 Program because at the time of the Program's formulation that was the latest year for which TRI data were available.[7] In 1988 the 12,000 TRI facilities reported 1.4 billion pounds of the 17 Program chemicals that were either released to the environment or transferred off-site for waste management. The 33/50 Program goal is to reduce this amount by *at least* 50 percent — 700 million pounds — in five years, making maximum use of pollution prevention strategies.[8]

In January 1991 the EPA Administrator sent letters to the CEOs of the "Top 600" companies, inviting them to join the 33/50 Program. The facilities of these so-called "first-round" companies accounted for more than 75 percent of the total 1988 releases and transfers of the 17 Program chemicals. A series of meetings were also held with executives of different manufacturing sectors to discuss the Program's implementation. Representatives from the American Petroleum Institute, American Paper Institute, Chemical Manufacturers Association, and Dow Chemical Company, as well as the Environmental Defense Fund, were key participants in these meetings. The 33/50 Program was publicly announced in February 1991.

Within two months 322 of the "first-round" companies had committed to the Program. In July letters of invitation were sent to the 5,400 "second-round" companies. As of May 1994, subsequent mailings to more than 8,700 companies has resulted in a total of 1,242 companies committing to the Program.

Program Implementation

With a relatively modest annual budget of $400,000 and a staff that includes six at headquarters and two full-time equivalent regional staff, EPA implemented the four elements that comprise the 33/50 Program:

- outreach to recruit corporate participation,
- public recognition of companies for their participation,
- pollution prevention technical assistance to corporate participants, and
- program evaluation.

Recruiting Companies

EPA solicits companies for participation in the Program on a continuing basis. The Agency contacts companies via written communications and meetings. Companies are contacted as they report to TRI for the first time or as corporate affiliations change. A 33/50 representative in each EPA region solicits new Program participants and maintains contacts with participating parent companies. In addition, the 33/50 Program staff publicizes about the Program through press releases, articles, and conference presentations.

Public Recognition

Company participation and progress has been publicized through five "Progress Updates" (the sixth is in progress). Companies that agree to participate receive a formal certificate of participation from EPA. Reduction commitment information is available to the public. EPA sponsors awards programs to highlight companies' reduction efforts.

Technical Assistance and Technology Transfer

While direct technical assistance is not a part of the 33/50 Program, EPA "funnels" information between state technical assistance programs and among corporations through the Pollution Prevention Information Clearinghouse. EPA provides industry-specific publications prepared by the Agency's Office of Research and Development (three of which were sponsored through the 33/50 Program itself); these focus on ways to reduce the 17 Program chemicals at the source. In addition, the Agency prepares and distributes company profiles describing reduction activities implemented by Program participants.

Program Evaluation

EPA evaluates 33/50 Program progress first by looking at overall reductions in releases and transfers of the 17 chemicals. It also compares aggregate releases and transfers of the 17 Program chemicals from all facilities of participating parent companies with releases and transfers from all facilities of parent companies choosing not to participate in the Program. EPA counts as party of the Program participation total releases and transfers from *all* facilities of participating companies, regardless of whether there is a commitment covering each facility.

INFORM's Research Findings on the 33/50 Program

The Importance of Studying 33/50

The 33/50 Program is the first major experiment in taking a new, voluntary approach to traditional government regulations. Such regulations, particularly those setting prescriptive standards for treatment and disposal of waste, have proven increasingly costly for government and industry; both have expressed need for a new and more collaborative approach to solving toxics problems. But even before its effectiveness has been thoroughly examined, the 33/50 Program is being used as a model for numerous other programs throughout EPA. Therefore, the Agency approached INFORM to serve as an outside evaluator of the Program and its unique mix of voluntary participation and public recognition in accelerating the pace of reduction in the releases and transfers of a set of TRI chemicals.

Although EPA recognizes all reductions achieved through a wide variety of methods (from source reduction to end-of-pipe waste treatment), a key Program goal was to encourage participating companies to use source reduction as the preferred means for meeting the Program's 33- and 50-percent release-and-transfer reduction goals. Hence, INFORM particularly seeks to examine the effectiveness of this voluntary approach in spurring new source reduction action.

Since the mid-1980s, leaders in the environmental movement, government agencies, academia, and various industries have recognized the need to shift the paradigm of industrial waste management from end-of-pipe waste treatment and disposal to strategies that recycle — but most of all prevent — pollution at its source (i.e., source reduction). There has been increasing agreement about several aspects of the source reduction approach. First, there is agreement that government-imposed prescriptive technical standards are not an effective way to maximize source reduction. Operations in plants making or using chemicals are often unique, even among facilities of the same industry sector, due to their particular mix of raw materials, operating environments, customers, suppliers, products, age of the facility, etc. In these distinct industrial environments, process operations personnel familiar with the materials and phases of operation are best suited to identify source reduction opportunities. Second, public and private sector leaders have agreed that source reduction, unlike end-of-pipe strategies, often increases production efficiency and saves companies money. Finally, INFORM's own case-study research (*Cutting Chemical Wastes*, 1986, and *Environmental Dividends: Cutting More Chemical Wastes*, 1992) shows that the obstacles to source reduction are largely institutional — an absence of programs in place that systematically identify sources of waste, that train and reward employees for finding source reduction opportunities, that establish high level plant leadership for source reduction progress, or that charge the cost of waste back to the process generating it.

Since government-imposed prescriptive standards are clearly not the best path to promoting source reduction, a voluntary program seems to be one alternative offering businesses the chance to step forward to identify and make waste-reducing plant changes, many of which would be in their direct economic interest and would also generate favorable publicity.

INFORM's Evaluation Goals

Beginning three years from implementation of the 33/50 Program (and five years from the Program's 1988 baseline of TRI data), INFORM's interest is in gaining insight into several questions, by taking a detailed look at the 33/50 Program and its companies and facilities:

- Is the Program meeting its national goals?
- Has this type of completely voluntary initiative with its element of public recognition spurred reductions in releases and transfers of the 17 Program chemicals greater than would have occurred without 33/50?
- How have Program participants met their goals — has the Program stimulated major initiatives in source reduction, or have participants relied on recycling and end-of-pipe waste management and disposal strategies?
- Can modifications of the program be identified that might lead to greater participation from the private sector and more impact?
- Does the 33/50 Program history and experience shed light on the potential effectiveness of other voluntary programs?

Because there are only two years of TRI data available since the 33/50 Program began, INFORM's research findings are clearly preliminary. Most differences and trends can only be hinted at so far. Continuing these analyses with future years' data will shed further light on the value of the program.

INFORM Methodology

INFORM's evaluation of 33/50 takes a four-pronged approach:

- examining the TRI database from 1988 through 1995 (this report uses data through 1992) to see how much releases and transfers were reduced and, from the 1991 and later data (additional data elements required under the federal Pollution Prevention Act), how much waste was reduced and what strategies were used,

- scanning EPA's 33/50 Program materials and correspondence with corporations as part of assessing the dynamics of Program relationships, and to understand the commitments companies are making and the strategies they are planning,
- conducting a survey of participating and non-participating parent companies and facilities to get an overview of whether or not they are going beyond regulatory compliance, and
- conducting in-depth, on-site interviews of participating and non-participating parent companies and facilities to gain more insight on these questions and on whether and how participation in the Program may have led to greater cooperation between government and industry.

The INFORM study of the TRI data is conducted by a method called a matched-pair analysis — a method designed to isolate 33/50 Program impact from other factors reported on the TRI Form R that influence decreases in releases and transfers (e.g., the state where the TRI facility is located, the amount of each chemical reported, whether or not energy recovery, recycling, or source reduction was reported for the chemical, the class of chemical, the production index from 1990 to 1991, the type of activity/use reported for the chemical, the maximum amount of each chemical on site during the year, and the SIC code or codes reported for the operations involving each chemical). Criteria for setting up the matched pairs arise are generated by a statistical method called an analysis of variance. Both the matched pair analysis and the analysis of variance are described in detail at the end of this chapter.

For this report, the matched-pair analysis had been done for the TRI 1992 data. Some pilot surveys and on-site interviews had been conducted. INFORM will complete and analyze a large pool of surveys and on-site interviews for its 33/50 Program report next year, as well as expand the matched-pair analysis to include 1993 TRI data.

Summary of Findings

Below is a summary of the results of INFORM's first year of 33/50 Program research. Following the summary is a discussion and illustration of these preliminary results.

Industry's Overall Response to the 33/50 Program

- Of the 8,091 parent companies that had been invited to participate in the 33/50 Program at the time of this report, 1,242 (15 percent of all eligible companies) agreed to participate.
  - — Among the 1,242 parent companies participating in the Program, 754 parent companies made numerical pledges measurable against the 1988 TRI baseline. Of these, 520 made pledges greater than reductions already achieved (for an additional 161 million

pounds), and 234 made pledges for reductions they had already achieved since 1988.

— 295 of the participating parent companies made numerical reduction pledges not measurable against the 1988 TRI baseline. These pledges include use reduction goals, goals for non-33/50 Program chemicals, and reduction goals with non-1988 baselines.

— 193 of the participating parent companies made no numerical reduction pledges at all.

- Of the 8,091 parent companies invited to participate in the 33/50 Program at the time of this report, 6,553 (81 percent) did not respond at all.
- 217 parent companies declined EPA's invitation to participate for some reason, including outright declines, the existence of companies' own reduction programs, or previous reductions made independently of the 33/50 Program.
- At the time of this report, 43 parent companies had written to EPA that they were undecided about participating in the 33/50 Program.
- Although many companies did not respond to EPA's invitation, the 15 percent that became participants account for 62 percent of the 1988 releases and transfers of 33/50 Program chemicals.
- The 33/50 Program attracted a considerable number of companies that had not made as great an effort to reduce releases and transfers of 33/50 Program chemicals as had others before the 33/50 Program began.

Reductions Associated with Commitment to the 33/50 Program

- After initiation of the 33/50 Program, the pace of reductions of the 17 Program chemicals at facilities not covered by a commitment slowed, while the pace of reductions was maintained at facilities covered by a commitment.
- Commitment to the 33/50 Program appears to have stimulated reduction of chemicals outside the Program's intended scope.
- Simply being contacted by EPA about joining the 33/50 Program appears to have stimulated reductions of chemicals outside the Program's intended scope.

How Reductions Were Achieved

- Facilities covered by a commitment to the 33/50 Program appear to have relied predominantly on end-of-pipe treatment technologies or on-site recycling and energy recovery, rather than on source reduction, to achieve reductions in their releases and transfers of the 17 Program chemicals.
- Among facilities that reported implementing a "pioneering" source reduction activity (one that goes beyond simple housekeeping or operations changes) in 1991 or 1992, there is no difference, visible to date, in the percent reduction achieved by those facilities covered by a commitment from those not covered by a commitment.

Reductions Stimulated by Factors Other than the 33/50 Program

- On average, TRI facilities reported significant reductions in releases and transfers of the 17 Program chemicals from 1988 to 1991. So far, added reductions achieved by facilities covered by a commitment to the 33/50 Program do not appear to be much greater than reductions that would have occurred had the Program not existed at all.
- Among the TRI facilities examined by INFORM whose use of one or more of the 17 targeted chemicals dropped below the reporting threshold in 1991 and 1992, no association is visible between this drop and their status as facilities covered or not covered by a commitment to the 33/50 Program.

The Overall Extent to which 33/50 Program Design Contributes to Program Goals

- The constantly changing make-up of parent companies makes it difficult to ensure that all have been contacted and encouraged to participate. To achieve maximum possible participation, the Program would need to include systematic contacts at the facility level.
- EPA's exclusive use of TRI data to measure 33/50 reductions precludes measuring how much of the reduction was due to source reduction, the other goal of the Program. Source reduction amounts are not reported to TRI and would have to be reported separately by the companies and facilities.

Releases and Transfers of 33/50 Program Chemicals, 1988-1992

The goal of a 50-percent reduction in releases and transfers of the 17 Program chemicals by 1995 was considered quite ambitious at the time the 33/50 Program was established. According to EPA, industry leaders, discussing the design of the program, considered the 50-percent-by-1995 goal reasonable, but expressed concern about attaining the interim goal of 33 percent by 1992.

While industry and EPA agreed on Program goals and strategies, many environmental organizations stated that, given what was known at the time about the benefits of source reduction and the need for special incentives to promote industry use of this strategy, and the passage of the Federal Pollution Prevention Act, EPA should have made pollution prevention at the source the required strategy for achieving the Program's goals. Two major reports published in 1986, in fact, concluded that such a goal could probably be achieved by aggressive use of source reduction strategies alone: U.S. Congressional Office of Technology Assessment (OTA), in *Serious Reduction of Hazardous Waste,* forecast that U.S. industry could reduce waste generation at its source roughly 10 percent a year for five years by using readily available technologies that would often save money through increased production efficiency. INFORM's study, *Cutting*

Chemical Wastes (involving case studies of the practices of 29 chemical plants), found that source reduction efforts by plants often cut waste streams containing toxic chemicals by 50 percent or more.

In 1994 the national environmental community emphasized in a letter to EPA's administrator the importance of a focus on source reduction and urged that an awards program, if any, should recognize only true pollution prevention progress by participating companies.[9]

EPA's Evaluation of 33/50 Program Progress

Overall, releases and transfers of the 17 targeted chemicals from all facilities making or using them in quantities that trigger TRI reporting (regardless of 33/50 Program participation status) were reduced 40 percent between 1988 and 1992. EPA's 1992 interim goal of a 33-percent reduction was exceeded, and the goal of a 50-percent reduction by 1995 is close to being met. The question remains, how much of the reduction that has occurred is due directly to the existence of the 33/50 Program?

Both EPA's own evaluation and that by INFORM attempt to shed light on this question. But it is important to distinguish the differences in approach taken by EPA and by INFORM. EPA's evaluation compares aggregate releases and transfers of the 17 Program chemicals from all facilities of participating parent companies with all facilities of parent companies choosing not to participate in the Program. INFORM's evaluation compares facilities "covered by a commitment" to the 33/50 Program with facilities that are not. Facilities that are covered by a commitment are facilities whose parent company has made a commitment for all of its facilities or whose parent company has made a commitment that specifically covers that facility or for which the facility itself has made a commitment to the 33/50 Program. (See Box 11-B.)

The two cases in which EPA's approach differs from INFORM's are:

- where only one facility of a company has made a commitment to the Program but the parent company itself has not. In this case, INFORM includes *only* the releases and transfers from this facility towards the Program's goals, but not the releases and transfers from the company's other facilities. EPA, on the other hand, includes the releases and transfers from *all* facilities belonging to the parent company.
- where the parent company has made a commitment that specifically excludes some of its facilities. In this case, EPA counts the releases and transfers from *all* facilities belonging to the parent company towards the Program's goals, even including those specifically excluded from the companies commitment. INFORM does not.

To distinguish this difference in approaches, this report refers to EPA's designation as "participation" and to INFORM's designation as "covered by a commitment."

EPA's evaluation of "participating" companies led to a number

Box 11-B. Key Terms Used in This Chapter

TRI: EPA's Toxics Release Inventory: an annually updated database of release quantities of about 300 chemicals and chemical categories into the nation's air, water, and land, and transfers to off-site locations for treatment, or disposal since 1987, and for recycling and energy recovery since 1991..

TRI facility: any industrial facility meeting the threshold criteria (10 or more employees, manufacture at least 25,000 pounds or otherwise use at least 10,000 pounds of a given TRI chemical in a calendar year) triggering reporting release and transfer information for that year to EPA.

Form R: the report form completed and submitted to EPA by all TRI facilities for each chemical on the TRI list.

33/50 Program chemical: any of 17 chemicals and chemical categories targeted by EPA's 33/50 Program. (See Appendix P.)

Non-program chemical: any TRI chemical other than the 17 chemicals and chemical categories targeted by EPA's 33/50 Program.

Facility reporting at least one Program chemical: any TRI facility reporting any of the 17 chemicals targeted by the 33/50 Program.

Facility not reporting Program chemicals: any TRI facility not reporting any of the 17 chemicals targeted by the 33/50 Program. A parent company owning only these facilities would not have been contacted by EPA about joining the 33/50 Program.

Facilities covered by a commitment: facilities reporting at least one program chemical and who have made a commitment to participate in the program or whose parent company made a commitment that covers all of its facilities or a set of its facilities that includes this one.

Facilities not covered by a commitment: facilities reporting at least one program chemical whose parent company was contacted by EPA but neither the parent company, nor the facility, has made a commitment to participate in the program that included the facility.

Releases and transfers: all media releases and off-site transfers, not including transfers to recycling or energy recovery reported in 1991 and later years.

of conclusions, three of the major ones being:

- "Between 1991 and 1992, facilities owned by Program participants reduced releases and transfers of the 17 Program chemicals by 15 percent, nearly twice the rate of reduction achieved by facilities owned by non-participating companies.
- Participating companies accounted for 80 percent of the reduction in 33/50 Program chemical releases and transfers in the last year.
- Since 1988, participating companies have almost halved their releases and transfers of 33/50 Program chemicals (48%)."

How much of this progress that can be attributed to the existence of the 33/50 Program is a complicated question. A wide variety of factors may motivate changes on the part of a company, such as the impact of regulations and economic costs, attitudes of communities in which companies are located, stories in the media, investor pressure, and positive incentives like the 33/50 Program. Different combinations of these factors may lead to changes, and all may be a real part of achieving environmental progress in one form or another.

INFORM's research specifically seeks to distinguish participation in the Program from other factors that might influence reported reductions in releases and transfers of the 17 chemicals targeted by the Program. As of this first report, the impact of the 33/50 Program is not clear. Preliminary perspectives gained so far are based on analysis of matched sets of facilities similar in many basic ways except their commitment to the 33/50 Program. Each matched set includes between 4,000 and 8,000 individual facilities. INFORM compared percent reduction in releases and transfers from 1988 levels for both groups of facilities in each matched set. Moreover, because there are only two years of TRI data available since initiation of the Program, any association between commitment to the Program and reduction in releases and transfers can only be hinted at. Repeated analyses with future years' TRI data, along with the results of a broad set of INFORM surveys and interviews, will provide a more solid basis for firm conclusions.

Figure 11-1.

TRI Releases and Transfers of 33/50 Program Chemicals, 1988-1992

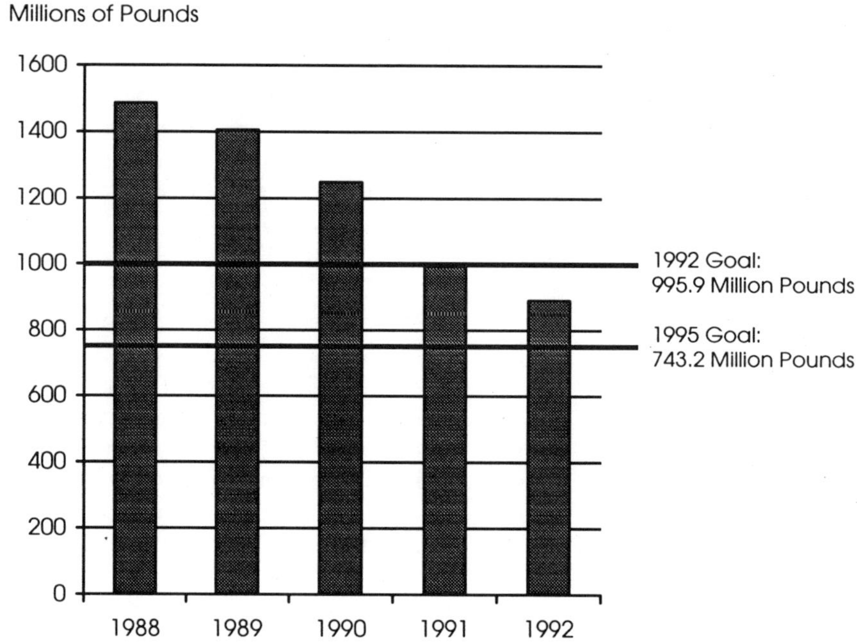

Amounts for recycling and energy recovery reported for 1991 and 1992 are not included

INFORM's Evaluation of 33/50 Program Progress

Industry's Overall Response to the 33/50 Program

Finding: The progress reported by the 33/50 participating companies toward the Program's goals has been substantial, but suggests that these goals were not as ambitious as was thought at the outset. (See Figure 11-1.)

Finding: Among the 754 parent companies making numerical pledges measurable against the 1988 baseline, 520 made pledges greater than reductions already achieved (for an additional 161 million pounds), and 234 made pledges for quantities they had already reduced since 1988. (See Figure 11-2.)

Evaluating the effectiveness of the Program depends to a large extent on the data facilities routinely submit to TRI. EPA does not require any additional data to be submitted by participating companies. While reductions made by most companies committing to the 33/50 Program can be measured against the 1988 base year, for others this is not possible. The flexible terms under which companies can join the 33/50 Program make measurement of some companies' progress in meeting their stated goals not possible. As noted earlier, the only requirement for participation is a letter of commitment. Companies committing to the Program have full

Figure 11-2.

Quantity of Release and Transfer Reductions Achieved and Pledged by 754 Participating Parent Companies

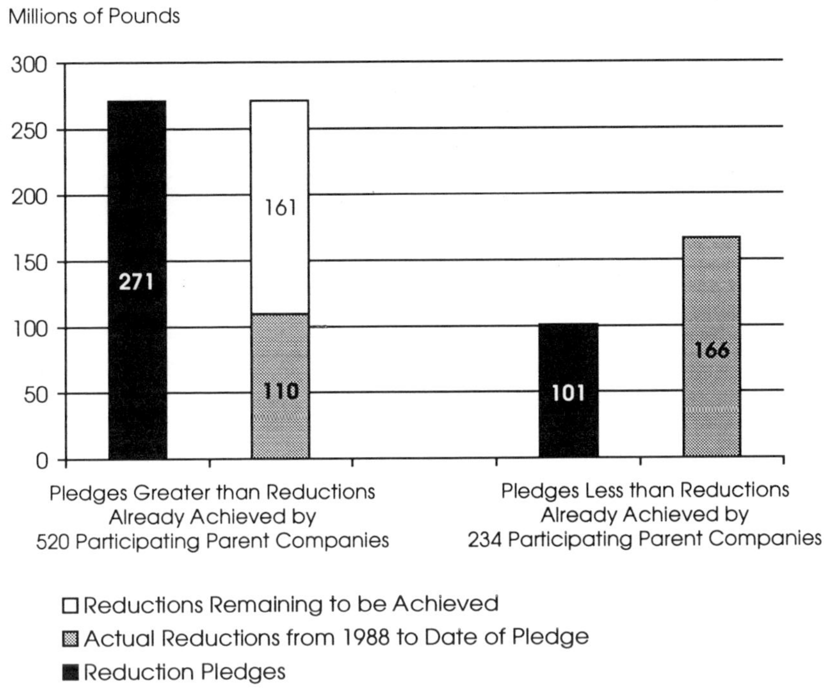

flexibility in selecting the chemicals that will be reduced (they can even choose chemicals other than the 17 targeted by 33/50), the amount and pace of reductions, and the strategies they will use to achieve their reduction target.

Although 193 of the companies committing to the Program made no numerical pledges at all, a numerical pledge is not required to be counted as participating. Of those making numerical commitments, a significant portion cannot be quantified to the 1988 TRI baseline because of the type of reduction commitment made. For example, some companies commit to reducing the *use* of a chemical rather than to a reduction in releases and transfers. Other companies agree to reduce toxic wastes based on a production index; the amount of waste generated can decrease or *increase* depending on the level of activity at the plant. Others use a base year other than 1988 because they did not meet the reporting thresholds for the Program chemicals in 1988.

Of the eligible parent companies, 1,242 were participating in the 33/50 Program as of May 1994 (they accounted for 62 percent of releases and transfers of Program chemicals in 1988). Of these 1,242 participating parent companies, 754 (61 percent) made pledges quantifiable to the 1988 TRI baseline. The remaining pledges were not quantifiable to 1988.

Not all pledges are for reduction beyond what the company had

Figure 11-3.

Percent Change in Releases and Transfers of the 17 Program Chemicals since 1988

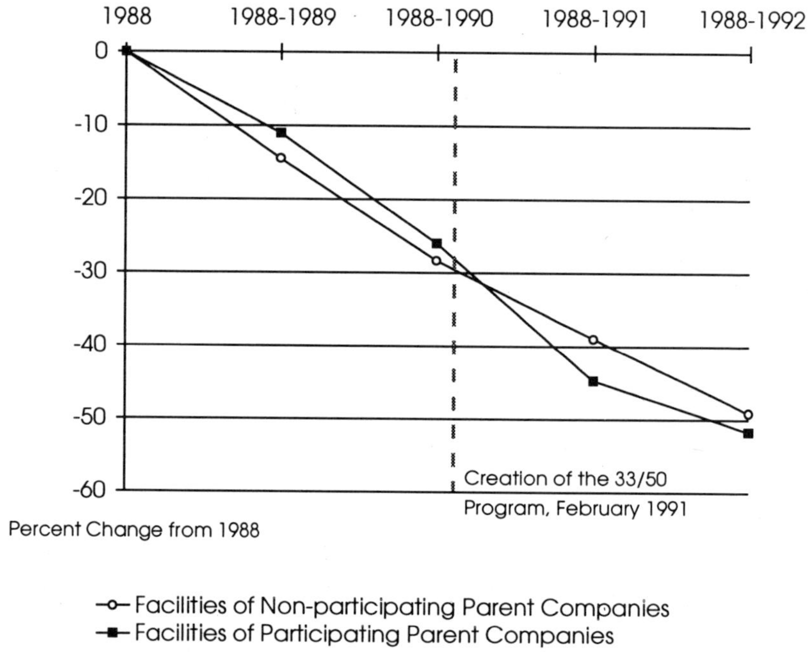

The steeper the downward slope of the line, the faster the rate of reduction.

already accomplished at the time of the pledge. This is possible because pledges were made starting in 1991 when each company already knew how much it had reduced releases and transfers since 1988. A total of 234 company pledges did not exceed reductions already made at the time the pledge was made. (See Figure 11-2.)

However, 69 percent of the companies making pledges quantifiable against the TRI 1988 baseline (520 out of 754) did make pledges that exceeded reductions already achieved at the time of the pledge. These 520 parent companies have pledged to achieve an additional 161 million pounds of reductions in releases and transfers by 1995. (See Figure 11-2.)

Finding: The 33/50 Program attracted some facilities of parent companies not making as great an effort to reduce as others before the Program began. (See Figure 11-3.)

While one would think, intuitively, that parent companies signing up first for the 33/50 Program would be those having made the most progress in reducing their TRI wastes, INFORM's analyses found this not to be true. In fact, facilities covered by a commitment had smaller percentage reductions from 1988 to 1991, the time the program began, of releases and transfers of the 17 target chemicals than facilities not covered by a commitment .

After 1991 it appears that this trend may be reversing, with facilities covered by a commitment showing somewhat larger reductions in 1991 and 1992.

Reductions Associated with Commitment to the 33/50 Program

Finding: After initiation of the 33/50 Program, the pace of reductions at facilities not covered by a commitment seems to have slowed, while the pace of reductions was maintained at facilities covered by a commitment. (See Figure 11-3.)

Prior to 1991, the percent reduction of the 17 Program chemicals achieved by facilities that were to become covered by a commitment to the 33/50 Program was less than the percent reduction of facilities not covered by a commitment. This trend was reversed in 1991, however, when facilities not covered by a commitment slowed their pace of reduction while facilities covered by a commitment surpassed the percent reduction achieved by their non-committing counterparts. (See Figure 11-3.)

The 3,196 matched pairs used in this part of the analysis represent 34 percent of all 1988 TRI forms for facilities covered by a commitment and 20 percent of forms for facilities not covered by a commitment. (See Figure 11-3.) Releases and transfers of the 17 Program chemicals reported by the matched pairs amount to 25 percent of total releases and transfers for these chemicals from facilities covered by a commitment and 28 percent of releases and transfers from facilities not covered by a commitment.

Finding: Commitment to the 33/50 Program appears to have stimulated reduction of chemicals outside the Program's intended scope. (See Figure 11-4.)

Facilities covered by a commitment reported a faster rate of reduction of TRI chemicals outside the scope of the 33/50 Program after initiation of the 33/50 Program than facilities that did not report using any of the 17 Program chemicals.

By looking at changes in releases and transfers of non-Program chemicals, INFORM sought to gain insight into the breadth of Program impact, if any, at facilities reporting Program chemicals and covered by a commitment to the Program . There appears to be an association between commitment to the Program and improvement in the rate of reduction in releases and transfers of *non*-Program chemicals. While the rate of change increased, however, facilities covered by a commitment consistently had lower percent reductions for non-Program chemicals than did facilities not reporting any 33/50 Program chemicals.

Between 1988 and 1990, releases and transfers of non-Program chemicals actually increased at facilities that were to become covered by a commitment to the 33/50 Program and decreased at facilities not reporting any Program chemicals. By 1991, however, facilities covered by a commitment

Figure 11-4.

Percent Change in Releases and Transfers of Non-Program Chemicals for 2,421 Matched Pairs

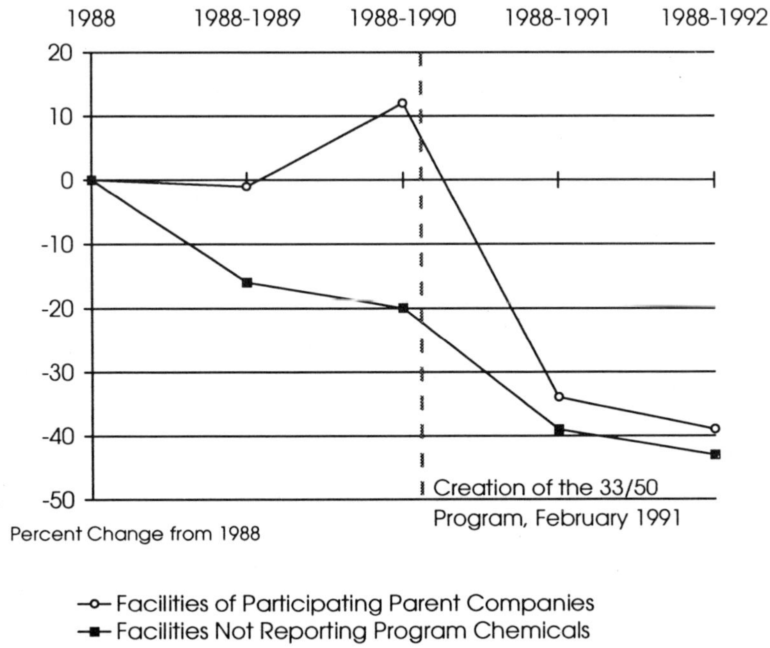

The steeper the downward slope of the line, the faster the rate of reduction.

began reporting decreasing releases and transfers of their non-Program chemicals. In 1992 these decreases were occurring at a rate great enough to bring them close to, but not exceed, the percent decrease achieved by facilities not reporting any Program chemicals. (See Figure 11-4.)

The 2,421 matched pairs used in this part of the analysis represent 15 percent of all 1988 TRI forms for facilities covered by a commitment and 13 percent of forms for facilities not reporting any Program chemicals. Releases and transfers of non-Program chemicals amount to 6 percent of total releases and transfers for these chemicals from facilities covered by a commitment and 14 percent of releases and transfers from facilities not reporting any Program chemicals. (See Figure 11-4.)

Finding: Simply being contacted by EPA about joining the 33/50 Program appears to have stimulated reductions of chemicals outside the scope of the Program. (See Figure 11-5.)

Since EPA's announcement of the Program, facilities not covered by a commitment (facilities of parent companies who had been contacted by EPA but chose not to participate) reported consistent reductions in releases and transfers of TRI chemicals outside the scope of the 33/50 Program. By contrast, releases and transfers of these same chemicals increased between 1991 and 1992 at facilities that do not report using any of the 17 Program chemicals. (See Figure 11-5.) TRI data for 1993 through 1995, when available, will help determine whether or not this is indeed a trend.

Figure 11-5.

Percent Change in Releases and Transfers of Non-Program Chemicals for Matched Pairs

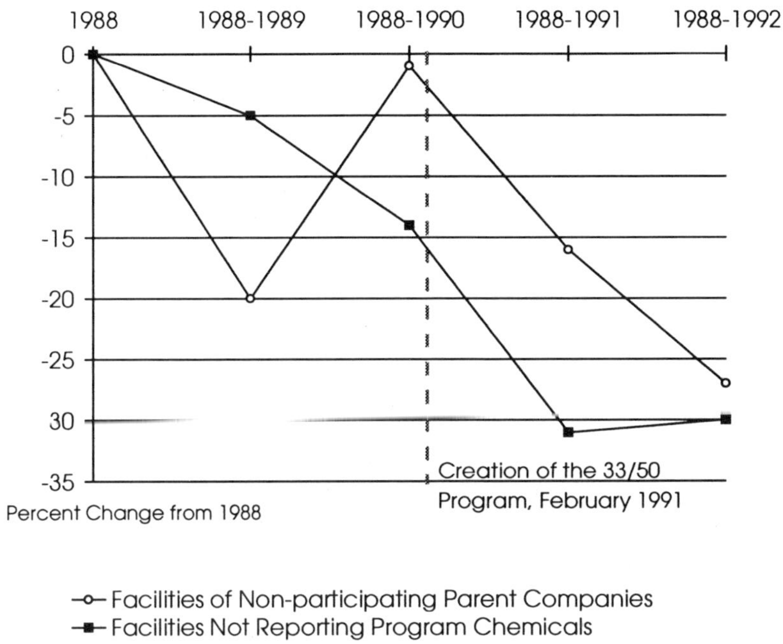

The steeper the downward slope of the line, the faster the rate of reduction.

The TRI data offer some preliminary evidence that EPA's contacting parent companies that subsequently chose not to commit to the Program may , in and of itself, have stimulated a steady decrease in releases and transfers of non-Program chemicals at their facilities. However, the percent change is consistently less than that reported by facilities not reporting any Program chemicals (parent companies owning only facilities that do not report Program chemicals would not have been contacted by EPA regarding the 33/50 Program). While releases and transfers of non-Program chemicals at facilities reporting at least one Program chemical but not covered by a commitment varied wildly between 1988 and 1990, a steady rate of decrease began in 1990 and continued to 1992. Meanwhile, facilities not reporting any Program chemicals have been steadily decreasing releases and transfers of non-Program chemicals since 1988, but showed a slight increase in 1992. (See Figure 11-5.) Tracking 1993 through 1995 TRI data for these matched pairs will provide greater insight into the trends associated with commitment to the 33/50 Program.

The 2,160 matched pairs used in this part of the analysis represent 13 percent of all 1988 TRI forms for facilities reporting at least one Program chemical but not covered by a commitment and 11 percent of forms for facilities not reporting any Program chemicals. Releases and transfers of non-Program chemicals from the matched pairs amount to 10 percent of total releases and transfers for these chemicals from all facilities reporting at least one Program chemical but not covered by a commitment and 9.0 percent of releases and transfers all from facilities not reporting any Program chemicals. (See Figure 11-5.)

How Release and Transfer Reductions Were Achieved

Pollution prevention, as defined in the federal Pollution Prevention Act of 1990, is synonymous with source reduction — that is, avoiding the creation of waste in the first place. Indeed, from the outset EPA has strongly emphasized source reduction as the primary means of achieving the reduction goals of the 33/50 Program. INFORM sought to assess the extent to which commitment to the 33/50 Program has promoted source reduction.

TRI data indicate that overall there has *not* been a reduction in the total amount of the 17 Program chemicals generated as waste by TRI facilities. In response to the federal Pollution Prevention Act of 1990, EPA collects information on the quantity of waste generated prior to recycling, treatment or disposal — a term currently referred to as "total production-related waste." Total production-related waste for the 17 Program chemicals increased slightly between 1991 and 1992. Industry projects, however, that its generation of production-related waste of the 17 Program chemicals will decrease in 1993 and 1994, while it projects an increase in total waste generation of all other TRI chemicals.

Although total production-related waste could be reduced through source reduction, it could also be reduced by other methods that are reported by TRI facilities — such as lowering production levels, terminating production processes at a facility, or exporting production units to facilities outside the United States. While EPA requires TRI facilities to indicate what type of source reduction activity, if any, was implemented during the reporting year, the Office of Management and Budget (OMB) did not allow EPA to require TRI facilities to report on Form R the *amount* of waste reduced through source reduction in the reporting year. Therefore, using only TRI data, INFORM cannot directly relate commitment to the Program with the amount of the 17 Program chemicals reduced through source reduction each year. INFORM can, however, use TRI data to examine possible association between commitment to the 33/50 Program and reduction in releases and transfers at those facilities reporting source reduction activities in 1991 or 1992 and those not reporting source reduction activities during those years.

The following three figures show the results of a matched-pair analysis of facilities that did or did not report using source reduction for at least one Program chemical in 1991 or 1992 (the 1991 reporting year was the first year that facilities were required to report this information to EPA). It is important to emphasize again that any associations between source reduction achievement and commitment to the 33/50 Program suggested here are preliminary since the data can only indicate possible impacts from those source reduction activities that were identified and implemented early on. TRI data for 1993-1995 will show more clearly what impact the Program might be having on implementation of source reduction actions.

Figure 11-6.

Percent Change in Releases and Transfers on Matched Forms Reporting Source Reduction Activity in 1991 and 1992

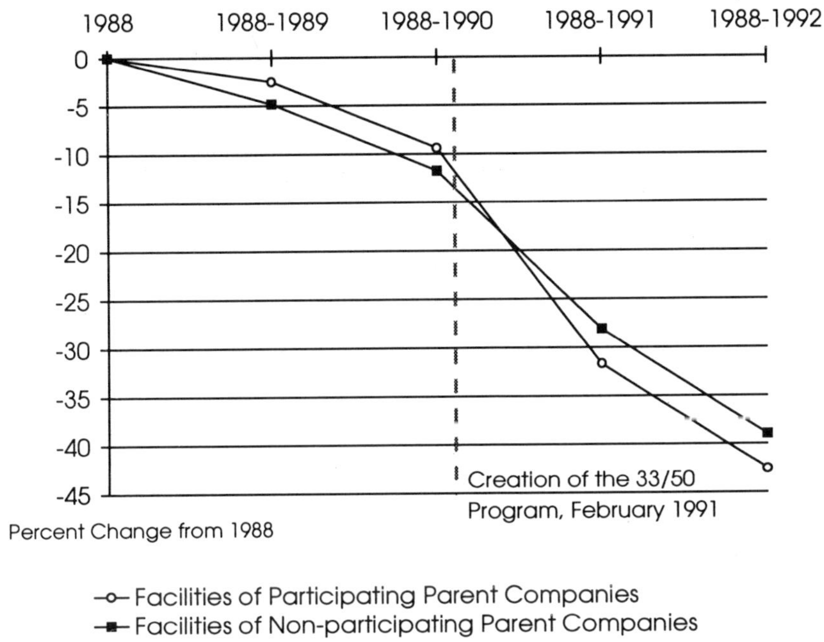

The steeper the downward slope of the line, the faster the rate of reduction.

Source Reduction Achievements

Finding: Facilities covered by a commitment to the 33/50 Program appear to have relied on end-of-pipe treatment technologies or on-site recycling and energy recovery, rather than source reduction, to achieve reductions in their releases and transfers of the 17 Program chemicals. (See Figures 11-6 and 11-7.)

The trend in achieving reduction of releases and transfers among those matched pairs that reported source reduction in either 1991 or 1992 is similar to the trend for all facilities reporting Program chemicals (discussed earlier). That is, the percent reduction achieved by facilities covered by a commitment surpassed that of facilities not covered by a commitment after initiation of the 33/50 Program. Although these facilities reported implementing at least one source reduction activity in the reporting year, INFORM cannot evaluate the extent to which source reduction has contributed to the percent reduction shown here because TRI does not require facilities to report the amount of waste reduced through source reduction. (See Figure 11-6.)

By 1990 the percent reduction of the 17 Program chemicals at facilities covered by a commitment but *not* reporting source reduction in 1991 or 1992 appears to be much greater than that of facilities not covered by a commitment . This suggests that commitment to the 33/50 Program is more strongly associated with greater reductions at facilities not implementing source

Figure 11-7.

Percent Change in Releases and Transfers on Matched Forms Not Reporting Source Reduction Activity

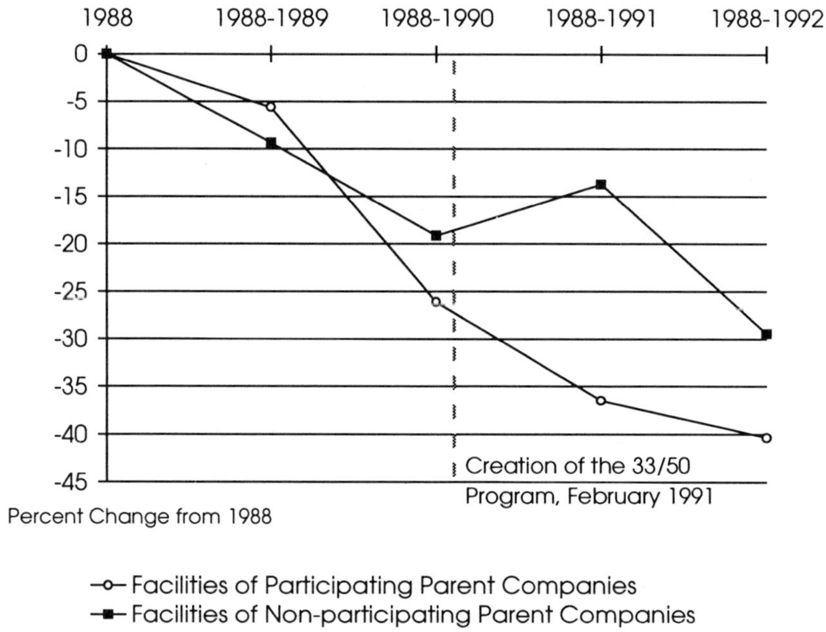

The steeper the downward slope of the line, the faster the rate of reduction.

reduction in 1991 or 1992 than for facilities that did report source reduction. Because these facilities did not report source reduction in 1991 or 1992 (and since INFORM's variance analysis shows that, for TRI facilities, changes in the production index have not shown a significant impact on quantities of releases and transfers), the percent reductions in releases and transfers reported in those years can be more likely attributed to end-of-pipe waste management methods than to source reduction. (See Figure 11-7.)

Finding: For facilities that reported implementing a "pioneering" source reduction activity in 1991 or 1992, there is essentially no difference in the percent reduction achieved by those facilities covered by a commitment from those not covered by a commitment. (See Figure 11-8.)

For 33/50 facilities reporting the implementation of "pioneering" source reduction activities, both those covered by a commitment and those not covered by a commitment both show a steady decrease in releases and transfers of the 17 Program chemicals between 1988 and 1992. As previously stated, because TRI does not require facilities to report the amount of waste reduced through source

Figure 11-8.

Percent Change in Releases and Transfers on Forms Reporting "Pioneering" Source Reduction Activity in 1991 or 1992

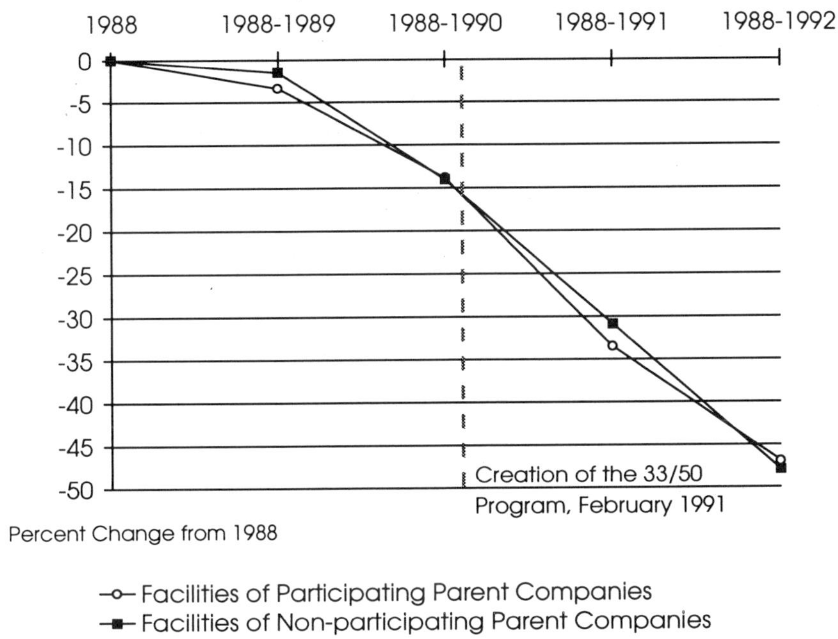

The steeper the downward slope of the line, the faster the rate of reduction.

reduction, INFORM cannot evaluate the extent to which source reduction contributed to the percent reduction shown here. (See Figure 11-8.)

INFORM defines pioneering source reduction activities as those that go beyond the straightforward housekeeping, maintenance, equipment, and operational changes that companies often find to increase the efficiency of their production processes (80 percent of the source reduction activities documented in INFORM's 1992 report, *Environmental Dividends: Cutting More Chemical Wastes*, were efficiency changes.) Pioneering source reduction activities include substituting less- or non-toxic or hazardous raw materials in place of presently used materials, finding new production processes or chemical syntheses for producing currently marketed products, and reformulating or changing to products that are less- or non-toxic or hazardous yet serve the same market. For the purpose of this analysis, INFORM considers the following source reduction activity codes reported on Section 8.10 of TRI Form R to be pioneering:

- W42, substituted raw materials,
- W53, different process catalysts,
- W73, substituted coating materials,
- W81, changed product specifications,
- W82, modified design or composition, and
- W89, other product modifications.

Figure 11-9.

Percent Change in Releases and Transfers for Forms Not Reporting this Chemical in 1991 or 1992

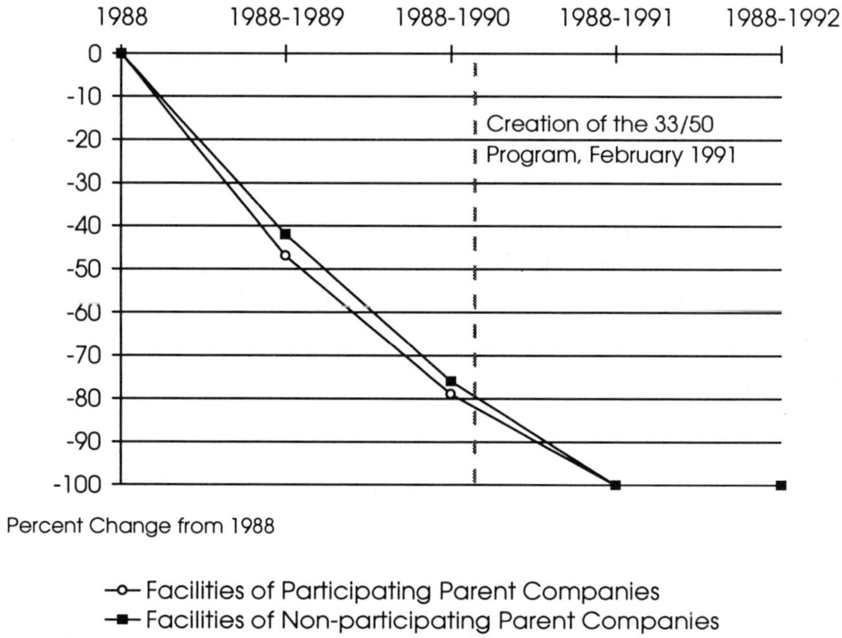

Reductions Stimulated by Factors Other than the 33/50 Program

Finding: On average, TRI facilities have reported large reductions in releases and transfers of the 17 Program chemicals since 1988. So far, reductions achieved by facilities covered by a commitment to the 33/50 Program do not appear to be much greater than reductions that would have occurred had the Program not existed at all. (See Figure 11-3.)

Finding: There appears to be a general trend among TRI facilities to bring TRI chemical use levels below the threshold requiring that the chemical be reported to TRI. This trend does not, however, appear to be associated with commitment to the 33/50 Program. (See Figure 11-9.)

Use of the 17 Program chemicals at some facilities fell below the reporting threshold in 1991 and 1992. Therefore, these facilities were not required to submit Form Rs in 1991 and 1992. (See Figure 11-9.)

The Overall Extent to which 33/50 Program Design Makes Effective Assessment of the Program's Impact on Industry Progress Possible

Finding: The constantly changing make-up of parent companies makes it difficult to ensure that all have been contacted and encouraged to participate. To achieve maximum possible participation, the Program would need to include systematic contacts at the facility level.

The 33/50 Program focuses on parent company performance rather than on individual facilities (where reductions actually take place). As facilities are bought and sold, this adds to the difficulty of ensuring that all companies have been contacted about participating in the Program. Tracking reduction progress over time is similarly complicated by the problems of determining which specific facilities of any given parent are participating in any given year. For example, in determining progress of a participating company, EPA counts releases and transfers of the 17 Program chemicals from all of a company's facilities even if only one of its facilities has made a commitment to the Program but the parent itself has not. If the facility that made the commitment was sold, then the parent company counted as participating is no longer counted as participating because the only commitment identified with that parent company was for a facility that no longer belongs to the parent company. Releases and transfers for the entire company are, then, switched from participation to non-participation status.

Finding: EPA's exclusive use of TRI data to measure 33/50 reductions precludes measuring how much of the reduction was due to source reduction, the other goal of the Program.

Source reduction amounts are not reported to TRI and would have to be reported separately by the companies and facilities.

The 33/50 Program does not ask companies or facilities to provide information on the amount of waste reduced due to source reduction activities each year on a systematic basis. Also, TRI does not collect this data. Therefore, this aspect of the Program cannot be measured nor progress assessed. In surveying facilities as an ongoing part of its evaluation, INFORM will ask companies to provide these data.

Evaluation Method

The goal of the INFORM evaluation of the 33/50 Program is essentially to know whether the Program has made a difference. The goals of the Program are to reduce releases and transfers of 17 TRI chemicals and to encourage achieving this reduction through pollution prevention (source reduction). Many factors at work may combine to result in reduction in releases and transfers at a particular facility, aside from the 33/50 Program. Determining whether or not releases and transfers were reduced more at 33/50 participating facilities and at such facilities reporting source reduction does not reveal whether or not the reduction was the result of the 33/50 Program because other factors leading to reductions may happen to be prevalent at 33/50 participating facilities. Such factors might be changes in production levels, the industry or state the facility is in, how much of the chemical is used during the year, or what type of chemical it is.

One way to learn whether the 33/50 Program led to the reductions, rather than some other factor, would be to ask the facility. INFORM is doing this, as part of the evaluation, in the form of questionnaires and interviews. However, there are more than 12,000 facilities reporting at least one Program chemical and 23,000 TRI facilities, and it is not possible to question them all. Therefore, this report uses statistical analysis to evaluate the probable impact of the 33/50 Program in the face of these other factors.

Analysis of Variance

Statistical analysis compares 33/50 participating facilities with non-33/50 participating facilities in subsets of facilities where other factors are the same. This analysis looks at factors reported to TRI, such as the amount of waste reported, the industry sector, the types of uses to which the chemical is put, the type of chemical itself, whether production has increased/ decreased, whether recycling and/ or energy recovery is practiced on site, to see if these are associated with differences in the amounts of releases and transfers and total production waste reported. It looks at facilities with all but one factor the same to see if, on average, the releases/transfers/wastes are different when the one factor is different. For example, Facility A and Facility B, both located in Delaware, manufacture toluene for use on site and have about 1,000 pounds maximum on site during the year. One may expect the reported waste of Facility A to be about the same as that of Facility B. However, the analysis of variance shows that if the two facilities are in different industries even with all these other factors the same — for instance, if Facility A was a chemical company which manufactured toluene and Facility B used toluene as a solvent in its metal-finishing operations — then we should expect the reported waste to be significantly different. The evaluation would then have to be sure to match Facility A with another facility that was also in the same industry.

The purpose of the analysis of variance is to identify those factors of the facility and/or chemical as reported to TRI that may be associated with different levels of wastes generated and to identify, therefore, how to match pairs of facilities so they can be tracked in future years of TRI data to see how their comparative reported wastes and releases and transfers differ. First, the analysis of variance will identify significant factors. Then, each facility falling under the commitment of a participating parent company will be matched with a facility that belongs to a parent company that is not participating, either because it reports none of the 17 Program chemicals or because it does not fall within a 33/50 commitment. The matches will take the first 33/50 Program facility and find a second facility that has the same characteristics, except that it is a non-participating facility. The 1992 and later releases and transfers of these two groups of facilities will then be compared to see if the first, 33/50 participating, group reported lower releases and transfers.

An analysis of variance was performed on the TRI data as reported for calendar year 1991. These data include expanded information on recycling, energy recovery, and treatment and source reduction activities, which was not required to be reported in previous years.

Model Factors

A general linear model was used with no interactive terms. That is, changes in reported waste were assumed to be linearly related to the factors without significant relations occurring between factors. For example, it is assumed that, on average, chemical plants are not all located in one state or that toluene is not manufactured at all facilities reporting its use, independent of the amount of reported waste.

The factors, independent variables, included in this model are:

- size as determined by the amount of waste reported,
- whether or not energy recovery takes place on site,
- whether or not recycling takes place on site,
- whether or not source reduction was reported for the chemical,
- the class of chemical,
- the production index (from 1990 to 1991),
- the type of activity/use,
- the maximum amount on site during the year,
- the SIC code(s) reported from the operations involving the chemical, and

for the facility:

- the state where the facility is located.

The size factor was incorporated by defining two groups based on the total amount of waste reported for 1990 and 1991 and running the model for each group separately (see below).

The dependent variables, the elements whose variation may be explained by the above factors, include:

- the reported waste for 1990, 1991, and 1993 (projected),
- the quantity released as reported for 1990, 1991, and 1993 (projected),
- the difference in the wastes between 1990 and 1991 and as projected between 1990 and 1993,
- the difference in the quantity released between 1990 and 1991 and as projected between 1990 and 1993.
- the total releases and transfers in 1988 and 1991, and
- the difference in total releases and transfers between 1988 and 1991.

The models incorporating the dependent variable against the common group of independent variables were run separately for small waste reporters and large waste reporters (see below).

The Data

Because 1991 was the first year for which waste data were reported, several subsets of the data had to be eliminated from the analysis. First, only the consistent TRI data records were used. Consistent records were those for which data were reported in the same manner for each of the four years (the four years being prior, current, following-year projection and second-year projection, which are reported on the same form each year). That is, if one year had a number or zero for the amount, then each of the other three years also had to have a number or zero and could not have been left blank. If all four years on the form were left blank, then that was also considered a consistent record. The total number of consistent records is 44,969 out of 80,123 TRI forms. Second, any form with both 1990 and 1991 total production-related waste of zero was removed from the analysis. There were 5,016 such forms, or 11 percent.

All forms with 1990 or 1991 waste greater than 100,000 pounds were analyzed as a separate group. These large waste reporters (8,624 forms) represent 19 percent of the forms but more than 97 percent of the amounts of waste. The subset of forms having total production-related waste in both 1990 and 1991 less than or equal to 100,000 pounds, the small waste reporters, contains 31,329 forms representing 70 percent of the consistent data forms, but 2 percent of the waste. With such a skewed distribution of pounds, any analysis that included the large waste reporters could not detect anything about the other 80 percent of forms. Therefore, the analysis was done on two subsets of the data: small waste reporters and large waste reporters.

In addition, each form was matched to the form the facility reported for that chemical in 1988 to obtain the total amount of releases and transfers in 1988. If no form was found, the 1988 amount was assumed to be zero. Because off-site transfers to energy recovery and recycling were not required to be reported in 1988, the amounts for energy recovery and recycling were excluded from total releases and transfers for 1991 for comparison with the total for 1988.

Model Results

In addition to size, the factors that turn out to be significant — that can be said to be associated with different levels of the dependent variable if they are different — are:

- chemical class,
- activity/use category,
- maximum amount category, and
- industry category.

The factor significant in most, but not all, cases was:

- state location of facility

The factors significant in a few cases only were:

- source reduction reported,
- energy recovery on site, and
- recycling on site.

The factor that was not significant in any case was:

- production index.

The model was run for both small and large waste reporters. The model is not as good at explaining the variation among the large reporters, primarily because the variation in waste is quite large for this group just as it was for all TRI facilities as a whole. However, where factors are significant for large reporters, they tend to be the same as those for the group of small reporters.

The model was also run against the TRI Sections 5 and 6 data of total releases and transfers. By definition, this number differs from the "quantity released" of Section 8 by including all off-site transfers and not just those transferred off site for disposal. Again, the model is not as good at explaining total releases and transfers especially for large waste reporters but no factors are significant here that were not also significant in the other runs of the model.

Facility Matching and Tracking

As a result of this analysis, facilities were matched on the following factors:

- amount of reported total production-related waste,
- the class of chemical,
- the type of activity/use,
- the maximum amount on site,
- the industry (SIC code), and
- state location.

Where there were not enough large waste reporters to make a match, then the industry criteria was dropped for this group.

Limitations

Such analysis cannot establish cause and effect. It shows associations. That is, for the group of facilities analyzed, the differences are as found, and with the large numbers of facilities one can infer with reasonable confidence that the differences are significant without having to question or interview each facility.

The analysis looks at facilities, and the 33/50 Program is aimed at parent companies. This analysis has assumed that where a parent company has committed to participating in the Program, each of its facilities has the same degree of commitment. This, of course, is not always true, and to the extent it is not, the analysis will show less of an effect for the 33/50 Program.

Matched-Pair Analysis

Matching Forms for the 17 Program Chemicals from 1988

The purpose of the analysis of variance described above was to identify those factors of the facility and/or chemical as reported to TRI that may be associated with different levels of wastes generated and to identify, therefore, how to match pairs of facilities so they can be tracked using future years of TRI data to see how their comparative reported wastes and releases and transfers differ. Each facility falling under the commitment of a participating parent company was matched with a facility that belongs to a parent company that is not participating, either because it reports none of the 17 Program chemicals or because it does not fall within a 33/50 commitment. The forms were matched based on:

- amount of total TRI releases and transfers,
- the class of chemical,
- the type of activity/use,
- the maximum amount on site,
- the industry (SIC code), and
- state location.

The facilities that reported to TRI for at least one of the 17 Program chemicals in 1988 were divided into two groups:

- Group A: those facilities that are covered by a commitment to the 33/50 Program, and
- Group B: those facilities that are not covered by a commitment to the 33/50 Program.

"Covered by a commitment" means that the facility's parent company has made a commitment for all of its facilities or the parent company has made a commitment for a set of its facilities including this one or that the facility itself has made a commitment. This differs from EPA's designation of commitments in that EPA counts parent companies and adds releases and transfers from all of the companies' facilities, regardless of whether there is a commitment covering each facility. This analysis will not include a facility as covered by a commitment where only one facility of a company has made a commitment and the parent company has not or where the parent company made a commitment for a subset of its facilities but not for all of them. In these cases, EPA does include the releases and transfers from the other facilities not covered by a commitment in overall totals for participating parent companies.

Each TRI form for a Program chemical from a facility in Group A was matched, where possible, according to the above six criteria. That is, a form from among Group B that was for the same chemical, maximum amount range, activity/use code, SIC code, location state, and total releases and transfers, constituted a match.

Three of these criteria differ somewhat from the actual TRI Form R: activity/use category, SIC code, and total releases and transfers.

The activity/use categories used in the matching are:

- chemical produced/imported for sale/distribution,
- chemical produced/imported for on-site use/processing,
- chemical imported for other activities,
- chemical produced for other activities,
- chemical processed but not produced/imported, and
- chemical otherwise used only.

The amounts of total releases and transfers were first matched within 50 percent, that is a match was successful if the matching form from Group B had reported total releases and transfers within plus-50 percent or minus-50 percent of the total releases and transfers of the form from Group A. The remaining forms were then matched to within plus- or minus-75 percent, and then within one order of magnitude. Finally, for the forms in Group A that remained unmatched and that had total releases and transfers greater than 100,000 pounds, the criteria of SIC code was dropped and the forms were matched for total releases and transfers within one order of magnitude. This was done because the previous analysis of variance showed that for forms with large amounts the industry category was not significant.

The TRI facilities report all 4-digit SIC codes that are applicable to their use of TRI chemicals. Therefore, more than one 2-digit SIC code may be reported for a TRI chemical form. In these cases, the 2-digit SIC code for matching purposes was designated a "multiple" SIC code, and matches were made to other "multiple" SIC codes but not on the specific 4-digit SIC codes reported.

Where more than one form from Group B matched a form from Group A, one form from Group B was randomly picked. No form in Group B was picked more than once.

Then, for each pair of matched forms, the amounts of total releases and transfers reported to TRI for that chemical from that facility in each of the years 1989 through 1992 were obtained from TRI.

The data are from the three years 1988, 1989, and 1990 before the start of the 33/50 Program and the two years of 1991 and 1992 after the Program began. Any conclusions from these data are preliminary because there are only two years under the 33/50 Program.

Matching Non-Program Chemical Forms from 1988

A second matching exercise was performed taking each facility in the 33/50 Program and matching its forms for non-Program chemicals with forms from facilities that are not part of the 33/50 Program because they have not reported a Program chemical to TRI since 1988. Thus, all forms in Group A were matched with forms in this third group, and all forms in Group B were matched with forms in the third group as well. They were randomly matched according to the same criteria. No form in the third group was matched more than once.

---

1 U.S. Environmental Protection Agency, *1992 Toxics Release Inventory Public Data Release,* EPA 745-R-94-001, April 1994.

2 EPA, *1992 Toxics Release Inventory Public Data Release,* April 1994.

3 U.S. Environmental Protection Agency, *EPA's 33/50 Program Third Progress Update,* EPA 745-R-93-001, 1993.

4 U.S. Environmental Protection Agency, *EPA's 33/50 Program, A Progress Report,* July 1991.

5 U.S. Environmental Protection Agency, Fact Sheet for the 33/50 Project, 1991.

6 56FR7849, February 26, 1991; EPA, Fact Sheet, 1991.

7 U.S. Environmental Protection Agency, *EPA's 33/50 Program Fifth Progress Update,* EPA 745-R-94-002, 1994.

8 EPA, *EPA's 33/50 Program,* July 1991.

9 Letter to Carol Browner, U.S. Environmental Protection Agency Administrator, from environmental organizations (National Environmental Law Center, Sierra Club, U.S. Public Interest Research Group, Greenpeace, Citizen Action, World Wildlife Fund, Environmental Action, Working Group on Community Right-to-Know, and Environmental Defense Fund), May 10, 1994, regarding awards to companies for making large reductions in releases and transfers of 33/50 Program chemicals.

Appendices

Reporting Systems

A Toxics Release Inventory (TRI) Form R
B Methods of Calculating On-Site Recycling
C Toxics Release Inventory (TRI) Chemicals Added for 1995
D Biennial Reporting System (BRS) Forms IC and GM, with Waste Minimization Instructions
E Resource Conservation and Recovery Act (RCRA) Toxic Waste Codes
F Environmental Reporting Systems and Corporate Environmental Reports

Chemical Data

G Chemicals in the Environment: Additional Data
H Chemicals in Commerce: Additional Toxic Substances Control Act (TSCA) Data for Halogenated Compounds
I Toxics Release Inventory (TRI) Chemicals: Classifications, with Release/Disposal and Waste Data
J Chemicals in Waste: Additional Toxics Release Inventory (TRI) Data
K Chemicals in Waste: Additional Biennial Reporting System (BRS) Data

Industry Data

L Standard Industrial Classification (SIC) Codes
M Industry Profiles
N Industry and Waste: Additional Toxics Release Inventory (TRI) Data
O Environmental Management of Toxics Release Inventory (TRI) Waste by Parent Companies: Total Waste, Carcinogens, Ozone Depleters

33/50 Program Evaluation

P 33/50 Program Chemicals

Additional Information

Q Database Access

Appendix A

Toxics Release Inventory (TRI) Form R

(IMPORTANT: Type or print; read instructions before completing form)

Form Approved OMB Number: 2070-0093
Approval Expires: 11/92

EPA United States Environmental Protection Agency

FORM R TOXIC CHEMICAL RELEASE INVENTORY REPORTING FORM

Section 313 of the Emergency Planning and Community Right-to-Know Act of 1986, also known as Title III of the Superfund Amendments and Reauthorization Act

TRI FACILITY ID NUMBER

Toxic Chemical, Category, or Generic Name

WHERE TO SEND COMPLETED FORMS:

1. EPCRA Reporting Center
P.O. Box 3348
Merrifield, VA 22116-3348
ATTN: TOXIC CHEMICAL RELEASE INVENTORY

2. APPROPRIATE STATE OFFICE
(See instructions in Appendix F)

Enter "X" here if this is a revision

For EPA use only

IMPORTANT: See instructions to determine when "Not Applicable (NA)" boxes should be checked.

PART I. FACILITY IDENTIFICATION INFORMATION

SECTION 1. REPORTING YEAR

19 ____

SECTION 2. TRADE SECRET INFORMATION

2.1	Are you claiming the toxic chemical identified on page 3 trade secret? ☐ Yes (Answer question 2.2; Attach substantiation forms) ☐ No (Do not answer 2.2; Go to Section 3)
2.2	If yes in 2.1, is this copy: ☐ Sanitized ☐ Unsanitized

SECTION 3. CERTIFICATION (Important: Read and sign after completing all form sections.)

I hereby certify that I have reviewed the attached documents and that, to the best of my knowledge and belief, the submitted information is true and complete and that the amounts and values in this report are accurate based on reasonable estimates using data available to the preparers of this report.

Name and official title of owner/operator or senior management official

Signature

Date Signed

SECTION 4. FACILITY IDENTIFICATION

4.1

Facility or Establishment Name

TRI Facility ID Number

Street Address

City

County

State

Zip Code

Mailing Address (if different from street address)

City

State

Zip Code

PUT LABEL HERE

EPA Form 9350-1 (Rev. 12/4/92) - Previous editions are obsolete.

EPA
United States Environmental Protection Agency

EPA FORM R

PART I. FACILITY IDENTIFICATION INFORMATION (CONTINUED)

TRI FACILITY ID NUMBER
Toxic Chemical, Category, or Generic Name

SECTION 4. FACILITY IDENTIFICATION (Continued)

4.2	This report contains information for: **(Important: check only one)**	a. ☐ An entire facility			b. ☐ Part of a facility		
4.3	**Technical Contact**	Name			Telephone Number (include area code)		
4.4	**Public Contact**	Name			Telephone Number (include area code)		
4.5	**SIC Code (4-digit)**	a.	b.	c.	d.	e.	f.
4.6	**Latitude and Longitude**	Latitude			Longitude		
		Degrees	Minutes	Seconds	Degrees	Minutes	Seconds

4.7	**Dun & Bradstreet Number(s) (9 digits)**	a.
		b.
4.8	**EPA Identification Number(s) (RCRA I.D. No.) (12 characters)**	a.
		b.
4.9	**Facility NPDES Permit Number(s) (9 characters)**	a.
		b.
4.10	**Underground Injection Well Code (UIC) I.D. Number(s) (12 digits)**	a.
		b.

SECTION 5. PARENT COMPANY INFORMATION

5.1	Name of Parent Company ☐ NA	
5.2	Parent Company's Dun & Bradstreet Number ☐ NA	**(9 digits)**

EPA United States Environmental Protection Agency

EPA FORM R

PART II. CHEMICAL-SPECIFIC INFORMATION

TRI FACILITY ID NUMBER
Toxic Chemical, Category, or Generic Name

SECTION 1. TOXIC CHEMICAL IDENTITY	(Important: DO NOT complete this section if you complete Section 2 below.)
1.1	CAS Number (Important: Enter only one number exactly as it appears on the Section 313 list. Enter category code if reporting a chemical category.)
1.2	Toxic Chemical or Chemical Category Name (Important: Enter only one name exactly as it appears on the Section 313 list.)
1.3	Generic Chemical Name (Important: Complete **only** if Part I, Section 2.1 is checked "yes." Generic Name must be structurally descriptive.)

SECTION 2. MIXTURE COMPONENT IDENTITY	(Important: DO NOT complete this section if you complete Section 1 above.)
2.1	Generic Chemical Name Provided by Supplier (Important: Maximum of 70 characters, including numbers,letters, spaces, and punctuation.)

SECTION 3. ACTIVITIES AND USES OF THE TOXIC CHEMICAL AT THE FACILITY (Important: Check all that apply.)

3.1	**Manufacture the toxic chemical:**	a. ☐ Produce b. ☐ Import	If produce or import: c. ☐ For on-site use/processing d. ☐ For sale/distribution e. ☐ As a byproduct f. ☐ As an impurity
3.2	**Process the toxic chemical:**	a. ☐ As a reactant b. ☐ As a formulation component	c. ☐ As an article component d. ☐ Repackaging
3.3	**Otherwise use the toxic chemical:**	a. ☐ As a chemical processing aid b. ☐ As a manufacturing aid	c. ☐ Ancillary or other use

SECTION 4. MAXIMUM AMOUNT OF THE TOXIC CHEMICAL ON-SITE AT ANY TIME DURING THE CALENDAR YEAR

4.1	☐ (Enter two-digit code from instruction package.)

EPA Form 9350-1(Rev. 12/4/92) - Previous editions are obsolete.

EPA
United States
Environmental Protection
Agency

EPA FORM R

PART II. CHEMICAL-SPECIFIC INFORMATION (CONTINUED)

TRI FACILITY ID NUMBER
Toxic Chemical, Category, or Generic Name

SECTION 5. RELEASES OF THE TOXIC CHEMICAL TO THE ENVIRONMENT ON-SITE

			A. Total Release (pounds/year) (enter range code from instructions or estimate)	B. Basis of Estimate (enter code)	C. % From Stormwater
5.1	Fugitive or non-point air emissions	☐ NA			
5.2	Stack or point air emissions	☐ NA			
5.3	Discharges to receiving streams or water bodies (enter one name per box)				
5.3.1	Stream or Water Body Name				
5.3.2	Stream or Water Body Name				
5.3.3	Stream or Water Body Name				
5.4	Underground injections on-site	☐ NA			
5.5	Releases to land on-site				
5.5.1	Landfill	☐ NA			
5.5.2	Land treatment/ application farming	☐ NA			
5.5.3	Surface impoundment	☐ NA			
5.5.4	Other disposal	☐ NA			

☐ **Check here only if additional Section 5.3 information is provided on page 5 of this form.**

EPA Form 9350-1 (Rev. 12/4/92) - Previous editions are obsolete.

Range Codes: A = 1 - 10 pounds; B = 11 - 499 pounds; C = 500 - 999 pounds.

EPA
United States
Environmental Protection
Agency

EPA FORM R

PART II. CHEMICAL-SPECIFIC INFORMATION (CONTINUED)

TRI FACILITY ID NUMBER
Toxic Chemical, Category, or Generic Name

SECTION 5.3 ADDITIONAL INFORMATION ON RELEASES OF THE TOXIC CHEMICAL TO THE ENVIRONMENT ON-SITE				
5.3	**Discharges to receiving streams or water bodies** (enter one name per box)	**A. Total Release** (pounds/ year) (enter range code from instructions or estimate)	**B. Basis of Estimate** (enter code)	**C. % From Stormwater**
5.3.__	**Stream or Water Body Name**			
5.3.__	**Stream or Water Body Name**			
5.3.__	**Stream or Water Body Name**			

SECTION 6. TRANSFERS OF THE TOXIC CHEMICAL IN WASTES TO OFF-SITE LOCATIONS

6.1 DISCHARGES TO PUBLICLY OWNED TREATMENT WORKS (POTW)

6.1.A Total Quantity Transferred to POTWs and Basis of Estimate

6.1.A.1 Total Transfers (pounds/year) (enter range code or estimate)	**6.1.A.2** Basis of Estimate (enter code)

6.1.B POTW Name and Location Information

6.1.B.__ POTW Name		**6.1.B.__** POTW Name	
Street Address		Street Address	
City	County	City	County
State	Zip Code	State	Zip Code

If additional pages of Part II, Sections 5.3 and/or 6.1 are attached, indicate the total number of pages in this box ☐ and indicate which Part II, Sections 5.3/6.1 page this is, here. ☐
(example: 1, 2, 3, etc.)

EPA Form 9350-1 (Rev. 12/4/92) - Previous editions are obsolete.

Range Codes: A = 1 - 10 pounds; B = 11 - 499 pounds; C = 500 - 999 pounds.

EPA
United States
Environmental Protection
Agency

EPA FORM R

PART II. CHEMICAL-SPECIFIC INFORMATION (CONTINUED)

TRI FACILITY ID NUMBER
Toxic Chemical, Category, or Generic Name

SECTION 6.2 TRANSFERS TO OTHER OFF-SITE LOCATIONS

6.2.__ Off-site EPA Identification Number (RCRA ID No.)

Off-Site Location Name

Street Address

City | County

State | Zip Code | Is location under control of reporting facility or parent company? ☐ Yes ☐ No

A. Total Transfers (pounds/year) (enter range code or estimate)	B. Basis of Estimate (enter code)	C. Type of Waste Treatment/Disposal/ Recycling/Energy Recovery (enter code)
1.	1.	1. M
2.	2.	2. M
3.	3.	3. M
4.	4.	4. M

SECTION 6.2 TRANSFERS TO OTHER OFF-SITE LOCATIONS

6.2.__ Off-site EPA Identification Number (RCRA ID No.)

Off-Site Location Name

Street Address

City | County

State | Zip Code | Is location under control of reporting facility or parent company? ☐ Yes ☐ No

A. Total Transfers (pounds/year) (enter range code or estimate)	B. Basis of Estimate (enter code)	C. Type of Waste Treatment/Disposal/ Recycling/Energy Recovery (enter code)
1.	1.	1. M
2.	2.	2. M
3.	3.	3. M
4.	4.	4. M

If additional pages of Part II, Section 6.2 are attached, indicate the total number of pages in this box ☐ and indicate which Part II, Section 6.2 page this is, here. ☐ (example: 1, 2, 3, etc.)

Range Codes: A = 1 - 10 pounds; B = 11 - 499 pounds;
C = 500 - 999 pounds.

EPA
United States Environmental Protection Agency

EPA FORM R

PART II. CHEMICAL-SPECIFIC INFORMATION (CONTINUED)

TRI FACILITY ID NUMBER
Toxic Chemical, Category, or Generic Name

SECTION 7A. ON-SITE WASTE TREATMENT METHODS AND EFFICIENCY

☐ **Not Applicable (NA) - Check here if no on-site waste treatment is applied to any waste stream containing the toxic chemical or chemical category.**

a. General Waste Stream (enter code)	b. Waste Treatment Method(s) Sequence [enter 3-character code(s)]	c. Range of Influent Concentration	d. Waste Treatment Efficiency Estimate	e. Based on Operating Data?
7A.1a	**7A.1b** 1 ☐ 2 ☐ 3 ☐ 4 ☐ 5 ☐ 6 ☐ 7 ☐ 8 ☐	**7A.1c**	**7A.1d** %	**7A.1e** Yes ☐ No ☐
7A.2a	**7A.2b** 1 ☐ 2 ☐ 3 ☐ 4 ☐ 5 ☐ 6 ☐ 7 ☐ 8 ☐	**7A.2c**	**7A.2d** %	**7A.2e** Yes ☐ No ☐
7A.3a	**7A.3b** 1 ☐ 2 ☐ 3 ☐ 4 ☐ 5 ☐ 6 ☐ 7 ☐ 8 ☐	**7A.3c**	**7A.3d** %	**7A.3e** Yes ☐ No ☐
7A.4a	**7A.4b** 1 ☐ 2 ☐ 3 ☐ 4 ☐ 5 ☐ 6 ☐ 7 ☐ 8 ☐	**7A.4c**	**7A.4d** %	**7A.4e** Yes ☐ No ☐
7A.5a	**7A.5b** 1 ☐ 2 ☐ 3 ☐ 4 ☐ 5 ☐ 6 ☐ 7 ☐ 8 ☐	**7A.5c**	**7A.5d** %	**7A.5e** Yes ☐ No ☐

If additional copies of page 7 are attached, indicate the total number of pages in this box ☐ and indicate which page 7 this is, here. ☐ (example: 1, 2, 3, etc.)

EPA Form 9350-1 (Rev. 12/4/92) - Previous editions are obsolete.

EPA United States Environmental Protection Agency	**EPA FORM R** **PART II. CHEMICAL-SPECIFIC INFORMATION (CONTINUED)**	TRI FACILITY ID NUMBER
		Toxic Chemical, Category, or Generic Name

SECTION 7B. ON-SITE ENERGY RECOVERY PROCESSES

☐ Not Applicable (NA) - Check here if no on-site energy recovery is applied to any waste stream containing the toxic chemical or chemical category.

Energy Recovery Methods [enter 3-character code(s)]

1	2	3	4

SECTION 7C. ON-SITE RECYCLING PROCESSES

☐ Not Applicable (NA) - Check here if no on-site recycling is applied to any waste stream containing the toxic chemical or chemical category.

Recycling Methods [enter 3-character code(s)]

1	2	3	4	5
6	**7**	**8**	**9**	**10**

EPA United States Environmental Protection Agency

EPA FORM R

PART II. CHEMICAL-SPECIFIC INFORMATION (CONTINUED)

TRI FACILITY ID NUMBER
Chemical, Category, or Generic Name

SECTION 8. SOURCE REDUCTION AND RECYCLING ACTIVITIES

All quantity estimates can be reported using up to two significant figures.		Column A 1991 (pounds/year)	Column B 1992 (pounds/year)	Column C 1993 (pounds/year)	Column D 1994 (pounds/year)
8.1	Quantity released *				
8.2	Quantity used for energy recovery on-site				
8.3	Quantity used for energy recovery off-site				
8.4	Quantity recycled on-site				
8.5	Quantity recycled off-site				
8.6	Quantity treated on-site				
8.7	Quantity treated off-site				
8.8	Quantity released to the environment as a result of remedial actions, catastrophic events, or one-time events not associated with production processes (pounds/year)				
8.9	Production ratio or activity index				

8.10	Did your facility engage in any source reduction activities for this chemical during the reporting year? If not, enter "NA" in Section 8.10.1 and answer Section 8.11.			
	Source Reduction Activities [enter code(s)]	Methods to Identify Activity (enter codes)		
8.10.1		a.	b.	c.
8.10.2		a.	b.	c.
8.10.3		a.	b.	c.
8.10.4		a.	b.	c.

8.11	Is additional optional information on source reduction, recycling, or pollution control activities included with this report? (Check one box)	YES ☐	NO ☐

* Report releases pursuant to EPCRA Section 329(8) including "any spilling, leaking, pumping, pouring, emitting, emptying, discharging, injecting, escaping, leaching, dumping, or disposing into the environment." Do not include any quantity treated on-site or off-site.

EPA Form 9350 - 1 (Rev. 12/4/92) - Previous editions are obsolete.

Appendix B

Methods of Calculating On-site Recycling

For illustrative purposes, it is useful to think of the manufacturing process and recycling process as pieces of equipment with input and output streams. The manufacturing process has inputs of fresh feed (A) and recycled feed (B) and outputs of a recycling stream (C) and a product stream (D). The recycling process has the recycling stream (C) as its input and the recycled feed (B) and the recycling remains (E) as outputs. The remains may be used elsewhere in the plant or subjected to further on- or off-site waste management. The split stream (B′) represents material added or removed before the recycled feed is added to the manufacturing process. (See Figure B-1.)

For these examples, let n equal the amount of the TRI chemical of interest in stream N. The capital letter for the stream is also equal to the total number of pounds of all material including the TRI chemical, other chemicals, water, etc., in that stream per unit time (say, per minute). Thus, a is equal to the number of pounds of the chemical in the fresh feed stream (stream A) per minute. By mass balance:

$A + B \pm B' = C + D$ for the manufacturing process, and

$C = B + E$ for the recycling process.

Since TRI reporting is chemical specific, facilities are supposed to report only the amounts of the chemical of interest recycled on site. Some facilities, however, report the entire quantity of the recycling stream (C times the number of minutes of operation per year) as the amount recycled on site on TRI Form R Section 8. First Chemical Corporation of Pascagoula, Mississippi, uses this method to calculate on-site recycling of sulfuric acid. In 1992 the facility reported recycling 4.0 billion pounds of sulfuric acid on site. This figure actually represents the total pounds of sulfuric acid and water sent to the acid regeneration unit rather than just the acid constituent portion of the stream. Calculating on-site recycling in this manner makes First Chemical's total production-related waste 11 percent of the nation's total.

Depending on a facility's definition of on-site recycling, the quantity may be calculated and reported to TRI in four ways:

1) c times the number of minutes of operation per year. This number is the total amount of the chemical of interest put through on-site recycling in the year. Using the sulfuric acid regeneration example,

Figure B-1.

On-Site Recycling

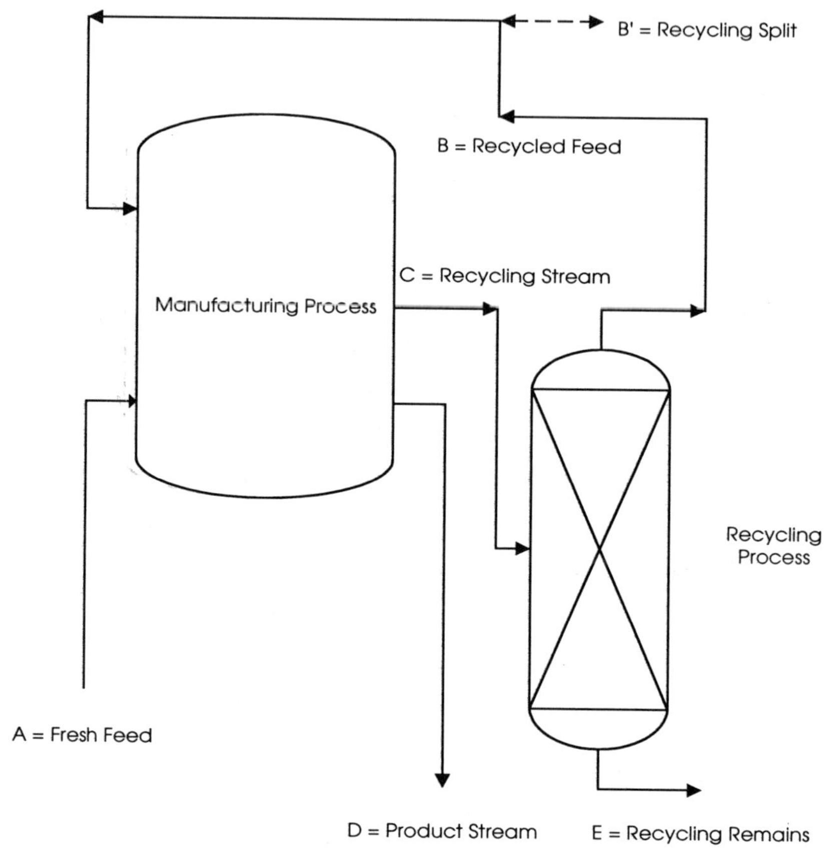

this calculation would include only the acid constituent portion of the regenerator stream. If First Chemical's acid regeneration stream contained only 25 percent acid by weight, the facility would have reported 1 billion pounds of on-site recycling, rather than 4 billion pounds, using this calculation method.

2) *d* is the amount of the chemical of interest that leaves as product per minute, and *a* is the amount of that chemical fed into the process per minute from fresh stock. The difference (*d* minus *a*) multiplied by the minutes of operation per year yields the amount of recycled chemical that ends up in the product. This *can* be reported as the amount of on-site recycling of the chemical if the recycling stream is not split (B′ = 0, so no material is added or removed before the recycled feed reenters the process) *and* none of the chemical is present in the recycled remains ($e = 0$). For First Chemical, this quantity would be the amount of concentrated sulfuric acid generated by recycling used in production for the year. It is also possible that some of the regenerated acid would be used to make an entirely different product or could itself be sold as product, in which case this calculation method could not be used.

3) *b*, which is the amount of the chemical leaving the recycling loop, can be used as the total quantity of on-site recycling for that particular chemical. Any chemical present in the recycled remains (*e*) would have to be counted elsewhere (e.g., released, transferred off-site, etc.). If First Chemical put 1 billion pounds of pure sulfuric acid into the regenerator during the year, and removed 80 percent of it as pure sulfuric acid (whether or not the acid was returned to the manufacturing process), then the facility would report 800 million pounds of on-site recycling for sulfuric acid.

4) The entire recycling process can also be considered an integral part of the manufacturing process, in which case no on-site recycling will be reported. In this report, this type of on-site recycling is called in-process recovery. If First Chemical considered its acid regeneration to be in-process recovery, the plant would have reported zero pounds of on-site recycling for sulfuric acid in 1992. Facilities may also sell the recycled material as product and consider the recycling loop to be a production process and, therefore, not report any of the recycled material as waste generated.

Appendix C

Toxics Release Inventory (TRI) Chemicals Added for 1995

Chemicals

71751-41-2	Abamectin [Avermectin B1]
30560-19-1	Acephate (Acetylphosphoramidothioic acid O,S-dimethyl ester)
62476-59-9	Acifluorfen, sodium salt [5-(2-Chloro-4-(triflouromethyl)phenoxy)-2-nitro-benzoic acid, sodium salt]
15972-60-8	Alachlor
116-06-3	Aldicarb
28057-48-9	d-trans-Allethrin [d-trans-Chrysanthemic acid of d-allethrone]
107-11-9	Allylamine
20859-73-8	Aluminum phosphide
834-12-8	Ametryn (N-Ethyl-N'-(1-methylethyl)-6-(methylthio)-1,3,5,-triazine-2,4-diamine)
33089-61-1	Amitraz
101-05-3	Anilazine [4,6-dichloro-N-(2-chlorophenyl)-1,3,5-triazin-2-amine]
1912-24-9	Atrazine (6-Chloro-N-ethyl-N'-(1-methylethyl)-1,3,5,-triazine-2,4-diamine)
22781-23-3	Bendiocarb [2,2-Dimethyl-1,3-benzodioxol-4-ol methylcarbamate]
1861-40-1	Benfluralin (N-Butyl-N-ethyl-2,6-dinitro-4-(trifluoromethyl)benzenamine)
17804-35-2	Benomyl
82657-04-3	Bifenthrin
56-35-9	Bis(tributylin) oxide
10294-34-5	Boron trichloride
7637-07-2	Boron trifluoride
314-40-9	Bromacil (5-Bromo-6-methyl-3-(1-methylpropyl)-2,4-(1H,3H)-pyrimidinedione)
53404-19-6	Bromacil, lithium salt [2,4-(1H,3H)-Pyrimidinedione, 5-bromo-6-methyl-3-(1-methylpropyl), lithium salt]
7726-95-6	Bromine
35691-65-7	1-Bromo-1-(bromomethyl)-1,3-propanedicarbonitrile
52-51-7	2-Bromo-2-nitropropane-1,3-diol (Bronopol)
1689-84-5	Bromoxynil (3,5-Dibromo-4-hydroxybenzonitrile)
1689-99-2	Bromoxynil octanoate (Octanoic acid, 2,6-dibromo-4-cyanophenyl ester)
357-57-3	Brucine
6459-94-5	C.I. Acid Red 114
28407-37-6	C.I. Direct Blue 218
1563-66-2	Carbofuran
5234-68-4	Carboxin (5,6-Dihydro-2-methyl-N-phenyl-1,4-oxathiin-3-carboxamide)
2439-01-2	Chinomethionat [6-Methyl-1,3-dithiolo[4,5-b]quinoxalin-2-one]
115-28-6	Chlorendic acid
90982-32-4	Chlorimuron ethyl [Ethyl-2-[[[(4-chloro-6-methoxyprimidin-2-yl)-carbonyl]-amino]sulfonyl]benzoate]
4080-31-3	1-(3-Chloroallyl)-3,5,7-triaza-1-azoniaadamantane chloride
106-47-8	p-Chloroaniline
563-47-3	3-Chloro-2-methyl-1-propene
104-12-1	p-Chlorophenyl isocyanate
76-06-2	Chloropicrin
542-76-7	3-Chloropropionitrile

95-69-2	p-Chloro-o-toluidine
75-88-7	2-Chloro-1,1,1-trifluoro-ethane (HCFC-133a)
75-72-9	Chlorotrifluoromethane (CFC-13)
460-35-5	3-Chloro-1,1,1-trifluoro-propane (HCFC-253fb)
5598-13-0	Chlorpyrifos methyl [O,O-dimethyl-O-(3,5,6-trichloro-2-pyridyl)phosphorothioate
64902-72-3	Chlorsulfuron [2-chloro-N-[[4-methoxy-6-methyl-1,3,5-triazin-2-yl)amino]carbonyl]benzenesulfonamide]
4170-30-3	Crotonaldehyde
21725-46-2	Cyanazine
1134-23-2	Cycloate
108-93-0	Cyclohexanol
68359-37-5	Cyfluthrin [3-(2,2-Dichloroethenyl)-2,2-dimethylcyclopropanecarboxylic acid, cyano(4-fluoro-3-phenoxyphenyl)methyl ester]
68085-85-8	Cyhalothrin [3-(2-Chloro-3,3,3-trifluoro-1-propenyl)-2,2-dimethylcyclopropanecarboxylic acid cyano(3-phenoxyphenyl)methyl ester]
533-74-4	Dazomet(Tetrahydro-3,5-dimethyl-2H-1,3,5-thiadiazine-2-thione)
53404-60-7	Dazomet, sodium salt [Tetrahydro-3,5-dimethyl-2H-1,3,5-thiadiazine-2-thione, ion(1-), sodium]
94-82-6	2,4,-DB
1929-73-3	2,4-D butoxyethyl ester
94-80-4	2,4-D butyl ester
2971-38-2	2,4-D chlorocrotyl ester
13684-56-5	Desmedipham
1928-43-4	2,4-D 2-ethylhexyl ester
53404-37-8	2,4-D 2-ethyl-4-methylpentyl ester
333-41-5	Diazinon
10222-01-2	2,2-Dibromo-3-nitrilopropionamide
1918-00-9	Dicamba (3,6-Dichloro-2-methyoxybenzoic acid)
99-30-9	Dichloran [2,6-Dichloro-4-nitroaniline]
612-83-9	3,3'-Dichlorobenzidine dihydrochloride
64969-34-2	3,3'-Dichlorobenzidine sulfate
110-57-6	trans-1,4-Dichloro-2-butene
1649-08-7	1,2-Dichloro-1,1-difluoroethane (HCFC-132b)
75-43-4	Dichlorofluoromethane (HCFC-21)
127564-92-5	Dichloropentafluoropropane
13474-88-9	1,1-dichloro-1,2,2,3,3-pentafluoropropane (HCFC-225cc)
111512-56-2	1,1-dichloro-1,2,3,3,3-pentafluoropropane (HCFC-225eb)
422-44-6	1,2-dichloro-1,1,2,3,3-pentafluoropropane (HCFC-225bb)
431-86-7	1,2-dichloro-1,1,3,3,3-pentafluoropropane (HCFC-225da)
507-55-1	1,3-dichloro-1,1,2,2,3-pentafluoropropane (HCFC-225cb)
136013-79-1	1,3-dichloro-1,1,2,3,3-pentafluoropropane (HCFC-225ea)
128903-21-9	2,2-dichloro-1,1,1,3,3-pentafluoropropane (HCFC-225aa)
422-48-0	2,3-dichloro-1,1,1,2,3-pentafluoropropane (HCFC-225ba)
422-56-0	3,3-dichloro-1,1,1,2,2-pentafluoropropane (HCFC-225ca)
97-23-4	Dichlorophene [2,2'-Methylene-bis(4-chlorophenol)]
10061-02-6	trans-1,3-Dichloropropene
51338-27-3	Diclofop methyl [2-[4-(2,4-Dichlorophenoxy)phenoxy]propanoic acid, methyl ester]
77-73-6	Dicyclopentadiene
38727-55-8	Diethatyl ethyl
35367-38-5	Diflubenzuron
101-90-6	Diglycidyl resorcinol ether
55290-64-7	Dimethipin [2,3,-Dihydro-5,6-dimethyl-1,4-dithiin-1,1,4,4-tetraoxide]
60-51-5	Dimethoate
20325-40-0	3,3'-Dimethoxybenzidine dihydrochloride (o-Dianisidine dihydrochloride)
111984-09-9	3,3'-Dimethoxybenzidine hydrochloride (o-Dianisidine hydrochloride)
124-40-3	Dimethylamine
2300-66-5	Dimethylamine dicamba
612-82-8	3,3'-Dimethylbenzidine dihydrochloride (o-Tolidine dihydrochloride)
41766-75-0	3,3'-Dimethylbenzidine dihydrofluoride (o-Tolidine dihydrofluoride)
2524-03-0	Dimethyl chlorothiophosphate
75-78-5	Dimethyldichlorosilane

68-12-2	N,N-Dimethylformamide
576-26-1	2,6-Dimethylphenol
88-85-7	Dinitrobutyl phenol (Dinoseb)
39300-45-3	Dinocap
957-51-7	Diphenamid
122-39-4	Diphenylamine
2164-07-0	Dipotassium endothall [7-Oxabicyclo(2.2.1)heptane-2,3-dicarboxylic acid, dipotassium salt]
136-45-8	Dipropyl isocinchomeronate
138-93-2	Disodium cyanodithioimidocarbonate
94-11-1	2,4-D isopropyl ester
541-53-7	2,4-Dithiobiuret
330-54-1	Diuron
2439-10-3	Dodine [Dodecylguanidine monoacetate]
120-36-5	2,4,-DP
1320-18-9	2,4-D propylene glycol butyl ether ester
2702-72-9	2,4-D sodium salt
13194-48-4	Ethoprop [Phosphorodithioic acid O-ethyl S,S-dipropyl ester]
759-94-4	Ethyl dipropylthiocarbamate [EPTC]
52-85-7	Famphur
60168-88-9	Fenarimol [.alpha.-(2-Chlorophenyl)-.alpha.-4-chlorophenyl)-5-pyrimidinemethanol]
13356-08-6	Fenbutatin oxide (Hexakis(2-methyl-2-phenyl-propyl)distannoxane)
66441-23-4	Fenoxaprop ethyl [2-(4-((6-Chloro-2-benzoxazolylen)oxy)phenoxy)propanoic acid,ethyl ester]
72490-01-8	Fenoxycarb [2-(4-Phenoxyphenoxy)ethyl]carbamic acid ethyl ester]
39515-41-8	Fenpropathrin [2,2,3,3-Tetramethylcyclopropane carboxylic acid cyano(3-phenoxy-phenyl)methyl ester]
55-38-9	Fenthion [O,O-Dimethyl O-[3-methyl-4-(methylthio)phenyl]ester, phosphorothioic acid]
51630-58-1	Fenvalerate [4-Chloro-alpha-(1-methylethyl)benzeneacetic acid cyano(3-phenoxyphenyl)methyl ester]
14484-64-1	Ferbam [Tris(dimethylcarbamo-dithioato-S,S')iron]
69806-50-4	Fluazifop-butyl [2-[4-[[5-(Trifluoromethyl)-2-pyridinyl]oxy]-phenoxy]propanoic acid, butyl ester]
7782-41-4	Fluorine
51-21-8	Fluorouracil (5-Fluorouracil)
69409-94-5	Fluvalinate [N-[2-Chloro-4-(trifluoromethyl)phenyl]-DL-valine(+)-cyano (3-phenoxyphenyl)methyl ester]
133-07-3	Folpet
72178-02-0	Fomesafen [5-(2-Chloro-4-(trifluoromethyl)phenoxy)-N-methylsulfonyl)-2-nitrobenzamide]
319-84-6	alpha-Hexachlorocyclohexane
110-54-3	n-Hexane
51235-04-2	Hexazinone
67485-29-4	Hydramethylnon [Tetrahydro-5,5-dimethyl-2(1H)-pyrimidinone[3-[4-(trifluoromethyl)phenyl]-1-[2-[4-(trifluoromethyl)phenyl]ethenyl]-2-propenylidene]hydrazone]
35554-44-0	Imazalil [1-[2-(2,4-Dichlorophenyl)-2-(2-propenyloxy)ethyl]-1H-imidazole]
55406-53-6	3-Iodo-2-propynyl butylcarbamate
13463-40-6	Iron pentacarbonyl
465-73-6	Isodrin
25311-71-1	Isofenphos [2-[[Ethoxyl[(1-methylethyl)amino]phosphinothioyl]oxy]benzoic acid 1-methylethyl ester]
77501-63-4	Lactofen [5-(2-Chloro-4-(trifluoromethyl)phenoxy)-2-nitro-2-ethoxy-1- methyl-2-oxoethyl ester]
330-55-2	Linuron
554-13-2	Lithium carbonate
121-75-5	Malathion
93-65-2	Mecoprop
149-30-4	2-Mercaptobenzothiazole (MBT)
150-50-5	Merphos
137-42-8	Metham sodium (Sodium methyldithiocarbamate)

20354-26-1	Methazole [2-(3,4-Dichlorophenyl)-4-methyl-1,2,4-oxadiazolidine-3,5-dione]
2032-65-7	Methiocarb
94-74-6	Methoxone (4-Chloro-2-methylphenoxy) acetic acid (MCPA))
3653-48-3	Methoxone-sodium salt ((4-chloro-2-methylphenoxy) acetate sodium salt)
556-61-6	Methyl isothiocyanate [Isothiocyanatomethane]
75-86-5	2-Methyllactonitrile
924-42-5	N-Methylolacrylamide
298-00-0	Methyl parathion
872-50-4	N-Methyl-2-pyrrolidone
75-79-6	Methyltrichlorosilane
9006-42-2	Metiram
21087-64-5	Metribuzin
7786-34-7	Mevinphos
2212-67-1	Molinate (1H-Azepine-1-carbothioic acid, hexahydro-S-ethyl ester)
150-68-5	Monuron
88671-89-0	Myclobutanil [.alpha.-Butyl-.alpha.-(4-chlorophenyl)-1H-1,2,4-triazole-1-propanenitrile]
142-59-6	Nabam
300-76-5	Naled
1929-82-4	Nitrapyrin (2-Chloro-6-(trichloromethyl) pyridine)
100-01-6	p-Nitroaniline
27314-13-2	Norflurazon [4-Chloro-5-(methylamino)-2-[3-(trifluoromethyl)phenyl]-3(2H)-pyridazinone]
19044-88-3	Oryzalin [4-(Dipropylamino)-3,5-dinitrobenzenesulfonamide]
301-12-2	Oxydemeton methyl [S-(2-(ethylsulfinyl)ethyl) o,o-dimethyl ester phosphorothioic acid]
19666-30-9	Oxydiazon [3-[2,4-Dichloro-5-(1-methylethoxy)phenyl]-5-(1,1-dimethylethyl)-1,3,4-oxadiazol-2(3H)-one]
42874-03-3	Oxyfluorfen
10028-15-6	Ozone
1910-42-5	Paraquat dichloride
1114-71-2	Pebulate [Butylethylcarbamothioic acid S-propyl ester]
40487-42-1	Pendimethalin [N-(1-Ethylpropyl)-3,4-dimethyl-2,6-dinitrobenzenamine]
57-33-0	Pentobarbital sodium
594-42-3	Perchloromethyl mercaptan
52645-53-1	Permethrin [3-(2,2-Dichloroethenyl)-2,2-dimethylcyclopropanecarboxylic acid, (3-phenoxyphenyl)methyl ester]
85-01-8	Phenanthrene
26002-80-2	Phenothrin [2,2-Dimethyl-3-(2-methyl-1-propenyl)cyclopropanecarboxylic acid (3-phenoxyphenyl)methyl ester]
95-54-5	1,2-Phenylenediamine
108-45-2	1,3-Phenylenediamine
615-28-1	1,2-Phenylenediamine dihydrochloride
624-18-0	1,4-Phenylenediamine dihydrochloride
57-41-0	Phenytoin
7803-51-2	Phosphine
1918-02-1	Picloram
51-03-6	Piperonyl butoxide
29232-93-7	Pirimiphos methyl [O-(2-(Diethylamino)-6-methyl-4-pyrimidinyl)-O,O-dimethylphosphorothioate]
7758-01-2	Potassium bromate
128-03-0	Potassium dimethyldithiocarbamate
137-41-7	Potassium N-methyldithiocarbamate
41198-08-7	Profenofos [O-(4-Bromo-2-chlorophenyl)-O-ethyl-S-propyl phosphorothioate]
7287-19-6	Prometryn [N,N'-Bis(1-methylethyl)-6-methylthio-1,3,5-triazine-2,4-diamine]
1918-16-7	Propachlor [2-Chloro-N-(1-methylethyl)-N-phenylacetamide]
709-98-8	Propanil [N-(3,4-Dichlorophenyl)propanamide]
2312-35-8	Propargite
107-19-7	Propargyl alcohol
31218-83-4	Propetamphos [3-[[(Ethylamino)methoxyphosphinothioyl]oxy]-2-butenoic acid, 1-methylethyl ester]
60207-90-1	Propiconazole [1-[2-(2,4-Dichlorophenyl)-4-propyl-1,3-dioxolan-2-yl]- methyl-1H-1,2,4,-triazole]

76578-14-8	Quizalofop-ethyl [2-[4-[(6-Chloro-2-quinoxalinyl)oxy]phenoxy]propanoic acid ethyl ester]
10453-86-8	Resmethrin [[5-(Phenylmethyl)-3-furanyl]methyl 2,2-dimethyl-3-(2-methyl-1-propenyl)cyclopropanecarboxylate]]
74051-80-2	Sethoxydim [2-[1-(Ethoxyimino)butyl]-5-[2-(ethylthio)propyl]-3-hydroxy-2-cyclohexen-1-one]
122-34-9	Simazine
26628-22-8	Sodium azide
1982-69-0	Sodium dicamba [3,6-Dichloro-2-methoxybenzoic acid, sodium salt]
128-04-1	Sodium dimethyldithiocarbamate
62-74-8	Sodium fluoroacetate
7632-00-0	Sodium nitrite
131-52-2	Sodium pentachlorophenate
132-27-4	Sodium o-phenylphenoxide
2699-79-8	Sulfuryl fluoride [Vikane]
35400-43-2	Sulprofos [O-Ethyl O-[4-(methylthio)phenyl]phosphorodithioic acid S-propyl ester]
34014-18-1	Tebuthiuron [N-[5-(1,1-Dimethylethyl)-1,3,4-thiadiazol-2-yl)-N,N′-dimethylurea]
3383-96-8	Temephos
5902-51-2	Terbacil [5-Chloro-3-(1,1-dimethylethyl)-6-methyl-2,4(1H,3H)-pyrimidinedione]
354-11-0	1,1,1,2-Tetrachloro-2-fluoroethane (HCFC-121a)
354-14-3	1,1,2,2-Tetrachloro-1-fluoroethane (HCFC-121)
64-75-5	Tetracycline hydrochloride
7696-12-0	Tetramethrin [2,2-Dimethyl-3-(2-methyl-1-propenyl)cyclopropanecarboxylic acid (1,3,4,5,6,7-hexahydro-1,3-dioxo-2H-isoindol-2-yl)methyl ester]
148-79-8	Thiabendazole [2-(4-Thiazolyl)-1H-benzimidazole]
28249-77-6	Thiobencarb [Carbamic acid, diethylthio-, s-(p-chlorobenzyl)]
59669-26-0	Thiodicarb
23564-06-9	Thiophanate ethyl [[1,2-Phenylenebis(iminocarbonothioyl)]bis carbamic acid diethyl ester]
23564-05-8	Thiophanate-methyl
79-19-6	Thiosemicarbazide
43121-43-3	Triadimefon [1-(4-Chlorophenoxy)-3,3-dimethyl-1-(1H-1,2,4-triazol-1-yl)-2-butanone]
2303-17-5	Triallate
101200-48-0	Tribenuron methyl [2-(((((4-Methoxy-6-methyl-1,3,5-triazin-2-yl)-methylamino)carbonyl)amino)sulfonyl)-, methyl ester]
1983-10-4	Tributyltin fluoride
2155-70-6	Tributyltin methacrylate
78-48-8	S,S,S-Tributyltrithiophosphate (DEF)
76-02-8	Trichloroacetyl chloride
96-18-4	1,2,3-Trichloropropane
57213-69-1	Triclopyr, triethylammonium salt
121-44-8	Triethylamine
26644-46-2	Triforine [N,N′-[1,4-Piperazinediyl-bis(2,2,2-trichloroethylidene)] bisformamide]
75-77-4	Trimethylchlorosilane
2655-15-4	2,3,5-Trimethylphenyl methylcarbamate
639-58-7	Triphenyltin chloride
76-87-9	Triphenyltin hydroxide
50471-44-8	Vinclozolin [3-(3,5-Dichlorophenyl)-5-ethenyl-5-methyl-2,4-oxazolidinedione]

Categories

Diisocyanates

38661-72-2	1,3-Bis(methylisocyanate)cyclohexane
10347-54-3	1,4-Bis(methylisocyanate)cyclohexane
2556-36-7	1,4-Cyclohexane diisocyanate
134190-37-7	Diethyldiisocyanatobenzene
4128-73-8	4,4'-Diisocyanatodiphenyl ether
75790-87-3	2,4'-Diisocyanatodiphenyl sulfide
91-93-0	3,3'-Dimethoxybenzidine-4,4'-diisocyanate
91-97-4	3,3'-Dimethyl-4,4'-diphenylene diisocyanate
139-25-3	3,3'-Dimethyldiphenylmethane-4,4'-diisocyanate
822-06-0	Hexamethylene-1,6-diisocyanate
4098-71-0	lsophorone diisocyanate
75790-84-0	4-Methyldiphenylmethane-3,4-diisocyanate
5124-30-1	1,1-Methylene bis(4-isocyanatocyclohexane)
101-68-8	Methylenebis(phenylisocyanate) (MDI)
3173-72-6	1,5-Naphthalene diisocyanate
123-61-5	1,3-Phenylene diisocyanate
104-49-4	1,4-Phenylene diisocyanate
9016-87-9	Polymeric diphenylmethane diisocyanate
16938-22-0	2,2,4-Trimethylhexamethylene diisocyanate
15646-96-5	2,4,4-Trimethylhexamethylene diisocyanate

Nicotine and salts

Nitrate compounds (water dissociable; reportable only when in aqueous solution)

Polychlorinated alkanes

Includes those chemicals defined by the following formula:

$$C_xH_{2x-y}Cl_y$$

where x = 10 to 13; y = 3 to 12; and where the average chlorine content ranges from 40-70% with the limiting molecular formulas $C_{10}H_{19}Cl_3$ and $C_{13}H_{16}Cl_{12}$.

Polycyclic aromatic compounds (PACs)

56-55-3	Benz(a)anthracene
218-01-9	Benzo(a)phenanthrene
50-32-8	Benzo(a)pyrene
205-99-2	Benzo(b)fluoranthene
205-82-3	Benzo(i)fluoranthene
207-08-9	Benzo(k)fluoranthene
189-55-9	Benzo(rst)pentaphene
226-36-8	Dibenz(a,h)acridine
224-42-0	Dibenz(a,j)ac6dine
53-70-3	Dibenzo(a,h)anthracene
5385-75-1	Dibenzo(a,e)fluoranthene
192-65-4	Dibenzo(a,e)pyrene
189-64-0	Dibenzo(a,h)pyrene
191-30-0	Dibenzo(a,l)pyrene
194-59-2	7H-Dibenzo(c,g)carbazole
57-97-6	7,12-Dimethylbenz(a)anthracene
193-39-5	Indeno[1,2,3-cd]pyrene
3697-24-3	5-Methylchrysene
5522-43-0	1-Nitropyrene

Strychnine and salts

Source: 59FR61432, November 30, 1994.

Appendix D

Biennial Reporting System Forms IC and GM, with Waste Minimization Instructions

OMB#: 2050-0024 Expires 9/30/92

BEFORE COPYING FORM, ATTACH SITE IDENTIFICATION LABEL OR ENTER:

SITE NAME ______________________

EPA ID NO. |_|_|_|_|_|_|_|_|_|_|_|_|

U.S. ENVIRONMENTAL PROTECTION AGENCY

1991 Hazardous Waste Report

FORM IC

IDENTIFICATION AND CERTIFICATION

INSTRUCTIONS: Read the detailed instructions beginning on page 6 of the 1991 Hazardous Waste Report booklet before completing this form.

SEC. I Site name and location address. Complete items A through H. Check the box ☒ in items A, C, E, F, G, and H if same as label; if different, enter corrections. If label is absent, enter information. Instruction page 6

A. EPA ID No. Same as label ☐ or →

B. County

C. Site/company name Same as label ☐ or →

D. Has the site name associated with this EPA ID changed since 1989? ☐ 1 Yes ☐ 2 No

E. Street name and number. If not applicable, enter industrial park, building name or other physical location description. Same as label ☐ or →

F. City, town, village, etc. Same as label ☐ or →

G. State Same as label ☐

H. Zip Code Same as label ☐

SEC. II Mailing address of site. Instruction page 6

A. Is the mailing address the same as the location address? ☐ 1 Yes (SKIP TO SEC. III) ☐ 2 No (GO TO BOX B)

B. Number and street name of mailing address

C. City, town, village, etc.

D. State

E. Zip Code

SEC. III Name, title, and telephone number of the person who should be contacted if questions arise regarding this report. Instruction page 6

A. Please print: Last name First name M.I.

B. Title

C. Telephone

Extension

SEC. IV Enter the Standard Industrial Classification (SIC) Code that describes the principal products, group of products, produced or distributed, or the services rendered at the site's physical location. Enter more than one SIC Code only if no one industry description includes the combined activities of the site. Instruction page 7

A. B. C. D.

SEC. V "I certify under penalty of law that this document and all attachments were prepared under my direction or supervision in accordance with a system designed to assure that qualified personnel properly gather and evaluate the information submitted. Based on my inquiry of the person or persons who manage the system, or those persons directly responsible for gathering the information, the information submitted is, to the best of my knowledge and belief, true, accurate and complete. I am aware that there are significant penalties under Section 3008 of the Resource Conservation and Recovery Act for submitting false information, including the possibility of fine and imprisonment for knowing violations."

A. Please print: Last name First name M.I.

B. Title

C. Signature

D. Date of signature MO. DAY YR.

Page 1 of ______

EPA Form 8700-13A/B (Revised 8-91)

OVER -->

FORM IC

Sec. VI - Generator Status

EPA ID NO. [ ]

A. 1991 RCRA generator status
Instruction page 7
(CHECK ONE BOX BELOW)

- ☐ 1 LQG
- ☐ 2 SQG (SKIP TO SEC. VII)
- ☐ 3 CESQG
- ☐ 4 Non generator (CONTINUE TO BOX B)

B. Reason for not generating
Page 9
(CHECK ALL THAT APPLY)

- ☐ 1 Never generated
- ☐ 2 Out of business
- ☐ 3 Only excluded or delisted waste
- ☐ 4 Only non-hazardous waste
- ☐ 5 Periodic or occasional generator
- ☐ 6 Waste minimization activity
- ☐ 7 Other (SPECIFY COMMENTS IN BOX BELOW)

Sec. VII - On-Site Waste Management Status

A. RCRA permitted or interim status storage
Instruction page 10
[ ]

B. RCRA permitted or interim status treatment, disposal, or recycling
Page 10
[ ]

C. RCRA-exempt treatment, disposal, or recycling
Page 11
[ ]

Sec. VIII - Waste Minimization Activity during 1990 or 1991

A. Did this site begin or expand a source reduction activity during 1990 or 1991?
Instruction page 11

- ☐ 1 Yes
- ☐ 2 No

B. Did this site begin or expand a recycling activity during 1990 or 1991?
Page 12

- ☐ 1 Yes
- ☐ 2 No

C. Did this site systematically investigate opportunities for source reduction or recycling during 1990 or 1991?
Page 12

- ☐ 1 Yes
- ☐ 2 No

D. Did any of the factors listed below delay or limit this site's ability to initiate new or additional source reduction activities in 1990 or 1991?
Page 12
(CHECK YES OR NO FOR EACH ITEM)

Yes	No		
☐1	☐ 2	a.	Insufficient capital to install new source reduction equipment or implement new source reduction practices
☐1	☐ 2	b.	Lack of technical information on source reduction techniques applicable to the specific production processes
☐1	☐ 2	c.	Source reduction is not economically feasible: cost savings in waste management or production will not recover the capital investment
☐1	☐ 2	d.	Concern that product quality may decline as a result of source reduction
☐1	☐ 2	e.	Technical limitations of the production processes
☐1	☐ 2	f.	Permitting burdens
☐1	☐ 2	g.	Source reduction previously implemented -- additional reduction does not appear to be technically feasible
☐1	☐ 2	h.	Source reduction previously implemented - additional reduction does not appear to be economically feasible
☐1	☐ 2	i.	Source reduction previously implemented - additional reduction does not appear to be feasible due to permitting requirements
☐1	☐ 2	j.	Other (SPECIFY COMMENTS IN BOX BELOW)

E. Did any of the factors listed below delay or limit this site's ability to initiate new or additional on-site or off-site recycling activities during 1990 or 1991?
Page 12
(CHECK YES OR NO FOR EACH ITEM)

Yes	No		
☐1	☐ 2	a.	Insufficient capital to install new recycling equipment or implement new recycling practice
☐1	☐ 2	b.	Lack of technical information on recycling techniques applicable to this site's specific production processes
☐1	☐ 2	c.	Recycling is not economically feasible: cost savings in waste management or production will not recover the capital investment
☐1	☐ 2	d.	Concern that product quality may decline as a result of recycling
☐1	☐ 2	e.	Requirements to manifest wastes inhibit shipments off site for recycling
☐1	☐ 2	f.	Financial liability provisions inhibit shipments off site for recycling
☐1	☐ 2	g.	Technical limitations of production processes inhibit shipments off site for recycling
☐1	☐ 2	h.	Technical limitations of production processes inhibit on-site recycling
☐1	☐ 2	i.	Permitting burdens inhibit recycling
☐1	☐ 2	j.	Lack of permitted off-site recycling facilities
☐1	☐ 2	k.	Unable to identify a market for recyclable materials
☐1	☐ 2	l.	Recycling previously implemented -- additional recycling does not appear to be technically feasible
☐1	☐ 2	m.	Recycling previously implemented -- additional recycling does not appear to be economically feasible
☐1	☐ 2	n.	Recycling previously implemented - additional recycling does not appear to be feasible due to permitting requirements
☐1	☐ 2	o.	Other (SPECIFY COMMENTS IN BOX BELOW)

Comments:

Page 2 of ____

BEFORE COPYING FORM, ATTACH SITE IDENTIFICATION LABEL
OR ENTER:

SITE NAME ______________________

EPA ID NO.

U.S. ENVIRONMENTAL PROTECTION AGENCY

1991 Hazardous Waste Report

FORM **GM**

WASTE GENERATION AND MANAGEMENT

INSTRUCTIONS: Read the detailed instructions beginning on page 13 of the 1991 Hazardous Waste Report booklet before completing this form.

Sec. I

A. Waste description
Instruction Page 15

B. EPA hazardous waste code
Page 15

C. State hazardous waste code
Page 15

D. SIC code
Page 16

E. Origin code
Page 16
System type M

F. Source code
Page 17
A

G. Point of measurement
Page 17

H. Form code
Page 17
B

I. RCRA-radioactive mixed
Page 17

J. Reported TRI constituent
Page 18

K. CAS numbers
Page 18
1. 2. 3. 4. 5.

Sec. II

A. Quantity generated in 1990
instruction Page 18

B. Quantity generated in 1991
Page 18

C. UOM Density
Page 19
☐ 1 lbs/gal ☐ 2 sg

D. Did this site do any of the following to this waste: treat on site, dispose on site, recycle on site, or discharge to a sewer/POTW?
Page 19
☐ 1 Yes (CONTINUE TO SYSTEM 1)
☐ 2 No (SKIP TO SEC. III)

ON-SITE SYSTEM 1
On-site system type
Page 19
M
Quantity treated, disposed or recycled on site in 1991

ON-SITE SYSTEM 2
On-site system type
Page 19
M
Quantity treated, disposed or recycled on site in 1991

Sec. III

A. Was any of this waste shipped off site in 1991?
Instruction Page 20
☐ 1 Yes (CONTINUE TO BOX B)
☐ 2 No (SKIP TO SEC. IV)

Site 1
B. EPA ID No. of facility waste was shipped to
Page 20
C. System type shipped to
Page 20
M
D. Off-site availability code
Page 21
E. Total quantity shipped in 1991
Page 21

Site 2
B. EPA ID No. of facility waste was shipped to
Page 20
C. System type shipped to
Page 20
M
D. Off-site availability code
Page 21
E. Total quantity shipped in 1991
Page 21

Sec. IV

A. Did new activities in 1991 result in minimization of this waste?
Instruction Page 22
☐ 1 Yes (CONTINUE TO BOX B)
☐ 2 No (THIS FORM IS COMPLETE)

B. Activity
Page 22
W W
W W

C. Other effects
Page 22
☐ 1 Yes
☐ 2 No

D. Quantity recycled in 1991 due to new activities
Page 23

E. Activity/production index
Page 23

F. 1991 Source reduction quantity
Page 24

Comments:

Page ____ of ____

Instructions for Form GM, Section IV (part)

Section IV: New Waste Minimization Activities in 1991

Section IV requests information on any **new** activities undertaken during 1991 that resulted in waste minimization. This information is collected to obtain a national cross section of waste minimization activity in 1991. It is not intended to provide a chronology of activity at your site. Detailed definitions of waste minimization and its component parts, source reduction and recycling, are provided below.

Source reduction means the reduction or elimination of hazardous waste stream at the source, usually within a process. Source reduction measures include process modifications, feedstock substitutions, improvements in feedstock purity, housekeeping and management practices, increases in the efficiency of machinery, and recycling within a process. Source reduction implies any action that reduces the toxicity or the amount of waste exiting a process.

Recycling means the use or reuse of waste as an effective substitute for a commercial product, or as an ingredient or feedstock in an industrial process. It also refers to the reclamation of useful constituent fractions within a waste material or the removal of contaminants from a waste to allow it to be reused. As used in this report, recycling implies use, reuse, or reclamation of a waste, either on site or off site, after it has been generated.

Waste minimization means the reduction, to the extent feasible, of hazardous waste that is generated or subsequently treated, stored, or disposed. Waste minimization includes any source reduction or recycling activity undertaken by a generator that results in: (1) the reduction of total volume or quantity of hazardous waste stream; (2) the reduction of toxicity of hazardous waste stream; or (3) both, as long as the reduction is consistent with the goal of minimizing present and future threats to human health and the environment.

FORM GM

Section IV (Continued)

Box A: Did new activities in 1991 result in minimization of this waste?
During 1991, did you implement any new activities that resulted in minimization of the waste described in Section I, Box A?

> **NOTE:** Treatment (including burning and incineration) of the waste after it has exited the process is not considered waste minimization activity. The following are examples of activities that should not be reported here as waste minimization.
>
> - Sending waste off site for management (other than recycling)
> - Treatment to reduce volume (after the waste exits the process in which it was generated)
> - Treatment to reduce toxicity (after the waste exits the process in which it was generated)
> - Installation of filter press to reduce water content and volume
> - Installation of equipment to comply with Clean Water Act
>
> Bankruptcy or reduction in production volume due to economic factors are not waste minimization activities.

> **Continue with Box B** if you checked "Yes".
> **This form is complete** if you checked "No".

Box B: Activity
What activities were implemented in 1991 to achieve the waste minimization results for the waste described in Section I?

Review the list beginning on page 92 and select the codes representing activities undertaken for this waste. Response spaces are provided for up to four activities. If more than four codes are required, continue the entry in Comments, referencing Section IV, Box B. If fewer than four codes are applicable, enter "NA" in the remaining fields. See definitions of waste minimization, source reduction, and recycling on page 21.

> Activity Codes, page 92.

Box C: Other effects
Check "Yes" if the activities that resulted in minimization of the waste either:

- Increased the toxicity of the waste or
- Increased the quantity or toxicity of emissions into air, water, or land.

FORM GM

Section IV (Continued)

Box D: Quantity recycled in 1991 due to new activities
Enter the quantity of hazardous waste that was recycled during 1991 because of new recycling activities. Count both on-site and off-site recycling, but do not include quantities recycled in systems operational before 1991. Do not include closed-loop recycling, as that is to be reported as a source reduction activity. Enter "NA" if no hazardous waste stream was recycled because of new recycling activities.

Box E: Activity/production index
The activity/production index is a measure of changes in economic and other factors that affected the quantity of hazardous waste stream generated in 1991, compared to 1990. The index is used to distinguish inter-year quantity changes that resulted from waste minimization activity from those that are attributable to economic or other factors.

The EPA understands that some sites may find it impractical to calculate a meaningful activity/production index. If you cannot calculate an index for your site, enter "NA" in Box E.

Use the worksheet on page 24 to calculate the activity/production index. Determine the most appropriate measure of production or activity, using product manufactured, raw materials used, number of hours the plant was in operation, the total number of employee hours worked, sales, budget, and any other factor that is appropriate for the waste stream. Divide the value of that measure for 1991 by the comparable value for 1990.

Example 1:
If the firm manufactures tools using a process that generated a hazardous waste stream, the activity/production index would indicate the change in the number of tools produced in 1991 compared to 1990.

1,200 tools were produced in 1991, and 1,000 tools were produced in 1990. The activity/production index equals 1,200 divided by 1,000.

$$\frac{\text{(1991 production)}}{\text{(1990 production)}} \quad \frac{1{,}200}{1{,}000} = 1.2 \text{ (activity/production index)}$$

The number "1.2" would be entered in Box E.

Example 2:
If a firm that manufactures stainless steel food containers is losing market share to competitors making plastic containers, its production might have declined between 1990 and 1991.

88,000 containers were produced in 1991 and 110,000 containers were produced in 1990. The activity/production index equals 88,000 divided by 110,000.

$$\frac{\text{(1991 production)}}{\text{(1990 production)}} \quad \frac{88{,}000}{110{,}000} = 0.8 \text{ (activity/production index)}$$

The number "0.8" would be entered in Box E.

(Continued on next page)

FORM GM

Section IV (Continued)

Example 3:
If a firm is a dry cleaner that cleaned 2,200 garments in 1991 and 2,000 garments in 1990, the activity/production index would indicate the change in the number of garments cleaned. The activity/production index equals 2,200 divided by 2,000.

$$\frac{(1991\ \text{production})\quad 2{,}200}{(1990\ \text{production})\quad 2{,}000} = 1.1\ \text{(activity/production index)}$$

The number "1.1" would be entered in Box E.

Activity/Production Index Worksheet

Units produced or units of service provided in 1991		(____________)
divided by	÷	
Units produced or units of service provided in 1990		(____________)
Enter activity/production index in Box E	=	___._

Box F: 1991 Source reduction quantity
If you reported a source reduction activity in Box B (codes W11 through W99), enter your best estimate of the reduction in 1991 quantity generated that resulted from the source reduction activities. Report the quantity in the unit of measure reported in Section II, Box C. Enter "NA" in this space if:

- You did not report a source reduction activity or
- The source reduction activity you reported resulted only in a reduction in toxicity and not a reduction in quantity of waste.

If you completed Section II, Boxes A and B, and Section IV, Box E, calculate "Source Reduction Quantity" using the method described in the examples that follow.

If you did not complete the information requested in Section II, Boxes A and B, and Section IV, Box E, you may estimate the quantity of hazardous waste stream prevented in 1991 using another method. Review the three examples that follow to consider which approach your site might utilize. If you do not use this method, you must describe your computation in the Comments section at the end of the form. Reference Section IV, Box F. A blank Source Reduction Quantity Worksheet is included on page 28.

(Continued on next page)

FORM GM

Section IV (Continued)

Example 1:
A firm manufactures tools using a process that generates a hazardous waste stream. In 1990, the firm produced 1,000 tools and generated 2,000 gallons of waste. In 1991, the firm produced 1,200 tools and generated 1,800 gallons of waste. The activity/production index for the firm is 1.2. In 1991, the firm introduced a new process to minimize the quantity of hazardous waste it generated.

$$\frac{\text{(1991 production)}}{\text{(1990 production)}} \quad \frac{1{,}200}{1{,}000} = 1.2 \text{ (activity/production index)}$$

Source Reduction Quantity Worksheet

Step 1: Multiply the waste quantity generated in 1990 by the activity/production index.

	2,000	Quantity generated in 1990 (from Sec. II, Box A)
x	1.2	Times activity/production index (from Sec. IV, Box E)
=	2,400	Equals quantity that would have been generated without source reduction

Step 2: Subtract the 1991 waste quantity (Sec. II, Box B) from the quantity that would have been generated without source reduction (Total from Step 1).

	2,400	Quantity without source reduction
-	1,800	Minus quantity generated in 1991 (from Sec. II, Box B)
=	600	Equals quantity of generation prevented by source reduction (enter in Box F)

Step 3: Enter source reduction quantity in Box F.

Sec. II	A. Quantity generated in 1990 Instruction Page 18	B. Quantity generated in 1991 Page 18	C. UOM Page 19	Density	D. Did this site do any of the following to this waste: treat on site, dispose on site, recycle on site, or discharge to a sewer/POTW? Page 19
	2000.0	1800.0	5	8.34 [X] 1 lbs/gal [ ] 2 sg	[ ] 1 Yes (CONTINUE TO SYSTEM 1) [X] 2 No (SKIP TO SEC. III)

Sec. IV	A. Did new activities in 1991 result in minimization of this waste? Instruction Page 22	[X] 1 Yes (CONTINUE TO BOX B) [ ] 2 No (THIS FORM IS COMPLETE)			
B. Activity Page 22	C. Other effects Page 22	D. Quantity recycled in 1991 due to new activities Page 23	E. Activity/production index Page 23	F. 1991 Source reduction quantity Page 24	
W512 WNA WNA WNA	[ ] 1 Yes [X] 2 No	NA.	1.2	600.0	

Appendix E

Resource Conservation and Recovery Act (RCRA) Toxic Waste

Appendix E-1. Methodology for Analysis of RCRA Toxic Waste

In this *Toxics Watch* report, RCRA toxic waste is any waste that exhibits the characteristic of toxicity designated by the July 1, 1993, Federal Code of Regulations (40 CFR Parts 261.24 through 261.33) or that contains TRI constituents.[a] This excludes a RCRA hazardous waste that is corrosive, ignitable, or reactive unless the waste contained toxic constituents, as defined above.

For all waste stream reports, one number for "waste generated" is reported to the Biennial Reporting System (on Form GM, Section II.B). That is the figure used in this report as the total waste generated under BRS.

RCRA Regulated and RCRA Exempt Waste

When looking at how a waste is managed, the total waste is generally divided into two categories: RCRA managed and RCRA exempt. RCRA-managed waste includes waste that was subsequently managed in treatment units subject to RCRA permitting standards or transportation regulations. Waste that was subsequently managed in units exempt from RCRA permitting standards, such as closed wastewater treatment systems, are counted as RCRA-exempt wastes.

These two categories, however, are not reported as such to the BRS. Instead, how a waste is managed is reported under a series of codes, and assumptions must be made as to whether or not the codes represent RCRA-exempt treatment units. In this report, waste directly discharged to a POTW or to surface water under a National Pollutant Discharge Elimination System permit is considered exempt (codes M135 and M136 on Form GM, Section III.C.). For wastes managed on-site, the waste is considered a RCRA-exempt waste unless the regulatory status code (as reported on Form PS, Section I.C.) is for a RCRA-regulated system or a system that includes both RCRA-regulated and RCRA-exempt units (that is, codes 01, 05, and 06). If there is no indication of the specific type of system (that is, no Form PS), then the waste is considered a RCRA waste unless the facility reports that there are no RCRA permitted treatment, disposal, or recycling units at the site (on Form IC, Section VII).

EPA publishes a Biennial RCRA Hazardous Waste Report for each reporting year. That report concerns only the RCRA-regulated waste reported and, for the most part, includes in its summary tables the confidential business information. The numbers in this report differ from the EPA BRS report for the year 1991 in several respects.

All wastes reported under toxic waste codes are included in this *Toxics Watch* report, including both RCRA regulated and RCRA exempt.

Assumptions and Calculation Methodology

Confidential business information is not included. The total for the confidential business informa-

[a] That is, if a TRI CAS number is reported for the waste stream.

tion claims is approximately 36 billion pounds (18 million tons) managed in RCRA regulated units as reported in 1991.[b] There is no breakdown available for the amount of toxic BRS waste generated that is confidential.

The amount of waste managed as RCRA-exempt is a calculated number, based on certain assumptions. Two specific assumptions used for this report differ from those used by EPA in its report summarizing BRS data. One is that, if more than one type of treatment unit is reported (on Form PS) and one is exempt and one is regulated, the amount of waste reported in *Toxics Watch* is proportioned between the two types of units. The EPA report assumes that all the waste is managed in the RCRA-regulated unit.[c] Second is that, if the regulatory status of a treatment unit is "exempt from all Federal RCRA and other permitting regulations and from State-only regulation" (Form PS, Section I.C. code 08), this report assumes the waste managed is RCRA exempt, while the EPA report includes the waste as RCRA regulated.[d]

This second assumption accounts for a difference in the classification of wastes of about 37 billion pounds (18.4 million tons) between the two reports. Three petroleum refineries and a chemical plant report significant amounts of their RCRA wastes under waste code D018 (benzene characteristic waste) as discharged to POTWs under regulatory status code 08 on the Form PS (exempt from all federal RCRA and other permitting regulations and from state-only regulation). These amounts are assumed to be RCRA exempt in this report and are assumed to be RCRA regulated in the EPA report. The facilities and the amount of waste classified differently are:

— Arco Products Co., Ferndale, Washington, 5,110,000 tons

— Chevron, Pascagoula, Mississippi, 6,575,256 tons

— Mobil Chemical Co., Beaumont,Texas, 3,421,550 tons

— Shell Oil Company, Anacortes, Washington, 3,340,000 tons

Appendix E-2 lists all RCRA waste codes included as "toxic" in this report.

[b] John Sagar of EPA's Office of Solid Waste provided this estimate.
[c] Assumptions used by EPA are found in the Technical User Guide, Biennial Reporting System, Office of Solid Waste, United States Environmental Protection Agency, June 1994, p. 67.
[d] John Sager of EPA's Office of Solid Waste confirmed this assumption as used by EPA.

Appendix E-2. RCRA Toxic Waste Codes

Characteristic Hazardous Waste

D004 Arsenic
D005 Barium
D006 Cadmium
D007 Chromium
D008 Lead
D009 Mercury
D010 Selenium
D011 Silver
D012 Endrin(1,2,3,4,10,10-hexachloro-1,7-epoxy-1,4,4a,5,6,7,8,8a-octahydro-1,4-endo, endo-5,8-dimeth-ano-naphthalene)
D013 Lindane (1,2,3,4,5,6-hexa-chloro-cyclohexane, gamma isomer)
D014 Methoxychlor (1,1,1-trichloro-2,2-bis [pmethoxyphenyl] ethane)
D015 Toxaphene (C10 H10 ClN, Technical chlorinated camphene, 67-69 percent chlorine)
D016 2,4-D (2,4-Dichlorophenoxyacetic acid)
D017 2,4,5-TP Silvex (2,4,5-Trichloro-phenoxypropionic acid)
D018 Benzene
D019 Carbon tetrachloride
D020 Chlordane
D021 Chlorobenzene
D022 Chloroform
D023 o-Cresol
D024 m-Cresol
D025 p-Cresol
D026 Cresol
D027 1,4-Dichlorobenzene
D028 1,2-Dichloroethane
D029 1,1-Dichloroethylene
D030 2,4-Dinitrotoluene
D031 Heptachlor (and its epoxide)
D032 Hexachlorobenzene
D033 Hexachlorobutadiene
D034 Hexachloroethane
D035 Methyl ethyl ketone
D036 Nitrobenzene
D037 Pentachlorophenol
D038 Pyridine
D039 Tetrachloroethylene
D040 Trichloroethylene
D041 2,4,5-Trichlorophenol
D042 2,4,6-Trichlorophenol
D043 Vinyl chloride

Hazardous Waste from Nonspecific Sources

F001 The following spent halogenated solvents used in degreasing: Tetrachloroethylene, trichlor-ethylene, methylene chloride, 1,1,1trichloroethane, carbon tetrachloride and chlorinated fluorocarbons; all spent solvent mixtures/blends used in degreasing containing, before use, a total of ten percent or more (by volume) of one or more of the above halogenated solvents or those solvents listed in F002, F004, and F005; and still bottoms from the recovery of these spent solvents and spent solvent mixtures.

F002 The following spent halogenated solvents: Tetrachloroethylene, methylene chloride, trichloro-ethylene, 1,1,1-trichloroethane, chlorobenzene, 1,1,2-trichloro-1,2,2-trifluoroethane, ortho-dichloro-benzene, trichlorofluoromethane, and 1,1,2, trichloroethane; all spent solvent mixtures/blends containing, before use, a total of ten percent or more (by volume) of one or more of the above halogenated solvents or those solvents listed in F001, F004, and F005; and still bottoms from the recovery of these spent solvents and spent solvent mixtures.

F003 The following spent non-halogenated solvents: Xylene, acetone, ethyl acetate, ethyl benzene, ethyl ether, methyl isobutyl ketone, n-butyl alcohol, cyclohexanone, and methanol; all spent solvent mixtures/blends containing, before use, only the above spent non-halogenated solvents; and all spent solvent mixtures/blends containing, before use, one or more of the above non-halogenated solvents, and a total of ten percent or more (by volume) of one or more of those solvents listed in F001, F002, F004, and F005; and still bottoms from the recovery of these spent solvents and spent solvent mixtures.

F004 The following spent non-halogenated solvents: cresols, cresylic acid, and nitrobenzene; all spent solvent mixtures/blends containing, before use, a total of ten percent or more (by volume) of one or more of the above non-halogenated solvents or those solvents listed in F001, F002, and

F005; and still bottoms from the recovery of these spent solvents and spent solvent mixtures.

F005 The following spent non-halogenated solvents: toluene, methyl ethyl ketone, carbon disulfide, isobutanol, pyridine, benzene, 2-ethoxyethanol, and 2nitropropane; all spent solvent mixtures/blends containing, before use, a total of ten percent or more (by volume) of one or more of the above nonhalogenated solvents or those solvents listed in F001, F002, or F004; and still bottoms from the recovery of these spent solvents and spent solvent mixtures.

F006 Wastewater treatment sludges from electroplating operations except from the following processes: (I) sulfuric acid anodizing of aluminum; (2) tin plating on carbon steel; (3) zinc plating (segregated basis) on carbon steel; (4) aluminum or zinc-aluminum plating on carbon steel; (5) cleaning/stripping associated with tin, zinc, and aluminum plating on carbon steel; and (6) chemical etching and milling of aluminum.

F007 Spent cyanide plating bath solutions from electroplating operations.

F008 Plating bath residues from the bottom of plating baths from electroplating operations in which cyanides are used in the process.

F009 Spent stripping and cleaning bath solutions from electroplating operations in which cyanides are used in the process.

F010 Quenching bath residues from oil baths from metal heat treating operations in which cyanides are used in the process.

F011 Spent cyanide solutions from salt bath pot cleaning from metal heat treating operations.

F012 Quenching wastewater treatment sludges from metal heat treating operations in which cyanides are used in the process.

F019 Wastewater treatment sludges from the chemical conversion coating of aluminum except from zirconium phosphating in aluminum can washing when such phosphating is an exclusive conversion coating process.

F020 Wastes (except wastewater and spent carbon from hydrogen chloride purification) from the production or manufacturing use (as a reactant, chemical intermediate, or component in a formulating process) of tri- or tetrachlorophenol or of intermediates used to produce their pesticide derivatives. (This listing does not include wastes from the production of hexachlorophene from highly purified 2,4,5-trichlorophenol.)

F021 Wastes (except wastewater and spent carbon from hydrogen chloride purification) from the production or manufacturing use (as a reactant, chemical intermediate, or component in a formulating process) of pentachlorophenol, or of intermediates used to produce derivatives.

F022 Wastes (except wastewater and spent carbon from hydrogen chloride purification) from the manufacturing use (as a reactant, chemical intermediate, orcomponent in a formulating process) of tetra-, penta-, or hexachlorobenzenes under alkaline conditions.

F023 Wastes (except wastewater and spent carbon from hydrogen chloride purification) from the production of materials on equipment previously used for the production or manufacturing use (as a reactant, chemical intermediate, or component in a formulating process) of tri- and tetrachlorophenols. (This listing does not include wastes from equipment used only for the production or use of hexachlorophene from highly purified 2,4,5-trichlorophenol.)

F024 Process wastes including, but not limited to, distillation residues, heavy ends, tars, and reactor clean-out wastes, from the production of certain chlorinated aliphatic hydrocarbons by free radical catalyzed processes. These chlorinated aliphatic hydrocarbons are those having carbon chain lengths ranging from one to and including five, with varying amounts and positions of chlorine substitution. (This listing does not include wastewaters, wastewater treatment sludges, spent catalysts, and wastes listed in Sections 261.31. or 261.32)

F025 Condensed light ends, spent filters and filter aids, and spent desiccant wastes from the production of certain chlorinated aliphatic hydrocarbons, by free radical catalyzed processes. These chlorinated aliphatic hydrocarbons are those having carbon chain lengths ranging from one, to and including five, with varying amounts and positions of chlorine substitution.

Appendix E-2. RCRA Toxic Waste Codes (cont'd.)

F026 Wastes (except wastewater and spent carbon from hydrogen chloride purification) from the production of materials on equipment previously used for the manufacturing use (as a reactant, chemical intermediate, or component in a formulating process) of tetra-, penta-, or hexachlorobenzene under alkaline conditions.

F027 Discarded unused formulations containing tri-, tetra-, or pentachlorophenol or discarded unused formulations containing compounds derived from these chlorophenols. (This listing does not include formulations containing hexachlorophene synthesized from prepurified 2,4,5-trichlorophenol as the sole component.)

F028 Residues resulting from the incineration or thermal treatment of soil contaminated with EPA hazardous waste nos. F020, F021, F022, F023, F026, and F027.

F032 Wastewaters, process residuals, preservative drippage, and spent formulations from wood preserving processes generated at plants that currently use, or have previously used, chlorophenolic formulations [except potentially cross-contaminated wastes that have had the F032 waste code deleted in accordance with Section 261.35 (i.e., the newly promulgated equipment cleaning or replacement standards), and where the generator does not not resume or initiate use of chlorophenolic formulations]. This listing does not include K001 bottom sediment sludge from the treatment of wastewater from wood preserving processes that use creosote and/or pentachlorophenol.

F034 Wastewaters, process residuals, preservative drippage, and spent formulations from wood preserving processes generated at plants that use creosote formulations. This listing does not include K001 bottom sediment sludge from the treatment of wastewater from wood preserving processes that use creosote and/or pentachlorophenol.

F035 Wastewaters, process residuals, preservative drippage, and spent formulations from wood preserving processes generated at plants that use inorganic preservatives containing arsenic or chromium. This listing does not include K001 bottom sediment sludge from the treatment of wastewater from wood preserving processes that use creosote and/or pentachlorophenol.

F037 Petroleum refinery primary oil/water/solids separation sludge - Any sludge generated from the gravitational separation of oil/water/solids during the storage or treatment of process wastewaters and oily cooling wastewaters from petroleum refineries. Such sludges include, but are not limited to, those generated in oil/water/solids separators; tanks and impoundments; ditches and other conveyances; sumps; and storm water units receiving dry weather flow. Sludges generated in storm water units that do not receive dry weather flow, sludges generated in aggressive biological treatment units as defined in Section 261.31(b)(2) (including sludges generated in one or more additional units after wastewaters have been treated in aggressive biological treatment units), and K051 wastes are exempted from this listing.

F038 Petroleum refinery secondary (emulsified) oil/water/solids separation sludge - Any sludge and/or float generated from the physical and/or chemical separation of oil/water/solids in process wastewaters and oily cooling wastewaters from petroleum refineries. Such wastes include, but are not limited to, all sludges and floats generated in induced air flotation (IAF) units, tanks and impoundments, and all sludges generated in DAF units. Sludges generated in stormwater units that do not receive dry weather flow, sludges generated in aggressive biological treatment units as defined in Section 261.31(b)(2) (including sludges generated in one or more additional units after wastewaters have been treated in aggressive biological treatment units), and F037, K048, and K051 wastes are exempted from this listing.

F039 Leachate resulting from the treatment, storage, or disposal of wastes classified by more than one waste code under Subpart D, or from a mixture of wastes classified under Subparts C and D of this part. (Leachate resulting from the management of one or more of the following EPA Hazardous Wastes and no other hazardous wastes retains its hazardous waste code(s): F020, F021, F022, F023, F026, F027, and/or F028.)

Hazardous Waste from Specific Sources

K001 Bottom sediment sludge from the treatment of wastewaters from wood preserving processes that use creosote and/or pentachlorophenol.

K002 Wastewater treatment sludge from the production of chrome yellow and orange pigments.

K003 Wastewater treatment sludge from the production of molybdate orange pigments.

K004 Wastewater treatment sludge from the production of zinc yellow pigments.

K005 Wastewater treatment sludge from the production of chrome green pigments.

K006 Wastewater treatment sludge from the production of chrome oxide green pigments (anhydrous and hydrated).

K007 Wastewater treatment sludge from the production of iron blue pigments.

K008 Oven residue from the production of chrome oxide green pigments.

K009 Distillation bottoms from the production of acetaldehyde from ethylene.

K010 Distillation side cuts from the production of acetaldehyde from ethylene.

K011 Bottom stream from the wastewater stripper in the production of acrylonitrile.

K013 Bottom stream from the acetonitrile column in the production of acrylonitrile.

K014 Bottoms from the acetonitrile purification column in the production of acrylonitrile.

K015 Still bottoms from the distillation of benzyl chloride.

K016 Heavy ends or distillation residues from the production of carbon tetrachloride.

K017 Heavy ends (still bottoms) from the purification column in the production of epichlorohydrin.

K018 Heavy ends from the fractionation column in ethyl chloride production.

K019 Heavy ends from the distillation of ethylene dichloride in ethylene dichloride production.

K020 Heavy ends from the distillation of vinyl chloride in vinyl chloride monomer production.

K021 Aqueous spent antimony catalyst waste from fluoromethanes production.

K022 Distillation bottom tars from the production of phenol/acetone from cumene.

K023 Distillation light ends from the production of phthalic anhydride from naphthalene.

K024 Distillation bottoms from the production of phthalic anhydride from naphthalene.

K025 Distillation bottoms from the production of nitrobenzene by the nitration of benzene.

K026 Stripping still tails from the production of methyl ethyl pyridines.

K027 Centrifuge and distillation residues from toluene diisocyanate production.

K028 Spent catalyst from the hydrochlorinator reactor in the production of 1,1,1-trichloroethane.

K029 Waste from the product steam stripper in the production of 1,1,1-trichloroethane.

K030 Column bottoms or heavy ends from the combined production of trichloroethylene and perchloroethylene.

K031 By-product salts generated in the production of MSMA and cacodylic acid.

K032 Wastewater treatment sludge from the production of chlordane.

K033 Wastewater and scrub water from the chlorination of cyclopentadiene in the production of chlordane.

K034 Filter solids from the filtration of hexachlorocyclopentadiene in the production of chlordane.

K035 Wastewater treatment sludges generated in the production of creosote.

K036 Still bottoms from toluene reclamation distillation in the production of disulfoton.

K037 Wastewater treatment sludges from the production of disulfoton.

K038 Wastewater from the washing and stripping of phorate production.

K039 Filter cake from the filtration of diethylphosphorodithioic acid in the production of phorate.

K040 Wastewater treatment sludge from the production of phorate.

K041 Wastewater treatment sludge from the production of toxaphene.

K042 Heavy ends or distillation residues from the distillation of tetrachlorobenzene in the production of 2,4,5-T,

K043 2,6-dichlorophenol waste from the production of 2,4-D.

Appendix E-2. RCRA Toxic Waste Codes (cont'd.)

K046 Wastewater treatment sludges from the manufacturing, formulation, and loading of lead-based initiating compounds.

K048 Dissolved air flotation (DAF) float from the petroleum refining industry.

K049 Slop oil emulsion solids from the petroleum refining industry.

K050 Heat exchanger bundle cleaning sludge from the petroleum refining industry.

K051 API separator sludge from the petroleum refining industry.

K052 Tank bottoms (leaded) from the petroleum refining industry.

K060 Ammonia still lime sludge from coking operations.

K061 Emission control dust/sludge from the primary production of steel in electric furnaces.

K062 Spent pickle liquor generated by steel finishing operations of facilities within the iron and steel industry (SIC Codes 331 and 332).

K064 Acid plant blowdown slurry/sludge resulting from the thickening of blowdown slurry from primary copper production.

K065 Surface impoundment solids contained in and dredged from surface impoundments at primary lead smelting facilities.

K066 Sludge from treatment of process wastewater and/or acid plant blowdown from primary zinc production.

K069 Emission control dust/sludge from secondary lead smelting.

K071 Brine purification muds from the mercury cell process in chlorine production, in which separately prepurified brine is not used.

K073 Chlorinated hydrocarbon waste from the purification step of the diaphragm cell process using graphite anodes in chlorine production.

K083 Distillation bottoms from aniline production.

K084 Wastewater treatment sludges generated during the production of veterinary pharmaceuticals from arsenic or organoarsenic compounds.

K085 Distillation or fractionation column bottoms from the production of chlorobenzenes.

K086 Solvent washes and sludges, caustic washes and sludges, or water washes and sludges from cleaning tubs and equipment used in the formulation of ink from pigments, driers, soaps, and stabilizers containing chromium and lead.

K087 Decanter tank tar sludge from coking operations.

K088 Spent potliners from primary aluminum reduction.

K090 Emission control dust or sludge from ferrochromiumsilicon production.

K091 Emission control dust or sludge from ferrochromium production.

K093 Distillation fight ends from the production of phthalic anhydride from ortho-xylene.

K094 Distillation bottoms from the production of phthalic anhydride from ortho-xylene.

K095 Distillation bottoms from the production of 1,1,1-trichloroethane.

K096 Heavy ends from the heavy ends column from the production of 1,1,1-trichloroethane.

K097 Vacuum stripper discharge from the chlordane chlorinator in the production of chlordane.

K098 Untreated process wastewater from the production of toxaphene.

K099 Untreated wastewater from the production of 2,4-D.

K100 Waste leaching solution from acid leaching of emission control dust/sludge from secondary lead smelting.

K101 Distillation tar residues from the distillation of aniline-based compounds in the production of veterinary pharmaceuticals from arsenic or organoarsenic compounds.

K102 Residue from the use of activated carbon for decolorization in the production of veterinary pharmaceuticals from arsenic or organoarsenic compounds.

K103 Process residues from aniline extraction from the production of aniline.

K104 Combined wastewater streams generated from nitrobenzene/aniline production.

K105 Separated aqueous stream from the reactor product washing step in the production of chlorobenzenes.

K106 Wastewater treatment sludge from the mercury cell process in chlorine production.

K107 Column bottoms from product separation from the production of 1,1-dimethylhydrazine (UDMH) from carboxylic acid hydrazines.

K108 Condensed column overheads from product separation and condensed reactor vent gases from the production of 1,1-dimethylhydrazine (UDMH) from carboxylic acid hydrazides.

K109 Spent filter cartridges from product purification from the production of 1,1-dimethylhydrazine (UDMH) from carboxylic acid hydrazides.

K110 Condensed column overheads from intermediate separation from the production of 1,1-dimethylhydrazine (UDMH) from carboxylic acid hydrazides.

K111 Product washwaters from the production of dinitrotoluene via nitration of toluene.

K112 Reaction by-product water from the drving column in the production of toluenediamine via hydrogenation of dinitrotoluene.

K113 Condensed liquid light ends from purification of toluenediamine in production of toluenediamine via hydrogenation of dinitrotoluene.

K114 Vicinals from the purification of toluenediamine in production of toluenediamine via hvdrogenation of dinitrotoluene.

K115 Heavy ends from purification of toluenediamine in the production of toluenediamine via hydrogenation of dinitrotoluene.

K116 Organic condensate from the solvent recovery column in the production of toluene diisocyanate via phosgenation of toluenediamine.

K117 Wastewater from the reactor vent gas scrubber in the production of ethylene dibromide via bromination of ethene.

K118 Spent adsorbent solids from purification of ethylene dibromide in the production of ethylene dibromide via bromination of ethene.

K123 Process wastewater (including supernates, filtrates, and washwaters) from the production of ethylenebisdithiocarbamic acid and its salt.

K124 Reactor vent scrubber water from the production of ethylenebisdithiocarbamic acid and its salts.

K125 Filtration, evaporation, and centrifugation solids from the production of ethylenebisdithiocarbamic acid and its salts.

K126 Baghouse dust and floor sweepings in milling and packaging operations from production or formulation of ethylenebisdithiocarbamic acid and its salts.

K131 Wastewater from the reactor and spent sulfuric acid from the acid dryer from the production of methyl bromide.

K132 Spent absorbent and wastewater separator solids from the production of methyl bromide.

K136 Still bottoms from the purification of ethylene dibromide in the production of ethylene dibromide via bromination of ethene.

Discarded Commercial Chemical Products, Off-specification Species, Container Residuals, and Spill Residues Thereof —Acute Hazardous Waste

P001 2H-1-Benzopyran-2-one, 4-hydroxy-3-(3oxo-l-phenylbutyl)-, & salts, when present at concentrations greater than 0.3%

P001 Warfarin, & salts, when present at concentrations greater than 0.3%

P002 1-Acetyl-2-thiourea

P002 Acetamide, N-(aminothioxomethyl)-

P003 2-Propenal

P003 Acrolein

P004 1,4,5,8-Dimethanonaphthalene, 1,2,3,4,10,10-hexa-chloro-1,4,4a,5,8,8a,hexahydro, (lalpha, 4alpha, 4abeta, 5alpha, 8alpha, 8abeta)-

P004 Aldrin

P005 2-Propen-l-ol

P005 Allyl alcohol

P006 Aluminum phosphide

P007 3(2H)-Isoxazolone, 5-(aminomethyl)-

P007 5-(Aminomethyl)-3-isoxazolol

P008 4-Aminopyridine

P008 4-Pyridinamine

P010 Arsenic acid H3AsO4

P011 Arsenic oxide As205

P011 Arsenic pentoxide

P012 Arsenic oxide As203

P012 Arsenic trioxide

P013 Barium cyanide

P014 Benzenethiol

P014 Thiophenol

P015 Beryllium

P016 Dichloromethyl ether

P016 Methane, oxybis[chloro-

P017 2-Propanone, 1-bromo-

Appendix E-2. RCRA Toxic Waste Codes (cont'd.)

P017	Bromoacetone
P018	Brucine
P018	Strychnidin-10-one, 2,3-dimethoxy-
P020	Dinoseb
P020	Phenol, 2-(l-methylpropyl)-4,6-dinitro-
P021	Calcium cyanide
P021	Calcium cyanide Ca(CN)2
P022	Carbon disulfide
P023	Acetaldehyde, chloro-
P023	Chloroacetaldehyde
P024	Benzenamine, 4-chloro-
P024	p-Chloroaniline
P026	1-(o-Chlorophenyl)thiourea
P026	Thiourea, (2-chlorophenyl)-
P027	3-Chloropropionitrile
P027	Propanenitrile, 3-chloro-
P028	Benzene, (chloromethyl)-
P028	Benzyl chloride
P029	Copper cyanide
P029	Copper cyanide Cu(CN)
P030	Cyanides (soluble cyanide salts), not otherwise specified
P031	Cyanogen
P031	Ethanedinitrile
P033	Cyanogen chloride
P033	Cyanogen chloride (CN)Cl
P034	2-Cyclohexyl-4,6-dinitrophenol
P034	Phenol, 2-cyclohexyl-4,6-dinitro-
P036	Arsonous dichloride, phenyl-
P036	Dichlorophenylarsine
P037	2,7:3,6-Dimethanonaphth[2,3-b]oxirene, 3,4,5,6,9,9-hexachloro- 1 a,2,2a,3,6,6a,7,7a-octahydro-, (1aalpha, 2beta, 2aalpha, 3beta, 6beta, 6aalpha, 7beta, 7aalpha)-
P037	Dieldrin
P038	Arsine, diethyl-
P038	Diethylarsine
P039	Disulfoton
P039	Phosphorodithioic acid, O,O-diethyl S-[2(ethylthio)ethyll ester
P040	O,O-Diethyl O-pyrazinyl phosphorothioate
P040	Phosphorothioic acid, O,O-diethyl Opyrazinyl ester
P041	Diethyl-p-nitrophenyl phosphate
P041	Phosphoric acid, diethyl 4-nitrophenyl ester
P042	1,2-Benzenediol, 4-[l-hydroxy-2-(methylamino)ethyl]-, (R)-
P042	Epinephrine
P043	Diisopropylfluorophosphate (DFP)
P043	Phosphorofluoridic acid, bis(l-methylethyl) ester
P044	Dimethoate
P044	Phosphorodithioic acid, O,O-dimethyl S[2-(methylamino)-2-oxoethyl] ester
P045	2-Butanone,3,3-dimethyl-l-(methylthio)-,O-[methylamino)carbonyl] oxime
P045	Thiofanox
P046	alpha,alpha-Dimethylphenethylamine
P046	Benzeneethanamine, alpha, alpha-dimethyl-
P047	4,6-Dinitro-o-cresol, & salts
P047	Phenol, 2-methyl-4,6-dinitro-, & salts
P048	2,4-Dinitrophenol
P048	Phenol, 2,4-dinitro-
P049	Dithiobiuret
P049	Thioimidodicarbonic diamide [(H2N)C(S)]2NH
P050	6,9-Methano-2,4,3-benzodioxathiepin,6,7,8,9,10,10-hexachloro-1,5,5a,6,9,9a-hexahydro-,3oxide
P050	Endosulfan
P051	2,7:3,6-Dimethanonaphth[2,3-b]oxirene, 3,4,5,6,9,9-hexachloro-1a,2,2a,3,6,6a,7,7aoctahydro-, (1aalpha, 2beta, 2abeta, 3alpha, 6alpha, 6abeta, 7beta, 7aalpha)- & metabolites
P051	Endrin
P051	Endrin, & metabolites
P054	Aziridine
P054	Ethyleneimine
P056	Fluorine
P057	Acetamide, 2-fluoro-
P057	Fluoroacetamide
P058	Acetic acid, fluoro-, sodium salt
P058	Fluoroacetic acid, sodium salt
P059	4,7-Methano-1H-indene, 1,4,5,6,7,8,8heptachloro-3a,4,7,7a-tetrahydro-
P059	Heptachlor
P060	1,4,5,8-Dimethanonaphthalene, 1,2,3,4,10,10-hexa-chloro-1,4,4a,5,8,8a,-hexahydro-, (lalpha, 4alpha, 4abeta, -5bcta, 8beta, 8abeta)-
P060	Isodrin
P062	Hexaethyl tetraphosphate
P062	Tetraphosphoric acid, hexaethyl ester
P063	Hydrocyanic acid
P063	Hydrogen cyanide
P064	Methane, isocyanato-
P064	Methyl isocyanate
P065	Fulminic acid, mercury(2+) salt
P065	Mercury fulminate
P066	Ethanimidothioic acid, N-[[(methylamino)carbonyl]oxy]-, methyl ester

P066 Methomyl
P067 1,2-Propylenimine
P067 Aziridine, 2-methyl-
P068 Hydrazine, methyl-
P068 Methyl hydrazine
P069 2-Methyllactonitrile
P069 Propanenitrile, 2-hydroxy-2-methyl-
P070 Aldicarb
P070 Propanal, 2-methyl-2-(methylthio)-, O-[(methylamino)carbonyl]oxime
P071 Methyl parathion
P071 Phosphorothioic acid, O,O,-dimethyl O-(4nitrophenyl) ester
P072 alpha-Naphthylthiourea
P072 Thiourea, 1-naphthalenyl-
P073 Nickel carbonyl
P073 Nickel carbonyl Ni(CO)4, (T-4)-
P074 Nickel cyanide
P074 Nickel cyanide Ni(CN)2
P075 Nicotine, & salts
P075 Pyridine, 3-(l-methyl-2-pyrrolidinyl)-,(S)-, & salts
P076 Nitric oxide
P076 Nitrogen oxide NO
P077 Benzenamine, 4-nitro-
P077 p-Nitroaniline
P078 Nitrogen dioxide
P078 Nitrogen oxide N02
P081 1,2,3-Propanetriol, trinitrate
P081 Nitroglycerine
P082 Methanimine, N-methyl-N-nitroso-
P082 N-Nitrosodimethylamine
P084 N-Nitrosomethylvinylamine
P084 Vinylamine, N-methyl-N-nitroso-
P085 Diphosphoramide, octamethyl-
P085 Octamethylpyrophosphoramide
P087 Osmium oxide OsO4, (T-4)-
P087 Osmium tetroxide
P088 7-Oxabicyclo[2.2.1]heptane-2,3-dicarboxylic acid
P088 Endothall
P089 Parathion
P089 Phosphorothioic acid, O,O-diethyl-O-(4nitrophenyl) ester
P092 Mercury, (acetato-O)phenyl-
P092 Phenylmercury acetate
P093 Phenylthiourea
P093 Thiourea, phenyl-
P094 Phorate
P094 Phosphorodithioic acid, O,O-diethyl S-[(ethylthio)methyl] ester
P095 Carbonic dichloride
P095 Phosgene
P096 Hydrogen phosphide
P096 Phosphine
P097 Famphur
P097 Phosphorothioic acid O-[4-[(dimethylamino)sulfonyl]phenyll O,O-dimethyl ester
P098 Potassium cyanide
P098 Potassium cyanide K(CN)
P099 Argentate (1-), bis(cyano-C)-, potassium
P099 Potassium silver cyanide
P101 Ethyl cyanide
P101 Propanenitrile
P102 2-Propyn-l-ol
P102 Propargyl alcohol
P103 Selenourea
P104 Silver cyanide
P104 Silver cyanide Ag(CN)
P105 Sodium azide
P106 Sodium cyanide
P106 Sodium cyanide Na(CN)
P107 Strontium sulfide SrS
P108 Strychnidin-10-one, & salts
P108 Strychnine, & salts
P109 Tetraethyldithiopyrophosphate
P109 Thiodiphosphoric acid, tetraethyl ester
P110 Plumbane, tetraethyl-
P110 Tetraethyl lead
P111 Diphosphoric acid, tetraethyl ester
P111 Tetraethyl pyrophosphate
P113 Thallic oxide
P113 Thallium oxide Tl2O3
P114 Selenious acid, dithallium (1+) salt
P114 Thallium(I) selenite
P115 Sulfuric acid, dithallium (1+) salt
P115 Thallium(I) sulfate
P116 Hydrazinecarbothioamide
P116 Thiosemicarbazide
P118 Methanethiol, trichloro-
P118 Trichloromethanethiol
P119 Ammonium vanadate
P119 Vanadic acid, ammonium salt
P120 Vanadium oxide V2O5
P120 Vanadium pentoxide
P121 Zinc cyanide
P121 Zinc cyanide Zn(CN)2
P122 Zinc phosphide Zn3P2, when present at concentrations greater than 10%
P123 Toxaphene

Appendix E-2. RCRA Toxic Waste Codes (cont'd.)

Discarded Commercial Chemical Products, Off-specification Species, Container Residues, and Spill Residues Thereof—Toxic Wastes

	2,3,4,6-Tetrachlorophenol
	2,4,5-T
	2,4,5-Trichlorophenol
	2,4,6-Trichlorophenol
	Acetic acid, (2,4,5-trichlorophenoxy)-
	Pentachlorophenol
See	Phenol, 2,3,4,6-tetrachloro-
F027	Phenol, 2,4,5-trichloro-
	Phenol, 2,4,6-trichloro-
	Phenol, pentachloro-
	Propanoic acid, 2-(2,4,5-trichloro-phenoxy)-
	Silvex (2,4,5-TP)
U001	Acetaldehyde
U001	Ethanal
U002	2-Propanone
U002	Acetone
U003	Acetonitrile
U004	Acetophenone
U004	Ethanone, 1-phenyl-
U005	2-Acetylaminofluorene
U005	Acetamide, N-9H-fluoren-2-yl
U006	Acetyl chloride
U007	2-Propenamide
U007	Acrylamide
U008	2-Propenoic acid
U008	Acrylic acid
U009	2-Propenenitrile
U009	Acrylonitrile
U010	Azirino [2',3':3,4]pyrrolo[1,2-alindole-4,7-dione, 6-amino-8-[[(aminocarbonyl)oxy] methyl]l,la,2,8,8a,8b-hexahydro-8a-methoxy-5-methyl-, [laS-(laalpha, 8beta, 8aalpha, 8balpha)]-
U010	Mitomycin C
U011	1H-1,2,4-Triazol-3-amine
U011	Amitrole
U012	Aniline
U012	Benzenamine
U014	Auramine
U014	Benzenamine, 4,4'-carbonimidoyl-bis[N,N-dimethyl-
U015	Azaserine
U015	L-Serine, diazoacetate (ester)
U016	Benz[c]acridine
U017	Benzal chloride
U017	Benzene, (dichloromethyl)-
U018	Benz[a]anthracene
U019	Benzene
U021	[1,1'-Biphenyl]-4,4'-diamine
U021	Benzidine
U022	Benzo[a]pyrene
U023	Benzene, (trichloromethyl)-
U023	Benzotrichloride
U024	Dichloromethoxy ethane
U024	Ethane, 1,1'-[methyl-enebis(oxy)]bis[2-chloro-
U025	Dichloroethyl ether
U025	Ethane, 1,1'-oxybis[2-chloro-
U026	Chlornaphazin
U026	Naphthalenamine, N,N'-bis(2chloroethyl)-
U027	Dichloroisopropyl ether
U027	Propane, 2,2'-oxybis[2-chloro-
U028	1,2-Benzenedicarboxylic acid, bis(2-ethylhexyl) ester
U028	Diethylhexyl phthalate
U029	Methane, bromo-
U029	Methyl bromide
U030	4-Bromophenyl phenyl ether
U030	Benzene, 1-bromo-4-phenoxy-
U031	1-Butanol
U031	n-Butyl alcohol
U032	Calcium chromate
U032	Chromic acid H2CrO4, calcium salt
U033	Carbon oxyfluoride
U033	Carbonic difluoride
U034	Acetaldehyde, trichloro-
U034	Chloral
U035	Benzenebutanoic acid, 4-[bis(2-chloroethyl)amino]-
U035	Chlorambucil
U036	4,7-Methano-lH-indene, 1,2,4,5,6,7,8,8-octachloro-2,3,3a,4,7,7a-hexahydro-
U036	Chlordane, alpha & gamma isomers
U037	Benzene, chloro-
U037	Chlorobenzene
U038	Benzeneacetic acid, 4-chloro-alpha-(4-chlorophenyl)-alpha-hydroxy-, ethyl ester
U038	Chlorobenzilate
U039	p-Chloro-m-cresol
U039	Phenol, 4-chloro-3-methyl-
U041	Epichlorohydrin
U041	Oxirane, (chloromethyl)-
U042	2-Chloroethyl vinyl ether
U042	Ethene, (2-chloroethoxy)-
U043	Ethene, chloro-
U043	Vinyl chloride
U044	Chloroform
U044	Methane, trichloro-
U045	Methane, chloro-

U045 Methyl chloride
U046 Chloromethyl methyl ether
U046 Methane, chloromethoxy-
U047 beta-Chloronaphthalene
U047 Naphthalene, 2-chloro-
U048 o-Chlorophenol
U048 Phenol, 2-chloro-
U049 4-Chloro-o-toluidine, hydrochloride
U049 Benzenamine, 4-chloro-2-methyl-, hydrochloride
U050 Chrysene
U051 Creosote
U052 Cresol (Cresylic acid)
U052 Phenol, methyl-
U053 2-Butenal
U053 Crotonaldehyde
U055 Benzene, (1-methylethyl)-
U055 Cumene
U056 Benzene, hexahydro-
U056 Cyclohexane
U058 2H-1,3,2-Oxazaphosphorin-2-amine, N,N-bis(2-chloroethyl)tetrahydro-, 2-oxide
U058 Cyclophosphamide
U059 5,12-Naphthacenedione, 8-acetyl-10-[(3-amino-2,3,6-trideoxy)-alpha-L-lyxo-hexopyranosyl)oxy]-7,8,9,10-tetrahydro-6,8,11-trihydroxy-1-methoxy-, (8S-cis)-
U059 Daunomycin
U060 Benzene, 1,1'-(2,2-dichloro-ethylidene)bis[4-chloro-
U060 DDD
U061 Benzene, 1,1'-(2,2,2-trichloro-ethylidene)bis[4-chloro-
U061 DDT
U062 Carbamothioic acid, bis(l-methyl-ethyl)-, S-(2,3-dichloro-2-propenyl) ester
U062 Diallate
U063 Dibenz[a,h]anthracene
U064 Benzo[rst]pentaphene
U064 Dibenzo[a,i]pyrene
U066 1,2-Dibromo-3-chloropropane
U066 Propane, 1,2-dibromo-3-chloro-
U067 Ethane, 1,2-dibromo-
U067 Ethylene dibromide
U068 Methane, dibromo-
U068 Methylene bromide
U069 1,2-Benzenedicarboxylic acid, dibutyl ester
U069 Dibutyl phthalate
U070 Benzene, 1,2-dichloro-
U070 o-Dichlorobenzene
U071 Benzene, 1,3-dichloro-
U071 m-Dichlorobenzene
U072 Benzene, 1,4-dichloro-
U072 p-Dichlorobenzene
U073 [1,1'-Biphenyll-4,4'-diamine, 3,3'-dichloro-
U073 3,3'-Dichlorobenzidine
U074 1,4-Dichloro-2-butene
U074 2-Butene, 1,4-dichloro-
U075 Dichlorodifluoromethane
U075 Methane, dichlorodifluoro-
U076 Ethane, 1,1-dichloro-
U076 Ethylidene dichloride
U077 Ethane, 1,2-dichloro-
U077 Ethylene dichloride
U078 1,1-Dichloroethylene
U078 Ethene, 1,1-dichloro-
U079 1,2-Dichloroethylene
U079 Ethene, 1,2-dichloro-,(E)-
U080 Methane, dichloro-
U080 Methylene chloride
U081 2,4-Dichlorophenol
U081 Phenol, 2,4-dichloro-
U082 2,6-Dichlorophenol
U082 Phenol, 2,6-dichloro-
U083 Propane, 1,2-dichloro-
U083 Propylene dichloride
U084 1,3-Dichloropropene
U084 1-Propene, 1,3-dichloro-
U085 1,2:3,4-Diepoxybutane
U085 2,2'-Bioxirane
U086 Hydrazine, 1,2-diethyl-
U086 N,N'-Diethylhydrazine
U087 O,O-Diethyl S-methyl dithio-phosphate
U087 Phosphorodithioic acid, O,O-diethyl S-methyl ester
U088 1,2-Benzenedicarboxylic acid, diethyl ester
U088 Diethyl phthalate
U089 Diethylstilbesterol
U089 Phenol, 4,4'-(1,2-diethyl-1,2-ethenediyl)bis, (E)-
U090 1,3-Benzodioxole, 5-propyl-
U090 Dihydrosafrole
U091 [1,1'-Biphenyl]-4,4'-diamine, 3,3'-dimethoxy-
U091 3,3'-Dimethoxybenzidine
U093 Benzenamine, N,N-dimethyl-4-(phenylazo)-
U093 p-Dimethylaminoazobenzene
U094 7,12-Dimethylbenz[a]anthracene
U094 Benz[a]anthracene, 7,12-dimethyl-
U095 [1,1'-Biphenyl]-4,4'-diamine, 3,3'-dimethyl-
U095 3,3'-Dimethylbenzidine

Appendix E-2. RCRA Toxic Waste Codes (cont'd.)

U096	alpha,alpha-Dimethylbenzyl-hydroperoxide
U096	Hydroperoxide, 1-methyl-1-phenylethyl-
U097	Carbamic chloride, dimethyl-
U097	Dimethylcarbamoyl chloride
U098	1,1-Dimethylhydrazine
U098	Hydrazine, 1,1-dimethyl-
U099	1,2-Dimethylhydrazine
U099	Hydrazine, 1,2-dimethyl-
U101	2,4-Dimethylphenol
U101	Phenol, 2,4-dimethyl-
U102	1,2-Benzenedicarboxylic acid, dimethyl ester
U102	Dimethyl phthalate
U103	Dimethyl sulfate
U103	Sulfuric acid, dimethyl ester
U105	2,4-Dinitrotoluene
U105	Benzene, 1-methyl-2,4-dinitro-
U106	2,6-Dinitrotoluene
U106	Benzene, 2-methyl-1,3-dinitro-
U107	1,2-Benzenedicarboxylic acid, dioctyl ester
U107	Di-n-octyl phthalate
U108	1,4-Diethyleneoxide
U108	1,4-Dioxane
U109	1,2-Diphenylhydrazine
U109	Hydrazine, 1,2-diphenyl-
U111	1-Propanamine, N-nitroso-N-propyl-
U111	Di-n-propylnitrosamine
U113	2-Propenoic acid, ethyl ester
U113	Ethyl acrylate
U114	Carbamodithioic acid, 1,2-ethane-diylbis-, salts & esters
U114	Ethylenebisdithiocarbamic acid, salts & esters
U115	Ethylene oxide
U115	Oxirane
U116	2-Imidazolidinethione
U116	Ethylenethiourea
U118	2-Propenoic acid, 2-methyl-, ethyl ester
U118	Ethyl methacrylate
U119	Ethyl methanesulfonate
U119	Methanesulfonic acid, ethyl ester
U120	Fluoranthene
U121	Methane, trichlorofluoro-
U121	Trichloromonofluoromethane
U122	Formaldehyde
U123	Formic acid
U126	Glycidylaldehyde
U126	Oxiranecarboxyaldehyde
U127	Benzene, hexachloro-
U127	Hexachlorobenzene
U128	1,3-Butadiene, 1,1,2,3,4,4-hexachloro-
U128	Hexachlorobutadiene
U129	Cyclohexane, 1,2,3,4,5,6-hexachloro-, (lalpha, 2alpha, 3beta, 4alpha, 5alpha, 6beta)-
U129	Lindane
U130	1,3-Cyclopentadiene, 1,2,3,4,5,5-hexachloro-
U130	Hexachlorocyclopentadiene
U131	Ethane, hexachloro-
U131	Hexachloroethane
U132	Hexachlorophene
U132	Phenol, 2,2'-methylenebis[3,4,6-trichloro-
U133	Hydrazine
U134	Hydrofluoric acid
U134	Hydrogen fluoride
U135	Hydrogen sulfide
U135	Hydrogen sulfide H2S
U136	Arsinic acid, dimethyl-
U136	Cacodylic acid
U137	Indeno[1,2,3-cd]pyrene
U138	Methane, iodo-
U138	Methyl iodide
U140	1-Propanol, 2-methyl-
U140	Isobutyl alcohol
U141	1,3-Benzodioxole, 5-(1-propenyl)-
U141	Isosafrole
U142	1,3,4-Metheno-2H-cyclobuta[cd]-pentalen2-one, l,la,3,3a,4,5,5,5a,5b,6-decachlorooctahydro-
U142	Kepone
U143	2-Butenoic acid, 2-methyl-, 7-[[2,3dihydroxy-2-(1-methoxyethyl) -3-methyl- 1 oxobutoxy]methyl]-2,3,5,7a-tetrahydro-lHpyrrolizin-1-yl ester, [lS-[lalpha(Z), 7(2S*,3R*), 7aalpha]]-
U143	Lasiocarpine
U144	Acetic acid, lead(2+) salt
U144	Lead acetate
U145	Lead phosphate
U145	Phosphoric acid, lead(2+) salt (2:3)
U146	Lead subacetate
U146	Lead, bis(acetato-O)tetrahydroxytri-
U147	2,5-Furandione
U147	Maleic anhydride
U148	3,6-Pyridazinedione, 1,2-dihydro-
U148	Maleic hydrazide
U149	Malononitrile
U149	Propanedinitrile
U150	L-Phenylalanine, 4-[bis(2-chloro-ethyl)amino]-
U150	Melphalan
U151	Mercury
U152	2-Propenenitrile, 2-methyl-
U152	Methacrylonitrile

U153 Methanethiol
U153 Thiomethanol
U154 Methanol
U154 Methyl alcohol
U155 1,2-Ethanediamine, N,N-dimethyl-N′-2-pyridinyl-N′-(2-thienylmethyl)-
U155 Methapyrilene
U156 Carbonochloridic acid, methvl ester,
U156 Methyl chlorocarbonate
U157 3-Methylcholanthrene
U157 Benz[j]aceanthrylene, 1,2-dihydro-3-methyl-
U158 4,4'-Methylenebis(2-chloroaniline)
U158 Benzenamine, 4,4'-methylenebis[2-chloro-
U159 2-Butanone
U159 Methyl ethyl ketone (MEK)
U160 2-Butanone, peroxide
U160 Methyl ethyl ketone peroxide
U161 4-Methyl-2-pentanone
U161 Methyl isobutyl ketone
U161 Pentanol, 4-methyl-
U162 2-Propenoic acid, 2-methyl-, methyl ester
U162 Methyl methacrylate
U163 Guanidine, N-methyl-N′-nitro-N-nitroso-
U163 MNNG
U164 4(1H)-Pyrimidinone, 2,3-dihydro-6methyl-2-thioxo-
U164 Methylthiouracil
U165 Naphthalene
U166 1,4-Naphthalenedione
U166 1,4-Naphthoquinone
U167 1-Napthalenamine
U167 alpha-Naphthylamine
U168 2-Napthalenamine
U168 beta-Naphthylamine
U169 Benzene, nitro-
U169 Nitrobenzene
U170 p-Nitrophenol
U170 Phenol, 4-nitro-
U171 2-Nitropropane
U171 Propane, 2-nitro-
U172 1-Butanamine, N-butyl-N-nitroso-
U172 N-Nitrosodi-n-butylamine
U173 Ethanol, 2,2'-(nitrosoimino)bis-
U173 N-Nitrosodiethanolamine
U174 Ethanamine, N-ethyl-N-nitroso-
U174 N-Nitrosodiethylamine
U176 N-Nitroso-N-ethylurea
U176 Urea, N-ethyl-N-nitroso-
U177 N-Nitroso-N-methylurea
U177 Urea, N-methyl-N-nitroso-
U178 Carbamic acid, methylnitroso-, ethyl ester
U178 N-Nitroso-N-methylurethane
U179 N-Nitrosopiperidine
U179 Piperidine, 1-nitroso-
U180 N-Nitrosopyrrolidine
U180 Pyrrolidine, 1-nitroso-
U181 5-Nitro-o-toluidine
U181 Benzenamine, 2-methyl-5-nitro
U182 1,3,5-Trioxane, 2,4,6-trimethyl-
U182 Paraldehyde
U183 Benzene, pentachloro-
U183 Pentachlorobenzene
U184 Ethane, pentachloro-
U184 Pentachloroethane
U185 Benzene, pentachloronitro-
U185 Pentachloronitrobenzene (PCNB)
U187 Acetamide, N-(4-ethoxyphenyl)-
U187 Phenacetin
U188 Phenol
U190 1,3-Isobenzofurandione
U190 Phthalic anhydride
U191 2-Picoline
U191 Pyridine, 2-methyl-
U192 Benzamide, 3,5-dichloro-N-(1,1-dimethyl-2-propynyl)-
U192 Pronamide
U193 1,2-Oxathiolane, 2,2-dioxide
U193 1,3-Propane sultone
U194 1-Propanamine
U194 n-Propylamine
U196 Pyridine
U197 2,5-Cyclohexadiene-1,4-dione
U197 p-Benzoquinone
U200 Reserpine
U200 Yohimban-16-carboxylic acid, 11,17dimethoxy-18-[(3,4,5-trimethoxybenzoyl)oxy]-, methyl ester, (3beta, 16beta, 17alpha, 18beta, 20alpha)-
U201 1,3-Benzenediol
U201 Resorcinol
U202 1,2-Benzisothiazol-3(2H)-one, 1,1-dioxide, & salts
U202 Saccharin, & salts
U203 1,3-Benzodioxole, 5-(2-propenyl)-
U203 Safrole
U204 Selenious acid
U204 Selenium dioxide
U205 Selenium sulfide
U205 Selenium sulfide SeS2
U206 D-Glucose, 2-deoxy-2-[[(methyl-nitrosoamino)-carbonyl]amino]-
U206 Glucopyranose, 2-deoxy-2-(3-methyl-3-nitrosoureido)-,D-

Appendix E-2. RCRA Toxic Waste Codes (cont'd.)

U206	Streptozotocin
U207	1,2,4,5-Tetrachlorobcnzene
U207	Benzene, 1,2,4,5-tetrachloro-
U208	1,1,1,2-Tetrachloroethane
U208	Ethane, 1,1,1,2-tetrachloro-
U209	1,1,2,2-Tetrachloroethane
U209	Ethane, 1,1,2,2-tetrachloro-
U210	Ethene, tetrachloro-
U210	Tetrachloroethylene
U211	Carbon tetrachloride
U211	Methane, tetrachloro-
U214	Acetic acid, thallium(l+) salt
U214	Thallium(I) acetate
U215	Carbonic acid, dithallium(1+) salt
U215	Thallium(I) carbonate
U216	Thallium chloride Tlcl
U216	Thallium(I) chloride
U217	Nitric acid, thallium(1+) salt
U217	Thallium(I) nitrate
U218	Ethanethioamide
U218	Thioacetamide
U219	Thiourea
U220	Benzene, methyl-
U220	Toluene
U221	Benzenediamine, ar-methyl-
U221	Toluenediamine
U222	Benzenamine, 2-methyl-, hydrochloride
U222	o-Toluidine hydrochloride
U223	Benzene, 1,3-diisocyanatomethyl-
U223	Toluene diisocyanate
U225	Bromoform
U225	Methane, tribromo-
U226	Ethane, 1,1,1-trichloro-
U226	Methyl chloroform
U227	1,1,2-Trichloroethane
U227	Ethane, 1,1,2-trichloro-
U228	Ethene, trichloro-
U228	Trichloroethylene
U234	1,3,5-Trinitrobenzene
U234	Benzene, 1,3,5-trinitro-
U235	1-Propanol, 2,3-dibromo-, phosphate (3:1)
U235	Tris(2,3,-dibromopropyl) phosphate
U236	2,7-Naphthalenedisulfonic acid,3,3'-[(3,3'-dimethyl[1,1'-biphenyl]-4,4'-diyl)bis(azo)bis[5-amino-4-hydroxy]-, tetrasodium salt
U236	Trypan blue
U237	2,4-(1H,3H)-Pyrimidinedione, 5-[bis(2chloroethvl)amino]-
U237	Uracil mustard
U238	Carbamic acid, ethyl ester
U238	Ethyl carbamate (urethane)
U239	Benzene, dimethyl-
U239	Xylene
U240	2,4-D, salts & esters
U240	Acetic acid, (2,4-dichlorophenoxy)-, salts & esters
U243	1-Propene, 1,1,2,3,3,3-hexachloro-
U243	Hexachloropropene
U244	Thioperoxydicarbonic diamide [(H2N)C(S)]2S2, tetramethyl-
U244	Thiram
U246	Cyanogen bromide (CN)Br
U247	Benzene, 1,1'-(2,2,2-trichloroethylidene)bis[4-methoxy-
U247	Methoxychlor
U248	2H-1-Benzopyran-2-one, 4-hydroxy-3-(3-oxo-l-phenyl-butyl)-, & salts, when present at concentrations of 0.3% or less
U248	Warfarin, & salts, when present at concentrations of 0.3% or less
U249	Zinc phosphide Zn3P2, when present at concentrations of 10% or less
U328	Benzenamine, 2-methyl-
U328	o-Toluidine
U353	Benzenamine, 4-methyl-
U353	p-Toluidine
U359	Ethanol, 2-ethoxy-
U359	Ethylene glycol monoethyl ether

Appendix F

Environmental Reporting Systems and Corporate Environmental Reports

This Appendix is taken from a World Wildlife Fund/Hampshire Research Institute study of national and state environmental reporting systems and corporate environmental reports. Data contained in these reporting systems and corporate reports are compared to an environmental reporting model, or benchmark, that allows a wide range of possible analyses. This Appendix lists the data elements that appear in each system and a few corporate reports as compared to the benchmark, with comments explaining special circumstances. (See Table F-1.) Reporting systems and guidelines and corporate reports analyzed in the complete study are also itemized here.

Table F-1. Data Elements in Proposed Environmental Reporting Model Compared to Data Elements Currently Reported

Type	Primary Data Categories	Specific Data Elements
Identification		
	Facility	Facility name and address
		Technical/public contact person
		Industrial classification (e.g. Standard Industrial Classification code)
		Latitude and longitude
		Related permits
		Facility identification number
	Parent Company	Name of parent company
		Parent company identification number
	Trade Secret	Notification of omitted data
		Company's justification of the need for confidentiality
		Signature of company official documenting need
	Reporting Year	Year for which data are being reported/submission date
		Indication if plant began or ceased operation in that year
	Chemical	Chemical name
		Chemical identification number (e.g. Chemical Abstracts Service number)
	Data Precision and Units	Units of measurement/roundoff (significant figures)
	Related Production	Amount/units
	Worker Exposure	Number of workers exposed
		Duration and level of exposure
Energy and Water Use		
	Energy Use	BTUs per year
	Water Use	Water Use Liters per year

Key to symbols and comments follows the table.

Canada	*Comments*	**Massachusetts**	*Comments*	**Netherlands**	*Comments*	**New Jersey**	*Comments*	**Sweden**	*Comments*	**United Kingdom**	*Comments*	**United States (TRI)**	*Comments*	**Dow 1993**	*Comments*	**Henkel 1994**	*Comments*	**ICI 1993**	*Comments*
●		●		●		●		●		●		●		●	25	●	25	●	28
●		●		●		●		●		●		●		●					
●		●		●		●		●		●		●							
●				●		○	30					●							
●				●		●						●							
●		●		●		●						●							
●				●								●	1	●		●		●	
												●	1						
	13	●		●		●						●							
		●		●		●						●							
		●		●		●						●							
●		●		●		●						●		●		●		●	
●		○	9	●												●			
		●		●		●				●		●		●				●	
●		●		●		●				●		●		●					
●	2	●	2	●	2	●	2	●	2	●	2	●	29	●	2	●	2	●	2
○	15	○	10	○	3	●						○	3			○	20		
														●				●	26

Table F-1. Data Elements in Proposed Environmental Reporting Model Compared to Data Elements Currently Reported (cont'd.)

Type	Primary Data Categories	Specific Data Elements
Releases and Transfers of Chemical in Waste Stream		
	Environmental Releases	Releases to air, water, and land, by type
		Basis of estimates of releases
	One-time Non-Production Releases	Remedial actions
		Fires, floods, earthquakes
	Off-site Transfers in Waste	Amount of off-site recycling, by location and method
		Amount used for energy recovery off-site, by location
		Amount of waste treated off-site, by location and method
		Amount of off-site disposal, by location and method
	On-site Transfers in Waste	Amount of on-site recycling by method
		Amount used for energy recovery on-site
		Amount of waste treated on-site by method
	Total Nonproduct Releases and Transfers	Sum of Environmental Releases, Off-site Transfers of Waste, and On-site Transfers of Waste
	Source Reduction Actions	Amount of reduction due to each practice:
		Changes in operating practices
		Inventory control
		Spill and leak prevention
		Raw material modification
		Product modifications
		Process changes
		Cleaning practice changes
Transfers of Chemical in Product Stream		
	Use/Production	Amount brought on-site/physical state for each different use
		Amount produced on site
		Amount consumed on site
		Amount in product (by type) shipped
	Inventory	Maximum amount of substances on-site
		Amount at start and end of inventory
		Average daily inventory

Key to symbols and comments follows the table.

Canada	*Comments*	**Massachusetts**	*Comments*	**Netherlands**	*Comments*	**New Jersey**	*Comments*	**Sweden**	*Comments*	**United Kingdom**	*Comments*	**United States (TRI)**	*Comments*	**Dow 1993**	*Comments*	**Henkel 1994**	*Comments*	**ICI 1993**	*Comments*
●		●	10	●		●		●		●		●		○	17	●	21	●	
●	9	○	11			●						●							
●		○	12				7					○	4						
⊛		○	10			●		●				●		●	18	○	22		
⊛		○	10			●		●				●		●	18				
●		○	10	●	19	●				●	19	●		●	18				
⊛		○	10			●		●				●		●	18	○	22		
						●	31					●	5	●	18	○	22		
						●	31					●	5	●	18				
⊛						●	31	●				●	5	●	18	●		●	27
○	14	○	32			●						⊛		⊛	18	●		●	
				⊛	27														
○	15	○	10			●							6			○	23		
		○	10			○							6			○	23		
		○	10			●							6			○	23		
		○	10			●							6			○	23		
		○	10			●							6			○	23		
		○	10			○							6			○	23		
		○	10			●							6			○	23		
				●		○													
		●	16	●		●													
				●		●										●	24		
		●	8	●		●	8	●											
						●		●				●							
						●													
						●													

Key to Symbols and Comments

Symbols

● Data element included in reporting system / corporate report
❍ Data element available in some form
✇ Data element can be calculated from other data

Comments

1 There are issues with the parent company information for as many as 30 percent of reporting TRI facilities.
2 Units of measurement only
3 Production or activity index reported.
4 Non-production related waste reported as single number regardless of how managed.
5 Total quantity and methods reported but not quantity by method.
6 Methods undertaken but not total quantity or quantity by method.
7 Included in waste generation
8 Amount shipped as product is facility-wide, not product specific.
9 Facilities may explain if any chemicals reported the previous year are not reported in current year.
10 Some TRI Form R data provided. There is a process-level ratio of emissions (releases plus off-site transfers) to base-year emissions. A similar ratio is reported for waste, although actual amounts of emissions and reductions in waste by source reduction cannot be calculated. The process-level ratio for waste is intended to reflect percent reduction by source reduction only.
11 Facility must indicate if change of basis of estimate has changed quantity.
12 Included in waste generation, facilities may describe events
13 Facilities indicate confidentiality on form.
14 Releases and off-site transfers only
15 Facilities must explain changes in amounts of releases and off-site transfers which include changes in production and estimation methods; source reduction activities may be listed voluntarily.
16 Also report amount processed and otherwise used
17 Media percentages for global emissions, also global emissions by chemical by SARA 313 and 33/50 Program chemicals
18 Total for SARA 313 chemicals
19 POTWs
20 Sales percent by product sector, plus total production units
21 SO2, NOx air emissions; Ni, Cu, Cr releases to water
22 Total of on-site and off-site activities
23 Specific project descriptions
24 Solvents and chlorinated hydrocarbons
25 Some facility names given
26 Efficiency
27 Amount only
28 Company also provides individual facility reports with facility-specific data.
29 Units of measurement only, some range code reporting
30 New Jersey locator data given
31 Total amount regardless of method
32 On-site transfers to recycling not included.

Source: Frances H. Irwin, *et al., A Proposed Benchmark for Industrial Pollutant Release and Transfer Reporting,* World Wildlife Fund, January 1995.

Environmental Reporting Systems and Guidelines Analyzed

Canada National Pollutant Release Inventory
Massachusetts Toxics Use Reduction Act
Netherlands
New Jersey Pollution Prevention Act
Sweden
U.S. Toxics Release Inventory (TRI)
United Kingdom
Coalition for Environmentally Responsible Economies (CERES)
European Chemical Industry Council (CEFIC)
Public Environmental Reporting Initiative (PERI)

Corporate Environmental Reports Analyzed

Albright & Wilson (Tenneco)
Arco
AT&T
BASF
Baxter International, Inc.
Boehringer Ingelheim
BP
Bristol-Myers Squibb Co.
British Airways
Canadian Pacific Forest Products Ltd.
Ciba
Degussa
Dofasco
Dow
Dow Canada
Dow Corning
Dow Europe
DSM
Dupont
Elf Atochem
EniChem
Exxon
General Electric
Georgia Pacific
Gillette Company
Henkel
Hoechst Celanese
Huls
IBM
ICI
Johnson & Johnson
Kunert AG
Merck
MoDo
Monsanto Corporation
Montecatini
Neste
Nobel Industries
Noranda Forest Products
Noranda Minerals
Norsk Hydro
Northern Telecom
Novo Nordisk
Ontario Hydro
Phillips Petroleum
Polaroid Corporation
Rhone-Poulenc
Rockwell International
Rohm and Haas Europe
Sandoz
SC Johnson
Shell (Switzerland)
Shell (UK)
Shell Canada, Ltd.
Shell International
SmithKline Beecham
Solvay
Statoil
Sunoco
Texaco
Thyssen Stahl
Toyota
Union Carbide
Upjohn
Volkswagen
Waste Management, Inc.
Wessex Water

Appendix G

Chemicals in the Environment: Additional Data

Appendix G-1. Methodology for Estimating Population Exposed and Blood Levels of Lead, Chapter 2, Table 2-2

Elevated Blood Levels as follows:

Paint and Plumbing	> 15 mg/dl
Primary Smelters	≥ 25 mg/dl
Secondary Smelters	> 20 mg/dl
Food	"approaching" 10 mg/dl

Paint - 12 M = number under seven yrs. living in houses built before 1974, (potentially painted with lead paint). 6 M = number living in lead-painted houses built before 1940, 99 percent of which have >0.7 mg/cm² of lead.

Gasoline - 5.6 M – Estimated from 1984 Census Data for 100 largest US cities (11 percent of a total population of 50.6 million people are under 7 yrs). Assumes all children in these cities are/were potentially exposed to lead from automobile emissions and fall-out. 1.2M = number projected to have blood lead levels below 15ug/dL as a result of reductions in leaded gasoline.

Stationary Sources - Population of children living within an undefined radius around US smelters and lead acid battery plants. Number with elevated blood lead levels derived by applying prevalence rates from studies around specific smelter operations to population estimates.

Dust and Soil - Estimate equals the sum of the total potentially exposed to lead from stationary sources, paint and gasoline, the primary sources of lead in dust and soil. Since simultaneous exposure from all three sources is unlikely, this number overestimates the actual number.

Plumbing Fixtures and Solder - 21 M =Total 1983 US population of children <6 yrs. Reflects potential exposure to lead in fresh solder in new homes (4 percent), in older solder of buildings constructed from 1950 - 1984 (54 percent), iron pipes and related lead connectors and solder in homes built from 1920 - 1949 (24 percent), and lead pipes in homes built before 1920 (13 percent). 3.8M is derived by EPA = number of children under the age of six who are consumers of tap water from public systems that are expected to contain lead levels above 20 ug/l, the {proposed} EPA limit under the SDWA (estimated as 9 percent of the total 42 million consumers calculated by statistical regressional analyses.

Food - Estimated to be 5 percent of all children less than six years old expected to have blood lead levels approaching 10 ug/dl as a result of dietary lead.

Source: Developed from information reported in Paul Mushak and Annemarie F. Crocetti, "Determination of Numbers of Lead-Exposed American Children as a Function of Lead Source: Integrated Summary of a Report to the U.S. Congress on Childhood Lead Poisoning," *Environmental Research*, 50, no. 2 (1989): 210-229.

Appendix G-2. Calculation of Percentages from Range Data

When a data set is composed of ranges, rather than single numbers, the calculation of percentages requires caution. The easiest approach, using the mid-point of each range, can lead to serious inaccuracies. Similarly, it is not legitimate to calculate percentage ranges by comparing the low end of a range to the sum of all the low-end estimates, and the high end to the sum of all high-end estimates.

The simplified example below gives range estimates for three categories (A, B, and C). Category A has a value between 3 and 10; Category B between 7 and 25; Category C between 4 and 12.

Category	Minimum	Maximum	Percent of Total
Category A	3	10	?
Category B	7	25	?
Category C	4	12	?

The total of all categories in this example is therefore somewhere between 14 and 47. If Category A is 3, however, it is not safe to assume that Categories B and C are 7 and 4, respectively; they might be 25 and 12.

To calculate the range of possible percentages represented by Category A, one must consider all possibilities. At one extreme, the true value for Category A may be the minimum value of the stated range (3), while the true values for Categories B and C might be at their maximum values (25 and 12, respectively). In this case, Category A would represent 3 out of (3 + 25 + 12), or 7.5 percent. It is, however, equally possible that the true value for Category A is 10, while the true values for Categories B and C are 7 and 4, respectively (the minimum value of their respective ranges). In this case, Category A would represent 10 out of (10 + 7 + 4), or 47.6 percent. (See figure on following page.)

Category	Minimum	Maximum	Percent of Total
Category A	3	10	7.5 - 47.6
Category B	7	25	24.1 - 78.1
Category C	4	12	10.3 - 54.5

Appendix G-2. Calculation of Percentages from Range Data (cont'd.)

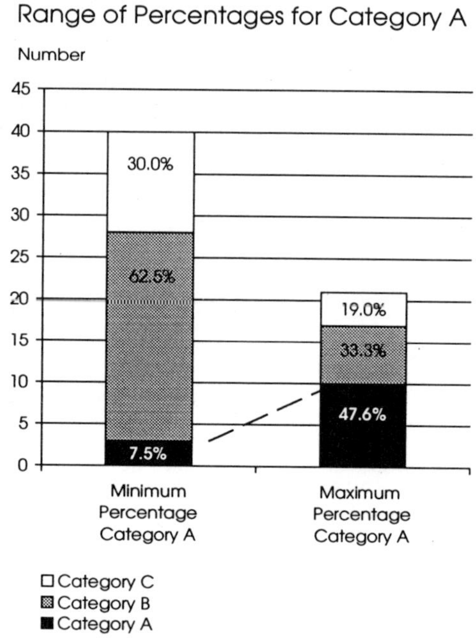

When, as in Table 2-4, one assembles categories into larger classes, a parallel problem exists. To calculate the percentage of emissions attributable to a given class, one must consider two extreme possibilities. On the one hand, the true value of every category within the class may be at the minimum value of the stated range, while the true value of every category that is outside the class may be at the maximum value of its stated range.

Class	Category	Minimum	Maximum	Percent of Total
Class 1	Category A	3	10	?
	Category B	7	25	
Class 2	Category C	4	12	?

In the example above, if Categories A and B are in Class 1, and Category C is in Class 2, Class 1 could represent as little as (3 + 7), while Class 2 could be as much as 12. In this case, Class 1 would represent 46 percent of the total. On the other hand, the true value of each member of Class 1 might be at the maximum of the range, while the true value of each member of Class 2 may be at its minimum. In this case, Class 1 would represent (10 + 25), while Class 2 would be 4. Accordingly, Class 1 could represent as much as 90 percent of the total.

Appendix G-2. Calculation of Percentages from Range Data (cont'd.)

Class	Category	Minimum	Percent of Maximum	Total
Class 1	Category A	3	10	45.5 - 89.7
	Category B	7	25	
Class 2	Category C	4	12	10.3 - 54.5

When, as in Table 2-4, a given category may reflect more than one class, one must additionally consider the range of possible contributions of each class to that category. In one extreme case, all of the emissions in a "U/P" designated category in that table might really be "U." The other extreme, in which all emissions are really "P," could also be true. The need to consider these possibilities is reflected in the broad range of percentages presented in Table 2-4 and its accompanying text.

Table G-3. Weighted Medians (ug/m3) for Air and Breath Concentrations of Selected Organic Compounds in New Jersey

Compound	Fall 1981 (128,600)* Daytime Air			Summer 1982 (109,400) Daytime Air			Winter 1983 (94,00) Daytime Air		
	Personal	Outdoor	Breath	Personal	Outdoor	Breath	Personal	Outdoor	Breath
Chloroform	3.1	0.6	1.8	0.8	0.1	2.3	2.2	0.1	0.1
1,1,1-Trichloroethane	17.0	4.8	6.6	6.6	5.5	5.2	26.0	1.5	2.3
Benzene	17.0	7.8	12.0	NC**	NC	NC	NC	NC	NC
Carbon Tetrachloride	1.5	0.9	0.7	0.4	0.8	0.2	NM***	NM	NM
Trichloroethylene	2.4	1.6	0.9	3.0	0.2	0.1	1.6	0.6	0.1
Tetrachloroethylene	8.4	3.6	6.8	5.4	3.3	4.3	9.7	8.0	4.5
Stryene	2.0	0.7	0.8	1.2	0.3	0.8	1.7	0.6	0.2
m,p-Dichlorobenzene	3.5	0.8	1.3	2.3	0.9	1.3	5.8	0.7	1.2
Ethylbenzene	7.9	3.2	2.9	4.2	1.9	1.7	8.2	4.1	1.3
o-Xylene	5.8	3.1	2.2	5.1	1.8	1.0	9.9	3.6	1.0
m,p-Xylene	18.0	8.2	6.4	13.0	5.9	3.2	25.0	10.0	3.0

* Population of Elizabeth and Bayonne for which estimates apply.
** Not calculated — cartridges contaminated.
*** Not measurable (most samples).

Source: Lance Wallce, *Project Summary: The Total Exposure Assessment Methodology (TEAM) Study*, Office of Acid Deposition, Environmental Monitoring and Quality Assurance, U.S. Environmental Protection Agency, Washington, DC EPA/600/S6-87/002 June 1987, 24.

Table G-4. Weighted Medians (ug/m3) for Air and Breath Concentrations of Prevalent Organic Compounds in Los Angeles and Contra Costa, California, 1984

Compounds	Los Angeles Winter			Los Angeles Summer			Contra Costa Summer		
		Daytime Air			Daytime Air			Daytime Air	
	Breath	Personal	Outdoor	Breath	Personal	Outdoor	Breath	Personal	Outdoor
m,p-Xylene	2.3	23	21	1.4	18	6.7	1.1	10	1.2
1,1,1-Trichloroethane	6.3	19	20	3.8	11	5.3	0.1	5.5	2.2
Tetrachloroethylene	5.8	8.2	9.0	4.0	3.4	1.7	2.0	2.2	0.2
Benzene	3.1	15	14	4.2	7.2	3.1	1.8	6.3	1.3
o-Xylene	0.7	10	7.9	0.5	4.0	2.2	0.4	3.6	0.4
Ethylbenzene	0.8	8.0	7.1	0.5	6.0	1.9	0.4	2.9	0.4
n-Octane	0.5	4.1	1.9	0.8	3.2	0.5	0.5	2.3	0.2
m,p-Dichlorobenzene	0.5	2.2	1.0	0.6	0.9	0.4	0.9	0.9	0.2
a-Pinene	0.9	1.9	0.2	0.9	1.6	0.3	0.3	1.0	0.0
n-Undecane	0.4	2.8	1.2	0.3	1.2	0.5	0.7	1.3	0.5
n-Decane	0.3	2.2	1.1	0.3	1.8	0.5	0.7	1.0	3.4
Trichloroethylene	0.2	2.2	0.5	0.2	1.2	0.0	0.2	0.5	0.1
Styrene	0.2	2.3	1.9	0.2	1.5	0.6	0.5	0.8	0.2
Sample Size	112-115	110-114	23-25	51	50-51	24	66-69	66-68	9-10

Source: *The Total Exposure Assessment Methodology (TEAM) Study: Selected Communities in Northern and Southern California*, Vol. III, Office of Acid Deposition, Environmental Monitoring and Quality Assurance, U.S. Environmental Protection Agency, Washington, D.C. EPA/600/6-87-/002c, June 1987, Table 6.

Table G-5. Source and Waste Characterizing National Prioirities List Sites from Three States

State and Site	HRS	Source	Site Type	Contaminants of Concern	Waste Type
Delaware					
Army Creek Landfill	69.92	▲/●	L	lead chromium arsenic organic compounds	municipal and hazardous waste disposal
Coker's Sanitation Service Landfills	52.15	▲	L	acrolein ethylbenzene bis (2-chloroethyl) ether	latex rubber sludges from latex plant
E.I. du Pont de Nemours (Newport Pigment Plant Landfill)	51.91	▲	M	heavy metals including: barium cadmium zinc trichloroethylene tetrachloroethylene	pigment plant—landfill for inorganically bonded metals, plant pigments, pigment sludges, magnetic tapes, low-level radioactive residues
Tybouts Corner Landfill	73.67	▲/●	L	hazardous organic and inorganic substances	landfill for municipal and industrial wastes
Michigan					
American Anodco	57.99	▲	M	nitric acid chromium aluminum copper nickel	cleaning, brightening, anodizing and sealing aluminum parts for the automotive industry - cooling and process water disposal in a lagoon.
Berlin & Farro	66.74	▲	L	C-56 liquids (pesticide byproduct) contaminated sludges	incinerator for liquified industrial wastes, landfill for disposal of crushed and empty drums
Bofors Nobel, Inc.	53.42	▲	M	benzidine DCB aniline benzene tetrachloroethylene 1,2-dichloroethane calcium sulfate	herbicide manufacturer [benzidine,3,3-dichloro benzidine (DCB), other compounds]
Butterworth #2 Landfill	50.31	●	L		landfill accepted industrial wastes including plating wastes, cyanides, and organic solvents
Gratiot County Landfill	53.65	▲	L	PBBs	Michigan Chemical Corp. disposed of various plant wastes including PBBs.
Liquid Disposal, Inc.	63.28	▲	L	PCBs	incinerator for liquid wastes, various industrial liquids and sludges
Northernaire Plating	57.93	▲/●	M	plating sludge liquefied plating solution chrome cyanide	electroplating facility

Table G-5. Source and Waste Characterizing National Prioirities List Sites from Three States (cont'd.)

State and Site	HRS	Source	Site Type	Contaminants of Concern	Waste Type
Michigan, cont'd.					
Ott/Story/Cordova Chemical Co.	53.41	▲	M	phosgene gas contaminated wastewater, soils, sludges organic chemicals	
Packaging Corp. of America	51.91	▲	M	heavy metals arsenic	untreated pulp mill black liquor and other process wastes from paper mill
Rockwell International Corp.	52.15	▲/●	M	emulsified oils ferric chloride sodium hydroxide polymer flocculent lead arsenic cyanide 4-methyl-2-pentanone heavy metals polynuclear aromatic hydrocarbons	manufacturing of universal joints for automotive industry, in residential neighborhood
Rose Township Dump	50.92	●	L	PCBs greases	liquid industrial wastes such as paint sludges, solvents, oils
Spiegelberg Landfill	53.61	●	L		open dump with paint sludges and liquid wastes
Springfield Township Dump	51.97	●	L	PCBs oils greases metals organic chemicals	liquid industrial wastes including paint sludges, solvents, PCBs, oils, greases
Thermo-Chem	53.36	●	R	methylene chloride C-66 (pesticide residue) carbon tetrachloride tetrachloroethylene 1,1,1-trichloroethane	plant for reclaiming solvents such as trichloroethylene, methylene chloride, paint wastes, and antifreeze
Velsicol Chemical Corp.	52.29	▲	M	polybrominated biphenyls TRIS	manufacturing of a variety of chemicals including polybrominated biphenyls and TRIS
New York					
Batvia Landfill	50.18	▲/●	L	industrial wastes including magnesium sludges, chromium hydroxide sludges, spent solvents and oil	

Table G-5. Source and Waste Characterizing National Prioirities List Sites from Three States (cont'd.)

State and Site	HRS	Source	Site Type	Contaminants of Concern	Waste Type
New York, cont'd.					
Circuitron Corp.	54.27	▲/●	M	metal-containing plating wastes—heavy metals chlorinated organic solvents 1,1,1-trichloroethane sulfuric acid sodium hydroxide caustic soda	manufactured circuit boards
General Electric Moreau Site (Caputo Landfill)	58.21	▲	M	liquid PCB wastes other chemical contamination	
Hooker (S Area)	51.62	▲	M	inorganic and organic wastes including: hexachlorobutadiene (C-46) hexachlorocyclopentadiene (C-56) chlorinated benzenes chlorinated toluenes trichlorophenols benzene toluene	chemical plant wastes (check description)
Hudson River PCBs	54.66	▲	M	PCBs	General Electric discharged 1.1 million pounds of PCBs into river
Jones Sanitation Site	52.52	▲/●	L	oils, greases, acids, alkalis, solvents, metals from plating operations, pigments, phenol, methylene chloride, chloroform, trichloroethylene, naphthalene, acetone	industrial and liquid wastes and sludges generated by Alfa-Laval, a manufacturer of mechanical separating equipment
Liberty Industrial Finishing	50.65	▲/●	M	heavy metals such as chromium and cadmium	electroplating, anodizing, and painting operations
LI Tungsten Corp.	50.00	▲	M	heavy metals, chlorides, sulfates, lead, cadmium, tungsten, chromium, arsenic, barium, silver, PCBs, cyanide, acids, alkalis, radium, thorium, uranium, asbestos fibers	tungsten smelter, producing tungsten carbide powder, tungsten wire, and welding rods
Love Canal	52.23	▲	L		16-acre landfill—dumping of various chemicals
Old Bethpage Landfill	58.83	▲	L		landfill for disposing of incinerator residue household trash, liquid and solid industrial process wastes, organic residues, metal hydroxide sludges

Table G-5. Source and Waste Characterizing National Prioirities List Sites from Three States (cont'd.)

State and Site	HRS	Source	Site Type	Contaminants of Concern	Waste Type
New York, cont'd.					
Onondaga Lake	50.00	▲	M	mercury contamination barium cadmium chromium cobalt lead benzene chlorobenzene total xylenes various polycyclic aromatic hydrocarbons pesticides PCBs	chemical manufacturing wastes. Allied manufactured numerous organic and inorganic chemicals, used a mercury cell process to produce chlorine, sodium hydroxide, potassium hydroxide,aqueous waste streams containing mercury, byproducts generated from soda ash production, wastes generated from acid washing of light oil
Pfohl Brothers Landfill	50.11	●	L	cyanides, plating sludge, waste paint and paint sludge, lithographic inks, pigments, organic solvents, liquid and solid PCB-contaminated wastes, sludge from distillation processes, petroleum wastes, phenol tar containing chlorinated benzenes and dioxins, benzene, phenol, chlorobenzene, dichlorobenzene, barium, manganese, mercury	municipal and industrial landfill
Pollution Abatement Services	70.80	▲/●	L	toxic, flammable, and explosive wastes including off-specification polymer gels, plating wastes, metal sludges, paint wastes, and laboratory chemicals	liquid waste incineration facility
Rosen Brothers Scrap Yard	51.35	●	L	1,1-dichloroethylene 1,1-dichloroethane 1,1,1-trichloroethane tetrachloroethylene trichloroethane fluorine di-n-butyl phthalate flouranthene pyrene di-n-octyl phthalate cadmium, chromium, lead, PCB-1242, chysene, anthracene, phenanthracene, pyrene	municipal and industrial waste dump, crushed cars and refrigerators
Sinclair Refinery	53.90	▲	M	cloth filters, fuller's earth, oil sludges, contaminated	refinery wastes

Table G-5. Source and Waste Characterizing National Prioirities List Sites from Three States (cont'd.)

State and Site	HRS	Source	Site Type	Contaminants of Concern	Waste Type
				soil, fly ash, mercury, PCBs, oil compounds	
Syosset Landfill	54.27	▲/●	L	heavy metals, industrial sludges, VOCs	municipal and industrial mixed waste landfill
Wide Beach Development	56.58	●	O	PCBs	subdivision of 66 homes, waste oils were spread on roads for dust control from 1940s-1978

Key:
- ▲ Process Waste
- ● Product Use
- ▲/● Both
- O Other
- L Landfill, dump, incinerator, or other disposal site
- M Manufacturing facility
- R Recycling facility
- HRS Hazard Ranking System score

Source: Derived from the National Priorities List database on RTK-Net.

Table G-6. Codes for Monitor Types in the Air Quality Subsystem (AQS) of Aerometric Information Retrieval System (AIRS)

Code	Description
A	Tribal Monitors
C	Non-EPA Federal Monitors
D	World Meteorological Organization
E	World Health Organization
0	Unknown
1	NAMS (National Air Monitoring System)
2	SLAMS (State and Local Air Monitoring System)
3	Other
4	Industrial Data
5	Index Sites
6	PAMS (Photochemical Air Monitoring Systems) Meteorological and VOC
7	PAM/NAMS for Criteria Pollutants
8	PAM/SLAMS for Criteria Pollutants
9	Secured

Table G-7. STORET Parameter Codes** for Chemicals in Search Set*

CAS Number	Chemical Name	Parameter Code(s)	
50-00-0	Formaldehyde	71880	
56-23-5	Carbon tetrachloride	32102	
60-57-1	Dieldrin	39380	
67-56-1	Methanol	77885	
67-66-3	Chloroform	32106	
67-72-1	Hexachloroethane	34396	
71-43-2	Benzene	34030	
71-55-6	1,1,1-Trichloroethane	34506	
74-87-3	Chloromethane	34418	
75-00-3	Chloroethane	34311	
75-01-4	Vinyl chloride	39175	
75-05-8	Acetonitrile	76997	
75-09-2	Dichloromethane	34423	
75-15-0	Carbon disulfide	77041	
75-25-2	Bromoform	32104	
75-69-4	Trichlorofluoromethane (CFC-11)	34488	
75-71-8	Dichlorodifluoromethane (CFC-12)	34668	
76-13-1	Freon 113	Not Found For Water	
78-87-5	1,2-Dichloropropane	34541	
78-93-3	Methyl ethyl ketone	81595	
79-00-5	1,1,2-Trichloroethane	34511	
79-01-6	Trichloroethylene	39180	
79-34-5	1,1,2,2-Tetrachloroethane	34516	
87-68-3	Hexachloro-1,3-butadiene	39702	
88-74-4	ortho-Nitroaniline	Not Found For Water	
95-50-1	1,2-Dichlorobenzene	34536	
100-41-4	Ethylbenzene	34371	
100-42-5	Styrene	77128	
106-46-7	1,4-Dichlorobenzene	34571	
106-93-4	1,2-Dibromoethane	77651	
106-99-0	1,3-Butadiene	81561	
107-02-8	Acrolein	34210	
107-06-2	1,2-Dichloroethane	32103	34531
107-21-1	Ethylene glycol	77023	81688
108-10-1	Methyl isobutyl ketone	78133	
108-88-3	Toluene	34010	
108-90-7	Chlorobenzene	34301	
117-81-7	Di-(2-ethylhexyl) phthalate	39100	
118-74-1	Hexachlorobenzene	39700	
120-12-7	Anthracene	34220	
120-82-1	1,2,4-Trichlorobenzene	34551	
127-18-4	Tetrachloroethylene	34475	
1024-57-3	Epoxyheptachlor	39420	
1330-20-7	Xylene (mixed isomers)	81551	
7439-92-1	Lead	1051	
7439-96-5	Manganese	1055	
7439-97-6	Mercury	71900	
7440-02-0	Nickel	1067	
7440-43-9	Cadmium	1027	
7440-47-3	Chromium	1034	
7647-01-0	Hydrochloric acid	438	
7723-14-0	Phosphorus (yellow or white)	665	
7782-50-5	Chlorine	50060	

* Storage and Retrieval of U.S. Waterways Parametric Data (STORET).

** There are multiple parameters for most chemicals; those selected represent total water concentrations, rather than dissolved or suspended fractions.

Appendix H

Chemicals in Commerce: Additional Data for Halo-organics

This Appendix consists of two types of tables.

Table H-1 presents the 100 chlorinated organic chemicals with the largest amount of production (and import) reported to the Toxic Substances Control Act Chemical Inventory Update of 1989. In this table, the production amount is the calculated mid-point of the broad ranges of production provided by EPA to prevent disclosure of data claimed confidential. This table also excludes an unknown number of chemicals whose identity was claimed as confidential when submitted. On this table, only the total for all chlorinated organics is a value received from EPA, not a mid-point calculated from a range.

The remaining tables in this Appendix provide the functions for the fluorinated, chlorinated, brominated, and iodinated organic chemicals introduced into commerce between 1979 and 1989 and produced and imported in the greatest amount. In these tables, the production amount provided for each function is the value as received from EPA.

Table H-1. Top 100 Chlorinated Organic Chemicals by Production Amount, on the TSCA Inventory Update, 1989*

Rank	CAS Number	Chemical	Count Mid-point Number	Production Mid-point Amount Pounds	Production Amount as Percent of Total** Percent
1	107-06-2	Ethane, 1,2-dichloro-	19	9,365,702,000	12.09
2	75-01-4	Ethene, chloro-	11	9,319,010,500	12.03
3	74-87-3	Methane, chloro-	12	965,027,150	1.25
4	71-55-6	Ethane, 1,1,1-trichloro-	13	764,931,200	0.99
5	75-78-5	Silane, dichlorodimethyl-	3	737,002,000	0.95
6	75-44-5	Carbonic dichloride	8	683,010,550	0.88
7	56-23-5	Methane, tetrachloro-	21	613,172,000	0.79
8	67-66-3	Methane, trichloro-	16	572,418,150	0.74
9	107-05-1	1-Propene, 3-chloro-	2	554,755,400	0.72
10	127-18-4	Ethene, tetrachloro-	11	552,743,350	0.71
11	75-45-6	Methane, chlorodifluoro-	12	431,787,200	0.56
12	106-89-8	Oxirane, (chloromethyl)-	8	421,291,150	0.54
13	75-09-2	Methane, dichloro-	17	407,563,650	0.53
14	75-71-8	Methane, dichlorodifluoro-	8	391,279,550	0.51
15	68390-96-5	Hydrocarbons, C3, chloro	2	336,899,200	0.44
16	108-90-7	Benzene, chloro-	4	331,053,200	0.43
17	75-34-3	Ethane, 1,1-dichloro-	2	325,287,575	0.42
18	760-23-6	1-Butene, 3,4-dichloro-	3	304,497,300	0.39
19	76-13-1	Ethane, 1,1,2-trichloro-1,2,2-trifluoro-	8	270,839,750	0.35
20	126-99-8	1,3-Butadiene, 2-chloro-	3	231,154,990	0.30
21	79-01-6	Ethene, trichloro-	6	199,506,300	0.26
22	79-00-5	Ethane, 1,1,2-trichloro-	5	192,118,050	0.25
23	25068-38-6	Phenol, 4,4'-(1-methylethylidene)bis-, polymer wit	3	163,754,295	0.21
24	616-23-9	1-Propanol, 2,3-dichloro-	3	146,407,925	0.19
25	110-57-6	2-Butene, 1,4-dichloro-, (E)-	3	141,004,190	0.18
26	75-35-4	Ethene, 1,1-dichloro-	2	136,953,935	0.18
27	106-46-7	Benzene, 1,4-dichloro-	3	118,746,590	0.15
28	75-69-4	Methane, trichlorofluoro-	13	113,063,150	0.15
29	75-00-3	Ethane, chloro-	6	108,434,160	0.14
30	87-90-1	s-Triazine-2,4,6(1H,3H,5H)-trione, trichloro-	3	91,462,635	0.12
31	100-44-7	Benzene, (chloromethyl)-	3	88,557,510	0.11
32	79-04-9	Acetyl chloride, chloro-	6	87,247,615	0.11
33	25168-05-2	Benzene, chloromethyl-	3	82,213,900	0.11
34	88-73-3	Benzene, 1-chloro-2-nitro-	3	73,678,880	0.10
35	75-79-6	Silane, trichloromethyl-	3	68,819,380	0.09
36	94-75-7	Acetic acid, (2,4-dichlorophenoxy)-	2	68,269,840	0.09
37	79-11-8	Acetic acid, chloro-	10	67,425,000	0.09
38	5216-25-1	Benzene, 1-chloro-4-(trichloromethyl)-	3	64,585,230	0.08
39	100-00-5	Benzene, 1-chloro-4-nitro-	2	63,443,565	0.08
40	96-23-1	2-Propanol, 1,3-dichloro-	3	62,287,450	0.08
41	78-87-5	Propane, 1,2-dichloro-	3	54,486,835	0.07
42	2702-72-9	Acetic acid, (2,4-dichlorophenoxy)-, sodium salt	3	44,391,040	0.06
43	2402-79-1	Pyridine, 2,3,5,6-tetrachloro-	3	44,178,850	0.06
44	764-41-0	2-Butene, 1,4-dichloro-	3	42,725,055	0.06
45	2524-04-1	Ethyl phosphorochloridothioate, ((EtO)2ClPS)	2	42,102,640	0.05
46	95-50-1	Benzene, 1,2-dichloro-	3	41,990,310	0.05
47	68002-59-5	Quaternary ammonium compounds, di-C14-18-alkyldime	2	40,656,640	0.05
48	1476-11-5	2-Butene, 1,4-dichloro-, (Z)-	3	39,401,045	0.05
49	95-49-8	Benzene, 1-chloro-2-methyl-	4	37,987,455	0.05
50	67-48-1	Ethanaminium, 2-hydroxy-N,N,N-trimethyl-, chloride	3	36,850,080	0.05
51	111-91-1	Ethane, 1,1'-[methylenebis(oxy)]bis[2-chloro-	3	35,715,510	0.05
52	120-82-1	Benzene, 1,2,4-trichloro-	5	34,509,745	0.04
53	2941-64-2	Carbonochloridothioic acid, S-ethyl ester	3	33,914,254	0.04
54	98-56-6	Benzene, 1-chloro-4-(trifluoromethyl)-	2	31,774,900	0.04
55	75-68-3	Ethane, 1-chloro-1,1-difluoro-	4	31,541,546	0.04
56	68411-72-3	Ethane, chloro derivs.	3	30,996,350	0.04

Count		Production	
Low Number	**High** Number	**Low** Pounds	**High** Pounds
7	31	3,015,844,000	15,715,560,000
3	18	4,772,391,000	13,865,630,000
6	18	225,758,300	1,704,296,000
8	17	221,954,400	1,307,908,000
1	4	147,352,000	1,326,652,000
4	12	179,630,100	1,186,391,000
12	30	185,725,000	1,040,619,000
9	23	124,734,300	1,020,102,000
1	3	313,303,300	796,207,500
3	19	243,002,000	862,484,700
6	17	279,879,200	583,695,200
5	10	140,488,700	702,093,600
11	22	186,748,600	628,378,700
2	14	199,387,800	583,171,300
1	3	246,399,600	427,398,800
2	5	206,000,800	456,105,600
1	3	82,669,150	567,906,000
1	4	74,720,600	534,274,000
3	12	166,848,700	374,830,800
2	4	51,642,880	410,667,100
1	10	147,385,600	251,627,000
1	8	101,881,400	282,354,700
1	4	74,879,790	252,628,800
1	4	41,976,750	250,839,100
1	4	45,811,280	236,197,100
1	3	61,103,070	212,804,800
1	4	80,493,380	156,999,800
8	18	36,294,800	189,831,500
3	9	36,397,520	180,470,800
1	5	30,408,470	152,516,800
1	4	62,475,920	114,639,100
3	8	27,717,630	146,777,600
1	4	45,855,600	118,572,200
1	4	46,502,760	100,855,000
1	4	45,854,240	91,784,520
1	3	49,511,900	87,027,780
3	16	28,499,900	106,350,100
1	4	27,829,660	101,340,800
1	3	20,614,430	106,272,700
1	4	19,225,700	105,349,200
1	4	15,074,480	93,899,190
1	4	11,033,040	77,749,040
1	4	30,382,280	57,975,420
1	4	29,122,330	56,327,780
1	3	29,388,050	54,817,230
1	5	10,068,440	73,912,180
1	3	26,528,420	54,784,860
1	4	13,415,380	65,386,710
2	5	21,937,000	54,037,910
1	4	16,208,720	57,491,440
1	4	16,600,970	54,830,050
3	6	22,295,420	46,724,070
1	4	7,937,228	59,891,280
1	3	10,052,250	53,497,550
1	6	8,881,801	54,201,290
1	4	12,950,700	49,042,000

Table H-1. Top 100 Chlorinated Organic Chemicals by Production Amount, on the TSCA Inventory Update, 1989 (cont'd.)*

Rank	CAS Number	Chemical	Count Mid-point Number	Production Mid-point Amount Pounds	Production Amount as Percent of Total** Percent
57	106-43-4	Benzene, 1-chloro-4-methyl-	3	29,651,836	0.04
58	3757-76-4	Phenol, 2,4-dichloro-, sodium deriv.	3	28,442,742	0.04
59	98-88-4	Benzoyl chloride	2	28,136,130	0.04
60	6358-85-6	Acetoacetanilide, 2,2''-(3,3'-dichloro-4,4'-biphen	15	28,071,230	0.04
61	68527-02-6	Alkenes, C12-24, chloro	2	27,974,025	0.04
62	120-83-2	Phenol, 2,4-dichloro-	3	27,796,330	0.04
63	99-54-7	Benzene, 1,2-dichloro-4-nitro-	3	27,680,980	0.04
64	61789-80-8	Quaternary ammonium compounds, bis(hydrogenated ta	5	26,031,386	0.03
65	37439-34-2	2(1H)-Pyridinone, 3,5,6-trichloro-, sodium salt	3	25,630,300	0.03
66	68606-33-7	Hydrocarbons, C1-6, chloro	3	25,014,630	0.03
67	26265-08-7	Phenol, 4,4'-(1-methylethylidene)bis[2,6-dibromo-,	3	24,727,580	0.03
68	2176-62-7	Pyridine, pentachloro-	2	23,756,290	0.03
69	63449-39-8	Paraffin waxes and Hydrocarbon waxes, chloro	6	23,431,306	0.03
70	100-20-9	1,4-Benzenedicarbonyl dichloride	3	23,140,811	0.03
71	98-07-7	Benzene, (trichloromethyl)-	2	23,054,744	0.03
72	72030-26-3	Cyclopentene, hexachloro-	3	22,482,007	0.03
73	96-18-4	Propane, 1,2,3-trichloro-	2	22,177,715	0.03
74	76-14-2	Ethane, 1,2-dichloro-1,1,2,2-tetrafluoro-	3	20,857,899	0.03
75	2893-78-9	1,3,5-Triazine-2,4,6(1H,3H,5H)-trione, 1,3-dichlor	3	20,856,055	0.03
76	108-77-0	1,3,5-Triazine, 2,4,6-trichloro-	4	20,810,830	0.03
77	77-47-4	1,3-Cyclopentadiene, 1,2,3,4,5,5-hexachloro-	3	19,416,815	0.03
78	75-54-7	Silane, dichloromethyl-	3	19,338,515	0.02
79	79-34-5	Ethane, 1,1,2,2-tetrachloro-	6	19,242,910	0.02
80	68938-79-4	Benzoic acid, 3,6-dichloro-2-hydroxy-, potassium s	3	19,022,310	0.02
81	563-47-3	1-Propene, 3-chloro-2-methyl-	7	18,643,872	0.02
82	2524-03-0	Methyl phosphorochloridothioate, ((MeO)2ClPS)	3	18,356,544	0.02
83	95-76-1	Benzenamine, 3,4-dichloro-	3	17,311,742	0.02
84	107-64-2	1-Octadecanaminium, N,N-dimethyl-N-octadecyl-, chl	3	17,260,595	0.02
85	75-77-4	Silane, chlorotrimethyl-	6	16,680,365	0.02
86	61788-76-9	Alkanes, chloro	3	16,475,893	0.02
87	76-15-3	Ethane, chloropentafluoro-	4	16,212,547	0.02
88	7398-69-8	Diallyldimethylammonium chloride	2	15,672,331	0.02
89	68938-81-8	Phenol, 2,5-dichloro-, potassium salt	3	14,637,442	0.02
90	68938-80-7	Benzoic acid, 3,6-dichloro-2-hydroxy-, dipotassium	3	13,536,825	0.02
91	99-63-8	1,3-Benzenedicarbonyl dichloride	3	13,533,010	0.02
92	630-20-6	Ethane, 1,1,1,2-tetrachloro-	3	13,236,389	0.02
93	56780-58-6	Starch, 2-hydroxy-3-(trimethylammonio)propyl ether	2	11,985,747	0.02
94	106-75-2	Formic acid, chloro-, diester with diethylene glyc	3	11,036,989	0.01
95	2431-50-7	1-Butene, 2,3,4-trichloro-	3	11,000,277	0.01
96	107-30-2	Methane, chloromethoxy-	2	10,744,221	0.01
97	594-42-3	Methanesulfenyl chloride, trichloro-	3	10,544,260	0.01
98	140-08-9	Ethanol, 2-chloro-, phosphite	2	9,473,389	0.01
99	1982-69-0	Benzoic acid, 3,6-dichloro-2-methoxy-, sodium salt	3	9,337,411	0.01
100	68955-37-3	Acid chlorides, tallow, hydrogenated	3	8,027,963	0.01
		Subtotal for Mid-point of Production of Top 100 Chlorinated Organics	438	31,191,080,899	40.28
		Total for Actual Production of All Chlorinated Organics		77,437,854,980	100.00

* Top 100 chlorinated organics by actual production amount as reported to TSCA Inventory Update, 1989. Rank is among 958 chlorinated organic chemical.

** Because mid-point production amounts for individual chemicals are compared to acutal production amount for all chlorinated organics, percentages can only be approximate. See introduction to this Appendix.

Count		**Production**	
Low Number	**High** Number	**Low** Pounds	**High** Pounds
1	4	7,008,192	52,295,480
1	4	8,998,093	47,887,390
1	3	12,248,380	44,023,880
6	24	14,908,080	41,234,380
1	3	5,592,969	50,355,080
1	4	8,915,719	46,676,940
1	4	15,285,040	40,076,920
3	6	8,133,351	43,929,420
1	4	14,152,660	37,107,940
1	4	15,788,100	34,241,160
1	4	18,238,200	31,216,960
1	3	17,521,810	29,990,770
2	10	5,550,401	41,312,210
2	4	9,242,051	37,039,570
1	3	5,781,718	40,327,770
1	4	5,826,094	39,137,920
1	3	11,902,960	32,452,470
1	5	8,100,118	33,615,680
1	4	7,069,440	34,642,670
1	6	13,681,890	27,939,770
1	4	6,833,440	32,000,190
2	4	12,875,170	25,801,860
4	8	13,233,560	25,252,260
1	4	10,718,380	27,326,240
3	10	8,744,554	28,543,190
1	4	8,159,337	28,553,750
1	4	7,122,084	27,501,400
2	4	12,391,830	22,129,360
3	8	4,658,930	28,701,800
1	4	5,665,905	27,285,880
1	6	6,669,874	25,755,220
1	3	5,426,262	25,918,400
1	4	8,926,903	20,347,980
1	4	4,458,789	22,614,860
1	4	4,028,569	23,037,450
1	4	3,467,517	23,005,260
1	3	3,106,043	20,865,450
2	4	3,539,907	18,534,070
1	4	6,281,584	15,718,970
1	3	2,371,401	19,117,040
1	4	3,427,889	17,660,630
1	3	2,876,247	16,070,530
1	4	3,033,962	15,640,860
1	4	2,608,045	13,447,880
203	673	12,741,648,187	49,640,513,610

Table H-2. New Fluorinated Organic Chemicals Entering Commerce, by Function, 1979-1993

Rank	Primary Function	PMNs Submitted Number	Notices of Commence-ment Number	PMN Expected Production Pounds	TSCA Inventory Update Production Pounds	TSCA Inventory Update Production as Percent of PMN Expected Production Percent	TSCA Inventory Update Production Cumula-tive Percent Percent
1	Blowing agents	5	4	46,183,225	46,112,605	99.85	22.67
2	Fluxing agents	4	2	28,925,600	28,867,300	99.80	36.86
3	Degreasers	1	1	28,864,000	28,864,000	100.00	51.06
4	Fire extinguishing agents	5	2	24,494,360	21,636,560	88.33	61.69
5	Pesticides	16	11	22,641,729	19,715,729	87.08	71.39
6	Additives / processing aids	3	3	17,701,200	17,701,200	100.00	80.09
7	Refrigerants	4	3	14,410,165	12,291,565	85.30	86.13
8	Herbicides	44	29	16,006,890	11,441,340	71.48	91.76
9	Intermediates	82	18	22,468,251	4,981,342	22.17	94.21
10	Solvents	7	6	2,297,350	2,264,350	98.56	95.32
11	Reactive dyes	32	18	1,409,855	1,121,536	79.55	95.87
12	Heat transfer agents	28	20	1,811,986	907,936	50.11	96.32
13	Surfactants	19	13	1,320,862	811,562	61.44	96.72
14	Soil release agents / soil retardants	12	7	940,280	766,480	81.52	97.09
15	Water repellent/proofing agents	8	5	1,303,496	588,280	45.13	97.38
16	Sizes	7	6	1,188,000	528,000	44.44	97.64
17	Functional fluids	31	24	1,182,826	527,226	44.57	97.90
18	Insecticides	5	5	460,746	460,746	100.00	98.13
19	Oil repellents	4	2	507,096	451,880	89.11	98.35
20	Agricultural chemicals (type unknown)	4	4	448,697	448,697	100.00	98.57
21	Metal treating agents	6	2	902,000	445,500	49.39	98.79
22	Dyes (type unknown)	16	13	428,602	426,226	99.45	99.00
23	Lubricating agents	9	2	290,758	264,000	90.80	99.13
24	Basic dyes	10	6	330,000	198,000	60.00	99.23
25	Acid dyes	4	4	192,544	192,544	100.00	99.32
26	Catalysts	8	5	182,292	152,900	83.88	99.40
27	Wetting agents	7	2	156,200	143,000	91.55	99.47
28	Dispersants	1	1	132,000	132,000	100.00	99.53
29	Safeners	6	4	178,486	122,870	68.84	99.59
30	Light stabilizers	1	1	110,000	110,000	100.00	99.65
31	Monomers	12	6	465,551	101,149	21.73	99.70
32	Curing agents	18	10	308,216	91,956	29.83	99.74
33	Polymer additives	4	2	163,643	81,767	49.97	99.78
34	Prepolymers	1	1	74,800	74,800	100.00	99.82
35	Antistaining agents	1	1	66,000	66,000	100.00	99.85
36	Photosensitive agents	11	9	71,496	62,146	86.92	99.88
37	Solvent dyes	1	1	44,000	44,000	100.00	99.90
38	Fillers / sealants	1	1	35,200	35,200	100.00	99.92
39	Not elsewhere classified	29	2	2,146,583	33,550	1.56	99.94
40	Electrolytes	3	2	100,331	25,531	25.45	99.95
41	Lubricant additives	2	1	23,980	23,100	96.33	99.96
42	Color former	6	3	80,960	14,960	18.48	99.97
43	Textile finishing agents	6	1	358,628	11,000	3.07	99.97
44	Luminescent agents	1	1	7,700	7,700	100.00	99.98
45	Initiators	6	3	81,556	6,596	8.09	99.98
46	Solder masks	4	1	24,420	5,940	24.32	99.98
47	Photographic chemicals (unspecified)	10	9	7,069	4,896	69.25	99.99
48	Resists	2	2	4,620	4,620	100.00	99.99
49	Surface coating additives	3	2	334,620	4,620	1.38	99.99
50	Reagents	6	1	23,227	2,970	12.79	99.99
51	Nucleating agents	4	4	2,665	2,665	100.00	99.99
52	Emulsifiers	2	1	11,440	2,640	23.08	100.00

Table H-2. New Fluorinated Organic Chemicals Entering Commerce, by Function, 1979-1993 (cont'd.)

Rank	Primary Function	PMNs Submitted Number	Notices of Commencement Number	PMN Expected Production Pounds	TSCA Inventory Update Production Pounds	TSCA Inventory Update Production as Percent of PMN Expected Production Percent	TSCA Inventory Update Production Cumulative Percent Percent
53	Antistatic agents	2	2	2,200	2,200	100.00	100.00
54	Ink additives	1	1	1,760	1,760	100.00	100.00
55	Sensitizing dyes	12	10	1,983	1,738	87.68	100.00
56	Adhesion promoters / adhesives	2	1	2,411	1,135	47.08	100.00
57	Defoamers	2	1	45,000	1,000	2.22	100.00
58	Coolants	2	1	2,970	990	33.33	100.00
59	Adhesive additives	1	1	550	550	100.00	100.00
60	Vat dyes	1	1	319	319	100.00	100.00
61	Liquid crystals	1	1	220	220	100.00	100.00
62	Polymerization inhibitors	1	1	110	110	100.00	100.00
63	Antihalation dyes	1	1	110	110	100.00	100.00
64	Corrosion inhibitors	1	0	2,200	0	0.00	100.00
65	Accelerators	1	0	499	0	0.00	100.00
66	Antioxidants	1	0	957,000	0	0.00	100.00
67	Binders	2	0	67,100	0	0.00	100.00
68	Pigments	1	0	2,200	0	0.00	100.00
69	Parting agents	5	0	5,445	0	0.00	100.00
70	Stabilizers	1	0	22,000	0	0.00	100.00
71	Antifogging agents	1	0	99,000	0	0.00	100.00
72	Diazo coupling agents	1	0	1,452	0	0.00	100.00
73	Phosphorescent agents	1	0	660	0	0.00	100.00
74	Fixatives (photography)	1	0	5,500	0	0.00	100.00
75	Fungicides	2	0	242,000	0	0.00	100.00
76	Frothers	2	0	143,000	0	0.00	100.00
77	Papermaking agents	3	0	387,200	0	0.00	100.00
	Total	571	308	243,899,087	203,393,310	83.39	
	Total Non-repeating	490	259	215,510,605	175,754,314	81.55	

This table lists all primary codes based on prorated maximum production ranges. Excludes those primary codes which are polymeric and those PMN cases condsidered by EPA to be invalid.

Table H-3. New Chlorinated Organic Chemicals Entering Commerce, by Function, 1979-1993

Rank	Primary Function	PMNs Submitted Number	Notices of Commencement Number	PMN Expected Production Pounds	TSCA Inventory Update Production Pounds	TSCA Inventory Update Production as Percent of PMN Expected Production Percent	TSCA Inventory Update Production Cumulative Percent Percent
1	Binders	9	3	85,316,000	64,801,000	75.95	13.20
2	Agricultural chemicals (type unknown)	16	10	67,794,096	60,615,496	89.41	25.55
3	Blowing agents	4	4	46,112,605	46,112,605	100.00	34.94
4	Bleaching assistants	3	2	49,280,000	36,740,000	74.55	42.43
5	Pesticides	31	23	35,529,008	34,136,408	96.08	49.38
6	Degreasers	1	1	28,864,000	28,864,000	100.00	55.26
7	Fluxing agents	1	1	28,864,000	28,864,000	100.00	61.14
8	Herbicides	74	44	45,007,466	21,486,034	47.74	65.52
9	Antiseize agents	3	3	17,046,920	17,046,920	100.00	68.99
10	Intermediates	142	65	43,352,590	15,581,459	35.94	72.16
11	Fuel additives	2	1	40,040,000	10,120,000	25.27	74.23
12	Photographic chemicals (unspecified)	49	34	11,138,901	10,072,663	90.43	76.28
13	Coagulants	2	1	9,768,000	9,108,000	93.24	78.13
14	Reactive dyes	244	128	34,613,346	7,429,048	21.46	79.65
15	Wet strength additives	4	2	7,431,600	7,414,000	99.76	81.16
16	Catalysts	95	43	12,152,510	6,514,809	53.61	82.48
17	Flame retardants	11	5	14,287,988	6,488,988	45.42	83.81
18	Initiators	9	4	23,325,265	5,775,319	24.76	84.98
19	Antistatic agents	9	7	6,147,592	5,721,892	93.08	86.15
20	Papermaking agents	10	3	11,746,803	4,809,999	40.95	87.13
21	Retention aids	6	3	8,794,500	4,367,000	49.66	88.02
22	Additives / processing aids	3	3	3,847,800	3,847,800	100.00	88.80
23	Heat stabilizers	3	2	3,825,800	3,806,000	99.48	89.58
24	Safeners	8	6	4,101,588	2,995,868	73.04	90.19
25	Emulsifiers	12	2	2,941,840	2,618,000	88.99	90.72
26	Prepolymers	4	2	2,939,999	2,499,999	85.03	91.23
27	Light stabilizers	6	5	3,005,200	2,433,200	80.97	91.73
28	Flocculating agents	4	3	4,525,400	2,325,400	51.39	92.20
29	Solvents	5	5	2,263,250	2,263,250	100.00	92.66
30	Fungicides	2	2	2,103,200	2,103,200	100.00	93.09
31	Swelling agents	1	1	1,980,000	1,980,000	100.00	93.49
32	Stabilizers	14	7	2,077,812	1,927,112	92.75	93.88
33	Pigments	33	21	3,561,888	1,863,048	52.31	94.26
34	Curing agents	25	16	3,150,070	1,834,690	58.24	94.64
35	Demulsifiers	5	3	1,966,998	1,815,000	92.27	95.01
36	Modifiers	8	5	4,591,488	1,786,444	38.91	95.37
37	Softeners	14	6	3,494,319	1,731,059	49.54	95.72
38	Oxidizers	2	2	1,650,000	1,650,000	100.00	96.06
39	Functional fluids	4	3	1,252,900	1,252,900	100.00	96.32
40	Coupling agents	38	32	2,100,175	1,243,715	59.22	96.57
41	Dewatering agents	9,473	1	1,100,000	1,100,000	100.00	96.79
42	Reagents	10	5	1,102,508	1,082,224	98.16	97.01
43	Viscosity adjustors	3	1	1,097,899	999,999	91.08	97.22
44	Fragrances	2	2	990,000	990,000	100.00	97.42
45	Soil release agents / soil retardants	2	2	990,000	990,000	100.00	97.62
46	Activators	5	5	847,689	847,689	100.00	97.79
47	Dyes (type unknown)	90	46	3,720,202	831,015	22.34	97.96
48	Disperse dyes	27	6	2,125,699	792,000	37.26	98.12
49	Adhesion promoters / adhesives	9	8	758,901	736,901	97.10	98.27
50	Scavengers	9	5	4,403,665	678,333	15.40	98.41

Table H-3. New Chlorinated Organic Chemicals Entering Commerce, by Function, 1979-1993 (cont'd.)

Rank	Primary Function	PMNs Submitted Number	Notices of Commence-ment Number	PMN Expected Production Pounds	TSCA Inventory Update Production Pounds	TSCA Inventory Update Production as Percent of PMN Expected Production Percent	TSCA Inventory Update Production Cumula-tive Percent Percent
51	Optical quenchers	2	2	654,500	654,500	100.00	98.55
52	Plasticizers	7	2	2,101,352	552,552	26.30	98.66
53	Water repellent/proofing agents	2	2	484,000	484,000	100.00	98.76
54	Photosensitive agents	14	10	951,667	467,645	49.14	98.85
55	Oil repellents	1	1	440,000	440,000	100.00	98.94
56	Ultraviolet absorbers	2	1	440,004	440,000	100.00	99.03
57	Color former	17	12	575,740	399,740	69.43	99.11
58	Corrosion inhibitors	7	3	3,348,400	367,400	10.97	99.19
59	Acid dyes	26	10	616,273	340,329	55.22	99.26
60	Insecticides	11	4	1,861,750	317,416	17.05	99.32
61	Lubricating agents	6	2	1,765,720	266,200	15.08	99.38
62	Monomers	14	6	2,453,000	264,770	10.79	99.43
63	Not elsewhere classified	12	7	6,543,934	229,934	3.51	99.48
64	Surfactants	16	5	4,055,278	224,017	5.52	99.52
65	Bleaching agents	12	3	4,182,640	222,640	5.32	99.57
66	Basic dyes	19	8	756,008	215,600	28.52	99.61
67	Antioxidants	3	1	315,333	198,000	62.79	99.65
68	Heat transfer agents	1	1	188,100	188,100	100.00	99.69
69	Surface coating additives	12	5	179,634	176,994	98.53	99.73
70	Adhesive additives	3	2	579,700	167,200	28.84	99.76
71	Dye coupling agents	6	1	701,074	165,000	23.54	99.79
72	Dispersants	7	6	204,490	164,890	80.63	99.83
73	Direct dyes	12	7	238,335	163,350	68.54	99.86
74	Clarifiers	2	2	102,723	102,723	100.00	99.88
75	Inhibitors	2	1	88,066	88,000	99.93	99.90
76	Nucleating agents	4	3	75,128	74,963	99.78	99.91
77	Ink additives	5	3	87,340	57,420	65.74	99.93
78	Brighteners	11	5	98,626	45,540	46.17	99.94
79	Dye leveling agents	2	1	138,600	41,800	30.16	99.94
80	Retarders (chemical processes)	2	1	85,096	35,200	41.37	99.95
81	Fluorescent agents	1	1	33,440	33,440	100.00	99.96
82	Azoic dyes	4	3	62,040	26,840	43.26	99.96
83	Thickeners	1	1	24,860	24,860	100.00	99.97
84	Gelling agents	1	1	24,860	24,860	100.00	99.97
85	Resists	3	1	44,000	22,000	50.00	99.98
86	Mordant dyes	1	1	19,800	19,800	100.00	99.98
87	Solvent dyes	2	2	12,540	12,540	100.00	99.98
88	Bluing agents	1	1	11,440	11,440	100.00	99.99
89	Biocides	3	2	64,099	9,099	14.20	99.99
90	Preservatives	1	1	8,800	8,800	100.00	99.99
91	Fillers / sealants	1	1	7,700	7,700	100.00	99.99
92	Textile finishing agents	2	1	41,800	6,600	15.79	99.99
93	Cosmetic ingredients	2	1	206,800	6,600	3.19	100.00
94	Sensitizing dyes	9	7	5,436	5,172	95.14	100.00
95	Refrigerants	1	1	5,005	5,005	100.00	100.00
96	Antihalation dyes	3	2	2,860	2,750	96.15	100.00
97	Pigment additives	4	1	113,256	2,640	2.33	100.00
98	Fluorescent dyes	1	1	2,200	2,200	100.00	100.00
99	Parting agents	2	1	3,960	1,980	50.00	100.00
100	Metal treating agents	9	1	382,140	1,980	0.52	100.00
101	Antifogging agents	3	2	1,327	887	66.83	100.00
102	Accelerators	3	1	5,720	660	11.54	100.00

Table H-3. New Chlorinated Organic Chemicals Entering Commerce, by Function, 1979-1993 (cont'd.)

Rank	Primary Function	PMNs Submitted Number	Notices of Commence-ment Number	PMN Expected Production Pounds	TSCA Inventory Update Production Pounds	TSCA Inventory Update Production as Percent of PMN Expected Production Percent	TSCA Inventory Update Production Cumula-tive Percent Percent
103	Developers (image formation)	1	1	440	440	100.00	100.00
104	Leuco dyes	2	2	321	321	100.00	100.00
105	Absorbents / adsorbents	1	0	16,830	0	0.00	100.00
106	Flotation agents	1	0	990,000	0	0.00	100.00
107	Hue modifier	2	0	14,520	0	0.00	100.00
108	Detackifiers	1	0	66,000	0	0.00	100.00
109	Sizes	3	0	1,474,000	0	0.00	100.00
110	Flavors	1	0	110,000	0	0.00	100.00
111	Polymer strippers	1	0	2,860,000	0	0.00	100.00
112	Antiscaling agents	3	0	442,200	0	0.00	100.00
113	Ion exchange agents	2	0	187,000	0	0.00	100.00
114	Polymerization inhibitors	1	0	2,200	0	0.00	100.00
115	Collectors / depressants	1	0	550,000	0	0.00	100.00
116	Diazo coupling agents	1	0	1,452	0	0.00	100.00
117	Milling aids	1	0	104,940	0	0.00	100.00
118	Drilling mud additives	1	0	220,000	0	0.00	100.00
119	Extraction agents	1	0	7,920	0	0.00	100.00
120	Cleaners	2	0	6,380,000	0	0.00	100.00
121	Fixing agents (textiles)	1	0	96,800	0	0.00	100.00
122	Deodorants	1	0	1,320,000	0	0.00	100.00
123	Solder masks	1	0	12,001	0	0.00	100.00
124	Fertilizers (micronutrients)	3	0	4,070,000	0	0.00	100.00
125	Complexing agents	3	0	1,485,000	0	0.00	100.00
126	Wetting agents	1	0	396,000	0	0.00	100.00
127	Vat dyes	1	0	11,000	0	0.00	100.00
128	Dye carriers	1	0	33,000	0	0.00	100.00
129	Leather processing agents	1	0	55,000	0	0.00	100.00
130	Lubricant additives	1	0	880	0	0.00	100.00
131	Polymer additives	1	0	2,200	0	0.00	100.00
	Total	1,413	748	755,435,776	490,889,021	64.98	
	Total Non-repeating	1,323	701	724,786,142	463,218,908	63.91	

This table lists all primary codes based on prorated maximum production ranges. Excludes those primary codes which are polymeric and those PMN cases condsidered by EPA to be invalid.

Table H-4. New Brominінated Organic Chemicals Entering Commerce, by Function, 1979-1993

Rank	Primary Function	PMNs Submitted Number	Notices of Commence-ment Number	PMN Expected Production Pounds	TSCA Inventory Update Production Pounds	TSCA Inventory Update Production as Percent of PMN Expected Production Percent	TSCA Inventory Update Production Cumula-tive Percent Percent
1	Flame retardants	40	13	132,406,790	39,911,482	30.14	64.69
2	Fire extinguishing agents	1	1	11,000,000	11,000,000	100.00	82.52
3	Pesticides	2	2	4,983,000	4,983,000	100.00	90.60
4	Antiscaling agents	1	1	999,999	999,999	100.00	92.22
5	Insecticides	1	1	866,800	866,800	100.00	93.62
6	Corrosion inhibitors	2	2	826,399	826,399	100.00	94.96
7	Herbicides	3	2	867,174	748,000	86.26	96.18
8	Photographic chemicals (unspecified)	20	16	505,685	490,732	97.04	96.97
9	Softeners	2	1	446,050	349,250	78.30	97.54
10	Color former	5	5	319,471	319,471	100.00	98.06
11	Intermediates	21	9	1,856,109	253,387	13.65	98.47
12	Papermaking agents	1	1	158,884	158,884	100.00	98.72
13	Catalysts	5	3	381,920	153,120	40.09	98.97
14	Curing agents	5	1	132,000	110,000	83.33	99.15
15	Bleaching agents	2	1	1,606,000	105,600	6.58	99.32
16	Disperse dyes	10	2	466,189	101,319	21.73	99.49
17	Not elsewhere classified	2	2	67,760	67,760	100.00	99.60
18	Fluxing agents	1	1	66,000	66,000	100.00	99.70
19	Dyes (type unknown)	7	5	290,356	43,956	15.14	99.77
20	Antioxidants	2	1	108,599	35,266	32.47	99.83
21	Monomers	13	1	1,181,675	21,120	1.79	99.87
22	Reactive dyes	4	1	102,467	18,867	18.41	99.90
23	Color enhancing dyes (contrast enhancers	1	1	16,500	16,500	100.00	99.92
24	Coupling agents	1	1	14,300	14,300	100.00	99.95
25	Fragrances	2	2	6,600	6,600	100.00	99.96
26	Ultraviolet absorbers	1	1	6,600	6,600	100.00	99.97
27	Safeners	1	1	4,532	4,532	100.00	99.97
28	Accelerators	1	1	3,300	3,300	100.00	99.98
29	Gelling agents	1	1	3,300	3,300	100.00	99.99
30	Photosensitive agents	5	3	25,318	2,939	11.61	99.99
31	Light stabilizers	1	1	2,200	2,200	100.00	99.99
32	Surface coating additives	3	3	1,210	1,210	100.00	100.00
33	Additives / processing aids	3	1	23,221	1,210	5.21	100.00
34	Binders	1	1	660	660	100.00	100.00
35	Initiators	1	1	139	139	100.00	100.00
36	Activators	1	1	139	139	100.00	100.00
37	Nucleating agents	1	1	110	110	100.00	100.00
38	Leuco dyes	1	1	101	101	100.00	100.00
39	Sensitizing dyes	1	1	101	101	100.00	100.00
40	Reagents	1	1	22	22	100.00	100.00
41	Antifogging agents	3	3	18	18	100.00	100.00
42	Sizes	2	0	541,992	0	0.00	100.00
43	Flavors	1	0	59	0	0.00	100.00
44	Plasticizers	1	0	4,400,000	0	0.00	100.00
45	Scavengers	2	0	87,083	0	0.00	100.00
46	Insect attractants	1	0	2,640	0	0.00	100.00
47	Phosphorescent agents	1	0	660	0	0.00	100.00
48	Antiplasticizers	1	0	13	0	0.00	100.00
49	Fixing agents (textiles)	1	0	96,800	0	0.00	100.00
50	Basic dyes	2	0	96,228	0	0.00	100.00
51	Polymer additives	1	0	22,000	0	0.00	100.00
	Total	193	98	164,995,172	61,694,392	37.39	
	Total Non-repeating	179	91	162,511,809	63,197,006	38.89	

This table lists all primary codes based on prorated maximum production ranges. Excludes those primary codes which are polymeric and those PMN cases condsidered by EPA to be invalid.

Table H-5. New Iodinated Organic Chemicals Entering Commerce, by Function, 1979-1993

Rank	Primary Function	PMNs Submitted Number	Notices of Commencement Number	PMN Expected Production Pounds	TSCA Inventory Update Production Pounds	TSCA Inventory Update Production as Percent of PMN Expected Production Percent	TSCA Inventory Update Production Cumulative Percent Percent
1	Catalysts	7	3	459,074	396,000	86.26	32.95
2	Corrosion inhibitors	2	2	469,997	469,997	100.00	72.05
3	Antiseize agents	1	1	169,998	169,998	100.00	86.19
4	Curing agents	3	3	41,998	41,998	100.00	89.69
5	Photosensitive agents	2	2	286	286	100.00	89.71
6	Initiators	2	1	1,830	986	53.85	89.79
7	Stabilizers	1	1	88,000	88,000	100.00	97.11
8	Heat stabilizers	1	0	4,950	0	0.00	97.11
9	Intermediates	3	0	67,110,296	0	0.00	97.11
10	Fungicides	1	0	24,948	0	0.00	97.11
11	Surfactants	1	1	22,000	22,000	100.00	98.94
12	Wetting agents	1	0	2,200	0	0.00	98.94
13	Dyes (type unknown)	2	2	240	240	100.00	98.96
14	Sensitizing dyes	5	4	10,721	10,703	99.84	99.85
15	Ink additives	1	1	1,760	1,760	100.00	100.00
	Total	33	21	68,408,298	1,201,968	1.76	
	Total Non-repeating	32	20	68,238,300	1,031,969	1.51	

This table lists all primary codes based on prorated maximum production ranges. Excludes those primary codes which are polymeric and those PMN cases condsidered by EPA to be invalid.

Appendix I

Toxics Release Inventory (TRI) Chemicals: Classifications, with Release/Disposal and Waste Data

Table I-1. TRI Chemicals by Classifications and Special Groups, with Quantity Released/ Disposed Of and Total Production-Related Waste, 1992

		Chemical Classsifications							Special Groups				
CAS Number	Chemical	Organics (Non-halogenated)	Acids/Bases/Salts	Metals	Halo-organics	Non-metallic Inorganics	Mixtures	Trade Secrets	Carcinogens	Ozone Depleters	Chloro-organics	Quantity Released/ Disposed of Pounds	Total Production-related Waste Pounds
75-07-0	Acetaldehyde	✔							✖			8,431,379	31,834,013
60-35-5	Acetamide	✔							✖			101,001	144,319
67-64-1	Acetone	✔										139,039,676	672,068,269
75-05-8	Acetonitrile	✔										21,429,372	2,581,322,698
53-96-3	2-Acetylaminofluorene	✔							✖			0	0
107-02-8	Acrolein	✔										135,163	3,305,840
79-06-1	Acrylamide	✔							✖			4,275,321	4,840,323
79-10-7	Acrylic acid	✔										5,074,341	61,790,567
107-13-1	Acrylonitrile	✔							✖			5,442,217	46,537,679
309-00-2	Aldrin				✔				✖		✖	0	0
107-18-6	Allyl alcohol	✔										229,952	2,083,277
107-05-1	Allyl chloride				✔						✖	122,224	5,196,542
7429-90-5	Aluminum (fume or dust)			✔								5,967,550	131,824,600
1344-28-1	Aluminum oxide (fibrous forms)			✔								1,308,827	3,661,010
117-79-3	2-Aminoanthraquinone	✔							✖			0	0
60-09-3	4-Aminoazobenzene	✔							✖			250	250
92-67-1	4-Aminobiphenyl	✔							✖			3	73,003
82-28-0	1-Amino-2-methyl-anthraquinone	✔							✖			0	0
7664-41-7	Ammonia					✔						455,599,635	1,383,853,783
6484-52-2	Ammonium nitrate (solution)		✔									49,700,242	150,857,399
7783-20-2	Ammonium sulfate (solution)		✔									29,261,313	77,217,088
62-53-3	Aniline	✔							✖			1,783,054	21,628,202
90-04-0	o-Anisidine	✔							✖			2,637	13,633
104-94-9	p-Anisidine	✔										55	1,128
134-29-2	o-Anisidine hydrochloride				✔				✖		✖	0	0
120-12-7	Anthracene	✔										569,044	12,272,595
7440-36-0	Antimony			✔								161,643	5,268,714
	Antimony compounds			✔								4,054,705	22,690,828
7440-38-2	Arsenic					✔			✖			1,857,786	2,348,508
	Arsenic compounds					✔						4,106,260	11,335,468
1332-21-4	Asbestos (friable)					✔			✖			4,949,097	8,395,583
7440-39-3	Barium			✔								966,414	1,137,580
	Barium compounds			✔								18,462,353	46,622,415
98-87-3	Benzal chloride				✔						✖	973	41,916
55-21-0	Benzamide	✔										0	0
71-43-2	Benzene	✔							✖			13,390,673	145,101,986
92-87-5	Benzidine	✔							✖			0	0
98-07-7	Benzoic trichloride				✔				✖		✖	6,070	296,071
98-88-4	Benzoyl chloride				✔						✖	14,308	1,257,053
94-36-0	Benzoyl peroxide	✔										19,671	220,347
100-44-7	Benzyl chloride				✔				✖		✖	45,254	707,884
7440-41-7	Beryllium			✔					✖			37,213	63,402
	Beryllium compounds			✔								52,126	75,106
92-52-4	Biphenyl	✔										1,258,180	6,976,630

Table I-1. TRI Chemicals by Classifications and Special Groups, with Quantity Released/ Disposed Of and Total Production-Related Waste, 1992 (cont'd.)

CAS Number	Chemical	Chemical Classsifications: Organics (Non-halogenated)	Acids/Bases/Salts	Metals	Halo-organics	Non-metallic Inorganics	Mixtures	Trade Secrets	Special Groups: Carcinogens	Ozone Depleters	Chloro-organics	Quantity Released/ Disposed of Pounds	Total Production-related Waste Pounds
111-44-4	Bis(2-chloroethyl) ether				✔				✖		✖	13,798	1,199,590
542-88-1	Bis(chloromethyl) ether				✔				✖		✖	310	331
108-60-1	Bis(2-chloro-1-methyl-ethyl)ether				✔						✖	11,300	12,859,300
103-23-1	Bis(2-ethylhexyl) adipate	✔										611,877	3,004,862
353-59-3	Bromochlorodifluoro-methane (Halon 1211)				✔					✖	✖	16,749	61,749
75-25-2	Bromoform				✔				✖			14,100	20,500
74-83-9	Bromomethane				✔					✖		3,005,194	3,582,339
75-63-8	Bromotrifluoromethane (Halon 1301)				✔					✖		110,445	168,545
106-99-0	1,3-Butadiene	✔							✖			4,046,531	453,627,237
141-32-2	Butyl acrylate	✔										351,856	4,726,036
71-36-3	n-Butyl alcohol	✔										32,300,656	152,896,118
78-92-2	sec-Butyl alcohol	✔										710,251	16,970,329
75-65-0	tert-Butyl alcohol	✔										2,606,556	76,907,238
85-68-7	Butyl benzyl phthalate	✔										734,483	4,976,181
106-88-7	1,2-Butylene oxide	✔										87,072	791,678
123-72-8	Butyraldehyde	✔										624,770	3,238,895
4680-78-8	C.I. Acid Green 3	✔										0	0
569-64-2	C.I. Basic Green 4	✔										23,327	28,353
989-38-8	C.I. Basic Red 1	✔										382	691
1937-37-7	C.I. Direct Black 38	✔							✖			0	0
2602-46-2	C.I. Direct Blue 6	✔							✖			0	0
16071-86-6	C.I. Direct Brown 95			✔					✖			0	0
2832-40-8	C.I. Disperse Yellow 3	✔										1,231	3,360
3761-53-3	C.I. Food Red 5	✔							✖			0	0
81-88-9	C.I. Food Red 15	✔										2	1,702
3118-97-6	C.I. Solvent Orange 7	✔										0	0
97-56-3	C.I. Solvent Yellow 3	✔										0	0
842-07-9	C.I. Solvent Yellow 14	✔										0	0
492-80-8	C.I. Solvent Yellow 34	✔							✖			0	0
128-66-5	C.I. Vat Yellow 4	✔										0	0
7440-43-9	Cadmium			✔					✖			153,619	1,656,952
	Cadmium compounds			✔								468,220	13,924,917
156-62-7	Calcium cyanamide	✔										38,405	88,405
133-06-2	Captan	✔							✖			17,097	34,439
63-25-2	Carbaryl	✔										37,436	525,739
75-15-0	Carbon disulfide	✔										93,554,822	127,135,361
56-23-5	Carbon tetrachloride				✔				✖	✖	✖	1,426,570	39,136,449
463-58-1	Carbonyl sulfide	✔										16,163,428	25,507,349
120-80-9	Catechol	✔										363,130	70,041,383
133-90-4	Chloramben				✔						✖	0	0
57-74-9	Chlordane				✔				✖		✖	1,700	12,590
7782-50-5	Chlorine					✔						71,168,030	430,848,879
10049-04-4	Chlorine dioxide					✔						3,112,849	37,034,637
79-11-8	Chloroacetic acid				✔						✖	16,746	1,012,286
532-27-4	2-Chloroacetophenone				✔						✖	0	0

Table I-1. TRI Chemicals by Classifications and Special Groups, with Quantity Released/ Disposed Of and Total Production-Related Waste, 1992 (cont'd.)

		Chemical Classsifications							Special Groups				
CAS Number	Chemical	Organics (Non-halogenated)	Acids/Bases/Salts	Metals	Halo-organics	Non-metallic Inorganics	Mixtures	Trade Secrets	Carcinogens	Ozone Depleters	Chloro-organics	Quantity Released/ Disposed of Pounds	Total Production-related Waste Pounds
108-90-7	Chlorobenzene				✔						✖	2,475,509	16,979,055
510-15-6	Chlorobenzilate				✔				✖		✖	0	0
75-00-3	Chloroethane				✔						✖	2,758,993	44,803,130
67-66-3	Chloroform				✔				✖		✖	17,802,805	56,079,423
74-87-3	Chloromethane				✔						✖	5,779,134	14,505,784
107-30-2	Chloromethyl methyl ether				✔				✖		✖	1,301	36,159
	Chlorophenols				✔				✖		✖	146,232	2,329,719
126-99-8	Chloroprene				✔						✖	1,559,346	12,411,912
1897-45-6	Chlorothalonil				✔				✖		✖	181,152	204,943
7440-47-3	Chromium			✔					✖			5,395,166	104,832,861
	Chromium compounds			✔								35,745,584	171,072,379
7440-48-4	Cobalt			✔								128,158	8,037,603
	Cobalt compounds			✔								557,487	3,823,812
7440-50-8	Copper			✔								29,512,497	675,138,852
	Copper compounds			✔								46,462,501	502,456,962
8001-58-9	Creosote	✔							✖			2,153,138	17,554,499
120-71-8	p-Cresidine	✔							✖			6,725	31,520
1319-77-3	Cresol (mixed isomers)	✔										960,567	13,382,788
108-39-4	m-Cresol	✔										566,861	3,322,007
95-48-7	o-Cresol	✔										541,166	1,129,641
106-44-5	p-Cresol	✔										305,048	1,944,861
98-82-8	Cumene	✔										3,715,939	320,391,682
80-15-9	Cumene hydroperoxide	✔										360,020	932,174
135-20-6	Cupferron	✔							✖			10	79
	Cyanide compounds		✔									4,241,284	14,910,262
110-82-7	Cyclohexane	✔										14,061,768	94,716,569
94-75-7	2,4-D (acetic acid)				✔						✖	57,207	200,669
1163-19-5	Decabromodiphenyl oxide				✔							1,157,192	2,849,268
2303-16-4	Diallate	✔							✖			0	0
615-05-4	2,4-Diaminoanisole	✔							✖			0	0
39156-41-7	2,4-Diaminoanisole sulfate	✔							✖			0	0
101-80-4	4,4'-Diaminodiphenyl ether	✔							✖			1,768	24,083
25376-45-8	Diaminotoluene (mixed isomers)	✔							✖			29,760	5,696,903
95-80-7	2,4-Diaminotoluene	✔							✖			1,941	12,329
334-88-3	Diazomethane	✔										0	0
132-64-9	Dibenzofuran	✔										96,995	5,217,842
96-12-8	1,2-Dibromo-3-chloropropane				✔				✖		✖	294	294
106-93-4	1,2-Dibromoethane				✔				✖			36,874	141,237
124-73-2	Dibromotetrafluoroethane (Halon 2402)				✔					✖		0	0
84-74-2	Dibutyl phthalate	✔										342,347	1,103,627
25321-22-6	Dichlorobenzene (mixed isomers)				✔				✖		✖	3,842	637,200
95-50-1	1,2-Dichlorobenzene				✔						✖	482,566	11,478,802
541-73-1	1,3-Dichlorobenzene				✔						✖	5,022	87,313

Table I-1. TRI Chemicals by Classifications and Special Groups, with Quantity Released/ Disposed Of and Total Production-Related Waste, 1992 (cont'd.)

		Chemical Classsifications							Special Groups				
CAS Number	Chemical	Organics (Non-halogenated)	Acids/Bases/Salts	Metals	Halo-organics	Non-metallic Inorganics	Mixtures	Trade Secrets	Carcinogens	Ozone Depleters	Chloro-organics	Quantity Released/ Disposed of Pounds	Total Production-related Waste Pounds
106-46-7	1,4-Dichlorobenzene				✔				✖		✖	351,236	1,330,116
91-94-1	3,3'-Dichlorobenzidine				✔				✖		✖	5,700	27,887
75-27-4	Dichlorobromomethane				✔				✖		✖	194	195
75-71-8	Dichlorodifluoromethane (CFC-12)				✔					✖	✖	11,359,695	13,168,673
107-06-2	1,2-Dichloroethane				✔				✖		✖	3,127,466	221,813,665
540-59-0	1,2-Dichloroethylene				✔						✖	23,222	8,669,998
75-09-2	Dichloromethane				✔				✖		✖	75,729,079	286,593,104
120-83-2	2,4-Dichlorophenol				✔						✖	10,312	107,961
78-87-5	1,2-Dichloropropane				✔				✖		✖	620,279	68,342,373
78-88-6	2,3-Dichloropropene				✔						✖	160,756	4,728,756
542-75-6	1,3-Dichloropropylene				✔				✖		✖	41,720	17,695,797
76-14-2	Dichlorotetrafluoro-ethane (CFC-114)				✔					✖	✖	1,080,021	2,152,419
62-73-7	Dichlorvos				✔				✖		✖	1,455	4,622
115-32-2	Dicofol				✔						✖	209	613
1464-53-5	Diepoxybutane	✔							✖			0	0
111-42-2	Diethanolamine	✔										1,561,157	4,836,156
117-81-7	Di-(2-ethylhexyl) phthalate	✔							✖			2,131,979	10,665,724
84-66-2	Diethyl phthalate	✔										161,598	1,960,282
64-67-5	Diethyl sulfate	✔							✖			3,706	5,012,924
119-90-4	3,3'-Dimethoxybenzidine	✔							✖			8	87
60-11-7	4-Dimethylamino-azobenzene	✔							✖			0	0
119-93-7	3,3'-Dimethylbenzidine	✔							✖			0	0
79-44-7	Dimethylcarbamyl chloride	✔							✖			0	0
57-14-7	1,1-Dimethyl hydrazine	✔							✖			251	17,077
105-67-9	2,4-Dimethylphenol	✔										135,578	851,832
131-11-3	Dimethyl phthalate	✔										85,416	931,854
77-78-1	Dimethyl sulfate	✔							✖			6,026	1,121,560
99-65-0	m-Dinitrobenzene	✔										1,241	854,241
528-29-0	o-Dinitrobenzene	✔										157	224,400
100-25-4	p-Dinitrobenzene	✔										130	30,130
534-52-1	4,6-Dinitro-o-cresol	✔										5,648	472,763
51-28-5	2,4-Dinitrophenol	✔										45,964	787,676
121-14-2	2,4-Dinitrotoluene	✔										1,863	107,850
606-20-2	2,6-Dinitrotoluene	✔										549	63,423
25321-14-6	Dinitrotoluene (mixed isomers)	✔										66,431	946,545
123-91-1	1,4-Dioxane	✔							✖			1,134,027	5,783,622
122-66-7	1,2-Diphenylhydrazine	✔							✖			0	0
106-89-8	Epichlorohydrin				✔				✖		✖	525,985	18,581,697
110-80-5	2-Ethoxyethanol	✔										377,400	2,602,442
140-88-5	Ethyl acrylate	✔							✖			221,369	8,423,314
100-41-4	Ethylbenzene	✔										10,857,715	96,538,764
541-41-3	Ethyl chloroformate				✔						✖	1,953	129,377
74-85-1	Ethylene	✔										35,854,137	1,180,225,916
107-21-1	Ethylene glycol	✔										20,109,179	561,144,278

Table I-1. TRI Chemicals by Classifications and Special Groups, with Quantity Released/ Disposed Of and Total Production-Related Waste, 1992 (cont'd.)

		Chemical Classsifications							Special Groups				
CAS Number	Chemical	Organics (Non-halogenated)	Acids/Bases/Salts	Metals	Halo-organics	Non-metallic Inorganics	Mixtures	Trade Secrets	Carcinogens	Ozone Depleters	Chloro-organics	Quantity Released/ Disposed of Pounds	Total Production-related Waste Pounds
151-56-4	Ethyleneimine	✔							✖			0	0
75-21-8	Ethylene oxide	✔							✖			1,435,389	8,201,743
96-45-7	Ethylene thiourea	✔							✖			12,919	14,983
2164-17-2	Fluometuron	✔										2,808	11,028
50-00-0	Formaldehyde	✔							✖			16,913,837	298,670,590
76-13-1	Freon 113				✔					✖	✖	23,906,231	289,662,188
	Glycol ethers	✔										49,847,660	131,379,713
76-44-8	Heptachlor				✔				✖		✖	210	108,210
118-74-1	Hexachlorobenzene				✔				✖		✖	50,210	4,116,741
87-68-3	Hexachloro-1,3-butadiene				✔						✖	6,534	8,906,178
77-47-4	Hexachlorocyclopentadiene				✔						✖	10,915	296,207
67-72-1	Hexachloroethane				✔						✖	32,183	3,232,680
1335-87-1	Hexachloronaphthalene				✔						✖	0	0
680-31-9	Hexamethylphosphoramide	✔							✖			0	0
302-01-2	Hydrazine					✔			✖			25,608	168,820
10034-93-2	Hydrazine sulfate		✔						✖			120,002	120,002
7647-01-0	Hydrochloric acid		✔									298,900,276	2,475,552,419
74-90-8	Hydrogen cyanide		✔									3,123,903	37,573,237
7664-39-3	Hydrogen fluoride		✔									10,860,641	243,107,876
123-31-9	Hydroquinone	✔										285,943	1,169,940
78-84-2	Isobutyraldehyde	✔										406,607	6,168,559
67-63-0	Isopropyl alcohol (manufacturing)	✔										1,222,666	4,822,449
80-05-7	4,4'-Isopropylidenediphenol	✔										817,736	10,290,693
120-58-1	Isosafrole	✔										0	0
7439-92-1	Lead			✔					✖			5,880,827	260,778,713
	Lead compounds			✔								26,999,354	1,107,360,694
58-89-9	Lindane				✔				✖		✖	427	2,440
108-31-6	Maleic anhydride	✔										460,619	36,880,348
12427-38-2	Maneb			✔								13,980	14,364
7439-96-5	Manganese			✔								20,320,149	92,712,389
	Manganese compounds			✔								75,565,406	237,882,578
7439-97-6	Mercury			✔								45,054	1,705,168
	Mercury compounds			✔								188,996	338,898
67-56-1	Methanol	✔										259,001,005	2,238,505,652
72-43-5	Methoxychlor				✔						✖	178	431
109-86-4	2-Methoxyethanol	✔										1,817,780	17,941,981
96-33-3	Methyl acrylate	✔										270,844	3,080,550
1634-04-4	Methyl tert-butyl ether	✔										2,903,712	7,106,790
101-14-4	4,4'-Methylenebis (2-chloroaniline)				✔				✖		✖	33,233	38,346
101-61-1	4,4'-Methylenebis(N,N-dimethyl) benzeneamine	✔							✖			0	0
101-68-8	Methylenebis (phenylisocyanate)	✔										2,040,760	3,633,780
74-95-3	Methylene bromide				✔							37,612	2,738,197
101-77-9	4,4'-Methyenedianiline	✔							✖			26,608	234,442

Table I-1. TRI Chemicals by Classifications and Special Groups, with Quantity Released/Disposed Of and Total Production-Related Waste, 1992 (cont'd.)

CAS Number	Chemical	Chemical Classsifications: Organics (Non-halogenated)	Acids/Bases/Salts	Metals	Halo-organics	Non-metallic Inorganics	Mixtures	Trade Secrets	Special Groups: Carcinogens	Ozone Depleters	Chloro-organics	Quantity Released/ Disposed of Pounds	Total Production-related Waste Pounds
78-93-3	Methyl ethyl ketone	✔										88,491,478	465,413,844
60-34-4	Methyl hydrazine	✔										1	1
74-88-4	Methyl iodide				✔							34,230	79,303
108-10-1	Methyl isobutyl ketone	✔										25,840,592	350,963,788
624-83-9	Methyl isocyanate	✔										7,654	167,238
80-62-6	Methyl methacrylate	✔										2,823,047	13,704,586
90-94-8	Michler's ketone	✔							✖			0	0
1313-27-5	Molybdenum trioxide			✔								720,580	10,315,038
76-15-3	Monochloropentafluoro-ethane (CFC-115)				✔					✖	✖	419,169	491,599
505-60-2	Mustard gas	✔							✖			0	0
91-20-3	Naphthalene	✔										3,922,572	60,045,613
134-32-7	alpha-Naphthylamine	✔							✖			2	2
91-59-8	beta-Naphthylamine	✔							✖			0	0
7440-02-0	Nickel			✔					✖			6,051,436	87,495,571
	Nickel compounds			✔					✖			4,293,605	63,460,089
7697-37-2	Nitric acid		✔									29,559,498	310,850,709
139-13-9	Nitrilotriacetic acid	✔							✖			6,773	807,090
99-59-2	5-Nitro-o-anisidine	✔							✖			39	84
98-95-3	Nitrobenzene	✔										916,765	5,262,783
92-93-3	4-Nitrobiphenyl	✔							✖			0	0
1836-75-5	Nitrofen	✔							✖			0	0
51-75-2	Nitrogen mustard	✔							✖			0	0
55-63-0	Nitroglycerin	✔										41,802	507,407
88-75-5	2-Nitrophenol	✔										47	24,170
100-02-7	4-Nitrophenol	✔										2,530	742,718
79-46-9	2-Nitropropane	✔							✖			173,791	1,072,782
156-10-5	p-Nitrosodiphenylamine	✔										4,924	28,424
121-69-7	N,N-Dimethylaniline	✔										86,805	1,380,283
924-16-3	N-Nitrosodi-n-butylamine	✔							✖			0	0
55-18-5	N-Nitrosodiethylamine	✔							✖			0	0
62-75-9	N-Nitrosodimethylamine	✔							✖			0	0
86-30-6	N-Nitrosodiphenylamine	✔							✖			0	500,000
621-64-7	N-Nitrosodi-n-propylamine	✔							✖			0	0
4549-40-0	N-Nitrosomethyl-vinylamine	✔							✖			0	0
59-89-2	N-Nitrosomorpholine	✔							✖			0	0
759-73-9	N-Nitroso-N-ethylurea	✔							✖			0	0
684-93-5	N-Nitroso-N-methylurea	✔							✖			0	0
16543-55-8	N-Nitrosonornicotine	✔							✖			0	0
100-75-4	N-Nitrosopiperidine	✔							✖			0	0
2234-13-1	Octochloronaphthalene				✔						✖	0	0
20816-12-0	Osmium tetroxide			✔								0	0
56-38-2	Parathion	✔										482	783
87-86-5	Pentachlorophenol				✔				✖		✖	101,020	330,398
79-21-0	Peracetic acid	✔										7,840	63,069
108-95-2	Phenol	✔										15,654,693	176,366,012
106-50-3	p-Phenylenediamine	✔										9,426	233,277

Table I-1. TRI Chemicals by Classifications and Special Groups, with Quantity Released/ Disposed Of and Total Production-Related Waste, 1992 (cont'd.)

CAS Number	Chemical	Chemical Classsifications: Organics (Non-halogenated)	Acids/Bases/Salts	Metals	Halo-organics	Non-metallic Inorganics	Mixtures	Trade Secrets	Special Groups: Carcinogens	Ozone Depleters	Chloro-organics	Quantity Released/ Disposed of Pounds	Total Production-related Waste Pounds
90-43-7	2-Phenylphenol	✔										25,913	265,706
75-44-5	Phosgene				✔						✖	5,219	9,580,825
7664-38-2	Phosphoric acid		✔									196,807,410	682,122,515
7723-14-0	Phosphorus (yellow or white)					✔						359,033	1,277,536
85-44-9	Phthalic anhydride	✔										927,214	32,913,247
88-89-1	Picric acid	✔										1,068,681	1,649,918
	Polybrominated biphenyls				✔				✖			500	500
1336-36-3	Polychlorinated biphenyls (PCBs)				✔				✖		✖	48,499	843,892
1120-71-4	Propane sultone	✔							✖			120	120
57-57-8	beta-Propiolactone	✔							✖			0	0
123-38-6	Propionaldehyde	✔										752,998	4,256,832
114-26-1	Propoxur	✔										100	961
115-07-1	Propylene	✔										21,295,605	1,615,374,591
75-55-8	Propyleneimine	✔							✖			398	398
75-56-9	Propylene oxide	✔							✖			1,425,929	16,373,703
110-86-1	Pyridine	✔										665,418	8,332,731
91-22-5	Quinoline	✔										98,177	490,360
106-51-4	Quinone	✔										24,029	35,247
82-68-8	Quintozene	✔										1,742	175,433
81-07-2	Saccharin (manufacturing)	✔							✖			1,429	19,988
94-59-7	Safrole	✔							✖			0	0
7782-49-2	Selenium					✔						4,477	43,964
	Selenium compounds					✔						166,384	758,934
7440-22-4	Silver			✔								16,745	1,669,418
	Silver compounds			✔								63,392	4,354,356
100-42-5	Styrene	✔							✖			33,687,236	256,580,387
96-09-3	Styrene oxide	✔							✖			329	91,020
7664-93-9	Sulfuric acid		✔									187,976,508	10,269,925,138
79-34-5	1,1,2,2-Tetra-chloroethane				✔						✖	56,561	25,213,478
127-18-4	Tetrachloroethylene				✔				✖		✖	12,552,614	132,195,977
961-11-5	Tetrachlorvinphos				✔						✖	105,320	313,105
7440-28-0	Thallium			✔								0	0
	Thallium compounds			✔								1,170	83,575
62-55-5	Thioacetamide	✔							✖			0	0
139-65-1	4,4'-Thiodianiline	✔							✖			0	0
62-56-6	Thiourea	✔							✖			23,491	41,316
1314-20-1	Thorium dioxide			✔								64,000	64,010
7550-45-0	Titanium tetrachloride			✔								153,747	39,816,191
108-88-3	Toluene	✔										186,681,857	1,323,162,737
584-84-9	Toluene-2,4-diiso-cyanate	✔							✖			13,189	116,675
91-08-7	Toluene-2,6-diiso-cyanate	✔							✖			2,874	28,133
26471-62-5	Toluenediisocyanate (mixed isomers)	✔							✖			51,305	6,453,015

Table I-1. TRI Chemicals by Classifications and Special Groups, with Quantity Released/ Disposed Of and Total Production-Related Waste, 1992 (cont'd.)

		Chemical Classsifications							Special Groups				
CAS Number	Chemical	Organics (Non-halogenated)	Acids/Bases/Salts	Metals	Halo-organics	Non-metallic Inorganics	Mixtures	Trade Secrets	Carcinogens	Ozone Depleters	Chloro-organics	Quantity Released/ Disposed of Pounds	Total Production-related Waste Pounds
95-53-4	o-Toluidine	✔							✖			45,829	2,154,329
636-21-5	o-Toluidine hydrochloride				✔				✖		✖	0	0
8001-35-2	Toxaphene				✔				✖		✖	0	0
68-76-8	Triaziquone	✔										0	0
52-68-6	Trichlorfon				✔						✖	116	3,661
120-82-1	1,2,4-Trichlorobenzene				✔						✖	513,864	2,829,122
71-55-6	1,1,1-Trichloroethane				✔					✖	✖	112,587,880	323,014,728
79-00-5	1,1,2-Trichloroethane				✔						✖	567,677	72,736,223
79-01-6	Trichloroethylene				✔						✖	28,162,324	271,892,548
75-69-4	Trichlorofluoromethane (CFC-11)				✔					✖	✖	9,647,521	66,695,343
95-95-4	2,4,5-Trichlorophenol				✔						✖	0	0
88-06-2	2,4,6-Trichlorophenol				✔				✖		✖	86	800,189
1582-09-8	Trifluralin	✔										36,718	95,841
95-63-6	1,2,4-Trimethylbenzene	✔										6,042,898	45,193,640
126-72-7	Tris(2,3-dibromopropyl) phosphate				✔				✖			0	0
51-79-6	Urethane	✔							✖			6,486	17,586
7440-62-2	Vanadium (fume or dust)			✔								45,379	740,537
108-05-4	Vinyl acetate	✔										7,155,692	39,544,444
593-60-2	Vinyl bromide				✔				✖			33,300	129,300
75-01-4	Vinyl chloride				✔				✖		✖	1,086,384	222,432,306
75-35-4	Vinylidene chloride				✔						✖	242,823	6,872,928
1330-20-7	Xylene (mixed isomers)	✔										108,789,871	549,893,102
108-38-3	m-Xylene	✔										1,348,989	3,897,942
95-47-6	o-Xylene	✔										2,068,548	55,564,796
106-42-3	p-Xylene	✔										3,985,990	5,807,344
87-62-7	2,6-Xylidine	✔										50	1,508
7440-66-6	Zinc (fume or dust)			✔								15,854,563	103,631,113
	Zinc compounds			✔								120,490,959	470,171,187
12122-67-7	Zineb			✔								0	0
	Mixtures and other trade name products						✔					1,694,943	8,982,491
	Trade secrets							✔				4,110	692,321
	Total											3,401,386,170	37,333,775,624

Appendix J

Chemicals in Waste: Additional Toxics Release Inventory (TRI) Data

Table J-1. The 25 TRI Chemicals with the Largest Increases in Waste Released/Disposed of, 1991-1992

		Released/Disposed Of			
CAS Number	Chemical	1991 Pounds	1992 Pounds	1991-1992 Net Difference Pounds	1991-1992 Percent Change Percent
7664-38-2	Phosphoric acid	165,636,708	196,807,410	31,170,702	18.82
7664-93-9	Sulfuric acid	175,031,446	187,976,508	12,945,062	7.40
7647-01-0	Hydrochloric acid	286,910,132	298,900,276	11,990,144	4.18
75-15-0	Carbon disulfide	88,651,226	93,554,822	4,903,596	5.53
7783-20-2	Ammonium sulfate (solution)	24,853,450	29,261,313	4,407,863	17.74
100-42-5	Styrene	29,439,694	33,687,236	4,247,542	14.43
	Glycol ethers	46,939,998	49,847,660	2,907,662	6.19
108-95-2	Phenol	14,034,817	15,654,693	1,619,876	11.54
	Mixtures and other trade names	416,801	1,694,943	1,278,142	306.66
100-41-4	Ethylbenzene	9,657,843	10,857,715	1,199,872	12.42
7697-37-2	Nitric acid	28,449,136	29,559,498	1,110,362	3.90
7664-39-3	Hydrogen fluoride	9,937,143	10,860,641	923,498	9.29
74-90-8	Hydrogen cyanide	2,218,562	3,123,903	905,341	40.81
75-05-8	Acetonitrile	20,597,262	21,429,372	832,110	4.04
95-63-6	1,2,4-Trimethylbenzene	5,515,959	6,042,898	526,939	9.55
1163-19-5	Decabromodiphenyl oxide	694,834	1,157,192	462,358	66.54
95-48-7	o-Cresol	96,437	541,166	444,729	461.16
75-65-0	tert-Butyl alcohol	2,199,073	2,606,556	407,483	18.53
120-12-7	Anthracene	162,927	569,044	406,117	249.26
	Chromium compounds	35,341,562	35,745,584	404,022	1.14
98-95-3	Nitrobenzene	517,441	916,765	399,324	77.17
107-21-1	Ethylene glycol	19,718,138	20,109,179	391,041	1.98
95-47-6	o-Xylene	1,678,783	2,068,548	389,765	23.22
	Antimony compounds	3,673,377	4,054,705	381,328	10.38
1634-04-4	Methyl tert-butyl ether	2,564,838	2,903,712	338,874	13.21

Total Production-related Waste			
1991 Pounds	**1992** Pounds	**1991-1992 Net Difference** Pounds	**1991-1992 Percent Change** Percent
603,067,696	682,122,515	79,054,819	13.11
10,289,832,954	10,269,925,138	-19,907,816	-0.19
2,252,607,074	2,475,552,419	222,945,345	9.90
122,010,312	127,135,361	5,125,049	4.20
69,278,447	77,217,088	7,938,641	11.46
258,689,499	256,580,387	-2,109,112	-0.82
127,247,161	131,379,713	4,132,552	3.25
187,951,700	176,366,012	-11,585,688	-6.16
7,233,363	8,982,491	1,749,128	24.18
109,707,080	96,538,764	-13,168,316	-12.00
300,703,408	310,850,709	10,147,301	3.37
236,839,170	243,107,876	6,268,706	2.65
34,822,062	37,573,237	2,751,175	7.90
2,482,839,851	2,581,322,698	98,482,847	3.97
30,677,914	45,193,640	14,515,726	47.32
2,229,722	2,849,268	619,546	27.79
752,746	1,129,641	376,895	50.07
73,537,790	76,907,238	3,369,448	4.58
10,956,484	12,272,595	1,316,111	12.01
146,729,962	171,072,379	24,342,417	16.59
4,680,197	5,262,783	582,586	12.45
589,066,620	561,144,278	-27,922,342	-4.74
49,121,344	55,564,796	6,443,452	13.12
37,692,503	22,690,828	-15,001,675	-39.80
4,210,372	7,106,790	2,896,418	68.79

Table J-2. The 25 TRI Chemicals with the Largest Decreases in Waste Released/Disposed of, 1991-1992

		Released/Disposed Of			
CAS Number	Chemical	1991 Pounds	1992 Pounds	1991-1992 Net Difference Pounds	1991-1992 Percent Change Percent
67-56-1	Methanol	277,209,655	259,001,005	-18,208,650	-6.57
67-64-1	Acetone	157,048,181	139,039,676	-18,008,505	-11.47
	Zinc compounds	137,583,588	120,490,959	-17,092,629	-12.42
79-10-7	Acrylic acid	19,381,455	5,074,341	-14,307,114	-73.82
7664-41-7	Ammonia	469,340,497	455,599,635	-13,740,862	-2.93
71-55-6	1,1,1-Trichloroethane	125,928,847	112,587,880	-13,340,967	-10.59
78-93-3	Methyl ethyl ketone	100,294,177	88,491,478	-11,802,699	-11.77
108-88-3	Toluene	193,808,129	186,681,857	-7,126,272	-3.68
76-13-1	Freon 113	30,913,989	23,906,231	-7,007,758	-22.67
	Manganese compounds	81,886,362	75,565,406	-6,320,956	-7.72
7782-50-5	Chlorine	77,141,781	71,168,030	-5,973,751	-7.74
	Copper compounds	51,502,778	46,462,501	-5,040,277	-9.79
71-43-2	Benzene	17,951,313	13,390,673	-4,560,640	-25.41
75-09-2	Dichloromethane	79,759,180	75,729,079	-4,030,101	-5.05
79-01-6	Trichloroethylene	31,623,552	28,162,324	-3,461,228	-10.95
75-71-8	Dichlorodifluoro-methane (CFC-12)	14,481,048	11,359,695	-3,121,353	-21.55
110-82-7	Cyclohexane	16,871,884	14,061,768	-2,810,116	-16.66
127-18-4	Tetrachloroethylene	15,321,406	12,552,614	-2,768,792	-18.07
1330-20-7	Xylene (mixed isomers)	111,545,206	108,789,871	-2,755,335	-2.47
67-66-3	Chloroform	20,484,275	17,802,805	-2,681,470	-13.09
7440-50-8	Copper	32,088,559	29,512,497	-2,576,062	-8.03
74-85-1	Ethylene	38,296,484	35,854,137	-2,442,347	-6.38
	Barium compounds	20,615,982	18,462,353	-2,153,629	-10.45
7439-96-5	Manganese	22,340,248	20,320,149	-2,020,099	-9.04
71-36-3	n-Butyl alcohol	34,165,017	32,300,656	-1,864,361	-5.46

Total Production-related Waste			
1991 Pounds	**1992** Pounds	**1991-1992 Net Difference** Pounds	**1991-1992 Percent Change** Percent
2,238,281,753	2,238,505,652	223,899	0.01
700,607,607	672,068,269	-28,539,338	-4.07
427,226,586	470,171,187	42,944,601	10.05
72,265,961	61,790,567	-10,475,394	-14.50
1,119,514,284	1,383,853,783	264,339,499	23.61
356,623,272	323,014,728	-33,608,544	-9.42
450,131,409	465,413,844	15,282,435	3.40
1,279,580,712	1,323,162,737	43,582,025	3.41
270,240,491	289,662,188	19,421,697	7.19
140,917,370	237,882,578	96,965,208	68.81
464,999,928	430,848,879	-34,151,049	-7.34
333,371,700	502,456,962	169,085,262	50.72
262,822,660	145,101,986	-117,720,674	-44.79
286,651,384	286,593,104	-58,280	-0.02
266,856,336	271,892,548	5,036,212	1.89
16,288,900	13,168,673	-3,120,227	-19.16
206,535,537	94,716,569	-111,818,968	-54.14
145,625,193	132,195,977	-13,429,216	-9.22
545,003,803	549,893,102	4,889,299	0.90
60,034,145	56,079,423	-3,954,722	-6.59
720,952,763	675,138,852	-45,813,911	-6.35
1,160,221,358	1,180,225,916	20,004,558	1.72
48,899,762	46,622,415	-2,277,347	-4.66
101,360,514	92,712,389	-8,648,125	-8.53
156,302,561	152,896,118	-3,406,443	-2.18

Table J-3. The 25 TRI Chemicals with the Largest Projected Increases in Waste Released/Disposed of, 1992-1994

		Released/Disposed Of			
CAS Number	**Chemical**	**1992** Pounds	**Projected 1994** Pounds	**1992-1994 Net Difference** Pounds	**1992-1994 Percent Change** Percent
7439-96-5	Manganese	20,320,149	44,552,489	24,232,340	119.25
8001-58-9	Creosote	2,153,138	22,319,174	20,166,036	936.59
	Copper compounds	46,462,501	54,239,783	7,777,282	16.74
75-56-9	Propylene oxide	1,425,929	3,709,231	2,283,302	160.13
75-15-0	Carbon disulfide	93,554,822	95,789,803	2,234,981	2.39
	Chromium compounds	35,745,584	37,633,952	1,888,368	5.28
7440-50-8	Copper	29,512,497	30,888,823	1,376,326	4.66
1344-28-1	Aluminum oxide (fibrous forms)	1,308,827	2,235,173	926,346	70.78
7440-02-0	Nickel	6,051,436	6,800,250	748,814	12.37
	Cadmium compounds	468,220	1,003,373	535,153	114.30
7429-90-5	Aluminum (fume or dust)	5,967,550	6,453,556	486,006	8.14
101-68-8	Methylenebis(phenyl-isocyanate)	2,040,760	2,299,239	258,479	12.67
	Nickel compounds	4,293,605	4,493,703	200,098	4.66
75-65-0	tert-Butyl alcohol	2,606,556	2,737,977	131,421	5.04
7440-62-2	Vanadium (fume or dust)	45,379	169,295	123,916	273.07
74-90-8	Hydrogen cyanide	3,123,903	3,233,449	109,546	3.51
25321-14-6	Dinitrotoluene (mixed isomers)	66,431	116,722	50,291	75.70
141-32-2	Butyl acrylate	351,856	401,409	49,553	14.08
1319-77-3	Cresol (mixed isomers)	960,567	997,810	37,243	3.88
103-23-1	Bis(2-ethylhexyl) adipate	611,877	647,847	35,970	5.88
121-69-7	N,N-Dimethylaniline	86,805	112,067	25,262	29.10
123-38-6	Propionaldehyde	752,998	773,300	20,302	2.70
25376-45-8	Diaminotoluene (mixed isomers)	29,760	49,314	19,554	65.71
107-05-1	Allyl chloride	122,224	140,936	18,712	15.31
140-88-5	Ethyl acrylate	221,369	235,803	14,434	6.52

Total Production-related Waste

1992 Pounds	Projected 1994 Pounds	1992-1994 Net Difference Pounds	1992-1994 Percent Change Percent
92,712,389	120,121,294	27,408,905	29.56
17,554,499	36,321,427	18,766,928	106.91
502,456,962	571,914,778	69,457,816	13.82
16,373,703	19,626,118	3,252,415	19.86
127,135,361	138,053,167	10,917,806	8.59
171,072,379	176,722,744	5,650,365	3.30
675,138,852	699,355,443	24,216,591	3.59
3,661,010	5,494,389	1,833,379	50.08
87,495,571	94,681,819	7,186,248	8.21
13,924,917	7,163,462	-6,761,455	-48.56
131,824,600	146,523,078	14,698,478	11.15
3,633,780	3,697,321	63,541	1.75
63,460,089	59,308,203	-4,151,886	-6.54
76,907,238	83,195,617	6,288,379	8.18
740,537	507,524	-233,013	-31.47
37,573,237	37,094,078	-479,159	-1.28
946,545	993,575	47,030	4.97
4,726,036	5,124,672	398,636	8.43
13,382,788	12,765,870	-616,918	-4.61
3,004,862	2,992,055	-12,807	-0.43
1,380,283	844,630	-535,653	-38.81
4,256,832	3,930,276	-326,556	-7.67
5,696,903	5,489,714	-207,189	-3.64
5,196,542	5,306,996	110,454	2.13
8,423,314	8,491,742	68,428	0.81

Table J-4. The 25 TRI Chemicals with the Largest Projected Decreases in Waste Released/Disposed of, 1992-1994

		Released/Disposed Of			
CAS Number	**Chemical**	**1992** Pounds	**Projected 1994** Pounds	**1992-1994 Net Difference** Pounds	**1992-1994 Percent Change** Percent
7664-93-9	Sulfuric acid	187,976,508	77,025,966	-110,950,542	-59.02
7664-38-2	Phosphoric acid	196,807,410	90,560,171	-106,247,239	-53.99
7647-01-0	Hydrochloric acid	298,900,276	214,873,655	-84,026,621	-28.11
7664-41-7	Ammonia	455,599,635	382,191,371	-73,408,264	-16.11
71-55-6	1,1,1-Trichloroethane	112,587,880	40,271,208	-72,316,672	-64.23
67-56-1	Methanol	259,001,005	217,375,989	-41,625,016	-16.07
108-88-3	Toluene	186,681,857	147,254,594	-39,427,263	-21.12
	Manganese compounds	75,565,406	52,062,162	-23,503,244	-31.10
75-09-2	Dichloromethane	75,729,079	53,606,274	-22,122,805	-29.21
76-13-1	Freon 113	23,906,231	5,362,738	-18,543,493	-77.57
67-64-1	Acetone	139,039,676	122,254,178	-16,785,498	-12.07
78-93-3	Methyl ethyl ketone	88,491,478	71,944,001	-16,547,477	-18.70
6484-52-2	Ammonium nitrate (solution)	49,700,242	39,481,110	-10,219,132	-20.56
79-01-6	Trichloroethylene	28,162,324	18,955,105	-9,207,219	-32.69
1330-20-7	Xylene (mixed isomers)	108,789,871	100,073,685	-8,716,186	-8.01
75-69-4	Trichlorofluoromethane (CFC-11)	9,647,521	2,878,370	-6,769,151	-70.16
74-85-1	Ethylene	35,854,137	29,784,076	-6,070,061	-16.93
75-71-8	Dichlorodifluoromethane (CFC-12)	11,359,695	5,546,012	-5,813,683	-51.18
127-18-4	Tetrachloroethylene	12,552,614	7,375,482	-5,177,132	-41.24
108-95-2	Phenol	15,654,693	11,307,252	-4,347,441	-27.77
108-10-1	Methyl isobutyl ketone	25,840,592	21,673,572	-4,167,020	-16.13
67-66-3	Chloroform	17,802,805	13,663,473	-4,139,332	-23.25
115-07-1	Propylene	21,295,605	17,395,434	-3,900,171	-18.31
110-82-7	Cyclohexane	14,061,768	10,994,248	-3,067,520	-21.81
75-05-8	Acetonitrile	21,429,372	18,392,575	-3,036,797	-14.17

Total Production-related Waste			
1992 Pounds	**Projected 1994** Pounds	**1992-1994 Net Difference** Pounds	**1992-1994 Percent Change** Percent
10,269,925,138	10,105,682,279	-164,242,859	-1.60
682,122,515	671,015,987	-11,106,528	-1.63
2,475,552,419	2,500,236,268	24,683,849	1.00
1,383,853,783	1,117,353,318	-266,500,465	-19.26
323,014,728	181,774,090	-141,240,638	-43.73
2,238,505,652	2,208,777,616	-29,728,036	-1.33
1,323,162,737	1,352,847,744	29,685,007	2.24
237,882,578	219,001,881	-18,880,697	-7.94
286,593,104	243,432,591	-43,160,513	-15.06
289,662,188	357,062,513	67,400,325	23.27
672,068,269	712,213,956	40,145,687	5.97
465,413,844	474,948,294	9,534,450	2.05
150,857,399	145,121,720	-5,735,679	-3.80
271,892,548	248,825,195	-23,067,353	-8.48
549,893,102	602,185,559	52,292,457	9.51
66,695,343	3,296,804	-63,398,539	-95.06
1,180,225,916	1,101,144,575	-79,081,341	-6.70
13,168,673	6,610,680	-6,557,993	-49.80
132,195,977	115,628,649	-16,567,328	-12.53
176,366,012	176,827,504	461,492	0.26
350,963,788	352,439,138	1,475,350	0.42
56,079,423	51,580,787	-4,498,636	-8.02
1,615,374,591	1,528,395,048	-86,979,543	-5.38
94,716,569	220,680,731	125,964,162	132.99
2,581,322,698	3,079,499,079	498,176,381	19.30

Table J-5. The 25 TRI Chemicals with Largest Quantities of Total Recycled Waste, 1992

CAS Number	Chemical	Total Recycled Pounds	Total Energy Recovery Pounds	Total Treated Pounds	Quantity Released/ Disposed of Pounds	Total Production-related Waste Pounds	Non-Production-related Waste Pounds
7664-93-9	Sulfuric acid	7,068,452,870	103,428	3,013,392,332	187,976,508	10,269,925,138	3,522,137
75-05-8	Acetonitrile	2,511,466,278	34,186,005	14,241,043	21,429,372	2,581,322,698	12,758
	Lead compounds	1,042,138,350	41,842	38,181,148	26,999,354	1,107,360,694	1,287,095
108-88-3	Toluene	654,476,356	338,027,884	143,976,640	186,681,857	1,323,162,737	479,129
7440-50-8	Copper	639,505,240	20,819	6,100,296	29,512,497	675,138,852	491,213
67-56-1	Methanol	490,776,751	399,689,097	1,089,038,799	259,001,005	2,238,505,652	639,753
107-21-1	Ethylene glycol	448,479,915	13,602,675	78,952,509	20,109,179	561,144,278	198,170
115-07-1	Propylene	343,447,371	744,713,119	505,918,496	21,295,605	1,615,374,591	183,465
106-99-0	1,3-Butadiene	322,753,595	77,256,906	49,570,205	4,046,531	453,627,237	137,163
	Zinc compounds	313,101,884	272,899	36,305,445	120,490,959	470,171,187	1,374,675
	Copper compounds	311,575,763	52,758	144,365,940	46,462,501	502,456,962	930,700
98-82-8	Cumene	308,424,694	5,631,601	2,619,448	3,715,939	320,391,682	12,065
7439-92-1	Lead	248,617,895	3,013,173	3,266,818	5,880,827	260,778,713	61,729
108-10-1	Methyl isobutyl ketone	243,664,202	68,661,970	12,797,024	25,840,592	350,963,788	27,958
79-01-6	Trichloroethylene	233,867,939	2,306,044	7,556,241	28,162,324	271,892,548	71,831
67-64-1	Acetone	231,073,609	173,458,645	128,496,339	139,039,676	672,068,269	257,235
7664-41-7	Ammonia	229,573,826	53,556,096	645,124,226	455,599,635	1,383,853,783	1,366,277
74-85-1	Ethylene	197,286,622	497,793,629	449,291,528	35,854,137	1,180,225,916	687,169
78-93-3	Methyl ethyl ketone	196,269,075	123,915,256	56,738,035	88,491,478	465,413,844	121,088
71-55-6	1,1,1-Trichloroethane	194,945,111	9,517,631	5,964,106	112,587,880	323,014,728	103,973
7647-01-0	Hydrochloric acid	189,945,296	57,973	1,986,648,874	298,900,276	2,475,552,419	221,897
75-01-4	Vinyl chloride	176,167,910	17,766,157	27,411,855	1,086,384	222,432,306	54,340
100-42-5	Styrene	174,164,405	33,801,464	14,927,282	33,687,236	256,580,387	106,470
50-00-0	Formaldehyde	169,362,610	10,794,444	101,599,699	16,913,837	298,670,590	29,434
	Manganese compounds	156,574,649	28,180	5,714,343	75,565,406	237,882,578	11,393
	Subtotal	17,096,112,216	2,608,269,695	8,568,198,671	2,245,330,995	30,517,911,577	12,389,117
	Percent of Total	88.32	73.08	77.86	66.01	81.74	36.47
	All Others	2,261,977,181	960,907,018	2,436,924,673	1,156,055,175	6,815,864,047	21,580,706
	Total	19,358,089,397	3,569,176,713	11,005,123,344	3,401,386,170	37,333,775,624	33,969,823

Table J-6. The 25 TRI Chemicals with the Largest Quantities of Waste Used for Total Energy Recovery, 1992

CAS Number	Chemical	Total Recycled Pounds	Total Energy Recovery Pounds	Total Treated Pounds	Quantity Released/ Disposed of Pounds	Total Production-related Waste Pounds	Non-Production-related Waste Pounds
115-07-1	Propylene	343,447,371	744,713,119	505,918,496	21,295,605	1,615,374,591	183,465
74-85-1	Ethylene	197,286,622	497,793,629	449,291,528	35,854,137	1,180,225,916	687,169
67-56-1	Methanol	490,776,751	399,689,097	1,089,038,799	259,001,005	2,238,505,652	639,753
108-88-3	Toluene	654,476,356	338,027,884	143,976,640	186,681,857	1,323,162,737	479,129
1330-20-7	Xylene (mixed isomers)	149,455,573	238,887,500	52,760,158	108,789,871	549,893,102	661,016
67-64-1	Acetone	231,073,609	173,458,645	128,496,339	139,039,676	672,068,269	257,235
78-93-3	Methyl ethyl ketone	196,269,075	123,915,256	56,738,035	88,491,478	465,413,844	121,088
106-99-0	1,3-Butadiene	322,753,595	77,256,906	49,570,205	4,046,531	453,627,237	137,163
75-65-0	tert-Butyl alcohol	36,943	70,684,077	3,579,662	2,606,556	76,907,238	670
108-10-1	Methyl isobutyl ketone	243,664,202	68,661,970	12,797,024	25,840,592	350,963,788	27,958
7664-41-7	Ammonia	229,573,826	53,556,096	645,124,226	455,599,635	1,383,853,783	1,366,277
100-41-4	Ethylbenzene	24,322,506	50,020,968	11,337,575	10,857,715	96,538,764	204,372
95-47-6	o-Xylene	2,895,775	49,661,868	938,605	2,068,548	55,564,796	981
71-43-2	Benzene	59,500,031	41,051,269	31,160,013	13,390,673	145,101,986	122,584
120-80-9	Catechol	303,911	39,333,748	30,040,594	363,130	70,041,383	245
71-36-3	n-Butyl alcohol	58,123,363	34,526,819	27,945,280	32,300,656	152,896,118	116,654
75-05-8	Acetonitrile	2,511,466,278	34,186,005	14,241,043	21,429,372	2,581,322,698	12,758
100-42-5	Styrene	174,164,405	33,801,464	14,927,282	33,687,236	256,580,387	106,470
107-06-2	1,2-Dichloroethane	145,656,072	33,728,659	39,301,468	3,127,466	221,813,665	47,278
	Glycol ethers	18,814,965	29,968,634	32,748,454	49,847,660	131,379,713	204,006
74-90-8	Hydrogen cyanide	184,712	23,473,083	10,791,539	3,123,903	37,573,237	1,152
108-95-2	Phenol	31,347,870	20,841,707	108,521,742	15,654,693	176,366,012	39,447
108-05-4	Vinyl acetate	1,393,558	18,379,131	12,616,063	7,155,692	39,544,444	8,047
79-10-7	Acrylic acid	1,508,359	18,176,568	37,031,299	5,074,341	61,790,567	6,884
75-01-4	Vinyl chloride	176,167,910	17,766,157	27,411,855	1,086,384	222,432,306	54,340
	Subtotal	6,264,663,638	3,231,560,259	3,536,303,924	1,526,414,412	14,558,942,233	5,486,141
	Percent of Total	32.36	90.54	32.13	44.88	39.00	16.15
	All Others	13,093,425,759	337,616,454	7,468,819,420	1,874,971,758	22,774,833,391	28,483,682
	Total	19,358,089,397	3,569,176,713	11,005,123,344	3,401,386,170	37,333,775,624	33,969,823

Table J-7. The 25 TRI Chemicals with the Largest Quantities of Total Treated Waste, 1992

CAS Number	Chemical	Total Recycled Pounds	Total Energy Recovery Pounds	Total Treated Pounds	Quantity Released/ Disposed of Pounds	Total Production-related Waste Pounds	Non-Production-related Waste Pounds
7664-93-9	Sulfuric acid	7,068,452,870	103,428	3,013,392,332	187,976,508	10,269,925,138	3,522,137
7647-01-0	Hydrochloric acid	189,945,296	57,973	1,986,648,874	298,900,276	2,475,552,419	221,897
67-56-1	Methanol	490,776,751	399,689,097	1,089,038,799	259,001,005	2,238,505,652	639,753
7664-41-7	Ammonia	229,573,826	53,556,096	645,124,226	455,599,635	1,383,853,783	1,366,277
115-07-1	Propylene	343,447,371	744,713,119	505,918,496	21,295,605	1,615,374,591	183,465
74-85-1	Ethylene	197,286,622	497,793,629	449,291,528	35,854,137	1,180,225,916	687,169
7664-38-2	Phosphoric acid	90,922,816	8,898	394,383,391	196,807,410	682,122,515	12,122,137
7782-50-5	Chlorine	108,816,142	77,503	250,787,204	71,168,030	430,848,879	35,581
7697-37-2	Nitric acid	44,113,139	538	237,177,534	29,559,498	310,850,709	56,138
76-13-1	Freon 113	33,838,374	338,224	231,579,359	23,906,231	289,662,188	20,170
	Copper compounds	311,575,763	52,758	144,365,940	46,462,501	502,456,962	930,700
108-88-3	Toluene	654,476,356	338,027,884	143,976,640	186,681,857	1,323,162,737	479,129
67-64-1	Acetone	231,073,609	173,458,645	128,496,339	139,039,676	672,068,269	257,235
7664-39-3	Hydrogen fluoride	122,163,546	730,121	109,353,568	10,860,641	243,107,876	11,428
108-95-2	Phenol	31,347,870	20,841,707	108,521,742	15,654,693	176,366,012	39,447
50-00-0	Formaldehyde	169,362,610	10,794,444	101,599,699	16,913,837	298,670,590	29,434
107-21-1	Ethylene glycol	448,479,915	13,602,675	78,952,509	20,109,179	561,144,278	198,170
	Chromium compounds	77,577,722	111,291	57,637,782	35,745,584	171,072,379	1,272,980
78-93-3	Methyl ethyl ketone	196,269,075	123,915,256	56,738,035	88,491,478	465,413,844	121,088
1330-20-7	Xylene (mixed isomers)	149,455,573	238,887,500	52,760,158	108,789,871	549,893,102	661,016
106-99-0	1,3-Butadiene	322,753,595	77,256,906	49,570,205	4,046,531	453,627,237	137,163
75-09-2	Dichloromethane	147,972,768	15,080,526	47,810,731	75,729,079	286,593,104	56,850
7783-20-2	Ammonium sulfate (solution)	1,856,214	0	46,099,561	29,261,313	77,217,088	3,100
7550-45-0	Titanium tetrachloride	0	0	39,662,444	153,747	39,816,191	1,798
107-06-2	1,2-Dichloroethane	145,656,072	33,728,659	39,301,468	3,127,466	221,813,665	47,278
	Subtotal	11,807,193,895	2,742,826,877	10,008,188,564	2,361,135,788	26,919,345,124	23,101,540
	Percent of Total	60.99	76.85	90.94	69.42	72.10	68.01
	All Others	7,550,895,502	826,349,836	996,934,780	1,040,250,382	10,414,430,500	10,868,283
	Total	19,358,089,397	3,569,176,713	11,005,123,344	3,401,386,170	37,333,775,624	33,969,823

Table J-8. The 25 TRI Chemicals with the Largest Quantities of Waste Released/Disposed of, 1992

CAS Number	**Chemical**	**Total Recycled** Pounds	**Total Energy Recovery** Pounds	**Total Treated** Pounds	**Quantity Released/ Disposed of** Pounds	**Total Production-related Waste** Pounds	**Non-Production-related Waste** Pounds
7664-41-7	Ammonia	229,573,826	53,556,096	645,124,226	455,599,635	1,383,853,783	1,366,277
7647-01-0	Hydrochloric acid	189,945,296	57,973	1,986,648,874	298,900,276	2,475,552,419	221,897
67-56-1	Methanol	490,776,751	399,689,097	1,089,038,799	259,001,005	2,238,505,652	639,753
7664-38-2	Phosphoric acid	90,922,816	8,898	394,383,391	196,807,410	682,122,515	12,122,137
7664-93-9	Sulfuric acid	7,068,452,870	103,428	3,013,392,332	187,976,508	10,269,925,138	3,522,137
108-88-3	Toluene	654,476,356	338,027,884	143,976,640	186,681,857	1,323,162,737	479,129
67-64-1	Acetone	231,073,609	173,458,645	128,496,339	139,039,676	672,068,269	257,235
	Zinc compounds	313,101,884	272,899	36,305,445	120,490,959	470,171,187	1,374,675
71-55-6	1,1,1-Trichloroethane	194,945,111	9,517,631	5,964,106	112,587,880	323,014,728	103,973
1330-20-7	Xylene (mixed isomers)	149,455,573	238,887,500	52,760,158	108,789,871	549,893,102	661,016
75-15-0	Carbon disulfide	18,175,988	5,733,207	9,671,344	93,554,822	127,135,361	10,587
78-93-3	Methyl ethyl ketone	196,269,075	123,915,256	56,738,035	88,491,478	465,413,844	121,088
75-09-2	Dichloromethane	147,972,768	15,080,526	47,810,731	75,729,079	286,593,104	56,850
	Manganese compounds	156,574,649	28,180	5,714,343	75,565,406	237,882,578	11,393
7782-50-5	Chlorine	108,816,142	77,503	250,787,204	71,168,030	430,848,879	35,581
	Glycol ethers	18,814,965	29,968,634	32,748,454	49,847,660	131,379,713	204,006
6484-52-2	Ammonium nitrate (solution)	69,715,921	0	31,441,236	49,700,242	150,857,399	218,130
	Copper compounds	311,575,763	52,758	144,365,940	46,462,501	502,456,962	930,700
74-85-1	Ethylene	197,286,622	497,793,629	449,291,528	35,854,137	1,180,225,916	687,169
	Chromium compounds	77,577,722	111,291	57,637,782	35,745,584	171,072,379	1,272,980
100-42-5	Styrene	174,164,405	33,801,464	14,927,282	33,687,236	256,580,387	106,470
71-36-3	n-Butyl alcohol	58,123,363	34,526,819	27,945,280	32,300,656	152,896,118	116,654
7697-37-2	Nitric acid	44,113,139	538	237,177,534	29,559,498	310,850,709	56,138
7440-50-8	Copper	639,505,240	20,819	6,100,296	29,512,497	675,138,852	491,213
7783-20-2	Ammonium sulfate (solution)	1,856,214	0	46,099,561	29,261,313	77,217,088	3,100
	Subtotal	11,833,266,068	1,954,690,675	8,914,546,860	2,842,315,216	25,544,818,819	25,070,288
	Percent of Total	61.13	54.77	81.00	83.56	68.42	73.80
	All Others	7,524,823,329	1,614,486,038	2,090,576,484	559,070,954	11,788,956,805	8,899,535
	Total	19,358,089,397	3,569,176,713	11,005,123,344	3,401,386,170	37,333,775,624	33,969,823

Table J-9. The 25 TRI Chemicals with the Largest Quantities of Non-production-related Waste, 1992

CAS Number	Chemical	Total Recycled Pounds	Total Energy Recovery Pounds	Total Treated Pounds	Quantity Released/ Disposed of Pounds	Total Production-related Waste Pounds	Non-Production-related Waste Pounds
7664-38-2	Phosphoric acid	90,922,816	8,898	394,383,391	196,807,410	682,122,515	12,122,137
7664-93-9	Sulfuric acid	7,068,452,870	103,428	3,013,392,332	187,976,508	10,269,925,138	3,522,137
	Nickel compounds	56,602,655	5,883	2,557,946	4,293,605	63,460,089	2,173,457
	Zinc compounds	313,101,884	272,899	36,305,445	120,490,959	470,171,187	1,374,675
7664-41-7	Ammonia	229,573,826	53,556,096	645,124,226	455,599,635	1,383,853,783	1,366,277
	Lead compounds	1,042,138,350	41,842	38,181,148	26,999,354	1,107,360,694	1,287,095
	Chromium compounds	77,577,722	111,291	57,637,782	35,745,584	171,072,379	1,272,980
	Copper compounds	311,575,763	52,758	144,365,940	46,462,501	502,456,962	930,700
7440-66-6	Zinc (fume or dust)	83,872,166	77,054	3,827,330	15,854,563	103,631,113	777,619
74-85-1	Ethylene	197,286,622	497,793,629	449,291,528	35,854,137	1,180,225,916	687,169
1330-20-7	Xylene (mixed isomers)	149,455,573	238,887,500	52,760,158	108,789,871	549,893,102	661,016
67-56-1	Methanol	490,776,751	399,689,097	1,089,038,799	259,001,005	2,238,505,652	639,753
87-68-3	Hexachloro-1,3-butadiene	1,124,000	0	7,775,644	6,534	8,906,178	540,364
7440-50-8	Copper	639,505,240	20,819	6,100,296	29,512,497	675,138,852	491,213
108-88-3	Toluene	654,476,356	338,027,884	143,976,640	186,681,857	1,323,162,737	479,129
1332-21-4	Asbestos (friable)	717,992	0	2,728,494	4,949,097	8,395,583	374,618
67-64-1	Acetone	231,073,609	173,458,645	128,496,339	139,039,676	672,068,269	257,235
127-18-4	Tetrachloroethylene	92,042,225	10,216,146	17,384,992	12,552,614	132,195,977	237,639
7647-01-0	Hydrochloric acid	189,945,296	57,973	1,986,648,874	298,900,276	2,475,552,419	221,897
6484-52-2	Ammonium nitrate (solution)	69,715,921	0	31,441,236	49,700,242	150,857,399	218,130
75-71-8	Dichlorodifluoro-methane (CFC-12)	1,250,454	2,121	556,403	11,359,695	13,168,673	211,980
100-41-4	Ethylbenzene	24,322,506	50,020,968	11,337,575	10,857,715	96,538,764	204,372
	Glycol ethers	18,814,965	29,968,634	32,748,454	49,847,660	131,379,713	204,006
107-21-1	Ethylene glycol	448,479,915	13,602,675	78,952,509	20,109,179	561,144,278	198,170
7440-47-3	Chromium	96,492,170	335	2,945,190	5,395,166	104,832,861	188,015
	Subtotal	12,579,297,647	1,805,976,575	8,377,958,671	2,312,787,340	25,076,020,233	30,641,783
	Percent of Total	64.98	50.60	76.13	68.00	67.17	90.20
	All Others	6,778,791,750	1,763,200,138	2,627,164,673	1,088,598,830	12,257,755,391	3,328,040
	Total	19,358,089,397	3,569,176,713	11,005,123,344	3,401,386,170	37,333,775,624	33,969,823

Table J-10. The Five Chemicals in Each Chemical Class with the Largest Quantities of Total Production-related Waste, 1992

CAS Number	Class	Total Recycled Pounds	Total Energy Recovery Pounds	Total Treated Pounds	Quantity Released/ Disposed of Pounds	Total Production-Related Wastes Pounds	Non-Production-Related Wastes Pounds
Non-halogenated Organics							
75-05-8	Acetonitrile	2,511,466,278	34,186,005	14,241,043	21,429,372	2,581,322,698	12,758
67-56-1	Methanol	490,776,751	399,689,097	1,089,038,799	259,001,005	2,238,505,652	639,753
115-07-1	Propylene	343,447,371	744,713,119	505,918,496	21,295,605	1,615,374,591	183,465
108-88-3	Toluene	654,476,356	338,027,884	143,976,640	186,681,857	1,323,162,737	479,129
74-85-1	Ethylene	197,286,622	497,793,629	449,291,528	35,854,137	1,180,225,916	687,169
	Subtotal	4,197,453,378	2,014,409,734	2,202,466,506	524,261,976	8,938,591,594	2,002,274
	Total	6,815,399,071	3,291,670,114	3,285,596,495	1,301,048,144	14,693,713,824	5,287,754
Acids/Bases/Salts							
7664-93-9	Sulfuric acid	7,068,452,870	103,428	3,013,392,332	187,976,508	10,269,925,138	3,522,137
7647-01-0	Hydrochloric acid	189,945,296	57,973	1,986,648,874	298,900,276	2,475,552,419	221,897
7664-38-2	Phosphoric acid	90,922,816	8,898	394,383,391	196,807,410	682,122,515	12,122,137
7697-37-2	Nitric acid	44,113,139	538	237,177,534	29,559,498	310,850,709	56,138
7664-39-3	Hydrogen fluoride	122,163,546	730,121	109,353,568	10,860,641	243,107,876	11,428
	Subtotal	7,515,597,667	900,958	5,740,955,699	724,104,333	13,981,558,657	15,933,737
	Total	7,588,016,487	24,718,641	5,838,950,440	810,551,077	14,262,236,645	16,156,485
Metals							
	Lead compounds	1,042,138,350	41,842	38,181,148	26,999,354	1,107,360,694	1,287,095
7440-50-8	Copper	639,505,240	20,819	6,100,296	29,512,497	675,138,852	491,213
	Copper compounds	311,575,763	52,758	144,365,940	46,462,501	502,456,962	930,700
	Zinc compounds	313,101,884	272,899	36,305,445	120,490,959	470,171,187	1,374,675
7439-92-1	Lead	248,617,895	3,013,173	3,266,818	5,880,827	260,778,713	61,729
	Subtotal	2,554,939,132	3,401,491	228,219,647	229,346,138	3,015,906,408	4,145,412
	Total	3,363,585,794	4,350,318	380,742,365	426,203,405	4,174,881,882	8,689,602
Halo-organics							
71-55-6	1,1,1-Trichloro-ethane	194,945,111	9,517,631	5,964,106	112,587,880	323,014,728	103,973
76-13-1	Freon 113	33,838,374	338,224	231,579,359	23,906,231	289,662,188	20,170
75-09-2	Dichloromethane	147,972,768	15,080,526	47,810,731	75,729,079	286,593,104	56,850
79-01-6	Trichloroethylene	233,867,939	2,306,044	7,556,241	28,162,324	271,892,548	71,831
75-01-4	Vinyl chloride	176,167,910	17,766,157	27,411,855	1,086,384	222,432,306	54,340
	Subtotal	786,792,102	45,008,582	320,322,292	241,471,898	1,393,594,874	307,164
	Total	1,241,493,116	189,317,231	565,856,670	320,535,332	2,317,202,349	1,865,579
Non-metallic Inorganics							
7664-41-7	Ammonia	229,573,826	53,556,096	645,124,226	455,599,635	1,383,853,783	1,366,277
7782-50-5	Chlorine	108,816,142	77,503	250,787,204	71,168,030	430,848,879	35,581
10049-04-4	Chlorine dioxide	2,013,000	0	31,908,788	3,112,849	37,034,637	966
	Arsenic compounds	6,235,500	2	993,706	4,106,260	11,335,468	40,407
1332-21-4	Asbestos (friable)	717,992	0	2,728,494	4,949,097	8,395,583	374,618
	Subtotal	347,356,460	53,633,601	931,542,418	538,935,871	1,871,468,350	1,817,849
	Total	349,085,115	53,635,155	931,996,683	541,349,159	1,876,066,112	1,862,524
	Mixtures	440,667	5,011,254	1,835,627	1,694,943	8,982,491	87,879
	Trade secrets	69,147	474,000	145,064	4,110	692,321	20,000
	Grand Total	19,358,089,397	3,569,176,713	11,005,123,344	3,401,386,170	37,333,775,624	33,969,823

Table J-11. The 25 Carcinogens with the Largest Quantities of Total Production-related Waste, 1992

CAS Number	Chemical	Total Recycled Pounds	Total Energy Recovery Pounds	Total Treated Pounds	Quantity Released/ Disposed of Pounds	Total Production-Related Waste Pounds	Non-Production-Related Waste Pounds
106-99-0	1,3-Butadiene	322,753,595	77,256,906	49,570,205	4,046,531	453,627,237	137,163
50-00-0	Formaldehyde	169,362,610	10,794,444	101,599,699	16,913,837	298,670,590	29,434
75-09-2	Dichloromethane	147,972,768	15,080,526	47,810,731	75,729,079	286,593,104	56,850
7439-92-1	Lead	248,617,895	3,013,173	3,266,818	5,880,827	260,778,713	61,729
100-42-5	Styrene	174,164,405	33,801,464	14,927,282	33,687,236	256,580,387	106,470
75-01-4	Vinyl chloride	176,167,910	17,766,157	27,411,855	1,086,384	222,432,306	54,340
107-06-2	1,2-Dichloroethane	145,656,072	33,728,659	39,301,468	3,127,466	221,813,665	47,278
71-43-2	Benzene	59,500,031	41,051,269	31,160,013	13,390,673	145,101,986	122,584
127-18-4	Tetrachloroethylene	92,042,225	10,216,146	17,384,992	12,552,614	132,195,977	237,639
7440-47-3	Chromium	96,492,170	335	2,945,190	5,395,166	104,832,861	188,015
7440-02-0	Nickel	78,402,208	14,343	3,027,584	6,051,436	87,495,571	6,611
78-87-5	1,2-Dichloro-propane	46,537,442	16,800,000	4,384,652	620,279	68,342,373	0
	Nickel compounds	56,602,655	5,883	2,557,946	4,293,605	63,460,089	2,173,457
67-66-3	Chloroform	7,771,704	7,037,330	23,467,584	17,802,805	56,079,423	46,723
107-13-1	Acrylonitrile	21,232,672	3,648,141	16,214,649	5,442,217	46,537,679	4,477
56-23-5	Carbon tetra-chloride	16,973,929	4,895,825	15,840,125	1,426,570	39,136,449	83,930
75-07-0	Acetaldehyde	120,252	10,421,593	12,860,789	8,431,379	31,834,013	153
62-53-3	Aniline	8,959,535	5,876,717	5,008,896	1,783,054	21,628,202	40,844
106-89-8	Epichlorohydrin	4,383,879	3,592,794	10,079,039	525,985	18,581,697	1,866
542-75-6	1,3-Dichloro-propylene	3,871,000	13,340,000	443,077	41,720	17,695,797	0
8001-58-9	Creosote	14,446,500	116,746	838,115	2,153,138	17,554,499	77,840
75-56-9	Propylene oxide	14,734	5,877,096	9,055,944	1,425,929	16,373,703	989
117-81-7	Di-(2-ethylhexyl) phthalate	7,112,689	709,972	711,084	2,131,979	10,665,724	5,776
140-88-5	Ethyl acrylate	43,540	7,117,436	1,040,969	221,369	8,423,314	3,726
1332-21-4	Asbestos (friable)	717,992	0	2,728,494	4,949,097	8,395,583	374,618
	Subtotal	1,899,920,412	322,162,955	443,637,200	229,110,375	2,894,830,942	3,862,512
	Total for All Carcinogens	1,913,253,682	337,823,560	464,227,493	239,763,102	2,955,067,837	4,015,146
	Percent of Grand Total	9.88	9.47	4.22	7.05	7.92	11.82
	Grand Total	19,358,089,397	3,569,176,713	11,005,123,344	3,401,386,170	37,333,775,624	33,969,823

Table J-12. TRI Waste of Ozone Depleters, 1992*

CAS Number	Chemical	Total Recycled Pounds	Total Energy Recovery Pounds	Total Treated Pounds	Quantity Released/ Disposed of Pounds	Total Production-Related Waste Pounds	Non-Production-Related Waste Pounds
71-55-6	1,1,1-Trichloroethane	194,945,111	9,517,631	5,964,106	112,587,880	323,014,728	103,973
76-13-1	Freon 113	33,838,374	338,224	231,579,359	23,906,231	289,662,188	20,170
75-69-4	Trichlorofluoromethane (CFC-11)	55,781,209	573,340	693,273	9,647,521	66,695,343	18,832
56-23-5	Carbon tetrachloride	16,973,929	4,895,825	15,840,125	1,426,570	39,136,449	83,930
75-71-8	Dichlorodifluoromethane (CFC-12)	1,250,454	2,121	556,403	11,359,695	13,168,673	211,980
74-83-9	Bromomethane	458,200	29,900	89,045	3,005,194	3,582,339	0
76-14-2	Dichlorotetrafluoroethane (CFC-114)	824,121	0	248,277	1,080,021	2,152,419	6,633
76-15-3	Monochloropentafluoroethane (CFC-115)	53,300	0	19,130	419,169	491,599	900
75-63-8	Bromotrifluoromethane (Halon 1301)	58,000	0	100	110,445	168,545	0
353-59-3	Bromochlorodifluoromethane (Halon 1211)	45,000	0	0	16,749	61,749	0
124-73-2	Dibromotetrafluoroethane (Halon 2402)	0	0	0	0	0	0
	Total for Ozone Depleters	304,227,698	15,357,041	254,989,818	163,559,475	738,134,032	446,418
	Percent of Grand Total	1.57	0.43	2.32	4.81	1.98	1.31
	Grand Total	19,358,089,397	3,569,176,713	11,005,123,344	3,401,386,170	37,333,775,624	33,969,823

* In descending order by amount of total production-related waste.

Table J-13. The 25 TRI Chloro-organics with the Largest Quantities of Production-related Waste, 1992

CAS Number	Chemical	Total Recycled Pounds	Total Energy Recovery Pounds	Total Treated Pounds	Quantity Released/ Disposed of Pounds	Total Production-Related Waste Pounds	Non-Production-Related Waste Pounds
71-55-6	1,1,1-Trichloroethane	194,945,111	9,517,631	5,964,106	112,587,880	323,014,728	103,973
76-13-1	Freon 113	33,838,374	338,224	231,579,359	23,906,231	289,662,188	20,170
75-09-2	Dichloromethane	147,972,768	15,080,526	47,810,731	75,729,079	286,593,104	56,850
79-01-6	Trichloroethylene	233,867,939	2,306,044	7,556,241	28,162,324	271,892,548	71,831
75-01-4	Vinyl chloride	176,167,910	17,766,157	27,411,855	1,086,384	222,432,306	54,340
107-06-2	1,2-Dichloroethane	145,656,072	33,728,659	39,301,468	3,127,466	221,813,665	47,278
127-18-4	Tetrachloroethylene	92,042,225	10,216,146	17,384,992	12,552,614	132,195,977	237,639
79-00-5	1,1,2-Trichloroethane	31,387,219	16,481,220	24,300,107	567,677	72,736,223	40
78-87-5	1,2-Dichloropropane	46,537,442	16,800,000	4,384,652	620,279	68,342,373	0
75-69-4	Trichlorofluoro-methane (CFC-11)	55,781,209	573,340	693,273	9,647,521	66,695,343	18,832
67-66-3	Chloroform	7,771,704	7,037,330	23,467,584	17,802,805	56,079,423	46,723
75-00-3	Chloroethane	2,765,746	16,355,223	22,923,168	2,758,993	44,803,130	126
56-23-5	Carbon tetrachloride	16,973,929	4,895,825	15,840,125	1,426,570	39,136,449	83,930
79-34-5	1,1,2,2-Tetrachloro-ethane	14,528,192	53,600	10,575,125	56,561	25,213,478	0
106-89-8	Epichlorohydrin	4,383,879	3,592,794	10,079,039	525,985	18,581,697	1,866
542-75-6	1,3-Dichloropropylene	3,871,000	13,340,000	443,077	41,720	17,695,797	0
108-90-7	Chlorobenzene	6,016,570	1,891,168	6,595,808	2,475,509	16,979,055	22,720
74-87-3	Chloromethane	452,437	4,553,164	3,721,049	5,779,134	14,505,784	21,547
75-71-8	Dichlorodifluoro-methane (CFC-12)	1,250,454	2,121	556,403	11,359,695	13,168,673	211,980
108-60-1	Bis(2-chloro-1-methyl-ethyl)ether	2,400,000	5,590,000	4,858,000	11,300	12,859,300	0
126-99-8	Chloroprene	1,469,500	73,026	9,310,040	1,559,346	12,411,912	10,177
95-50-1	1,2-Dichlorobenzene	4,111,558	824,332	6,060,346	482,566	11,478,802	130,708
75-44-5	Phosgene	0	615,410	8,960,196	5,219	9,580,825	46
87-68-3	Hexachloro-1,3-butadiene	1,124,000	0	7,775,644	6,534	8,906,178	540,364
540-59-0	1,2-Dichloroethylene	2,570,330	1,378,993	4,697,453	23,222	8,669,998	33
	Subtotal	1,227,885,568	183,010,933	542,249,841	312,302,614	2,265,448,956	1,681,173
	Total for All Chloro-organics	1,236,959,099	189,273,878	565,154,298	316,105,885	2,307,493,160	1,864,995
	Percent of Grand Total	6.39	5.30	5.14	9.29	6.18	5.49
	Grand Total	19,358,089,397	3,569,176,713	11,005,123,344	3,401,386,170	37,333,775,624	33,969,823

Appendix K

Chemicals in Waste: Additional Biennial Reporting System (BRS) Data

Facilities report amounts of waste generated and managed on site to BRS. Waste management methods fall into two categories: RCRA units and exempt units, depending on whether or not the waste management method requires a RCRA permit. Facilities also report on waste minimization (identified as WM), in the form of quantities of waste recycled and quantities of waste reduced by source reduction.

Individual waste streams reported to BRS are identified by means of waste codes which designate the waste by chemical, production process, or chemical properties (see Chapter 4). A waste stream may be designated by more than one waste code, due to mixing of waste from various sources prior to waste management. This appendix lists the amounts of all toxic waste reported to BRS in 1991 by waste code except for those data that are confidential. Single and multiple waste code waste streams are listed separately.

Appendix E contains a key identifying all individual waste codes *except* for those based exclusively on chemical properties. These are ignitable waste (waste code D001), corrosive waste (D002), and reactive waste (D003). The amounts identified by these codes included here are only the waste streams for which a TRI chemical was identified as a constituent in the waste.

Table K-1. Quantities of Waste Reported to BRS by Waste Code, 1991

RCRA Hazardous Waste Code	Reports Number	1991 Toxic Waste Generated Pounds	1991 Toxic Waste Managed Pounds
No code	551	6,877,547,100	6,931,230,000
Multiple Waste Code Waste Streams*			
D	44,943	161,166,964,300	168,768,377,660
DF	53,857	47,005,620,200	47,906,604,960
DFK	141	61,586,697,880	61,539,335,380
DFL**	48	60,440	21,500
DFP	240	4,681,714,520	4,678,475,320
DFPK	6	75,812,340	75,721,840
DFPU	343	7,209,260	3,546,700
DFPUK	21	117,508,740	77,877,880
DFU	2,052	1,266,198,040	1,049,140,240
DFUK	77	10,261,751,860	10,235,416,420
DFUL**	17	2,678,680	0
DK	497	23,437,307,800	25,028,600,820
DL**	63	26,000	60
DP	1,691	188,891,160	174,275,000
DPL**	6	400	120
DPU	1,272	59,102,740	51,997,320
DPUK	13	4,730,759,280	4,716,510,480
DPUL**	2	220	0
DU	5,732	739,627,000	680,086,680
DUK	19	48,241,340	11,162,000
DUL**	11	21,400	0
F	9,277	112,772,218,560	113,855,428,800
FK	56	1,010,434,820	1,006,030,980
FL**	5	840	0
FP	60	15,516,580	14,836,240
FPK	1	7,720	0
FPL**	1	60	0
FPU	29	10,155,140	1,815,600
FPUK	11	1,767,373,520	1,412,488,160
FU	533	797,025,900	745,005,240
FUK	19	175,030,300	64,358,220
K	153	3,714,990,680	3,482,026,540
P	384	102,350,800	100,577,220
PK	1	2,376,224,400	3,391,225,400
PL**	27	10,700	0
PU	319	110,318,280	250,544,620
PUK	3	1,420,961,860	1,426,840,240
PUL**	3	100	0
U	867	3,455,021,760	3,256,428,960
UK	18	1,060,370,340	1,052,545,600
UL**	10	4,900	0
Subtotal	122,828	444,164,210,860	455,057,302,200

Quantity Managed			Quantity Recycled due to WM****	WM Source Reduction Quantity****
in RCRA Units Pounds	**in Exempt Units** Pounds	**by Storage** Pounds	Pounds	Pounds
449,197,300	6,482,031,980	0	2,380,980	138,622,360
106,061,877,080	62,482,835,120	223,665,460	61,955,100	1,681,875,280
16,658,264,120	30,959,399,640	288,941,200	34,269,440	156,569,380
61,128,228,900	410,776,960	329,520	0	331,120
21,500	0	0	0	0
4,659,482,440	18,992,880	0	21,040	5,620
75,706,840	0	15,000	0	0
3,526,840	0	19,860	5,600	17,580
77,200,280	0	677,600	0	0
728,645,980	299,833,040	20,661,220	1,228,660	2,828,760
9,991,308,580	241,286,600	2,821,240	0	500,000
0	0	0	0	0
8,257,966,540	16,763,284,760	7,349,520	26,228,260	983,342,260
60	0	0	0	0
86,140,360	87,947,580	187,060	417,120	53,554,600
120	0	0	0	0
44,554,160	6,255,780	1,187,380	600	135,140
43,396,900	4,587,203,240	85,910,340	0	0
0	0	0	0	0
428,485,500	249,863,160	1,738,020	171,340	30,531,800
11,108,000	0	54,000	0	3,620
0	0	0	0	0
7,494,018,960	106,361,137,360	272,480	4,110,600	3,581,568,680
960,098,400	30,972,580	14,960,000	1,104,600	1,948,500
0	0	0	0	0
14,796,320	16,000	23,920	0	86,340
0	0	0	0	0
0	0	0	0	0
1,815,600	0	0	140	480
1,287,072,160	125,416,000	0	0	0
28,620,920	716,343,300	41,020	5,740	610,640
62,756,960	11,300	1,589,960	0	0
2,211,149,820	1,267,869,300	3,007,420	10,163,800	13,138,800
14,848,080	85,718,540	10,600	0	1,471,060
2,376,189,400	0	1,015,036,000	0	0
0	0	0	0	40
306,660	250,197,060	40,900	80	67,260
1,426,821,380	0	18,860	0	0
0	0	0	0	0
105,355,540	3,150,333,200	740,220	40	49,554,800
1,705,600	1,050,840,000	0	0	0
0	0	0	0	0
224,241,470,000	229,146,533,400	1,669,298,800	139,682,160	6,558,141,760

Table K-1. Quantities of Waste Reported to BRS by Waste Code, 1991 (cont'd.)

RCRA Hazardous Waste Code	Reports Number	1991 Toxic Waste Generated Pounds	1991 Toxic Waste Managed Pounds
Single Waste Code Waste Streams			
D001	1,848	325,749,320	124,047,700
D002	2,048	57,440,625,620	56,845,444,960
D003	86	113,957,340	113,564,480
D004	1,337	229,039,720	59,287,300
D005	931	167,003,520	52,657,440
D006	1,514	4,406,580,360	2,286,506,960
D007	6,229	44,881,635,640	45,490,125,940
D008	7,462	11,282,068,080	17,873,294,940
D009	3,485	1,593,406,940	2,765,907,340
D010	228	27,833,340	4,178,600
D011	1,826	598,191,420	584,598,760
D012	13	1,375,660	0
D013	56	315,520	246,140
D014	25	33,380	2,140
D015	21	108,060	0
D016	109	3,464,780	2,801,780
D017	10	3,380	920
D018***	3,079	321,775,894,200	318,881,333,120
D019***	81	333,195,900	330,839,780
D020***	33	1,152,080	0
D021***	30	667,700,740	664,396,340
D022***	225	12,654,940	902,700
D023***	10	736,500	0
D024***	14	679,780	0
D025***	13	3,410,820	933,200
D026***	116	17,742,320	10,627,080
D027***	33	290,180	1,200
D028***	81	2,227,242,840	2,218,712,840
D029***	36	15,687,800	901,560
D030***	26	4,508,875,820	4,506,523,260
D031***	9	147,840	1,107,500
D032***	23	12,265,140	148,140
D033***	6	500	0
D034***	5	5,120	0
D035***	793	360,514,560	21,036,660
D036***	37	136,468,460	125,716,480
D037***	42	963,980	0
D038***	34	349,905,180	344,246,060
D039***	270	30,132,480	13,046,880
D040***	171	83,963,220	200,682,620
D041***	7	18,240	0
D042***	8	1,220,840	1,188,460
D043***	56	1,342,479,560	1,337,400,920
F001	10,915	380,666,820	3,419,137,320
F002	9,188	549,783,860	1,677,771,620
F003	6,516	563,619,020	410,546,040

Quantity Managed			Quantity Recycled due to WM****	WM Source Reduction Quantity****
in RCRA Units Pounds	**in Exempt Units** Pounds	**by Storage** Pounds	Pounds	Pounds
88,579,340	35,468,360	0	1,898,140	17,444,440
8,544,995,560	48,300,449,400	0	9,143,540	3,084,028,320
61,361,100	52,203,380	0	122,840	9,414,840
24,912,400	34,371,340	3,560	191,800	2,277,660
40,547,080	12,028,360	82,000	326,780	1,076,160
1,126,126,020	1,160,318,680	62,260	1,428,260	75,126,500
15,564,574,940	29,924,600,720	950,280	16,444,560	662,670,400
9,981,589,020	5,742,145,760	2,149,560,160	27,436,240	78,970,020
1,337,800,380	1,428,092,780	14,180	87,880	65,171,440
3,200	4,175,400	0	921,000	103,560
3,519,020	581,049,440	30,300	240,600	295,220
0	0	0	0	0
246,140	0	0	0	80
300	0	1,840	0	920
0	0	0	0	0
2,612,620	189,160	0	0	10,640
0	0	920	0	200
189,941,116,740	128,744,456,880	195,759,500	23,233,880	226,396,000
2,005,400	328,781,360	53,020	10,400	71,320
0	0	0	0	20
539,616,340	124,780,000	0	0	0
18,660	884,040	0	400	20
0	0	0	0	0
0	0	0	0	0
3,200	930,000	0	0	3,239,800
10,001,200	625,880	0	21,200	482,820
1,200	0	0	0	0
955,884,440	1,262,828,000	400	0	0
901,560	0	0	0	0
526,309,060	3,980,214,200	0	0	1,600
0	1,107,500	0	1,080,900	0
600	0	147,540	0	280
0	0	0	0	0
0	0	0	0	0
4,495,160	16,175,640	365,860	0	315,860
125,707,340	9,140	0	0	124,711,360
0	0	0	160	277,200
0	344,246,060	0	0	0
95,520	12,891,420	59,940	85,220	74,960
2,080	200,680,540	0	23,120	457,160
0	0	0	0	0
1,188,460	0	0	0	0
1,337,400,920	0	0	507,580	635,520
9,332,660	3,409,757,340	47,320	2,277,180	12,561,660
1,482,349,180	195,224,200	198,240	1,486,520	7,848,540
127,086,980	282,073,400	1,385,660	5,664,980	122,457,800

Table K-1. Quantities of Waste Reported to BRS by Waste Code, 1991 (cont'd.)

RCRA Hazardous Waste Code	Reports Number	1991 Toxic Waste Generated Pounds	1991 Toxic Waste Managed Pounds
F004	88	401,300	96,000
F005	3,527	323,763,060	246,277,000
F006	3,363	8,539,220,060	6,112,822,380
F007	598	1,859,115,020	1,839,268,200
F008	249	49,046,280	25,469,000
F009	222	358,474,880	355,895,460
F010	15	18,460	0
F011	27	236,720	0
F012	4	5,660	0
F019	255	179,769,500	164,331,960
F020	25	613,860	78,320
F021	1	0	0
F024	11	3,697,340	195,600
F025***	4	937,020	843,400
F027	89	302,260	426,738,520
F032***	41	92,584,760	540,973,040
F034***	9	8,871,760	6,759,820
F035***	8	490,120	365,900
F037***	78	416,411,220	390,144,840
F038***	16	15,117,220	72,000
F039***	311	19,099,237,960	21,204,547,900
K001	79	9,975,140	43,243,180
K002	4	18,341,460	16,050,120
K004	1	100,800,000	100,800,000
K009	1	500,656,200	500,656,200
K010	1	16,808,600	4,585,600
K011	4	1,593,268,000	1,593,062,000
K013	4	1,425,209,320	1,419,594,000
K014	1	13,002,000	13,002,000
K015	1	4,168,060	0
K016	2	1,834,080	1,719,000
K017	3	17,393,340	21,700
K018	2	153,800	0
K019	5	9,813,000	8,356,800
K022	8	102,731,440	100,348,460
K027	6	37,641,980	31,160,560
K030	1	711,860	0
K035	6	868,640	154,400
K037	1	3,200	0
K046	9	1,615,660	597,260
K048	39	580,413,880	600,944,300
K049	29	79,836,680	92,106,440
K050	72	5,681,920	939,780
K051	96	115,875,140	194,574,160
K052	34	1,586,900	372,320
K060	1	25,476,700	25,476,700
K061	179	1,040,558,960	225,303,700
K062	193	2,798,683,760	2,309,515,440

Quantity Managed			Quantity Recycled due to WM****	WM Source Reduction Quantity****
in RCRA Units Pounds	in Exempt Units Pounds	by Storage Pounds	Pounds	Pounds
95,840	0	160	920	151,560
127,464,160	118,698,720	114,120	1,350,100	3,274,280
1,211,134,520	4,900,461,700	1,226,160	3,921,060	183,600,960
169,976,180	1,669,276,200	15,820	10,440	107,755,040
5,600	25,435,420	27,980	0	133,100
309,720	355,582,380	3,360	11,140	11,460,500
0	0	0	0	0
0	0	0	0	0
0	0	0	0	0
78,537,120	85,758,760	36,080	20,000	678,600
0	78,320	0	0	0
0	0	0	0	0
195,600	0	0	0	0
695,800	0	147,600	0	0
0	426,738,520	0	0	169,440
21,344,780	519,628,260	0	7,060	32,380
4,200	6,755,620	0	0	0
365,900	0	0	0	340
38,179,000	200,614,640	151,351,200	1,809,240	28,108,120
72,000	0	0	0	0
16,027,404,540	5,169,143,360	8,000,000	0	11,250,940
0	43,243,180	0	0	506,940
13,109,000	2,941,120	0	0	8,987,000
0	100,800,000	0	0	0
500,656,200	0	0	0	0
4,371,600	0	214,000	0	0
925,292,000	667,770,000	0	0	95,835,400
602,958,000	816,636,000	0	0	0
0	13,002,000	0	0	0
0	0	0	0	0
1,719,000	0	0	0	0
0	0	21,700	0	0
0	0	0	0	0
0	0	8,356,800	0	0
87,119,280	12,424,180	805,000	0	0
31,160,560	0	0	0	0
0	0	0	0	0
150,000	0	4,400	75,000	75,000
0	0	0	0	0
597,260	0	0	0	0
439,757,500	118,392,460	42,794,340	1,399,720	47,379,800
15,948,840	27,813,600	48,344,000	151,200	32,260
150,800	117,360	671,620	163,360	263,920
128,919,380	64,537,900	1,116,880	23,432,660	9,204,200
157,200	163,400	51,720	345,400	0
0	25,476,700	0	0	0
84,552,080	140,737,620	14,000	23,663,140	13,151,920
133,606,100	2,169,260,580	6,648,760	20,417,720	40,201,040

Table K-1. Quantities of Waste Reported to BRS by Waste Code, 1991 (cont'd.)

RCRA Hazardous Waste Code	**Reports** Number	**1991 Toxic Waste Generated** Pounds	**1991 Toxic Waste Managed** Pounds
K069	7	5,545,000	3,967,000
K071	19	58,204,400	54,535,500
K073	1	0	0
K083	8	8,538,300	3,668,840
K084	4	258,303,000	257,681,400
K085	8	2,424,340	1,472,240
K086	54	1,766,440	18,780
K087	16	119,493,860	78,546,360
K088	839	171,462,220	5,194,200
K091	1	260	0
K093	2	732,140	0
K094	4	2,183,000	0
K096	1	178,400	178,400
K099	1	0	0
K104	2	633,887,600	631,338,000
K106	11	3,357,340	0
K111	2	684,194,800	684,086,000
K112	3	692,355,280	692,355,280
K113	2	3,275,380	3,197,340
K114	2	3,545,140	3,545,140
K115	1	1,837,420	0
K118	3	18,860	0
K123	1	0	0
K132***	5	7,454,460	0
LABP**	70	1,093,560	0
P001	29	68,560	10,440
P002	4	5,260	0
P003	37	203,820	0
P004	17	1,420	60
P005	22	3,260	0
P006	8	20	0
P007	2	100	0
P008	11	136,600	0
P010	14	3,020	0
P011	18	13,080	0
P012	80	13,700	0
P013	1	20	0
P014	17	1,960	0
P015	34	9,540	80
P018	22	110,660	0
P020	86	4,568,220	1,183,480
P021	17	2,020	0
P022	57	824,180	124,500
P023	2	300	0
P024	27	6,954,940	0
P027	1	20	0
P028	19	44,680	1,000
P029	55	18,898,480	12,284,480

Quantity Managed in RCRA Units Pounds	Quantity Managed in Exempt Units Pounds	Quantity Managed by Storage Pounds	Quantity Recycled due to WM**** Pounds	WM Source Reduction Quantity**** Pounds
180,520	3,786,480	0	0	0
54,535,500	0	0	0	7,900,000
0	0	0	0	0
3,553,180	89,260	26,400	0	570,280
0	257,681,400	0	0	0
0	1,472,240	0	0	0
18,780	0	0	0	1,280
5,697,000	72,849,360	0	0	0
5,194,200	0	0	0	60,720
0	0	0	0	0
0	0	0	0	0
0	0	0	0	0
178,400	0	0	0	0
0	0	0	0	0
631,338,000	0	0	0	0
0	0	0	0	280,460
0	684,086,000	0	0	0
5,104,000	687,251,280	0	0	13,362,060
3,197,340	0	0	0	52,660
3,545,140	0	0	0	0
0	0	0	0	0
0	0	0	0	38,200
0	0	0	0	0
0	0	0	0	0
0	0	0	0	13,620
220	10,220	0	0	0
0	0	0	0	0
0	0	0	0	0
60	0	0	0	0
0	0	0	0	0
0	0	0	0	0
0	0	0	0	0
0	0	0	0	0
0	0	0	0	0
0	0	0	0	0
0	0	0	0	11,080
0	0	0	0	0
0	0	0	0	0
0	80	0	0	0
0	0	0	0	0
11,460	1,172,020	0	0	0
0	0	0	0	0
0	124,500	0	0	615,280
0	0	0	0	0
0	0	0	0	0
0	0	0	0	0
0	1,000	0	0	0
100	12,284,380	0	0	20

Table K-1. Quantities of Waste Reported to BRS by Waste Code, 1991 (cont'd.)

RCRA Hazardous Waste Code	Reports Number	1991 Toxic Waste Generated Pounds	1991 Toxic Waste Managed Pounds
P030	258	29,238,200	29,158,460
P031	1	20	0
P033	4	120	0
P034	1	0	0
P037	17	10,800	0
P038	1	280	0
P039	24	155,160	86,000
P040	3	4,000	0
P041	6	18,860	18,720
P042	72	3,720	0
P043	6	2,080	20
P044	24	22,920	0
P046	1	0	0
P047	9	88,480	0
P048	53	305,840	0
P050	19	28,980	0
P051	10	2,140	0
P054	2	80	0
P057	2	120	0
P058	3	80	0
P059	11	5,560	7,680
P060	1	0	0
P063	8	967,640	966,420
P064	9	1,300	0
P066	19	224,080	20
P068	9	32,660	0
P069	3	20	0
P070	22	299,740	20
P071	21	55,480	22,320
P073	1	0	0
P074	3	0	0
P075	48	64,320	0
P076	3	20	0
P077	38	16,000	0
P078	9	4,140	0
P081	9	296,000	0
P082	4	260	40
P087	77	3,640	0
P088	6	8,700	1,260
P089	44	23,120	0
P092	21	780	0
P093	7	40	0
P094	17	380,400	0
P095	3	200	0
P096	4	100	0
P097	4	820	0
P098	207	790,960	0
P099	4	40	0

Quantity Managed			Quantity Recycled due to WM****	WM Source Reduction Quantity****
in RCRA Units Pounds	in Exempt Units Pounds	by Storage Pounds	Pounds	Pounds
20,016,680	9,141,780	0	0	7,960
0	0	0	0	0
0	0	0	0	0
0	0	0	0	0
0	0	0	0	0
0	0	0	0	0
86,000	0	0	0	0
0	0	0	0	0
0	18,720	0	0	0
0	0	0	0	0
20	0	0	0	0
0	0	0	0	0
0	0	0	0	0
0	0	0	0	0
0	0	0	100,000	0
0	0	0	0	1,160
0	0	0	0	0
0	0	0	0	0
0	0	0	0	0
0	0	0	0	0
0	7,680	0	0	0
0	0	0	0	0
966,420	0	0	0	0
0	0	0	0	0
20	0	0	0	6,760
0	0	0	0	0
0	0	0	0	0
0	20	0	0	133,060
0	0	22,320	0	80
0	0	0	0	0
0	0	0	0	0
0	0	0	0	0
0	0	0	0	0
0	0	0	0	0
0	0	0	0	100
0	0	0	0	0
40	0	0	0	0
0	0	0	0	0
0	0	1,260	0	0
0	0	0	0	0
0	0	0	0	0
0	0	0	0	0
0	0	0	0	0
0	0	0	0	0
0	0	0	0	0
0	0	0	0	0
0	0	0	0	0
0	0	0	0	0

Table K-1. Quantities of Waste Reported to BRS by Waste Code, 1991 (cont'd.)

RCRA Hazardous Waste Code	**Reports** Number	**1991 Toxic Waste Generated** Pounds	**1991 Toxic Waste Managed** Pounds
P101	4	60	0
P102	8	22,700	22,480
P104	15	3,440	0
P105	210	124,500	13,840
P106	192	1,121,820	104,680
P108	24	3,060	0
P109	4	0	0
P110	7	3,600	45,000
P111	6	340	0
P112	5	20	0
P113	6	40	0
P114	1	0	0
P115	11	204,620	34,540
P116	7	80	0
P119	45	2,400	0
P120	50	170,040	0
P121	13	2,408,440	2,402,000
P122	7	20	0
P123	16	8,560	0
U001	30	190,851,880	188,075,860
U002	84	7,215,520	151,160
U003	35	1,126,620	591,400
U004	3	300	0
U006	9	120	0
U007	70	501,540	167,580
U008	21	225,720	54,560
U009	35	1,254,980	32,700
U010	13	97,960	0
U011	9	580	0
U012	65	385,860	8,460
U014	1	0	0
U016	1	2,200	0
U017	2	160	0
U018	3	20	0
U019	51	562,360	4,660
U020	3	160	0
U021	19	320	40
U022	4	71,560	0
U024	3	0	0
U025	1	60	0
U028	72	29,882,060	44,466,420
U029	10	500	0
U030	2	960	0
U031	21	9,480	40
U032	7	31,280	200
U034	5	320	0
U035	2	0	0
U036	113	7,200	1,400

Quantity Managed in RCRA Units Pounds	Quantity Managed in Exempt Units Pounds	Quantity Managed by Storage Pounds	Quantity Recycled due to WM**** Pounds	WM Source Reduction Quantity**** Pounds
0	0	0	0	0
0	0	22,480	0	0
0	0	0	0	0
240	13,600	0	0	0
300	10,700	93,680	0	15,380
0	0	0	0	0
0	0	0	0	0
0	0	45,000	0	0
0	0	0	0	0
0	0	0	0	0
0	0	0	0	0
0	0	0	0	0
4,500	30,040	0	0	3,480
0	0	0	0	0
0	0	0	0	60
0	0	0	0	0
0	2,402,000	0	0	0
0	0	0	0	0
0	0	0	0	40
188,075,860	0	0	0	0
45,380	105,780	0	0	1,400
591,400	0	0	0	0
0	0	0	0	0
0	0	0	0	0
167,580	0	0	0	0
54,560	0	0	0	0
32,700	0	0	0	1,060
0	0	0	0	0
0	0	0	0	0
8,460	0	0	20	0
0	0	0	0	0
0	0	0	0	0
0	0	0	0	0
0	0	0	0	0
4,300	360	0	0	20
0	0	0	0	0
40	0	0	0	0
0	0	0	0	0
0	0	0	0	0
0	0	0	0	0
2,690,120	41,776,300	0	0	6,020
0	0	0	0	0
0	0	0	0	0
40	0	0	0	920
200	0	0	0	0
0	0	0	0	0
0	0	0	0	0
940	460	0	0	200

Table K-1. Quantities of Waste Reported to BRS by Waste Code, 1991 (cont'd.)

RCRA Hazardous Waste Code	**Reports** Number	**1991 Toxic Waste Generated** Pounds	**1991 Toxic Waste Managed** Pounds
U037	19	80,700	38,620
U038	1	0	0
U039	5	20	0
U041	10	21,020	0
U044	120	990,820	56,660
U045	4	0	0
U046	2	0	0
U047	4	0	0
U048	8	7,140	0
U050	3	60	0
U051	79	9,572,060	0
U052	32	114,480	0
U053	4	20	0
U055	8	157,040	0
U056	19	19,460	0
U057	9	5,960	0
U058	14	13,340	0
U059	2	0	0
U060	6	78,000	0
U061	84	4,570,560	20
U062	1	74,400	0
U063	1	0	0
U066	7	4,740	0
U067	14	660	0
U068	1	0	0
U069	47	433,180	280
U070	33	26,420	20
U071	3	580	0
U072	25	2,240	0
U073	4	10,300	0
U075	85	17,460	0
U076	3	1,280	860
U077	34	2,214,780	15,180
U078	4	66,900	14,360
U079	2	180	0
U080	234	1,561,140	104,080
U081	14	2,026,800	2,096,680
U082	2	0	0
U083	5	31,200	29,880
U084	7	1,016,480	698,320
U085	2	20	0
U086	1	0	0
U087	5	1,140	0
U088	21	980	1,200
U091	4	0	0
U092	5	3,000	0
U093	3	40	0
U094	2	40	40

Quantity Managed in RCRA Units Pounds	Quantity Managed in Exempt Units Pounds	Quantity Managed by Storage Pounds	Quantity Recycled due to WM**** Pounds	WM Source Reduction Quantity**** Pounds
38,620	0	0	0	0
0	0	0	0	0
0	0	0	0	0
0	0	0	0	0
56,660	0	0	0	9,900
0	0	0	0	0
0	0	0	0	0
0	0	0	0	160
0	0	0	0	0
0	0	0	0	0
0	0	0	0	15,980
0	0	0	0	700
0	0	0	0	0
0	0	0	0	0
0	0	0	0	0
0	0	0	0	0
0	0	0	0	0
0	0	0	0	0
0	0	0	0	0
0	20	0	0	0
0	0	0	0	0
0	0	0	0	0
0	0	0	0	0
0	0	0	0	0
0	0	0	0	0
280	0	0	0	0
20	0	0	0	0
0	0	0	0	0
0	0	0	0	0
0	0	0	0	17,420
0	0	0	0	0
0	0	860	0	0
14,880	0	300	0	363,560
14,360	0	0	0	0
0	0	0	0	0
68,700	35,380	0	0	199,060
2,009,740	0	86,940	0	0
0	0	0	0	0
29,880	0	0	0	0
698,320	0	0	305,560	128,920
0	0	0	0	0
0	0	0	0	0
0	0	0	0	0
1,200	0	0	0	28,000
0	0	0	0	0
0	0	0	0	2,080
0	0	0	0	0
40	0	0	0	0

Table K-1. Quantities of Waste Reported to BRS by Waste Code, 1991 (cont'd.)

RCRA Hazardous Waste Code	**Reports** Number	**1991 Toxic Waste Generated** Pounds	**1991 Toxic Waste Managed** Pounds
U095	19	560	0
U096	6	8,340	0
U097	1	0	0
U098	3	28,920	0
U101	9	580	0
U102	23	35,640	0
U103	24	460	0
U105	5	38,160	38,140
U106	3	20	0
U107	44	128,120	820
U108	35	31,880	0
U109	2	20	0
U110	3	0	0
U112	32	100,820	280
U113	24	131,840	2,020
U114	15	23,120	20
U115	15	7,140	0
U116	11	12,600	0
U117	44	2,340	0
U118	7	780	0
U119	5	20	0
U121	61	117,360	0
U122	505	3,335,440	154,240
U123	32	5,840	0
U124	5	320	0
U125	12	4,700	0
U127	4	420	0
U128	7	540	0
U129	44	28,426,620	28,250,480
U130	3	440	0
U131	3	1,220	0
U132	11	580	0
U133	110	153,380	3,240
U134	58	215,169,260	215,141,180
U135	29	3,700	0
U136	18	5,060	0
U137	2	60	0
U138	12	360	0
U139	1	100	0
U140	6	22,660	0
U141	2	0	0
U142	5	360	0
U144	31	40,880	0
U145	3	860	0
U146	6	40	0
U147	66	118,660	180
U148	3	340	0
U149	3	0	0

Quantity Managed in RCRA Units Pounds	Quantity Managed in Exempt Units Pounds	Quantity Managed by Storage Pounds	Quantity Recycled due to WM**** Pounds	WM Source Reduction Quantity**** Pounds
0	0	0	0	0
0	0	0	0	0
0	0	0	0	0
0	0	0	0	0
0	0	0	0	0
0	0	0	0	0
0	0	0	0	0
38,140	0	0	0	0
0	0	0	0	0
820	0	0	0	0
0	0	0	0	0
0	0	0	0	0
0	0	0	0	0
280	0	0	0	460
2,020	0	0	0	0
20	0	0	0	0
0	0	0	0	20
0	0	0	0	0
0	0	0	0	40
0	0	0	0	0
0	0	0	0	0
0	0	0	0	100
18,080	45,100	91,060	0	10,020
0	0	0	0	60
0	0	0	0	0
0	0	0	0	0
0	0	0	0	0
0	0	0	0	0
0	28,250,480	0	0	0
0	0	0	0	0
0	0	0	0	0
0	0	0	0	0
340	660	2,240	0	5,040
3,080	215,138,100	0	0	100
0	0	0	0	0
0	0	0	0	0
0	0	0	0	0
0	0	0	0	0
0	0	0	0	0
0	0	0	0	0
0	0	0	0	0
0	0	0	0	0
0	0	0	0	0
0	0	0	0	0
0	0	0	0	0
180	0	0	0	15,420
0	0	0	0	0
0	0	0	0	0

Table K-1. Quantities of Waste Reported to BRS by Waste Code, 1991 (cont'd.)

RCRA Hazardous Waste Code	**Reports** Number	**1991 Toxic Waste Generated** Pounds	**1991 Toxic Waste Managed** Pounds
U150	1	0	0
U151	189	146,000	1,820
U153	4	155,020	0
U154	88	789,360	118,040
U155	2	80	0
U156	3	60	0
U157	3	80	0
U158	17	18,380	7,040
U159	59	1,653,020	5,840
U160	22	55,100	53,400
U161	12	17,680	0
U162	44	1,887,220	1,284,200
U163	9	20	0
U164	1	20	0
U165	81	2,967,040	1,800
U166	2	0	0
U167	14	1,040	0
U168	4	80	0
U169	31	12,100	11,300
U170	34	2,012,120	0
U171	7	111,440	0
U172	1	5,360	0
U176	1	0	0
U177	8	60	0
U180	2	340	0
U182	4	0	0
U183	1	2,520	0
U184	1	0	0
U185	19	4,940	0
U186	5	420	0
U187	5	3,400	0
U188	368	5,300,280	860,880
U189	8	8,400	0
U190	71	2,645,540	36,240
U191	7	440	80
U192	3	8,880	0
U193	3	0	0
U194	2	840	0
U196	30	3,100	660
U197	13	6,080	0
U200	3	2,580	0
U201	51	62,180	0
U202	17	42,560	0
U203	1	0	0
U204	17	80	0
U205	2	0	0
U206	1	0	0
U207	5	24,200	2,100

Quantity Managed in RCRA Units Pounds	Quantity Managed in Exempt Units Pounds	Quantity Managed by Storage Pounds	Quantity Recycled due to WM**** Pounds	WM Source Reduction Quantity**** Pounds
0	0	0	0	0
100	1,000	720	120	5,100
0	0	0	0	0
54,040	64,000	0	303,520	10,020
0	0	0	0	0
0	0	0	0	0
0	0	0	0	0
0	0	7,040	0	6,740
5,840	0	0	0	841,120
53,400	0	0	0	0
0	0	0	0	0
160	1,276,540	7,500	0	11,520
0	0	0	0	0
0	0	0	0	0
1,320	480	0	0	0
0	0	0	0	0
0	0	0	0	0
0	0	0	0	0
500	10,800	0	0	0
0	0	0	0	0
0	0	0	0	0
0	0	0	0	0
0	0	0	0	0
0	0	0	0	0
0	0	0	0	0
0	0	0	0	0
0	0	0	0	0
0	0	0	0	0
0	0	0	0	0
0	0	0	0	0
0	0	0	0	0
839,080	0	21,800	0	103,240
0	0	0	0	0
2,040	0	34,200	0	31,460
80	0	0	0	0
0	0	0	0	0
0	0	0	0	0
0	0	0	0	0
660	0	0	0	0
0	0	0	0	600
0	0	0	0	0
0	0	0	0	0
0	0	0	0	0
0	0	0	0	0
0	0	0	0	0
0	0	0	0	0
0	0	0	0	0
2,100	0	0	0	0

Table K-1. Quantities of Waste Reported to BRS by Waste Code, 1991 (cont'd.)

RCRA Hazardous Waste Code	**Reports** Number	**1991 Toxic Waste Generated** Pounds	**1991 Toxic Waste Managed** Pounds
U208	5	7,780	0
U209	4	20	0
U210	108	7,258,300	29,420
U211	71	221,160	4,100
U213	62	31,880	0
U214	10	60	0
U215	2	0	0
U216	3	0	0
U217	7	35,580	34,800
U218	7	60	0
U219	50	11,300	0
U220	153	15,626,980	1,819,540
U221	19	1,629,800	0
U222	6	140	0
U223	185	1,061,920	703,200
U225	12	1,680	0
U226	434	8,079,520	4,981,860
U227	17	35,060	300
U228	97	1,487,580	18,000
U234	6	480	0
U235	2	20	0
U236	5	3,500	3,500
U238	11	700	0
U239	142	4,383,260	1,535,360
U240	65	3,699,360	3,672,080
U243	1	0	0
U244	30	84,120	0
U246	24	680	0
U247	7	40	0
U248	18	280	0
U249	6	42,000	42,000
U328	22	7,842,060	0
U353	5	0	0
U359	33	102,260	5,320
Subtotal	78,187	497,201,992,260	501,929,034,820
Total	201,566	948,243,750,220	963,917,566,300

* "D" indicates that the waste stream contains at least two "D" waste codes. "DF" indicates that the waste stream contains at least one "D" and one "F" waste code, etc.
** "L" and "ABP" denote laboratory waste.
*** Waste code added for 1991 BRS reports and not required in 1989 reports.
**** WM refers to waste minimization.

Quantity Managed in RCRA Units Pounds	Quantity Managed in Exempt Units Pounds	Quantity Managed by Storage Pounds	Quantity Recycled due to WM**** Pounds	WM Source Reduction Quantity**** Pounds
0	0	0	0	0
0	0	0	0	0
29,220	0	200	0	1,140
4,100	0	0	0	155,400
0	0	0	0	0
0	0	0	0	0
0	0	0	0	0
0	0	0	0	0
0	34,800	0	0	0
0	0	0	0	0
0	0	0	0	0
140	1,819,400	0	500	14,280
0	0	0	0	13,500
0	0	0	0	0
703,200	0	0	0	45,360
0	0	0	0	0
680	4,977,100	4,080	3,320	6,380
0	300	0	0	0
18,000	0	0	0	2,520
0	0	0	0	0
0	0	0	0	0
3,500	0	0	0	0
0	0	0	0	0
100	1,535,260	0	0	0
3,672,080	0	0	0	0
0	0	0	0	0
0	0	0	0	237,540
0	0	0	0	0
0	0	0	0	0
0	0	0	0	0
0	42,000	0	0	0
0	0	0	0	0
0	0	0	0	0
0	5,320	0	0	0
253,420,079,280	245,889,798,780	2,619,156,760	170,124,380	5,083,741,380
478,110,746,580	481,518,364,160	4,288,455,560	312,187,520	11,780,505,500

Appendix L

Standard Industrial Classification (SIC) Codes

Manufacturing

Major Groups		*Abbreviated for This Report*
20	Food and kindred products	Food
21	Tobacco products	Tobacco
22	Textile mill products	Textiles
23	Apparel and other finished products made from fabrics and similar materials	Apparel
24	Lumber and wood products, except furniture	Lumber
25	Furniture and fixtures	Furniture
26	Paper and allied products	Paper
27	Printing, publishing, and allied industries	Printing
28	Chemicals and allied products	Chemicals
29	Petroleum refining and related industries	Petroleum
30	Rubber and miscellaneous plastics products	Plastics
31	Leather and leather products	Leather
32	Stone, clay, glass, and concrete products	Stone/Clay/Glass
33	Primary metal industries	Primary Metals
34	Fabricated metal products, except machinery and transportation equipment	Fabricated Metals
35	Industrial and commercial machinery and computer equipment	Machinery
36	Electronic and other electrical equipment and components, except computer equipment	Electrical
37	Transportation equipment	Transportation
38	Measuring, analyzing, and controlling instruments; photographic, medical and optical goods; watches and clocks	Measuring/ Photographic
39	Miscellaneous manufacturing industries	Miscellaneous Manufacturing
		Multiple Codes (20-39)
		No Codes (20-39)

Source: Executive Office of the President, Office of Management and Budget, *Standard Industrial Classification Manual*, 1987.

Appendix M

Industry Profiles

For both the Toxics Release Inventory (TRI) and the Biennial Reporting System, facilities report the Standard Industrial Classification (SIC) code or codes under which their operations fall. Under TRI facilities report all the applicable manufacturing SIC codes (codes ranging from 20 through 39), while under BRS the primary SIC code for the facility is reported.

The following Profiles collect both TRI and BRS information for SIC codes 20 through 39 and compare TRI and BRS data. In addition, for TRI data only, a Profile is included for facilities that have reported more than one SIC code in the range 20 to 39 (called multiple SIC codes in this report). While some facilities in both systems report no SIC code at all or no SIC code in the 20 through 39 range, this category is not detailed in this Appendix.

The Profiles emphasize production-related waste generated. They show, for facilities reporting under the specific SIC codes:

- Amounts of reported production-related toxic waste generation for 1991 for BRS, for 1991 and 1992 for TRI, and as projected for 1993 and 1994 for TRI. For BRS this is the amount of all materials in the waste stream, the total waste generated, under toxic waste codes as reported on Form GM, Section II.B. For TRI this is the amount of the toxic chemical in waste generated as reported in Sections 8.1 through 8.7 on TRI Form R.
- Amounts of TRI production-related waste for special groups of toxic chemicals for the year 1992. The special groups are carcinogens, ozone depleters, chloro-organics, metals, and halo-organics. The amounts are from facilities reporting under the SIC code.
- Amounts of TRI production-related waste for the five TRI chemicals with the largest amount of production-related waste reported to TRI in 1992. The amounts are from facilities reporting under the SIC code.
- The five facilities that reported the largest amount of TRI production-related waste from all TRI chemicals in 1992.
- The five facilities that reported the largest amount of waste generated under toxic waste codes to BRS for the year 1991.
- The one facility that reported the largest amount of increase in TRI production-related waste from 1991 to 1992.

- The one facility that reported the largest amount of decrease in TRI production-related waste from 1991 to 1992.
- The one facility that projected the largest amount of increase in TRI production-related waste from 1992 to 1994.
- The one facility that projected the largest amount of decrease in TRI production-related waste from 1992 to 1994.
- A bar chart showing total production-related waste for all TRI facilities under that SIC code. Total production-related waste is broken down into the types of waste management practiced, including recycled, used for energy recovery, treated, and released/disposed of, without a further breakdown to on- and off-site management.
- A pie chart showing the breakdown in releases of TRI chemicals of total air emissions, surface water discharges, underground injection, and on-site releases to land.

Industry Profile: SIC 20 Food

Reported Production-related Toxic Waste Generation

Reporting Year/Source	Pounds	Rank**
1991 BRS	88,710,920	18
1991 TRI	380,691,966	11
1992 TRI	389,637,145	11
1993 TRI*	408,264,525	11
1994 TRI*	382,807,750	11

Special Groups, 1992 TRI	Pounds	Rank**
Carcinogens	2,004,102	16
Ozone depleters	1,141,494	16
Chloro-organics	942,818	19
Metals	1,909,191	15
Halo-organics	1,439,795	19

Top 5 Chemicals, 1992 TRI

		Pounds
7647-01-0	Hydrochloric acid	143,319,526
7664-93-9	Sulfuric acid	87,459,044
7664-41-7	Ammonia	67,701,279
7664-38-2	Phosphoric acid	24,595,401
7783-20-2	Ammonium sulfate (solution)	19,534,220

Top 5 Facilities, 1992 TRI

Archer Daniels Midland, Decatur, IL	51,708,075
Archer Daniels Midland, Cedar Rapids, IA	50,390,534
Corn Products & Best Foods, Bedford Park, IL	22,275,200
Kraft Food Ingredients Corp., Memphis, TN	21,113,100
A. E. Staley Manufacturing Co., Decatur, IL	16,693,997

Top 5 Facilities, 1991 BRS

Anheuser-Busch Inc., Van Nuys, CA	65,106,740
Nestle, Fulton, NY	18,951,500
Owensboro Grain Company, Owensboro, KY	500,000
Fries and Fries Inc., Cincinnati, OH	413,760
Caschem Inc., Bayonne, NJ	348,260

TRI Production-related Waste, 1991-1994*

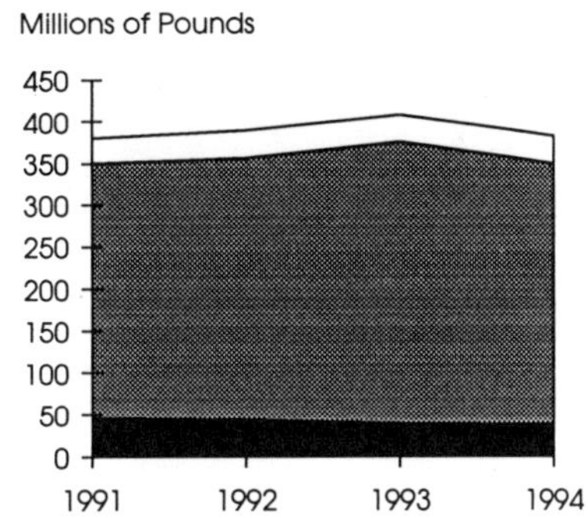

Total TRI Releases, 1992

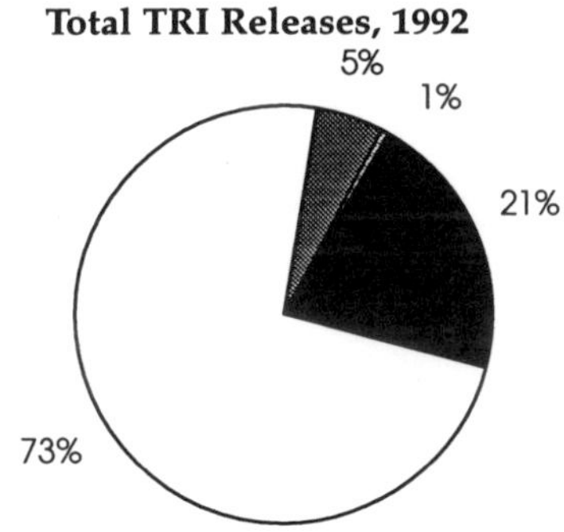

Total: 39.1 Million Pounds

Total Air Emissions	73%
Surface Water Discharges	5%
Underground Injection	1%
Releases to Land	21%

	Pounds	Pounds	Pounds
Facility with Largest Reported TRI Increase	**1991**	**1992**	**Increase**
Corn Products & Best Foods, Bedford Park, IL	16,143,400	22,275,200	6,131,800
Facility with Largest Reported TRI Decrease	**1991**	**1992**	**Decrease**
Archer Daniels Midland, Cedar Rapids, IA	55,297,231	50,390,534	-4,906,697
Facility with Largest Projected TRI Increase	**1992**	**1994***	**Increase**
Archer Daniels Midland, Cedar Rapids, IA	50,390,534	57,357,119	6,966,585
Facility with Largest Projected TRI Decrease	**1992**	**1994***	**Decrease**
Kraft Food Ingredients Corp., Memphis, TN	21,113,100	16,252,700	-4,860,400

*Projected ** Rank out of 20 industries (BRS) or 22 industries (TRI)

Industry Profile: SIC 21 Tobacco

Reported Production-related Toxic Waste Generation

Reporting Year/Source	Pounds	Rank**
1991 BRS	343,200	20
1991 TRI	55,046,792	19
1992 TRI	60,185,440	19
1993 TRI*	4,188,411	21
1994 TRI*	3,754,369	21

Special Groups, 1992 TRI	Pounds	Rank**
Carcinogens	0	21
Ozone depleters	56,544,743	4
Chloro-organics	56,544,743	8
Metals	6,826	21
Halo-organics	56,544,743	8

Top 5 Chemicals, 1992 TRI

		Pounds
75-69-4	Trichlorofluoromethane (CFC-11)	56,506,244
7664-41-7	Ammonia	2,086,931
7647-01-0	Hydrochloric acid	437,603
7664-93-9	Sulfuric acid	428,652
91-20-3	Naphthalene	386,601

Top 5 Facilities, 1992 TRI

R. J. Reynolds Tobacco Co., Winston-Salem, NC	55,480,275
Philip Morris USA, Richmond, VA	1,189,100
R. J. Reynolds Tobacco Co., Winston-Salem, NC	867,797
Liggett Group Inc., Durham, NC	671,867
American Tobacco Co., Reidsville, NC	461,250

Top 5 Facilities, 1991 BRS

Liggett Group Inc., Durham, NC	123,360
T. Hasegawa U.S.A. Inc., Cerritos, CA	71,220
Philip Morris USA, Richmond, VA	51,200
Brown & Williamson Tobacco, Macon, GA	39,420
Brown & Williamson Co., Louisville, KY	24,880

TRI Production-related Waste, 1991-1994*

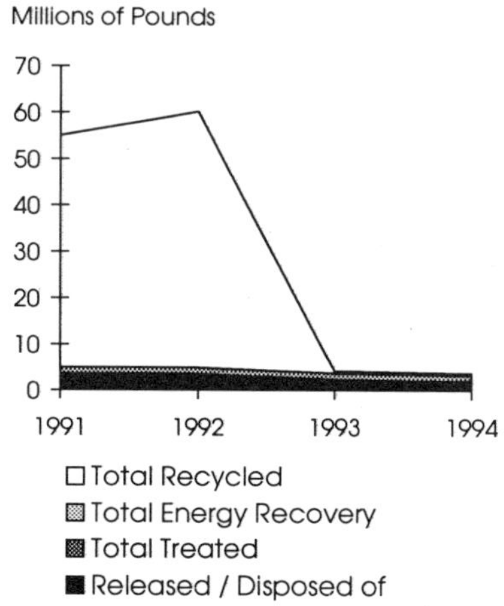

Total TRI Releases, 1992

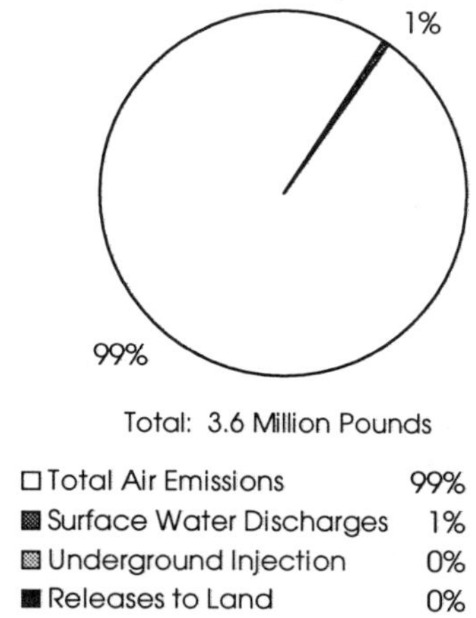

	Pounds 1991	Pounds 1992	Pounds Increase
Facility with Largest Reported TRI Increase			
R. J. Reynolds Tobacco Co., Winston-Salem, NC	50,231,281	55,480,275	5,248,994
Facility with Largest Reported TRI Decrease	**1991**	**1992**	**Decrease**
Philip Morris USA, Richmond, VA	1,358,900	1,189,100	-169,800
Facility with Largest Projected TRI Increase	**1992**	**1994***	**Increase**
R. J. Reynolds Tobacco Co., Winston-Salem, NC	867,797	955,020	87,223
Facility with Largest Projected TRI Decrease	**1992**	**1994***	**Decrease**
R. J. Reynolds Tobacco Co., Winston-Salem, NC	55,480,275	0	-55,480,275

*Projected ** Rank out of 20 industries (BRS) or 22 industries (TRI)

Industry Profile: SIC 22 Textiles

Reported Production-related Toxic Waste Generation

Reporting Year/Source	Pounds	Rank**
1991 BRS	1,079,880,480	11
1991 TRI	98,220,702	16
1992 TRI	100,223,930	16
1993 TRI*	93,406,235	16
1994 TRI*	84,499,332	16

Special Groups, 1992 TRI		
Carcinogens	2,387,176	15
Ozone depleters	1,727,390	15
Chloro-organics	7,580,873	13
Metals	1,339,066	16
Halo-organics	7,798,625	13

Top 5 Chemicals, 1992 TRI

		Pounds
7664-93-9	Sulfuric acid	41,396,987
78-93-3	Methyl ethyl ketone	11,151,163
108-88-3	Toluene	9,969,832
67-64-1	Acetone	4,147,727
7664-38-2	Phosphoric acid	4,089,159

Top 5 Facilities, 1992 TRI

Avondale Mills Inc., Sylacauga, AL	10,901,400
Galey & Lord Inc., Society Hill, SC	8,834,900
Gencorp Polymer Products, Columbus, MS	7,457,866
Wellman Inc., Johnsonville, SC	4,709,879
Magnolia Finishing Plant, Blacksburg, SC	3,767,859

Top 5 Facilities, 1991 BRS

Bekaert Corp., Rome, GA	1,003,205,100
Advanced Fiber Technologies, Hackensack, NJ	52,404,320
Malden Mills Industries Inc., Lawrence, MA	5,945,760
Gencorp Polymer Products, Columbus, MS	5,200,540
Columbus Coated Fabrics, Columbus, OH	1,425,340

TRI Production-related Waste, 1991-1994*

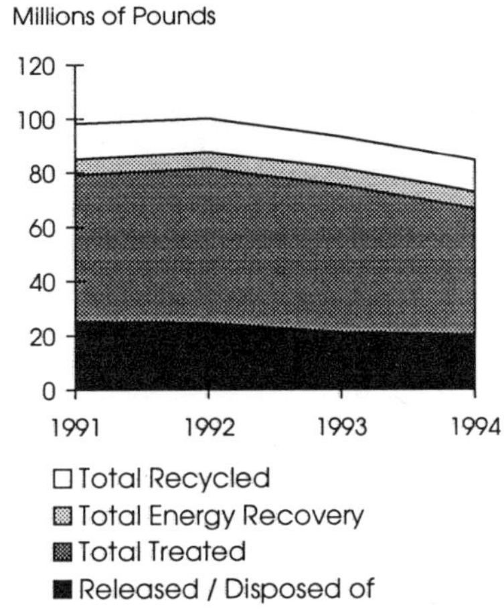

Total TRI Releases, 1992

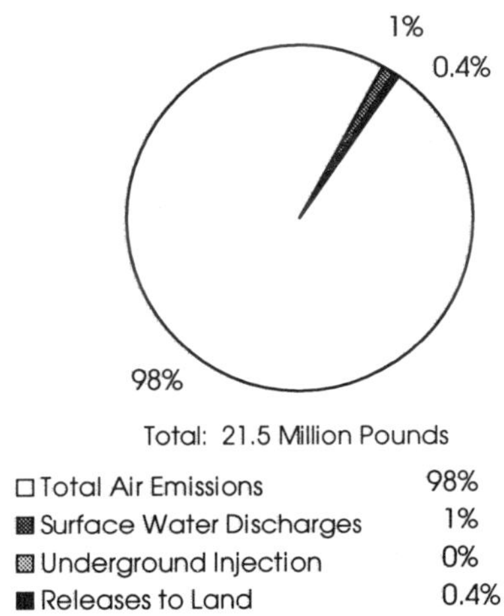

	Pounds	Pounds	Pounds
Facility with Largest Reported TRI Increase	**1991**	**1992**	**Increase**
U.S. Finishing, Greenville, SC	236	1,682,000	1,681,764
Facility with Largest Reported TRI Decrease	**1991**	**1992**	**Decrease**
Galey & Lord Inc., Society Hill, SC	11,189,200	8,834,900	-2,354,300
Facility with Largest Projected TRI Increase	**1992**	**1994***	**Increase**
Galey & Lord Inc., Society Hill, SC	8,834,900	10,160,400	1,325,500
Facility with Largest Projected TRI Decrease	**1992**	**1994***	**Decrease**
Avondale Mills Inc., Sylacauga, AL	10,901,400	3,201,400	-7,700,000

*Projected ** Rank out of 20 industries (BRS) or 22 industries (TRI)

Industry Profile: SIC 23 Apparel

Reported Production-related Toxic Waste Generation

Reporting Year/Source	Pounds	Rank**
1991 BRS	68,752,020	19
1991 TRI	2,883,172	22
1992 TRI	3,146,914	22
1993 TRI*	2,606,173	22
1994 TRI*	2,020,519	22

Special Groups, 1992 TRI	Pounds	Rank**
Carcinogens	341,782	20
Ozone depleters	354,974	20
Chloro-organics	548,267	20
Metals	116,897	20
Halo-organics	548,267	20

Top 5 Chemicals, 1992 TRI		Pounds
67-64-1	Acetone	694,509
78-93-3	Methyl ethyl ketone	611,786
108-10-1	Methyl isobutyl ketone	416,323
71-55-6	1,1,1-Trichloroethane	354,974
108-88-3	Toluene	192,912

Top 5 Facilities, 1992 TRI	Pounds
Forbo Industries Inc., Hazleton, PA	806,800
Chrysler Corp., Sandusky, OH	418,976
Glenmore Plastic Industries, Brooklyn, NY	303,986
Resistol Hats, Garland, TX	255,220
Burrell-Leder Beltech Inc., Skokie, IL	196,000

Top 5 Facilities, 1991 BRS	Pounds
Squibb Manufacturing Inc., Humacao, PR	64,697,800
YKK USA, Macon, GA	2,977,480
Handcraft Textile Print Co., Plainfield, CT	336,800
Economy Color Card Co. Inc., Elizabeth, NJ	156,860
Shieldalloy Metallurgical, Newfield, NJ	113,800

TRI Production-related Waste, 1991-1994*

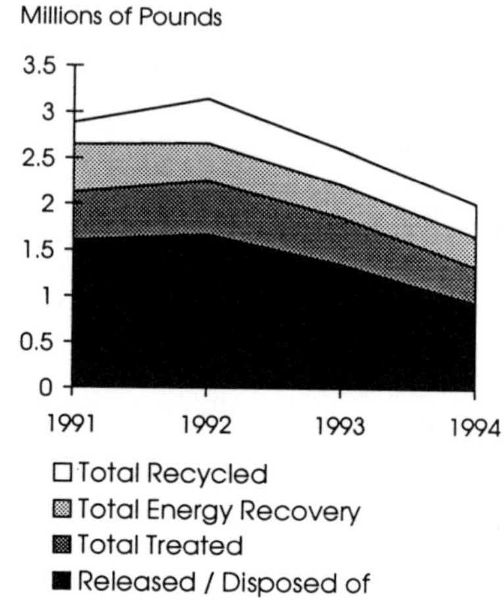

Total TRI Releases, 1992

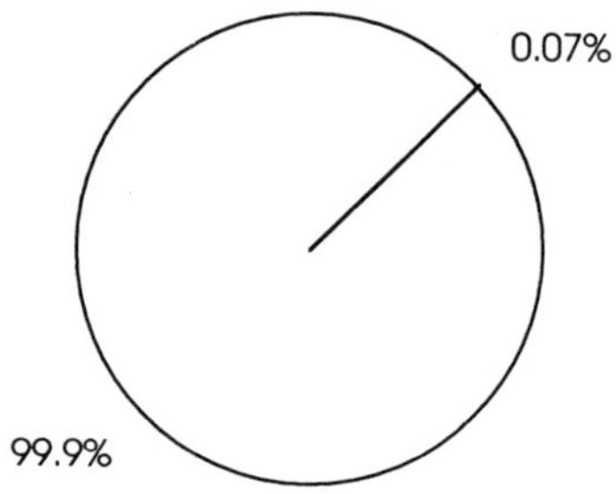

Total: 1.6 Million Pounds

Total Air Emissions	99.9%
Surface Water Discharges	0.07%
Underground Injection	0%
Releases to Land	0%

	Pounds	Pounds	Pounds
Facility with Largest Reported TRI Increase	**1991**	**1992**	**Increase**
Forbo Industries Inc., Hazleton, PA	713,800	806,800	93,000
Facility with Largest Reported TRI Decrease	**1991**	**1992**	**Decrease**
Champion Products Inc., Perry, NY	113,580	39,706	-73,874
Facility with Largest Projected TRI Increase	**1992**	**1994***	**Increase**
Franklin Shoe Co., Farmington, ME	136,825	158,000	21,175
Facility with Largest Projected TRI Decrease	**1992**	**1994***	**Decrease**
Resistol Hats, Garland, TX	255,220	6,420	-248,800

*Projected ** Rank out of 20 industries (BRS) or 22 industries (TRI)

Industry Profile: SIC 24 Lumber

Reported Production-related Toxic Waste Generation

Reporting Year/Source	Pounds	Rank**
1991 BRS	335,354,620	14
1991 TRI	67,834,787	17
1992 TRI	63,091,614	18
1993 TRI*	82,183,306	17
1994 TRI*	75,824,342	17

Special Groups, 1992 TRI	Pounds	Rank**
Carcinogens	24,277,415	13
Ozone depleters	792,589	19
Chloro-organics	1,608,686	17
Metals	610,651	19
Halo-organics	1,608,686	17

Top 5 Chemicals, 1992 TRI

		Pounds
8001-58-9	Creosote	17,152,121
108-88-3	Toluene	10,974,778
1330-20-7	Xylene (mixed isomers)	8,383,683
50-00-0	Formaldehyde	4,537,813
78-93-3	Methyl ethyl ketone	3,790,563

Top 5 Facilities, 1992 TRI

Kerr-Mcgee Chemical Corp., Columbus, MS	5,750,016
Kerr-Mcgee Chemical Corp., Madison, IL	3,683,909
Celotex Corp., Marrero, LA	2,045,549
Northway Cabinetry Div.,Nortak, Rensselaer, IN	1,755,200
Abtco Inc., Toledo, OH	1,522,560

Top 5 Facilities, 1991 BRS

Koppers Industries Inc., Florence, SC	52,855,260
Rolscreen Company, Pella, IA	49,188,860
Koppers Industries Inc., Montgomery, AL	33,434,820
Marley Cooling Tower Co., Stockton, CA	29,796,800
Koppers Industries Inc., Tie Plant, MS	28,257,780

TRI Production-related Waste, 1991-1994*

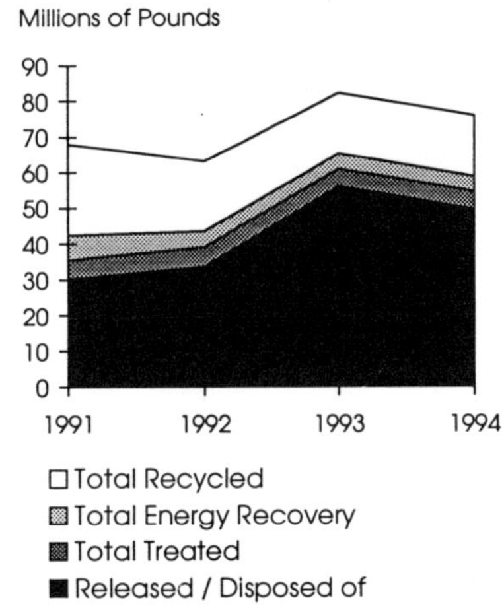

Total TRI Releases, 1992

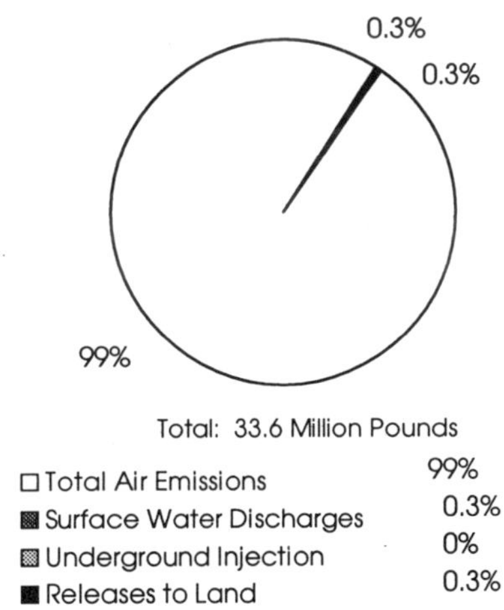

	Pounds 1991	Pounds 1992	Pounds Increase
Facility with Largest Reported TRI Increase	**1991**	**1992**	**Increase**
Kerr-Mcgee Chemical Corp., Columbus, MS	2,530,336	5,750,016	3,219,680
Facility with Largest Reported TRI Decrease	**1991**	**1992**	**Decrease**
Medite, Las Vegas, NM	6,774,903	578,031	-6,196,872
Facility with Largest Projected TRI Increase	**1992**	**1994***	**Increase**
Kerr-Mcgee Chemical Corp., Columbus, MS	5,750,016	26,000,000	20,249,984
Facility with Largest Projected TRI Decrease	**1992**	**1994***	**Decrease**
Sanderson Plumbing Products, Columbus, MS	1,119,577	0	-1,119,577

*Projected ** Rank out of 20 industries (BRS) or 22 industries (TRI)

Industry Profile: SIC 25 Furniture

Reported Production-related Toxic Waste Generation

Reporting Year/Source	Pounds	Rank**
1991 BRS	199,752,520	17
1991 TRI	62,729,636	18
1992 TRI	66,227,908	17
1993 TRI*	64,395,101	18
1994 TRI*	62,853,431	18

Special Groups, 1992 TRI	Pounds	Rank**
Carcinogens	1,311,081	17
Ozone depleters	3,574,437	12
Chloro-organics	4,362,920	16
Metals	1,041,725	17
Halo-organics	4,362,920	16

Top 5 Chemicals, 1992 TRI

		Pounds
108-88-3	Toluene	18,480,158
1330-20-7	Xylene (mixed isomers)	11,872,947
67-56-1	Methanol	9,412,773
78-93-3	Methyl ethyl ketone	6,195,566
67-64-1	Acetone	4,492,140

Top 5 Facilities, 1992 TRI

Steelcase Inc., Grand Rapids, MI	3,554,640
Bassett Furniture Industries, Dublin, GA	1,623,480
Meridian Inc., Spring Lake, MI	1,241,175
Madix Inc., Goodwater, AL	1,193,386
Steelcase Inc., Kentwood, MI	1,098,148

Top 5 Facilities, 1991 BRS

Graber Industries Inc., Middleton, WI	89,367,060
Daystrom Furniture, South Boston, VA	29,670,060
Cal-Style Furniture Mfg. Co., Compton, CA	28,263,100
Steelcase Inc., Grand Rapids, MI	10,742,480
Virco Manufacturing Corp., San Luis, AZ	2,773,600

TRI Production-related Waste, 1991-1994*

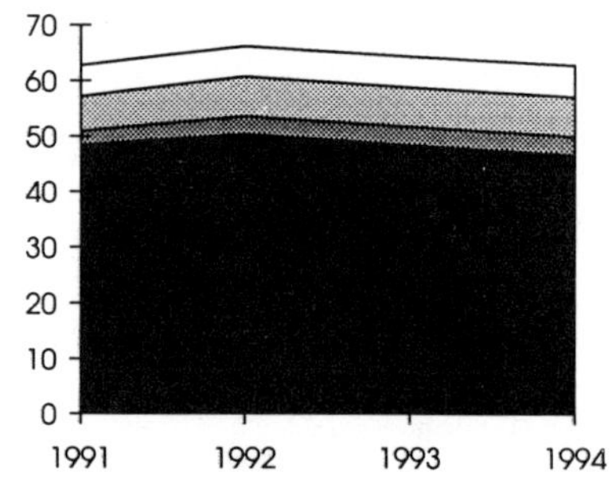

Total TRI Releases, 1992

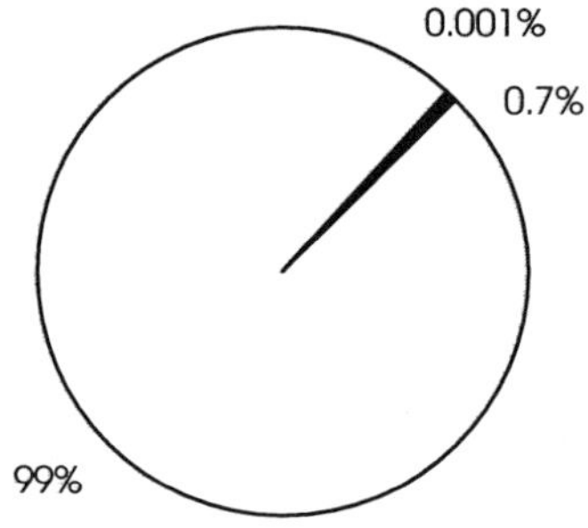

Total: 55.0 Million Pounds

Total Air Emissions	99%
Surface Water Discharges	0.001%
Underground Injection	0%
Releases to Land	0.7%

	Pounds	Pounds	Pounds
Facility with Largest Reported TRI Increase	**1991**	**1992**	**Increase**
Steelcase Inc., Grand Rapids, MI	3,216,419	3,554,640	338,221
Facility with Largest Reported TRI Decrease	**1991**	**1992**	**Decrease**
Meridian Inc., Spring Lake, MI	1,532,148	1,241,175	-290,973
Facility with Largest Projected TRI Increase	**1992**	**1994***	**Increase**
Peters-Revington Furniture, Delphi, IN	676,810	1,090,600	413,790
Facility with Largest Projected TRI Decrease	**1992**	**1994***	**Decrease**
Madix Inc., Goodwater, AL	1,193,386	416,640	-776,746

*Projected ** Rank out of 20 industries (BRS) or 22 industries (TRI)

Industry Profile: SIC 26 Paper

Reported Production-related Toxic Waste Generation

Reporting Year/Source	Pounds	Rank**
1991 BRS	3,993,351,820	9
1991 TRI	2,491,445,311	5
1992 TRI	2,537,521,812	4
1993 TRI*	2,468,038,359	4
1994 TRI*	2,445,343,962	4

Special Groups, 1992 TRI	Pounds	Rank**
Carcinogens	26,012,567	11
Ozone depleters	1,085,758	17
Chloro-organics	21,005,011	12
Metals	5,373,492	14
Halo-organics	21,029,095	12

Top 5 Chemicals, 1992 TRI

		Pounds
67-56-1	Methanol	992,617,878
7664-93-9	Sulfuric acid	728,265,728
7647-01-0	Hydrochloric acid	278,237,947
108-88-3	Toluene	139,600,704
7782-50-5	Chlorine	77,412,622

Top 5 Facilities, 1992 TRI

Alabama River Pulp Co. Inc., Claiborne, AL	74,917,400
Boise Cascade Corp., De Ridder, LA	58,668,900
Union Camp Corp., Franklin, VA	52,784,610
International Paper, Mobile, AL	50,580,250
Federal Paper Board Co. Inc., Riegelwood, NC	50,467,060

Top 5 Facilities, 1991 BRS

Williamette Industries, Johnsonburg, PA	3,855,217,360
Nashua Corp., Merrimack, NH	79,389,120
Napanoch Paper Mill, Napanoch, NY	13,619,660
3M Co., St Paul, MN	2,144,240
Graphics Technology International, South Hadley, MA	2,138,620

TRI Production-related Waste, 1991-1994*

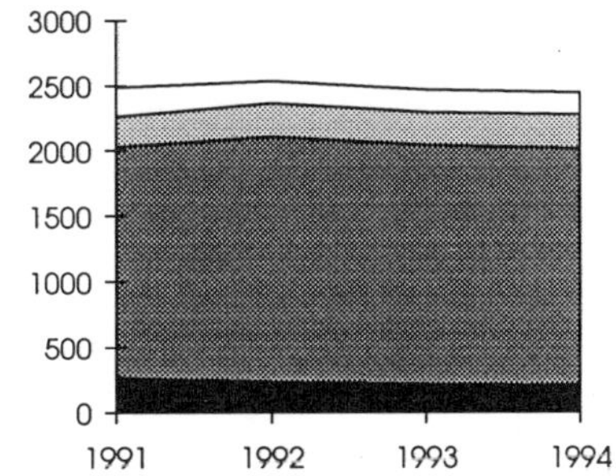

Total TRI Releases, 1992

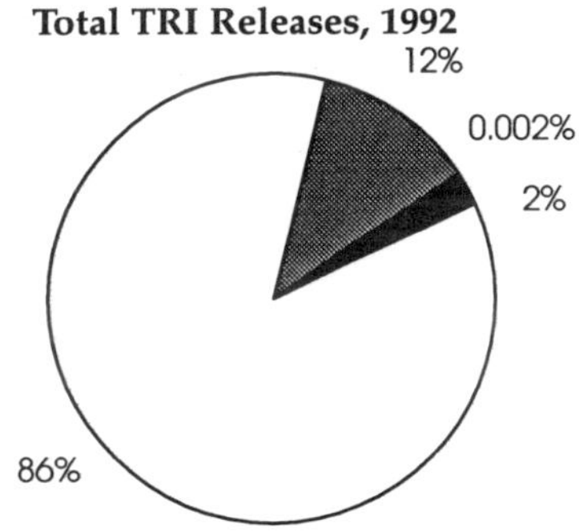

Total: 233.0 Million Pounds

Total Air Emissions	86%
Surface Water Discharges	12%
Underground Injection	0.002%
Releases to Land	2%

	Pounds	Pounds	Pounds
Facility with Largest Reported TRI Increase	**1991**	**1992**	**Increase**
International Paper, Mobile, AL	17,823,330	50,580,250	32,756,920
Facility with Largest Reported TRI Decrease	**1991**	**1992**	**Decrease**
ITT Rayonier Inc., Jesup, GA	85,727,750	23,432,105	-62,295,645
Facility with Largest Projected TRI Increase	**1992**	**1994***	**Increase**
International Paper, Texarkana, TX	47,361,460	54,112,200	6,750,740
Facility with Largest Projected TRI Decrease	**1992**	**1994***	**Decrease**
Stone Savannah River Pulp, Port Wentworth, GA	31,535,267	0	-31,535,267

*Projected ** Rank out of 20 industries (BRS) or 22 industries (TRI)

Industry Profile: SIC 27 Printing

Reported Production-related Toxic Waste Generation

Reporting Year/Source	Pounds	Rank**
1991 BRS	217,093,120	15
1991 TRI	266,876,401	12
1992 TRI	274,812,686	12
1993 TRI*	270,814,103	12
1994 TRI*	264,199,957	12

Special Groups, 1992 TRI	Pounds	Rank**
Carcinogens	949,106	18
Ozone depleters	3,475,254	14
Chloro-organics	4,484,150	15
Metals	968,350	18
Halo-organics	4,484,150	15

Top 5 Chemicals, 1992 TRI

		Pounds
108-88-3	Toluene	237,056,662
1330-20-7	Xylene (mixed isomers)	9,603,260
7664-93-9	Sulfuric acid	7,124,183
78-93-3	Methyl ethyl ketone	6,125,379
71-55-6	1,1,1-Trichloroethane	3,439,954

Top 5 Facilities, 1992 TRI

Quad Graphics Inc., Lomira, WI	25,456,981
Quebecor Printing Inc., Dickson, TN	25,078,317
Ringier America Inc., Corinth, MS	23,758,688
Ringier America Inc., Evans, GA	22,859,340
Brown Printing Co., Franklin, KY	18,756,857

Top 5 Facilities, 1991 BRS

R R Donnelley & Sons Co., Chicago, IL	33,794,760
Toppan Interamerica Inc., McDonough, GA	20,651,740
Quebecor Printing Dickson Inc., Dickson, TN	19,107,560
R.R. Donnelley & Sons Co., Warsaw, IN	15,258,040
Roto Cylinders, Palmyra, NJ	12,073,320

TRI Production-related Waste, 1991-1994*

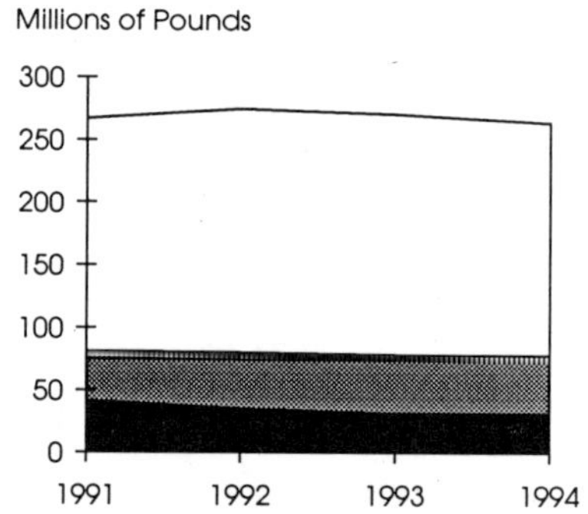

Total TRI Releases, 1992

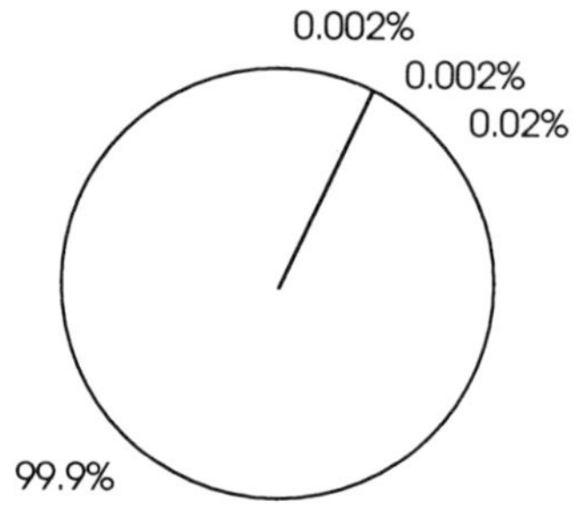

Total: 40.5 Million Pounds

Total Air Emissions	99.9%
Surface Water Discharges	0.002%
Underground Injection	0.002%
Releases to Land	0.02%

Facility with Largest Reported TRI Increase	Pounds 1991	Pounds 1992	Pounds Increase
Ringier America Inc., Corinth, MS	18,151,757	23,758,688	5,606,931
Facility with Largest Reported TRI Decrease	**1991**	**1992**	**Decrease**
Graphic Packaging Corp., Franklin, OH	6,035,869	760,959	-5,274,910
Facility with Largest Projected TRI Increase	**1992**	**1994***	**Increase**
Quad Graphics Inc., Lomira, WI	25,456,981	33,603,547	8,146,566
Facility with Largest Projected TRI Decrease	**1992**	**1994***	**Decrease**
World Color Press, Salem, IL	8,228,255	3,026,180	-5,202,075

*Projected ** Rank out of 20 industries (BRS) or 22 industries (TRI)

Industry Profile: SIC 28 Chemicals

Reported Production-related Toxic Waste Generation

Reporting Year/Source	Pounds	Rank**
1991 BRS	388,570,517,800	1
1991 TRI	19,672,469,407	1
1992 TRI	19,897,327,333	1
1993 TRI*	20,293,688,270	1
1994 TRI*	20,058,858,183	1

Special Groups, 1992 TRI	Pounds	Rank**
Carcinogens	2,025,855,111	1
Ozone depleters	293,828,498	1
Chloro-organics	1,368,191,432	1
Metals	147,576,757	6
Halo-organics	1,375,083,971	1

Top 5 Chemicals, 1992 TRI

CAS No.	Chemical	Pounds
7664-93-9	Sulfuric acid	6,302,550,254
75-05-8	Acetonitrile	2,579,262,739
7647-01-0	Hydrochloric acid	1,471,593,195
67-56-1	Methanol	1,001,317,467
7664-41-7	Ammonia	756,477,509

Top 5 Facilities, 1992 TRI

Facility	Pounds
First Chemical Corp., Pascagoula, MS	4,046,638,711
Goodyear Tire & Rubber Co., Beaumont, TX	2,526,855,525
Solvay Polymers Inc., Deer Park, TX	412,262,000
Goodyear Tire & Rubber Co., Houston, TX	319,906,880
Kemira Inc., Savannah, GA	316,522,270

Top 5 Facilities, 1991 BRS

Facility	Pounds
Dow Chemical Company, Midland, MI	60,274,801,720
DuPont-Chambers Works, Deepwater, NJ	48,842,136,960
Shell Oil Company, Deer Park, TX	38,728,552,500
Amoco Chemical Company, Alvin, TX	16,492,217,040
Rhone-Poulenc Ag Company, Institute, WV	13,313,468,980

TRI Production-related Waste, 1991-1994*

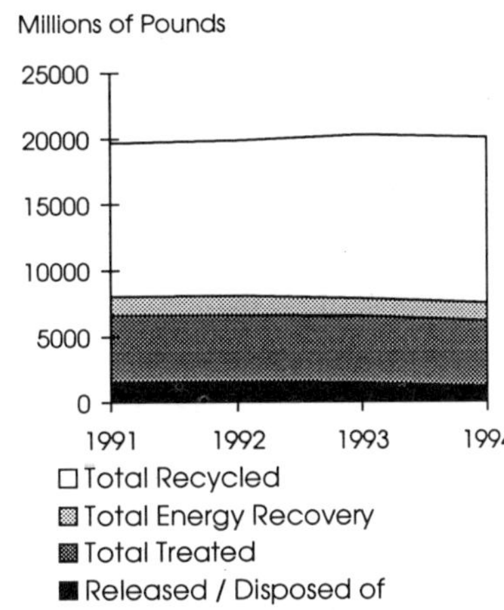

Total TRI Releases, 1992

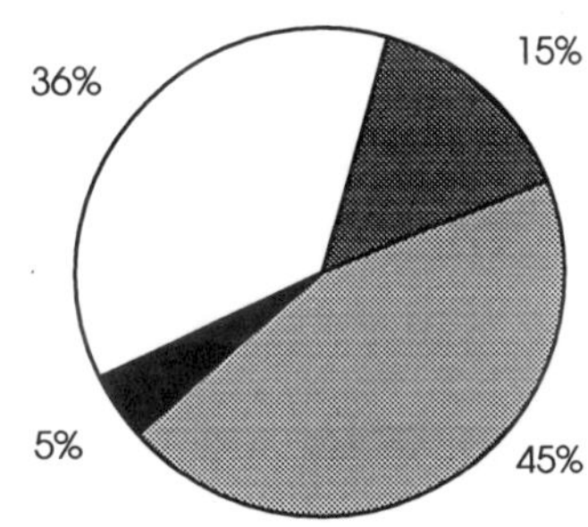

Total: 1.5 Billion Pounds

Total Air Emissions	36%
Surface Water Discharges	15%
Underground Injection	45%
Releases to Land	5%

	Pounds	Pounds	Pounds
Facility with Largest Reported TRI Increase	**1991**	**1992**	**Increase**
Goodyear Tire & Rubber Co., Beaumont, TX	2,423,678,742	2,526,855,525	103,176,783
Facility with Largest Reported TRI Decrease	**1991**	**1992**	**Decrease**
DuPont Chambers Works, Deepwater, NJ	243,531,644	69,782,276	-173,749,368
Facility with Largest Projected TRI Increase	**1992**	**1994***	**Increase**
Goodyear Tire & Rubber Co., Beaumont, TX	2,526,855,525	3,027,332,113	500,476,588
Facility with Largest Projected TRI Decrease	**1992**	**1994***	**Decrease**
SCM Chemicals, Baltimore, MD	287,807,796	36,808,552	-250,999,244

*Projected ** Rank out of 20 industries (BRS) or 22 industries (TRI)

Industry Profile: SIC 29 Petroleum

Reported Production-related Toxic Waste Generation

Reporting Year/Source	Pounds	Rank**
1991 BRS	270,856,101,200	2
1991 TRI	2,562,915,297	3
1992 TRI	2,945,379,328	3
1993 TRI*	2,797,582,295	3
1994 TRI*	2,900,069,882	3

Special Groups, 1992 TRI

Carcinogens	47,503,164	7
Ozone depleters	925,789	18
Chloro-organics	1,486,136	18
Metals	8,327,454	11
Halo-organics	1,497,781	18

Top 5 Chemicals, 1992 TRI

		Pounds
7664-93-9	Sulfuric acid	1,016,916,812
115-07-1	Propylene	861,019,767
74-85-1	Ethylene	322,434,685
108-88-3	Toluene	157,872,385
7664-41-7	Ammonia	157,029,178

Top 5 Facilities, 1992 TRI

Uno-Ven Co., Lemont, IL	488,229,292
National Cooperative Refinery, Mc Pherson, KS	312,856,711
Amoco Oil Co., Whiting, IN	226,785,956
Quaker State Corp., Newell, WV	200,377,755
Star Enterprises Inc., Port Arthur, TX	150,327,643

Top 5 Facilities, 1991 BRS

Amoco Oil Company Refinery, Texas City, TX	52,275,017,600
Citgo Petroleum Corporation, Lake Charles, LA	27,121,056,040
Chevron USA Products Company, Philadelphia, PA	24,434,042,460
Shell Oil Co., Martinez, CA	21,547,730,200
Shell Oil Co., Roxana, IL	18,882,321,460

TRI Production-related Waste, 1991-1994*

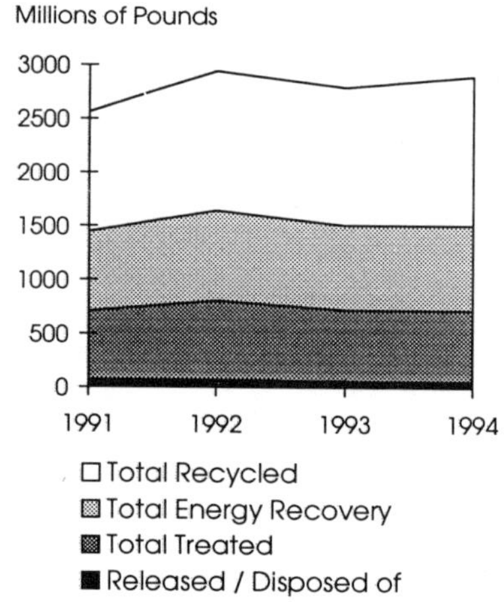

Total TRI Releases, 1992

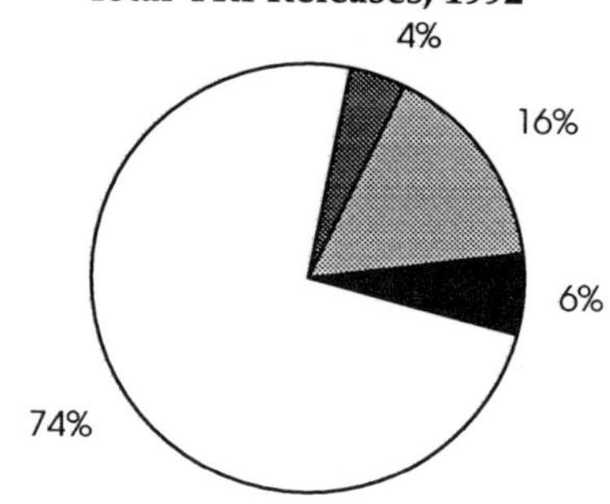

Total: 83.2 Million Pounds

Total Air Emissions	74%
Surface Water Discharges	4%
Underground Injection	16%
Releases to Land	6%

	Pounds	Pounds	Pounds
Facility with Largest Reported TRI Increase	**1991**	**1992**	**Increase**
ARCO Cherry Point Refinery, Ferndale, WA	14,020,197	95,392,864	81,372,667
Facility with Largest Reported TRI Decrease	**1991**	**1992**	**Decrease**
Fina Oil & Chemical Co., Port Arthur, TX	140,704,719	83,207,724	-57,496,995
Facility with Largest Projected TRI Increase	**1992**	**1994***	**Increase**
Indian Refining L.P., Lawrenceville, IL	50,138,064	126,754,039	76,615,975
Facility with Largest Projected TRI Decrease	**1992**	**1994***	**Decrease**
Uno-Ven Co., Lemont, IL	488,229,292	430,066,615	-58,162,677

*Projected ** Rank out of 20 industries (BRS) or 22 industries (TRI)

Industry Profile: SIC 30 Plastics

Reported Production-related Toxic Waste Generation

Reporting Year/Source	Pounds	Rank**
1991 BRS	376,091,940	12
1991 TRI	508,051,776	9
1992 TRI	567,294,382	9
1993 TRI*	536,392,585	9
1994 TRI*	422,046,257	10

Special Groups, 1992 TRI	Pounds	Rank**
Carcinogens	60,744,615	5
Ozone depleters	24,705,907	8
Chloro-organics	66,419,787	7
Metals	238,049,575	5
Halo-organics	66,915,432	7

Top 5 Chemicals, 1992 TRI

CAS No.	Chemical	Pounds
	Lead compounds	221,101,808
108-88-3	Toluene	57,653,930
7664-93-9	Sulfuric acid	42,873,525
75-09-2	Dichloromethane	38,462,338
67-64-1	Acetone	30,702,487

Top 5 Facilities, 1992 TRI

Facility	Pounds
Gates Rubber Co., Iola, KS	219,486,444
Flexel Inc., Tecumseh, KS	38,956,600
Flexel Indiana Inc., Covington, IN	19,712,020
Ametek Inc., Wurtland, KY	10,956,000
3M Co., Nevada, MO	8,710,698

Top 5 Facilities, 1991 BRS

Facility	Pounds
Windsor Plastics Inc., Evansville, IN	193,168,220
Evanite Fiber Corp., Corvallis, OR	53,468,180
Lear Plastics Corp., Mendon, MI	11,841,840
Baxter Healhcare, Pharmaseal Div., Toa Alta, PR	9,391,260
3M Co., Nevada, MO	7,278,060

TRI Production-related Waste, 1991-1994*

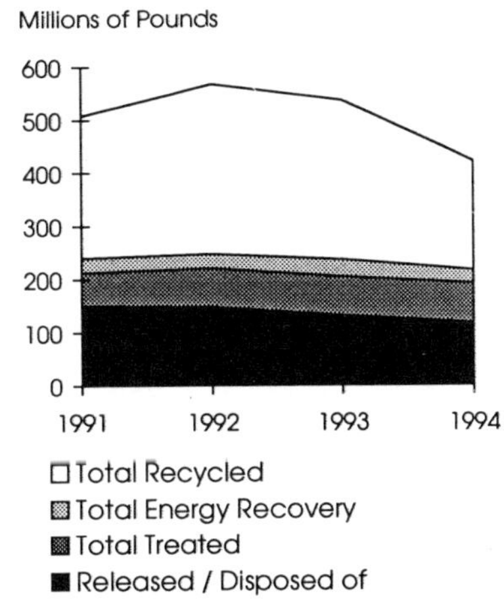

Total TRI Releases, 1992

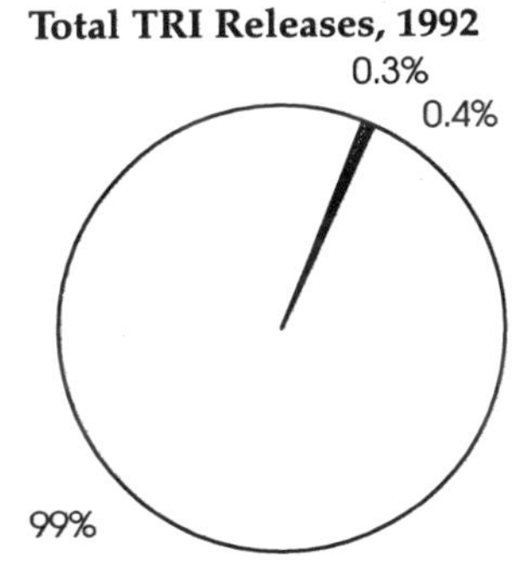

Total: 138.2 Million Pounds

Total Air Emissions	99%
Surface Water Discharges	0.3%
Underground Injection	0%
Releases to Land	0.4%

	Pounds	Pounds	Pounds
Facility with Largest Reported TRI Increase	**1991**	**1992**	**Increase**
Gates Rubber Co., Iola, KS	177,302,326	219,486,444	42,184,118
Facility with Largest Reported TRI Decrease	**1991**	**1992**	**Decrease**
Viskase Corp., Bedford Park, IL	7,547,931	5,841,440	-1,706,491
Facility with Largest Projected TRI Increase	**1992**	**1994***	**Increase**
Toray Plastics America Inc., North Kingstown, RI	5,317,556	10,635,077	5,317,521
Facility with Largest Projected TRI Decrease	**1992**	**1994***	**Decrease**
Gates Rubber Co., Iola, KS	219,486,444	100,339,220	-119,147,224

*Projected ** Rank out of 20 industries (BRS) or 22 industries (TRI)

Industry Profile: SIC 31 Leather

Reported Production-related Toxic Waste Generation

Reporting Year/Source	Pounds	Rank**
1991 BRS	203,725,540	16
1991 TRI	44,987,787	21
1992 TRI	52,480,219	21
1993 TRI*	50,035,879	19
1994 TRI*	52,167,105	19

Special Groups, 1992 TRI

Special Groups, 1992 TRI	Pounds	Rank**
Carcinogens	567,290	19
Ozone depleters	315,016	21
Chloro-organics	514,628	21
Metals	8,082,478	12
Halo-organics	514,628	21

Top 5 Chemicals, 1992 TRI

CAS	Chemical	Pounds
7664-93-9	Sulfuric acid	24,119,555
	Chromium compounds	7,427,443
7664-41-7	Ammonia	5,102,832
	Glycol ethers	3,511,817
108-88-3	Toluene	2,730,139

Top 5 Facilities, 1992 TRI

Facility	Pounds
Blueside Co. Inc., Saint Joseph, MO	11,268,466
Pfister & Vogel Leather Co., Milwaukee, WI	7,145,027
JRB Co. Inc., Akron, OH	4,771,103
Garden State Tanning, Fleetwood, PA	3,559,276
Seton Co., Newark, NJ	1,695,471

Top 5 Facilities, 1991 BRS

Facility	Pounds
Diceon Electronics Inc., Irvine, CA	190,158,460
Polaroid Corporation, Waltham, MA	8,615,680
Seton Company, Leather Div., Saxton, PA	1,940,220
Eagle Ottawa Leather Co., Grand Haven, MI	695,240
Garden State Tanning, Fleetwood, PA	629,500

TRI Production-related Waste, 1991-1994*

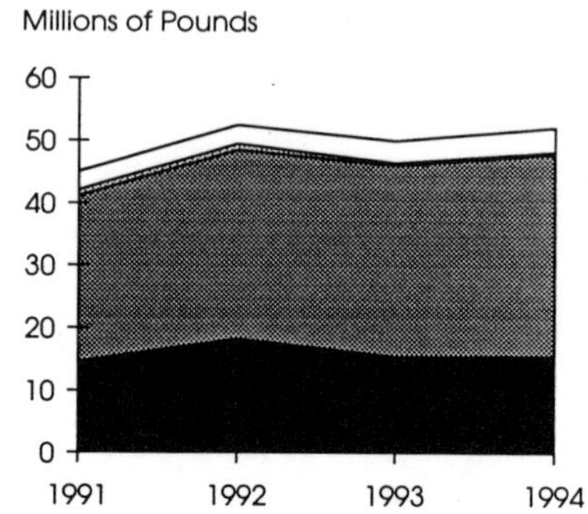

Total TRI Releases, 1992

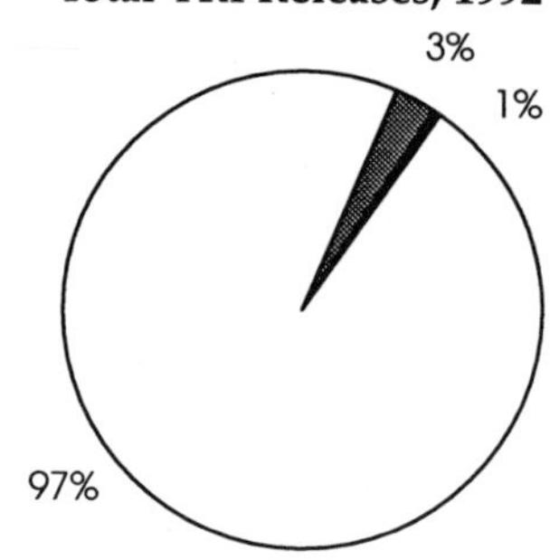

Total: 10.5 Million Pounds

Total Air Emissions	97%
Surface Water Discharges	3%
Underground Injection	0%
Releases to Land	1%

	Pounds	Pounds	Pounds
Facility with Largest Reported TRI Increase	**1991**	**1992**	**Increase**
Garden State Tanning, Fleetwood, PA	1,460,043	3,559,276	2,099,233
Facility with Largest Reported TRI Decrease	**1991**	**1992**	**Decrease**
Pfister & Vogel Leather Co., Milwaukee, WI	7,957,560	7,145,027	-812,533
Facility with Largest Projected TRI Increase	**1992**	**1994***	**Increase**
JRB Co. Inc., Akron, OH	4,771,103	7,456,866	2,685,763
Facility with Largest Projected TRI Decrease	**1992**	**1994***	**Decrease**
Garden State Tanning, Fleetwood, PA	3,559,276	401,000	-3,158,276

*Projected ** Rank out of 20 industries (BRS) or 22 industries (TRI)

Industry Profile: SIC 32 Stone/Clay/Glass

Reported Production-related Toxic Waste Generation

Reporting Year/Source	Pounds	Rank**
1991 BRS	362,430,800	13
1991 TRI	999,977,077	6
1992 TRI	935,576,617	8
1993 TRI*	1,039,486,747	6
1994 TRI*	1,165,083,734	6

Special Groups, 1992 TRI	Pounds	Rank**
Carcinogens	38,208,260	9
Ozone depleters	7,958,026	11
Chloro-organics	28,706,049	11
Metals	106,170,657	8
Halo-organics	28,714,049	11

Top 5 Chemicals, 1992 TRI

		Pounds
108-88-3	Toluene	191,075,266
7664-93-9	Sulfuric acid	177,005,161
1330-20-7	Xylene (mixed isomers)	139,102,672
	Lead compounds	72,104,511
78-93-3	Methyl ethyl ketone	49,044,304

Top 5 Facilities, 1992 TRI

Material Service Corp., Chicago, IL	99,982,822
Paulding Co., Paulding, OH	73,346,746
Material Service Corp., Chicago, IL	67,804,533
Systech Environmental Corp., Fredonia, KS	64,347,324
Systech Environmental Corp., Demopolis, AL	60,355,837

Top 5 Facilities, 1991 BRS

G T E Products Corp Sylvania, Central Falls, RI	174,315,980
Saint George Crystal, Ltd., Jeanette, PA	28,496,880
Corning Inc., Corning, NY	16,930,020
United Oil Recovery Inc., Meriden, CT	14,715,740
3M Co., Prairie Du Chien, WI	14,192,980

TRI Production-related Waste, 1991-1994*

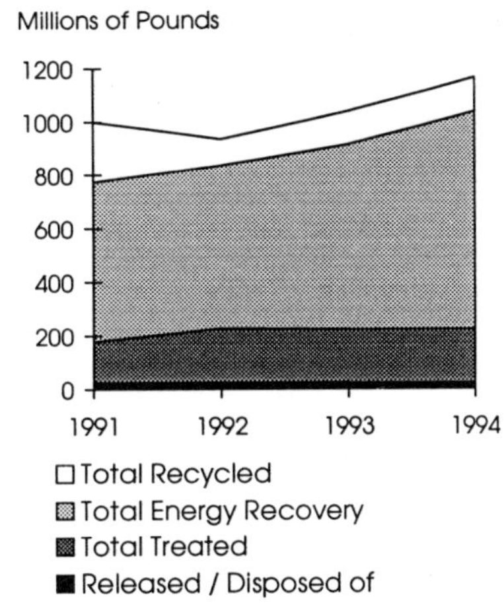

Total TRI Releases, 1992

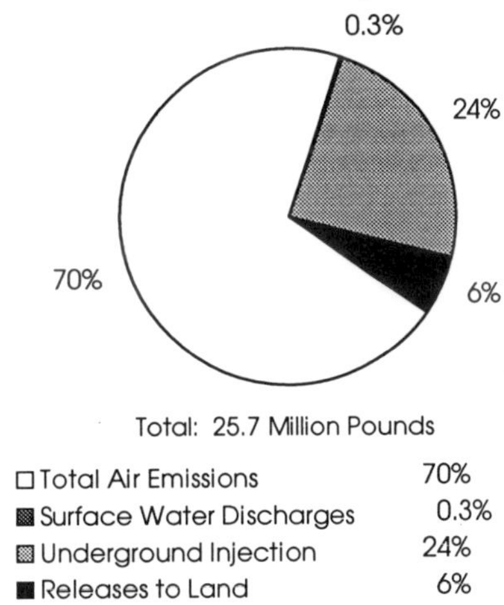

	Pounds	Pounds	Pounds
Facility with Largest Reported TRI Increase	**1991**	**1992**	**Increase**
Material Service Corp., Chicago, IL	59,067,966	99,982,822	40,914,856
Facility with Largest Reported TRI Decrease	**1991**	**1992**	**Decrease**
Corning Asahi Video Products, State College, PA	163,842,990	21,869,850	-141,973,140
Facility with Largest Projected TRI Increase	**1992**	**1994***	**Increase**
Corning Asahi Video Products, State College, PA	21,869,850	44,711,100	22,841,250
Facility with Largest Projected TRI Decrease	**1992**	**1994***	**Decrease**
Systech Environmental Corp., Demopolis, AL	60,355,837	57,566,125	-2,789,712

*Projected ** Rank out of 20 industries (BRS) or 22 industries (TRI)

Industry Profile: SIC 33 Primary Metals

Reported Production-related Toxic Waste Generation

Reporting Year/Source	Pounds	Rank**
1991 BRS	30,608,272,760	6
1991 TRI	3,654,952,230	2
1992 TRI	4,044,002,976	2
1993 TRI*	4,111,972,546	2
1994 TRI*	4,345,464,739	2

Special Groups, 1992 TRI	Pounds	Rank**
Carcinogens	254,905,265	2
Ozone depleters	20,473,548	9
Chloro-organics	40,301,025	10
Metals	2,172,137,413	1
Halo-organics	40,367,207	10

Top 5 Chemicals, 1992 TRI

		Pounds
7664-93-9	Sulfuric acid	976,143,527
7440-50-8	Copper	382,310,171
	Lead compounds	379,885,754
	Zinc compounds	333,009,909
7647-01-0	Hydrochloric acid	264,915,702

Top 5 Facilities, 1992 TRI

Cyprus Miami Mining Corp., Claypool, AZ	394,955,000
Doe Run Co., Boss, MO	231,500,858
Elkem Metals Co., Marietta, OH	118,624,331
Magnesium Corp. of America, Rowley, UT	117,492,861
Timken Co., Canton, OH	97,000,000

Top 5 Facilities, 1991 BRS

Armco Inc., Lyndora, PA	4,931,192,360
J&L Specialty Products Corp., Midland, PA	4,657,012,480
Carpenter Technology Corp., Reading, PA	2,570,861,600
Quanex Corp. Michigan Seamless, South Lyon, MI	1,784,240,860
Zinc Corporation of America, Bartlesville, OK	1,606,431,540

TRI Production-related Waste, 1991-1994*

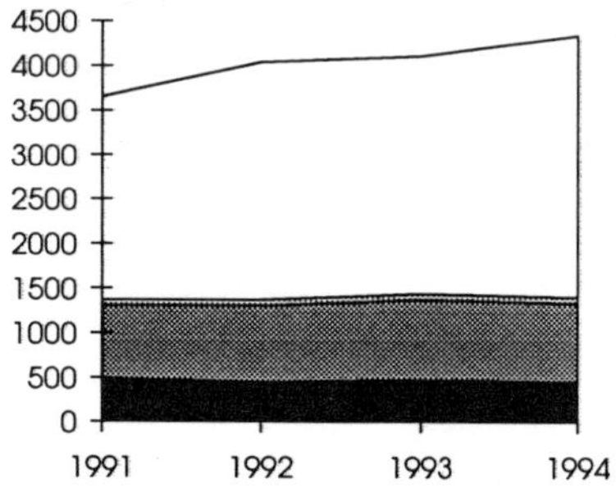

Total TRI Releases, 1992

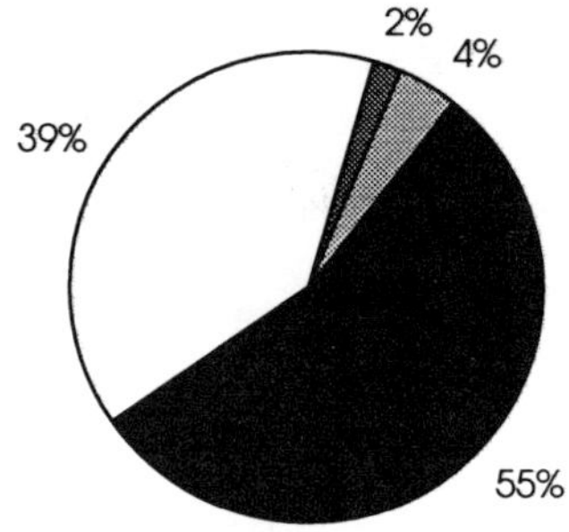

Total: 345.3 Million Pounds

Total Air Emissions	39%
Surface Water Discharges	2%
Underground Injection	4%
Releases to Land	55%

	Pounds	Pounds	Pounds
Facility with Largest Reported TRI Increase	**1991**	**1992**	**Increase**
Doe Run Co., Boss, MO	50,358,284	231,500,858	181,142,574
Facility with Largest Reported TRI Decrease	**1991**	**1992**	**Decrease**
GNB Inc., Frisco, TX	72,883,740	4,179,363	-68,704,377
Facility with Largest Projected TRI Increase	**1992**	**1994***	**Increase**
Inmetco, Ellwood City, PA	4,652,464	178,342,323	173,689,859
Facility with Largest Projected TRI Decrease	**1992**	**1994***	**Decrease**
Doe Run Co., Boss, MO	231,500,858	125,151,200	-106,349,658

*Projected ** Rank out of 20 industries (BRS) or 22 industries (TRI)

Industry Profile: SIC 34 Fabricated Metals

Reported Production-related Toxic Waste Generation

Reporting Year/Source	Pounds	Rank**
1991 BRS	40,687,820,920	4
1991 TRI	919,137,839	8
1992 TRI	962,656,507	7
1993 TRI*	939,002,061	7
1994 TRI*	971,522,127	7

Special Groups, 1992 TRI	Pounds	Rank**
Carcinogens	47,019,162	8
Ozone depleters	107,690,937	2
Chloro-organics	257,421,043	2
Metals	263,253,688	4
Halo-organics	257,427,703	2

Top 5 Chemicals, 1992 TRI

		Pounds
79-01-6	Trichloroethylene	141,774,611
7664-93-9	Sulfuric acid	105,289,102
71-55-6	1,1,1-Trichloroethane	98,057,649
7440-50-8	Copper	94,555,209
	Zinc compounds	70,509,976

Top 5 Facilities, 1992 TRI

Uniform Tubes Inc., Trappe, PA	74,099,262
Warner-Lambert Co., Milford, CT	70,150,930
Keystone Cement Co., Bath, PA	51,499,385
Signet Systems Inc., Harrodsburg, KY	48,281,595
Double Eagle Steel Coating Co., Dearborn, MI	39,295,000

Top 5 Facilities, 1991 BRS

General Motors Corp., Detroit, MI	3,572,176,980
Buckbee-Mears Cortland, Cortland, NY	2,101,036,060
U.S. Steel Corp., Fairless Hills, PA	2,015,340,400
Blount Inc., Lewiston, ID	1,029,266,320
GTE Products Corp., Warren, PA	994,362,360

TRI Production-related Waste, 1991-1994*

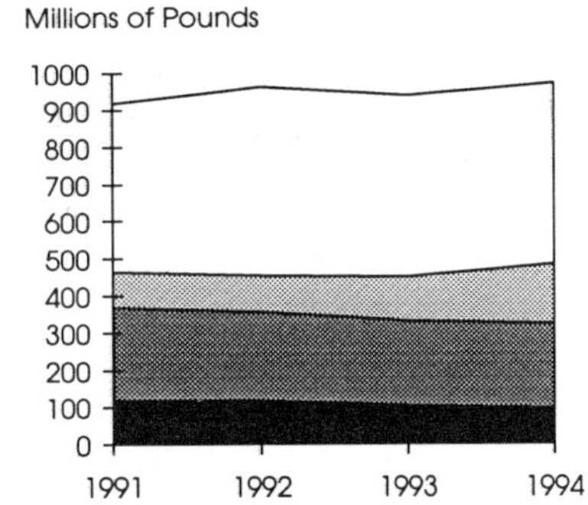

Total TRI Releases, 1992

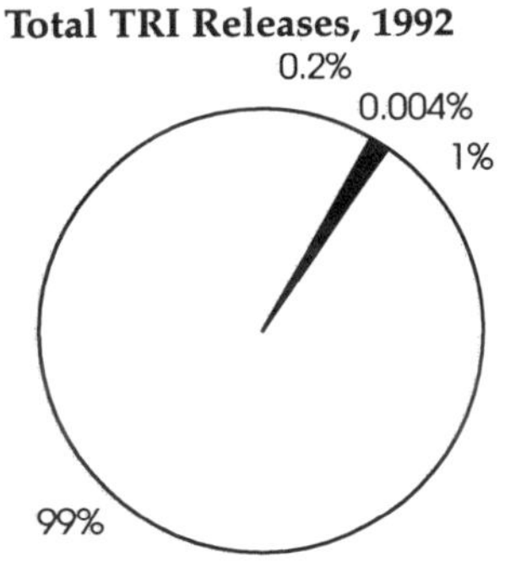

Total: 102.0 Million Pounds

Total Air Emissions	99%
Surface Water Discharges	0.2%
Underground Injection	0.004%
Releases to Land	1%

	Pounds	Pounds	Pounds
Facility with Largest Reported TRI Increase	**1991**	**1992**	**Increase**
Double Eagle Steel Coating Co., Dearborn, MI	31,893,000	39,295,000	7,402,000
Facility with Largest Reported TRI Decrease	**1991**	**1992**	**Decrease**
Midstates Wire, Crawfordsville, IN	29,268,549	3,284,591	-25,983,958
Facility with Largest Projected TRI Increase	**1992**	**1994***	**Increase**
Keystone Cement Co., Bath, PA	51,499,385	115,213,876	63,714,491
Facility with Largest Projected TRI Decrease	**1992**	**1994***	**Decrease**
Delta Faucet Co., Greensburg, IN	20,104,210	12,932,775	-7,171,435

*Projected ** Rank out of 20 industries (BRS) or 22 industries (TRI)

Industry Profile: SIC 35 Machinery

Reported Production-related Toxic Waste Generation

Reporting Year/Source	Pounds	Rank**
1991 BRS	2,910,808,380	10
1991 TRI	211,347,793	13
1992 TRI	207,000,051	13
1993 TRI*	191,487,495	14
1994 TRI*	174,373,640	14

Special Groups, 1992 TRI

Carcinogens	27,189,438	10
Ozone depleters	59,626,428	3
Chloro-organics	112,659,974	3
Metals	45,804,309	9
Halo-organics	112,659,974	3

Top 5 Chemicals, 1992 TRI

		Pounds
71-55-6	1,1,1-Trichloroethane	53,673,430
79-01-6	Trichloroethylene	46,487,268
7664-93-9	Sulfuric acid	12,133,818
7440-50-8	Copper	11,165,472
7440-47-3	Chromium	10,573,293

Top 5 Facilities, 1992 TRI

Amana Refrigeration Inc., Fayetteville, TN	33,355,915
Thermo King De Puerto Rico, Arecibo, PR	17,316,209
Thermo King Corp., Louisville, GA	10,339,134
Modine Manufacturing Co., Lawrenceburg, TN	9,778,137
Modine Heat Transfer Inc., Camdenton, MO	4,798,338

Top 5 Facilities, 1991 BRS

IBM Corp., Yorktown, NY	1,166,579,100
Carrier Corp., Syracuse, NY	300,208,800
IBM Corp., Owego, NY	272,561,520
Alcoa Technical Center, Alcoa Center, PA	195,790,720
Control Data Corp., Bloomington, MN	124,758,400

TRI Production-related Waste, 1991-1994*

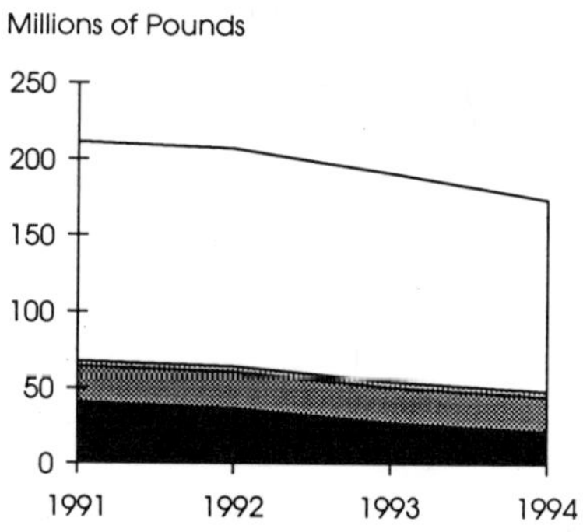

Total TRI Releases, 1992

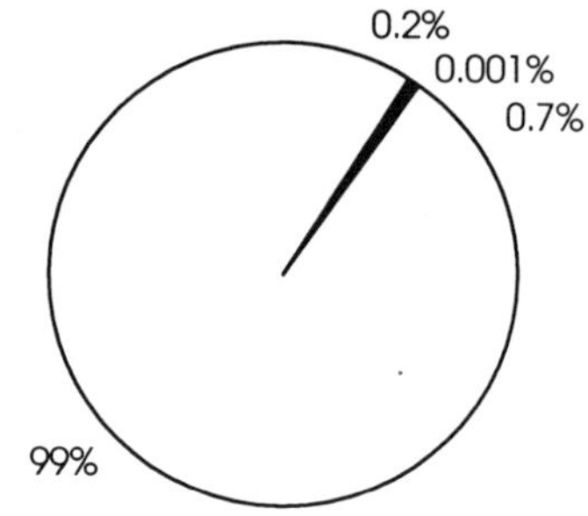

Total: 34.1 Million Pounds

Total Air Emissions	99%
Surface Water Discharges	0.2%
Underground Injection	0.001%
Releases to Land	0.7%

	Pounds	Pounds	Pounds
Facility with Largest Reported TRI Increase	**1991**	**1992**	**Increase**
Aeroquip Corp., New Haven, IN	39,260	3,798,920	3,759,660
Facility with Largest Reported TRI Decrease	**1991**	**1992**	**Decrease**
Modine Heat Transfer Inc., Camdenton, MO	7,258,305	4,798,338	-2,459,967
Facility with Largest Projected TRI Increase	**1992**	**1994***	**Increase**
Modine Heat Transfer Inc., Camdenton, MO	4,798,338	7,975,074	3,176,736
Facility with Largest Projected TRI Decrease	**1992**	**1994***	**Decrease**
Thermo King Corp., Louisville, GA	10,339,134	5,153,005	-5,186,129

*Projected ** Rank out of 20 industries (BRS) or 22 industries (TRI)

Industry Profile: SIC 36 Electrical

Reported Production-related Toxic Waste Generation

Reporting Year/Source	Pounds	Rank**
1991 BRS	33,679,602,720	5
1991 TRI	994,456,225	7
1992 TRI	963,576,363	6
1993 TRI*	865,330,352	8
1994 TRI*	850,486,153	8

Special Groups, 1992 TRI		
Carcinogens	62,889,640	4
Ozone depleters	50,749,648	6
Chloro-organics	107,094,552	4
Metals	480,164,916	2
Halo-organics	108,321,355	4

Top 5 Chemicals, 1992 TRI		Pounds
	Lead compounds	383,993,987
7664-93-9	Sulfuric acid	205,352,805
7440-50-8	Copper	43,568,800
7647-01-0	Hydrochloric acid	40,718,112
71-55-6	1,1,1-Trichloroethane	32,529,180

Top 5 Facilities, 1992 TRI	
Johnson Controls Inc., Garland, TX	52,472,277
Johnson Controls Inc., Geneva, IL	41,691,018
IBM Corp., Endicott, NY	41,265,792
Exide Corp., Frankfort, IN	32,191,543
Valmont Industries Inc., Valley, NE	28,010,331

Top 5 Facilities, 1991 BRS	
National Semiconductor Corp., Santa Clara, CA	2,905,245,660
American Telephone & Telegraph, Richmond, VA	2,035,166,820
National Semi Conductor, West Jordan, UT	1,739,225,980
Zycon Corp., Santa Clara, CA	1,640,436,620
IBM Corp., Austin, TX	1,410,272,360

TRI Production-related Waste, 1991-1994*

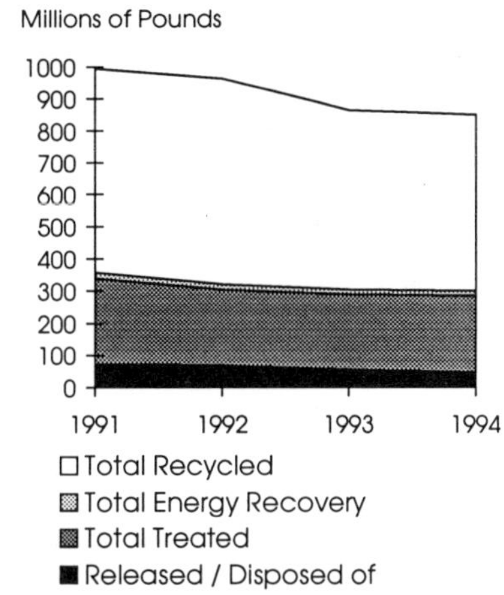

Total TRI Releases, 1992

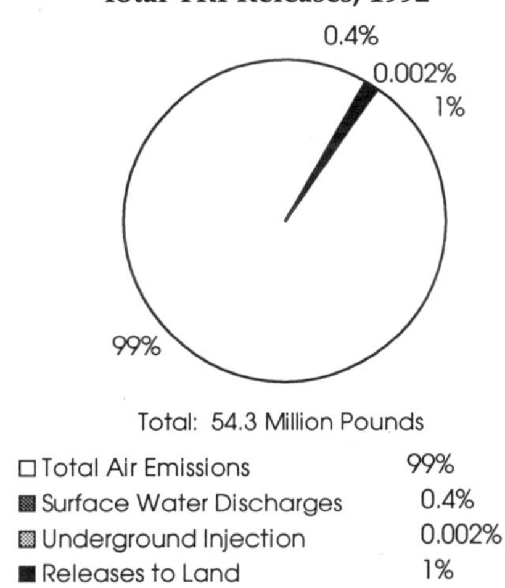

	Pounds	Pounds	Pounds
Facility with Largest Reported TRI Increase	**1991**	**1992**	**Increase**
Johnson Controls Inc., Garland, TX	9,888,204	52,472,277	42,584,073
Facility with Largest Reported TRI Decrease	**1991**	**1992**	**Decrease**
IBM Corp., Endicott, NY	61,239,649	41,265,792	-19,973,857
Facility with Largest Projected TRI Increase	**1992**	**1994***	**Increase**
Exide Corp., Frankfort, IN	32,191,543	42,714,704	10,523,161
Facility with Largest Projected TRI Decrease	**1992**	**1994***	**Decrease**
Johnson Controls Inc., Garland, TX	52,472,277	9,242,208	-43,230,069

*Projected ** Rank out of 20 industries (BRS) or 22 industries (TRI)

Industry Profile: SIC 37 Transportation Equipment

Reported Production-related Toxic Waste Generation

Reporting Year/Source	Pounds	Rank**
1991 BRS	18,618,250,440	7
1991 TRI	459,765,222	10
1992 TRI	471,959,721	10
1993 TRI*	453,602,281	10
1994 TRI*	435,593,168	9

Special Groups, 1992 TRI		
Carcinogens	58,346,397	6
Ozone depleters	51,026,163	5
Chloro-organics	93,943,894	5
Metals	130,068,832	7
Halo-organics	93,985,394	5

TRI Production-related Waste, 1991-1994*

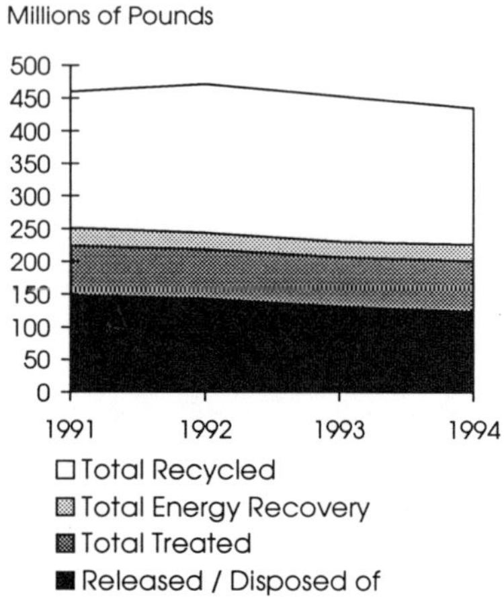

Top 5 Chemicals, 1992 TRI		Pounds
1330-20-7	Xylene (mixed isomers)	56,511,146
71-55-6	1,1,1-Trichloroethane	39,930,493
7440-50-8	Copper	38,058,029
7664-93-9	Sulfuric acid	36,796,484
79-01-6	Trichloroethylene	34,656,366

Total TRI Releases, 1992

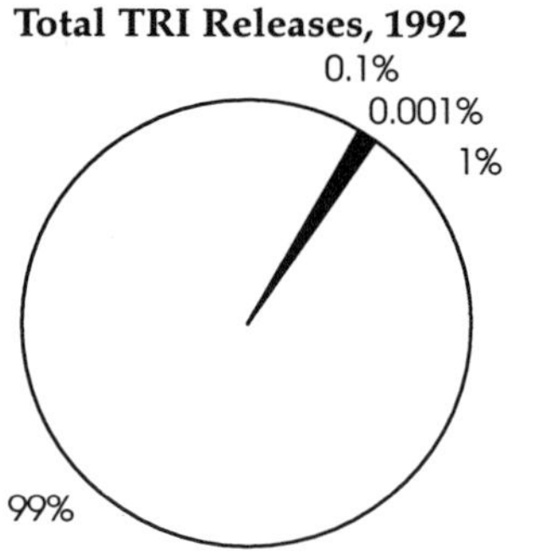

Total: 137.1 Million Pounds

Total Air Emissions	99%
Surface Water Discharges	0.1%
Underground Injection	0.001%
Releases to Land	1%

Top 5 Facilities, 1992 TRI	
Preferred Technical Group Inc., Mitchell, IN	22,410,718
Saturn Corp., Spring Hill, TN	21,565,599
Blairsville Machine Products, Blairsville, PA	15,171,760
General Motors Corp., Warren, OH	14,674,830
Honda of America Mfg. Inc., Marysville, OH	8,190,572

Top 5 Facilities, 1991 BRS	
Pratt & Whitney Aircraft Group, East Hartford, CT	3,366,820,700
LTV Aerospace & Defense Co., Dallas, TX	2,516,839,500
Inland Fisher Guide, Anderson, IN	1,061,842,160
Monroe Auto Equipment Co., Cozad, NE	756,054,120
Douglas Aircraft Company, Los Angeles, CA	747,945,560

	Pounds	Pounds	Pounds
Facility with Largest Reported TRI Increase	**1991**	**1992**	**Increase**
Saturn Corp., Spring Hill, TN	3,895,260	21,565,599	17,670,339
Facility with Largest Reported TRI Decrease	**1991**	**1992**	**Decrease**
Blairsville Machine Products, Blairsville, PA	18,206,112	15,171,760	-3,034,352
Facility with Largest Projected TRI Increase	**1992**	**1994***	**Increase**
Saturn Corp., Spring Hill, TN	21,565,599	32,327,530	10,761,931
Facility with Largest Projected TRI Decrease	**1992**	**1994***	**Decrease**
Modine Manufacturing Co., Logansport, IN	6,781,204	545,352	-6,235,852

*Projected ** Rank out of 20 industries (BRS) or 22 industries (TRI)

Industry Profile: SIC 38 Measurement/Photographic Equipment

Reported Production-related Toxic Waste Generation

Reporting Year/Source	Pounds	Rank**
1991 BRS	85,061,296,940	3
1991 TRI	122,969,517	15
1992 TRI	125,739,677	15
1993 TRI*	112,676,843	15
1994 TRI*	103,299,566	15

Special Groups, 1992 TRI	Pounds	Rank**
Carcinogens	25,222,958	12
Ozone depleters	20,143,780	10
Chloro-organics	43,562,915	9
Metals	6,879,680	13
Halo-organics	43,577,607	9

Top 5 Chemicals, 1992 TRI

		Pounds
67-56-1	Methanol	18,662,240
75-09-2	Dichloromethane	17,433,320
67-64-1	Acetone	16,910,165
76-13-1	Freon 113	9,742,822
71-55-6	1,1,1-Trichloroethane	7,557,325

Top 5 Facilities, 1992 TRI

Eastman Kodak Co., Rochester, NY	52,110,960
Polaroid Corp., Waltham, MA	8,992,217
Du Pont Towanda Plant, Towanda, PA	6,404,125
3M Co., Hartford City, IN	4,416,795
Zimmer Inc., Warsaw, IN	3,872,898

Top 5 Facilities, 1991 BRS

Kodak Park, Rochester, NY	83,225,844,980
Polaroid Corporation, New Bedford, MA	410,014,040
General Electric Co., Somersworth, NH	301,114,980
Polaroid Corporation, Norwood, MA	245,829,920
Schlumberger Industries, West Union, SC	182,590,280

TRI Production-related Waste, 1991-1994*

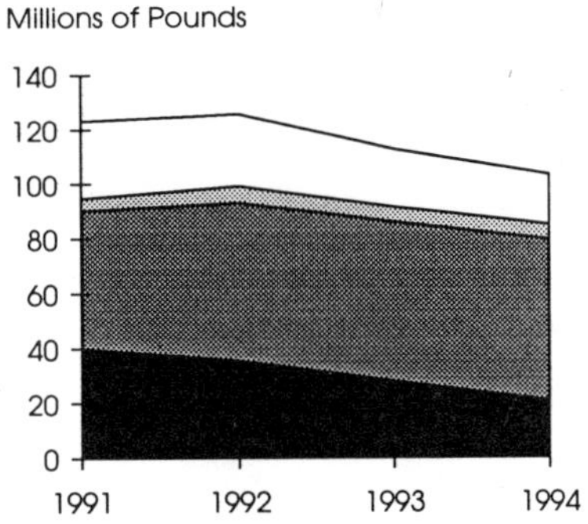

Total TRI Releases, 1992

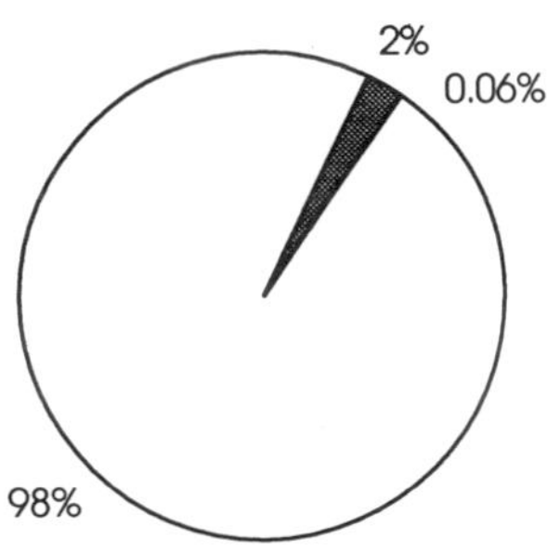

Total: 35.3 Million Pounds

Total Air Emissions	98%
Surface Water Discharges	2%
Underground Injection	0%
Releases to Land	0.06%

	Pounds 1991	Pounds 1992	Pounds Increase
Facility with Largest Reported TRI Increase	**1991**	**1992**	**Increase**
Eastman Kodak Co., Rochester, NY	45,717,433	52,110,960	6,393,527
Facility with Largest Reported TRI Decrease	**1991**	**1992**	**Decrease**
International Paper Co., Binghamton, NY	3,197,275	853,380	-2,343,895
Facility with Largest Projected TRI Increase	**1992**	**1994***	**Increase**
Baxter Healthcare Corp., Aibonito, PR	565,700	862,600	296,900
Facility with Largest Projected TRI Decrease	**1992**	**1994***	**Decrease**
Zimmer Inc., Warsaw, IN	3,872,898	22,942	-3,849,956

*Projected ** Rank out of 20 industries (BRS) or 22 industries (TRI)

Industry Profile: SIC 39 Miscellaneous

Reported Production-related Toxic Waste Generation

Reporting Year/Source	Pounds	Rank**
1991 BRS	6,002,867,540	8
1991 TRI	51,696,646	20
1992 TRI	55,014,507	20
1993 TRI*	43,397,018	20
1994 TRI*	41,498,672	20

Special Groups, 1992 TRI		
Carcinogens	6,283,617	14
Ozone depleters	3,558,952	13
Chloro-organics	6,962,007	14
Metals	12,848,514	10
Halo-organics	6,970,872	14

Top 5 Chemicals, 1992 TRI

		Pounds
108-88-3	Toluene	10,947,621
7440-50-8	Copper	7,144,064
78-93-3	Methyl ethyl ketone	5,212,889
85-68-7	Butyl benzyl phthalate	3,653,400
71-55-6	1,1,1-Trichloroethane	2,864,486

Top 5 Facilities, 1992 TRI

Armstrong World Industries, Lancaster, PA	3,993,347
Oneida Ltd., Sherrill, NY	3,403,948
YKK USA National Mfg. Center, Macon, GA	3,197,862
Kurz-Hastings Inc., Philadelphia, PA	3,170,000
American Biltrite Inc., Trenton, NJ	2,308,810

Top 5 Facilities, 1991 BRS

3M Co., Cottage Grove, MN	5,336,152,080
Scovill Fasteners Inc., Clarkesville, GA	294,509,040
Ribco Manufacturing Inc., Pawtucket, RI	78,694,740
RI Buckle Co. Inc., Providence, RI	70,965,980
Talon Inc., Meadville, PA	53,645,280

TRI Production-related Waste, 1991-1994*

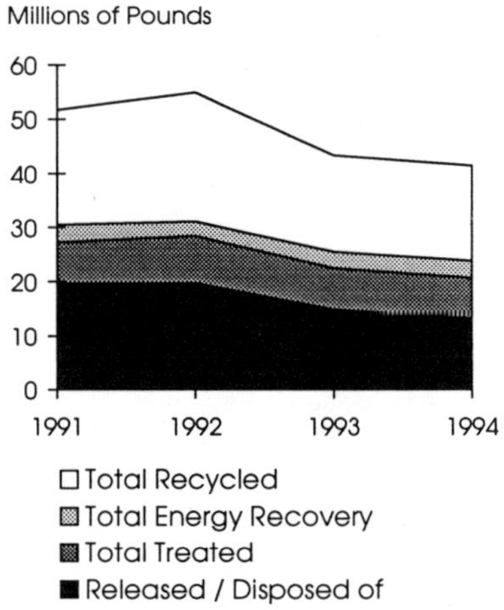

Total TRI Releases, 1992

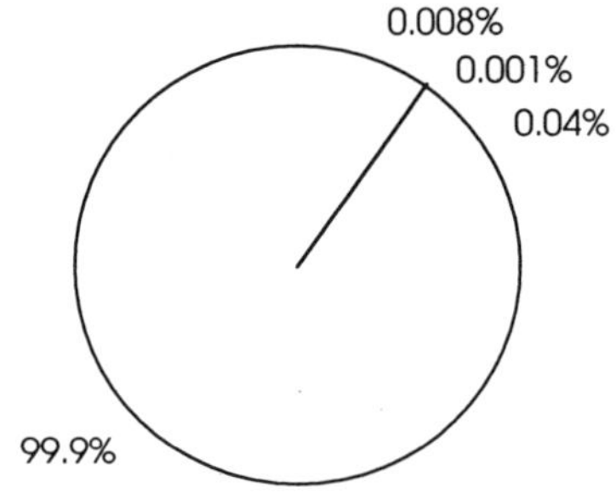

Total: 18.4 Million Pounds

Total Air Emissions	99.9%
Surface Water Discharges	0.008%
Underground Injection	0.001%
Releases to Land	0.04%

	Pounds	Pounds	Pounds
Facility with Largest Reported TRI Increase	**1991**	**1992**	**Increase**
Armstrong World Industries, Lancaster, PA	2,536,677	3,993,347	1,456,670
Facility with Largest Reported TRI Decrease	**1991**	**1992**	**Decrease**
NER Data Products Inc., Blytheville, AR	862,021	109,547	-752,474
Facility with Largest Projected TRI Increase	**1992**	**1994***	**Increase**
YKK USA, Macon, GA	1,756,241	2,157,444	401,203
Facility with Largest Projected TRI Decrease	**1992**	**1994***	**Decrease**
Oneida Ltd., Sherrill, NY	3,403,948	0	-3,403,948

*Projected ** Rank out of 20 industries (BRS) or 22 industries (TRI)

Industry Profile: SIC 20-39 Multiple Codes

Reported Production-related Toxic Waste Generation

Reporting Year/Source	Pounds	Rank**
1991 BRS	N/A	N/A
1991 TRI	2,530,599,122	4
1992 TRI	2,412,177,342	5
1993 TRI*	2,378,251,462	5
1994 TRI*	2,370,238,092	5

Special Groups, 1992 TRI		
Carcinogens	240,432,348	3
Ozone depleters	27,539,480	7
Chloro-organics	81,234,176	6
Metals	389,958,948	3
Halo-organics	81,387,526	6

Top 5 Chemicals, 1992 TRI		Pounds
7664-93-9	Sulfuric acid	479,951,275
98-82-8	Cumene	291,154,263
7664-41-7	Ammonia	263,042,630
7647-01-0	Hydrochloric acid	180,982,908
67-56-1	Methanol	146,159,463

Top 5 Facilities, 1992 TRI	
Texaco Refining & Marketing, El Dorado, KS	357,281,731
Citgo Petroleum Corp., Lake Charles, LA	257,397,209
Hoechst-Celanese Corp., Spartanburg, SC	183,100,691
Star Enterprises Inc., Union, LA	180,304,951
East Penn Manufacturing Co., Lyon Station, PA	127,434,250

Top 5 Facilities, 1991 BRS

Not applicable -
only one SIC code is reported per waste stream to the BRS database.

TRI Production-related Waste, 1991-1994*

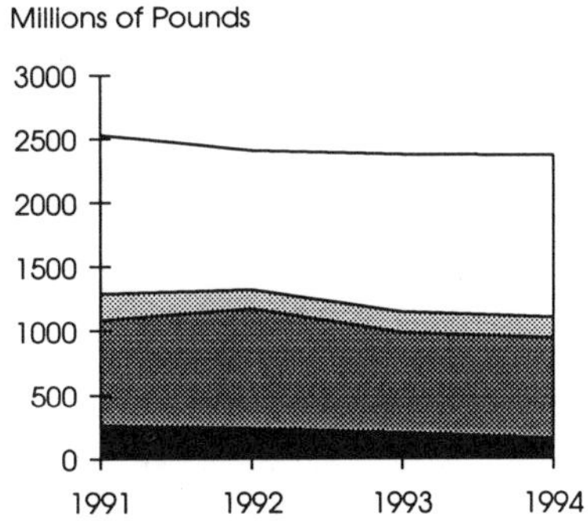

Total TRI Releases, 1992

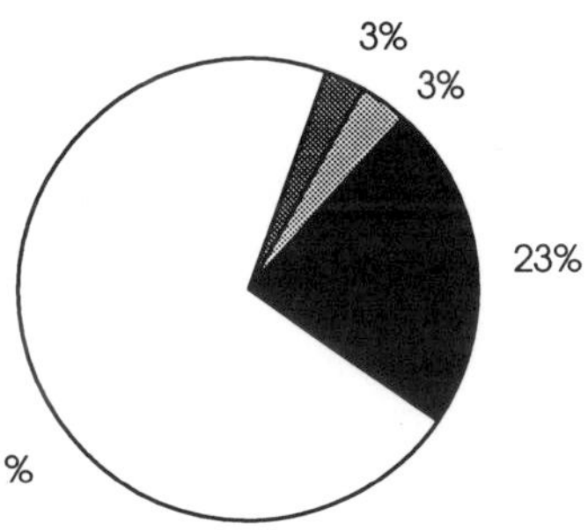

Total: 218.7 Million Pounds

Total Air Emissions	71%
Surface Water Discharges	3%
Underground Injection	3%
Releases to Land	23%

	Pounds	Pounds	Pounds
Facility with Largest Reported TRI Increase	**1991**	**1992**	**Increase**
Star Enterprises Inc., Union, LA	9,652,137	180,304,951	170,652,814
Facility with Largest Reported TRI Decrease	**1991**	**1992**	**Decrease**
Phillips 66 Co., Sweeny, TX	154,483,279	21,901,036	-132,582,243
Facility with Largest Projected TRI Increase	**1992**	**1994***	**Increase**
Phillips 66 Co., Sweeny, TX	21,901,036	136,858,900	114,957,864
Facility with Largest Projected TRI Decrease	**1992**	**1994***	**Decrease**
Star Enterprises Inc., Union, LA	180,304,951	18,289,731	-162,015,220

*Projected ** Rank out of 20 industries (BRS) or 22 industries (TRI)

Industry Profile: National Summary

Reported Production-related Toxic Waste Generation

Reporting Year/Source	Pounds	Rank**
1991 BRS	948,243,750,120	
1991 TRI	36,316,963,077	
1992 TRI	37,333,775,624	
1993 TRI*	37,445,906,395	
1994 TRI*	37,460,411,532	

Special Groups, 1992 TRI	
Carcinogens	2,955,067,837
Ozone depleters	738,134,032
Chloro-organics	2,307,493,160
Metals	4,174,881,882
Halo-organics	2,317,202,349

Top 5 Chemicals, 1992 TRI		Pounds
7664-93-9	Sulfuric acid	10,269,925,138
75-05-8	Acetonitrile	2,581,322,698
7647-01-0	Hydrochloric acid	2,475,552,419
67-56-1	Methanol	2,238,505,652
115-07-1	Propylene	1,615,374,591

Top 5 Facilities, 1992 TRI	
First Chemical Corp., Pascagoula, MS	4,046,638,711
Goodyear Tire & Rubber Co., Beaumont, TX	2,526,855,525
Uno-Ven Co., Lemont, IL	488,229,292
Solvay Polymers Inc., Deer Park, TX	412,262,000
Cyprus Miami Mining Corp., Claypool, AZ	394,955,000

Top 5 Facilities, 1991 BRS	
Kodak Park, Rochester, NY	83,225,844,980
Dow Chemical Company, Midland, MI	60,274,801,720
Amoco Oil Company Refinery, Texas City, TX	52,275,053,600
DuPont-Chambers Works, Deepwater, NJ	48,843,789,760
Shell Oil Company, Deer Park, TX	38,738,555,340

TRI Production-related Waste, 1991-1994*

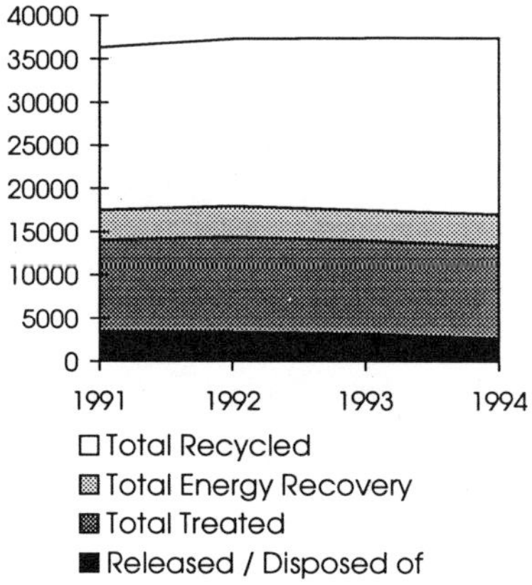

Total TRI Releases, 1992

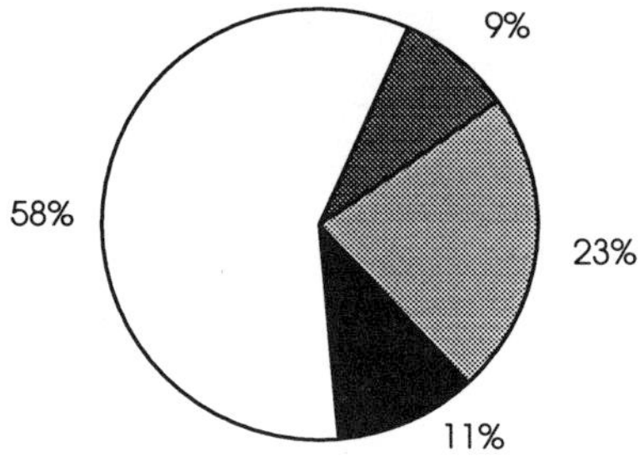

Total: 3,181.6 Million Pounds

Total Air Emissions	58%
Surface Water Discharges	9%
Underground Injection	23%
Releases to Land	11%

	Pounds	Pounds	Pounds
Facility with Largest Reported TRI Increase	**1991**	**1992**	**Increase**
Doe Run Co., Boss, MO	50,358,284	231,500,858	181,142,574
Facility with Largest Reported TRI Decrease	**1991**	**1992**	**Decrease**
DuPont Chambers Works, Deepwater, NJ	243,531,644	69,782,276	-173,749,368
Facility with Largest Projected TRI Increase	**1992**	**1994***	**Increase**
Goodyear Tire & Rubber Co., Beaumont, TX	2,526,855,525	3,027,332,113	500,476,588
Facility with Largest Projected TRI Decrease	**1992**	**1994***	**Decrease**
SCM Chemicals, Baltimore, MD	287,807,796	36,808,552	-250,999,244

*Projected ** Rank out of 20 industries (BRS) or 22 industries (TRI)

Appendix N

Industry and Waste: Additional Toxics Release Inventory (TRI) Data

Table N-1. TRI Production-related Waste on Forms Reporting and Not Reporting Source Reduction Activity, by Industry, 1991-1994

	Recycled On-site				
SIC Code Industry	**1991** Pounds	**1992** Pounds	**Change 1991-1992** Percent	**Projected 1994** Pounds	**Projected Change 1992-1994** Percent
On Forms Reporting No Source Reduction Activity					
20 Food	20,949,835	21,586,237	3.0	20,455,357	-5.2
21 Tobacco	0	0	—	0	—
22 Textiles	7,825,610	6,935,667	-11.4	7,011,619	1.1
23 Apparel	139,732	162,303	16.2	108,794	-33.0
24 Lumber	12,777,839	15,621,710	22.3	14,238,718	-8.9
25 Furniture	1,379,165	1,140,990	-17.3	1,245,096	9.1
26 Paper	167,086,903	106,209,137	-36.4	103,565,741	-2.5
27 Printing	85,865,661	88,033,887	2.5	90,788,240	3.1
28 Chemicals	9,335,609,236	9,499,279,500	1.8	10,202,868,500	7.4
29 Petroleum	324,697,775	366,287,241	12.8	367,790,109	0.4
30 Plastics	216,896,359	261,421,086	20.5	141,357,981	-45.9
31 Leather	816,676	875,117	7.2	1,032,089	17.9
32 Stone/Clay	168,897,621	35,205,562	-79.2	57,877,235	64.4
33 Primary Metals	1,231,931,110	1,420,206,559	15.3	1,575,069,163	10.9
34 Fabr. Metals	39,554,420	49,417,537	24.9	36,698,039	-25.7
35 Machinery	18,409,383	16,267,331	-11.6	18,212,195	12.0
36 Electrical	174,731,641	151,940,607	-13.0	134,196,630	-11.7
37 Transportation	38,716,032	39,494,091	2.0	33,555,416	-15.0
38 Measure./Photo.	4,750,695	3,447,359	-27.4	3,420,811	-0.8
39 Miscellaneous	6,272,537	8,471,095	35.1	6,570,542	-22.4
Multiple codes 20-39	750,455,461	573,849,108	-23.5	819,635,112	42.8
No codes 20-39	10,399,204	5,557,624	-46.6	30,584,058	450.3
Subtotal	12,618,162,895	12,671,409,748	0.4	13,666,281,445	7.9
On Forms Reporting Source Reduction Activity					
20 Food	8,296,368	10,115,489	21.9	11,152,707	10.3
21 Tobacco	50,077,709	55,317,334	10.5	416,844	-99.2
22 Textiles	3,882,262	4,012,075	3.3	3,725,020	-7.2
23 Apparel	25,998	34,925	34.3	19,628	-43.8
24 Lumber	11,557,021	2,984,014	-74.2	1,962,845	-34.2
25 Furniture	1,450,972	1,140,926	-21.4	1,426,502	25.0
26 Paper	58,217,561	63,327,751	8.8	63,720,139	0.6
27 Printing	94,885,936	102,120,073	7.6	91,724,652	-10.2
28 Chemicals	1,841,318,866	1,794,107,855	-2.6	1,878,314,676	4.7
29 Petroleum	14,408,122	19,174,885	33.1	19,119,261	-0.3
30 Plastics	37,168,071	40,260,802	8.3	44,529,316	10.6
31 Leather	72,086	41,889	-41.9	42,593	1.7
32 Stone/Clay	54,706,393	61,222,659	11.9	67,124,648	9.6
33 Primary Metals	361,049,612	380,441,193	5.4	441,324,446	16.0
34 Fabr. Metals	200,785,911	209,468,891	4.3	202,761,654	-3.2
35 Machinery	85,338,731	82,073,839	-3.8	64,088,499	-21.9
36 Electrical	147,461,183	138,604,739	-6.0	111,153,693	-19.8
37 Transportation	32,311,810	24,910,939	-22.9	7,971,845	-68.0
38 Measure./Photo.	5,793,620	5,978,938	3.2	903,130	-84.9
39 Miscellaneous	3,380,859	2,390,377	-29.3	1,994,556	-16.6
Multiple codes 20-39	222,065,096	214,786,226	-3.3	231,814,609	7.9
No codes 20-39	265,305	269,321	1.5	277,303	3.0
Subtotal	3,234,519,492	3,212,785,140	-0.7	3,245,568,566	1.0

Recyled Off-site				
1991 Pounds	**1992** Pounds	**Change 1991-1992** Percent	**Projected 1994** Pounds	**Projected Change 1992-1994** Percent
1,041,214	950,393	-8.7	1,089,449	14.6
0	0	—	0	—
229,782	313,684	36.5	258,550	-17.6
71,620	283,877	296.4	223,297	-21.3
863,109	816,866	-5.4	772,461	-5.4
1,039,967	1,508,815	45.1	1,354,106	-10.3
2,562,817	2,360,514	-7.9	1,044,188	-55.8
1,968,966	1,719,794	-12.7	1,102,819	-35.9
358,128,246	396,981,224	10.8	384,092,654	-3.2
484,023,995	564,009,195	16.5	574,775,827	1.9
7,273,068	11,395,504	56.7	15,185,434	33.3
1,484,122	1,760,100	18.6	2,446,389	39.0
1,570,825	1,974,527	25.7	1,578,773	-20.0
496,305,710	661,048,476	33.2	545,459,691	-17.5
175,633,593	212,888,288	21.2	214,112,675	0.6
29,642,424	34,638,998	16.9	36,478,175	5.3
172,727,979	169,320,123	-2.0	168,088,128	-0.7
104,132,938	128,831,565	23.7	130,926,577	1.6
7,457,766	8,735,490	17.1	8,138,266	-6.8
8,792,461	10,187,032	15.9	6,599,451	-35.2
237,932,413	268,948,632	13.0	184,589,400	-31.4
7,288,256	6,261,791	-14.1	6,115,172	-2.3
2,100,171,271	2,484,934,888	18.3	2,284,431,482	-8.1
72,349	379,848	425.0	122,544	-67.7
3,917	1,914	-51.1	0	-100.0
1,050,641	1,254,766	19.4	790,199	-37.0
990	1,300	31.3	1,300	0.0
245,340	211,449	-13.8	159,972	-24.3
1,670,855	1,609,780	-3.7	1,662,617	3.3
1,119,776	889,100	-20.6	658,841	-25.9
3,152,084	2,697,571	-14.4	2,402,666	-10.9
107,179,378	107,380,237	0.2	99,718,536	-7.1
293,904,169	353,379,975	20.2	426,741,789	20.8
6,910,270	6,317,099	-8.6	4,390,144	-30.5
498,178	294,793	-40.8	298,675	1.3
1,687,869	1,126,700	-33.2	855,144	-24.1
189,430,688	205,296,086	8.4	377,413,960	83.8
38,066,514	37,201,949	-2.3	33,937,878	-8.8
10,227,130	9,598,597	-6.1	6,967,401	-27.4
142,069,201	181,914,347	28.0	137,685,324	-24.3
33,286,376	34,801,362	4.6	36,118,824	3.8
10,201,154	8,481,313	-16.9	6,219,076	-26.7
2,711,416	2,836,910	4.6	2,429,731	-14.4
33,055,924	33,193,394	0.4	31,568,658	-4.9
96,839	91,131	-5.9	80,215	-12.0
876,641,058	988,959,621	12.8	1,170,223,494	18.3

Table N-1. TRI Production-related Waste on Forms Reporting and Not Reporting Source Reduction Activity, by Industry, 1991-1994 (cont'd.)

SIC Code Industry	Energy Recovery On-site 1991 Pounds	1992 Pounds	Change 1991-1992 Percent	Projected 1994 Pounds	Projected Change 1992-1994 Percent
On Forms Reporting No Source Reduction Activity					
20 Food	156,802	146,277	-6.7	237,496	62.4
21 Tobacco	0	0	—	0	—
22 Textiles	328,793	451,088	37.2	452,088	0.2
23 Apparel	0	0	—	0	—
24 Lumber	69,509	91,810	32.1	139,687	52.1
25 Furniture	7,062	4,325	-38.8	4,360	0.8
26 Paper	201,273,704	224,389,783	11.5	235,632,252	5.0
27 Printing	618,907	551,101	-11.0	58,800	-89.3
28 Chemicals	746,240,110	791,532,287	6.1	707,583,424	-10.6
29 Petroleum	456,707,187	447,500,658	-2.0	432,742,644	-3.3
30 Plastics	12,351,857	11,117,867	-10.0	9,462,210	-14.9
31 Leather	0	0	—	0	—
32 Stone/Clay	307,515,100	303,995,979	-1.1	441,504,002	45.2
33 Primary Metals	31,686,503	29,997,836	-5.3	28,216,194	-5.9
34 Fabr. Metals	73,000,972	63,680,957	-12.8	129,376,899	103.2
35 Machinery	166,600	250,950	50.6	250,950	0.0
36 Electrical	4,245,353	5,162,529	21.6	1,890,850	-63.4
37 Transportation	1,127,999	457,302	-59.5	428,079	-6.4
38 Measure./Photo.	291,000	633,644	117.7	580,000	-8.5
39 Miscellaneous	0	0	—	0	—
Multiple codes 20-39	136,702,617	78,290,662	-42.7	93,921,530	20.0
No codes 20-39	4,003,700	0	-100.0	0	—
Subtotal	1,976,493,775	1,958,255,055	-0.9	2,082,481,465	6.3
On Forms Reporting Source Reduction Activity					
20 Food	9,616	9,805	2.0	14,000	42.8
21 Tobacco	0	0	—	0	—
22 Textiles	3,341,116	4,210,058	26.0	4,479,101	6.4
23 Apparel	0	0	—	0	—
24 Lumber	4,442,316	1,620,644	-63.5	1,586,867	-2.1
25 Furniture	28,418	36,125	27.1	39,988	10.7
26 Paper	24,433,398	26,192,856	7.2	23,470,205	-10.4
27 Printing	158,877	113,479	-28.6	28,000	-75.3
28 Chemicals	343,961,789	319,702,326	-7.1	316,270,132	-1.1
29 Petroleum	128,409,257	235,416,044	83.3	196,608,952	-16.5
30 Plastics	3,270,148	3,564,617	9.0	4,460,522	25.1
31 Leather	0	0	—	0	—
32 Stone/Clay	280,462,900	300,972,565	7.3	369,322,400	22.7
33 Primary Metals	14,613,363	18,374,718	25.7	19,531,902	6.3
34 Fabr. Metals	12,261,823	18,496,564	50.8	17,832,468	-3.6
35 Machinery	16,926	5,092	-69.9	47	-99.1
36 Electrical	1,193,949	1,619,353	35.6	2,023,788	25.0
37 Transportation	1,978,925	1,611,002	-18.6	1,856,530	15.2
38 Measure./Photo.	219,570	433,456	97.4	390,000	-10.0
39 Miscellaneous	599,786	666,634	11.1	1,339,400	100.9
Multiple codes 20-39	46,181,987	49,255,606	6.7	49,424,204	0.3
No codes 20-39	380,000	666,114	75.3	524,400	-21.3
Subtotal	865,964,164	982,967,058	13.5	1,009,202,906	2.7

Energy Recovery Off-site				
1991 Pounds	**1992** Pounds	**Change 1991-1992** Percent	**Projected 1994** Pounds	**Projected Change 1992-1994** Percent
124,718	121,653	-2.5	116,825	-4.0
0	0	—	0	—
1,050,220	841,831	-19.8	737,945	-12.3
515,800	402,783	-21.9	328,897	-18.3
757,037	1,278,802	68.9	1,198,240	-6.3
3,563,527	4,570,862	28.3	4,579,999	0.2
3,529,787	3,636,538	3.0	3,330,313	-8.4
2,546,399	2,814,787	10.5	2,359,308	-16.2
190,122,247	227,226,025	19.5	208,127,270	-8.4
760,458	1,964,086	158.3	1,095,786	-44.2
6,129,366	6,476,344	5.7	6,078,296	-6.1
74,696	110,666	48.2	5,335	-95.2
7,305,237	2,979,966	-59.2	2,416,159	-18.9
1,873,938	6,393,767	241.2	6,433,978	0.6
7,802,858	8,625,955	10.5	7,900,304	-8.4
2,177,376	2,575,060	18.3	2,685,149	4.3
5,138,539	5,442,544	5.9	5,141,981	-5.5
10,092,546	10,120,342	0.3	9,079,546	-10.3
2,684,466	3,250,448	21.1	2,915,314	-10.3
1,938,826	1,376,719	-29.0	1,390,974	1.0
5,566,577	6,553,497	17.7	6,075,219	-7.3
594,212	600,498	1.1	314,237	-47.7
254,348,830	297,363,173	16.9	272,311,075	-8.4
3,140	2,608	-16.9	2,105	-19.3
7,193	6,882	-4.3	21	-99.7
1,344,259	575,673	-57.2	510,676	-11.3
47	2,213	4608.5	2,000	-9.6
1,734,844	1,442,256	-16.9	1,353,575	-6.1
2,617,106	2,524,986	-3.5	2,445,806	-3.1
3,783,881	3,992,932	5.5	3,215,656	-19.5
1,981,976	1,997,388	0.8	1,405,610	-29.6
107,732,225	115,436,475	7.2	102,434,107	-11.3
149,435,909	147,898,741	-1.0	155,291,570	5.0
5,106,596	5,481,550	7.3	4,532,638	-17.3
865,427	856,001	-1.1	293,667	-65.7
343,473	384,589	12.0	556,060	44.6
11,001,064	12,384,806	12.6	10,160,458	-18.0
4,249,135	5,445,046	28.1	4,746,393	-12.8
1,038,536	868,222	-16.4	623,177	-28.2
6,536,747	5,755,574	-12.0	4,351,874	-24.4
13,951,048	12,586,698	-9.8	13,377,992	6.3
1,518,994	1,666,200	9.7	1,276,854	-23.4
716,909	635,925	-11.3	474,944	-25.3
12,308,191	10,533,847	-14.4	10,459,801	-0.7
84,741	112,815	33.1	8,108	-92.8
326,361,441	330,591,427	1.3	317,523,092	-4.0

Table N-1. TRI Production-related Waste on Forms Reporting and Not Reporting Source Reduction Activity, by Industry, 1991-1994 (cont'd.)

	Treated On-site				
SIC Code Industry	**1991** Pounds	**1992** Pounds	**Change 1991-1992** Percent	**Projected 1994** Pounds	**Projected Change 1992-1994** Percent
On Forms Reporting No Source Reduction Activity					
20 Food	239,472,316	247,360,662	3.3	253,128,000	2.3
21 Tobacco	1,321,157	1,260,317	-4.6	1,337,700	6.1
22 Textiles	30,956,725	31,594,962	2.1	30,278,886	-4.2
23 Apparel	386,343	397,538	2.9	323,523	-18.6
24 Lumber	2,568,504	2,853,874	11.1	2,924,331	2.5
25 Furniture	1,062,040	1,690,846	59.2	2,094,650	23.9
26 Paper	1,377,098,340	1,584,508,958	15.1	1,556,426,588	-1.8
27 Printing	7,555,542	10,172,197	34.6	5,605,578	-44.9
28 Chemicals	2,952,722,763	2,923,434,220	-1.0	2,678,108,349	-8.4
29 Petroleum	282,634,816	373,531,324	32.2	316,607,220	-15.2
30 Plastics	33,998,086	42,607,421	25.3	45,725,605	7.3
31 Leather	20,986,402	24,379,779	16.2	26,825,845	10.0
32 Stone/Clay	127,763,863	181,923,488	42.4	182,526,571	0.3
33 Primary Metals	411,855,285	427,447,211	3.8	446,768,237	4.5
34 Fabr. Metals	189,030,012	175,938,599	-6.9	175,877,171	-0.0
35 Machinery	17,060,745	16,712,293	-2.0	16,499,799	-1.3
36 Electrical	180,949,600	161,335,357	-10.8	165,796,442	2.8
37 Transportation	45,515,525	50,066,199	10.0	54,129,837	8.1
38 Measure./Photo.	13,737,394	16,002,422	16.5	18,133,769	13.3
39 Miscellaneous	4,408,691	5,285,293	19.9	4,795,308	-9.3
Multiple codes 20-39	616,664,362	732,982,971	18.9	577,610,745	-21.2
No codes 20-39	114,697,803	163,175,788	42.3	191,112,001	17.1
Subtotal	6,672,446,314	7,174,661,719	7.5	6,752,636,155	-5.9
On Forms Reporting Source Reduction Activity					
20 Food	29,114,455	27,850,026	-4.3	24,165,507	-13.2
21 Tobacco	0	0	—	0	—
22 Textiles	17,202,789	18,057,682	5.0	10,896,493	-39.7
23 Apparel	210	306	45.7	337	10.1
24 Lumber	1,743,649	1,634,889	-6.2	1,592,902	-2.6
25 Furniture	519,211	465,837	-10.3	466,317	0.1
26 Paper	338,132,977	229,706,208	-32.1	190,304,527	-17.2
27 Printing	25,051,586	28,029,520	11.9	35,851,702	27.9
28 Chemicals	1,787,250,484	1,800,175,794	0.7	2,032,135,842	12.9
29 Petroleum	347,221,024	359,973,354	3.7	341,095,213	-5.2
30 Plastics	23,605,870	25,283,188	7.1	24,304,991	-3.9
31 Leather	947,429	1,161,841	22.6	1,025,781	-11.7
32 Stone/Clay	20,808,148	14,569,753	-30.0	16,322,665	12.0
33 Primary Metals	281,775,488	334,170,367	18.6	349,375,982	4.6
34 Fabr. Metals	36,781,245	35,654,959	-3.1	33,508,139	-6.0
35 Machinery	2,774,337	2,970,248	7.1	2,688,825	-9.5
36 Electrical	66,601,906	55,102,743	-17.3	57,287,399	4.0
37 Transportation	13,837,349	11,976,060	-13.5	11,030,763	-7.9
38 Measure./Photo.	30,778,997	35,606,850	15.7	35,488,109	-0.3
39 Miscellaneous	1,803,192	1,863,422	3.3	1,675,073	-10.1
Multiple codes 20-39	166,747,096	164,412,181	-1.4	172,869,937	5.1
No codes 20-39	3,003,147	3,422,547	14.0	2,936,145	-14.2
Subtotal	3,195,700,589	3,152,087,775	-1.4	3,345,022,649	6.1

Treated Off-site				
1991 Pounds	**1992** Pounds	**Change 1991-1992** Percent	**Projected 1994** Pounds	**Projected Change 1992-1994** Percent
27,586,149	28,734,510	4.2	25,479,859	-11.3
2,144	1,822	-15.0	20	-98.9
3,174,785	5,269,136	66.0	3,564,738	-32.3
103,474	141,259	36.5	59,345	-58.0
595,121	629,309	5.7	295,857	-53.0
424,071	493,315	16.3	355,701	-27.9
46,741,174	49,326,259	5.5	48,860,444	-0.9
567,737	534,833	-5.8	539,781	0.9
228,106,113	253,541,711	11.2	222,335,181	-12.3
5,017,328	3,310,301	-34.0	3,638,766	9.9
2,064,181	2,818,024	36.5	2,735,037	-2.9
4,175,364	4,226,677	1.2	4,127,653	-2.3
1,361,361	3,357,486	146.6	1,527,688	-54.5
52,568,338	58,187,558	10.7	55,746,378	-4.2
15,430,442	20,369,126	32.0	14,517,169	-28.7
2,612,777	3,275,473	25.4	2,885,418	-11.9
14,266,815	12,757,017	-10.6	12,050,605	-5.5
11,891,051	10,126,645	-14.8	9,303,077	-8.1
4,264,658	4,430,057	3.9	3,558,358	-19.7
526,603	553,575	5.1	351,345	-36.5
24,196,649	26,480,106	9.4	21,246,213	-19.8
1,378,838	1,847,844	34.0	1,540,290	-16.6
447,055,173	490,412,043	9.7	434,718,923	-11.4
7,991,255	8,089,536	1.2	8,914,342	10.2
5,650	3,150	-44.2	3,310	5.1
2,470,552	2,021,433	-18.2	1,456,973	-27.9
31,202	47,166	51.2	6,693	-85.8
245,582	283,281	15.4	82,976	-70.7
509,895	542,389	6.4	413,607	-23.7
6,395,858	5,721,739	-10.5	5,788,297	1.2
963,712	358,484	-62.8	238,882	-33.4
98,250,490	93,378,928	-5.0	83,707,929	-10.4
2,335,155	1,684,544	-27.9	1,706,330	1.3
1,852,636	1,897,607	2.4	1,417,203	-25.3
430,352	477,144	10.9	393,032	-17.6
1,265,254	1,718,913	35.9	464,636	-73.0
74,517,007	37,464,516	-49.7	30,882,385	-17.6
6,269,792	6,512,500	3.9	4,586,951	-29.6
1,245,784	1,296,655	4.1	958,996	-26.0
4,952,808	4,932,965	-0.4	3,306,561	-33.0
4,328,324	3,294,811	-23.9	2,714,279	-17.6
1,145,027	1,564,974	36.7	1,319,779	-15.7
874,375	964,179	10.3	593,445	-38.5
15,950,184	14,457,442	-9.4	13,785,562	-4.6
1,282,031	1,249,451	-2.5	1,154,749	-7.6
233,312,925	187,961,807	-19.4	163,896,917	-12.8

Table N-1. TRI Production-related Waste on Forms Reporting and Not Reporting Source Reduction Activity, by Industry, 1991-1994 (cont'd.)

SIC Code Industry	Releases and Off-site Disposal				
	1991 Pounds	**1992** Pounds	**Change 1991-1992** Percent	**Projected 1994** Pounds	**Projected Change 1992-1994** Percent
On Forms Reporting No Source Reduction Activity					
20 Food	33,543,739	34,154,421	1.8	30,358,046	-11.1
21 Tobacco	2,131,157	1,923,258	-9.8	1,987,570	3.3
22 Textiles	14,141,819	14,526,626	2.7	13,108,213	-9.8
23 Apparel	1,301,037	1,447,775	11.3	775,193	-46.5
24 Lumber	17,127,328	20,742,569	21.1	39,599,728	90.9
25 Furniture	26,254,446	29,579,880	12.7	27,551,851	-6.9
26 Paper	206,777,723	190,993,143	-7.6	173,999,328	-8.9
27 Printing	20,714,139	19,438,160	-6.2	18,535,844	-4.6
28 Chemicals	787,854,232	835,223,866	6.0	670,152,374	-19.8
29 Petroleum	49,567,861	50,648,925	2.2	45,518,735	-10.1
30 Plastics	76,903,715	79,491,856	3.4	68,074,431	-14.4
31 Leather	8,361,793	11,690,066	39.8	12,020,383	2.8
32 Stone/Clay	15,980,519	16,962,244	6.1	15,734,391	-7.2
33 Primary Metals	288,151,988	282,030,164	-2.1	302,979,023	7.4
34 Fabr. Metals	75,384,000	80,429,150	6.7	67,678,118	-15.9
35 Machinery	19,960,564	19,863,952	-0.5	13,955,473	-29.7
36 Electrical	39,725,910	42,908,880	8.0	32,369,687	-24.6
37 Transportation	80,836,636	85,910,543	6.3	75,792,445	-11.8
38 Measure./Photo.	14,061,051	13,372,631	-4.9	6,356,238	-52.5
39 Miscellaneous	11,401,922	12,243,161	7.4	8,401,481	-31.4
Multiple codes 20-39	166,634,227	152,544,975	-8.5	99,282,425	-34.9
No codes 20-39	11,823,799	13,447,420	13.7	12,347,732	-8.2
Subtotal	1,968,639,605	2,009,573,665	2.1	1,736,578,709	-13.6
On Forms Reporting Source Reduction Activity					
20 Food	12,330,010	10,135,680	-17.8	7,571,513	-25.3
21 Tobacco	1,497,865	1,670,763	11.5	8,904	-99.5
22 Textiles	11,221,349	10,159,249	-9.5	7,228,831	-28.8
23 Apparel	306,719	225,469	-26.5	171,512	-23.9
24 Lumber	13,107,588	12,880,141	-1.7	9,916,183	-23.0
25 Furniture	22,202,901	20,918,832	-5.8	19,212,831	-8.2
26 Paper	54,291,412	46,266,894	-14.8	35,327,443	-23.6
27 Printing	20,844,879	16,231,412	-22.1	13,558,075	-16.5
28 Chemicals	787,993,228	739,926,885	-6.1	473,009,209	-36.1
29 Petroleum	23,792,241	20,600,055	-13.4	17,337,680	-15.8
30 Plastics	74,521,553	69,161,417	-7.2	49,792,449	-28.0
31 Leather	6,275,262	6,606,146	5.3	3,655,663	-44.7
32 Stone/Clay	10,308,514	9,182,186	-10.9	7,273,362	-20.8
33 Primary Metals	208,192,136	170,559,719	-18.1	156,102,942	-8.5
34 Fabr. Metals	44,887,122	38,526,986	-14.2	27,988,269	-27.4
35 Machinery	20,676,480	16,603,341	-19.7	8,079,536	-51.3
36 Electrical	33,854,594	26,779,585	-20.9	15,143,191	-43.5
37 Transportation	67,758,663	57,772,162	-14.7	49,307,958	-14.7
38 Measure./Photo.	26,065,125	22,135,895	-15.1	14,599,862	-34.0
39 Miscellaneous	8,269,069	7,540,185	-8.8	4,882,422	-35.2
Multiple codes 20-39	96,138,338	85,888,695	-10.7	57,954,677	-32.5
No codes 20-39	2,610,497	2,040,808	-21.8	1,412,142	-30.8
Subtotal	1,547,145,545	1,391,812,505	-10.0	979,534,654	-29.6

Total Production-related Waste				
1991 Pounds	**1992** Pounds	**Change 1991-1992** Percent	**Projected 1994** Pounds	**Projected Change 1992-1994** Percent
322,874,773	333,054,153	3.2	330,865,032	-0.7
3,454,458	3,185,397	-7.8	3,325,290	4.4
57,707,734	59,932,994	3.9	55,412,039	-7.5
2,518,006	2,835,535	12.6	1,819,049	-35.8
34,758,447	42,034,940	20.9	59,169,022	40.8
33,730,278	38,989,033	15.6	37,185,763	-4.6
2,005,070,448	2,161,424,332	7.8	2,122,858,854	-1.8
119,837,351	123,264,759	2.9	118,990,370	-3.5
14,598,782,947	14,927,218,833	2.2	15,073,267,752	1.0
1,603,409,420	1,807,251,730	12.7	1,742,169,087	-3.6
355,616,632	415,328,102	16.8	288,618,994	-30.5
35,899,053	43,042,405	19.9	46,457,694	7.9
630,394,526	546,399,252	-13.3	703,164,819	28.7
2,514,372,872	2,885,311,571	14.8	2,960,672,664	2.6
575,836,297	611,349,612	6.2	646,160,375	5.7
90,029,869	93,584,057	3.9	90,967,159	-2.8
591,785,837	548,867,057	-7.3	519,534,323	-5.3
292,312,727	325,006,687	11.2	313,214,977	-3.6
47,247,030	49,872,051	5.6	43,102,756	-13.6
33,341,040	38,116,875	14.3	28,109,101	-26.3
1,938,152,306	1,839,649,951	-5.1	1,802,360,644	-2.0
150,185,812	190,890,965	27.1	242,013,490	26.8
26,037,317,863	27,086,610,291	4.0	27,229,439,254	0.5
57,817,193	56,582,992	-2.1	51,942,718	-8.2
51,592,334	57,000,043	10.5	429,079	-99.2
40,512,968	40,290,936	-0.5	29,087,293	-27.8
365,166	311,379	-14.7	201,470	-35.3
33,076,340	21,056,674	-36.3	16,655,320	-20.9
28,999,358	27,238,875	-6.1	25,667,668	-5.8
486,374,863	376,097,480	-22.7	322,485,108	-14.3
147,039,050	151,547,927	3.1	145,209,587	-4.2
5,073,686,460	4,970,108,500	-2.0	4,985,590,431	0.3
959,505,877	1,138,127,598	18.6	1,157,900,795	1.7
152,435,144	151,966,280	-0.3	133,427,263	-12.2
9,088,734	9,437,814	3.8	5,709,411	-39.5
369,582,551	389,177,365	5.3	461,918,915	18.7
1,140,579,358	1,158,691,405	1.6	1,384,792,075	19.5
343,301,542	351,306,895	2.3	325,361,752	-7.4
121,317,924	113,415,994	-6.5	83,406,481	-26.5
402,670,388	414,709,306	3.0	330,951,830	-20.2
167,452,495	146,953,034	-12.2	122,378,191	-16.7
75,722,487	75,867,626	0.2	60,196,810	-20.7
18,355,606	16,897,632	-7.9	13,389,571	-20.8
592,446,816	572,527,391	-3.4	567,877,448	-0.8
7,722,560	7,852,187	1.7	6,393,062	-18.6
10,279,645,214	10,247,165,333	-0.3	10,230,972,278	-0.2

Table N-2. TRI Production-related Waste on All Forms, by Industry, 1991-1994

SIC Code Industry	Recycled On-site 1991 Pounds	1992 Pounds	Change 1991-1992 Percent	Projected 1994 Pounds	Projected Change 1992-1994 Percent
20 Food	29,246,203	31,701,726	8.4	31,608,064	-0.3
21 Tobacco	50,077,709	55,317,334	10.5	416,844	-99.2
22 Textiles	11,707,872	10,947,742	-6.5	10,736,639	-1.9
23 Apparel	165,730	197,228	19.0	128,422	-34.9
24 Lumber	24,334,860	18,605,724	-23.5	16,201,563	-12.9
25 Furniture	2,830,137	2,281,916	-19.4	2,671,598	17.1
26 Paper	225,304,464	169,536,888	-24.8	167,285,880	-1.3
27 Printing	180,751,597	190,153,960	5.2	182,512,892	-4.0
28 Chemicals	11,176,928,102	11,293,387,355	1.0	12,081,183,176	7.0
29 Petroleum	339,105,897	385,462,126	13.7	386,909,370	0.4
30 Plastics	254,064,430	301,681,888	18.7	185,887,297	-38.4
31 Leather	888,762	917,006	3.2	1,074,682	17.2
32 Stone/Clay	223,604,014	96,428,221	-56.9	125,001,883	29.6
33 Primary Metals	1,592,980,722	1,800,647,752	13.0	2,016,393,609	12.0
34 Fabr. Metals	240,340,331	258,886,428	7.7	239,459,693	-7.5
35 Machinery	103,748,114	98,341,170	-5.2	82,300,694	-16.3
36 Electrical	322,192,824	290,545,346	-9.8	245,350,323	-15.6
37 Transportation	71,027,842	64,405,030	-9.3	41,527,261	-35.5
38 Measure./Photo.	10,544,315	9,426,297	-10.6	4,323,941	-54.1
39 Miscellaneous	9,653,396	10,861,472	12.5	8,565,098	-21.1
Multiple codes 20-39	972,520,557	788,635,334	-18.9	1,051,449,721	33.3
No codes 20-39	10,664,509	5,826,945	-45.4	30,861,361	429.6
Total	15,852,682,387	15,884,194,888	0.2	16,911,850,011	6.5

SIC Code Industry	Energy Recovery On-site 1991 Pounds	1992 Pounds	Change 1991-1992 Percent	Projected 1994 Pounds	Projected Change 1992-1994 Percent
20 Food	166,418	156,082	-6.2	251,496	61.1
21 Tobacco	0	0	—	0	—
22 Textiles	3,669,909	4,661,146	27.0	4,931,189	5.8
23 Apparel	0	0	—	0	—
24 Lumber	4,511,825	1,712,454	-62.0	1,726,554	0.8
25 Furniture	35,480	40,450	14.0	44,348	9.6
26 Paper	225,707,102	250,582,639	11.0	259,102,457	3.4
27 Printing	777,784	664,580	-14.6	86,800	-86.9
28 Chemicals	1,090,201,899	1,111,234,613	1.9	1,023,853,556	-7.9
29 Petroleum	585,116,444	682,916,702	16.7	629,351,596	-7.8
30 Plastics	15,622,005	14,682,484	-6.0	13,922,732	-5.2
31 Leather	0	0	—	0	—
32 Stone/Clay	587,978,000	604,968,544	2.9	810,826,402	34.0
33 Primary Metals	46,299,866	48,372,554	4.5	47,748,096	-1.3
34 Fabr. Metals	85,262,795	82,177,521	-3.6	147,209,367	79.1
35 Machinery	183,526	256,042	39.5	250,997	-2.0
36 Electrical	5,439,302	6,781,882	24.7	3,914,638	-42.3
37 Transportation	3,106,924	2,068,304	-33.4	2,284,609	10.5
38 Measure./Photo.	510,570	1,067,100	109.0	970,000	-9.1
39 Miscellaneous	599,786	666,634	11.1	1,339,400	100.9
Multiple codes 20-39	182,884,604	127,546,268	-30.3	143,345,734	12.4
No codes 20-39	4,383,700	666,114	-84.8	524,400	-21.3
Total	2,842,457,939	2,941,222,113	3.5	3,091,684,371	5.1

Recyled Off-site

1991 Pounds	1992 Pounds	Change 1991-1992 Percent	Projected 1994 Pounds	Projected Change 1992-1994 Percent
1,113,563	1,330,241	19.5	1,211,993	-8.9
3,917	1,914	-51.1	0	-100.0
1,280,423	1,568,450	22.5	1,048,749	-33.1
72,610	285,177	292.8	224,597	-21.2
1,108,449	1,028,315	-7.2	932,433	-9.3
2,710,822	3,118,595	15.0	3,016,723	-3.3
3,682,593	3,249,614	-11.8	1,703,029	-47.6
5,121,050	4,417,365	-13.7	3,505,485	-20.6
465,307,624	504,361,461	8.4	483,811,190	-4.1
777,928,164	917,389,170	17.9	1,001,517,616	9.2
14,183,338	17,712,603	24.9	19,575,578	10.5
1,982,300	2,054,893	3.7	2,745,064	33.6
3,258,694	3,101,227	-4.8	2,433,917	-21.5
685,736,398	866,344,562	26.3	922,873,651	6.5
213,700,107	250,090,237	17.0	248,050,553	-0.8
39,869,554	44,237,595	11.0	43,445,576	-1.8
314,797,180	351,234,470	11.6	305,773,452	-12.9
137,419,314	163,632,927	19.1	167,045,401	2.1
17,658,920	17,216,803	-2.5	14,357,342	-16.6
11,503,877	13,023,942	13.2	9,029,182	-30.7
270,988,337	302,142,026	11.5	216,158,058	-28.5
7,385,095	6,352,922	-14.0	6,195,387	-2.5
2,976,812,329	3,473,894,509	16.7	3,454,654,976	-0.6

Energy Recovery Off-site

1991 Pounds	1992 Pounds	Change 1991-1992 Percent	Projected 1994 Pounds	Projected Change 1992-1994 Percent
127,858	124,261	-2.8	118,930	-4.3
7,193	6,882	-4.3	21	-99.7
2,394,479	1,417,504	-40.8	1,248,621	-11.9
515,847	404,996	-21.5	330,897	-18.3
2,491,881	2,721,058	9.2	2,551,815	-6.2
6,180,633	7,095,848	14.8	7,025,805	-1.0
7,313,668	7,629,470	4.3	6,545,969	-14.2
4,528,375	4,812,175	6.3	3,764,918	-21.8
297,854,472	342,662,500	15.0	310,561,377	-9.4
150,196,367	149,862,827	-0.2	156,387,356	4.4
11,235,962	11,957,894	6.4	10,610,934	-11.3
940,123	966,667	2.8	299,002	-69.1
7,648,710	3,364,555	-56.0	2,972,219	-11.7
12,875,002	18,778,573	45.9	16,594,436	-11.6
12,051,993	14,071,001	16.8	12,646,697	-10.1
3,215,912	3,443,282	7.1	3,308,326	-3.9
11,675,286	11,198,118	-4.1	9,493,855	-15.2
24,043,594	22,707,040	-5.6	22,457,538	-1.1
4,203,460	4,916,648	17.0	4,192,168	-14.7
2,655,735	2,012,644	-24.2	1,865,918	-7.3
17,874,768	17,087,344	-4.4	16,535,020	-3.2
678,953	713,313	5.1	322,345	-54.8
580,710,271	627,954,600	8.1	589,834,167	-6.1

Table N-2. TRI Production-related Waste on All Forms, by Industry, 1991-1994 (cont'd.)

SIC Code Industry	1991 Pounds	1992 Pounds	Change 1991-1992 Percent	Projected 1994 Pounds	Projected Change 1992-1994 Percent
Treated On-site					
20 Food	268,586,771	275,210,688	2.5	277,293,507	0.8
21 Tobacco	1,321,157	1,260,317	-4.6	1,337,700	6.1
22 Textiles	48,159,514	49,652,644	3.1	41,175,379	-17.1
23 Apparel	386,553	397,844	2.9	323,860	-18.6
24 Lumber	4,312,153	4,488,763	4.1	4,517,233	0.6
25 Furniture	1,581,251	2,156,683	36.4	2,560,967	18.7
26 Paper	1,715,231,317	1,814,215,166	5.8	1,746,731,115	-3.7
27 Printing	32,607,128	38,201,717	17.2	41,457,280	8.5
28 Chemicals	4,739,973,247	4,723,610,014	-0.3	4,710,244,191	-0.3
29 Petroleum	629,855,840	733,504,678	16.5	657,702,433	-10.3
30 Plastics	57,603,956	67,890,609	17.9	70,030,596	3.2
31 Leather	21,933,831	25,541,620	16.4	27,851,626	9.0
32 Stone/Clay	148,572,011	196,493,241	32.3	198,849,236	1.2
33 Primary Metals	693,630,773	761,617,578	9.8	796,144,219	4.5
34 Fabr. Metals	225,811,257	211,593,558	-6.3	209,385,310	-1.0
35 Machinery	19,835,082	19,682,541	-0.8	19,188,624	-2.5
36 Electrical	247,551,506	216,438,100	-12.6	223,083,841	3.1
37 Transportation	59,352,874	62,042,259	4.5	65,160,600	5.0
38 Measure./Photo.	44,516,391	51,609,272	15.9	53,621,878	3.9
39 Miscellaneous	6,211,883	7,148,715	15.1	6,470,381	-9.5
Multiple codes 20-39	783,411,458	897,395,152	14.5	750,480,682	-16.4
No codes 20-39	117,700,950	166,598,335	41.5	194,048,146	16.5
Total	9,868,146,903	10,326,749,494	4.6	10,097,658,804	-2.2
Releases and Off-site Disposal					
20 Food	45,873,749	44,290,101	-3.5	37,929,559	-14.4
21 Tobacco	3,629,022	3,594,021	-1.0	1,996,474	-44.5
22 Textiles	25,363,168	24,685,875	-2.7	20,337,044	-17.6
23 Apparel	1,607,756	1,673,244	4.1	946,705	-43.4
24 Lumber	30,234,916	33,622,710	11.2	49,515,911	47.3
25 Furniture	48,457,347	50,498,712	4.2	46,764,682	-7.4
26 Paper	261,069,135	237,260,037	-9.1	209,326,771	-11.8
27 Printing	41,559,018	35,669,572	-14.2	32,093,919	-10.0
28 Chemicals	1,575,847,460	1,575,150,751	-0.0	1,143,161,583	-27.4
29 Petroleum	73,360,102	71,248,980	-2.9	62,856,415	-11.8
30 Plastics	151,425,268	148,653,273	-1.8	117,866,880	-20.7
31 Leather	14,637,055	18,296,212	25.0	15,676,046	-14.3
32 Stone/Clay	26,289,033	26,144,430	-0.6	23,007,753	-12.0
33 Primary Metals	496,344,124	452,589,883	-8.8	459,081,965	1.4
34 Fabr. Metals	120,271,122	118,956,136	-1.1	95,666,387	-19.6
35 Machinery	40,637,044	36,467,293	-10.3	22,035,009	-39.6
36 Electrical	73,580,504	69,688,465	-5.3	47,512,878	-31.8
37 Transportation	148,595,299	143,682,705	-3.3	125,100,403	-12.9
38 Measure./Photo.	40,126,176	35,508,526	-11.5	20,956,100	-41.0
39 Miscellaneous	19,670,991	19,783,346	0.6	13,283,903	-32.9
Multiple codes 20-39	262,772,565	238,433,670	-9.3	157,237,102	-34.1
No codes 20-39	14,434,296	15,488,228	7.3	13,759,874	-11.2
Total	3,515,785,150	3,401,386,170	-3.3	2,716,113,363	-20.1

Treated Off-site

1991 Pounds	1992 Pounds	Change 1991-1992 Percent	Projected 1994 Pounds	Projected Change 1992-1994 Percent
35,577,404	36,824,046	3.5	34,394,201	-6.6
7,794	4,972	-36.2	3,330	-33.0
5,645,337	7,290,569	29.1	5,021,711	-31.1
134,676	188,425	39.9	66,038	-65.0
840,703	912,590	8.6	378,833	-58.5
933,966	1,035,704	10.9	769,308	-25.7
53,137,032	55,047,998	3.6	54,648,741	-0.7
1,531,449	893,317	-41.7	778,663	-12.8
326,356,603	346,920,639	6.3	306,043,110	-11.8
7,352,483	4,994,845	-32.1	5,345,096	7.0
3,916,817	4,715,631	20.4	4,152,240	-11.9
4,605,716	4,703,821	2.1	4,520,685	-3.9
2,626,615	5,076,399	93.3	1,992,324	-60.8
127,085,345	95,652,074	-24.7	86,628,763	-9.4
21,700,234	26,881,626	23.9	19,104,120	-28.9
3,858,561	4,572,128	18.5	3,844,414	-15.9
19,219,623	17,689,982	-8.0	15,357,166	-13.2
16,219,375	13,421,456	-17.3	12,017,356	-10.5
5,409,685	5,995,031	10.8	4,878,137	-18.6
1,400,978	1,517,754	8.3	944,790	-37.8
40,146,833	40,937,548	2.0	35,031,775	-14.4
2,660,869	3,097,295	16.4	2,695,039	-13.0
680,368,098	678,373,850	-0.3	598,615,840	-11.8

Total Production-related Waste

1991 Pounds	1992 Pounds	Change 1991-1992 Percent	Projected 1994 Pounds	Projected Change 1992-1994 Percent
380,691,966	389,637,145	2.3	382,807,750	-1.8
55,046,792	60,185,440	9.3	3,754,369	-93.8
98,220,702	100,223,930	2.0	84,499,332	-15.7
2,883,172	3,146,914	9.1	2,020,519	-35.8
67,834,787	63,091,614	-7.0	75,824,342	20.2
62,729,636	66,227,908	5.6	62,853,431	-5.1
2,491,445,311	2,537,521,812	1.8	2,445,343,962	-3.6
266,876,401	274,812,686	3.0	264,199,957	-3.9
19,672,469,407	19,897,327,333	1.1	20,058,858,183	0.8
2,562,915,297	2,945,379,328	14.9	2,900,069,882	-1.5
508,051,776	567,294,382	11.7	422,046,257	-25.6
44,987,787	52,480,219	16.7	52,167,105	-0.6
999,977,077	935,576,617	-6.4	1,165,083,734	24.5
3,654,952,230	4,044,002,976	10.6	4,345,464,739	7.5
919,137,839	962,656,507	4.7	971,522,127	0.9
211,347,793	207,000,051	-2.1	174,373,640	-15.8
994,456,225	963,576,363	-3.1	850,486,153	-11.7
459,765,222	471,959,721	2.7	435,593,168	-7.7
122,969,517	125,739,677	2.3	103,299,566	-17.8
51,696,646	55,014,507	6.4	41,498,672	-24.6
2,530,599,122	2,412,177,342	-4.7	2,370,238,092	-1.7
157,908,372	198,743,152	25.9	248,406,552	25.0
36,316,963,077	37,333,775,624	2.8	37,460,411,532	0.3

Appendix O

Environmental Management of Toxics Release Inventory (TRI) Waste by Parent Companies: Total Waste, Carcinogens, Ozone Depleters

For this *Toxics Watch* report, data for parent companies were aggregated from facility TRI Section 8 data reported for 1992. Facilities are required to report their parent companies to TRI. Some facilities do not report any parent company, however, even if the facilities are not independent operating entities. In addition, some facilities may report a subsidiary parent rather than an ultimate parent company. Information available from Dun and Bradstreet was used to supplement parent company identification for facilities reporting to TRI in 1992.

Some caveats apply when aggregating data for parent companies. The 1991 TRI data used here are data that were reported on the 1992 forms.[a] This assumes that an individual facility had the same parent company for both 1991 and 1992, which may not have been the case. The same is true for facility projections for 1993 and 1994: Projections for parent companies in these tables are based on the 1992 parent company affiliations as identified for this report. Finally, since the Dun and Bradstreet data are updated periodically, they may represent affiliations formed since 1992 rather than the actual parent-facility relationship as it existed in 1992.

Tables O-1 through O-12 present aggregated parent company data for production-related waste, amounts of waste management, and releases and transfers to disposal. The data track changes in these quantities for 1991-1992, as well as projections for 1992-1994. Aggregate data for all TRI chemicals are presented, as well as data for ozone depleters and carcinogens as defined in Chapter 5.

[a] The TRI data used for this report were made available to the public by EPA in April 1994. EPA accepts revisions to TRI data continuously, and facilities may have revised their parent company affiliation since that time.

*Table O-1. 1992 Production-related Waste for the 100 TRI Parent Companies with Largest Total Production-related Waste in 1991**

Total Production-related Waste Rank* 1991 Rank	1992 Rank	Parent Company	1992 Total Production-related Waste Pounds	Recycling Percent	Energy Recovery Percent	Treated Percent	Released/ Disposed of Percent
				Type of Waste Management as Percent of Total Production-related Waste			
59	52	3M Minnesota Mining & Mfg Co	142,532,844	32.50	18.57	24.98	23.95
91	86	Albemarle Corporation	84,721,007	55.02	3.67	33.32	7.99
15	10	Allied-Signal Inc	393,304,084	30.96	2.13	63.77	3.13
78	82	Aluminum Company of America	92,774,032	33.09	10.18	46.77	9.96
24	20	American Cyanamid	292,663,520	30.14	4.58	13.64	51.64
26	65	American Petrofina Holding Co	116,650,527	9.32	13.09	75.29	2.31
58	147	American Telephone & Telgraph	49,782,766	55.51	1.04	38.76	4.69
18	14	Amoco Corporation	332,195,627	77.73	1.75	16.47	4.06
64	59	Archer Daniels Midland	129,950,718	12.47	0.00	86.05	1.48
67	64	Armco Inc	117,001,724	56.91	3.74	33.79	5.56
28	23	Asarco Incorporated	274,577,841	71.85	0.00	1.96	26.19
21	13	Atlantic Richfield Company	348,950,397	1.53	89.34	6.66	2.47
80	91	BASF Corporation	81,442,291	12.70	32.42	49.47	5.41
73	75	Boise Cascade Corporation	104,802,992	0.43	5.51	88.02	6.04
57	55	BP America Inc	138,890,631	22.79	20.27	17.80	39.15
25	28	Bristol-Myers Squibb Company	254,755,612	89.81	0.42	7.93	1.84
55	83	Cargill Incorporated	89,972,643	19.51	1.48	70.99	8.02
48	71	Champion International Corp	111,459,868	0.06	11.98	78.55	9.41
79	32	Chevron Corporation	230,084,763	30.44	2.19	62.67	4.71
76	70	Ciba-Geigy Corporation	111,885,784	22.43	1.73	73.03	2.80
29	27	Citgo Petroleum Corporation	257,398,721	88.20	0.00	9.45	2.34
75	50	Copper Range Company Inc	148,266,000	0.00	0.00	94.53	5.47
42	191	Corning Inc	33,013,240	78.95	0.36	7.56	13.13
22	24	Coulton Chemical Corp	273,469,050	99.10	0.05	0.83	0.02
39	39	Courtaulds United States Inc	199,372,005	69.69	0.66	7.57	22.08
7	9	Cyprus Minerals Company	406,802,516	99.16	0.00	0.00	0.84
9	6	Dow Chemical Company	517,495,767	18.54	17.21	60.85	3.40
96	114	Dow Corning Corporation	62,533,092	30.97	8.13	58.53	2.37
88	176	DSM Finance USA Inc	37,579,273	9.49	2.20	83.57	4.74
3	4	DuPont	781,956,864	7.05	10.85	51.29	30.81
77	61	East Penn Manufacturing Co Inc	127,434,250	98.80	0.00	0.95	0.25
11	34	Eastman Kodak Company	221,067,151	2.00	17.73	54.87	25.40
31	53	EC Acquisition Inc	141,554,974	42.94	0.00	55.72	1.34
12	18	Elf Aquitaine Inc	310,500,972	7.64	0.33	84.83	7.20
83	73	Eli Lilly and Company	105,701,269	3.59	0.01	88.37	8.04
84	79	Exxon Corporation	103,727,602	0.55	15.62	71.32	12.51
95	115	Farmland Industries Inc	61,778,149	52.37	12.16	16.04	19.43
1	1	First Mississippi Corporation	4,054,298,758	99.71	0.18	0.00	0.11
50	40	Ford Motor Company	193,092,838	67.90	1.40	15.30	15.40
90	88	Formosa Plastics Corp USA	82,648,902	39.47	20.85	38.96	0.72
44	46	Freeport-McMoran Inc	166,929,776	0.11	2.13	4.67	93.09
40	33	Gates Corporation	229,743,060	98.86	0.19	0.44	0.51
68	43	General Dynamics Corporation	171,466,568	0.61	0.08	98.45	0.87
53	48	General Electric Company	156,380,585	15.79	3.48	71.06	9.67
33	37	General Motors Corporation	205,303,728	59.34	3.29	15.54	21.83
94	108	Georgia Gulf Corporation	69,409,964	11.18	59.38	28.81	0.63
23	22	Georgia-Pacific Corporation	286,216,696	3.94	8.00	80.15	7.91
2	2	Goodyear Tire & Rubber Co	2,864,512,848	99.42	0.17	0.15	0.26
51	47	Hercules Incorporated	159,313,623	54.10	1.01	36.08	8.81
20	12	HM Anglo-American Ltd	349,598,460	2.15	0.21	95.20	2.44

* Top 100 parent companies with largest total production-related waste in 1991, listed alphabetically. Rank is among total of 10,840 parent companies.

Table O-1. 1992 Production-related Waste for the 100 TRI Parent Companies with Largest Total Production-related Waste in 1991 (cont'd.)*

Total Production-related Waste Rank* 1991 Rank	1992 Rank	Parent Company	1992 Total Production-related Waste Pounds	Type of Waste Management as Percent of Total Production-related Waste: Recycling Percent	Energy Recovery Percent	Treated Percent	Released/ Disposed of Percent
5	5	Hoechst Celanese Corporation	695,043,839	69.72	14.87	10.27	5.14
56	49	Holdernam Inc	152,788,233	0.02	99.92	0.00	0.06
87	112	IBM	64,804,317	70.37	3.81	24.52	1.29
13	11	International Paper Company	393,119,070	18.02	10.37	65.12	6.49
74	158	ITT Corporation	45,567,386	27.60	8.98	44.85	18.58
66	63	James River Corp Virginia	119,696,995	0.88	4.89	87.82	6.42
38	29	Johnson Controls Inc	248,804,407	99.07	0.17	0.56	0.20
14	15	Kemira Holdings Inc	316,522,270	82.14	0.00	17.55	0.31
27	26	Lafarge Corporation	272,588,945	0.00	99.74	0.18	0.09
54	116	Lyondell Petrochemical Co	61,142,072	0.99	34.82	61.60	2.59
69	68	Maxwell Communication Corp	112,364,873	89.76	0.55	0.09	9.60
93	103	Mead Corporation	72,966,918	10.14	1.80	79.31	8.74
43	51	Mobil Corporation	143,543,010	20.86	3.12	68.27	7.75
17	19	Monsanto Company	305,224,967	13.36	9.24	52.35	25.04
16	16	National Cooperative Refinery	312,856,711	0.00	99.75	0.10	0.15
85	95	Novacor Chemicals Inc	76,802,325	92.73	7.13	0.04	0.10
10	17	Occidental Petroleum Corp	310,551,333	19.97	10.77	60.75	8.52
92	92	Olin Corporation	81,244,608	27.32	0.06	69.69	2.93
47	157	Pacific Dunlop Holdings Inc	46,030,080	72.84	0.05	23.52	3.59
72	77	Pfizer Inc	104,309,696	80.42	3.54	11.64	4.40
34	99	Phillips Petroleum Company	75,822,794	51.83	11.45	28.38	8.34
19	21	PPG Industries Inc	286,962,296	61.64	6.21	30.09	2.06
97	105	Procter & Gamble Company	71,649,886	0.56	8.24	78.30	12.90
82	74	PVS Chemicals Inc	105,579,793	98.63	0.00	1.33	0.04
36	38	Quaker State Corporation	200,443,094	99.78	0.01	0.02	0.19
37	94	Reilly Industries Inc	77,653,080	90.14	7.71	1.72	0.43
60	57	Renco Group Inc	132,870,622	11.60	0.11	41.48	46.82
65	56	Rhone-Poulenc Inc	137,846,308	40.54	14.38	43.32	1.76
62	60	Rohm and Haas Company	128,840,024	5.51	13.54	78.83	2.12
99	89	Scott Paper Company	82,463,376	3.64	13.23	74.31	8.82
35	36	Shell Petroleum Inc	207,535,270	16.33	16.38	59.04	8.25
52	44	Shintech Inc	169,928,062	99.91	0.00	0.00	0.09
6	8	Solvay America Inc	413,270,803	96.18	0.14	3.49	0.18
70	58	Sterling Chemicals Inc	130,742,106	0.01	60.24	11.30	28.45
49	45	Stone Container Corporation	168,606,473	3.47	10.93	78.64	6.96
100	97	Tenneco Inc	76,486,963	13.07	10.68	67.41	8.85
4	3	Texaco Inc	850,779,190	66.75	8.22	24.07	0.96
86	84	Texas Olefins Company	86,059,770	39.51	51.32	8.82	0.35
41	41	Timken Co	190,028,461	48.09	0.00	51.46	0.45
98	102	U T I Corporation	74,152,474	98.84	0.00	0.09	1.08
71	72	Union Camp Corporation	109,937,394	0.68	19.50	70.20	9.63
45	31	Union Carbide Corporation	231,052,269	26.58	7.86	60.34	5.21
8	7	Uno-Ven Company	488,229,292	1.17	31.23	67.58	0.02
46	35	Upjohn Company	214,667,954	82.21	9.97	3.83	3.99
61	66	Vista Chemical Company	113,919,792	13.47	8.18	77.64	0.71
89	87	Warner-Lambert Company	82,916,356	88.81	5.11	1.69	4.40
63	67	Westinghouse Electric Corp	113,217,242	76.63	2.20	14.88	6.29
32	42	Weyerhaeuser Company	185,370,540	5.03	4.06	86.60	4.31
81	78	Witco Corporation	104,014,625	68.29	0.41	24.90	6.41
30	25	Zeneca Holdings Inc	272,952,202	2.64	1.72	86.07	9.57
		Subtotal	25,796,936,938	56.09	9.37	28.12	6.42
		Percent of Total	69.10				
		Total	37,333,775,624	51.85	9.56	29.48	9.11

Table O-2. The 100 TRI Parent Companies with Largest Total Production-related Waste in 1991: Change 1991-1992*

Total Production-related Waste Rank* 1991 Rank	1992 Rank	TRI Parent Company	Facilities Number	Change in Total Production-related Waste 1991 to 1992 Percent	Total Production-related Waste 1991 Pounds	1992 Pounds
59	52	3M Minnesota Mining & Mfg Co	49	6.93	133,295,212	142,532,844
91	86	Albemarle Corporation	4	7.18	79,048,168	84,721,007
15	10	Allied-Signal Inc	82	20.19	327,224,403	393,304,084
78	82	Aluminum Company of America	42	-9.21	102,182,930	92,774,032
24	20	American Cyanamid	31	8.88	268,790,236	292,663,520
26	65	American Petrofina Holding Co	7	-55.66	263,065,287	116,650,527
58	147	American Telephone & Telgraph	22	-63.30	135,648,848	49,782,766
18	14	Amoco Corporation	42	9.93	302,200,939	332,195,627
64	59	Archer Daniels Midland	44	4.64	124,189,340	129,950,718
67	64	Armco Inc	25	-1.36	118,617,631	117,001,724
28	23	Asarco Incorporated	12	18.91	230,912,617	274,577,841
21	13	Atlantic Richfield Company	11	21.98	286,073,412	348,950,397
80	91	BASF Corporation	41	-19.53	101,211,504	81,442,291
73	75	Boise Cascade Corporation	10	-3.37	108,455,786	104,802,992
57	55	BP America Inc	58	0.28	138,497,229	138,890,631
25	28	Bristol-Myers Squibb Company	15	-3.64	264,382,024	254,755,612
55	83	Cargill Incorporated	74	-37.37	143,667,165	89,972,643
48	71	Champion International Corp	19	-29.09	157,177,353	111,459,868
79	32	Chevron Corporation	27	126.53	101,570,843	230,084,763
76	70	Ciba-Geigy Corporation	16	6.82	104,743,646	111,885,784
29	27	Citgo Petroleum Corporation	3	11.73	230,374,230	257,398,721
75	50	Copper Range Company Inc	1	39.25	106,477,000	148,266,000
42	191	Corning Inc	23	-80.77	171,656,190	33,013,240
22	24	Coulton Chemical Corp	1	0.32	272,609,056	273,469,050
39	39	Courtaulds United States Inc	13	1.26	196,889,648	199,372,005
7	9	Cyprus Minerals Company	8	-9.57	449,838,157	406,802,516
9	6	Dow Chemical Company	26	29.32	400,178,093	517,495,767
96	114	Dow Corning Corporation	9	-17.11	75,438,320	62,533,092
88	176	DSM Finance USA Inc	7	-55.28	84,028,643	37,579,273
3	4	DuPont	82	-10.30	871,763,023	781,956,864
77	61	East Penn Manufacturing Co Inc	1	23.40	103,268,982	127,434,250
11	34	Eastman Kodak Company	22	-41.02	374,792,471	221,067,151
31	53	EC Acquisition Inc	14	-33.04	211,416,430	141,554,974
12	18	Elf Aquitaine Inc	29	-13.95	360,822,594	310,500,972
83	73	Eli Lilly and Company	13	14.03	92,694,642	105,701,269
84	79	Exxon Corporation	24	12.03	92,592,229	103,727,602
95	115	Farmland Industries Inc	16	-18.92	76,190,934	61,778,149
1	1	First Mississippi Corporation	7	0.04	4,052,567,255	4,054,298,758
50	40	Ford Motor Company	52	23.18	156,762,332	193,092,838
90	88	Formosa Plastics Corp USA	3	1.61	81,340,909	82,648,902
44	46	Freeport-McMoran Inc	4	-1.52	169,503,206	166,929,776
40	33	Gates Corporation	19	23.44	186,119,501	229,743,060
68	43	General Dynamics Corporation	16	44.95	118,295,917	171,466,568
53	48	General Electric Company	135	2.30	152,867,098	156,380,585
33	37	General Motors Corporation	131	1.69	201,885,284	205,303,728
94	108	Georgia Gulf Corporation	4	-9.03	76,296,837	69,409,964
23	22	Georgia-Pacific Corporation	68	5.36	271,657,667	286,216,696
2	2	Goodyear Tire & Rubber Co	37	5.64	2,711,678,031	2,864,512,848
51	47	Hercules Incorporated	32	3.22	154,342,904	159,313,623
20	12	HM Anglo-American Ltd	45	22.06	286,415,645	349,598,460

* Top 100 parent companies with largest total production-related waste in 1991, listed alphabetically. Rank is among total of 10,840 parent companies.

Change from 1991 to 1992 in:

Recycling Percent	**Energy Recovery** Percent	**Treated** Percent	**Released/ Disposed of** Percent
63.94	-5.68	18.47	-27.26
13.98	-14.05	9.12	-21.88
27.08	16.22	19.20	-10.43
-5.37	17.48	-15.78	-9.21
8.87	12.04	38.33	2.85
-75.98	-23.27	-55.13	23.61
-75.60	-5.65	2.54	-23.15
12.74	-15.59	9.77	-18.14
-8.57	—	7.79	-29.40
-9.67	45.22	7.55	26.75
32.29	—	143.15	-9.62
36.99	30.63	-32.68	-4.32
6.68	-19.83	-5.11	-72.67
9.95	7.01	-3.16	-14.42
22.12	-12.14	27.10	-11.00
-2.18	-51.38	-8.46	-24.62
-6.18	-17.43	-45.26	8.12
440.11	41.02	-36.15	-0.85
76.76	52.44	194.92	11.05
-0.90	-53.21	13.39	-2.26
10.65	-78.54	70.10	-44.53
—	—	39.93	28.43
-84.18	54.25	5.81	-3.91
-0.03	0.00	71.67	-0.01
0.48	-5.87	7.89	1.84
-9.52	—	—	-14.62
34.40	-3.55	44.54	-5.33
-41.09	19.44	0.61	-23.05
24.36	-27.67	-59.95	11.33
-68.12	24.27	0.70	3.69
24.02	—	-14.10	-5.49
-96.87	20.18	-9.35	-16.80
-9.88	—	-44.65	29.90
7.75	27.49	-16.87	5.76
-34.16	-62.56	17.03	19.60
443.92	18.33	15.88	-13.22
-25.97	5.02	-8.23	-17.44
0.08	-1.08	—	-25.24
19.04	-3.31	122.83	-2.73
-5.72	-9.54	18.15	36.04
-19.63	-20.28	-48.48	3.82
23.07	192.83	227.82	4.55
-22.98	4.40	47.60	-39.30
0.72	16.60	7.55	-25.73
14.87	-25.93	-3.29	-16.57
4.21	-13.76	-1.98	-33.30
-6.65	23.12	5.72	-5.60
5.58	41.31	13.06	4.52
-13.20	-23.10	36.38	29.83
-23.93	18.17	22.20	140.02

Table O-2. The 100 TRI Parent Companies with Largest Total Production-related Waste in 1991: Change 1991-1992 (cont'd.)*

Total Production-related Waste Rank*				Change in Total Production-related Waste	Total Production-related Waste	
1991 Rank	1992 Rank	TRI Parent Company	Facilities Number	1991 to 1992 Percent	1991 Pounds	1992 Pounds
5	5	Hoechst Celanese Corporation	32	4.63	664,260,025	695,043,839
56	49	Holdernam Inc	5	10.27	138,557,559	152,788,233
87	112	IBM	14	-24.59	85,938,259	64,804,317
13	11	International Paper Company	75	9.85	357,861,789	393,119,070
74	158	ITT Corporation	36	-57.55	107,342,178	45,567,386
66	63	James River Corp Virginia	33	0.64	118,931,873	119,696,995
38	29	Johnson Controls Inc	28	26.30	197,001,615	248,804,407
14	15	Kemira Holdings Inc	1	-5.93	336,468,720	316,522,270
27	26	Lafarge Corporation	12	10.48	246,731,180	272,588,945
54	116	Lyondell Petrochemical Co	2	-58.82	148,467,787	61,142,072
69	68	Maxwell Communication Corp	11	-0.91	113,391,152	112,364,873
93	103	Mead Corporation	12	-4.38	76,305,530	72,966,918
43	51	Mobil Corporation	30	-15.39	169,661,117	143,543,010
17	19	Monsanto Company	29	-4.18	318,539,891	305,224,967
16	16	National Cooperative Refinery	1	-3.22	323,281,992	312,856,711
85	95	Novacor Chemicals Inc	3	-16.60	92,093,529	76,802,325
10	17	Occidental Petroleum Corp	37	-18.06	378,978,357	310,551,333
92	92	Olin Corporation	30	5.80	76,794,324	81,244,608
47	157	Pacific Dunlop Holdings Inc	21	-70.82	157,758,502	46,030,080
72	77	Pfizer Inc	18	-4.08	108,746,663	104,309,696
34	99	Phillips Petroleum Company	16	-62.33	201,285,528	75,822,794
19	21	PPG Industries Inc	41	-2.51	294,347,709	286,962,296
97	105	Procter & Gamble Company	33	-3.97	74,614,794	71,649,886
82	74	PVS Chemicals Inc	5	6.38	99,246,319	105,579,793
36	38	Quaker State Corporation	4	0.01	200,427,416	200,443,094
37	94	Reilly Industries Inc	6	-60.65	197,345,362	77,653,080
60	57	Renco Group Inc	6	2.98	129,026,395	132,870,622
65	56	Rhone-Poulenc Inc	41	13.83	121,100,436	137,846,308
62	60	Rohm and Haas Company	19	1.69	126,694,078	128,840,024
99	89	Scott Paper Company	14	12.86	73,063,787	82,463,376
35	36	Shell Petroleum Inc	20	3.54	200,444,529	207,535,270
52	44	Shintech Inc	1	10.95	153,156,611	169,928,062
6	8	Solvay America Inc	11	-11.00	464,330,610	413,270,803
70	58	Sterling Chemicals Inc	1	16.08	112,634,697	130,742,106
49	45	Stone Container Corporation	15	7.43	156,939,166	168,606,473
100	97	Tenneco Inc	31	4.81	72,973,720	76,486,963
4	3	Texaco Inc	23	25.15	679,817,476	850,779,190
86	84	Texas Olefins Company	1	-5.33	90,902,428	86,059,770
41	41	Timken Co	17	9.97	172,795,626	190,028,461
98	102	U T I Corporation	2	0.09	74,087,204	74,152,474
71	72	Union Camp Corporation	12	0.17	109,751,012	109,937,394
45	31	Union Carbide Corporation	21	37.90	167,547,040	231,052,269
8	7	Uno-Ven Company	1	13.30	430,919,553	488,229,292
46	35	Upjohn Company	4	33.77	160,474,577	214,667,954
61	66	Vista Chemical Company	7	-11.14	128,205,102	113,919,792
89	87	Warner-Lambert Company	6	1.02	82,076,027	82,916,356
63	67	Westinghouse Electric Corp	49	-10.02	125,827,984	113,217,242
32	42	Weyerhaeuser Company	25	-8.51	202,608,033	185,370,540
81	78	Witco Corporation	41	4.04	99,979,164	104,014,625
30	25	Zeneca Holdings Inc	59	21.04	225,500,012	272,952,202
		Subtotal	2,438	-0.50	25,926,952,238	25,796,936,938
		Percent of Total	10.32		71.39	69.10
		Total	23,630	2.80	36,316,963,077	37,333,775,624

Change from 1991 to 1992 in:

Recycling Percent	**Energy Recovery** Percent	**Treated** Percent	**Released/ Disposed of** Percent
4.64	1.42	13.73	-2.06
-9.06	10.28	—	6.38
-29.12	-0.64	-11.67	-25.28
3.00	11.88	13.83	-8.09
-83.35	7.05	-0.59	13.53
26.72	-3.49	3.07	-23.59
27.41	36.99	-48.36	-7.31
-7.14	—	-0.38	36.63
—	10.40	116.82	-2.69
-6.47	1.04	-69.75	-29.56
0.30	-28.53	-23.31	-8.85
5.37	229.99	-8.60	14.60
25.89	-33.62	-21.75	-19.91
-23.06	-34.07	8.92	0.53
—	-3.25	12.52	1.57
-16.98	-11.15	-53.14	-9.00
0.69	93.22	-30.30	-10.10
14.04	-93.22	6.20	-27.17
-76.95	21.11	3.20	-6.50
-1.83	15.89	-20.90	-3.60
-76.91	4.03	31.51	-0.53
7.87	-21.61	-15.29	3.70
26.81	7.01	-4.59	-7.42
6.21	—	21.12	-1.36
-0.01	65.63	0.00	6.31
-63.77	467.92	7.98	-81.87
-9.12	-14.97	21.29	-6.41
4.28	15.71	23.30	24.62
-10.18	-21.07	7.78	11.24
0.29	3.55	17.36	-0.62
55.57	-5.07	-3.69	9.61
10.97	—	—	-5.46
-10.18	1.71	-29.39	-4.72
-42.68	23.18	24.01	1.20
-2.50	131.29	0.82	2.51
9.82	22.78	2.59	-2.82
11.31	-45.03	514.00	-10.41
0.00	-20.76	793.82	-4.56
13.90	-37.27	6.66	-2.98
0.02	—	1.32	6.99
-38.48	0.12	1.58	-5.20
789.94	-26.55	14.15	-12.53
4639.78	30.97	5.03	-58.54
42.22	25.01	-10.86	-14.65
-22.83	183.73	-14.81	-33.21
0.16	11.09	2.84	7.62
-12.61	15.70	1.75	-9.24
35.10	-3.45	-10.36	-9.57
13.45	85.66	-10.85	-17.62
9.96	36.91	26.33	-11.58
-2.52	4.87	3.05	-4.77
2.81	4.27	4.33	-3.25

Table O-3. The 100 TRI Parent Companies with Largest Amount Released/Disposed of in 1991: Actual and Projected Change 1991-1994*

Released/Disposed of Rank*			1991 Released/Disposed of	Change in Amount Released/Disposed of 1991 to 1992		Change in Projected Amount Released/Disposed of 1992 to 1994	
1991 Rank	1992 Rank	Parent Company	Pounds	Pounds	Percent	Pounds	Percent
10	15	3M Minnesota Mining & Mfg Co	46,918,373	-12,788,372	-27.26	-13,615,757	-39.89
41	221	Ahlstrom Filtration Inc	13,719,000	-11,490,400	-83.76	-1,000	-0.04
90	101	Air Products and Chemicals	7,192,226	-882,825	-12.27	-2,596,568	-41.15
76	89	Albemarle Corporation	8,662,806	-1,895,694	-21.88	-171,403	-2.53
40	42	Allied-Signal Inc	13,740,395	-1,433,390	-10.43	-4,087,589	-33.21
64	60	Aluminum Company of America	10,173,958	-937,229	-9.21	-818,225	-8.86
3	3	American Cyanamid	146,937,759	4,186,326	2.85	-106,373,108	-70.39
94	87	American National Can Company	7,030,693	53,306	0.76	-536,753	-7.58
33	36	Amoco Corporation	16,462,547	-2,987,013	-18.14	-485,998	-3.61
15	9	Arcadian Corporation	36,187,699	18,377,871	50.78	-9,016,778	-16.52
81	114	Armco Steel Company LP	8,042,935	-2,677,970	-33.30	-323,620	-6.03
4	5	Asarco Incorporated	79,567,915	-7,654,308	-9.62	-13,515,804	-18.79
74	64	Atlantic Richfield Company	9,000,161	-388,878	-4.32	-1,002,992	-11.65
34	131	BASF Corporation	16,126,029	-11,718,316	-72.67	-1,327,042	-30.11
66	62	Bethlehem Steel Corporation	10,104,255	-1,110,756	-10.99	-1,018,786	-11.33
55	77	Boeing Company	11,193,169	-3,349,536	-29.92	-2,915,401	-37.17
86	99	Boise Cascade Corporation	7,392,435	-1,066,186	-14.42	-11,784	-0.19
8	10	BP America Inc	61,096,520	-6,718,822	-11.00	-6,140,850	-11.29
23	16	Cabot Corporation	23,839,689	9,184,513	38.53	-4,761,013	-14.42
99	85	Cargill Incorporated	6,676,311	541,829	8.12	-508,060	-7.04
71	66	CF Industries Inc	9,368,384	-825,171	-8.81	1,630	0.02
62	55	Champion International Corp	10,581,732	-89,672	-0.85	-1,013,480	-9.66
70	51	Chevron Corporation	9,762,220	1,078,748	11.05	-869,967	-8.02
58	104	Citgo Petroleum Corporation	10,857,744	-4,834,694	-44.53	-3,386,200	-56.22
61	33	Coastal Corporation	10,610,783	4,252,803	40.08	-8,626,828	-58.04
11	12	Courtaulds United States Inc	43,231,126	794,365	1.84	-3,149,679	-7.15
73	72	Crown Cork & Seal Company	9,098,194	-961,775	-10.57	-244,863	-3.01
32	96	Doe Run Company	16,988,973	-10,376,507	-61.08	3,094,594	46.80
29	27	Dow Chemical Company	18,601,720	-990,822	-5.33	351,462	2.00
1	1	DuPont	232,304,835	8,583,353	3.69	-37,813,922	-15.70
87	88	E R Carpenter Company Inc	7,371,424	-330,583	-4.48	-838,644	-11.91
6	8	Eastman Kodak Company	67,501,537	-11,342,928	-16.80	-2,280,544	-4.06
25	25	Elf Aquitaine Inc	21,133,862	1,216,728	5.76	-8,700,471	-38.93
91	68	Eli Lilly and Company	7,104,027	1,392,462	19.60	-4,592,274	-54.05
31	30	Elkem Metals Company	17,599,964	-819,623	-4.66	-130,000	-0.77
92	92	Emerald Acquisition Corp	7,088,353	-355,579	-5.02	-21,119	-0.31
36	38	Exxon Corporation	14,950,399	-1,976,636	-13.22	-2,009,439	-15.49
37	45	Farmland Industries Inc	14,536,546	-2,535,517	-17.44	151,400	1.26
17	18	Ford Motor Company	30,569,399	-834,913	-2.73	390,314	1.31
2	2	Freeport-McMoran Inc	149,683,106	5,714,466	3.82	-105,264,967	-67.74
98	103	Gencorp Inc	6,686,913	-519,835	-7.77	-838,396	-13.59
27	32	General Electric Company	20,370,488	-5,241,980	-25.73	-3,460,312	-22.87
9	11	General Motors Corporation	53,713,427	-8,900,894	-16.57	-1,038,522	-2.32
22	23	Georgia-Pacific Corporation	23,986,125	-1,344,255	-5.60	-2,975,121	-13.14
93	83	Goodyear Tire & Rubber Co	7,064,917	319,280	4.52	-1,133,892	-15.36
89	121	Great Lakes Chemical Corp	7,285,274	-2,541,160	-34.88	-208,251	-4.39
46	37	Harrisons & Crosfield America	12,749,394	647,274	5.08	8,296	0.06
59	34	Hercules Incorporated	10,809,926	3,224,634	29.83	-3,245,609	-23.13
14	14	Hoechst Celanese Corporation	36,448,835	-751,100	-2.06	-6,046,523	-16.94
84	94	IBP Inc	7,760,104	-1,104,325	-14.23	4,661,610	70.04

* Top 100 parent companies with largest total amount released/disposed of in 1991, listed alphabetically. Rank is among total of 10,840 parent companies.

Table O-3. The 100 TRI Parent Companies with Largest Amount Released/Disposed of in 1991: Actual and Projected Change 1991-1994 (cont'd.)*

Released/Disposed of Rank*				Change in Amount Released/Disposed of 1991 to 1992		Change in Projected Amount Released/Disposed of 1992 to 1994	
1991 Rank	1992 Rank	Parent Company	1991 Released/ Disposed of Pounds	Pounds	Percent	Pounds	Percent
65	35	IMC Fertilizer Group Inc	10,108,758	3,673,235	36.34	-5,670,229	-41.14
54	70	Imcera Group Inc	11,235,659	-2,936,974	-26.14	-406,994	-4.90
16	17	Inland Steel Industries Inc	33,194,154	-1,656,302	-4.99	-27,052,312	-85.78
96	105	Inspiration Resources Corp	6,955,830	-964,880	-13.87	-2,659,860	-44.40
20	21	International Paper Company	27,743,313	-2,244,765	-8.09	126,420	0.50
85	69	ITT Corporation	7,457,749	1,008,736	13.53	-1,026,041	-12.12
67	79	James River Corp Virginia	10,054,220	-2,371,538	-23.59	-2,808,720	-36.56
53	48	Kerr-Mcgee Corporation	11,239,879	24,591	0.22	18,691,242	165.93
26	26	Lenzing Fibers Corp	21,022,210	499,905	2.38	3,500,000	16.26
100	73	Leviton Manufacturing Co Inc	6,519,456	1,599,872	24.54	1,478,162	18.21
51	50	Louisiana-Pacific Corporation	11,828,054	-789,625	-6.68	-3,475,494	-31.49
78	43	LTV Steel Co Inc	8,332,450	3,962,105	47.55	-5,108,972	-41.55
24	24	Magma Copper Company	23,680,400	-1,109,300	-4.68	-196,600	-0.87
50	52	Maxwell Communication Corp	11,833,506	-1,046,914	-8.85	1,269,217	11.77
42	31	MGF Industries	13,336,400	2,533,600	19.00	-11,853,000	-74.69
60	78	Miles Inc	10,721,147	-2,974,989	-27.75	-1,530,632	-19.76
49	47	Mississippi Chemical Corp	11,882,272	-479,703	-4.04	-6,433,536	-56.42
38	49	Mobil Corporation	13,887,719	-2,765,075	-19.91	-1,241,079	-11.16
5	4	Monsanto Company	76,030,994	401,415	0.53	876,771	1.15
43	56	NKK USA Corporation	13,304,860	-2,961,445	-22.26	1,644,442	15.90
47	39	Northwestern Steel & Wire Co	11,900,590	1,045,340	8.78	402,220	3.11
19	19	Occidental Petroleum Corp	29,419,283	-2,972,316	-10.10	-5,769,526	-21.82
21	22	Phelps Dodge Corporation	26,621,209	-3,381,707	-12.70	5,507,022	23.70
69	59	Procter & Gamble Company	9,981,099	-740,332	-7.42	-2,617,613	-28.33
79	82	Quantum Chemical Corporation	8,167,844	-750,115	-9.18	-1,407,900	-18.98
45	57	R R Donnelley & Sons Company	12,900,090	-2,804,616	-21.74	-890,537	-8.82
7	6	Renco Group Inc	66,465,019	-4,259,219	-6.41	2,946,801	4.74
44	58	Reynolds Metals Company	13,056,853	-3,296,586	-25.25	-384,027	-3.93
63	40	RTZ America Inc	10,297,605	2,344,000	22.76	1,868,800	14.78
88	84	Scott Paper Company	7,316,861	-45,106	-0.62	920,725	12.66
35	29	Shell Petroleum Inc	15,615,362	1,500,302	9.61	-5,267,775	-30.78
97	110	Sibv/Ms Holdings Inc	6,873,680	-1,139,805	-16.58	100,747	1.76
77	75	Simpson Investment Company	8,559,272	-515,655	-6.02	-5,186,988	-64.49
13	13	Sterling Chemicals Inc	36,751,872	441,078	1.20	-1,132,635	-3.05
52	46	Stone Container Corporation	11,448,015	287,218	2.51	-1,443,088	-12.30
95	90	Tenneco Inc	6,962,145	-196,375	-2.82	-131,453	-1.94
72	71	Texaco Inc	9,143,221	-951,562	-10.41	-626,642	-7.65
57	54	Union Camp Corporation	11,163,662	-579,995	-5.20	-404,370	-3.82
39	44	Union Carbide Corporation	13,770,629	-1,725,275	-12.53	48,550	0.40
56	53	Uniroyal Chemical Corporation	11,170,525	-435,998	-3.90	752,555	7.01
28	41	Unocal Corporation	20,311,967	-8,002,818	-39.40	-2,335,312	-18.97
68	65	Upjohn Company	10,046,824	-1,471,460	-14.65	-437,179	-5.10
82	61	USX Corporation	8,010,661	1,058,743	13.22	141,305	1.56
12	7	Vulcan Materials Company	41,457,797	19,152,444	46.20	-52,661,201	-86.88
83	86	Westinghouse Electric Corp	7,843,318	-724,649	-9.24	-614,379	-8.63
30	28	Westvaco Corporation	17,712,365	-544,855	-3.08	-2,443,669	-14.23
75	76	Weyerhaeuser Company	8,844,354	-846,800	-9.57	43,227	0.54
48	63	Wheeling-Pittsburgh Corp	11,889,180	-3,101,265	-26.08	-948,873	-10.80
80	93	Witco Corporation	8,094,981	-1,426,303	-17.62	-229,924	-3.45
18	20	Zeneca Holdings Inc	29,548,944	-3,422,948	-11.58	-9,117,141	-34.90
		Subtotal	2,267,598,863	-90,314,392	-3.98	-481,653,743	-21.24
		Percent of Total	64.50	78.95		70.29	
		Total	3,515,785,150	-114,398,980	-3.25	-685,272,807	-20.15

Table O-4. Rank of TRI Parent Companies for Production-related Waste and Releases and Transfers for Disposal, Actual 1991 to Projected 1994*

Parent Company	1991 Released/ Disposed of Rank	1991 Total Waste Rank	1992 Released/ Disposed of Rank	1992 Total Waste Rank	Projected 1993 Released/ Disposed of Rank	Projected 1993 Total Waste Rank	Projected 1994 Released/ Disposed of Rank	Projected 1994 Total Waste Rank
3M Minnesota Mining & Mfg Co	10	59	15	52	18	55	23	52
Abbott Laboratories	148	199	160	220	162	215	183	208
Acme Metals Inc	242	207	442	188	383	180	357	176
Ahlstrom Filtration Inc	41	209	221	262	203	266	188	266
Air Products and Chemicals	90	152	101	161	118	163	135	156
Akzo Nobel Inc	203	145	207	155	193	151	184	152
Albemarle Corporation	76	91	89	86	93	87	81	90
Alcan Aluminum Corp	279	201	272	209	253	195	238	194
Allegheny Ludlum Corporation	548	148	566	160	539	155	496	157
Allied-Signal Inc	40	15	42	10	54	11	60	7
Aluminum Company of America	64	78	60	82	65	81	58	82
Amax Inc	180	107	167	81	168	80	165	81
Amerada Hess Corporation	244	133	116	93	198	111	156	98
American Brands Inc	172	262	183	245	202	242	193	234
American Cyanamid	3	24	3	20	3	25	9	40
American National Can Company	94	243	87	233	94	255	82	250
American Petrofina Holding Co	228	26	186	65	231	76	271	76
American Tape Co	165	254	141	242	124	238	139	238
American Telephone & Telg Co	185	58	214	147	287	147	389	155
Ametek Inc	823	292	906	300	1047	282	984	270
Amoco Corporation	33	18	36	14	42	18	33	17
Arcadian Corporation	15	162	9	123	7	115	8	146
Archer Daniels Midland	201	64	233	59	260	58	245	53
Aristech Chemical Corporation	108	120	117	132	139	131	143	130
Armco Inc	123	67	97	64	78	67	73	66
Armco Steel Company LP	81	169	114	202	111	199	105	201
Arvin Industries Inc	325	265	325	366	300	367	275	348
Asarco Incorporated	4	28	5	23	6	28	4	25
Ash Grove Cement Company	656	245	842	267	752	220	709	213
Ashland Oil Inc	234	180	226	125	216	144	199	150
Atlantic Richfield Company	74	21	64	13	68	12	70	13
Avery Dennison Corporation	135	249	158	243	181	263	214	282
B F Goodrich Company	226	128	248	121	254	116	263	112
BASF Corporation	34	80	131	91	145	105	153	105
Batus Holdings Inc	554	276	573	252	474	233	444	230
Beaumont Methanol Holding Co	7802	239	8081	229	7590	228	7175	226
Bessemer Capital Partners LP	417	125	394	134	398	133	394	137
Bethlehem Steel Corporation	66	151	62	120	71	139	65	143
Blairsville Machine Products	8535	259	8965	292	8978	313	8981	307
Boeing Company	55	258	77	301	90	318	109	331
Boise Cascade Corporation	86	73	99	75	95	75	88	74
Borden Chemicals & Plastics LP	181	135	195	133	185	132	177	138
Borden Inc	151	260	136	249	157	261	161	265
Bowater Incorporated	131	136	119	144	134	161	138	164
BP America Inc	8	57	10	55	9	59	7	58
Bridgestone/Firestone Inc	204	290	199	290	194	293	230	299
Bristol-Myers Squibb Company	107	25	125	28	122	27	126	28
Buffalo Color Corporation	696	273	648	269	618	276	573	274
Cabot Corporation	23	156	16	131	16	134	17	153
Cargill Incorporated	99	55	85	83	82	85	77	87
Castle Energy Corporation	867	114	1383	145	946	95	665	60

* Top 300 parent companies with largest total production-related waste in 1991, listed alphabetically. Rank is among total of 10,840 parent companies.

Table O-4. Rank of TRI Parent Companies for Production-related Waste and Releases and Transfers for Disposal, Actual 1991 to Projected 1994 (cont'd.)*

Parent Company	1991 Released/ Disposed of Rank	1991 Total Waste Rank	1992 Released/ Disposed of Rank	1992 Total Waste Rank	Projected 1993 Released/ Disposed of Rank	Projected 1993 Total Waste Rank	Projected 1994 Released/ Disposed of Rank	Projected 1994 Total Waste Rank
CF Industries Inc	71	248	66	337	66	381	57	384
Champion International Corp	62	48	55	71	55	68	52	75
Charter Power Systems Inc	4929	193	4194	195	3697	184	3403	181
Chattem Chemicals	255	261	322	268	295	265	270	254
Chevron Corporation	70	79	51	32	52	45	47	42
Chrysler Corporation	117	269	108	275	96	271	84	264
Ciba-Geigy Corporation	171	76	168	70	170	63	166	62
Citgo Petroleum Corporation	58	29	104	27	189	26	174	24
Coastal Corporation	61	103	33	90	64	96	90	106
Consolidated Papers Inc	218	288	144	178	144	192	142	195
Contran Corporation	308	266	358	286	422	288	453	287
Cookson America Inc	280	268	227	254	221	252	227	258
Copper Range Company Inc	104	75	74	50	67	42	59	34
Corning Inc	133	42	134	191	132	123	129	128
Coulton Chemical Corp	2707	22	2773	24	2495	20	2300	19
Courtaulds United States Inc	11	39	12	39	10	39	11	35
CPC International Inc	193	252	193	223	184	222	176	216
Crown Central Petroleum Corp	506	221	378	228	418	225	404	222
Crown Cork & Seal Company	73	246	72	247	70	250	68	252
Cyprus Minerals Company	145	7	156	9	126	7	100	8
D X Holding Company Inc	478	130	515	127	475	128	473	135
Degussa Corporation	149	137	145	129	135	121	122	122
Diamond Shamrock Inc	399	141	288	140	273	138	256	141
DIC Americas Inc	129	179	115	175	112	166	107	166
Doe Run Company	32	108	96	30	57	51	49	48
Douglas Battery Mfg Co	5928	150	6666	225	6128	214	5633	200
Dover Corporation	332	212	338	325	515	1042	501	1061
Dow Chemical Company	29	9	27	6	28	6	25	6
Dow Corning Corporation	251	96	286	114	312	112	312	109
DSM Finance USA Inc	283	88	249	176	238	245	226	245
DuPont	1	3	1	4	2	3	1	5
East Penn Manufacturing Co Inc	824	77	836	61	786	56	748	55
Eastman Kodak Company	6	11	8	34	8	32	5	30
EC Acquisition Inc	299	31	234	53	192	47	232	45
El Paso Refinery LP	1487	191	2727	98	2167	169	1662	95
Elf Aquitaine Inc	25	12	25	18	30	14	30	14
Eli Lilly and Company	91	83	68	73	110	94	132	97
Elkem Metals Company	31	237	30	62	31	64	27	64
Emerald Acquisition Corp	92	274	92	285	83	285	76	285
Equion Corporation	1124	147	1096	150	994	146	971	151
Ethyl Corporation	446	232	408	227	375	224	455	219
Exxon Corporation	36	84	38	79	46	77	42	77
Farmland Industries Inc	37	95	45	115	41	114	34	117
Federal Paper Board Company	127	183	112	96	107	98	115	126
Ferro Corporation	315	175	256	153	262	152	613	159
First Mississippi Corporation	110	1	129	1	115	1	110	1
Flexel Inc	166	127	153	122	143	119	131	121
FLS Holdings Inc	585	286	604	278	538	278	503	271
FMC Corporation	297	270	341	303	342	309	413	308
Ford Motor Company	17	50	18	40	15	41	13	39
Formosa Plastics Corp USA	677	90	556	88	594	93	542	94
Freeport-McMoran Inc	2	44	2	46	1	31	6	125
Gates Corporation	361	40	345	33	365	35	360	73
General Dynamics Corporation	213	68	285	43	367	46	502	44

Table O-4. Rank of TRI Parent Companies for Production-related Waste and Releases and Transfers for Disposal, Actual 1991 to Projected 1994 (cont'd.)*

	1991		1992		Projected 1993		Projected 1994	
Parent Company	**Released/ Disposed of** Rank	**Total Waste** Rank	**Released/ Disposed of** Rank	**Total Waste** Rank	**Released/ Disposed of** Rank	**Total Waste** Rank	**Released/ Disposed of** Rank	**Total Waste** Rank
General Electric Company	27	53	32	48	36	49	39	51
General Motors Corporation	9	33	11	37	11	34	10	31
General Tire Inc	566	116	486	110	455	107	499	107
Georgia Gulf Corporation	529	94	676	108	689	109	669	108
Georgia-Pacific Corporation	22	23	23	22	26	23	24	22
Giant Group Ltd	6515	115	6576	136	6010	103	5261	67
Gilman Investment Company Inc	191	278	222	296	341	305	338	301
Goodyear Tire & Rubber Co	93	2	83	2	79	2	89	2
Great Lakes Chemical Corp	89	182	121	186	123	193	117	197
Green Bay Packaging Inc	651	271	728	274	654	273	601	269
Gruner Jahr USA Prtg & Pubg Co	714	295	541	257	457	235	428	237
GTE Corporation	132	121	138	126	138	124	136	139
Gulfmet Holdings Corporation	1625	236	1696	253	1602	260	1491	244
Hampshire Chemical Corp	268	223	434	219	393	264	375	251
Handy & Harman	456	267	544	272	700	283	712	284
Hanlin Group Inc	643	219	2540	208	3439	203	3484	204
Harlan Castle Inc	208	122	266	128	3123	130	1034	133
Harrisons & Crosfield America	46	293	37	306	37	311	31	305
Hercules Incorporated	59	51	34	47	40	54	43	50
HM Anglo-American Ltd	157	20	67	12	105	13	102	79
Hoechst Celanese Corporation	14	5	14	5	14	5	15	4
Hoffman-La Roche	498	144	636	170	607	188	555	186
Holdernam Inc	1769	56	1720	49	1554	48	1436	46
Holly Corporation	2294	166	1354	119	1202	117	1103	119
Huntsman Chemical Corporation	716	282	694	282	642	290	598	286
IBM	357	87	441	112	527	159	608	203
IBP Inc	84	222	94	232	47	182	41	182
ICI Explosives Holdings Inc	493	161	601	205	560	210	528	236
Imcera Group Inc	54	184	70	163	72	167	67	172
Inco United States Inc	366	240	561	238	494	227	441	37
Inland Steel Industries Inc	16	160	17	172	20	202	118	361
International Paper Company	20	13	21	11	19	10	18	12
ITT Corporation	85	74	69	158	76	157	74	160
Ivaco	637	233	589	250	520	251	510	317
James River Corp Virginia	67	66	79	63	109	66	112	63
Johnson Controls Inc	607	38	625	29	731	37	753	32
Kemira Holdings Inc	500	14	386	15	491	16	457	15
Kerr-Mcgee Corporation	53	134	48	118	13	91	14	99
Kimberly-Clark Corporation	169	225	173	258	173	268	162	268
Koch Industries Inc	196	189	198	198	214	187	213	180
Krueger Acquisition Corp	679	158	651	156	627	158	586	162
Kyowa Hakko Kogyo Ltd	5114	202	5411	224	5311	221	4922	215
Lafarge Corporation	986	27	997	26	871	24	825	20
Laroche Holdings Inc	139	155	157	142	161	148	168	169
Lenzing Fibers Corp	26	200	26	215	24	206	19	193
Lincoln Group Inc	109	218	80	206	186	231	178	223
Lo Nidy Company Inc	1088	109	1408	109	1353	99	1162	91
Lone Star Industries Inc	2737	174	2622	148	2193	118	3683	115
Longview Fibre Company	509	275	335	294	315	286	277	277
Lorin Industries	2231	210	2062	259	1687	239	1386	212
Louisiana-Pacific Corporation	51	287	50	309	85	386	72	341
Lubrizol Corp	398	106	216	107	229	100	334	113
Lukens Inc	289	119	627	117	548	113	596	116
Lyondell Petrochemical Co	225	54	269	116	237	120	243	120

Table O-4. Rank of TRI Parent Companies for Production-related Waste and Releases and Transfers for Disposal, Actual 1991 to Projected 1994 (cont'd.)*

Parent Company	1991		1992		Projected 1993		Projected 1994	
	Released/ Disposed of Rank	Total Waste Rank	Released/ Disposed of Rank	Total Waste Rank	Released/ Disposed of Rank	Total Waste Rank	Released/ Disposed of Rank	Total Waste Rank
Macmillan Bloedel Inc	363	203	357	212	324	208	303	206
Magma Copper Company	24	170	24	171	22	165	21	168
Marine Shale Processors Inc	155	194	212	251	307	246	285	246
Mascotech	105	196	95	197	99	211	95	221
Maxwell Communication Corp	50	69	52	68	49	69	36	69
Mead Corporation	116	93	98	103	113	108	104	100
Merck & Co Inc	134	112	174	130	175	140	212	158
MGF Industries	42	217	31	194	33	186	128	232
Midstates Wire	2606	204	2566	605	2324	586	2151	586
Miles Inc	60	101	78	85	88	83	91	111
Mississippi Chemical Corp	49	105	47	76	114	50	108	47
Mitsubishi Metal America Corp	5572	178	5694	1384	5063	1085	4576	1049
Mobil Corporation	38	43	49	51	50	52	48	54
Modine Manufacturing Company	381	171	439	203	478	198	702	231
Monsanto Company	5	17	4	19	4	15	2	16
Moore Business Forms	839	241	287	256	248	232	229	229
Morton International Inc	323	142	273	151	306	145	307	145
Motorola Inc	215	250	149	331	188	349	255	330
National Cement Company Inc	6926	224	7571	273	6828	243	6279	225
National Cooperative Refinery	657	16	649	16	601	19	562	18
National Material LP	5510	220	7243	213	6773	204	6342	202
Neste Corporate Holding Inc	352	138	417	141	380	136	379	140
Nippon Mining U S Inc	384	257	265	239	213	247	167	247
Nitram Inc	265	242	313	263	288	270	246	248
NKK USA Corporation	43	186	56	200	45	197	37	198
North American Philips Corp	190	211	191	241	200	257	191	256
Northwestern Steel & Wire Co	47	205	39	196	38	189	32	188
Novacor Chemicals Inc	1835	85	1965	95	2241	84	2092	88
Nucor Corporation	328	195	324	164	715	156	656	154
Occidental Petroleum Corp	19	10	19	17	23	21	22	21
Oi-Neg TV Products Inc	725	208	873	187	748	181	1565	174
Olin Corporation	167	92	209	92	191	79	192	86
Owens-Illinois Inc	376	253	368	261	340	259	330	260
P H Glatfelter Co	227	176	213	181	195	176	194	175
P M C Inc	113	140	111	139	103	143	96	144
Pacific Dunlop Holdings Inc	267	47	260	157	226	153	210	149
Parker Hannifin Corporation	454	255	455	260	637	267	1241	262
Parsons & Whittemore Enterp	752	149	445	101	401	102	382	103
PCL Group Inc	338	181	532	165	512	160	506	163
Pechiney Corporation	176	281	171	299	160	298	154	293
Pegasus Holdings Inc	153	143	170	162	29	122	50	123
Pennzoil Company	103	226	126	217	120	213	114	210
Pfizer Inc	130	72	127	77	129	74	137	68
Phelps Dodge Corporation	21	131	22	152	17	125	16	129
Philip Morris Companies Inc	128	172	130	177	127	194	121	196
Phillips Petroleum Company	102	34	100	99	92	38	86	38
Pope & Talbot Inc	492	297	529	355	518	364	514	363
Potlatch Corporation	160	213	196	221	197	219	186	214
Powerine Oil Company Holdings	1028	230	1252	214	1391	253	1019	253
PPG Industries Inc	114	19	107	21	106	22	111	23
PQ Corporation	573	285	277	283	219	279	205	276
Printing Holdings LP	290	251	276	234	258	234	237	272
Procter & Gamble Company	69	97	59	105	80	110	80	110
PVS Chemicals Inc	2859	82	2921	74	2578	70	2391	71

Table O-4. Rank of TRI Parent Companies for Production-related Waste and Releases and Transfers for Disposal, Actual 1991 to Projected 1994 (cont'd.)*

Parent Company	1991 Released/ Disposed of Rank	1991 Total Waste Rank	1992 Released/ Disposed of Rank	1992 Total Waste Rank	Projected 1993 Released/ Disposed of Rank	Projected 1993 Total Waste Rank	Projected 1994 Released/ Disposed of Rank	Projected 1994 Total Waste Rank
Quad Graphics Inc	1306	234	1274	222	1061	201	911	187
Quaker State Corporation	795	36	738	38	664	40	676	36
Quanex Corporation	963	294	768	297	930	300	900	298
Quantum Chemical Corporation	79	104	82	69	91	71	94	72
R R Donnelley & Sons Company	45	277	57	324	60	353	56	353
Raytheon Company	245	157	263	173	388	173	433	190
Reading Tube Corp	4032	198	4052	193	3360	178	3111	179
Reilly Industries Inc	259	37	807	94	723	90	651	89
Renco Group Inc	7	60	6	57	5	57	3	56
Republic Engineered Steels	659	291	646	270	534	262	495	261
Rexene Corporation	197	197	179	398	167	406	209	420
Reynolds Metals Company	44	190	58	179	58	179	54	177
Rhone-Poulenc Inc	247	65	206	56	210	53	195	49
Riverwood International USA	125	192	154	137	159	137	164	142
RJR Nabisco Holdings Corp	183	117	190	111	208	368	189	369
Rohm and Haas Company	212	62	184	60	180	62	173	61
RTZ America Inc	63	118	40	113	34	92	29	93
Rubicon Inc	115	300	81	295	61	277	53	273
Sandoz Corporation	252	229	229	207	236	216	251	209
Scancem Industries Inc	4101	146	2199	185	2484	135	2244	131
Schuylkill Metals Corp.	865	231	779	390	677	350	637	346
Scott Paper Company	88	99	84	89	77	86	61	85
Seafab Metal Corp	7089	244	7301	237	8761	237	8776	239
Shell Petroleum Inc	35	35	29	36	44	33	38	29
Sherwin-Williams Company	320	247	255	240	249	280	224	278
Shintech Inc	1300	52	1326	44	1133	43	1055	41
Shuford Industries Inc	342	283	301	289	305	294	284	288
Sibv/Ms Holdings Inc	97	164	110	166	100	168	98	171
Simpson Investment Company	77	110	75	124	146	170	159	189
Sinclair Oil Corporation	501	165	462	149	426	162	399	161
Sloan Valve Company	1059	296	971	298	962	328	948	327
Solite Corporation	504	123	701	199	492	174	364	124
Solvay America Inc	471	6	474	8	502	9	575	11
Specialty Coatings Group Inc	195	264	178	293	179	343	179	306
Specialty Materials Corp	545	185	473	168	430	164	405	167
Spectrum Ltd	397	228	278	216	243	223	233	217
Standard Chlorine Chemical Co	1038	215	1113	236	1006	212	870	184
Sterling Chemicals Inc	13	70	13	58	12	61	12	59
Stone Container Corporation	52	49	46	45	51	60	44	57
Sun Company Inc	298	187	321	183	310	240	289	241
Sybron Chemicals Inc	787	163	710	154	632	142	591	147
Tate & Lyle Inc	623	188	682	204	665	196	602	199
Teledyne Inc	233	154	228	169	290	171	409	173
Temple-Inland Inc	101	111	106	100	98	101	93	102
Tenneco Inc	95	100	90	97	84	97	79	96
Texaco Inc	72	4	71	3	73	4	71	3
Texas Industries Inc	385	167	3432	146	3025	129	2814	114
Texas Olefins Company	847	86	858	84	823	88	851	84
Textron Inc	142	263	155	280	147	301	155	315
Thomson Consumer Electronics	238	284	211	264	204	256	197	257
Timken Co	433	41	433	41	468	36	470	33
Tosco Corporation	189	238	161	308	154	324	148	319
Total Petroleum Inc	420	159	384	192	439	355	434	356
Tremont Corporation	1263	279	1481	246	1281	297	1421	429

Table O-4. Rank of TRI Parent Companies for Production-related Waste and Releases and Transfers for Disposal, Actual 1991 to Projected 1994 (cont'd.)*

Parent Company	1991 Released/ Disposed of Rank	1991 Total Waste Rank	1992 Released/ Disposed of Rank	1992 Total Waste Rank	Projected 1993 Released/ Disposed of Rank	Projected 1993 Total Waste Rank	Projected 1994 Released/ Disposed of Rank	Projected 1994 Total Waste Rank
U T I Corporation	490	98	459	102	396	106	347	104
Unilever United States Inc	292	256	359	315	410	295	485	297
Union Camp Corporation	57	71	54	72	53	78	45	78
Union Carbide Corporation	39	45	44	31	39	29	35	27
Union Texas Petroleum Holdings	649	289	659	226	695	304	627	300
Uniroyal Chemical Corporation	56	272	53	287	48	292	40	281
United Acquisition Corp	1227	227	1420	190	1226	191	1104	192
United Technologies Corp	120	129	135	135	152	149	182	170
Unocal Corporation	28	206	41	265	56	291	46	295
Uno-Ven Company	935	8	1597	7	1308	8	1268	9
Upjohn Company	68	46	65	35	63	30	62	26
USS-Posco Industries	1256	280	1802	184	1533	172	1322	165
USX Corporation	82	153	61	143	59	126	55	132
Valmont Industries Inc	1157	216	1788	210	1799	207	1668	207
Veba Corporation	435	299	475	211	1100	209	1350	211
Vista Chemical Company	336	61	452	66	547	65	566	65
Vulcan Materials Company	12	132	7	106	21	183	66	263
W R Grace & Co Inc	146	168	177	189	166	190	158	191
Walter Industries Inc	144	235	148	231	137	217	133	233
Warner-Lambert Company	162	89	147	87	156	89	185	92
Wellman Inc	575	124	806	138	727	127	686	127
Westinghouse Electric Corp	83	63	86	67	81	72	83	80
Westlake International Corp	3896	113	1882	54	1227	1211	1128	1192
Westlake Monomers Corp	512	177	1044	230	883	226	822	224
Westvaco Corporation	30	102	28	104	32	104	28	101
Weyerhaeuser Company	75	32	76	42	69	44	64	43
Wheeling-Pittsburgh Corp	48	214	63	244	75	244	69	242
Willamette Industries Inc	150	139	142	159	130	154	125	148
Witco Corporation	80	81	93	78	89	73	85	70
Wolverine Holding Company	580	126	535	174	524	175	529	183
Zeneca Holdings Inc	18	30	20	25	27	17	26	10
Zeon Chemicals USA	600	173	598	182	638	141	582	134
Zollner Pistons	5890	298	6062	312	5541	317	5113	310

*Table O-5. 1992 Production-related Waste for the 100 TRI Parent Companies with Largest Total Production-related Waste of Carcinogens in 1991**

Total Production-related Waste Rank*				Type of Waste Management as Percent of Total Production-related Waste			
1991 Rank	**1992** Rank	**Parent Company**	**1992 Total Production-related Waste** Pounds	**Recycling** Percent	**Energy Recovery** Percent	**Treated** Percent	**Released/ Disposed of** Percent
57	58	Abbott Laboratories	7,645,788	44.15	0.22	26.25	29.38
81	82	Allied-Signal Inc	4,601,826	80.96	0.12	11.01	7.91
32	32	American Cyanamid	15,851,503	39.78	2.38	39.36	18.48
100	133	American Petrofina Holding Co	2,178,931	0.17	64.77	13.82	21.24
49	45	Ametek Inc	11,503,416	98.64	0.00	0.00	1.36
63	52	Amoco Corporation	8,818,835	6.21	46.13	33.21	14.46
37	47	Armco Inc	11,207,476	95.02	0.29	0.29	4.40
24	20	Atlantic Richfield Company	29,245,288	0.47	75.77	20.02	3.75
26	22	B F Goodrich Company	25,792,452	57.43	2.87	37.81	1.89
48	50	BASF Corporation	9,810,252	1.16	68.46	24.06	6.32
71	72	Baxter International Inc	5,789,380	82.62	0.00	10.30	7.08
54	60	Blairsville Machine Products	7,585,880	100.00	0.00	0.00	0.00
97	97	Boeing Company	3,330,495	76.95	0.63	2.82	19.60
39	75	Borden Chem & Plas Ltd Partnr	5,461,878	0.00	0.00	98.91	1.09
44	43	BP America Inc	12,836,693	56.68	3.70	8.76	30.86
60	59	Bridgestone/Firestone Inc	7,594,564	88.90	5.98	1.09	4.03
19	24	Bristol-Myers Squibb Company	23,902,640	84.14	0.11	13.86	1.89
62	57	Buffalo Color Corporation	7,764,020	96.63	0.00	2.65	0.72
70	69	Carpenter Technology Corp	6,059,573	98.93	0.02	0.00	1.05
74	35	Chevron Corporation	15,383,857	32.19	5.45	51.93	10.43
85	76	DIC Americas Inc	5,160,650	0.56	1.56	92.48	5.40
23	46	Dover Corporation	11,221,585	95.10	0.00	0.00	4.90
4	3	Dow Chemical Company	173,110,018	36.53	22.04	39.62	1.82
14	16	DuPont	38,773,727	13.61	16.48	57.12	12.79
86	157	Duriron Company Inc	1,627,514	96.58	0.00	0.04	3.37
78	95	Dynachem Inc	3,401,801	97.85	0.00	0.86	1.29
95	81	E R Carpenter Company Inc	4,644,071	0.26	0.37	0.61	98.76
6	5	East Penn Manufacturing Co Inc	110,496,839	99.90	0.00	0.00	0.10
40	28	Eastman Kodak Company	17,788,003	0.44	6.42	56.43	36.72
69	62	Elf Aquitaine Inc	7,292,648	90.33	2.17	5.82	1.68
35	23	Eli Lilly and Company	24,605,495	0.00	0.00	80.54	19.46
45	51	Exxon Corporation	9,586,874	2.78	27.22	61.10	8.90
21	18	Ferro Corporation	36,449,254	96.05	0.72	0.08	3.15
30	25	First Mississippi Corporation	20,060,564	95.16	4.64	0.00	0.20
83	79	Foamex LP	4,755,036	1.95	0.08	0.86	97.11
13	14	Formosa Plastics Corp USA	39,619,979	54.70	34.44	10.26	0.60
59	61	Franklin Smelting & Refining	7,371,983	91.29	0.00	8.58	0.13
33	40	General Electric Company	13,438,408	38.86	2.55	36.80	21.79
67	66	General Motors Corporation	6,777,005	79.13	0.84	4.34	15.69
65	94	General Smelting & Refining	3,497,800	94.84	0.00	3.00	2.16
10	9	General Tire Inc	67,085,263	99.44	0.01	0.00	0.55
27	26	Georgia Gulf Corporation	19,532,807	1.79	57.90	39.86	0.45
91	90	Georgia-Pacific Corporation	3,769,915	0.14	0.00	25.71	74.15
61	71	Glenbrook Nickel Co	5,893,001	63.32	0.00	0.00	36.68
1	1	Goodyear Tire & Rubber Co	345,442,975	98.76	0.63	0.34	0.26
88	85	Hercules Incorporated	4,116,610	2.69	0.03	52.02	45.27
2	2	Hoechst Celanese Corporation	202,027,880	82.13	4.61	10.23	3.03
76	42	Holdernam Inc	12,956,061	0.00	99.99	0.00	0.01
17	19	IBM Corp	29,548,779	95.13	0.70	3.55	0.62
87	64	Imcera Group Inc	7,192,882	30.09	32.69	5.06	32.16
42	39	Inco United States Inc	13,860,937	98.81	0.00	0.03	1.16

* Top 100 parent companies with largest total production-related waste of carcinogens in 1991, listed alphabetically. Rank is among total of 4,044 parent companies.

Table O-5. 1992 Production-related Waste for the 100 TRI Parent Companies with Largest Total Production-related Waste of Carcinogens in 1991 (cont'd.)*

Total Production-related Waste Rank*				Type of Waste Management as Percent of Total Production-related Waste			
1991 Rank	**1992** Rank	**Parent Company**	**1992 Total Production-related Waste** Pounds	**Recycling** Percent	**Energy Recovery** Percent	**Treated** Percent	**Released/ Disposed of** Percent
79	100	Johnson Controls Inc	3,170,208	91.42	0.00	2.55	6.03
51	38	Kerr-Mcgee Corporation	13,885,247	98.06	0.00	0.10	1.84
66	70	Lafarge Corporation	5,967,317	0.00	96.25	3.70	0.05
9	8	Lo Nidy Company Inc	67,425,425	99.81	0.00	0.00	0.19
38	27	Lukens Inc	18,756,432	97.63	0.00	1.24	1.12
29	31	Lyondell Petrochemical Co	16,265,600	0.00	14.76	82.21	3.03
93	93	Magma Copper Company	3,536,800	0.00	0.00	0.00	100.00
80	448	Maron Products Inc	275,010	100.00	0.00	0.00	0.00
64	290	Medite Corp	578,031	15.83	73.70	0.00	10.47
50	65	Merck & Co Inc	7,181,916	65.67	3.55	25.12	5.66
99	105	Miles Inc	3,017,900	0.51	10.31	59.61	29.58
84	112	Mobil Corporation	2,773,202	6.24	1.12	77.34	15.30
12	12	Monsanto Company	52,477,860	29.76	5.93	53.20	11.11
28	29	Moore Business Forms	17,093,086	99.28	0.07	0.02	0.63
89	89	Mosinee Paper Corporation	3,855,020	0.00	0.00	99.06	0.94
15	15	Neste Corporate Holding Inc	39,549,782	2.44	0.10	97.26	0.20
7	7	Novacor Chemicals Inc	75,394,550	92.98	6.89	0.04	0.10
8	13	Occidental Petroleum Corp	41,075,755	1.01	28.12	67.14	3.73
73	54	Olin Corporation	8,355,362	75.92	0.22	19.85	4.00
96	96	Owens-Corning Fiberglas Corp	3,376,417	3.43	0.69	63.60	32.28
25	1129	Pacific Dunlop Holdings Inc	47,074	34.69	0.00	58.26	7.05
41	34	Pfizer Inc	15,678,010	87.38	0.49	8.55	3.58
58	84	Phillips Petroleum Company	4,264,791	46.93	8.05	29.63	15.38
11	10	PPG Industries Inc	65,324,597	68.41	6.40	24.20	0.98
72	74	Precision Castparts Corp	5,601,185	97.93	0.00	0.02	2.05
46	41	Refined Metals Corp	13,413,302	90.21	0.00	0.00	9.79
5	121	Reilly Industries Inc	2,450,022	59.47	35.02	2.63	2.88
36	36	Rhone-Poulenc Inc	15,080,278	66.96	12.72	18.62	1.71
94	68	Rohm and Haas Company	6,444,566	0.58	10.29	84.49	4.64
56	56	Rubicon Inc	7,813,842	0.00	80.18	8.77	11.05
16	17	Shell Petroleum Inc	37,162,560	12.80	57.68	24.11	5.41
3	4	Shintech Inc	169,862,100	99.95	0.00	0.00	0.05
31	21	Specialty Materials Corp	27,041,596	96.96	0.00	0.79	2.24
52	53	Sterling Chemicals Inc	8,363,475	0.02	68.71	7.66	23.61
47	33	Sybron Chemicals Inc	15,763,060	99.02	0.00	0.43	0.55
75	63	Texas Olefins Company	7,268,913	0.00	72.07	25.69	2.24
82	73	Tomkins Corporation	5,664,831	43.65	0.60	0.32	55.42
55	55	Unilever United States Inc	7,828,802	96.36	0.00	2.43	1.21
53	48	Union Carbide Corporation	11,148,987	0.20	24.95	68.32	6.53
90	86	United Technologies Corp	4,066,411	87.77	0.89	3.12	8.23
18	6	Upjohn Company	79,803,489	91.09	0.02	4.24	4.65
34	37	Vista Chemical Company	14,429,990	60.32	0.40	37.95	1.33
92	87	Vulcan Materials Company	3,965,969	0.00	0.00	76.54	23.46
20	11	Westlake International Corp	63,862,803	0.00	99.38	0.58	0.04
22	30	Westlake Monomers Corp	16,940,855	12.75	84.37	2.56	0.32
68	67	Witco Corporation	6,556,389	97.24	0.00	1.63	1.13
98	92	Xerox Corporation	3,726,828	72.07	8.10	0.00	19.82
77	77	Zeon Chemicals USA	5,046,804	93.54	0.00	0.67	5.78
43	44	Zollner Pistons	12,488,413	99.99	0.00	0.00	0.01
		Subtotal	2,494,591,973	67.58	11.88	16.28	4.27
		Percent of Total	84.42				
		Total	2,955,067,837	64.74	19.66	26.74	8.11

Table O-6. The 100 TRI Parent Companies with Largest Total Production-related Waste of Carcinogens in 1991: Change 1991-1992*

Total Production-related Waste Rank* 1991 Rank	1992 Rank	Parent Company	TRI Facilities Number	Change in Total Production-related Waste 1991 to 1992 Percent	Total Production-related Waste 1991 Pounds	1992 Pounds
57	58	Abbott Laboratories	9	-10.17	8,511,044	7,645,788
81	82	Allied-Signal Inc	31	-7.80	4,991,289	4,601,826
32	32	American Cyanamid	20	-5.98	16,859,069	15,851,503
100	133	American Petrofina Holding Co	5	-38.98	3,570,913	2,178,931
49	45	Ametek Inc	4	6.21	10,831,217	11,503,416
63	52	Amoco Corporation	21	25.61	7,021,036	8,818,835
37	47	Armco Inc	18	-24.94	14,930,415	11,207,476
24	20	Atlantic Richfield Company	9	26.10	23,192,457	29,245,288
26	22	B F Goodrich Company	16	11.57	23,118,404	25,792,452
48	50	BASF Corporation	23	-12.88	11,260,825	9,810,252
71	72	Baxter International Inc	12	3.93	5,570,329	5,789,380
54	60	Blairsville Machine Products	1	-16.67	9,103,056	7,585,880
97	97	Boeing Company	1	-13.28	3,840,360	3,330,495
39	75	Borden Chemicals & Plastics LP	1	-62.86	14,705,043	5,461,878
44	43	BP America Inc	13	5.85	12,127,506	12,836,693
60	59	Bridgestone/Firestone Inc	6	3.21	7,358,493	7,594,564
19	24	Bristol-Myers Squibb Company	7	-20.62	30,110,715	23,902,640
62	57	Buffalo Color Corporation	1	10.47	7,028,200	7,764,020
70	69	Carpenter Technology Corp	4	6.05	5,713,868	6,059,573
74	35	Chevron Corporation	22	178.82	5,517,419	15,383,857
85	76	DIC Americas Inc	13	7.80	4,787,183	5,160,650
23	46	Dover Corporation	5	-57.80	26,593,721	11,221,585
4	3	Dow Chemical Company	16	14.35	151,387,737	173,110,018
14	16	DuPont	47	-14.32	45,252,705	38,773,727
86	157	Duriron Company Inc	3	-65.94	4,778,211	1,627,514
78	95	Dynachem Inc	1	-32.33	5,027,356	3,401,801
95	81	E R Carpenter Company Inc	9	14.30	4,063,187	4,644,071
6	5	East Penn Manufacturing Co Inc	1	14.91	96,157,109	110,496,839
40	28	Eastman Kodak Company	12	26.74	14,034,496	17,788,003
69	62	Elf Aquitaine Inc	12	26.16	5,780,319	7,292,648
35	23	Eli Lilly and Company	7	53.93	15,985,323	24,605,495
45	51	Exxon Corporation	16	-19.24	11,871,221	9,586,874
21	18	Ferro Corporation	10	33.51	27,301,307	36,449,254
30	25	First Mississippi Corporation	5	4.56	19,185,249	20,060,564
83	79	Foamex LP	18	-1.15	4,810,511	4,755,036
13	14	Formosa Plastics Corp USA	3	-12.70	45,383,316	39,619,979
59	61	Franklin Smelting & Refining	1	-0.54	7,412,005	7,371,983
33	40	General Electric Company	67	-18.39	16,467,102	13,438,408
67	66	General Motors Corporation	73	13.30	5,981,701	6,777,005
65	94	General Smelting & Refining	1	-47.53	6,665,846	3,497,800
10	9	General Tire Inc	2	15.16	58,251,884	67,085,263
27	26	Georgia Gulf Corporation	4	-13.77	22,650,863	19,532,807
91	90	Georgia-Pacific Corporation	47	-11.36	4,253,299	3,769,915
61	71	Glenbrook Nickel Co	2	-17.99	7,185,345	5,893,001
1	1	Goodyear Tire & Rubber Co	13	17.35	294,371,061	345,442,975
88	85	Hercules Incorporated	18	-10.89	4,619,880	4,116,610
2	2	Hoechst Celanese Corporation	21	12.18	180,100,372	202,027,880
76	42	Holdernam Inc	2	153.53	5,110,310	12,956,061
17	19	IBM Corp	7	-21.79	37,780,060	29,548,779
87	64	Imcera Group Inc	9	55.00	4,640,509	7,192,882

* Top 100 parent companies with largest total production-related waste of carcinogens in 1991, listed alphabetically. Rank is among total of 4,044 parent companies.

Change from 1991 to 1992 in:			
Recycling Percent	**Energy Recovery** Percent	**Treated** Percent	**Released/ Disposed of** Percent
17.11	18.08	-34.77	-11.47
3.21	9.75	-40.65	-30.38
-15.69	25.52	9.37	-13.20
—	-4.34	-81.88	6.86
6.71	—	0.00	-20.83
74.39	-0.27	141.95	-10.09
-25.89	175.00	-77.29	21.38
-11.56	26.84	33.62	-7.70
23.63	14.29	-0.65	-27.67
-1.55	-18.11	2.34	-2.70
5.78	—	63.68	-40.07
-16.67	—	—	—
-7.02	463.78	5,564.52	-39.49
—	—	-63.12	8.33
17.68	-9.39	52.84	-15.45
7.63	-12.21	-49.81	-24.09
-19.52	-58.32	-25.54	-25.93
10.29	—	0.10	177.21
6.08	-86.69	-32.14	15.77
1,153.57	63.40	123.41	55.30
—	-24.11	8.12	4.34
-58.81	-81.75	-95.34	-19.75
54.22	-3.95	2.16	-11.02
-34.80	-17.09	-2.95	-25.23
-66.92	—	-36.77	116.28
-32.66	—	-10.36	-14.98
23.91	-67.37	-62.07	16.82
14.92	—	—	8.31
-13.57	-21.26	80.44	-5.78
27.15	261.97	-0.23	-6.25
-100.00	—	61.61	57.86
305.30	-18.67	-24.86	6.47
34.54	-5.78	0.96	18.17
5.65	-14.50	—	39.70
-21.44	-93.69	-25.21	0.82
-17.29	-22.68	208.78	9.02
-2.60	—	28.16	11.76
-9.27	99.30	-4.46	-45.40
38.01	-68.35	-29.00	-29.21
-50.09	—	—	301.06
15.34	-94.68	-91.48	16.48
872.13	-20.85	-4.40	-51.94
—	-100.00	-9.77	-11.75
-15.66	—	—	-21.72
17.16	52.91	25.93	11.41
235.28	7,753.33	-16.44	-7.95
12.71	15.00	17.61	-15.08
—	153.52	—	495.65
-21.80	58.99	-30.10	-9.49
99.98	25.24	34.83	63.97

Table O-6. The 100 TRI Parent Companies with Largest Total Production-related Waste of Carcinogens in 1991: Change 1991-1992 (cont'd.)*

Total Production-related Waste Rank* 1991 Rank	1992 Rank	Parent Company	TRI Facilities Number	Change in Total Production-related Waste 1991 to 1992 Percent	Total Production-related Waste 1991 Pounds	1992 Pounds
42	39	Inco United States Inc	9	5.13	13,184,788	13,860,937
79	100	Johnson Controls Inc	8	-36.87	5,021,959	3,170,208
51	38	Kerr-Mcgee Corporation	12	30.71	10,622,967	13,885,247
66	70	Lafarge Corporation	9	-1.84	6,079,136	5,967,317
9	8	Lo Nidy Company Inc	1	2.98	65,477,036	67,425,425
38	27	Lukens Inc	5	25.89	14,899,330	18,756,432
29	31	Lyondell Petrochemical Co	1	-21.90	20,826,340	16,265,600
93	93	Magma Copper Company	1	-15.79	4,200,000	3,536,800
80	448	Maron Products Inc	1	-94.50	5,000,010	275,010
64	290	Medite Corp	1	-91.47	6,774,903	578,031
50	65	Merck & Co Inc	8	-33.36	10,776,985	7,181,916
99	105	Miles Inc	12	-19.32	3,740,382	3,017,900
84	112	Mobil Corporation	10	-42.19	4,796,806	2,773,202
12	12	Monsanto Company	17	9.12	48,092,136	52,477,860
28	29	Moore Business Forms	2	-19.59	21,257,049	17,093,086
89	89	Mosinee Paper Corporation	3	-15.52	4,563,010	3,855,020
15	15	Neste Corporate Holding Inc	8	0.26	39,447,260	39,549,782
7	7	Novacor Chemicals Inc	3	-16.69	90,499,500	75,394,550
8	13	Occidental Petroleum Corp	25	-50.96	83,762,217	41,075,755
73	54	Olin Corporation	10	51.08	5,530,484	8,355,362
96	96	Owens-Corning Fiberglas Corp	20	-13.56	3,906,189	3,376,417
25	1129	Pacific Dunlop Holdings Inc	7	-99.80	23,168,238	47,074
41	34	Pfizer Inc	3	17.32	13,362,900	15,678,010
58	84	Phillips Petroleum Company	11	-42.70	7,442,896	4,264,791
11	10	PPG Industries Inc	17	32.01	49,484,117	65,324,597
72	74	Precision Castparts Corp	8	1.14	5,538,073	5,601,185
46	41	Refined Metals Corp	2	15.85	11,578,013	13,413,302
5	121	Reilly Industries Inc	5	-97.97	120,461,701	2,450,022
36	36	Rhone-Poulenc Inc	16	-4.02	15,711,570	15,080,278
94	68	Rohm and Haas Company	13	56.92	4,106,802	6,444,566
56	56	Rubicon Inc	1	-8.65	8,554,061	7,813,842
16	17	Shell Petroleum Inc	17	-5.39	39,277,707	37,162,560
3	4	Shintech Inc	1	10.96	153,078,000	169,862,100
31	21	Specialty Materials Corp	3	45.41	18,596,383	27,041,596
52	53	Sterling Chemicals Inc	1	-18.39	10,248,630	8,363,475
47	33	Sybron Chemicals Inc	4	36.70	11,531,064	15,763,060
75	63	Texas Olefins Company	1	32.79	5,474,016	7,268,913
82	73	Tomkins Corporation	13	17.26	4,831,172	5,664,831
55	55	Unilever United States Inc	12	-9.95	8,693,440	7,828,802
53	48	Union Carbide Corporation	13	12.79	9,884,637	11,148,987
90	86	United Technologies Corp	27	-10.04	4,520,203	4,066,411
18	6	Upjohn Company	2	122.01	35,945,877	79,803,489
34	37	Vista Chemical Company	4	-11.74	16,349,445	14,429,990
92	87	Vulcan Materials Company	2	-6.36	4,235,561	3,965,969
20	11	Westlake International Corp	2	120.14	29,009,890	63,862,803
22	30	Westlake Monomers Corp	2	-36.82	26,813,317	16,940,855
68	67	Witco Corporation	19	10.22	5,948,508	6,556,389
98	92	Xerox Corporation	3	-0.62	3,750,153	3,726,828
77	77	Zeon Chemicals USA	2	-0.92	5,093,495	5,046,804
43	44	Zollner Pistons	1	0.00	12,488,413	12,488,413
		Subtotal	1,047	-0.09	2,496,887,615	2,494,591,973
		Percent of Total	23.77		85.34	84.42
		Total	4,404	1.00	2,925,828,260	2,955,067,837

Change from 1991 to 1992 in:

Recycling Percent	**Energy Recovery** Percent	**Treated** Percent	**Released/ Disposed of** Percent
5.47	—	5114.08	-18.92
-36.87	-100.00	18572.29	-55.48
31.06	-99.25	145.29	11.93
—	-5.38	3242.05	8.84
3.08	—	-30.56	-32.94
30.74	—	81.63	-72.42
—	0.00	-25.67	13.07
—	—	—	-15.79
-94.50	—	—	0.00
-97.46	-86.26	—	-19.22
-27.86	-25.88	-25.68	-72.32
480.94	-65.91	6.91	-21.86
-44.17	-87.40	-39.02	-41.29
21.81	-36.76	18.19	-13.33
-18.91	134.21	66.78	-66.83
—	—	-9.83	-88.99
18.79	52.00	-0.08	-29.42
-16.94	-12.75	-56.12	-13.95
27.58	539.99	-65.50	-9.71
119.01	-97.37	18.38	-35.59
-34.67	5.51	-17.67	-0.79
-99.93	—	5.98	-82.50
19.02	—	-20.04	219.20
6.70	15.35	-72.09	-11.44
35.82	1.59	38.27	-37.74
0.18	—	14.48	86.20
6.14	—	39.73	638.00
-98.79	1028.95	8.25	-49.15
-15.13	73.12	15.68	-7.67
-81.75	1.40	83.66	6.06
—	-11.56	174.55	-29.26
109.46	-16.84	1.08	-15.08
10.97	—	—	5.26
47.05	—	-31.52	34.13
-93.29	-25.05	11.92	-0.57
37.01	—	33.71	-1.94
—	5.43	413.78	15.04
0.14	-7.54	2.31	36.09
-9.97	—	25.06	-41.64
37.06	10.18	16.47	-9.47
-9.94	-11.48	2.25	-14.78
159.73	-89.41	29.26	-28.26
-25.09	-3.15	25.64	-38.38
-100.00	—	2.32	-23.83
—	120.11	114.67	515.03
-10.72	-40.61	154.05	-65.63
11.75	—	-36.17	-2.66
5.76	818.05	—	-37.26
-0.44	-97.52	-50.74	4.89
0.00	—	—	0.00
1.13	9.48	-7.80	-10.47
2.59	10.28	-6.15	-7.78

Table O-7. The 100 TRI Parent Companies with Largest Amount of Carcinogens Released/Disposed of in 1991: Actual and Projected Change 1991-1994*

Released/Disposed of Rank*				Change in Amount Released/Disposed of 1991 to 1992		Change in Projected Amount Released/Disposed of 1992 to 1994	
1991 Rank	1992 Rank	Parent Company	1991 Released/Disposed of Pounds	Pounds	Percent	Pounds	Percent
30	54	3M Minnesota Mining & Mfg Co	1,530,599	-658,737	-43.04	-1,126,426	-73.59
17	19	Abbott Laboratories	2,537,161	-290,925	-11.47	-1,191,715	-46.97
12	14	American Cyanamid	3,374,589	-445,591	-13.20	-579,410	-17.17
36	36	Amoco Corporation	1,417,753	-142,982	-10.09	-256,264	-18.08
51	113	Armco Steel Company LP	1,061,190	-612,235	-57.69	-902,635	-85.06
42	41	Atlantic Richfield Company	1,188,845	-91,541	-7.70	-177,912	-14.97
86	103	B F Goodrich Company	672,671	-186,145	-27.67	-234,715	-34.89
92	86	Barnhardt Manufacturing Co	620,450	-50,000	-8.06	-49,980	-8.06
91	80	BASF Corporation	636,751	-17,189	-2.70	-327,384	-51.41
85	121	Baxter International Inc	684,068	-274,083	-40.07	-516,188	-75.46
72	130	Bethlehem Steel Corporation	798,306	-419,556	-52.56	-561,044	-70.28
48	75	Boeing Company	1,078,900	-426,036	-39.49	-441,600	-40.93
53	69	Boise Cascade Corporation	1,054,024	-370,286	-35.13	-277,646	-26.34
7	8	BP America Inc	4,685,341	-723,683	-15.45	-895,047	-19.10
94	111	Bristol-Myers Squibb Company	610,335	-158,245	-25.93	-287,800	-47.15
23	22	Brunswick Corporation	2,068,658	63,144	3.05	-43,725	-2.11
100	58	Cairn Studio Ltd	569,000	272,000	47.80	309,000	54.31
28	20	Champion International Corp	1,915,550	308,114	16.08	-765,886	-39.98
55	31	Chevron Corporation	1,033,360	571,471	55.30	546,676	52.90
77	63	Coltec Industries Inc	762,407	-160	-0.02	-438,749	-57.55
73	48	Cone Mills Corporation	794,285	151,160	19.03	226,117	28.47
65	49	Cooper Industries Inc	845,999	87,219	10.31	-70,008	-8.28
26	29	Crain Industries Inc	1,981,763	-324,774	-16.39	-1,077,526	-54.37
84	91	Dover Corporation	684,974	-135,288	-19.75	-564,964	-82.48
11	11	Dow Chemical Company	3,536,256	-389,550	-11.02	1,529,000	43.24
89	62	Ducommun Incorporated	640,001	139,510	21.80	-489,901	-76.55
99	97	Duo-Fast Corp	570,953	-67,129	-11.76	-87,253	-15.28
4	4	DuPont	6,634,387	-1,673,664	-25.23	-3,820,104	-57.58
10	7	E R Carpenter Company Inc	3,926,179	660,294	16.82	287,515	7.32
2	1	Eastman Kodak Company	6,931,264	-400,287	-5.78	-1,910,986	-27.57
74	45	Echlin Inc	782,197	189,016	24.16	190,215	24.32
15	5	Eli Lilly and Company	3,033,006	1,754,889	57.86	-1,290,496	-42.55
71	57	Exxon Corporation	801,294	51,807	6.47	-153,236	-19.12
52	46	Federal Paper Board Company	1,060,000	-100,000	-9.43	-700,000	-66.04
60	39	Ferro Corporation	970,143	176,279	18.17	-865,697	-89.23
8	6	Foamex LP	4,580,482	37,357	0.82	-271,717	-5.93
87	71	Ford Motor Company	670,645	-10,214	-1.52	24,878	3.71
82	81	Future Foam Inc	712,747	-96,375	-13.52	-39,507	-5.54
5	15	General Electric Company	5,363,771	-2,435,205	-45.40	-2,544,571	-47.44
32	44	General Motors Corporation	1,501,994	-438,802	-29.21	-564,129	-37.56
95	83	Genuine Parts Company	592,063	3,093	0.52	-307,813	-51.99
14	16	Georgia-Pacific Corporation	3,167,506	-372,237	-11.75	-956,323	-30.19
16	21	Glenbrook Nickel Co	2,760,819	-599,541	-21.72	628,681	22.77
66	51	Goodyear Tire & Rubber Co	818,492	93,375	11.41	4,944	0.60
68	60	Great Lakes Chemical Corp	813,555	14,763	1.81	74,198	9.12
24	27	Hercules Incorporated	2,024,328	-160,884	-7.95	-939,117	-46.39
13	17	Hickory Springs Manufacturing Co	3,203,847	-649,548	-20.27	-1,855,320	-57.91
1	2	Hoechst Celanese Corporation	7,209,836	-1,087,150	-15.08	-3,065,724	-42.52
37	18	Imcera Group Inc	1,410,892	902,535	63.97	1,309,810	92.84
22	28	International Paper Company	2,073,349	-305,817	-14.75	-353,415	-17.05

* Top 100 parent companies with largest total amount of carcinogens released/disposed of in 1991, listed alphabetically. Rank is among total of 4,044 parent companies.

Table O-7. The 100 TRI Parent Companies with Largest Amount of Carcinogens Released/Disposed of in 1991: Actual and Projected Change 1991-1994 (cont'd.)*

Released/ Disposed of Rank*				Change in Amount Released/Disposed of 1991 to 1992		Change in Projected Amount Released/Disposed of 1992 to 1994	
1991 Rank	1992 Rank	Parent Company	1991 Released/ Disposed of Pounds	Pounds	Percent	Pounds	Percent
31	160	ISK Americas Inc	1,516,437	-1,220,856	-80.51	-1,245,139	-82.11
88	77	ITT Corporation	656,743	-8,717	-1.33	-133,359	-20.31
39	76	James River Corp Virginia	1,236,791	-587,553	-47.51	-817,626	-66.11
35	37	Koppers Holdings Corporation	1,459,695	-293,166	-20.08	-89,235	-6.11
59	35	Leggett & Platt Incorporated	978,771	298,061	30.45	506,303	51.73
33	30	Louisiana-Pacific Corporation	1,473,871	164,541	11.16	-127,660	-8.66
63	150	LTV Steel Co Inc	889,020	-567,355	-63.82	-648,358	-72.93
75	196	Lukens Inc	764,526	-553,700	-72.42	-561,300	-73.42
9	10	Magma Copper Company	4,200,000	-663,200	-15.79	-1,400,000	-33.33
62	84	Mcdonnell Douglas Corp	900,099	-311,329	-34.59	-701,193	-77.90
34	122	Merck & Co Inc	1,467,447	-1,061,281	-72.32	-1,239,302	-84.45
44	52	Miles Inc	1,142,398	-249,772	-21.86	-284,181	-24.88
81	117	Mobil Corporation	722,847	-298,485	-41.29	-457,029	-63.23
3	3	Monsanto Company	6,726,205	-896,477	-13.33	-2,215,683	-32.94
64	161	NKK USA Corporation	878,800	-584,940	-66.56	-502,990	-57.24
29	32	Occidental Petroleum Corp	1,695,615	-164,621	-9.71	-639,578	-37.72
19	12	Ohio Decorative Products Inc	2,336,534	803,943	34.41	-350,776	-15.01
58	38	Outboard Marine Corporation	1,000,340	147,691	14.76	782,666	78.24
46	42	Owens-Corning Fiberglas Corp	1,098,499	-8,658	-0.79	-17,114	-1.56
38	33	P M C Inc	1,270,227	83,325	6.56	319,136	25.12
78	95	Pennzoil Company	744,165	-228,147	-30.66	-164,695	-22.13
80	73	Phillips Petroleum Company	740,801	-84,733	-11.44	-61,504	-8.30
61	79	Potlatch Corporation	927,760	-303,413	-32.70	-448,970	-48.39
57	78	PPG Industries Inc	1,026,098	-387,277	-37.74	-774,190	-75.45
98	108	Quin-T Corp	575,000	-115,000	-20.00	-125,000	-21.74
96	67	Rexham Inc	591,800	93,870	15.86	209,800	35.45
41	56	Rubicon Inc	1,220,341	-357,019	-29.26	-376,521	-30.85
54	53	Schuller Corporation	1,047,765	-156,277	-14.92	-416,074	-39.71
90	66	Scot Forge Co	638,700	51,083	8.00	-418,700	-65.56
45	43	Scott Paper Company	1,132,315	-47,315	-4.18	32,185	2.84
79	574	Sebastiani Vineyards	742,854	-696,998	-93.83	-742,854	-100.00
18	24	Shell Petroleum Inc	2,366,783	-356,806	-15.08	-714,278	-30.18
70	61	Simpson Investment Company	804,242	-9,827	-1.22	-137,742	-17.13
76	98	Smithkline Beecham Americas	763,000	-261,320	-34.25	-479,090	-62.79
25	25	Sterling Chemicals Inc	1,985,960	-11,235	-0.57	-70,705	-3.56
67	72	Syntex USA Inc	817,817	-161,287	-19.72	-570,817	-69.80
47	59	T & N Inc	1,096,306	-259,780	-23.70	-51,602	-4.71
20	13	Tomkins Corporation	2,307,087	832,558	36.09	902,869	39.13
69	65	Union Carbide Corporation	804,249	-76,184	-9.47	27,362	3.40
83	136	Uniroyal Chemical Corporation	712,109	-344,705	-48.41	-341,963	-48.02
50	55	Uniroyal Goodrich Tire Company	1,064,532	-200,372	-18.82	-228,732	-21.49
6	9	Upjohn Company	5,170,340	-1,461,230	-28.26	-2,022,040	-39.11
49	145	USX Corporation	1,068,189	-738,578	-69.14	-796,334	-74.55
93	70	Vitafoam Incorporated	617,849	53,989	8.74	132,551	21.45
40	50	Vulcan Materials Company	1,221,305	-291,079	-23.83	-475,256	-38.91
21	23	Weyerhaeuser Company	2,103,506	-92,180	-4.38	153,850	7.31
56	151	Wheeling-Pittsburgh Corp	1,030,600	-712,400	-69.12	-971,000	-94.22
43	64	Xerox Corporation	1,177,460	-438,699	-37.26	-871,185	-73.99
97	89	Xerxes Corp	576,097	-20,699	-3.59	-23,297	-4.04
27	218	Yaffe Iron & Metal Inc	1,965,218	-1,778,033	-90.48	-1,770,474	-90.09
		Subtotal	167,852,098	-23,169,475	-13.80	-47,287,723	-28.17
		Percent of Total	64.56				
		Total	259,989,125	-20,226,023	-7.78	-42,704,084	-16.43

Table O-8. Rank of TRI Parent Companies for Production-related Waste and Releases and Transfers for Disposal for Carcinogens, Actual 1991 to Projected 1994*

Parent Company	1991		1992		Projected 1993		Projected 1994	
	Released/ Disposed of Rank	Total Waste Rank	Released/ Disposed of Rank	Total Waste Rank	Released/ Disposed of Rank	Total Waste Rank	Released/ Disposed of Rank	Total Waste Rank
3M Minnesota Mining & Mfg Co	30	142	54	185	87	227	97	228
Aarque Securities Corp	2098	284	1585	287	1458	267	1358	262
Abbott Laboratories	17	57	19	58	23	58	33	59
Acme Metals Inc	310	157	1085	146	976	142	878	132
Air Products and Chemicals	250	106	283	83	325	83	302	83
Akzo Nobel Inc	203	193	203	175	185	168	177	165
Alaska Pulp Corporation	149	292	126	276	123	297	590	456
Albemarle Corporation	113	131	132	140	115	135	107	138
Allied-Signal Inc	106	81	137	82	125	79	113	80
Aluminum Company of America	129	195	148	200	152	185	131	184
Amax Inc	1074	161	1134	142	1051	145	976	147
American Brands Inc	2418	272	1870	242	1723	251	1620	237
American Cyanamid	12	32	14	32	15	34	15	30
American Home Products Corp	402	188	346	166	316	158	355	155
American Honda Motor Co Inc	300	269	213	280	191	262	178	257
American Magotteaux Corp	240	138	288	144	276	134	262	131
American Petrofina Holding Co	124	100	107	133	131	138	130	129
American Telephone & Telegraph	115	172	123	182	187	252	274	312
Ametek Inc	218	49	245	45	205	40	182	37
Amoco Corporation	36	63	36	52	36	53	35	55
Aristech Chemical Corporation	138	124	162	147	157	146	154	143
Armada Corporation	229	231	289	258	407	290	564	311
Armco Inc	130	37	100	47	78	50	70	51
Armco Steel Company LP	51	179	113	230	217	219	204	215
Arvin Industries Inc	1219	145	1039	120	910	120	822	118
Asarco Incorporated	210	189	260	197	337	197	325	187
Asea Brown Boveri Inc	1336	251	334	440	322	421	378	440
Ash Grove Cement Company	2804	148	1578	174	1468	152	1395	149
Ashland Oil Inc	168	111	166	98	142	100	128	99
Atlantic Richfield Company	42	24	41	20	39	19	43	18
Auto-Tap Inc	432	174	418	546	392	583	364	571
Avesta Sheffield Holding Co	3934	184	3299	173	3127	144	3013	133
B F Goodrich Company	86	26	103	22	88	21	91	21
Baker Hughes Incorporated	667	143	761	109	707	86	695	84
Barnhardt Manufacturing Co	92	278	86	293	77	285	73	279
BASF Corporation	91	48	80	50	126	48	121	48
Baxter International Inc	85	71	121	72	161	67	191	66
Bekaert Corporation	928	293	1091	359	990	359	954	396
Bemis Company Inc	411	185	577	476	543	447	488	288
Benteler Industries Inc	2674	246	3256	243	3081	215	2978	211
Bethlehem Steel Corporation	72	239	130	329	169	433	151	427
Biocraft Laboratories Inc	1331	115	1418	88	1292	94	1211	91
Black & Decker Corporation	415	222	244	215	233	196	222	192
Blairsville Machine Products	3283	54	3301	60	3128	63	3020	64
Boeing Company	48	97	75	97	70	98	67	96
Boise Cascade Corporation	53	182	69	218	59	186	56	189
Borden Chemicals & Plastics LP	505	39	478	75	433	69	419	70
Borden Inc	209	162	185	156	173	160	152	154
Bowater Incorporated	119	237	112	244	117	237	137	255
BP America Inc	7	44	8	43	10	41	8	39
Bridgestone/Firestone Inc	131	60	155	59	166	59	180	58

* Top 300 parent companies with largest total production-related waste of carcinogens in 1991, listed alphabetically. Rank is among total of 4,044 parent companies.

Table O-8. Rank of TRI Parent Companies for Production-related Waste and Releases and Transfers for Disposal for Carcinogens, Actual 1991 to Projected 1994 (cont'd.)*

	1991		1992		Projected 1993		Projected 1994	
Parent Company	Released/ Disposed of Rank	Total Waste Rank	Released/ Disposed of Rank	Total Waste Rank	Released/ Disposed of Rank	Total Waste Rank	Released/ Disposed of Rank	Total Waste Rank
Bristol-Myers Squibb Company	94	19	111	24	100	22	115	40
Brunswick Corporation	23	132	22	127	21	124	19	124
Brush Wellman Inc	202	299	256	322	216	302	203	292
Buffalo Color Corporation	907	62	500	57	514	60	480	60
Cairn Studio Ltd	100	287	58	245	67	258	49	221
Carpenter Technology Corp	506	70	454	69	888	66	857	67
Champion International Corp	28	136	20	125	29	150	36	176
Chemetals Incorporated	2465	223	2579	223	2444	217	2350	213
Chevron Corporation	55	74	31	35	30	36	28	45
Ciba-Geigy Corporation	391	156	302	145	372	109	401	117
Coastal Corporation	272	113	198	102	188	101	188	100
Coastcast Corp	3477	227	3302	177	3126	174	3012	172
Coltec Industries Inc	77	233	63	241	89	270	114	334
Composites Cook & Polymers Co	301	259	114	246	127	259	116	258
Cone Mills Corporation	73	245	48	231	46	207	42	200
Cooper Industries Inc	65	107	49	103	57	105	57	114
Crain Industries Inc	26	144	29	151	49	213	46	216
Crucible Materials Corp	441	238	429	203	360	175	322	170
Dana Corporation	224	250	214	233	168	201	165	195
Dart Container Corp	2202	168	2232	158	2078	2858	1994	2763
Degussa Corporation	318	258	267	219	248	183	237	178
Dexter Corporation	439	167	576	152	520	127	860	123
DIC Americas Inc	178	85	167	76	171	74	163	74
Dover Corporation	84	23	91	46	261	486	249	474
Dow Chemical Company	11	4	11	3	4	4	2	4
Dow Corning Corporation	825	192	852	341	752	322	711	319
Driver-Harris Company	1207	116	690	138	586	123	3018	119
DSM Finance USA Inc	165	273	134	261	122	250	118	254
Ducommun Incorporated	89	236	62	196	93	216	213	244
Duo-Fast Corp	99	279	97	310	75	263	84	303
DuPont	4	14	4	16	9	18	13	19
Dura-Bond Bearing Co	3963	171	3300	150	3121	140	3014	139
Duriron Company Inc	810	86	509	157	482	154	458	152
Dynachem Inc	529	78	595	95	444	71	427	71
E R Carpenter Company Inc	10	95	7	81	6	82	6	85
East Penn Manufacturing Co Inc	346	6	317	5	283	5	270	5
Eastman Kodak Company	2	40	1	28	2	30	3	33
Eaton Corporation	256	234	312	213	286	184	289	179
Echlin Inc	74	175	45	165	43	159	44	160
Elf Aquitaine Inc	295	69	284	62	273	62	335	62
Eli Lilly and Company	15	35	5	23	16	28	24	41
Ellwood Group Inc	2514	235	2674	260	2501	231	2397	225
Emerson Electric Co	152	200	180	221	189	218	338	240
Equity Holdings Limited	117	120	164	239	178	247	172	263
Ethyl Corporation	688	165	497	179	593	157	557	150
Exxon Corporation	71	45	57	51	61	51	66	50
Federal Paper Board Company	52	197	46	209	50	195	105	343
Federal-Mogul Corporation	607	297	1209	232	1059	220	967	214
Ferro Corporation	60	21	39	18	41	17	273	16
First Mississippi Corporation	750	30	624	25	563	24	677	23
FMC Corporation	1086	221	1125	222	1049	226	983	260
Foamex LP	8	83	6	79	5	78	5	82
Ford Motor Company	87	140	71	149	65	147	62	146
Formosa Plastics Corp USA	201	13	183	14	194	14	171	14

Table O-8. Rank of TRI Parent Companies for Production-related Waste and Releases and Transfers for Disposal for Carcinogens, Actual 1991 to Projected 1994 (cont'd.)*

Parent Company	1991		1992		Projected 1993		Projected 1994	
	Released/ Disposed of Rank	Total Waste Rank	Released/ Disposed of Rank	Total Waste Rank	Released/ Disposed of Rank	Total Waste Rank	Released/ Disposed of Rank	Total Waste Rank
Franklin Smelting & Refining	1334	59	1343	61	1165	56	1077	56
Freudnberg Nnwovens LP	960	288	665	282	597	278	570	274
Fulcrum II Limited Partnership	997	204	1328	220	1237	190	1151	191
Future Foam Inc	82	252	81	273	69	254	64	251
GAF Corporation	347	261	351	237	331	221	317	229
Gates Corporation	132	228	102	236	114	228	103	222
General Electric Company	5	33	15	40	14	39	12	38
General Motors Corporation	32	67	44	66	47	61	45	61
General Smelting & Refining	953	65	397	94	2331	95	2249	97
General Tire Inc	158	10	135	9	110	9	153	9
Genuine Parts Company	95	262	83	270	111	323	126	382
Georgetown Industries Inc	1433	240	1529	248	1411	229	1332	224
Georgia Gulf Corporation	233	27	358	26	344	25	331	24
Georgia-Pacific Corporation	14	91	16	90	18	96	18	98
Glenbrook Nickel Co	16	61	21	71	12	45	9	43
Goodyear Tire & Rubber Co	66	1	51	1	51	1	54	1
Goulds Pumps Inc.	1040	202	1213	168	1086	155	971	148
Great Lakes Chemical Corp	68	203	60	183	53	172	48	175
Grumman Corporation	112	296	387	503	435	521	638	573
GTE Corporation	244	257	421	227	365	203	410	196
Hampshire Chemical Corp	146	137	224	115	199	108	186	126
Harlan Castle Inc	1408	135	1512	122	2877	116	1798	109
Harnischfeger Industries Inc	700	134	1064	159	940	141	813	140
Harrison Steel Castings Co Inc	416	180	432	189	366	173	328	163
Hauser Chemical Research Inc	377	249	168	49	135	43	111	36
Henkel of America Inc	270	294	174	262	266	244	281	242
Hercules Incorporated	24	88	27	85	27	87	37	94
Hickory Springs Manufacturing Co	13	109	17	117	20	131	31	171
Hoechst Celanese Corporation	1	2	2	2	3	2	7	2
Holdernam Inc	2586	76	2254	42	2101	42	2004	42
Huntsman Chemical Corporation	232	103	229	204	211	193	197	193
IBM Corp	213	17	220	19	231	26	318	49
Imcera Group Inc	37	87	18	64	17	54	16	52
Inco United States Inc	220	42	240	39	198	38	174	34
Ingersoll-Rand Company	221	207	547	252	564	232	529	230
Intermet Corporation	410	230	344	299	317	265	280	250
International Paper Company	22	112	28	113	26	113	25	116
Interspace/Concorde Battery	2982	242	3088	302	2918	272	2816	270
ISK Americas Inc	31	117	160	181	37	118	134	174
ITT Corporation	88	181	77	163	86	171	80	166
James River Corp Virginia	39	152	76	217	104	236	94	231
Johnson Controls Inc	126	79	211	100	721	128	2374	101
Kalamazoo Holdings Inc	324	268	406	584	304	264	283	266
Kanasco Ltd	1758	247	1997	278	3123	3502	3503	3550
Kaneka Texas Corp	552	298	527	284	448	256	370	220
Kerr-Mcgee Corporation	195	51	177	38	1	15	1	17
Koppers Holdings Corporation	35	153	37	176	35	170	30	159
Lafarge Corporation	1817	66	1838	70	1748	65	1642	63
Leggett & Platt Incorporated	59	216	35	184	34	164	29	157
Lo Nidy Company Inc	226	9	280	8	267	8	241	8
Lone Star Industries Inc	2205	276	2070	178	1903	151	2192	145
Louisiana-Pacific Corporation	33	173	30	153	33	163	32	169
LTV Steel Co Inc	63	224	150	408	149	429	149	447
Lubrizol Corp	1366	169	615	128	523	110	481	104

Table O-8. Rank of TRI Parent Companies for Production-related Waste and Releases and Transfers for Disposal for Carcinogens, Actual 1991 to Projected 1994 (cont'd.)*

Parent Company	1991		1992		Projected 1993		Projected 1994	
	Released/ Disposed of Rank	Total Waste Rank	Released/ Disposed of Rank	Total Waste Rank	Released/ Disposed of Rank	Total Waste Rank	Released/ Disposed of Rank	Total Waste Rank
Lukens Inc	75	38	196	27	167	27	170	25
Lyondell Petrochemical Co	123	29	99	31	94	31	82	28
M C Canfield Sons	1953	119	1908	101	3125	3495	3547	3531
Macalloy Corp.	3755	130	3303	136	3124	130	3015	125
Magma Copper Company	9	93	10	93	11	97	14	110
Mann Industries Inc	547	104	452	78	411	76	389	77
Maron Products Inc	2980	80	3087	448	2919	432	2819	426
Martin Roy'o Lumber Co Inc	198	199	807	445	718	428	683	422
Mascotech	228	248	128	216	109	191	99	186
Master Metals Inc	140	260	291	414	303	495	102	249
Mc Wane Inc	1209	265	1256	257	1175	238	1086	233
McDonnell Douglas Corp	62	166	84	207	165	273	173	316
Medite Corp	418	64	472	290	438	276	434	269
Merck & Co Inc	34	50	122	65	74	91	155	112
Merichem Company	101	275	90	253	80	233	74	227
Miles Inc	44	99	52	105	156	125	50	106
Mobil Corporation	81	84	117	112	138	129	136	130
Monsanto Company	3	12	3	12	7	11	4	11
Moore Business Forms	153	28	319	29	347	23	350	22
Morton International Inc	334	280	502	307	505	286	519	273
Mosinee Paper Corporation	151	89	673	89	789	88	749	87
MTM Americas Inc	366	208	480	118	587	133	674	134
Mylan Laboratories Inc	109	219	94	234	130	274	166	307
National Cement Company Inc	2709	191	3025	162	2713	169	2611	156
National-Standard Company	380	205	384	160	345	156	319	153
Neste Corporate Holding Inc	326	15	388	15	349	13	346	13
New Jersey Steel Corp	2124	290	2217	288	2060	279	1978	275
NKK USA Corporation	64	155	161	167	112	153	100	151
Nortek Inc	102	283	26	132	25	143	22	141
North American Philips Corp	164	264	165	249	145	234	129	235
Novacor Chemicals Inc	381	7	401	7	509	6	477	7
Nucor Corporation	1448	255	1649	305	1550	283	1462	277
Occidental Petroleum Corp	29	8	32	13	38	12	40	12
Ohio Decorative Products Inc	19	127	12	99	22	136	20	135
Olin Corporation	111	73	143	54	129	55	158	53
Oneida Ltd	1246	128	1374	135	2519	2849	2406	2728
Oshkosh Truck Corp	1203	281	1128	267	1484	288	2120	284
Outboard Marine Corporation	58	210	38	192	32	161	23	142
Owens-Corning Fiberglas Corp	46	96	42	96	44	99	38	92
Owens-Illinois Inc	181	254	189	264	176	301	162	294
P M C Inc	38	150	33	123	31	112	27	107
Pacific Dunlop Holdings Inc	948	25	1765	1129	1648	1020	1567	1002
Palos Verdes Building Corp	1300	266	1289	383	1331	332	1083	289
Parker Hannifin Corporation	937	163	885	164	807	165	785	161
Pearl River Wood Preserving Co	289	225	748	508	651	481	623	476
Pechiney Corporation	821	122	864	137	777	126	726	121
Pennzoil Company	78	232	95	169	82	162	72	158
Pfizer Inc	242	41	88	34	76	33	68	27
Phillips Petroleum Company	80	58	73	84	66	77	63	78
Polaroid Corporation	480	226	190	186	181	177	215	204
Potlatch Corporation	61	214	79	269	95	313	86	308
PPG Industries Inc	57	11	78	10	79	10	145	10
Precision Castparts Corp	472	72	299	74	268	73	255	73
Quaker Chemical Corporation	1488	105	1297	107	1166	104	1079	102

Table O-8. Rank of TRI Parent Companies for Production-related Waste and Releases and Transfers for Disposal for Carcinogens, Actual 1991 to Projected 1994 (cont'd.)*

	1991		1992		Projected 1993		Projected 1994	
Parent Company	**Released/ Disposed of** Rank	**Total Waste** Rank	**Released/ Disposed of** Rank	**Total Waste** Rank	**Released/ Disposed of** Rank	**Total Waste** Rank	**Released/ Disposed of** Rank	**Total Waste** Rank
Quanex Corporation	420	291	241	295	717	404	678	408
Quantum Chemical Corporation	136	129	133	250	137	249	299	335
Quin-T Corp	98	286	108	333	92	310	89	323
Rath Manufacturing Co Inc	570	270	614	286	1402	275	1320	268
Raytheon Company	1119	263	1583	291	1531	260	1443	243
Refined Metals Corp	238	46	34	41	71	46	39	31
Reilly Industries Inc	286	5	424	121	370	111	327	108
Rexene Corporation	200	123	249	229	227	214	214	210
Rexham Inc	96	229	67	238	73	223	55	199
Rhone-Poulenc Inc	173	36	176	36	170	37	157	35
Rockwell International Corp	145	241	270	324	870	576	966	1518
Rohm and Haas Company	170	94	158	68	140	72	125	75
Rosby Corporation	2203	256	2175	212	2025	188	1942	190
Rubicon Inc	41	56	56	56	55	57	51	57
S C Johnson & Son Inc	1804	183	1896	202	1733	179	1602	167
Sanders Lead Co Inc	1380	201	1348	205	1269	182	1319	183
Sandoz Corporation	207	133	371	131	335	117	323	115
Scancem Industries Inc	1980	108	1752	114	1571	85	1478	81
Schering-Plough Corporation	103	118	74	134	54	89	78	127
Schuller Corporation	54	198	53	190	62	200	69	212
Scot Forge Co	90	190	66	180	174	324	161	326
Scott Paper Company	45	194	43	193	42	178	34	173
Sebastiani Vineyards	79	253	574	761	3187	3468	3463	3540
Shell Petroleum Inc	18	16	24	17	28	16	26	15
Shintech Inc	409	3	376	4	328	3	312	3
Siegel-Robert Inc	2099	151	2077	139	1969	139	1886	137
Simpson Investment Company	70	211	61	194	64	194	65	202
Sloan Valve Company	889	218	723	198	715	211	675	208
Smithkline Beecham Americas	76	176	98	188	121	198	127	205
Solite Corporation	2340	170	2451	214	2281	192	2169	188
Special Metals & Technologies	1579	158	1753	161	1678	167	1590	164
Specialty Materials Corp	118	31	82	21	72	20	71	20
Sterling Chemicals Inc	25	52	25	53	24	49	21	47
Supradur Co Inc	375	186	1390	550	3143	3463	3453	3510
Sybron Chemicals Inc	372	47	361	33	307	32	277	29
Syndicate Systems Inc	2848	215	3036	235	2865	205	2770	185
Syntex USA Inc	67	160	72	172	107	202	148	218
T I C United Corp	1426	243	1336	271	1169	518	1160	1945
T & N Inc	47	147	59	143	45	132	41	128
Teledyne Inc	285	121	264	111	582	115	568	111
Tenneco Inc	379	154	47	119	52	121	47	120
Terex Corporation	1121	295	848	374	1094	357	1312	358
Texaco Inc	104	102	96	80	98	80	90	79
Texas Industries Inc	989	110	1742	108	1631	102	1547	90
Texas Instruments Incorporated	550	267	559	256	558	239	555	236
Texas Olefins Company	282	75	239	63	223	68	208	68
Textron Inc	215	146	197	126	214	137	221	144
Thomas Industries Inc	299	141	194	124	218	529	239	584
Thomas & Betts Corporation	156	274	152	251	147	255	117	259
Timken Co	271	212	251	206	224	180	229	182
Tomkins Corporation	20	82	13	73	13	70	10	69
Toyota Motor Sales USA Inc	1172	244	1237	294	1156	287	1019	256
Trinity American Corp	105	300	85	292	85	298	81	302
TRW Inc	157	289	104	247	1315	230	1235	217

Table O-8. *Rank of TRI Parent Companies* for Production-related Waste and Releases and Transfers for Disposal for Carcinogens, Actual 1991 to Projected 1994 (cont'd.)*

Parent Company	1991		1992		Projected 1993		Projected 1994	
	Released/ Disposed of Rank	Total Waste Rank	Released/ Disposed of Rank	Total Waste Rank	Released/ Disposed of Rank	Total Waste Rank	Released/ Disposed of Rank	Total Waste Rank
Tyco Laboratories Inc	1889	206	2064	154	2009	149	2074	168
U T I Corporation	923	178	935	170	800	166	714	162
Unilever United States Inc	258	55	340	55	348	47	329	46
Union Carbide Corporation	69	53	65	48	40	52	53	54
Uniroyal Chemical Corporation	83	177	136	191	113	187	101	203
Uniroyal Goodrich Tire Company	50	125	55	129	56	122	52	122
United Technologies Corp	135	90	142	86	179	93	220	95
Uno-Ven Company	524	149	1021	106	782	106	746	105
Upjohn Company	6	18	9	6	8	7	11	6
US Air Force	108	217	93	225	96	222	93	226
USX Corporation	49	164	145	208	146	199	133	197
Valero Energy Corporation	311	101	481	914	197	507	196	524
Vista Chemical Company	159	34	210	37	232	35	251	32
Vitafoam Incorporated	93	277	70	268	60	241	59	239
Vulcan Materials Company	40	92	50	87	58	90	60	89
Vygen Corp	594	196	593	187	550	176	531	177
W R Grace & Co Inc	212	282	350	308	340	295	326	285
Warner-Lambert Company	1294	220	1413	228	1283	208	1201	198
Westlake International Corp	1591	20	773	11	456	417	436	415
Westlake Monomers Corp	262	22	512	30	384	29	353	26
Westvaco Corporation	122	271	105	265	120	243	106	232
Weyerhaeuser Company	21	126	23	116	19	114	17	113
Wheeling-Pittsburgh Corp	56	209	151	412	434	921	420	905
Windway Capital Corp	3336	213	3304	201	3129	181	3017	180
Witco Corporation	414	68	400	67	404	64	381	65
Wolverine Holding Company	330	187	313	211	297	189	308	194
Wyman-Gordon Co	319	114	303	110	272	107	257	103
Xerox Corporation	43	98	64	92	68	84	123	93
Xerxes Corp	97	285	89	296	81	292	75	282
Yaffe Iron & Metal Inc	27	139	218	427	193	398	179	394
Zeneca Holdings Inc	107	159	109	141	99	148	143	136
Zeon Chemicals USA	174	77	163	77	132	75	119	72
Zollner Pistons	2000	43	2076	44	1942	44	1863	44

*Table O-9. 1992 Production-related Waste for the 100 TRI Parent Companies with Largest Total Production-related Waste of Ozone-depleting Chemicals in 1991**

Total Production-related Waste Rank*				Type of Waste Management as Percent of Total Production-related Waste			
1991 Rank	**1992** Rank	**Parent Company**	**1992 Total Production-related Waste** Pounds	**Recycling** Percent	**Energy Recovery** Percent	**Treated** Percent	**Released/ Disposed of** Percent
51	44	3M Minnesota Mining & Mfg Co	1,330,912	60.08	3.01	8.95	27.96
1	1	Allied-Signal Inc	233,220,397	0.33	0.01	98.64	1.02
91	156	Aluminum Company of America	382,135	13.89	2.19	1.82	82.10
30	26	American Honda Motor Co Inc	2,188,722	33.73	4.34	0.02	61.91
47	48	American Telephone & Telegraph	1,228,153	33.31	0.00	2.34	64.35
72	73	Amoco Corporation	738,289	0.04	0.00	3.54	96.42
82	111	Atlas Roofing Corporation	558,976	0.17	0.00	0.00	99.83
42	34	AVX Corporation	1,765,845	40.61	0.00	1.09	58.30
56	53	Baxter International Inc	1,094,745	44.99	0.00	5.48	49.53
14	12	Black & Decker Corporation	5,732,000	93.58	0.44	0.00	5.98
25	27	Boeing Company	2,187,093	13.88	2.35	1.83	81.94
35	52	Briggs & Stratton Corporation	1,122,015	26.69	0.00	0.00	73.31
28	17	Bristol-Myers Squibb Company	4,136,507	95.23	0.00	0.00	4.77
100	79	Brunswick Corporation	711,769	0.37	1.03	0.90	97.70
18	18	CF&I Steel Corp.	3,962,920	95.91	0.00	0.06	4.04
92	97	Champion Parts Inc	620,000	54.68	0.00	0.00	45.32
62	72	Chem-Tech Rubber Inc	762,920	0.00	0.00	0.04	99.96
85	120	Chevron Corporation	485,874	1.38	0.00	12.40	86.22
24	24	Chrysler Corporation	2,515,765	78.36	1.68	0.02	19.93
68	60	Coltec Industries Inc	876,206	17.10	2.22	2.78	77.90
60	80	Contran Corporation	708,000	12.15	0.00	0.00	87.85
84	134	Courtaulds Aerospace Inc	457,542	75.89	0.00	1.66	22.45
58	85	Dalton Foundries Inc	672,839	0.00	0.00	0.00	100.00
80	91	Deluxe Corporation	657,924	12.80	8.98	10.79	67.44
6	5	Dow Chemical Company	26,012,951	33.68	14.61	45.71	6.00
12	14	DuPont	5,478,718	4.99	0.00	22.86	72.14
19	25	E R Carpenter Company Inc	2,455,092	0.03	0.00	0.23	99.74
37	43	Eastman Kodak Company	1,353,219	0.00	1.92	20.14	77.94
61	82	Elf Aquitaine Inc	691,391	19.87	0.00	0.28	79.85
21	21	Emerson Electric Co	2,941,086	41.54	0.60	2.51	55.34
52	55	Ford Motor Company	980,064	13.59	1.41	3.57	81.43
22	59	Formosa Plastics Corp USA	903,307	31.46	54.34	1.11	13.09
53	49	Franklin Industries Inc	1,190,100	0.00	0.00	0.43	99.57
87	106	Future Foam Inc	577,000	0.00	0.00	0.00	100.00
27	32	General Dynamics Corporation	1,826,957	50.61	1.48	1.76	46.16
13	11	General Electric Company	5,778,415	28.40	1.40	10.31	59.89
8	10	General Motors Corporation	7,304,195	49.77	2.46	1.46	46.31
34	46	Great Western Foam Products Corp	1,319,053	6.54	0.00	0.00	93.46
93	93	Grede Foundries Inc	637,718	0.00	0.00	0.00	100.00
11	9	GTE Corporation	7,740,291	93.81	0.00	0.00	6.19
46	33	Hercules Incorporated	1,776,144	17.40	0.00	1.57	81.03
54	57	Hickory Springs Manufacturing Co	937,727	0.26	0.00	0.00	99.74
17	16	Holdernam Inc	4,200,290	0.00	99.99	0.00	0.01
43	41	Honeywell Inc	1,397,351	41.95	0.00	0.26	57.80
5	7	IBM Corp	15,117,496	97.28	0.24	0.44	2.04
40	30	International Controls Corp	1,861,801	22.56	22.56	22.56	32.32
50	50	ISK Americas Inc	1,165,667	0.00	0.00	90.31	9.69
67	104	ITT Corporation	585,949	23.32	0.05	2.72	73.90
65	152	Jasper Corp	391,462	0.00	0.00	13.66	86.34
75	98	Jones & Vining Incorporated	619,800	11.78	0.00	0.00	88.22

* Top 100 parent companies with largest total production-related waste of ozone-depleting chemicals in 1991, listed alphabetically. Rank is among total of 2,184 parent companies.

Table O-9. 1992 Production-related Waste for the 100 TRI Parent Companies with Largest Total Production-related Waste of Ozone-depleting Chemicals in 1991 (cont'd.)*

Total Production-related Waste Rank*				Type of Waste Management as Percent of Total Production-related Waste			
1991 Rank	1992 Rank	Parent Company	1992 Total Production-related Waste Pounds	Recycling Percent	Energy Recovery Percent	Treated Percent	Released/ Disposed of Percent
78	105	Lafarge Corporation	580,435	0.00	99.99	0.00	0.01
66	71	Leggett & Platt Incorporated	769,602	0.00	0.00	0.00	100.00
90	119	Lennox International Inc	489,400	22.48	0.00	6.42	71.11
95	113	Lincoln Electric Company	557,309	21.06	0.00	0.00	78.94
98	102	Litton Industries Inc	605,078	53.43	0.47	1.89	44.21
48	81	Lockheed Corporation	705,101	22.51	0.26	2.27	74.96
39	35	Marmon Group Inc	1,730,009	69.94	1.16	0.00	28.90
74	144	Martin Marietta Corporation	422,811	25.56	0.00	2.55	71.89
9	8	Mascotech	8,063,893	93.72	0.01	0.00	6.27
44	117	Matsushita Electric Corp America	517,411	92.01	0.00	0.00	7.99
31	36	Mcdonnell Douglas Corp	1,572,906	13.58	1.46	6.82	78.15
86	88	Miles Inc	664,929	0.00	0.00	61.91	38.09
7	6	Modine Manufacturing Company	17,029,666	96.73	0.03	0.01	3.22
57	77	Motorola Inc	719,105	24.12	1.29	0.60	73.98
79	110	National Cement Company Inc	560,021	0.00	100.00	0.00	0.00
33	28	National Machine Co.	2,011,694	99.57	0.00	0.00	0.43
36	38	Northrop Corporation	1,506,055	40.19	0.01	2.49	57.31
55	47	NSK Corporation	1,294,406	42.42	0.00	7.09	50.50
38	29	Occidental Petroleum Corp	1,942,164	2.62	10.01	57.41	29.96
76	54	Ohio Decorative Products Inc	1,018,809	0.00	5.96	0.00	94.04
26	13	Olin Corporation	5,531,047	90.82	0.00	1.75	7.42
83	67	Parker Hannifin Corporation	789,905	19.29	5.71	1.65	73.35
89	128	Pearson Inc	469,650	96.63	0.36	0.48	2.52
94	782	Praxair Inc	44,077	8.14	0.00	34.66	57.20
45	42	Raytheon Company	1,363,669	35.65	0.13	4.65	59.57
3	3	RJR Nabisco Holdings Corp	55,491,157	98.98	0.00	0.00	1.02
29	31	Rockwell International Corp	1,852,200	39.22	1.20	0.33	59.26
73	61	Rohr Industries Inc	870,873	11.02	0.00	0.23	88.75
97	165	SCI Systems Inc	362,711	20.21	4.95	8.98	65.87
88	198	S-Dip Corporation	299,124	0.00	0.00	0.00	100.00
69	101	Seagate Technology Inc	606,315	49.57	0.00	0.36	50.07
71	122	Sherwin-Williams Company	482,328	8.81	8.66	55.85	26.68
63	84	Siebe Industries Inc	673,069	19.98	0.00	3.53	76.49
99	69	Sundstrand Corporation	773,331	64.52	0.00	7.79	27.69
23	20	T & N Inc	3,172,918	92.41	0.00	0.00	7.59
49	40	Teledyne Inc	1,462,101	25.12	0.41	1.37	73.11
15	19	Textron Inc	3,910,549	78.93	0.30	0.63	20.14
32	37	Thiokol Corporation	1,525,354	16.82	0.21	0.07	82.91
59	58	Trinova Corporation	930,666	36.46	1.10	0.18	62.26
16	23	TRW Inc	2,537,374	92.31	0.20	0.10	7.39
2	2	U T I Corporation	72,592,526	98.93	0.00	0.03	1.05
64	167	UC Industries Inc	360,000	0.00	0.00	0.00	100.00
10	15	United Technologies Corp	4,873,680	68.18	0.57	0.54	30.71
20	39	US Department of Energy	1,503,683	55.66	0.00	0.05	44.28
41	63	US Surgical Corp	843,259	25.43	0.00	10.86	63.71
77	75	Vac Acquisition Corp	736,500	10.73	0.00	0.20	89.07
70	70	Veba Corporation	771,021	13.23	18.16	0.00	68.61
96	90	W R Grace & Co Inc	658,100	88.77	0.00	0.99	10.24
4	4	Westinghouse Electric Corp	30,626,377	96.53	0.35	0.02	3.10
81	440	Wheeling-Pittsburgh Corp	100,000	0.00	0.00	0.00	100.00
		Subtotal	602,335,160	44.85	1.92	41.35	11.88
		Percent of Total	80.63				
		Total	747,030,073	62.61	3.09	35.89	21.89

Table O-10. The 100 TRI Parent Companies with Largest Total Production-related Waste of Ozone-depleting Chemicals in 1991: Change 1991-1992*

Total Production-related Waste Rank*				Change in Total Production-related Waste	Total Production-related Waste	
1991 Rank	1992 Rank	Parent Company	TRI Facilities Number	1991 to 1992 Percent	1991 Pounds	1992 Pounds
51	44	3M Minnesota Mining & Mfg Co	8	-5.08	1,402,173	1,330,912
1	1	Allied-Signal Inc	43	17.87	197,865,214	233,220,397
91	156	Aluminum Company of America	9	-43.67	678,353	382,135
30	26	American Honda Motor Co Inc	3	-8.75	2,398,714	2,188,722
47	48	American Telephone & Telegraph	11	-21.51	1,564,685	1,228,153
72	73	Amoco Corporation	9	-12.02	839,201	738,289
82	111	Atlas Roofing Corporation	6	-25.77	752,988	558,976
42	34	AVX Corporation	3	5.41	1,675,169	1,765,845
56	53	Baxter International Inc	8	0.17	1,092,890	1,094,745
14	12	Black & Decker Corporation	9	-0.78	5,776,828	5,732,000
25	27	Boeing Company	13	-23.28	2,850,791	2,187,093
35	52	Briggs & Stratton Corporation	4	-39.19	1,845,111	1,122,015
28	17	Bristol-Myers Squibb Company	5	65.52	2,499,112	4,136,507
100	79	Brunswick Corporation	19	14.57	621,253	711,769
18	18	CF&I Steel Corp	1	15.11	3,442,670	3,962,920
92	97	Champion Parts Inc	3	-7.88	673,000	620,000
62	72	Chem-Tech Rubber Inc	1	-16.66	915,400	762,920
85	120	Chevron Corporation	8	-31.15	705,660	485,874
24	24	Chrysler Corporation	13	-17.73	3,057,878	2,515,765
68	60	Coltec Industries Inc	15	0.12	875,118	876,206
60	80	Contran Corporation	2	-31.32	1,030,800	708,000
84	134	Courtaulds Aerospace Inc	7	-35.67	711,270	457,542
58	85	Dalton Foundries Inc	1	-37.43	1,075,281	672,839
80	91	Deluxe Corporation	32	-14.31	767,779	657,924
6	5	Dow Chemical Company	8	3.45	25,145,966	26,012,951
12	14	DuPont	27	-18.24	6,700,696	5,478,718
19	25	E R Carpenter Company Inc	34	-28.62	3,439,513	2,455,092
37	43	Eastman Kodak Company	8	-26.01	1,828,861	1,353,219
61	82	Elf Aquitaine Inc	3	-26.25	937,443	691,391
21	21	Emerson Electric Co	29	-12.60	3,364,935	2,941,086
52	55	Ford Motor Company	32	-26.77	1,338,402	980,064
22	59	Formosa Plastics Corp USA	2	-72.48	3,282,745	903,307
53	49	Franklin Industries Inc	1	-4.63	1,247,900	1,190,100
87	106	Future Foam Inc	2	-18.16	705,000	577,000
27	32	General Dynamics Corporation	11	-29.06	2,575,509	1,826,957
13	11	General Electric Company	50	-10.26	6,439,314	5,778,415
8	10	General Motors Corporation	62	-9.04	8,030,223	7,304,195
34	46	Great Western Foam Products Corp	3	-32.46	1,952,923	1,319,053
93	93	Grede Foundries Inc	2	-1.89	650,000	637,718
11	9	GTE Corporation	11	14.68	6,749,329	7,740,291
46	33	Hercules Incorporated	8	12.56	1,578,002	1,776,144
54	57	Hickory Springs Manufacturing Co	23	-18.47	1,150,204	937,727
17	16	Holdernam Inc	1	20.01	3,500,088	4,200,290
43	41	Honeywell Inc	14	-14.48	1,633,974	1,397,351
5	7	IBM Corp	7	-41.33	25,767,696	15,117,496
40	30	International Controls Corp	4	10.75	1,681,081	1,861,801
50	50	ISK Americas Inc	1	-19.08	1,440,472	1,165,667
67	104	ITT Corporation	17	-33.76	884,610	585,949
65	152	Jasper Corp	11	-56.12	892,125	391,462
75	98	Jones & Vining Incorporated	1	-20.84	783,000	619,800
78	105	Lafarge Corporation	1	-24.64	770,183	580,435

* Top 100 parent companies with largest total production-related waste of ozone-depleting chemicals in 1991, listed alphabetically. Rank is among total of 2,184 parent companies.

Change from 1991 to 1992 in:			
Recycling Percent	Energy Recovery Percent	Treated Percent	Released/ Disposed of Percent
8.07	—	-24.54	-26.22
-45.35	-57.42	19.17	-29.16
-38.44	9.56	60.13	-45.92
-0.96	-2.18	-12.64	-12.90
-9.94	—	189.31	-28.18
135.71	-100.00	71.81	-13.35
-52.39	—	—	-25.70
10.42	—	-53.61	4.60
2.54	—	-15.27	0.09
2.32	-59.26	—	-27.49
-24.23	3,159.81	-48.21	-24.42
-28.30	—	—	-42.38
73.60	—	—	-14.25
-80.28	—	72.02	15.10
15.15	—	10.00	14.29
-12.18	—	—	-2.09
—	—	—	-16.69
—	—	—	-40.64
-7.43	-52.64	496.94	-40.22
6.68	247.77	141.30	-5.06
72.00	—	—	-36.58
-34.81	—	-50.92	-37.03
—	—	—	-37.43
-5.28	23.91	7.43	-21.49
-7.76	137.45	-1.80	-19.46
-72.72	-100.00	121.95	-22.89
175.09	—	70.84	-28.73
-100.00	3,900.00	-51.93	-16.36
11.26	—	-22.45	-31.97
-18.31	63.61	-22.48	-7.69
12.96	-51.58	158.56	-32.28
-21.69	-82.60	20.47	31.37
—	—	4.08	-4.67
—	—	—	-18.16
-18.42	439.72	-55.40	-38.23
-21.26	-39.42	75.01	-10.84
-5.33	106.79	4.74	-15.47
-28.73	—	—	-32.70
—	—	—	-1.89
16.07	—	0.00	-2.95
34.82	-100.00	6.00	9.26
—	—	—	-18.68
—	20.00	—	229.55
-5.98	—	61.75	-19.90
-41.48	-12.48	-59.71	-28.19
5.40	5.40	5.40	23.91
—	—	-15.59	-41.56
-37.48	-93.94	-26.64	-32.25
—	—	-40.35	-57.88
-20.22	—	—	-20.93
—	-24.63	-97.62	-7.59

Table O-10. The 100 TRI Parent Companies with Largest Total Production-related Waste of Ozone-Depleting Chemicals in 1991: Change 1991-1992 (cont'd.)*

Total Production-related Waste Rank* 1991 Rank	1992 Rank	TRI Parent Company	Facilities Number	Change in Total Production-related Waste 1991 to 1992 Percent	Total Production-related Waste 1991 Pounds	1992 Pounds
66	71	Leggett & Platt Incorporated	8	-13.47	889,438	769,602
90	119	Lennox International Inc	3	-29.22	691,400	489,400
95	113	Lincoln Electric Company	3	-13.70	645,789	557,309
98	102	Litton Industries Inc	14	-3.73	628,506	605,078
48	81	Lockheed Corporation	10	-54.49	1,549,437	705,101
39	35	Marmon Group Inc	2	1.94	1,697,055	1,730,009
74	144	Martin Marietta Corporation	9	-46.03	783,425	422,811
9	8	Mascotech	6	1.02	7,982,387	8,063,893
44	117	Matsushita Electric Corp America	2	-68.14	1,623,816	517,411
31	36	Mcdonnell Douglas Corp	11	-28.23	2,191,690	1,572,906
86	88	Miles Inc	4	-5.73	705,310	664,929
7	6	Modine Manufacturing Company	11	-23.03	22,125,762	17,029,666
57	77	Motorola Inc	12	-33.18	1,076,174	719,105
79	110	National Cement Company Inc	1	-27.27	770,001	560,021
33	28	National Machine Co	1	0.50	2,010,700	2,011,694
36	38	Northrop Corporation	8	-18.04	1,837,637	1,506,055
55	47	NSK Corporation	2	17.09	1,105,521	1,294,406
38	29	Occidental Petroleum Corp	13	14.14	1,701,580	1,942,164
76	54	Ohio Decorative Products Inc	5	31.24	776,291	1,018,809
26	13	Olin Corporation	12	103.75	2,714,610	5,531,047
83	67	Parker Hannifin Corporation	20	9.98	718,217	789,905
89	128	Pearson Inc	1	-32.41	694,806	469,650
94	782	Praxair Inc	5	-93.20	648,542	44,077
45	42	Raytheon Company	12	-14.90	1,602,356	1,363,669
3	3	RJR Nabisco Holdings Corp	3	10.45	50,242,431	55,491,157
29	31	Rockwell International Corp	18	-23.85	2,432,298	1,852,200
73	61	Rohr Industries Inc	4	9.21	797,438	870,873
97	165	SCI Systems Inc	8	-43.57	642,715	362,711
88	198	S-Dip Corporation	1	-57.11	697,372	299,124
69	101	Seagate Technology Inc	10	-29.85	864,288	606,315
71	122	Sherwin-Williams Company	5	-42.58	840,049	482,328
63	84	Siebe Industries Inc	11	-25.81	907,225	673,069
99	69	Sundstrand Corporation	11	24.12	623,045	773,331
23	20	T & N Inc	3	-1.99	3,237,278	3,172,918
49	40	Teledyne Inc	12	0.16	1,459,824	1,462,101
15	19	Textron Inc	21	-27.40	5,386,561	3,910,549
32	37	Thiokol Corporation	10	-27.73	2,110,615	1,525,354
59	58	Trinova Corporation	8	-12.80	1,067,321	930,666
16	23	TRW Inc	10	-47.54	4,836,491	2,537,374
2	2	U T I Corporation	1	0.60	72,551,945	72,592,526
64	167	UC Industries Inc	2	-60.00	900,000	360,000
10	15	United Technologies Corp	25	-28.05	6,773,975	4,873,680
20	39	US Department of Energy	6	-55.59	3,385,751	1,503,683
41	63	US Surgical Corp	3	-49.68	1,675,926	843,259
77	75	Vac Acquisition Corp	1	-4.94	774,800	736,500
70	70	Veba Corporation	2	-8.33	841,048	771,021
96	90	W R Grace & Co Inc	4	2.05	644,907	658,100
4	4	Westinghouse Electric Corp	18	-24.52	40,576,825	30,626,377
81	440	Wheeling-Pittsburgh Corp	1	-86.84	760,000	100,000
		Subtotal	979	-1.55	611,788,110	602,335,160
		Percent of Total	23.60		81.90	81.60
		Total	4,149	-1.19	747,030,073	738,134,032

Change from 1991 to 1992 in:

Recycling Percent	**Energy Recovery** Percent	**Treated** Percent	**Released/ Disposed of** Percent
—	—	—	-13.47
-29.49	—	1,208.33	-34.71
-26.92	—	—	-9.32
-4.68	1,040.00	9.67	-4.00
-34.14	-50.78	106.98	-59.25
13.08	17.65	-83.64	-18.03
-73.49	—	1.27	-16.76
0.03	-72.97	28.19	19.35
-70.09	—	—	28.33
-30.72	2.41	-1.47	-29.85
—	—	-4.66	-7.41
-22.78	-49.55	—	-29.77
-30.45	-32.12	-44.11	-33.94
—	-27.27	—	2,000.00
0.01	—	—	11.12
-17.96	-81.82	1,094.27	-21.23
27.53	—	340.55	-0.08
3.46	63,406.54	16.28	-16.05
—	-19.04	—	36.62
148.23	—	54.02	-34.60
51.91	5.49	207.84	1.49
-32.80	-21.92	-22.40	-17.34
-99.41	—	-25.75	42.93
9.54	-66.62	51.85	-26.91
10.45	—	—	10.28
1.76	-52.80	-51.77	-33.84
25.44	—	569.00	7.25
-66.00	36.90	-35.47	-34.29
—	—	—	-57.11
-20.30	—	1,176.47	-37.66
-86.13	1,007.64	-37.15	26.81
-24.10	—	-18.93	-26.53
37.76	-100.00	648.94	-15.30
0.95	—	-100.00	-25.41
27.57	229.44	-29.08	-6.40
-30.31	16.06	-63.77	-10.47
-8.18	-42.03	-68.72	-30.61
-21.44	-68.63	783.51	-3.83
-49.72	-22.82	-54.58	12.90
0.00	—	-24.81	6.57
—	—	—	-60.00
-24.37	5,820.34	-72.62	-34.48
-61.96	—	81,900.00	-43.82
-64.15	—	118.77	-48.14
189.38	—	-40.00	-11.95
-18.40	64.71	-56.25	-16.16
3.20	—	102.68	-10.85
-25.01	-14.98	-59.99	-6.46
—	—	—	-86.84
-8.99	4.34	17.56	-22.22
-10.13	4.49	16.21	-13.33

Table O-11. The 100 TRI Parent Companies with Largest Amount of Ozone-depleting Chemicals Released/Disposed of in 1991: Actual and Projected Change 1991-1994*

Released/ Disposed of Rank*			1991 Released/ Disposed of	Change in Amount Released/Disposed of 1991 to 1992		Change in Projected Amount Released/Disposed of 1992 to 1994	
1991 Rank	1992 Rank	Parent Company	Pounds	Pounds	Percent	Pounds	Percent
79	100	3M Minnesota Mining & Mfg Co	504,359	-132,227	-26.22	-450,568	-89.33
5	5	Allied-Signal Inc	3,354,181	-978,012	-29.16	-1,842,856	-54.94
66	119	Aluminum Company of America	580,142	-266,415	-45.92	-466,357	-80.39
70	51	American Brass & Iron Foundry	554,200	63,180	11.40	-276,379	-49.87
14	11	American Honda Motor Co Inc	1,555,597	-200,616	-12.90	-195,425	-12.56
26	31	American Telephone & Telegraph	1,100,524	-310,149	-28.18	-1,064,524	-96.73
39	40	Amoco Corporation	821,570	-109,711	-13.35	-17,450	-2.12
71	58	Ashland Oil Inc	547,128	29,840	5.45	-27,988	-5.12
45	61	Atlas Roofing Corporation	751,039	-192,991	-25.70	-751,039	-100.00
32	19	AVX Corporation	984,169	45,250	4.60	-984,169	-100.00
72	65	Baxter International Inc	541,800	479	0.09	-258,800	-47.77
65	82	Bethlehem Steel Corporation	594,900	-151,410	-25.45	-156,000	-26.22
87	114	Black & Decker Corporation	473,020	-130,039	-27.49	-443,020	-93.66
6	6	Boeing Company	2,371,300	-579,170	-24.42	-1,623,900	-68.48
91	77	Bridgestone/Firestone Inc	453,687	33,008	7.28	-453,482	-99.95
15	25	Briggs & Stratton Corporation	1,427,448	-604,911	-42.38	-1,427,448	-100.00
80	60	Brooke Group Ltd	498,919	65,800	13.19	-498,919	-100.00
63	41	Brunswick Corporation	604,148	91,240	15.10	-19,766	-3.27
94	38	Cargill Incorporated	440,255	277,445	63.02	201,545	45.78
34	35	Chem-Tech Rubber Inc	915,400	-152,800	-16.69	-651,400	-71.16
50	87	Chevron Corporation	705,660	-286,746	-40.64	-422,149	-59.82
38	75	Chrysler Corporation	838,700	-337,300	-40.22	-389,500	-46.44
48	42	Coltec Industries Inc	718,951	-36,407	-5.06	-378,111	-52.59
33	49	Contran Corporation	980,800	-358,800	-36.58	-980,800	-100.00
78	26	Crain Industries Inc	505,000	315,606	62.50	-255,000	-50.50
28	43	Dalton Foundries Inc	1,075,281	-402,442	-37.43	-1,075,281	-100.00
68	81	Deluxe Corporation	565,169	-121,467	-21.49	-563,139	-99.64
88	97	Dittler Brothers	462,600	-83,400	-18.03	-342,900	-74.12
8	8	Dow Chemical Company	1,938,932	-377,411	-19.46	-792,501	-40.87
1	1	DuPont	5,125,908	-1,173,386	-22.89	-2,326,016	-45.38
4	4	E R Carpenter Company Inc	3,435,916	-987,262	-28.73	-1,453,280	-42.30
19	18	Eastman Kodak Company	1,260,932	-206,239	-16.36	-339,833	-26.95
40	62	Elf Aquitaine Inc	811,457	-259,394	-31.97	-545,457	-67.22
11	7	Emerson Electric Co	1,763,251	-135,515	-7.69	-1,671,695	-94.81
77	27	Foamex LP	506,978	308,916	60.93	-279,861	-55.20
22	30	Ford Motor Company	1,178,442	-380,387	-32.28	-868,431	-73.69
20	15	Franklin Industries Inc	1,243,000	-58,000	-4.67	-763,000	-61.38
51	57	Future Foam Inc	705,000	-128,000	-18.16	-110,735	-15.71
16	24	General Dynamics Corporation	1,365,214	-521,913	-38.23	-1,287,848	-94.33
3	2	General Electric Company	3,881,113	-420,693	-10.84	-2,616,370	-67.41
2	3	General Motors Corporation	4,001,495	-619,097	-15.47	-2,988,645	-74.69
9	13	Great Western Foam Products Corp	1,831,923	-599,110	-32.70	-1,831,923	-100.00
58	47	Grede Foundries Inc	650,000	-12,282	-1.89	-650,000	-100.00
97	188	Grumman Corporation	428,463	-235,776	-55.03	-326,216	-76.14
81	78	GTE Corporation	493,564	-14,578	-2.95	-283,064	-57.35
76	98	Harley-Davidson Inc	507,300	-130,168	-25.66	-237,300	-46.78
17	10	Hercules Incorporated	1,317,196	122,038	9.26	-569,771	-43.26
23	22	Hickory Springs Manufacturing Co	1,150,204	-214,877	-18.68	-306,010	-26.60
31	29	Honeywell Inc	1,008,289	-200,688	-19.90	-717,942	-71.20
96	121	IBM Corp	429,100	-120,950	-28.19	-429,000	-99.98
85	52	International Controls Corp	485,683	116,118	23.91	-476,877	-98.19

* Top 100 parent companies with largest total amount of ozone-depleting chemicals released/disposed of in 1991, listed alphabetically. Rank is among total of 2,184 parent companies.

Table O-11. The 100 TRI Parent Companies with Largest Amount of Ozone-depleting Chemicals Released/Disposed of in 1991: Actual and Projected Change 1991-1994 (cont'd.)*

Released/ Disposed of Rank* 1991 Rank	1992 Rank	Parent Company	1991 Released/ Disposed of Pounds	Change in Amount Released/Disposed of 1991 to 1992 Pounds	Percent	Change in Projected Amount Released/Disposed of 1992 to 1994 Pounds	Percent
59	84	ITT Corporation	639,163	-206,146	-32.25	-616,663	-96.48
42	115	Jasper Corp	802,497	-464,494	-57.88	-802,497	-100.00
69	71	Johnson & Johnson	560,639	-36,549	-6.52	-252,639	-45.06
56	64	Jones & Vining Incorporated	691,500	-144,700	-20.93	-366,500	-53.00
99	91	JPS Textile Group Inc	423,000	-21,700	-5.13	-390,000	-92.20
100	85	Kato Spring of Georgia Inc	420,000	10,000	2.38	-420,000	-100.00
36	34	Leggett & Platt Incorporated	889,438	-119,836	-13.47	-876,013	-98.49
73	112	Lennox International Inc	533,000	-185,000	-34.71	-529,000	-99.25
86	83	Lincoln Electric Company	485,170	-45,238	-9.32	-485,170	-100.00
18	69	Lockheed Corporation	1,296,996	-768,456	-59.25	-942,496	-72.67
62	76	Marmon Group Inc	610,000	-110,000	-18.03	-110,000	-18.03
98	74	Mascotech	423,371	81,916	19.35	-235,991	-55.74
12	14	McDonnell Douglas Corp	1,752,131	-522,974	-29.85	-1,092,516	-62.35
43	63	Modine Manufacturing Company	781,941	-232,804	-29.77	-651,941	-83.37
41	67	Motorola Inc	805,300	-273,300	-33.94	-805,300	-100.00
74	50	N R G Barriers Inc	528,671	92,579	17.51	-528,671	-100.00
95	99	North American Philips Corp	439,136	-64,942	-14.79	-309,736	-70.53
27	23	Northrop Corporation	1,095,626	-232,566	-21.23	-451,626	-41.22
57	46	NSK Corporation	654,166	-539	-0.08	-654,166	-100.00
55	54	Occidental Petroleum Corp	693,122	-111,268	-16.05	-377,910	-54.52
52	20	Ohio Decorative Products Inc	701,291	256,798	36.62	-676,191	-96.42
61	89	Olin Corporation	627,981	-217,311	-34.60	-554,006	-88.22
67	55	Parker Hannifin Corporation	570,916	8,503	1.49	-540,216	-94.62
93	186	Pfizer Inc	450,017	-253,121	-56.25	-440,017	-97.78
90	53	Poly-Pak Industries Inc	458,182	123,673	26.99	-458,182	-100.00
84	79	Prestige Fabricators Inc	486,016	-26,566	-5.47	-36,016	-7.41
25	28	Raytheon Company	1,111,355	-299,075	-26.91	-1,058,045	-95.20
92	39	Reynolds Metals Company	453,540	259,000	57.11	-333,980	-73.64
75	59	RJR Nabisco Holdings Corp	512,961	52,723	10.28	-502,941	-98.05
13	16	Rockwell International Corp	1,658,869	-561,326	-33.84	-1,192,014	-71.86
47	33	Rohr Industries Inc	720,607	52,259	7.25	-351,607	-48.79
54	126	S-Dip Corporation	697,372	-398,248	-57.11	-386,163	-55.37
82	124	Seagate Technology Inc	487,027	-183,416	-37.66	-487,027	-100.00
53	73	Siebe Industries Inc	700,778	-185,916	-26.53	-580,778	-82.88
89	88	Stanley Works	462,147	-46,873	-10.14	-452,147	-97.84
24	17	Teledyne Inc	1,141,919	-73,031	-6.40	-1,049,589	-91.91
37	32	Textron Inc	879,492	-92,067	-10.47	-559,418	-63.61
10	12	Thiokol Corporation	1,822,455	-557,842	-30.61	-817,660	-44.87
64	56	Trinova Corporation	602,510	-23,095	-3.83	-565,510	-93.86
49	36	U T I Corporation	712,242	46,810	6.57	164,463	23.09
35	105	UC Industries Inc	900,000	-540,000	-60.00	-900,000	-100.00
7	9	United Technologies Corp	2,284,348	-787,561	-34.48	-1,914,458	-83.81
21	44	US Department of Energy	1,185,200	-519,337	-43.82	-508,500	-42.90
29	66	US Surgical Corp	1,035,894	-498,666	-48.14	-1,035,894	-100.00
46	45	VAC Acquisition Corp	745,000	-89,000	-11.95	-217,000	-29.13
60	68	Veba Corporation	631,000	-102,000	-16.16	-631,000	-100.00
83	72	Vulcan Materials Company	486,600	34,974	7.19	-103,400	-21.25
30	21	Westinghouse Electric Corp	1,015,204	-65,554	-6.46	-631,404	-62.19
44	329	Wheeling-Pittsburgh Corp	760,000	-660,000	-86.84	-760,000	-100.00
		Subtotal	99,271,097	-58,842,063	-59.27	-82,876,737	-83.49
		Percent of Total	75.87				
		Total	188,720,991	-25,161,516	-13.33	-129,765,490	-68.76

Table O-12. Rank of TRI Parent Companies for Production-related Waste and Releases and Transfers for Disposal for Ozone-depleting Chemicals, Actual 1991 to Projected 1994*

Parent Company	1991 Released/ Disposed of Rank	1991 Total Waste Rank	1992 Released/ Disposed of Rank	1992 Total Waste Rank	Projected 1993 Released/ Disposed of Rank	Projected 1993 Total Waste Rank	Projected 1994 Released/ Disposed of Rank	Projected 1994 Total Waste Rank
3M Minnesota Mining & Mfg Co	79	51	100	44	120	64	206	97
3V Inc	261	255	383	321	156	154	82	103
Abbott Laboratories	191	187	365	350	403	273	317	35
Acme-Cleveland Corporation	436	266	471	310	291	214	177	124
Albemarle Corporation	948	138	278	108	215	71	192	48
Alcotec Wire Co	709	111	657	107	1746	1885	2011	1886
Alliant Techsystems Inc	134	106	131	89	321	341	474	497
Allied-Signal Inc	5	1	5	1	5	1	3	1
Aluminum Company of America	66	91	119	156	101	156	104	150
America Hitachi Ltd	214	277	199	259	209	247	241	244
America Oki Inc	254	290	250	309	286	335	1161	1196
American Brands Inc	107	161	70	115	382	410	263	347
American Brass & Iron Foundry	70	117	51	99	35	69	48	83
American Home Products Corp	276	128	246	269	375	412	445	554
American Honda Motor Co Inc	14	30	11	26	8	22	4	14
American Telephone & Telegraph	26	47	31	48	92	100	257	289
Ames Industries Inc	357	219	264	185	196	140	211	131
Ametek Inc	298	233	280	248	684	613	1219	1244
Amoco Corporation	39	72	40	73	20	47	12	34
Amp-Akzo Corporation	371	211	487	220	332	160	1091	1126
Archer Daniels Midland	197	274	208	270	162	236	112	165
Armco Inc	194	270	150	233	113	186	80	136
Armstrong World Industries	106	127	109	142	127	158	602	720
Arrow Automotive Industries	385	186	86	83	51	55	38	63
Arrow International Inc	111	167	104	153	50	86	29	52
Artra Group Incorporated	190	264	143	221	175	246	828	928
Asea Brown Boveri Inc	209	224	184	227	282	224	1079	1258
Ashland Oil Inc	71	110	58	95	39	67	22	46
Astronautics Corp of America	354	246	336	289	227	210	142	130
Atlas Roofing Corporation	45	82	61	111	1190	1391	1573	1587
AVX Corporation	32	42	19	34	34	42	1107	1141
B F Goodrich Company	318	147	406	140	426	104	400	71
B W Freeman Heel Co	205	284	216	305	164	239	128	185
Bandag Incorporated	105	168	168	250	116	191	171	226
Barker Bros Inc	147	172	130	160	1743	1897	2017	1898
Baxter International Inc	72	56	65	53	70	43	47	29
Becton Dickinson and Company	250	153	90	103	149	169	174	195
Bethlehem Steel Corporation	65	102	82	136	46	85	28	56
Black & Decker Corporation	87	14	114	12	167	8	283	8
Boeing Company	6	25	6	27	6	24	14	26
Bridgestone/Firestone Inc	91	134	77	118	47	80	973	1046
Briggs & Stratton Corporation	15	35	25	52	61	79	1102	1136
Bristol-Myers Squibb Company	179	28	185	17	222	44	190	108
Brooke Group Ltd	80	129	60	109	43	82	1089	1124
Brunswick Corporation	63	100	41	79	23	52	20	44
C R Bard Inc	136	159	151	202	187	245	223	287
Calsonic International Inc	2136	189	2012	123	1742	103	1082	1185
Cargill Incorporated	94	151	38	74	25	53	18	39
Carnadmetalbox Investments USA	120	178	93	139	57	88	1105	1139
Caterpillar Inc	114	142	103	132	75	99	68	91
CF&I Steel Corp.	260	18	219	18	56	6	65	7

* Top 300 parent companies with largest total production-related waste of ozone-depleting chemicals in 1991, listed alphabetically. Rank is among total of 2,184 parent companies.

Table O-12. Rank of TRI Parent Companies for Production-related Waste and Releases and Transfers for Disposal for Ozone-depleting Chemicals, Actual 1991 to Projected 1994 (cont'd.)*

Parent Company	1991		1992		Projected 1993		Projected 1994	
	Released/ Disposed of Rank	Total Waste Rank	Released/ Disposed of Rank	Total Waste Rank	Released/ Disposed of Rank	Total Waste Rank	Released/ Disposed of Rank	Total Waste Rank
Champion Parts Inc	148	92	136	97	134	116	1078	1260
Chem-Tech Rubber Inc	34	62	35	72	32	66	53	88
Chevron Corporation	50	85	87	120	60	90	46	69
Chrysler Corporation	38	24	75	24	40	19	27	12
Ciba-Geigy Corporation	497	108	395	181	458	135	642	99
Collins & Aikman Holdings II	164	216	146	212	211	293	286	382
Coltec Industries Inc	48	68	42	60	38	62	37	61
Compaq Computer Corp	243	265	442	492	1511	1101	1411	1437
Cone Mills Corporation	180	244	113	175	67	118	134	191
Contran Corporation	33	60	49	80	88	128	1104	1142
Cooper Companies Inc	996	271	1603	472	1254	402	786	611
Cooper Industries Inc	146	144	180	161	377	274	829	809
Cordis Corp	137	170	125	148	144	175	163	184
Courtaulds Aerospace Inc	231	84	317	134	210	81	117	55
Crain Industries Inc	78	125	26	65	13	39	56	93
Crane Co	300	294	363	353	265	255	232	241
Crawford Fitting Company	230	250	247	277	362	391	1140	1174
Crucible Materials Corp	110	166	110	157	123	185	1076	1296
CTS Corporation	144	115	169	126	278	225	463	374
Cummins Engine Company Inc	128	158	134	163	560	326	999	844
Dalton Foundries Inc	28	58	43	85	104	177	1087	1122
Dana Corporation	201	212	226	223	390	318	395	333
Danaher Corporation	154	116	158	124	197	190	228	252
Datron Inc	181	181	205	207	135	143	106	119
Deluxe Corporation	68	80	81	91	168	150	783	831
Dittler Brothers	88	121	97	146	188	242	100	143
Donaldson Company Inc	550	140	504	62	346	51	1073	1360
Dover Corporation	264	249	223	208	631	465	1115	1149
Dow Chemical Company	8	6	8	5	9	4	6	3
Dow Corning Corporation	393	146	474	204	420	174	427	142
DuPont	1	12	1	14	1	10	1	9
E R Carpenter Company Inc	4	19	4	25	3	20	2	15
Eastman Kodak Company	19	37	18	43	14	34	9	24
Eaton Corporation	183	209	182	211	177	205	188	189
Echlin Inc	267	234	262	246	335	299	421	398
Electronics & Space Corp	257	298	436	425	329	329	252	261
Elf Aquitaine Inc	40	61	62	82	26	50	52	65
Eli Lilly and Company	308	226	270	224	230	164	173	113
Emerson Electric Co	11	21	7	21	33	36	132	90
Equity Holdings Limited	103	118	147	159	145	142	204	183
Essilor of America Inc	255	238	274	215	380	275	444	327
Ethox Corp.	249	139	366	178	240	113	138	70
FAG Holdings Corporation	259	184	242	192	270	198	534	624
Fleetwood Enterprises Inc	122	188	106	169	81	134	85	140
FMC Corporation	394	179	550	151	1180	115	996	82
Foamex LP	77	113	27	64	17	48	62	100
Ford Motor Company	22	52	30	55	45	73	43	78
Formosa Plastics Corp USA	404	22	282	59	213	56	119	31
Franklin Industries Inc	20	53	15	49	10	35	24	49
Future Foam Inc	51	87	57	106	31	65	19	45
Gaska Tape Inc	208	289	159	242	194	264	1106	1140
Gehl Co	141	135	177	188	151	179	169	179
Gencorp Inc	127	137	95	116	63	87	55	75
General Dynamics Corporation	16	27	24	32	68	49	159	156

Table O-12. Rank of TRI Parent Companies for Production-related Waste and Releases and Transfers for Disposal for Ozone-depleting Chemicals, Actual 1991 to Projected 1994 (cont'd.)*

	1991		1992		Projected 1993		Projected 1994	
Parent Company	Released/ Disposed of Rank	Total Waste Rank	Released/ Disposed of Rank	Total Waste Rank	Released/ Disposed of Rank	Total Waste Rank	Released/ Disposed of Rank	Total Waste Rank
General Electric Company	3	13	2	11	2	12	5	17
General Motors Corporation	2	8	3	10	4	15	7	22
Genicom Corp	408	263	348	282	476	561	470	524
Gentex Corporation	142	205	162	237	103	165	601	650
Goetze Corporation of America	150	182	164	219	128	192	260	320
Goody Products Inc	171	204	260	281	1197	1182	871	900
Grand Metropolitan Inc	177	248	173	253	1745	1889	2013	1890
Great Lakes Chemical Corp	199	267	249	293	160	141	84	126
Great Western Foam Products Corp	9	34	13	46	11	37	1086	1241
Grede Foundries Inc	58	93	47	93	183	256	1098	1132
Greif Bros Corporation	188	239	178	231	129	183	107	137
Grumman Corporation	97	141	188	241	152	203	115	151
GTE Corporation	81	11	78	9	66	14	64	76
Gulfstream Holdings Corp	175	203	141	158	93	132	61	87
Harley-Davidson Inc	76	112	98	145	59	92	50	77
Harris Corporation	309	185	377	314	366	304	468	335
Hercules Incorporated	17	46	10	33	7	27	13	28
Hewlett-Packard Company	133	130	198	179	423	343	1160	1229
Hickory Springs Manufacturing Co	23	54	22	57	16	45	11	33
HM Anglo-American Ltd	288	299	232	280	238	232	535	653
Hoechst Celanese Corporation	186	256	138	209	107	152	70	107
Holdernam Inc	1904	17	1906	16	1617	11	968	10
Honeywell Inc	31	43	29	41	27	41	45	50
Hydrosol Inc	1550	198	1529	274	1093	197	673	146
IBM Corp	96	5	121	7	235	9	998	1055
Inamed Corporation	372	292	179	174	108	114	77	80
Indiana Precision Tech	210	240	144	189	82	97	66	74
Inductotherm Industries Inc	104	163	37	76	811	842	792	841
Ingersoll-Rand Company	313	273	316	308	703	732	1218	1242
Inland Printing Company Inc	184	257	211	300	219	296	197	246
International Controls Corp	85	40	52	30	276	363	594	708
ISK Americas Inc	203	50	295	50	112	31	108	27
ITT Corporation	59	67	84	104	96	107	357	339
Jabil Circuit Co	418	236	314	218	363	258	859	822
Jasper Corp	42	65	115	152	191	204	1088	1123
Johnson & Johnson	69	107	71	112	58	89	44	72
Jones & Vining Incorporated	56	75	64	98	48	75	39	64
JPS Textile Group Inc	99	157	91	149	198	269	269	361
K & F Industries Inc	238	279	197	226	148	162	1094	1133
Kaman Aerospace Corp	302	251	300	272	237	215	191	161
Kato Spring of Georgia Inc	100	131	85	121	199	253	1095	1129
Kemet Electronics Corporation	200	252	132	193	110	172	135	170
Keystone Carbon Company	131	101	96	68	247	207	1092	467
Kimberly-Clark Corporation	364	269	484	442	925	1077	636	722
Knauf Fiber Glass Gmbh	126	192	341	444	281	372	627	695
Kohler Co	125	190	187	262	848	1010	714	807
Lafarge Corporation	1909	78	1957	105	1670	63	1014	37
Laroche Holdings Inc	112	150	120	176	71	108	73	112
La-Z-Boy Chair Company	129	194	108	170	161	235	193	245
Lefiell Manufacturing Co	172	242	207	296	246	327	168	224
Leggett & Platt Incorporated	36	66	34	71	54	96	482	587
Lennox International Inc	73	90	112	119	86	106	722	738
Lincoln Electric Company	86	95	83	113	100	137	1085	1128
Litton Industries Inc	151	98	139	102	131	95	102	92

Table O-12. Rank of TRI Parent Companies for Production-related Waste and Releases and Transfers for Disposal for Ozone-depleting Chemicals, Actual 1991 to Projected 1994 (cont'd.)*

	1991		1992		Projected 1993		Projected 1994	
Parent Company	**Released/ Disposed of** Rank	**Total Waste** Rank	**Released/ Disposed of** Rank	**Total Waste** Rank	**Released/ Disposed of** Rank	**Total Waste** Rank	**Released/ Disposed of** Rank	**Total Waste** Rank
Lockheed Corporation	18	48	69	81	55	70	36	53
Loctite Corporation	388	207	724	173	464	125	277	94
Loral Corporation	157	160	142	135	136	139	375	291
LTV Steel Co Inc	140	210	269	372	399	524	371	460
M & B Metal Products Co Inc	185	258	538	689	354	474	218	285
Magnetek Inc	547	230	413	186	1174	458	1116	1150
Marmon Group Inc	62	39	76	35	41	26	23	18
Marquette Tool & Die Co	189	202	217	184	115	102	71	68
Martin Marietta Corporation	115	74	123	144	89	123	67	96
Mascotech	98	9	74	8	69	13	69	111
Matsushita Electric Corp America	791	44	640	117	1231	288	1179	1192
Maytag Corporation	207	278	311	392	221	295	225	290
Mazda North America Inc	247	291	210	267	125	180	74	110
Mcdonnell Douglas Corp	12	31	14	36	15	38	16	32
Medline Industries Inc	170	109	107	78	106	101	1084	1146
Medtronic Inc	220	215	215	258	296	262	465	267
Meramec Group Inc	2078	272	48	66	214	201	215	155
Metromedia Company	438	197	429	162	740	178	924	258
Miles Inc	152	86	145	88	90	58	57	41
Millipore Corporation	166	193	194	201	279	265	680	707
Modine Manufacturing Company	43	7	63	6	62	5	88	5
Moog Inc	195	177	195	190	119	138	81	104
Motorola Inc	41	57	67	77	344	366	1182	1197
N R G Barriers Inc	74	120	50	96	283	376	1152	1186
Nashua Corp	155	174	231	256	205	219	1075	1306
National Cement Company Inc	1955	79	1979	110	1709	57	1048	36
National Machine Co.	1522	33	1503	28	1424	127	819	81
Neaton Auto Products Manufacturing	192	268	312	421	204	280	111	164
Nishikawa Standard Co	218	261	516	361	379	286	356	275
NMB USA Inc	135	152	149	168	255	241	1025	991
North American Philips Corp	95	114	99	127	95	129	90	127
Northrop Corporation	27	36	23	38	21	32	17	25
NSK Corporation	57	55	46	47	65	93	1096	1130
Occidental Petroleum Corp	55	38	54	29	42	25	41	19
Ohio Decorative Products Inc	52	76	20	54	83	126	318	417
Olin Corporation	61	26	89	13	91	7	166	6
Outboard Marine Corporation	167	222	116	172	114	181	1080	1233
Owens-Illinois Inc	176	228	154	225	97	146	63	98
Paccar Inc	121	175	101	154	53	84	59	85
Pace Industries Inc	124	183	248	343	308	411	1136	1164
Parker Hannifin Corporation	67	83	55	67	77	105	279	319
Paxar Corporation	215	297	318	416	218	282	327	413
Pearson Inc	1256	89	1354	128	922	145	603	148
Pechiney Corporation	206	235	245	278	260	249	278	273
Penn Engineering & Manufacturing	193	232	129	155	174	209	1100	1134
Pfizer Inc	93	119	186	244	289	276	544	544
Photocircuits Corporation	156	217	196	266	431	550	1247	1321
Pilkington Holdings Inc	101	103	118	141	85	109	162	178
Pitney Bowes Inc	169	105	224	125	1548	1574	1706	1706
Ply Gem Industries Inc	159	225	163	245	724	938	1312	1332
Poly-Pak Industries Inc	90	122	53	87	87	131	1097	1131
PPG Industries Inc	160	123	171	114	130	77	116	59
Pratt & Lambert Inc	788	281	815	531	507	336	350	221
Praxair Inc	1142	94	896	782	709	696	492	443

Table O-12. Rank of TRI Parent Companies for Production-related Waste and Releases and Transfers for Disposal for Ozone-depleting Chemicals, Actual 1991 to Projected 1994 (cont'd.)*

	1991		1992		Projected 1993		Projected 1994	
Parent Company	Released/ Disposed of Rank	Total Waste Rank	Released/ Disposed of Rank	Total Waste Rank	Released/ Disposed of Rank	Total Waste Rank	Released/ Disposed of Rank	Total Waste Rank
Precision Castparts Corp	119	145	166	203	201	202	378	445
Premix Inc	382	237	420	384	1005	966	1303	1314
Prestige Fabricators Inc	84	133	79	133	44	83	26	54
Pullman Holding Corp	149	208	117	177	78	120	60	95
Radiator Specialty Co	202	276	1100	255	1195	827	691	566
Raytheon Company	25	45	28	42	207	189	207	193
Reynolds Metals Company	92	126	39	56	49	72	101	153
RJR Nabisco Holdings Corp	75	3	59	3	930	1158	538	659
Rockwell International Corp	13	29	16	31	28	33	25	30
Rohr Industries Inc	47	73	33	61	29	59	33	58
Rostra Holding Inc	225	275	213	194	126	124	1108	1138
Russell Corp	173	241	155	238	99	166	72	114
Sabh US Inc	123	169	80	129	64	111	35	67
Sandberg Furniture Manufacturing	221	295	212	286	158	221	133	181
Sanden of America Inc	204	282	233	330	165	240	103	157
Sauer Inc	265	165	551	485	1760	1852	1835	1823
Scancem Industries Inc	1831	201	1817	92	1519	60	893	40
Schering-Plough Corporation	217	136	156	94	370	213	530	200
SCI Systems Inc	117	97	153	165	721	467	1119	632
S-Dip Corporation	54	88	126	198	73	122	42	79
Seagate Technology Inc	82	69	124	101	521	324	1167	1202
Senco Products Inc	108	162	172	252	153	226	172	225
Sequa Corporation	165	171	165	182	139	155	110	128
Sheldahl Inc	240	296	540	586	530	600	1240	1275
Sherwin-Williams Company	360	71	255	122	172	76	127	57
Sibv/Ms Holdings Inc	294	262	843	1000	1810	1854	1839	1831
Siebe Industries Inc	53	63	73	84	84	110	99	120
Siemens Corporation	178	200	176	206	459	408	1117	1151
SKF USA Inc	270	223	313	199	905	557	723	799
Sony USA Inc	299	285	332	283	1751	1634	1805	1811
Stanley Works	89	124	88	131	105	159	540	668
Steelcase Inc	109	154	92	137	111	168	418	512
Sundstrand Corporation	161	99	174	69	147	136	170	129
T & N Inc	130	23	152	20	94	18	91	11
Talley Industries Inc	317	253	548	419	843	695	670	612
Tecumseh Products Company	153	214	433	448	710	656	604	608
Teledyne Inc	24	49	17	40	37	46	129	116
Tenneco Inc	272	218	221	229	159	147	86	102
Texas Industries Inc	1950	283	1999	166	1710	98	1049	47
Texas Instruments Incorporated	162	199	181	230	137	182	151	167
Textron Inc	37	15	32	19	36	16	40	16
Therma-Tru Corp	174	245	148	234	122	194	113	166
Thiokol Corporation	10	32	12	37	12	30	8	23
Thomas & Betts Corporation	196	191	191	147	166	130	185	144
Ti Group Inc	168	180	128	138	80	91	49	60
Time Warner Inc	363	287	335	273	364	328	404	350
Timken Co	132	143	135	143	257	271	1187	1207
Trinova Corporation	64	59	56	58	118	121	255	201
Trutec Industries Inc	947	156	864	51	511	78	1101	1135
TRW Inc	228	16	193	23	256	28	480	396
Tyco Laboratories Inc	118	149	94	130	121	171	93	135
U T I Corporation	49	2	36	2	18	2	10	2
UC Industries Inc	35	64	105	167	1744	1895	2121	2106
Union City Body Company Inc	158	227	102	164	1747	1883	2073	2010

Table O-12. Rank of TRI Parent Companies for Production-related Waste and Releases and Transfers for Disposal for Ozone-depleting Chemicals, Actual 1991 to Projected 1994 (cont'd.)*

	1991		1992		Projected 1993		Projected 1994	
Parent Company	**Released/ Disposed of** Rank	**Total Waste** Rank	**Released/ Disposed of** Rank	**Total Waste** Rank	**Released/ Disposed of** Rank	**Total Waste** Rank	**Released/ Disposed of** Rank	**Total Waste** Rank
Unisys Corporation	116	148	137	171	140	173	541	599
United Musical Instruments USA	248	254	175	196	132	153	114	138
United Technologies Corp	7	10	9	15	19	17	32	38
US Air Force	211	259	200	251	228	270	175	215
US Department of Energy	21	20	44	39	22	29	15	20
US Navy	113	132	204	232	146	163	97	123
US Surgical Corp	29	41	66	63	102	94	1093	1127
Utility Trailer Mfg Co	198	260	240	327	203	259	140	182
Vac Acquisition Corp	46	77	45	75	30	54	21	43
Valeo Engine Cooling Inc	212	243	477	431	671	663	1241	1339
Varian Associates Inc	139	164	238	261	229	227	471	447
Veba Corporation	60	70	68	70	421	479	1166	1218
Vermont American Corporation	455	221	304	183	562	272	1183	1199
Vishay Intertechnology Inc	859	286	333	213	466	252	321	160
Vulcan Materials Company	83	104	72	100	52	74	31	51
W R Grace & Co Inc	457	96	448	90	449	68	521	73
Waltco Engineering Co	315	173	353	222	347	332	323	317
Walter Industries Inc	138	206	127	200	79	133	54	89
Walton Enterprises Inc	224	288	1329	1225	1852	1515	1636	1669
Watts Industries Inc	706	220	761	210	615	231	1077	1323
Weirton Steel Corporation	213	293	349	451	1198	1222	1443	1457
Weslock Co	237	280	272	364	185	234	124	158
Westinghouse Electric Corp	30	4	21	4	24	3	30	4
Wheeling-Pittsburgh Corp	44	81	329	440	1761	1865	1865	1865
Whirlpool Corporation	143	196	122	180	72	117	78	121
White Consolidated Industries	163	195	161	191	124	149	180	196
Whitman Corporation	305	300	452	460	520	617	307	364
Wolverine Holding Company	145	176	111	150	76	112	58	84
Woodward Governor Co	187	213	170	187	170	170	118	122
Xerox Corporation	373	229	236	205	1510	1555	1667	1667
Zeneca Holdings Inc	182	231	227	240	305	281	268	354
Zenith Electronics Corporation	102	155	133	195	1741	1903	2107	2078
Zexel USA Corp	303	247	431	320	725	605	1263	1329

Appendix P

33/50 Program Chemicals

Table P-1. Characteristics, Toxicity, Uses, and 1992 Releases and Transfers of 33/50 Program Chemicals

Chemical	Characteristics	Toxicity
Benzene	Clear, colorless, highly flammable liquid, characteristic odor, boiling point 80.1°C. Formed by coking coal (and petroleum refining?).	*Acute:* (from ingestion or inhalation) irritation of mucous membranes, restlessness, convulsions, excitement, depression. Death may follow from respiratory failure. *Chronic:* bone marrow depression and aplasia; rarely, leukemia. Harmful amounts may be absorbed through the skin. This substance has been listed as a carcinogen by EPA.
Cadmium and compounds	Silver-white, blue-tinged, lustrous metal; distorted hexagonal close-packed structure; easily cut with a knife; available in the form of bars, sheets, or wire or a gray, granular powder. Melting point 321°C, boiling point 765°C. (Found in zinc ores).	Cadmium and its salts are highly toxic. Ingestion of metal and soluble compounds causes increased salivation, choking, vomiting, abdominal pain, anemia, renal dysfunction, diarrhea, tenesmus. Inhalation (dust or fumes) causes throat dryness, cough, headache, vomiting, chest pains, extreme restlessness and irritability, pneumonitis, possibly bronchopneumonia. This substance and certain cadmium compounds have been listed as carcinogens by EPA.
Carbon tetrachloride	Colorless, clear, nonflammable, heavy liquid; characteritic odor, boiling point 76.7°C. Obtained from carbon disulfide and chlorine in the presence of a catalyst, or by the chlorination of hydrocarbons.	Poisoning by inhalation, ingestion or skin absorption. *Acute:* nausea, vomiting, diarrhea, headache, stupor, renal damage leading to anuria and azotemia, liver injury. Can be fatal. *Chronic:* primarily liver damage but kidney injury and visual disturbances also occur. Skin contact can lead to dermatitis through defatting action. This substance has been listed as a carcinogen by EPA.
Chloroform	Highly refractive, nonflammable, heavy, very volatile, sweet-tasting liquid; characteristic odor, boiling point 61-62°C. Made from acetone and bleaching powder by addition of sulfuric acid.	Inhalation of large doses may cause hypotension, respiratory and myocardial depression and death. Banned by FDA from use in drug, cosmetic and food packaging products in 1976. Carcinogen.
Chromium and compounds	Steel gray, lustrous metal; body-centered cubic structure; hard as corundum and less fusible than platinum. Takes a high polish; melting point 1900°C, boiling point 2642°C. Not oxidized by air even in the presence of moisture. Obtained from chromite ore by a silicothermic or aluminothermic.	Chromic acid or chromate salts constitute industrial hazards. Irritant effects on the skin and respiratory passages lead to ulceration. Oral ingestion may lead to severe irritation of the gastrointestinal tract, circulatory shock and renal damage. Chromium III compounds show little or no toxicity. Chromium VI and certain compounds are carcinogenic.
Cyanides:		
Sodium cyanide	White granules or fused pieces. Odorless when perfectly dry; somewhat deliquescent in damp air and emits slight odor of HCN, melting point 563°C.	Violent poison.

Industrial Uses	1992 Releases	1992 Transfers*
	Millions of Pounds	
Manufacture of medicinal chemicals, dyes and many other organic compounds, artificial leather, linoleum, oil, cloth, airplane dopes, varnishes, lacquers; as solvents for waxes, resins, oils, etc.	13.1	6.5
A constituent of easily fusible alloys; soft solder and solder for aluminum, electroplating (major use), deoxidizer in nickel plating; process engraving, electrodes for cadmium vapor lamps, photoelectric cells; photometry of UV sun-rays; in nickel-cadmium storage batteries.	0.1	3.0
As fire extinguisher; for cleaning clothing; rendering benzin nonflammable; as azeotropic drying agent for wet spark plugs in automobiles; as solvent for oils, fats, lacquers, seeds; exterminating destructive insects; solvent; starting material in manufacture of many organic compounds. (May form phosgene when used to put out electrical fires.)	1.4	1.2
Solvent for fats, oils, rubber, alkaloids, waxes, gutta-percha, resins; as cleansing agent; in fire extinguishers to lower freezing temperature of carbon tetrachloride; in rubber industry.	17.8	3.8
In manufacture of chrome-steel or chrome-nickel-steel alloys (stainless steel); for greatly increasing resistance and man-made ^{51}Cr isotope as tracer in various blood diseases and in the determination of blood volume (as the chloride or as sodium chromate).	25.4	115.7
Extracting gold and silver from ores; electroplating baths; fumigating citrus and other fruit trees, ships, railway cars, warehouses, etc.; manufacturing hydrocyanic acid and many other cyanides; case hardening of steel.	7.3	1.0

Table P-1. *Characteristics, Toxicity, Uses, and 1992 Releases and Transfers of 33/50 Program Chemicals (cont'd.)*

Chemical	Characteristics	Toxicity
Cyanides: (cont'd.)		
Hydrogen cyanide	Colorless gas or liquid; characteristic odor; very weakly acid; burns in air with a blue flame, melting point -13.4°C, boiling point 25.6°C. Prepared on a large scale by the catalytic oxidation of ammonia-methane mixtures.	Intensely poisonous, even when mixed with air. High concentrations produce tachypnea (causing increased intake of cyanide); then dyspnea, paralysis, unconsciousness, convulsions and respiratory arrest. Headache, vertigo, nausea and vomiting may occur with lesser concentrations. Chronic exposure over long periods may cause fatigue, weakness. Exposure to 150 ppm for 1/2 to 1 hour may endanger life. Death may result from a few minutes exposure to 300 ppm. Average fatal dose: 50-60 mg.
Dichloromethane	Colorless liquid; vapor is not flammable and when mixed with air is not explosive, boiling point 39.75°C (at 760 mm). Prepared through chlorination of methane.	Narcotic in high concentrations.
Lead and compounds	Occurs chiefly as sulfide in galena. Bluish-white, silvery-gray metal. Highly lustrous when freshly cut, tarnishes upon exposure to air. Very soft and malleable, easily melted, cast, rolled, and extruded. Prepared through recovery from ore and purification.	*Acute*: Most common in young children with history of pica; anorexia, vomiting, malaise, convulsions due to increased intracranial pressure. May leave permanent brain damage. *Chronic:* children show weight loss, weakness, anemia. Lead poisoning in adults is usually occupational, due mainly to inhalation of lead dust or fumes.
Mercury and compounds	Silver-white, heavy, mobile, liquid metal; slightly volatile at ordinary temperatures; solid mercury is a tin-white, ductile, malleable mass which may be cut with a knife, melting point -38.87°C, boiling point 356.72°C. Obtained by roasting cinnabar (mercuric sulfide). Mercury slats when heated with sodium carbonate yield metallic mercury and are reduced to metal by hydrogen peroxide in the presence of alkali hydroxide.	Readily absorbed via respiratory tract (elemental mercury vapor, mercury compound dusts), intact skin, and GI tract, although occasional incidental swallowing of metallic mercury is without harm. Spilled and heated elemental mercury is particularly hazardous. *Acute:* soluble salts have violent corrosive effects on skin and mucous membranes; severe nausea, vomiting, abdominal pain, bloody diarrhea; kidney damage; death usually within 10 days. *Chronic:* inflammation of mouth and gums, excessive salivation, loosening of teeth; kidney damage; muscle tremors, jerky gait, spasms of extremities; personality changes, depression, irritability, nervousness.
Methyl ethyl ketone	Flammable liquid, acetone-like odor, boiling point 79.6°C. Obtained by refluxing methyl acetoacetate and dilute sulfuric acid, or by the oxidation of secondary butyl alcohol; also by fermentation.	Exposure to MEK may occur through ingention, inhalation, and skin absorption. Short-term exposure to MEK can cause nose and throat irritation, nausea, vomiting, headaches, dizziness, and loss of coordination or bablance. May cause numbness in the fingers, arms, and legs, and unconsciousness. MEK volatalizes slowly in water and is mobile in soil. It is moderately toxic to aquatic life and contributes to smog formation. It does not cause any cumulative effects to aminal life.

Industrial Uses	1992 Releases	1992 Transfers
	Millions of Pounds	
Compressed gas is used for exterminating rodents and insects in ships and for killing insects on trees, etc.		
Solvent for cellulose acetate; degreasing and cleaning fluids; solvent in food processing.	75.4	46.2
Construction material for tank linings, piping, and other equipment handling corrosive gases and liquids used in the manufacture of sulfuric acid, petroleum refining, halogenation, sulfonation, extraction, condensation; for x-ray and atomic radiation protection; manufacture of tetraethyllead, pigments for paints, and other organic and inorganic lead compounds, bearing metal and alloys; storage batteries; in ceramics, plastics, and electronic devices; in building construction; in solder and other lead alloys; in the metallurgy of steel and other metals.	15.9	440.6
Used in barometers, thermometers, hydrometers, pyrometers; in mercury arc lamps producing UV rays; in switches, fluorescent lamps; in mercury boilers; manufacture all mercury salts; mirrors; as catalyst in oxidation of organic compounds; extracting gold and silver from ores; making amalgams, electric rectifiers, mercury fulminate; also in dentistry, in determining nitrogen, as cathode in electrolysis, electroanalysis, and many other uses. Also in pharmaceuticals, agricultural chemicals, antifouling paints.	0.02	0.3
As solvent; in the surface coating industry; manufacture smokeless powder; colorless synthetic resins.	91.3	72.3

Table P-1. Characteristics, Toxicity, Uses, and 1992 Releases and Transfers of 33/50 Program Chemicals (cont'd.)

Chemical	Characteristics	Toxicity
Methyl isobutyl ketone	Colorless liquid with a pleasant odor. Flammable liquid and a fire hazard.	Inhalation. Exposure to high concentrations can cause dizziness and fainting. Long-term exposure may damage the liver and kidneys. Breathing the vapor may cause loss of appetite, nausea, vomiting, and diarrhea. The vapor can irritate the eyes, nose, mouth, and throat. Contact can irritate the skin.
Nickel and compounds	Lustrous white, hard, ferromagnetic metal; face-centered cubic crystals, melting point 1555°C, boiling point 2837°C. Obtained by extraction and purification from many ores.	May cause dermatitis in sensitive individuals. Ingestion of soluble salts causes nausea, vomiting, diarrhea. Nickel and certain compounds have been listed as carcinogenic by EPA.
Tetrachloro-ethylene	Colorless, nonflammable liquid; ethereal odor, boiling point 121°C. Manufactured by catalytic oxidation of 1,1,2,2-tertrachloroethane.	Narcotic in high concentrations. Defatting action on skin can lead to dermatitis.
Toluene	Flammable, refractive liquid; benzene-like odor, boiling point 110.6°C. Obtained mainly from tar oil.	May cause mild macrocytic anemia but not leukopenia. Less toxic than benzene. Narcotic in high concentrations.
1,1,1-Trichloro-ethane	Nonflammable liquid, boiling point 74.1°C. (760mm). Prepared by action of chlorine on 1,1-dichloroethane; by catalytic addition of HCl to 1,1-dichloroethylene.	Irritating to eyes, mucous membranes, and in high concentrations, narcotic.
Trichloroethylene	Nonflammable, mobile liquid, characteristic odor resembling chloroform, boiling point 86.7°C (760mm). Usually prepared from *sym*-tetrachloroethane by elimination of HCl (by boiling with lime).	Moderate exposures can cause symptoms similar to alcohol inebriation. Higher concentrations can have narcotic effect. Deaths occurring after heavy exposure have been attributed to ventricular fibrillation. Liver injury is not definitely established in occupational exposures. Found to induce hepatocellular carcinomas in National Cancer Institute tests on mice.
Xylenes	Mobile, flammable colorless liquid, boiling point 137-140°C. Obtained from coal tar; manufactured from pseudocumene; by catalytic isomerization of a hydrocarbon fraction.	May be narcotic in high concentrations. Chronic toxicity not well defined, but is less toxic than benzene.

* Includes quantities sent off-site for energy recovery or recycling.

Source: Toxicity for methyl ethyl ketone (MEK) from *The Product Side of Pollution Prevention: Evaluating the Potential for Safe Substitutes,* Center for Clean Products and Clean Technologies, University of Tennessee, August 1994; characteristics, toxicity (except MEK), and use information from *Merck Index,* 10th Edition and NJ Fact Sheets; releases and transfers from U.S. Environmental Protection Agency, *1992 Toxics Release Inventory Public Data Release,* EPA 745-4-94-001, April 1994

Industrial Uses	1992 Releases	1992 Transfers
	Millions of Pounds	
As solvent.	26.3	40.0
Probably the largest use is in the manufacture of Monel metal, stainless steels, and nickel-chrome resistance wire; in alloys for electronic and space applications. Nickel plating; for various alloys such as new silver, Chinese silver, German silver; for coins, electrotypes, storage batteries; magnets, lightning-rod tips, electrical contacts and electrodes, spark plugs, machinery parts, catalyst for hydrogenation of oils and other organic substances.	5.0	91.8
Dry cleaning; degreasing metals; solvent.	12.3	10.7
In manufacture of benzoic acid, benzaldehyde, explosives, dyes, and many other organic compounds; as a solvent for paints, lacquers, gums, resins, in the extraction of various principles from plants; as gasoline additive.	193.4	130.7
In cold type metal cleaning, also in cleaning plastic molds.	115.0	31.9
Solvent for fats, waxes, resins, oils, rubber, paints, and varnishes. Solvent for cellulose esters and ethers. used for solvent extraction in many industries. In degreasing, in dry cleaning. In the manufacture of organic chemicals, pharmaceuticals, such as chloroacetic acid.	29.6	9.7
As solvent; raw material for production of benzoic acid, phthalic anhydride, isophthalic and terephthalic acids as well as their dimethyl esters used in the manufacture of polyester fibers; manufacture of dyes and other organics; sterilizing catgut; with Canada balsam as oil-immersion in microscopy; cleaning agent in microscopic technique.	118.8	115.1

Appendix Q

Database Access

This Appendix supplies information on access to databases discussed in *Toxics Watch 1995* (listed below). Some databases are available through U.S. EPA's National Computing Center. RTK-Net also provides on-line access to some databases.

Sources for electronic and printed media include the National Technical Information Service and the Government Printing Office. Information on these general sources appears at the end of this Appendix.

Air Quality Subsystem of the Aerometric Information Retrieval System (AQS/AIRS)

Biennial Reporting System (BRS)

Contract Laboratory Program (CLP) Analytical Result Database (CARD)

Chemicals In Commerce Information System (CICIS, data from Toxic Substances Control Act)

Chemical Update System (CUS, data from Toxic Substances Control Act — Inventory Update Rule)

Federal Reporting Data System II (to be changed to Safe Drinking Water Information System) (FRDS II)

Massachusetts Toxics Use Reduction Database, Form S and Form R (TURA)

New Jersey Release and Pollution Prevention Report Data

STOrage and RETrieval of U.S. Waterways Parametric Data (Water Quality System)

Toxics Release Inventory (TRI)

Database	*Air Quality Subsystem of the Aerometric Information Retrieval System*
Acronym	AQS/AIRS
Source	U.S. EPA
Contact	Virginia Ambrose, 919/541-5454 Information Management Division, EPA
Technical Support	AQS Hotline, 800/333-7909
Training	Jonathan Miller, 919/541-3330 AQS Bulletin Board (BBS) Helpline, 919/541-5384
Documentation	National Air Data Branch, EPA, 919/541-5447 919/541-7674 (Fax)
Access	*EPA's National Computer Center (NCC)* AIRS has three subsystems: Air Facility Subsystem (AFS), Air Quality Subsystem (AQS), and Air Mobile Subsystem (AMS), linked by a Geo-Common System (GCS). All subsystems are available once access to the system is made (only AQS data were analyzed for this *Toxics Watch*). *AIRS Electronic Bulletin Board* (BBS) 919/541-5742 or via Internet TTNBBS.RTPNC.EPA.GOV AIRS BBS provides useful information regarding contacts, manuals, and related software, as well as access to AIRS Executive (see below). The BBS supports access by personal computer and modem, at baud rates from 2400 to 14,400. Questions regarding problems or access can be directed to the AIRS BBS Helpline at 919/541-5384. *Airs Executive* In addition to the AIRS database maintained at the NCC, a personal computer application has been developed that provides summary information about air quality and about air emissions for criteria pollutants. This program, AIRS Executive, provides tabular and graphic display of data, as well as maps. Data are routinely updated. It may be accessed either via the AIRS BBS or through the Internet via a gopher or FTP connection.

Database	*Biennial Reporting System*
Acronym	BRS
Source	RTK-Net (see below)
	Final 1991 BRS data (available May 1994 from NCC) were scheduled to be available early in 1995 through RTK-Net.
Source	U.S. EPA NCC (see below)

Database	*Chemicals In Commerce Information System (data collected under the Toxic Substances Control Act)*
Acronym	CICIS
Source	U.S. EPA
Contact	TSCA Assistance Hotline 202/554-1404
Technical Support	John Sullivan, 202/260-3480
Documentation	TSCA Assistance Hotline or Technical Support (above)
Access	Copies of the public TSCA Inventory are available from the Government Printing Office (see below). Diskettes are available from the National Technical Information Service. Initiate non-confidential searches by submitting a written Freedom of Information Act (FOIA) request to U.S. EPA, Freedom of Information Office (A-101), 401 M Street, SW, Washington, DC 20460.

Database	*Chemical Update System (data collected under the Toxic Substances Control Act — Inventory Update Rule)*
Acronym	CUS
Source	U.S. EPA
Contact	TSCA Assistance Hotline 202/554-1404
Technical Support	John Sullivan, 202/260-0431
Documentation	TSCA Assistance Hotline or Technical Support (above)
Access	Initiate non-confidential searches by submitting a written Freedom of Information Act (FOIA) request to U.S. EPA, Freedom of Information Office (A-101), 401 M Street, SW, Washington, DC 20460. EPA is in the process of creating CUS information products, expected to be available in 1996.

Database	*Contract Laboratory Program (CLP) Analytical Result Database*
Acronym	CARD
Source	U.S. EPA
Contact	David Eng, CARD User Support, EPA, 703/603-8827 703/603-9112 (Fax)
Technical Support	Frederick Powers or Dona Brock, CARD/CADRE User Support Helpline, Computer Science Corporation, 702/735-1971 702/892-2521 (Fax)
Documentation	CARD User Support
Access	U.S. EPA NCC Preparation of special data extracts, on request At present, database access is generally limited to EPA staff and contractors. On-line direct access to CARD, as well as special requests for data extracts, will be granted upon approval from CARD user support. EPA contractors may apply through their EPA project officers.

Database	*Federal Reporting Data System II (to be changed to Safe Drinking Water Information System)*
Acronym	FRDS-II (to be changed to SDWIS)
Source	U.S. EPA
Contact	Abraham I. Siegel, Information Specialist, Office of Ground Water and Drinking Water, 202/260-2804
Technical Support	SDWIS User Group, EPA Systems Development Center, Science Applications International Corporation, 703/908-2460
Documentation	Office of Ground Water and Drinking Water, 202/260-2803
Access	U.S. EPA NCC To obtain access to FRDS-II Interactive System, the user must: • Obtain a TSO User ID and Account (see "EPA Guide to NCC Services Log-on Information"); • Contact the FRDS Technical Support Staff ; to become a member of the FRDS User File; • Receive a CLIST from technical support.

Database	*Massachusetts Toxics Use Reduction Database, Form S and Form R*
Acronym	TURA
Source	Commonwealth of Massachusetts, Department of Environmental Protection
Contact	Walter Hope, Massachusetts Department of Environmental Protection, 617/292-5982
Technical Support	Suzi Peck, Director, Toxics Use Reduction, Massachusetts Department of Environmental Protection, 617/292-5870
Access	Available (1990 through 1992) on diskette as ASCII files

Database	*New Jersey Release and Pollution Prevention Report Data*
Source	State of New Jersey, Department of Environmental Protection and Energy, Division of Environmental Safety, Health and Analytical Programs
Contact	Shirlee Schiffman, Chief, Bureau of Hazardous Substances Information, 609/292-6714
Technical Support	Same
Documentation	Same
Access	Available (1987 through 1992 data) on diskette as dBASE files; $50 for each year of data

Database	*STOrage and RETrieval of U.S. Waterways Parametric Data (Water Quality System)*
Acronym	STORET (WQS)
Source	U.S. EPA
Contact	STORET User Assistance, U.S. EPA, 800/424-9067
Tecnical Support	STORET User Assistance, U.S. EPA, 800/424-9067
Training	Louis Hoelman, 202/260-7050 202/260-1977 (Fax)
Documentation	STORET User Assistance, U.S. EPA, 800/424-9067
Access	U.S. EPA NCC State agencies may obtain access through the STORET points-of-contact in EPA Regional Offices.

Database	*Toxics Release Inventory*
Acronym	TRI
Source	National Library of Medicine TOXNET System
Contact	TRI Representative, Specialized Information Services, 301/496-6531
Technical Support	Same; also EPA's TRI User Support Service (TRI-US), 202/260-1531
Documentation	See Contact and Technical Support, above
Access	On-line access available at many EPA, federal depository, public, university, and medical libraries. Details for many locations available from TRI-US.
	TRI data are available for 1987 through 1992; public data release of 1993 data scheduled for March 1995
Additional Sources	RTK-Net (see below), on line
	National Technical Information Service (NTIS) for CD-ROM, diskettes, magnetic tapes
	U.S. Government Printing Office (GPO) for diskettes, magnetic tapes

General Sources

EPA National Computing Center (NCC)

Contact — National Technical Information Service (NTIS), to obtain account and user ID

Technical Support — Customer Call Center (CCC), 919/541-7862

EPA contractors or grantees may be able to arrange an account for work under the contract or grant through their Project Officers.

Detailed information on how to access the NCC mainframe, NCC VAX, National Environmental Supercomputer (NESC) systems is provided in the "Guide to NCC Services Log-on Information Reference." This document can be obtained from CCC (above) or on-line through Bookmanager. Bookmanager is an application available on the EPA mainframe accessible to users with NCC IDs.

RTK-Net

Technical Support — Unison Institute 202/797-7200 or OMB Watch 202/234-8494

Documentation — On-line RTK-Net Data Documentation

To obtain account: Register on-line. Accounts and connect time are free. To complete an application form on-line:

- Set parameters to: highest baud rate, 8, N, 1;
- Dial modem number 202/234-8570, or via Internet, telnet to rtknet.org;
- Users with a modem under 9600 baud may have to hit the break key when entering the system;
- At user-id prompt, type the word "public" in all lower case letters;
- Enter communications software type (type "h" for Help if regarding software abbreviations);
- At the Main Menu, cursor down to Registration Form;
- Follow the instructions on screen.

National Technical Information Service (NTIS)

National Technical Information Service
U.S. Department of Commerce
5285 Port Royal Road
Springfield, VA 22161
703/487-4850

Government Printing Office

Superintendent of Documents
Government Printing Office
Washington, DC 20402
202/783-3238

Glossary

33/50 Program: A voluntary program of the U.S. EPA encouraging reductions of TRI releases and transfers of 33 percent from 1988 to 1992 and 50 percent from 1988 to 1995 through pollution prevention or other means.

Activity index: See production ratio.

Area of Concern (AOC): Forty-three areas of chronic pollution within the Great Lakes basin, identified by the International Joint Commission, under the authority of the Great Lakes Water Quality Agreement of 1972.

Biennial Reporting System (BRS): Database maintained by the states and the U.S. EPA to which facilities generating waste streams that are toxic, corrosive, ignitable, or reactive and in amounts above certain thresholds must report.

Bioaccumulation: The uptake and retention of substances by an organism from its surrounding medium and from its food. Chemicals move through the food chain and tend to end up at higher concentrations in organisms at the upper end of the food chain such as predator fish, or in people or birds that eat these fish; the process of concentration of substances in living organisms.

Byproduct: The amount of a chemical that does not become a product and is not consumed or transformed during the production process. Generally, byproduct is all the "non-products" or wastes that leave the production process. This term, as used in the Massachusetts' Toxics Use Reduction Act reporting, however, excludes amounts generated as waste but reused or recycled (either on- of off-site) without any treatment or recovery. Byproduct includes air emissions, wastewaters, waste disposed of in landfills, transfers of waste to other energy recovery, treatment, or disposal facilities.

Carcinogen: A substance that can cause or contribute to the production of cancer.

Characteristic hazardous waste: A RCRA waste classified as hazardous because it is ignitable, corrosive, reactive, or toxic as determined by the Toxicity Characteristic Leachate Procedure (TCLP). It has an EPA waste code in the range "D001" to D043."

Chemical category: A group of closely-related individual chemicals that are counted together for purposes of TRI reporting threshold and release and transfer calculations. The chemicals are reported to TRI under a single name. The TRI list in effect at the time of the 1992 reporting included 20 chemical categories: 15 metal compound categories (such as lead compounds) and 5 organic compounds categories (such as glycol ethers).

Chloro-organics: Organic chemicals that contain at least one chlorine atom.

Chlorofluorocarbons (CFCs): A class of chemicals that depletes the ozone layer. They were used extensively in refrigeration, insulation, packaging materials, and aerosol propellants.

Commercial product use: The use of commercial products. In Chapter 2, refers sources of toxic chemical releases to the environment that are the deliberate result of product design, are inadvertently generated over the life of the product, or occur as products are discarded at the end of their useful lives.

Comprehensive Environmental Response, Compensation and Liability Act (CERCLA), otherwise known as Superfund. As amended by the Superfund Amendments and Reauthorization Act of 1986 (SARA), establishes a program to deal with the release of hazardous substances in spills and from uncontrolled, inactive, or abandoned disposal sites.

Corrosivity: A characteristic property of certain BRS waste streams as defined in 40 CFR 261.22 relating to pH levels and an ability to corrode as determined by standard testing methods.

DDT: 1,1,1-trichloro-2,2-bis(p-chlorophenyl) ethane. A pesticide.

Delisted: A chemical that previously appeared on the TRI list of chemicals and has been deleted because EPA has concluded that there is not sufficient evidence to establish any of the criteria for listing; reports on such chemicals are no longer required.

Disproportionate impact: A result of an environmental hazard that has a greater effect on one socioeconomic group than it has on the general population.

Energy recovery: The combustion or burning of a chemical to produce heat.

Environmental equity: The concept that the potential for exposure to environmental risks should be distributed evenly amongst the population and that no one group should bear a disproportionate burden.

Environmental justice movement: Grassroots and national groups in the United States that seek to promote social, economic, and/or environmental justice for people of color in the United States and abroad.

Environmental justice: The principle that fairness and equality should underlie efforts to protect individuals and communities from environmental hazards and that environmental protection should be adequate to safeguard human health.

Environmental management hierarchy: The types of waste management plus source reduction prioritized as to environmental desirability. In order of preference, the one most beneficial to the environment is source reduction, followed by recycling, energy recovery, treatment, and disposal as the least desirable option.

Environmental media: The air, water bodies such as oceans, rivers, lakes, and streams, and land areas to which environmental pollutants, including toxic chemicals, are released, discharged or disposed of.

Environmental racism: Racial discrimination in environmental policymaking and the enforcement of environmental regulations whether differential effects were intended or the unintended result of institutional practices.

EPA National Pretreatment Program: A program administered and implemented by EPA and approved states as a subset of the National Pollutant Discharge Elimination System program to control discharges of pollutants by industrial and commercial facilities to publicly owned sewage treatment plants (POTWs).

Facility: Defined for the purposes of TRI reporting as all buildings, equipment, structures, and other stationary items which are located on a single site or on contiguous or adjacent sites and which are owned or operated by the same entity. For the purposes of the BRS, each site with an EPA RCRA Identification Number is a facility.

Form GM: The BRS form that is completed by a facility for each of its hazardous waste streams. It contains information on the type of waste stream, the amount of the waste stream, and how it was managed during the year.

Form IC: The BRS form that is completed once for each facility reporting. It contains information on the name and address of the facility and whether or not waste minimization activity was undertaken at the facility during the years covered by the report.

Form R: The TRI form that must be completed by a facility for each of the chemicals on the TRI list that it used during the year above the threshold amounts.

Form S: The Massachusetts Toxics Use Reduction Act (TURA) reporting form that must be completed by a facility for each of the TURA-regulated chemicals used in excess of the reporting threshold. Facilities report amounts and types of chemical use, amounts of chemicals in products, and amounts in byproducts. They may also report qualitative data on source reduction.

Good operating practices: Source reduction activities such as inventory control, worker training, and housekeeping measures.

Great Lakes Water Quality Agreement of 1972: An agreement between the United States and Canada that commits environmental agencies from the two countries to develop and implement programs and other measures to restore and maintain the integrity of the waters of the Great Lakes Basin Ecosystem.

Group of Ten: The ten largest national environmental organizations in the United States: Environmental Defense Fund, Environmental Policy Institute/Friends of the Earth, Izaak Walton League, National Audubon Society, National Parks and Conservation Association, Natural Resources Defense Council, Sierra Club, and Sierra Club Legal Defense Fund.

Halo-organics: Organic chemicals containing at least one atom of any halogen.

Halogens: Chemical elements found in Group 17 of the Periodic Table of the Elements; namely fluorine, chlorine, bromine, iodine, and astatine.

Halogenated organics: See halo-organics.

Hazard Ranking System Score (HRS): A standard measure of the severity of contamination at hazardous waste sites, which EPA uses to prioritize sites. Scores are based on toxicity of contaminants present at the site, actual or potential pathways of human and environmental exposure.

Housekeeping measures: Source reduction activities related to better handling of materials.

Hydrochlorofluorocarbons (HCFCs): A class of chemicals that have been developed as temporary substitutes for CFCs and other ozone-depleting chemicals. They have a weaker effect on the ozone layer than the chemicals they were made to replace.

In-process or closed-loop recycling: Recycling that occurs within the production process, as opposed to being transported to another part of the facility or mixed with streams from other processes.

Incineration: The destruction of solid, liquid, or gaseous wastes by burning.

Industrial process waste: In Chapter 2, refers to a waste containing one or more toxic chemicals that is generated either deliberately or inadvertently as the direct result of the manufacture or processing of a toxic chemical or of a product containing a toxic chemical.

Ignitability: A characteristic property of certain BRS waste streams as defined in 40 CFR 261.21 relating to an ability to catch fire and burn vigorously.

Leachate: A liquid that has percolated through solid waste or other mediums and has extracted dissolved or suspended materials from it.

Materials accounting: See throughput data.

Materials balance: Calculations relating to an entire industrial process that "balance" inputs and outputs. If there were no waste stream, the amount of a chemical leaving a process or piece of equipment (output) would equal the amount entering (input). If wastes are generated, in order to balance, the calculations include waste plus outputs to equal inputs.

The 1987 Montreal Protocol on Substances that Deplete the Ozone Layer: An agreement adopted in 1987 by 25 countries requiring each party to freeze, and ultimately reduce production and consumption of chemicals known to deplete the ozone layer. The agreement has been revised and adopted by additional countries since 1987.

National Health and Nutrition Examination Surveys (NHANES): A series of ongoing studies by the National Center for Health Statistics/Centers for Disease Control and Prevention to ascertain the general state of health and nutrition in the U.S. population. Also Hispanic Health and Nutrition Examination Survey (HHANES).

National Pollutant Discharge Elimination System (NPDES): The national program established under the Federal Water Pollution Control Act, which requires all point source discharges into any body of water to be permitted by EPA or the designated state agency. Minimum pretreatment requirements for such discharges are established under the program.

National Priorities List (NPL): List of the most seriously contaminated hazardous waste sites in the country that EPA must identify, investigate, and remediate under CERCLA mandates.

Nonpoint Sources: The origin of pollution from broad areas through natural and human processes and activities that does not occur deliberately from a fixed discharge point.

Non-production-related waste: Waste that is generated as a one-time event, including large accidental spills, waste from a remedial action to clean up the environmental contamination from past disposal practices, or other wastes not occurring as a routine part of production operations. This does not include spills that occur as a routine part of the production operations that could be reduced or eliminated by improved handling, loading, or unloading procedures.

Normalization of production-related waste: Adjusting the amount of production-related waste at a facility to account for variations in production from year-to-year.

Off-site: Not at the site of the facility, including transfers of wastes sent to other facilities for recycling, energy recovery, treatment, or disposal.

On-site: Within the boundaries of the facility, including areas where wastes may be stored, treated or disposed of that are separate from the production processes but still within the boundaries of the reporting facility.

Organic: In chemistry, any compound that contains carbon atoms.

Ozone depleters: Chemicals that participate in photochemical reactions that lead to depletion of the ozone layer in the earth's upper atmosphere (stratosphere).

Ozone layer: The protective layer of ozone molecules that surrounds the earth and reduces the amount of high-energy ultraviolet radiation that reaches the earth's surface

Parent company: For the purposes of this report, a company that owns/ operates one or more TRI facilities.

Polychlorinated biphenyls (PCBs): A family of chemicals that, until banned from production and distribution in the United States, were used in a variety of products, notably as insulating fluid in electrical transformers; they are harmful to the liver and kidneys, and they accumulate in fat tissue.

Point sources: The origin of known or deliberate environmental releases from fixed points such as smokestacks and wastewater discharge pipes.

Pollution prevention: Source reduction (see below).

Polynuclear aromatic hydrocarbons (PAHs): A family of organic chemicals based on the chemical structure of benzene. This family includes a number of petroleum products and products of combustion processes.

Process level: In the data collected by the New Jersey Department of Environmental Protection, this term refers to the frame of reference for the mass balance calculation — in this case, around a single process rather than an entire facility.

Production ratio or activity index: In TRI, the ratio of production level in a reporting year to the previous year's level for each chemical reported. If a chemical is not manufactured but is "otherwise used," an activity index is defined by selecting a measure of use other than production and taking its ratio to the previous year.

Production-related waste: TRI chemical waste that is generated as a result of routine production and could be reduced or eliminated by improved handling, more efficient processes, change in product or product quality, or change in raw materials. This does not include spills resulting from large-scale accidents or waste from remedial actions to clean up contamination.

Projection of waste: TRI Form R includes projections of waste that indicate the amount of production-related waste that a facility expects to generate of each chemical in the two years following the report year. Separate projections are given for each of the two years for each of the amounts of recycling, energy recovery, treatment, and releases/ disposal.

Publicly owned treatment works (POTWs): A wastewater treatment plant that is owned by a state or municipality, including any devices used in the storage, treatment, recycling, and reclamation of domestic sewage or a combination of domestic and industrial wastewaters. The term also refers to the authority that has jurisdiction over discharges to and from such a treatment works.

Raw materials modifications: Switching from a toxic chemical to another chemical as a raw material. Raw materials modifications can be source reduction activities if a nontoxic substitute is chosen.

RCRA acute hazardous waste: Solid or liquid waste streams with properties as defined in 40 CFR denoted by waste codes beginning with "P."

RCRA exempt waste: Wastestreams generated at RCRA facilities that are managed in such a way that the type of waste management does not require a RCRA permit. Exempt types of waste management include wastewater treatment in tanks, regardless of the toxicity or hazard of the incoming waste stream, and closed-loop recycling units, which are units integral to the production process that recycle the chemical directly back into the production unit.

RCRA hazardous waste: Solid or liquid waste streams that are corrosive, ignitable, reactive, or toxic according to the RCRA definitions in 40 CFR.

RCRA managed waste: RCRA hazardous wastes that are not managed by exempt waste management techniques (see RCRA exempt waste).

RCRA toxic waste: For the purposes of this report, any RCRA wastes that exhibit the characteristic of toxicity designated by the July 1, 1993, Federal Code of Regulations (40 CFR Parts 261.24 through 261.33), or that contain TRI chemical constituents. This excludes RCRA hazardous wastes that are corrosive, ignitable, or reactive unless the waste contained toxic constituents as defined above.

Reactivity: A characteristic property of certain BRS waste streams as defined in 40 CFR 261.23 relating to chemical stability and an ability to react vigorously with water.

Recycling remains: Unused material from a recycling process. This material may be treated, used for energy recovery, released, disposed of, or transferred off-site.

Recycling: Extraction of a chemical from a manufacturing process stream that would otherwise have been waste, with the extracted chemical being reused in the original production process, in another production process, or sold as a separate product.

Released/disposed of: All TRI on-site releases and off-site transfers to disposal. This does not include off-site transfers to recycling, energy recovery, or treatment.

Releases: Annual quantities (in pounds) of a TRI chemical in waste released on site to air, water, underground injection, or land.

Remedial Action Plan (RAP): Documents called for under the Great Lakes Water Quality Amendments of 1987 that involve a three-part analysis to characterize the contamination in each Area of Concern, to identify the sources causing the contamination (stage I), to develop remedial strategies to restore beneficial uses by cleaning up contaminated areas and prevent further releases (stage II), and to confirm the restoration of beneficial uses (stage III).

Resource Conservation and Recovery Act (RCRA): The federal law enacted in 1976 by Congress that provides the basic structure for managing both hazardous and non-hazardous solid waste in the United States. This Act and its Hazardous and Solid Waste Amendments of 1984 (HSWA) prescribe activities designed to track hazardous waste from "cradle to grave" encouraging waste minimization, discouraging land disposal, and reducing the threat of hazardous waste (including certain wastewaters destined for land disposal), from generation to final disposition.

Smelter: A facility designed to melt or fuse ores to separate out the metallic components.

Source reduction activity: Equipment or technology modifications, process or procedure modifications, reformulations or redesign of products, substitution of raw materials, or improvements in housekeeping, maintenance, training, or inventory control that are undertaken to reduce the amount of waste generated during production.

Source reduction: Industrial source reduction is defined in the Pollution Prevention Act of 1990 as "any practice which 1) reduces the amount of hazardous substance, pollutant, or contaminant entering any waste stream or otherwise released into the environment (including fugitive emissions) prior to recycling treatment, or disposal; and 2) reduces the hazards to public health and the environment associated with the release of such substances, pollutants, or contaminants. The term includes equipment or technology modifications, process or procedure modifications, reformulations or redesign of products, substitution of raw materials, and improvements in housekeeping, maintenance, training, or inventory control."

Stratified Analysis: An analysis that involves separating a sample into several subsamples according to specific criteria such as age groups, socioeconomic status, etc.

Stratosphere: The part of the atmosphere that contains the ozone layer, located above the troposphere.

Throughput data: Data that describe the entire flow of a chemical in an industrial facility, including amount of the chemical brought on site, put into inventory or removed from inventory, amount produced, amount consumed or transformed during the production process, amount shipped as or in a product, and amount generated as waste.

Total Exposure Assessment Methodology (TEAM): A series of EPA studies to that were designed to characterize the degree of individual exposure to environmental pollutants and the sources of such exposure.

Total releases and transfers: The aggregate total in pounds of all TRI chemicals in waste released on site to the air, water, underground injection, or land, combined with transfers, which are sent to POTWs and other off-site locations for treatment, recycling, energy recovery, and/or disposal. This total may refer to overall nationwide TRI amounts or to a chemical, geographic area, industry, or single facility. If the reference is to data before 1991, then the total does not include off-site transfers to recycling or energy recovery.

Toxics Release Inventory (TRI): Annually updated database of release quantities of about 300 chemicals and chemical categories into the nation's air, water, and land, and transfers to off-site locations for treatment, or disposal since 1987, and for recycling and energy recovery since 1991.

Toxics use reduction: As defined by the Massachusetts Toxics Use Reduction Act, measures taken to reduce the use of toxic or hazardous substances by facilities. These include source reduction techniques as well as recycling, reuse, or extended use which is part of the production process (see in-process recycling).

Toxics Use Reduction Act (TURA): A Massachusetts act signed into law on July 24, 1989 (M.G.L. c.21I). Its essential goal is to promote toxics use reduction through establishment of a statewide goal of reducing toxic waste generated by 50% by 1997. Industries in Massachusetts are encouraged, but not required, to meet this goal by reducing production and use of toxic and hazardous substances. Eligible facilities report TURA data to the state on Form S.

Toxicity criteria: A characteristic property of certain BRS waste streams as defined in 40 CFR 261.24 for waste streams containing certain chemicals.

Transfers: TRI chemicals in waste that are sent from the reporting facility to a facility that recycles, treats, disposes of the chemical or burns the chemical for energy.

Treatment: A variety of processes that change the chemical in waste into another substance.

Treatment, Storage, and Disposal Facility (TSDF): Under RCRA, these facilities manage some or all of their wastes generated or transferred on site by RCRA permitted methods.

TRI facility: Any industrial facility meeting the threshold criteria (10 or more employees, manufacturing at least 25,000 pounds or otherwise using at least 10,000 pounds of a given TRI chemical in a calendar year) that trigger reporting release and transfer information for that year to EPA.

Ubiquitous: Found throughout the environment.

Use: The amount of a chemical that is used as input to or as a manufacturing aid during the production process or is produced at a facility. The New Jersey and Massachusetts databases collect pieces of information that are added together in this report to act as a surrogate for "use," which is not reported as a single number. For New Jersey, "use" is starting inventory minus ending inventory plus amount brought on site plus amount produced on site plus amount recycled. For Massachusetts, "use" is amount produced plus amount processed plus amount otherwise used.

Waste code: EPA identifiers consisting of one letter (D, F, P, U, or K) and three numbers that identify the type of hazardous waste stream being reported on the BRS report form.

Waste generated: On the BRS report form, the total amount of the waste stream, including the amount of the chemical constituent but also including any water, soil, or other material.

Waste managed: See RCRA-managed waste above.

Waste management: Activities undertaken by facilities to recycle, treat, or otherwise manage waste that has been generated. The activities include energy recovery and disposal in addition to recycling and treatment. They do not include source reduction activities, which take place before waste is generated.

Waste minimization: As reported to the BRS, source reduction and recycling.

Waste stream: Under RCRA, liquid or solid materials generated as waste and that contain hazardous materials.

Wastewater: Waste streams containing mostly water — either water used in processing or stormwater runoff.

Acronyms

AAEA	African American Environmentalist Association
AOC	Area of Concern
BIFs	Boilers and Industrial Furnaces
BRS	Biennial Reporting System
Btu	British Thermal Unit
CAAA	Clean Air Act Amendments
CDC	Center for Disease Control and Prevention
(CE)2	Center for Environment, Commerce, and Energy
CEC	Commission for Environmental Cooperation
CERCLA	Comprehensive Environmental Response, Compensation, and Liability Act of 1980
CERCLIS	Comprehensive Environmental, Response, Compensation, and Liability Information System
CFCs	Chlorofluorocarbons
CMA	Chemical Manufacturers Association
CWA	Clean Water Act
DDT	1,1,1-Trichloro-2,2-bis(p-chlorophenyl) ethane
DEP	Department of Environmental Protection
DOD	U.S. Department of Defense
DOE	U.S. Department of Energy
ECM-ID	Environmentally Conscious Manufacturing Integrated Demonstration
ECO	Environmental Career Organization
EHIA	Environmental High Impact Area
EnTA	Environmental Technology Assessment
EPA	U.S. Environmental Protection Agency
EU	European Union
GAO	U. S. General Accounting Office
GATT	General Agreement of Tariffs and Trade
GNP	Gross National Product
HAP	Hazardous Air Pollutant
HCFCs	Hydrochlorofluorocarbons
HHNES	Hispanic Health and Nutrition Examination Survey
HRS	Hazard Ranking System
ICOLP	International Cooperative for Ozone Layer Protection
ICPIC	International Cleaner Production Information Clearinghouse
IE/PAC	Industry & Environment Program Activity Centre
IETP	Integrated Environmental Target Plan
IPC	Integrated Pollution Prevention and Control
LDC	Less Developed Country
LEV	Low Emission Vehicle
LULU	Locally Undesirable Land Use
NAACP	National Association for the Advancement of Colored People
NAAEC	North American Agreement on Environmental Cooperation
NAFTA	North American Free Trade Agreement
NAM	National Association of Manufacturers
NAS	National Academy of Sciences; National Audubon Society
NCHS	National Center for Health Statistics
NDCEE	National Defense Center for Environmental Excellence
NECAG	Northeast Community Action Group
NEPP	National Environmental Policy Plan
NGOs	Non-Governmental Organizations
NHANES	National Health and Nutrition Examination Surveys
NOC	Notice of Commencement

NPDES	National Pollutant Discharge Elimination System
NPL	National Priorities List
NRDC	Natural Resources Defense Council
OECD	Organization of Economic Cooperation and Development
OEJ	Office of Environmental Justice
ORVR	Onboard Refueling Vapor Recovery
OSHA	Occupational Health and Safety Administration (or Act)
OSWER	Office of Solid Waste and Emergency Response
PAHs	Polynuclear Aromatic Hydrocarbons
PCBs	Polychlorinated Biphenyls
PMN	Premanufacture Notification
POTW	Publicly Owned Treatment Works
PRTR	Pollutant Release and Transfer Registers
RAP	Remedial Action Plan
RCRA	Resource Conservation and Recovery Act
R.I.S.E.	Residents Involved in Saving the Environment
ROD	Record of Decision
SIC	Standard Industrial Classification
SOCMI	Synthetic Organic Chemical Manufacturing Industry
SWDA	Solid Waste Disposal Act
SWOP	Southwest Organizing Project
TCLP	Toxicity Characteristic Leachate Procedure
TEAM	Total Exposure Assessment Methodology
TRI	Toxics Release Inventory
TSDF	Treatment, Storage and Disposal Facility
TURA	Toxics Use Reduction Act
UCCCRJ	United Church of Christ Commission for Racial Justice
UN	United Nations
UNEP	United Nations Environment Programme
UNITAR	United Nations Institute for Training and Research
VOC	Volatile Organic Compound
WTO	World Trade Organization
WWF	World Wildlife Fund

Index

A

B

C

F

G

H

I

J

K

L

M

N

O

P

Q

R

S

T

U

V

W

X

Y

—

Z

Contributors

Barbara F. Bass, Ph.D.

Barbara Bass is a toxicologist and policy analyst with expertise in a wide range of environmental issues. At Hampshire, she has coauthored national reports on the Toxics Release Inventory (TRI) and on pollution prevention. She has undertaken research ranging from drafting proposed neurotoxicity risk assessment guidelines identifying nontraditional measures of the effectiveness of EPA toxics and pesticides enforcement action. Dr. Bass has conducted human health risk assessments under Superfund provisions and other federal regulations. She received her Ph.D. in toxicology from the Johns Hopkins University.

Carroll L. Bastian

Carroll Bastian managed and coauthored *Toxics in the Community: National and Local Perspectives, 1989* and contributed to Hampshire's study for World Wildlife Fund of international toxic chemical inventories. She also has 15 years' experience in federal environmental policy positions. At EPA, she was deputy director for policy in the Office of International Activities, where she represented the United States in negotiations on CFCs and ozone and other toxic chemical issues and coordinated export policy for substances regulated under the Toxic Substances Control Act (TSCA), Resource Conservation and Recovery Act (RCRA), and other legislation. She has a master's degree in history from George Washington University.

Diane Benjamin

Diane Benjamin is a computer programmer and database specialist at Hampshire Research. She is on the development team for the Windows™ version of *RISK*ASSISTANT*™. She participates in preparation of TRI data for EPA's data release publications and for the 33/50 Program's case studies. Ms. Benjamin is a computer programmer/systems analyst in the U.S. Army Reserves, and she has completed her master's degree in computer systems management at the University of Maryland University College

Mark H. Dorfman

Mark Dorfman is senior research associate of INFORM's Chemical Hazards Prevention Program. He was lead author of *Preventing Pollution Through Technical Assistance: One State's Experience* and of *Environmental Dividends: Cutting More Chemical Wastes.* Current projects include the 33/50 Program evaluation and outreach in Louisiana, Ohio, and New Jersey. Mr.. Dorfman recently received an Asia Foundation Fellowship to conduct pollution prevention research and outreach in Kathmandu, Nepal, where he previously consulted for UNICEF, the Ministry of Health, and the German Technical Assistance Agency. He also worked as an analytical chemist in new York and was a member of a research team investigating ultraviolet disinfection of municipal wastewater in North Carolina. He has an M.S. in environmental chemistry from the University of North Carolina's School of Public Health at Chapel Hill.

John Howay

John Howay provides research assistance for this and other Hampshire projects, including verification of TRI data and updating of toxicity databases for *RISK*ASSISTANT.* Before joining Hampshire, he volunteered with the Toxic Trade Campaign of Greenpeace and edited the Greenpeace Inventory of Genetically Modified Organisms. His education includes a B.A. in ecology from Prescott College, Arizona, and graduate studies in soil science at the University of California, Davis.

Lois Lobo

Lois Lobo provided research assistance for *Toxics Watch* and for other studies including INFORM's *Stirring Up Innovation*. She has also researched international toxics release inventories, contributing to Hampshire studies on behalf of the World Wildlife Fund. Ms. Lobo holds a master's degree in international development from American University.

Sharon Martin

Sharon Martin performs desktop publishing and design and editing at Hampshire Research, including project management and production of annual TRI public data releases for EPA. She coauthored a Hampshire study on the TSCA Test Submissions database. Before joining Hampshire, she wrote and edited, with other responsibilities, for an economics firm, social justice organizations, and a legislative research group in the U.S. House of Representatives. She has an M.F.A. in writing poetry, from George Mason University.

Catherine G. Miller, Ph.D.

A consultant to both INFORM and Hampshire, Catherine Miller is Hampshire's senior data analyst, a senior environmental policy analysis, and a computer programmer. She has led Hampshire's policy analysis of all TRI, New Jersey Community Right-to-Know, RCRA hazardous waste, and 33/50 Program data. An expert in industrial source reduction, she is coauthor of *Cutting Chemical Wastes* and *Environmental Dividends*, INFORM's studies of pollution prevention practices, benefits, and motivations at organic chemical companies in the United States.

Dr. Miller previously worked for EPA (1971-75 and 1978-84), and she is the author of half a dozen EPA studies, including assessment of the economic benefits of municipal wastewater treatment and multimedia pollution control programs and the policy uses of air quality models and exposure assessment modeling. She has master's and doctoral degrees in public policy from the Kennedy School of Government at Harvard University along with an M.S. in mathematics from M.I.T.

Warren R. Muir, Ph.D.

President of Hampshire Research Institute and senior fellow of INFORM, Warren Muir is an internationally recognized authority on industrial pollution prevention, toxics release reporting, and toxic substances regulations. He directs Hampshire's involvement in encouraging other countries to develop pollutant release and transfer registries (akin to TRI) and is working with countries of the former Soviet Union on environmental concerns. He has been principal investigator and/or author on all of Hampshire's research in pollution prevention, toxics use reduction and hazardous waste. In addition to reports, articles, and testimony, Dr. Muir coauthored INFORM's *Cutting Chemical Wastes* and the follow-up study *Environmental Dividends.*

Dr. Muir has more than a decade of experience in senior environmental policy positions in the federal government and was EPA's first director of the Office of Toxic Substances (now the Office of Pollution Prevention and Toxics). He serves on the President's Council on Sustainable Development and on the Office of Technology Assessment's Advisory Group on New Approaches to Environmental Protection. He also teaches environmental health policy courses at the graduate level. Johns Hopkins School of Hygiene and Public Health. He has master's and doctoral degrees in chemistry from Northwestern University, with post-doctoral training in epidemiology at Johns Hopkins.

Thomas E. Natan, Jr., Ph.D.

Thomas Natan specializes at Hampshire in analysis of information related to industrial source reduction (pollution prevention). For a study with the World Wildlife Fund, he has analyzed national environmental reporting systems and the corporate environmental reports of more than 75 companies. In a project with the World Environment Center, he visited chemical plants in Poland, evaluating plans and progress toward waste reduction. Dr. Natan conducts data analysis, program-wide and an individual companies, for the 33/50 Program. He is the author of "Examples of Successful Pollution Prevention Programs," in *Industrial Pollution Prevention Handbook* (McGraw Hill, 1995). As food product development engineer for Procter and Gamble, he developed testing and standards to reduce waste (and costs) of raw materials and intermediates. He has an M.S. from the University of Cincinnati and a Ph.D. from Carnegie-Mellon University, both in chemical engineering.

Carolyn A. Nunley

Carolyn Nunley is a research associate in INFORM's Chemical Hazards Prevention Program. Her current research includes investigation of "substantial risk" notices submitted to EPA under TSCA, to assess their potential as a source of information on little-known health effects. She recently completed a series of workshops for community groups in the Great Lakes region. These workshops provided training to promote and evaluate industry progress in reducing waste at the source, using methodology and findings developed from INFORM's research on source reduction activities in the chemical industry. Prior to joining INFORM, Ms. Nunley worked for the State of Maryland Department of the Environment, managing the Health Assessment Division. She holds a Master's of Public Health, in environmental health, from the Yale School of Medicine.

Costas Pappas

Costas Pappas conducts case-study research for the 33/50 Program, analyzing company data and activities toward reducing environmental releases and transfers of chemicals targeted by the Program, including site visits. He is also participating in Hampshire's evaluation, for the State of New Jersey of the effectiveness of pollution prevention planning at industrial facilities. Mr. Pappas was formerly repair design and development engineer at General Electric Aircraft Engines. As a processes engineer at GE, he was responsible for design and implementation of a production facility utilizing hydrogen fluoride processes, now in use worldwide, that meet air, wastewater, and safety standards of EPA and OSHA. He has a master's degree in chemical engineering from the University of Cincinnati.

Bonnie A. Scarborough

Bonnie Scarborough conducts and assists research at Hampshire on topics as varied as environmental justice and data collected under TSCA. A coauthor of *Toxics Watch*, she is also participating in research, for Hampshire and INFORM, on "substantial risk" notices submitted to EPA under TSCA. As a research fellow at the Environmental and Energy Study Institute, she addressed topics of health effects of pollution and environmental justice issues. While at the University of Cambridge, she researched the Norwegian environmental movement. Ms. Scarborough holds an M.A. in political theory from New York University and an M.Phil in modern political philosophy from the University of Cambridge.

Hilary Sheevers, Ph.D.

For Hampshire Research, Hilary Sheevers has managed projects, participated in policy analysis, and coauthored studies on pollution prevention, hazardous waste reduction, and related topics. She participated in or led analyses of EPA information resources for hazardous waste reduction, evaluation of use of EPA's Office of Toxic Substances data by those outside the Office, regulatory reviews of New Jersey hazardous waste programs, and preliminary analysis and planning for public dissemination of the first TRI data. Dr. Sheevers is now a pharmacologist with the U.S. Food and Drug Administration. She has an M.S. in biology from American University and a Ph.D. in pharmacology and toxicology from the University of Arizona.

Daniel L. Tuttle II

Daniel Tuttle serves as project manager for Hampshire support of EPA's 33/50 Program, administering case-study research, data analysis, information system development, and EPA requests for Program information. He is undertaking research on efforts to stimulate voluntary reduction of greenhouse gas emissions, ascertaining the data needs for such programs. Mr. Tuttle previously served as senior study director for energy and environmental studies at Westat, where he managed projects involving complex surveys, systems and database development, and industry studies for EPA and the Department of Energy (DOE). He directed EPA's baseline RCRA hazardous waste study and DOE's Annual Survey of Oil and Gas Reserves and numerous other studies. He was also formerly an economist and energy specialist in EPA's Office of Policy Analysis. He holds an M.B.A. from New York University in economics.

John S. Young, Ph.D.

John Young, scientific director of Hampshire Research, is a toxicologist and risk assessor with extensive experience in toxic chemical policy issues. He has been manager and principal author of numerous studies for EPA. Dr. Young was lead author of INFORM's *Stirring Up Innovation: Environmental Improvements in Paints and Adhesives*. He served as chief scientist for the research effort that designed the *RISK* ASSISTANT* software system and continues that role in developing the Windows version of the software. He directs Hampshire's community technical assistance program, which provides scientific advice to citizens' groups. He is presently engaged in research on data needs and program prospects for voluntary reduction of greenhouse gases. Before joining Hampshire, Dr. Young served on the faculty of the Department of Environmental Health Sciences at the Johns Hopkins School of Hygiene and Public Health, specializing in sensory system toxicity. He has a Ph.D. in psychology from Brown University with post-doctoral training in neurobehavioral toxicology at Johns Hopkins.

Publications and Membership

Chemical Hazards Prevention: Selected Publications

Stirring Up Innovation: Environmental Improvements in Paints and Adhesives (John Young, Linda Ambrose, and Lois Lobo) 1994, 128 pp., $25.

Preventing Industrial Toxic Hazards: A Guide for Communities (Marian Wise and Lauren Kenworthy), 1993, 208 pp., $25.

Environmental Dividends: Cutting More Chemical Wastes (Mark H. Dorfman, Warren R. Muir, Ph.D., and Catherine G. Miller, Ph.D.), 1992, 288 pp., $75.

Tackling Toxics in Everyday Products: A Directory of Organizations (Nancy Lilienthal, Michele Ascione, and Adam Flint), 1992, 192 pp., $19.95.

Toward a More Informed Public: Recommendations for Improving the Toxics Release Inventory (Jacqueline B. Courteau and Nancy Lilienthal), 1991, 26 pp., $10.

Preventing Pollution Through Technical Assistance: One State's Experience (Mark H. Dorfman and John Riggio), 1990, 72 pp., $15.

Cutting Chemical Wastes: What 29 Organic Chemical Plants Are Doing to Reduce Hazardous Wastes (David J. Sarokin, Warren R. Muir, Ph.D., Catherine G. Miller, Ph.D., and Sebastian R. Sperber), 1986, 548 pp. $47.50.

Energy and Air Quality

Paving the Way to Natural Gas Vehicles (James S. Cannon), 1993, 192 pp., $25.

Sustainable Products and Practices: Selected Publications

Delivering the Goods: Benefits of Reusable Shipping Containers (David Saphire), 1994, 32 pp., $20.

Case Reopened: Reassessing Refillable Bottles (David Saphire), 1994, 366 pp., $25.

Germany, Garbage, and the Green Dot: Challenging the Throwaway Society (Bette K. Fishbein), 1994, 276 pp., $25.

Making Less Garbage: A Planning Guide for Communities (Bette K. Fishbein and Caroline Gelb), 1993, 192 pp. $30.

Business Recycling Manual (copublished with Recourse Systems, Inc.), 1991, 202 pp. $42.50.

Burning Garbage in the US: Practice vs. State of the Art (Marjorie J. Clarke, Maarten de Kadt, Ph.D., and David Saphire), 1991, 288 pp., $47.

Reducing Office Paper Waste (Robert Graff and Bette Fishbein), 1991, 28 pp., $15.

Garbage Management in Japan: Leading the Way (Allen Hershkowitz, Ph.D., and Eugene Salerni, Ph.D.), 1987, 152 pp., $5.

Other INFORM Publications

For a complete publications list, including materials on land and water conservation and a quarterly newsletter, or for more information, call or write to INFORM.

Sales Information

Payment, including shipping and handling charges, must be made in US funds drawn on a US bank and must accompany all orders. Please make checks payable to INFORM and mail to:

INFORM, Inc.
120 Wall Street
New York, NY 10005-4001

Please include a street address; UPS cannot deliver to a box number.

Shipping Fees

United States:	Add $3 for first book + $1 for each additional book. (4th class delivery; allow 4-6 weeks)
Canada:	Add $5 for first book + $3 for each additional book.
Foreign/surface:	Add $8 for first book + $4 each additional book.
Foreign/airmail:	Add $20 for first book + $10 each additional book.
Outside the US:	Allow additional shipping time.

Priority shipping is higher; please call for charges.

Discount Policy

Booksellers:	20% on 1-4 copies of same title 30% on 5 or more copies of same title
General bulk:	20% on 5 or more copies of same title

Students with ID; public interest and community groups with nonprofit federal ID:

	Price:
Books under $10:	No discount
Books $10-$15:	$10
Books $25 and up:	$15

Government, upon request:

Books $45 and under:	No discount
Books over $45	$45

Returns

Booksellers may return books, if in saleable condition, for full credit or cash refund up to 6 months from date of invoice. Books must be returned prepaid and include a copy of the invoice or packing list showing invoice number, date, list price, and original discount.

Membership

Individuals provide an important source of support to INFORM and receive the following benefits:

Member ($25):	A one-year subscription to *INFORM Reports,* INFORM's quarterly newsletter.
Friend ($50):	Member's benefits, plus advance notice of new publications.
Contributor ($100):	Friend's benefits, plus 10% discount on new INFORM studies.
Supporter ($250):	Friend's benefits, plus 20% discount on new INFORM studies.
Donor ($500):	Friend's benefits, plus 30% discount on new INFORM studies.
Associate ($1,000):	Friend's benefits, plus a complimentary copy of new INFORM studies.
Benefactor ($5,000):	Friend's benefits, plus a complimentary copy of new INFORM studies.

INFORM Board of Directors